Textbook of
Assisted Reproductive
Techniques

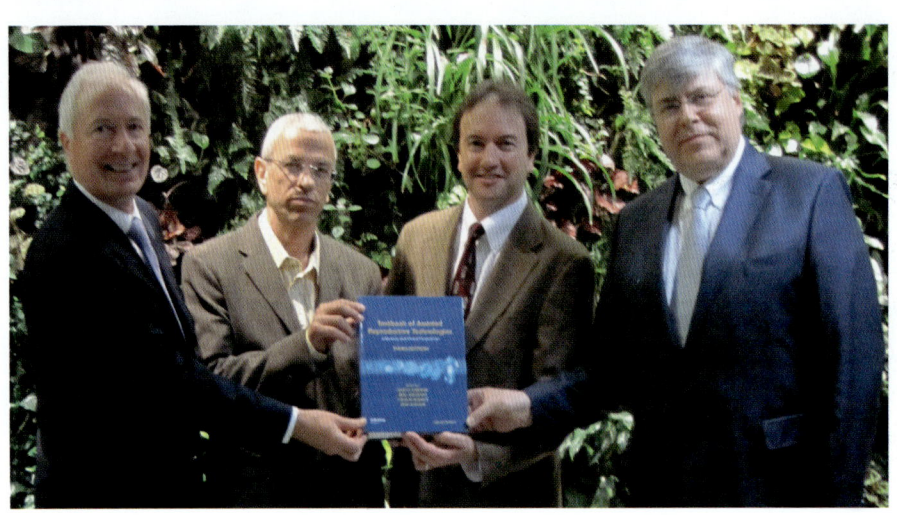

The editors (from left to right: Colin M. Howles, Ariel Weissman, David K. Gardner, and Zeev Shoham) at the annual meeting of ESHRE, Stockholm, July 2011

Textbook of Assisted Reproductive Techniques

Fourth Edition

Volume 1: Laboratory Perspectives

Edited by

David K. Gardner DPhil
Chair of Zoology, University of Melbourne, Melbourne, Australia

Ariel Weissman MD
Senior Physician, IVF Unit, Department of Obstetrics and Gynecology,
Edith Wolfson Medical Center, Holon and Sackler Faculty of Medicine,
Tel Aviv University, Tel Aviv, Israel

Colin M. Howles PhD, FRSM
Vice President, Regional Medical Affairs Fertility, External Scientific Affairs,
Global Development and Medical, Merck Serono SA, Geneva, Switzerland

Zeev Shoham MD
Director, Reproductive Medicine and Infertility Unit, Department of Obstetrics and
Gynecology, Kaplan Medical Center, Rehovot, Israel

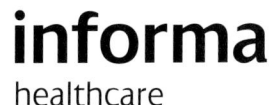

This edition published in 2012 by Informa Healthcare, 119 Farringdon Road, London EC1R 3DA, UK. Simultaneously published in the USA by Informa Healthcare, 52 Vanderbilt Avenue, 7th Floor, New York NY 10017, USA. Informa Healthcare is a trading division of Informa UK Ltd.

Registered Office: Informa House, 30–32 Mortimer Street, W1W 7RE. Registered in England and Wales number 1072954.

© 2012 Informa Healthcare, except as otherwise indicated.
No claim to original U.S. Government works.

All rights reserved. No part of this publication may be reproduced, stored in a retrieval system, or transmitted, in any form or by any means, electronic, mechanical, photocopying, recording, or otherwise, unless with the prior written permission of the publisher or in accordance with the provisions of the Copyright, Designs and Patents Act 1988 or under the terms of any licence permitting limited copying issued by the Copyright Licensing Agency Saffron House, 6–10 Kirby Street, London EC1N 8TS UK, or the Copyright Clearance Center, Inc., 222 Rosewood Drive, Danvers, MA 01923, USA (www.copyright.com or telephone +1 978-750-8400).

Reprinted material is quoted with permission. Although every effort has been made to ensure that all owners of copyright material have been acknowledged in this publication, we would be glad to acknowledge in subsequent reprints or editions any omissions brought to our attention. Product or corporate names may be trademarks or registered trademarks and are used only for identification and explanation without intent to infringe.

This book contains information from reputable sources, and although reasonable efforts have been made to publish accurate information, the publisher makes no warranties (either express or implied) as to the accuracy or fitness for a particular purpose of the information or advice contained herein. The publisher wishes to make it clear that any views or opinions expressed in this book by individual authors or contributors are their personal views and opinions and do not necessarily reflect the views/opinions of the publisher. Any information or guidance contained in this book is intended for use solely by medical professionals strictly as a supplement to the medical professional's own judgement, knowledge of the patient's medical history, relevant manufacturer's instructions, and the appropriate best practice guidelines. Because of the rapid advances in medical science, any information or advice on dosages, procedures, or diagnoses should be independently verified. This book does not indicate whether a particular treatment is appropriate or suitable for a particular individual. Ultimately it is the sole responsibility of the medical professional to make his or her own professional judgements, so as appropriately to advise and treat patients. Save for death or personal injury caused by the publisher's negligence and to the fullest extent otherwise permitted by law, neither the publisher nor any person engaged or employed by the publisher shall be responsible or liable for any loss, injury, or damage caused to any person or property arising in any way from the use of this book.

A CIP record for this book is available from the British Library.
Library of Congress Cataloging-in-Publication Data available on application.

Volume 1: ISBN 978-1-84184-970-6; eISBN 978-1-84184-971-3
Volume 2: ISBN 978-1-84184-972-0; eISBN 978-1-84184-973-7
Two volume set: 978-1-84184-974-4; eISBN 978-1-84184-975-1

Orders may be sent to: Informa Healthcare, Sheepen Place, Colchester, Essex CO3 3LP, UK
Telephone: +44 (0)20 7017 6682; Email: Books@Informa.com; www.informahealthcarebooks.com; www.informa.com

For corporate sales please contact: CorporateBooksIHC@informa.com
For foreign rights please contact: RightsIHC@informa.com
For reprint permissions please contact: PermissionsIHC@informa.com

Typeset by Exeter Premedia Services Pvt Ltd, India
Printed and bound in India by Replika Press Pvt Ltd

Contents

List of contributors — vii

The beginnings of human *in vitro* fertilization — x
Robert G. Edwards

Robert Edwards: The path to IVF — xxiii
Martin H. Johnson

I Establishing and Maintaining an IVF Laboratory

1. Setting up an ART laboratory — 1
   Jacques Cohen, Mina Alikani, Antonia Gilligan, and Tim Schimmel
2. Quality control: Maintaining stability in the laboratory — 9
   David H. McCulloh
3. The ART laboratory: Current standards — 31
   Cecilia Sjöblom

II Gamete Collection, Preparation and Selection

4. Evaluation of sperm — 48
   Kaylen M. Silverberg and Tom Turner
5. Sperm preparation techniques — 61
   Harold Bourne, Janell Archer, David H. Edgar, and H. W. Gordon Baker
6. Sperm chromatin assessment — 75
   Ashok Agarwal, Igor Tsarev, Juris Erenpreiss, and Rakesh Sharma
7. Oocyte retrieval and selection — 96
   Laura F. Rienzi and Filippo M. Ubaldi
8. Preparation and evaluation of oocytes for ICSI — 114
   Irit Granot and Nava Dekel
9. Hyaluronic acid binding-mediated sperm selection for ICSI — 122
   Gabor Huszar
10. Intracytoplasmic morphologically selected sperm injection — 135
    Monica Antinori
11. Use of in vitro maturation in a clinical setting: Patient populations and outcomes — 151
    Yoshiharu Morimoto, Aisaku Fukuda, and Manabu Satoh

III Micromanipulation

12. Micromanipulation — 163
    Frank L. Barnes
13. Intracytoplasmic sperm injection: Technical aspects — 172
    Queenie V. Neri, Devin Monahan, Zev Rosenwaks, and Gianpiero D. Palermo
14. Assisted hatching — 186
    Anna Veiga and Itziar Belil
15. Human embryo biopsy procedures — 197
    Alan R. Thornhill, Christian Ottolini, and Alan H. Handyside

IV Culture, Selection and Transfer of the Human Embryo

16. Analysis of fertilization — 212
    Thomas Ebner
17. Culture systems for the human embryo — 218
    David K. Gardner and Michelle Lane
18. Evaluation of embryo quality: Analysis of morphology and quantification of nutrient utilization and the metabolome — 240
    Denny Sakkas and David K. Gardner
19. Evaluation of embryo quality: Time-lapse imaging to assess embryo morphokinesis — 254
    Natalia Basile, Juan García-Velasco, and Marcos Meseguer
20. Evaluation of embryo quality: Proteomic strategies — 266
    Mandy Katz-Jaffe

V Cryopreservation

21. The human oocyte: Controlled rate cooling — 275
    Andrea Borini and Veronica Bianchi
22. The human oocyte: Vitrification — 285
    Masashige Kuwayama
23. The human embryo: Slow freezing — 293
    Nikica Zaninovic, Richard Bodine, Robert N. Clarke, Sam Jones, Ye Zhen, and Lucinda L. Veeck Gosden
24. The human embryo: Vitrification — 307
    Zsolt Peter Nagy, Ching-Chien Chang, and Gábor Vajta

VI Diagnosis of Genetic Disease in Preimplantation Embryos

25. Severe male factor: Genetic consequences and recommendations for genetic testing — 324
    Willy Lissens and Katrien Stouffs
26. Polar body biopsy and its clinical application — 336
    Markus Montag
27. Preimplantation genetic diagnosis for infertility — 346
    Dagan Wells and Elpida Fragouli
28. Genetic analysis of the embryo — 354
    Yuval Yaron, Veronica Gold, Sagit Peleg-Schalka, and Mira Malcov

VII Implantation

29. The analysis of endometrial receptivity — 366
    Tamara Garrido-Gomez, Francisco Domínguez, Maria Ruiz, Felip Vilella, and Carlos Simon

VIII Future Directions and Clinical Applications

30. Human embryonic stem cells — 380
    Rachel Eiges, Michal Avitzour, and Benjamin Reubinoff
31. Microfluidics in ART: Current progress and future directions — 396
    Jason E. Swain, Thomas B. Pool, Shuichi Takayama, and Gary D. Smith

Index — 415

List of contributors

Ashok Agarwal
Center for Reproductive Medicine, Glickman Urological and Kidney Institute, Cleveland, Ohio, USA
Obstetrics/Gynecology and Women's Health Institute, Cleveland Clinic, Cleveland, Ohio, USA

Mina Alikani
The Center for Human Reproduction, North Shore – Long Island Jewish Health System, Manhasset, New York, USA

Monica Antinori
International Associated Research Institute for Human Reproduction, RAPRUI Day Hospital, Rome, Italy

Janell Archer
Reproductive Services, The Royal Women's Hospital and Melbourne IVF, Melbourne, Victoria, Australia

Michal Avitzour
The Stem Cell Research Laboratory, Medical Genetics Institute, Shaare Zedek Medical Center affiliated with the Hebrew University School of Medicine, Jerusalem, Israel

H. W. Gordon Baker
University of Melbourne, Department of Obstetrics and Gynaecology, The Royal Women's Hospital and Melbourne IVF, Melbourne, Victoria, Australia

Frank L. Barnes
IVF Labs, LLC, Salt Lake City, Utah, USA

Natalia Basile
IVI Madrid, Madrid, Spain

Itziar Belil
Reproductive Medicine Service, Institut Universitari Dexeus, Barcelona, Spain

Veronica Bianchi
Tecnobios Procreazione Centre for Reproductive Health, Bologna, Italy

Richard Bodine
The Center for Reproductive Medicine, Weill Medical College of Cornell University, New York, New York, USA

Andrea Borini
Tecnobios Procreazione Centre for Reproductive Health, Bologna, Italy

Harold Bourne
Reproductive Services, The Royal Women's Hospital and Melbourne IVF, Melbourne, Victoria, Australia

Ching-Chien Chang
Reproductive Biology Associates, Atlanta, Georgia, USA

Robert N. Clarke
The Center for Reproductive Medicine, Weill Medical College of Cornell University, New York, New York, USA

Jacques Cohen
Tyho-Galileo Research Laboratories, Livingston, New Jersey, USA

Nava Dekel
Department of Biological Regulation, The Weizmann Institute of Science, Rehovot, Israel

Francisco Domínguez
Fundación IVI, Valencia University, INCLIVA, Valencia, Spain

Thomas Ebner
Landes- Frauen- und Kinderklinik, Kinderwunsch Zentrum, Linz, Austria

David H. Edgar
Reproductive Services, The Royal Women's Hospital and Melbourne IVF, Melbourne, Victoria, Australia

Robert G. Edwards
Duck End Farm, Dry Drayton, Cambridge, UK

Rachel Eiges
The Stem Cell Research Laboratory, Medical Genetics Institute, Shaare Zedek Medical Center affiliated with the Hebrew University School of Medicine, Jerusalem, Israel

Juris Erenpreiss
Andrology Laboratory, Riga Stradins University, Riga, Latvia

Elpida Fragouli
Reprogenetics UK, Institute of Reproductive Sciences, Oxford, UK
Nuffield Department of Obstetrics and Gynaecology, University of Oxford, Oxford, UK

List of Contributors

Aisaku Fukuda
IVF Osaka Clinic, Nagata Higashi, Higashi-Osaka, Osaka, Japan

Juan García-Velasco
IVI Madrid, Madrid, Spain

David K. Gardner
Department of Zoology, University of Melbourne, Melbourne, Victoria, Australia

Tamara Garrido-Gomez
Fundación IVI, Valencia University, INCLIVA, Valencia, Spain

Antonia Gilligan
Alpha Environmental, Emerson, New Jersey, USA

Veronica Gold
Sara Racine In Vitro Fertilization Unit, Tel Aviv Sourasky Medical Center, Tel Aviv, Israel

Irit Granot
IVF Unit, Department of Obstetrics and Gynecology, Kaplan Medical Center, Rehovot, Israel

Alan H. Handyside
The London Bridge Fertility, Gynaecology and Genetics Centre, London, and Faculty of Biological Sciences, University of Leeds, UK

Colin M. Howles
External Scientific Affairs, Global Development and Medical, Merck Serono SA, Geneva, Switzerland

Gabor Huszar
Sperm Physiology Laboratory and Male Fertility Program, Section of Reproductive Endocrinology, Department of Obstetrics, Gynecology and Reproductive Sciences, Yale University School of Medicine, New Haven, Connecticut, USA

Martin H. Johnson
The Anatomy School; Department of Physiology, Development and Neuroscience; The Centre for Trophoblast Research; University of Cambridge, Cambridge, UK

Sam Jones
The Center for Reproductive Medicine, Weill Medical College of Cornell University, New York, New York, USA

Mandy Katz-Jaffe
Colorado Center for Reproductive Medicine, Lone Tree, Colorado, USA

Masashige Kuwayama
Repro-Support Medical Research Centre, Shinjuku, Tokyo, Japan

Michelle Lane
Department of Obstetrics and Gynecology, University of Adelaide, Adelaide, South Australia, Australia
Repromed, Dulwich, South Australia, Australia

Willy Lissens
Center for Medical Genetics, UZ Brussel and Vrije Universiteit Brussel, Brussels, Belgium

Mira Malcov
Sara Racine In Vitro Fertilization Unit, Tel Aviv Sourasky Medical Center, Tel Aviv, Israel

David H. McCulloh
Department of Obstetrics, Gynecology and Women's Health, New Jersey Medical School, University of Medicine and Dentistry of New Jersey, Newark, New Jersey, USA

Marcos Meseguer
IVI Valencia, and Valencia University, Valencia, Spain

Devin Monahan
The Ronald O. Perelman & Claudia Cohen Center for Reproductive Medicine, Weill Cornell Medical College, New York, New York, USA

Markus Montag
Department of Gynaecological Endocrinology and Fertility Disorders, University of Heidelberg, Heidelberg, Germany

Yoshiharu Morimoto
IVF Namba Clinic, Minamihorie, Nishi-ku, Osaka-City, Osaka, Japan

Zsolt Peter Nagy
Reproductive Biology Associates, Atlanta, Georgia, USA

Queenie V. Neri
The Ronald O. Perelman & Claudia Cohen Center for Reproductive Medicine, Weill Cornell Medical College, New York, New York, USA

Christian Ottolini
The London Bridge Fertility, Gynaecology and Genetics Centre, London, and Department of Biosciences, University of Kent, Canterbury, UK

Gianpiero D. Palermo
The Ronald O. Perelman & Claudia Cohen Center for Reproductive Medicine, Weill Cornell Medical College, New York, New York, USA

Sagit Peleg-Schalka
Sara Racine In Vitro Fertilization Unit, Tel Aviv Sourasky Medical Center, Tel Aviv, Israel

Thomas B. Pool
Fertility Center of San Antonio, San Antonio, Texas, USA

Benjamin Reubinoff
IVF Unit, Department of Obstetrics and Gynecology, and Goldyne Savad Institute of Gene Therapy, Hadassah University Hospital, Jerusalem, Israel

Laura F. Rienzi
Genera Centre for Reproductive Medicine, Clinica Valle Giulia, Rome, Italy

Zev Rosenwaks
The Ronald O. Perelman & Claudia Cohen Center for Reproductive Medicine, Weill Cornell Medical College, New York, New York, USA

Maria Ruiz
Fundación IVI and IVIOMICS, Valencia University, INCLIVA, Valencia, Spain

Denny Sakkas
Department of Obstetrics and Gynecology, Yale University School of Medicine, New Haven, Connecticut, USA

Manabu Satoh
Department of Reproductive Technology, IVF Namba Clinic, Minamihorie, Nishi-ku, Osaka, Japan

Tim Schimmel
Tyho-Galileo Research Laboratories, Livingston, New Jersey, USA

Rakesh Sharma
Center for Reproductive Medicine, Glickman Urological and Kidney Institute, Cleveland, Ohio, USA
Obstetrics/Gynecology and Women's Health Institute, Cleveland Clinic, Cleveland, Ohio, USA

Zeev Shoham
Reproductive Medicine and Infertility Unit, Department of Obstetrics and Gynecology, Kaplan Medical Center, Rehovot, Israel

Kaylen M. Silverberg
Texas Fertility Center, Austin IVF, Austin, Texas, USA

Carlos Simon
Fundación IVI and IVIOMICS, Valencia University, INCLIVA, Valencia, Spain

Cecilia Sjöblom
Westmead Fertility Centre, University of Sydney, Western Clinical School, Westmead Hospital, Westmead, New South Wales, Australia

Gary D. Smith
Department of Obstetrics and Gynecology, and Department of Urology, and Molecular and Integrative Physiology, and Reproductive Medicine Program, University of Michigan, Ann Arbor, Michigan, USA

Katrien Stouffs
Center for Medical Genetics,
UZ Brussel and Vrije Universiteit Brussel, Brussels, Belgium

Jason E. Swain
Department of Obstetrics and Gynecology, and Reproductive Sciences Program, University of Michigan, Ann Arbor, Michigan, USA

Shuichi Takayama
Department of Biomedical Engineering, University of Michigan, Ann Arbor, Michigan, USA

Alan R. Thornhill
The London Bridge Fertility, Gynaecology and Genetics Centre, London, and Department of Biosciences, University of Kent, Canterbury, UK

Igor Tsarev
Center for Reproductive Medicine,
Glickman Urological and Kidney Institute, Cleveland, Ohio, USA
Obstetrics/Gynecology and Women's Health Institute, Cleveland Clinic, Cleveland, Ohio, USA

Tom Turner
Texas Fertility Center, Austin IVF, Austin, Texas, USA

Filippo M. Ubaldi
Centre for Reproductive Medicine, Clinica Valle Giulia, Rome, Italy

Gábor Vajta
BGI Shenzhen, Beishan Industrial Zone, Yantian District, Shenzhen, China

Lucinda L. Veeck Gosden
The Center for Reproductive Medicine, Weill Medical College of Cornell University, New York, New York, USA

Anna Veiga
Reproductive Medicine Service,
Institut Universitari Dexeus, Barcelona, Spain
Banc de Linies Cellulars, Centre de Medicina Regenerativa de Barcelona, Barcelona, Spain

Felip Vilella
Fundación IVI, Valencia University, INCLIVA, Valencia, Spain

Ariel Weissman
IVF Unit, Department of Obstetrics and Gynecology, Edith Wolfson Medical Center, Holon, Israel
Sackler Faculty of Medicine, Tel Aviv University, Tel Aviv, Israel

Dagan Wells
Reprogenetics UK, Institute of Reproductive Sciences, Oxford, UK
Nuffield Department of Obstetrics and Gynaecology, University of Oxford, Oxford, UK

Yuval Yaron
Prenatal Genetic Diagnosis Division, Genetic Institute; Department of Obstetrics and Gynecology, Lis Maternity Hospital, Tel Aviv Sourasky Medical Center; Sackler Faculty of Medicine, Tel Aviv University, Tel Aviv, Israel

Nikica Zaninovic
The Center for Reproductive Medicine, Weill Medical College of Cornell University, New York, New York, USA

Ye Zhen
The Center for Reproductive Medicine, Weill Medical College of Cornell University, New York, New York, USA

The beginnings of human *in vitro* fertilization

Robert G. Edwards

In vitro fertilization (IVF) and its derivatives in preimplantation diagnosis, stem cells, and the ethics of assisted reproduction continue to attract immense attention scientifically and socially. All these topics were introduced by 1970. Hardly a day passes without some public recognition of events related to this study, and clinics spread ever further worldwide. Now we must be approaching 1.5 million IVF births, it is time to celebrate what has been achieved by so many investigators, clinical, scientific, and ethical.

While much of this chapter "Introduction" covers the massive accumulation of events between 1960 and 2000, it also briefly discusses new perspectives emerging in the 21st century. Fresh advances also increase curiosity about how these fields of study began and how their ethical implications were addressed in earlier days. As for me, I am still stirred by recollections of those early days. Foundations were laid in Edinburgh, London, and Glasgow in the 1950s and early 1960s. Discoveries made then led to later days in Cambridge, working there with many PhD students. It also resulted in my working with Patrick Steptoe in Oldham. Our joint opening of Bourn Hall in 1980, which became the largest IVF clinic of its kind at the time, signified the end of the beginning of assisted human conception and the onset of dedicated applied studies.

INTRODUCTION

First of all, I must express in limited space my tributes to my teachers, even if inadequately. These include investigators from far-off days when the fundamental facts of reproductive cycles, surgical techniques, endocrinology, and genetics were elicited by many investigators. These fields began to move in the 20th century, and if one pioneer of these times should be saluted, it must be Gregory Pincus. Famous for the contraceptive pill, he was a distinguished embryologist, and part of his work dealt with the maturation of mammalian oocytes in vitro. He was the first to show how oocytes aspirated from their follicles would begin their maturation in vitro, and how a number matured and expelled a first polar body. I believe his major work was done in rabbits, where he found that the 10 to 11-hour timings of maturation in vitro accorded exactly with those occurring in vivo after an ovulatory stimulus to the female rabbit.

Pincus et al. also studied human oocytes (1). Extracting oocytes from excised ovaries, they identified chromosomes in a large number of oocytes and interpreted this as evidence of the completion of maturation in vitro. Many oocytes possessed chromosomes after 12 hours, the proportion remaining constant over the next 30 hours and longer. Twelve hours was taken as the period of maturation. Unfortunately, chromosomes were not classified for their meiotic stage. Maturing oocytes would be expected to display diakinesis or metaphase-I chromosome pairs. Fully mature oocytes would display metaphase-II chromosomes, signifying they were fully ripe and ready for fertilization. Nevertheless, it is well known that oocytes can undergo atresia in the ovary involving the formation of metaphase-II chromosomes in many of them. These oocytes complicated Pincus' estimates, even in controls, and were the source of his error which led later workers to inseminate human oocytes 12 hours after collection and culture in vitro (2,3). Work on human fertilization in vitro, and indeed comparable studies in animals, remained in abeyance from then and for many years. Progress in animal IVF had also been slow. After many relatively unsuccessful attempts in several species in the 1950s and 1960s, a virtual dogma arose that spermatozoa had to spend several hours in the female reproductive tract before acquiring the potential to bind to the zona pellucida and achieve fertilization. In the late 1960s, Austin and Chang independently identified the need for sperm capacitation, identified by a delay in fertilization after spermatozoa had entered the female reproductive tract (4,5). This discovery was taken by many investigators as the reason for the failure to achieve fertilization in vitro, and why spermatozoa had to be exposed to secretions of the female reproductive tract. At the same time, Chang reported that rabbit eggs that had fully matured in vitro failed to produce normal blastocysts, none of them implanting normally (6).

MODERN BEGINNINGS OF HUMAN IVF, PREIMPLANTATION GENETIC DIAGNOSIS, AND EMBRYO STEM CELLS

My PhD began at the Institute of Animal Genetics, Edinburgh University in 1952, encouraged by Professor Conrad Waddington, the inventor of epigenesis, and supervised by Dr Alan Beatty. At the time, capacitation transferred an hour or so after it became 8-cell. Their positive pregnancy test a few days after transfer was another milestone—surely nothing could now prevent their embryo developing to full term in a normal reproductive cycle, but those nine months lasted a very long time. Three more pregnancies were established using natural-cycle IVF as we abandoned the other approaches. A triploid embryo died in utero—more bad luck. A third pregnancy was lost through premature labor on a mountain walking holiday, two weeks after the mother's amniocentesis (32,33). It was a lovely, well-developed boy. Louise Brown's birth, and then Alistair's, proved to a waiting world that science and medicine had entered human conception. Our critics declared that the births were a fake, and advised against attending our presentation on the whole of the Oldham work at the Royal College of Obstetricians and Gynaecologists.

IVF WORLDWIDE

The Oldham period was over. Good facilities were now needed, with space for a large IVF clinic. Bourn Hall was an old Jacobean house in lovely grounds near Cambridge (Fig. I.7). Facilities on offer for IVF in Cambridge were far too small, so we purchased it mostly with venture capital. It was essential to conceive 100 or 1000 IVF babies to ensure that the method was safe and effective clinically. The immense delays in establishing Bourn Hall delayed our work by two years after Louise's birth. Finally, on minimal finance, Bourn Hall was opened in September 1980 on a shoestring, supported by our own cash and loans. The delay gave the rest of the world a chance to join in IVF. Alex Lopata delivered an IVF baby in Australia, and one or two others were born elsewhere. Natural-cycle IVF was chosen initially at Bourn Hall since it had proved successful in Oldham, and we became experts in it. Pregnancies flowed, at 15% per cycle. An Australian team of Alan Trounson and Carl Wood announced the establishment of several IVF pregnancies after stimulation by clomiphene and hCG and replacing two or three embryos (34), so they had moved ahead of us during the delayed opening of Bourn Hall. Our own effort now expanded prodigiously. Thousands of patients queued for IVF. Simon Fishel, Jacques Cohen, and Carol Fehilly joined the embryology team among younger trainees, and new clinicians joined Patrick and John Webster. Patients and pregnancies increased rapidly, and the world was left standing far behind. Howard and Georgeanna Jones began in Norfolk using gonadotropins for ovarian stimulation. Jean Cohen began in Paris, Wilfred Feichtinger and Peter Kemeter in Vienna, Klaus Diedrich and Hans van der Venn in Bonn, Lars Hamberger and Matts Wikland in Sweden, and Andre van Steirteghem and Paul Devroey in Brussels. IVF was now truly international.

The opening of Bourn Hall had not deterred our critics. They put up a fierce rearguard action against IVF, alongside LIFE, Society for the Unborn Child, individual gynecologists, and others.

Objections raised against IVF included low rates of pregnancy (no one mentioned the similar low rates of pregnancy with natural conception), the possibilities of oocyte and embryo donation, surrogate mothers, unmarried parents, one-sex parents, embryo cryopreservation, cloning, and endless other objections.

LIFE issued a legal action against me for the abortion of an embryo grown for 14 days and longer in vitro. Their action was rejected by the U.K. Attorney General since the laws of pregnancy began after implantation. We fully respected the intense ethical nature of our proceedings. We also recognized the need for research, and the necessity to protect or cryopreserve the best embryos for later replacement into their mothers. Those not replaced had to be used for research under strict controls, combined with open publication and discussion of our work.

Each year, 1000, rising to almost 2000, patients passed through Bourn Hall. Different stimulation regimens or new procedures could be tested in very little time.

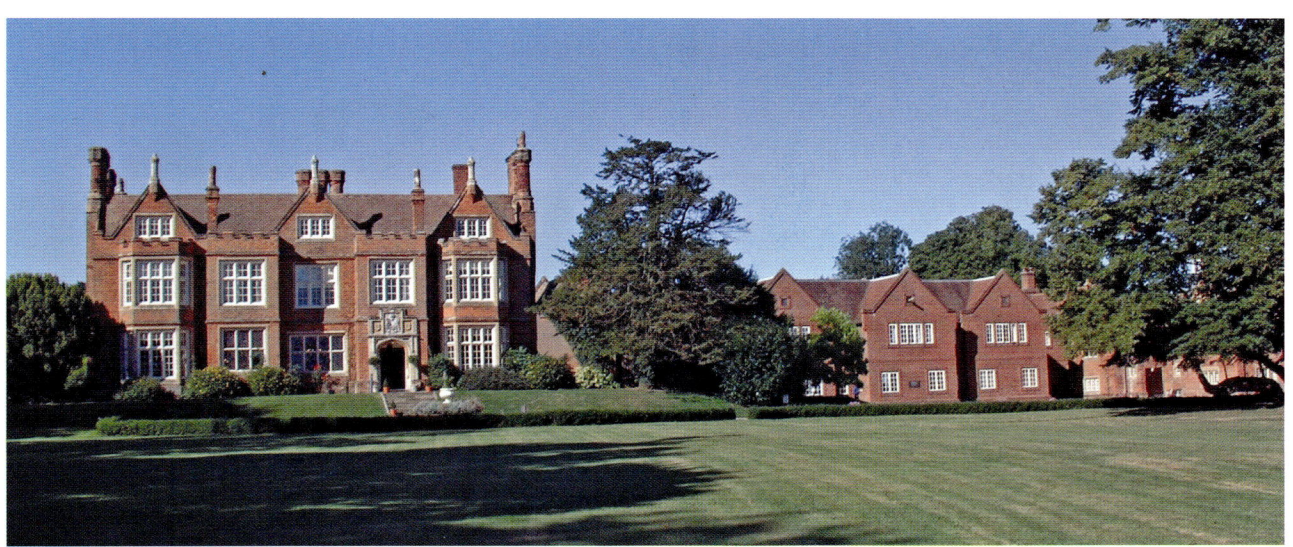

Figure I.7 Bourn Hall. *Source*: Courtesy of Dr P Brinsden.

Clomiphene/hMG was reintroduced. Bourn babies increased: 20, 50, 100 to 1000 after five to six years. This was far more than half of the world's entire IVF babies, including the first born in the United States, Germany, Italy, and many other countries. Detailed studies were performed on embryo culture, implantation, and abortion. We even tried aspirating epididymal spermatozoa for IVF, without achieving successful fertilization.

Among the immense numbers of patients, people with astonishingly varied conditions of infertility emerged. Some were poor responders in whom immense amounts of endocrine priming were essential, women with a natural menstrual cycle that was not as it should have been, previous misdiagnoses which had laid the cause of infertility on the wife when the husband had never even been investigated, and men bringing semen samples that we discovered had been obtained from a friend. The collaboration between nurses, clinicians, and scientists was remarkable. Yet trouble—ethical trouble—was never far away. I purchased a freezing machine to resume our Oldham work, but, unknown to me, Patrick talked to officers of the British Medical Association (BMA) and for some reason agreed to delay embryo cryopreservation. Apparently, the BMA felt it would be an unwelcome social development. I did not approve of these reservations: David Whittingham had shown how low-temperature cryostorage was successful with mouse embryos, without causing genetic damage. "Freezing and cloning" became a term of intense approbation at this time. I unwillingly curtailed our cryopreservation program.

One weekend, a major trouble erupted as a result of this difference between Patrick and me. My duties in Bourn Hall prevented me from attending a conference in London. Trying to be helpful, I telephoned my lecture to London. Reception at the other end was apparently so poor as to lead to misinterpretations of what I had said. Next morning, the press furore about my supposed practice of cryopreserving embryos after IVF was awful, so bad, indeed, that legal action had to be taken. Luckily, my lecture had been recorded, and listening to the tapes with a barrister revealed nothing contentious. I had said nothing improper in my lecture or during the question-answer session. That day, I issued seven libel actions against the cream of British society: the BMA and its secretary, the BBC, *The Times*, and other leading newspapers. There were seven in one day and another one later! If only one was lost, I could be ruined and disgraced. However, they were all won, even though it took several years with the BMA and its secretary. These legal actions had inhibited our research, the cryopreservation program being shut down for more than a year. Every single embryological note of mine from those days in Oldham and from Bourn Hall was examined in detail for my opponents by someone who was clearly an embryologist. Nothing was found to incriminate me.

That wretched period passed. The number of babies kept on growing, embryo cryopreservation was resumed, and Gerhard Dealmaker in The Netherlands beat us and the world to the first "ice" baby (35). Colin Howles and Mike McNamee joined us in endocrinology, and Mike Ashwood-Smith and Peter Holland's in embryology, as the old team faded away. Fascinating days had returned. Working with barristers, we designed consent forms which were far in advance of those used elsewhere. Oocyte donation and surrogacy by embryo transfer were introduced. The world's first paper on embryo stem cells appeared in *Science* in 1984, sent from Bourn Hall, and the world's first on human preimplantation diagnosis in 1987 appeared in *Human Reproduction*. However, embryo research faltered as all normal embryos were cryopreserved for their parents, so almost none were available for study. Alan Handyside, one of our Cambridge PhDs, joined Hammersmith Hospital in London to make major steps in introducing preimplantation genetic diagnosis (36). As we reached 1000 pregnancies, our data showed the babies to be as normal as those conceived in vivo.

Test-tube babies (an awful term) were no longer unique and were accepted worldwide, exactly as Patrick and I had hoped. Our work was being recognized (Fig. I.8). Clinics sprang up everywhere. Ultrasound was introduced to detect follicles for aspiration by the Scandinavians (37), making laparoscopy for oocyte recovery largely redundant. Artificial cycles were introduced in Australia and intracytoplasmic sperm injection (ICSI) in Belgium (38), and gonadotropin-releasing hormone agonists were used to inhibit the LH surge. Ian Craft in London showed how postmenopausal women aged 52 or more could establish pregnancies using oocyte donation and endocrine support. Women over 60 years of age conceived and delivered children. This breakthrough was especially welcome to me, since older women surely have the right to have children at ages almost the same as those possible for men.

Ethics continued side by side with advancing science and medicine. The U.K. governmental Warnock report recommended permitting embryo research and proposed a Licensing Authority for IVF. A year or so later, the U.K. House of Lords, in all its finery, responded with a 3:1 vote in favor, decisive support for all we had done in Mill

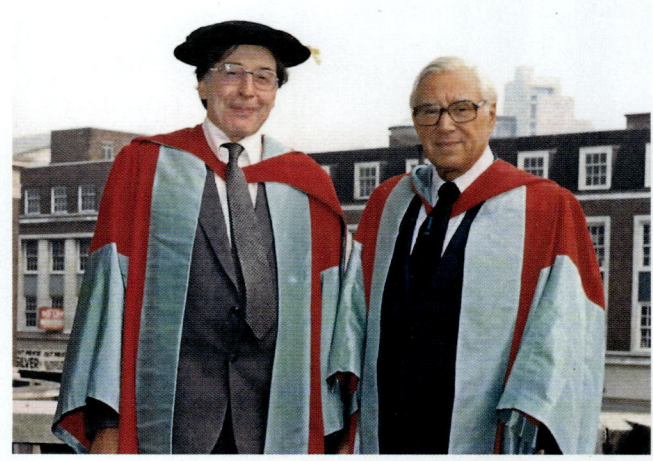

Figure I.8 A happy picture of Patrick and me, standing in our robes after being granted our Hon. DSc by Hull University.

Hill, Cambridge, and Oldham. What a wonderful day! The British House of Commons passed a liberal IVF law after intense debate, and so did the Spanish government, although elsewhere things were not so liberal. Ten years after the birth of Louise Brown, the British Parliament had therefore accepted IVF, research on human embryos until day 14, and establishing research embryos. Cloning and embryo stem cells still bothered the politicians in 1988, to re-emerge in 1998, gray shadows of my earlier times in Glasgow. IVF had also become fundamental to establish embryonic stem cells for organ repair, or cloning. During all this activity, tragedy struck all of us in Bourn Hall. Jean Purdy died in 1986 and Patrick Steptoe in 1988. They at least saw IVF come of age.

By the 1990s, burgeoning medical science was digging deeper into endless aspects of human conception in vitro. The intracytoplasmic injection of a single spermatozoon into an oocyte to achieve fertilization, ICSI, was one of the greatest advances since IVF was introduced. It transformed the treatment of male infertility, enabling severely oligozoospermic men to father their own children. It did not stop there, since epididymal spermatozoa and even those aspirated from the testis could be used for ICSI. Spermatids have also been used. ICSI became so simple that many clinics reduced IVF to fewer and fewer cases. New gonadotropin-releasing hormone antagonists introduced novel ways to control the cycle, enabling many oocytes to be stimulated by hMG and, subsequently, using recombinant human FSH. Treatment in the natural cycle could be improved, since these antagonists control LH levels and prevent premature LH surges. My own interests were returning to embryology, as the molecular biology revolution influenced our thinking. I am convinced that the oocyte and egg must be highly programmed, timewise, in embryonic polarities and integrating genetic systems such that the tight systems place every new gene product in its right place in the one-cell egg and cleaving embryo. This must be right; there can surely be no other explanations for the fabulous modification in embryonic growth in the first week or two of embryonic life. I have been delighted to work with Chris Hansis on identifying a gene (for hCG-β) in one blastomere of four- and eight-cell human embryos, providing evidence of blastomere differentiation at this early stage of embryogenesis (39).

This topic returns me to my scientific origins studying mouse embryos in the Institute of Animal Genetics in Edinburgh, where Waddington reported the amazing story of the gene *Aristapedia* in *Drosophila*, which he had induced to grow legs in place of eyes. These unusual flies then bred true, showing he had uncovered a gene that had been silenced for millions of years and how this could be an essential component of normal differentiation. He called it epigenesis, and we fear today that some aspects of IVF may lead to deleterious epigenetic changes in children such as Angelman or Beckwith–Wiedemann syndrome. Risks of epigenetic changes in cattle embryos and those of other species may be heightened by adding serum to media used to culture embryos to cause, for example large-calf syndrome. It would be wise to be well aware of these findings when practicing human IVF, for example by assessing the role of sera in human culture media.

IVF OUTLOOK

In one sense, opening up human conception in vitro was perhaps among the first examples of applied science in modern "hi tech." Human IVF has since spread throughout the world, with apparently more than 3.5 million babies born worldwide by 2008— yet Louise Brown is only just 30 years of age. The need for IVF and its derivatives is greater than ever, since up to 10% of couples may suffer from some form of infertility. Major advances in genetic technologies now identify hundreds of genes in a single cell, and diagnosing genetic disease in embryos promises to help avoid desperate genetic diseases in newborn children. Indeed, the ethics of this field have now become even more serious, since the typing of embryo genotypes provides detailed predictions of future life and health.

IVF has now combined closely with genetics to eliminate disease or disability genes, or lengthen the life span. But most of all, practicing IVF teaches a wider understanding of the desire and love for a child and a partner, the wonderful and ancient joys of parenthood, the pain of failure, the deep motivation needed in donating and receiving an urgently needed oocyte or a surrogate uterus. Parenthood is more responsible than ever before. Its complex choices are gathered before couples everywhere by the information revolution, placing family responsibilities on patients themselves, where it really matters. And IVF now reveals more and more about miracles preserved in embryogenesis from flies and frogs to humankind, over 600 million years of evolution.

The human genome project is now complete and will inevitably assist IVF since we will soon understand the genetic aspects of early embryo growth and how to detect abnormal genes in embryos. This textbook contains chapters which describe in detail the several advances and developments which have expanded the possibilities of treating diverse causes of human infertility as well as numerous genetic disorders.

Already it is clear that a staggering array of genes operates in preimplantation stages in mammalian including human embryos, and new methods are being introduced to deal with such highly multigenic embryonic systems. We are indeed enmeshed in a field embracing some of the most fundamental evolutionary stages of our existence as we pass from oocyte to blastocyst and to implantation.

REFERENCES

1. Pincus G, Saunders B. The comparative behavior of mammalian eggs in vivo and in vitro. VI. The maturation of human ovarian ova. Anat Rec 1939; 75: 537–45.
2. Menkin MF, Rock J. Am J Obstet Gynecol 1949; 55: 440.
3. Hayashi M. Seventh International Conference of the International Planned Parenthood Federation. Excerpta Medica, 1963: 505.

4. Austin CR. Adv Biosci 1969; 4: 5.
5. Chang M. Adv Biosci 1969; 4: 13.
6. Chang MC. The maturation of rabbit oocytes in culture and their maturation, activation, fertilization and subsequent development in the fallopian tubes. J Exp Zool 1955; 128: 379–405.
7. Runner M, Gates AH. Sterile, obese mothers. J Hered 1954; 45: 51–5.
8. Gates AH. Viability and developmental capacity of eggs from immature mice treated with gonadotrophins. Nature 1954; 177: 754–5.
9. Fowler RE, Edwards RG. Induction of superovulation and pregnancy in mature mice by gonadotrophins. J Endocrinol 1957; 15: 374–84.
10. Edwards RG, Gates AH. Timing of the stages of the maturation divisions, ovulation, fertilization and the first cleavage of eggs of adult mice treated with gonadotrophins. J Endocrinol 1959; 19: 292–304.
11. Edwards RG. Meiosis in ovarian oocytes of adult mammals. Nature (London) 1962; 196: 446–50.
12. Cole R, Edwards RG, Paul J. Cytodifferentiation and embryogenesis in cell colonies and tissue cultures derived from ova and blastocysts of the rabbit. Dev Biol 1966; 13: 385–407.
13. Edwards RG. Maturation in vitro of mouse, sheep, cow, pig, rhesus monkey and human ovarian oocytes. Nature 1965; 208: 349–51.
14. Edwards RG. Maturation in vitro of human ovarian oocytes. Lancet 1965; 2: 926–9.
15. Edwards RG, Donahue R, Baramki T, Jones H Jr. Preliminary attempts to fertilize human oocytes matured in vivo. Am J Obstet Gynecol 1966; 96: 192–200.
16. Yanagimachi R, Chang MC. J Exp Zool 1964; 156: 361–76.
17. Edwards RG, Talbert L, Israestam D, et al. Diffusion chamber for exposing spermatozoa to human uterine secretions. Am J Obstet Gynecol 1968; 102: 388–96.
18. Steptoe PC. Laparoscopy and ovulation. Lancet 1968; 2: 913.
19. Edwards RG, Bavister BD, Steptoe PC. Early stages of fertilisation in vitro of human oocytes matured in vitro. Nature (London) 1969; 221: 632–5.
20. Gardner RL, Edwards RG. Control of the sex ratio at full term in the rabbit by transferred sexed blastocysts. Nature (London) 1968; 218: 346–8.
21. Henderson SA, Edwards RG. Chiasma frequency and maternal age in mammals. Nature (London) 1968; 218: 22–8.
22. Edwards RG, Sharpe DJ. Social values and research in human embryology. Nature (London) 1971; 231: 81–91.
23. Palmer R. Acad Chir 1946; 72: 363.
24. Fragenheim H. Geburts Frauenheilkd 1964; 24: 740.
25. Steptoe PC. Laparoscopy in Gynaecology. Edinburgh: Livingstone, 1967.
26. Lunenfeld B. In: Inguilla W, Greenblatt RG, Thomas RB, eds. The Ovary. Springfield, IL: CC Thomas, 1969.
27. Steptoe PC, Edwards RG. Laparoscopic recovery of preovulatory human oocytes after priming of ovaries with gonadotrophins. Lancet 1970; 1: 683–9.
28. Edwards RG, Steptoe PC, Purdy JM. Fertilization and cleavage in vitro of preovulatory human oocytes. Nature (London) 1970; 227: 1307–9.
29. Steptoe PC, Edwards RG, Purdy JM. Human blastocysts grown in culture. Nature (London) 1971; 229: 132–3.
30. Edwards RG, Surani MAH. The primate blastocyst and its environment. Uppsala J Med Sci 1978; 22: 39–50.
31. Csapo AI, Pulkkinen MO, Kaihola HL. The relationship between the timing of luteectomy and the incidence of complete abortions. Am J Obstet Gycecol 1974; 118: 985–9.
32. Steptoe PC, Edwards RG. Reimplantation of a human embryo with subsequent tubal pregnancy. Lancet 1976; 1: 880–2.
33. Edwards RG, Steptoe PC, Purdy JM. Clinical aspects of pregnancies established with cleaving embryos grown in vivo. Br J Obstet Gynaecol 1980; 87: 757–68.
34. Trounson AO, Leeton JF, Wood C, et al. Pregnancies in humans by fertilization in vitro and embryo transfer in the controlled ovulatory cycle. Science 1981; 212: 681–2.
35. Zeilmaker GH, Alberda T, Gent I, et al. Two pregnancies following transfer of intact frozen–thawed embryos. Fertil Steril 1984; 42: 293–6.
36. Handyside A, Kontogianni EH, Hardy K, Winston RML. Pregnancies from biopsied human preimplantation embryos sexed by Y-specific DNA application. Nature (London) 1990; 344: 768–70.
37. Wikland M, Enk L, Hamberger L. Transvesical and transvaginal approaches for the aspiration of follicles by use of ultrasound. Ann NY Acad Sci 1985; 442: 182–94.
38. Palermo G, Joris H, Devroey P, et al. Pregnancies after intracytoplasmic injection of single spermatozoon into an oocyte. Lancet 1992; 340: 17–18.
39. Hansis C, Edwards RG. Cell differentiation in the preimplantation human embryo. Reprod BioMed Online 2003; 6: 215–20.

Robert Edwards: The path to IVF*

Martin H. Johnson

*This article is based on the research undertaken in preparation for the introductory lecture to the Nobel Symposium held in the Karolinska Institute, Stockholm, in December 2010 to celebrate the award of the Nobel Prize in Physiology or Medicine to Robert Geoffrey Edwards. An abbreviated account of the contents of this paper was published as "Robert Edwards: Nobel Laureate in Physiology and Medicine" in "Les Prix Nobel 2010," edited by Professor Karl Grandin, and published by the Nobel Foundation; this version is reproduced as published in Reproductive BioMedicine Online (2011) 23, 245–262, with the permission of the Editors and Publishers of Reproductive BioMedicine Online.

INTRODUCTION

Robert G Edwards was awarded the 2010 Nobel Prize for Physiology or Medicine "for the development of in vitro fertilization" (1). There is a variety of accounts of the events leading up to this discovery and its acceptance, most of them by participants (2), but historical scholarship is rarer. This account uses verifiable sources to produce a historical narrative of the path to in vitro fertilization (IVF) that differs in a number of places from the conventionally accepted version and adds further detail.

EDWARDS' LIFE HISTORY: SOURCES

Primary sources used were the publications by Edwards and Steptoe during the 1950s, 1960s, and 1970s; archives of the Royal Society of Medicine, Cambridge University, the Physiology Library at Cambridge, and the personal papers of RG Edwards (courtesy of Ruth Edwards); unpublished transcripts of interviews with RG Edwards, K Elder, and RL Gardner; personal recollections from the late 1970s by Edwards and Steptoe as recalled in interviews with Danny Abse for the autobiographical account "A Matter of Life" and on film with Peter Williams; members of RG Edwards' family and his colleagues and former students and staff members for clarificatory evidence about personal recollections by Edwards, for additional verifiable information and with whom to test some new interpretations.

CHILDHOOD BACKGROUND

Robert Geoffrey Edwards was born on September 27, 1925 in the small Yorkshire mill town of Batley, the year of the Batley deluge and "great flood." He arrived into a working-class family, and Edwards, who was known by his middle name of Geoff until he was 18, was the second of three brothers, with an older brother, Sammy and a younger one, Harry. These brothers he describes as competitive, "all determined to win or, if not to win, to go down fighting" (3). Sammy was named after his father, Samuel, who was frequently away from home working on the railways, maintaining the track in the Blea Moor tunnel on the Carlisle-Settle line. It was an unhealthy place to work, some 2600 m long and filled with coal-fired smoke that exacerbated Samuel's bronchitis, a consequence of being gassed in World War I. The one perk of working on the railways was the free rail pass for the family's annual holiday, which was regularly taken in far-away Southend-on-Sea, located near the mouth of the Thames and considered then to be a top-spot resort by working-class families.

Edwards' mother, Margaret, was a machinist in a local mill. She came originally from Manchester, to where the family relocated when Edwards was about five, having been offered the relative security of a council house at 25 Highgate Crescent in the suburb of Gorton. It was in Manchester that Edwards was to receive his education. In those days, bright working-class children could take a scholarship exam at age 10 or 11 to compete for the few coveted places at a grammar school: the potential pathway out of poverty and even to University. All three brothers passed the exam, but Sammy decided against grammar school, preferring to leave education as soon as he could to earn. His mother was reportedly furious at this wasted opportunity, and so when her two younger sons passed, there was no question that they would continue in education and it was with that that Geoff/Bob progressed in 1937 to Manchester Central Boy's High School (the building that now houses Shena Simon College in Whitworth Street), which also claims James Chadwick FRS (1891–1974) as an alumnus. Chadwick, like Edwards, was a Cambridge professor and the 1935 Nobel Laureate in Physics for discovering the neutron (4). The Edwards' summers were spent in the Yorkshire Dales, to where their mother took her sons to be closer to their father's place of work. There, Edwards labored on the farms and developed an enduring affection for the Dales.

These early experiences were formative. Edwards first became a life-long egalitarian, for five years a Labour Party Councillor (5), willing to listen to and talk with all and sundry, regardless of class, education, status, and background. Second, he developed an enduring curiosity about agricultural and natural history and especially the reproductive patterns among the Dales' sheep, pigs, and cattle. Finally, he claimed great pride in being a "Yorkshire man," traditionally having attributes of affability and generosity of spirit combined with no-nonsense blunt-speaking. Indeed, following his only meeting with Gregory Pincus [1903–1967; (6)] at a conference in Venice in May 1966, at which Edwards, the young pretender, clashed with the "father of the pill" over the timing of egg maturation in humans; he paid Pincus the biggest compliment he could imagine, saying "He would have made a fine Yorkshireman!" (3).

The intervention of World War II was to provide an unwelcome interruption to Edwards' education: when he left school in 1943, he was conscripted for war service into the British Army for almost four years (Fig. 1). To his surprise, as someone from a working-class family, he was identified as potential officer material and sent on an officer-training course, before being commissioned in 1946. However, his army experiences were broadly negative, the alien lifestyle of the officers' mess not being to his taste and reinforcing his socialist ideals. The one positive feature of his war service was the chance to travel overseas; particularly appreciated was his time in the Middle East. The years in the army were broken by nine months' compassionate leave back in the Yorkshire Dales, to which he was released to help and run a farm when his farmer friend there fell ill. So engaged did he become in farming life that, after discharge from the army in 1948, he returned home to Gorton, from where he applied to read agricultural sciences at the University College of North Wales at Bangor.

Having gained a place and a government grant to fund it, the six or so months that intervened were occupied in a government desk job in Salford, Greater Manchester, helping to organize the newly formed National Health Service. This office-work experience reinforced the anticipatory attractions of agricultural science. So his disappointment in the course offered at Bangor was acute. By that time, he was a relatively experienced 23-year-old, described by his impressionable 18-year-old public-school educated and self-described "unlikely" friend, John Slee (Fig. 2) (7), as being "both ambitious and flexible, and unusually confident in his own judgement." In Edwards' confident judgment, the course on offer was not "scientific," and he was bored through two tedious years of agricultural descriptions, after which he reported that his teachers were "glad to see the back of him" in Zoology for a year, a course much more to his style and led by the more intellectually challenging Rogers Brambell FRS [1901–1970; (8)]. However, that year was not enough to salvage his honors degree, and in 1951, aged 26 he gained a simple pass. Unbeknown to him at the time, he was not alone in this undistinguished academic embarrassment, as neither "Tibby" Marshall FRS [1878–1949; (9)], the founder of the Reproductive Sciences, nor Sir Alan Parkes FRS [1900–1990; (10)], the first Professor of Reproductive Sciences at Cambridge, who was later to recruit Edwards there, distinguished themselves as undergraduates. In 1951, however, Edwards "was disconsolate. It was a disaster. My grants were spent and I was in debt. Unlike some of the students I had no rich parents ... I could not write home, 'Dear Dad, please send me £100 as I did badly in the exams'" (3).

However, his low spirits did not last long. He learnt that John Slee had been accepted on a postgraduate diploma course in Animal Genetics at Edinburgh University under Conrad Waddington FRS [1905–1975; (11)], who had moved there in 1947 from Christ's College in Cambridge, home also to both Marshall and Parkes. Edwards applied, and, despite his pass degree and to his amazement, he was accepted. That summer, he worked in Yorkshire and

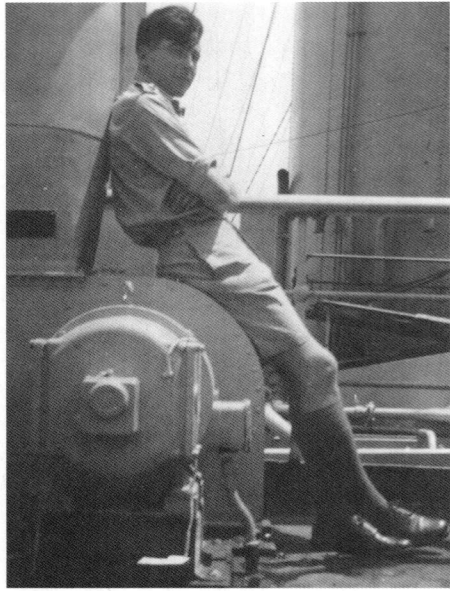

Figure 1 Edwards on National War Service in the 1940s. Source: Courtesy of Ruth Edwards.

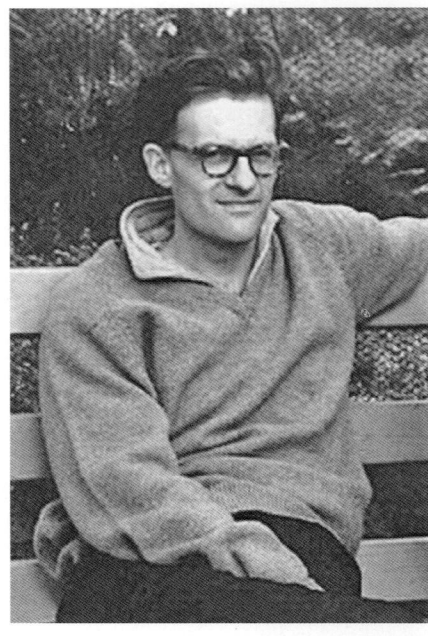

Figure 2 John Slee in the 1960s. Source: Courtesy of Ruth Edwards.

Wiltshire harvesting hay, as well as portering bananas and heaving sacks of flour in Manchester docks and taking a menial job with a newspaper, all to earn enough to pay his way in Edinburgh (3).

FAMILY LIFE

In Edinburgh, Edwards not only started to map out his scientific career, but importantly also met Ruth Fowler (Fig. 3), who was to become his life-long scientific collaborator and whom he was to marry in 1954, their five daughters arriving between 1959 and 1964: Caroline, Sarah, Jenny, and twins Anna and Meg. When they met, according to Edwards, in a statistics class, Ruth was studying for a genetics degree. Edwards claims that he was initially somewhat overwhelmed, even "intimidated" by Ruth's august family background. Her father, Sir Ralph Fowler FRS [1889–1944; (12)] and her maternal grandfather, Lord Ernest Rutherford FRS [1871–1937; (13)], were not only both "titled," but both also had the most impressive academic credentials imaginable: a world away from a working-class Northern family. Ralph Fowler was Plummer Professor of Mathematical Physics in Cambridge from 1932 to 1944. He was evidently an exceptionally talented mathematical physicist, a fine sportsman and "an inspirational teacher and leader of men" (12). Back in Cambridge in 1919 after World War I, he was stimulated to work with Rutherford, who had recently arrived there to take the chair of Experimental Physics. Rutherford was the first Nobel laureate in Ruth's family, having been awarded the 1908 Nobel Prize for Chemistry "for his investigations into the disintegration of the elements, and the chemistry of radioactive substances" (13).

Ralph Fowler not only worked under Rutherford, but in the course of doing so met his only daughter, Eileen, whom he married in 1921. They had four children, of whom Ruth was the last, born in December 1930. Tragically her mother died shortly afterwards and Ruth was to know only Mrs Phyllida Cook as her "mother"; both families moved into Cromwell House in Trumpington, Cambridge and were brought up together (12). Her father, although himself unwell, was to undertake grueling high security war work at the Ordnance Board and later at the Admiralty during World War II. His health deteriorated and he died at the relatively young age of 55 when Ruth was 13.

EDWARDS, THE RESEARCH SCIENTIST

The intellectual spirit of scientific enquiry that Edwards experienced in Edinburgh fitted his aptitudes well, for Waddington rewarded his Diploma year with a three-year PhD place (1952–55), followed by two years of postdoctoral research, and funded it to the princely sum of £240 per year (3). His chosen field of research was the developmental biology of the mouse. Edwards saw that to understand development involved engaging in an interdisciplinary mix, not just of embryology and reproduction, the conventional view at the time, but also of genetics. Given the scientific and social emphasis on genetics over the last 40 or so years, it is important to understand how advanced this view was in the 1950s, when genetic knowledge was still rudimentary and largely alien to the established developmental and reproductive biologists of the day, as Edwards himself was later to recall (14). For example, it was in the 1950s that DNA was established as the molecular carrier of genetic information (15–18), that it was first demonstrated that each cell of the body carried a full set of DNA/genes (19–21) and that genes were selectively expressed as mRNA to generate different cell phenotypes (22). Moreover, it was only by the late 1950s that cytogenetic studies led to the accepted human karyotype as 46 chromosomes (23,24), that agreement was reached on the Denver system of classification of human chromosomes (25) and that the chromosomal aneuploidies underlying developmental anomalies such as Down, Turner, and Klinefelter Syndromes were described (26–29).

The dates of these discoveries make Edwards' research between 1952 and 1957 all the more remarkable. Working under his supervisor Alan Beatty, he generated haploid, triploid, and aneuploid mouse embryos and studied their potential for development. In order to undertake what were, in effect, early attempts at "genetic engineering" in mammals, he needed to be able to manipulate the chromosomal composition of eggs, spermatozoa, and embryos. In mice, spermatozoa were abundant, and were studied in experiments mostly undertaken with a visiting Argentinean postdoc, Julio Sirlin (Fig. 4), whom Edwards describes as being "… the first man with whom I collaborated who was prepared to work at my pace" (3). Together they labeled spermatozoa radioactively in vivo in order to study the kinetics of spermatogenesis and then to follow the radioactive products post fertilization, thereby to demonstrate the fate of the male contributions to early development. They also exposed males and/or their spermatozoa to various agents, such as chemical mutagens and UV- or x-ray irradiation, and examined the effects on sperm-fertilizing capacity, and where it was shown to be present, how the treatment impacted on development. In some cases, sperm activation of the egg was evident, but in the absence of any functional sperm

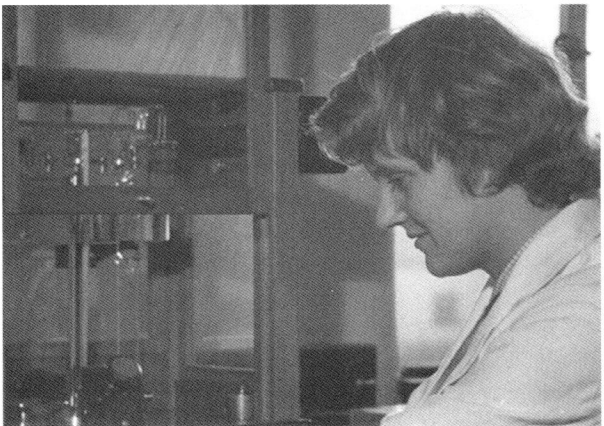

Figure 3 Ruth Fowler in the laboratory, Edinburgh in the 1950s.
Source: Courtesy of Ruth Edwards.

chromatin, and so gynogenetic embryos were formed. These experiments resulted in 14 papers, including four in *Nature*, between 1954 and 1959 (see ref. (30), for a full bibliographic record of Edwards).

Eggs and embryos were not as abundant as spermatozoa, and overcoming this problem led Edwards to two discoveries that proved to be of particular significance for his later IVF work. First, working with his wife Ruth, he devised ways of increasing the numbers of synchronized eggs recoverable from adult female mice through a series of papers, the first published in 1957 (31), on the control of ovulation induced by use of exogenous hormones. In doing so, they overturned the conventional wisdom that superovulation of adults was not possible. Second, working with an American postdoc, Alan Gates (Fig. 5) (32), Edwards described the remarkable timed sequence of egg chromosomal maturation events that led up to ovulation after injection of the ovulatory hormone, human chorionic gonadotropin.

His six years in Edinburgh, between 1951 and 1957, give an early taste of his prodigious energy, resulting in 38 papers (30). Indeed so productive was this period that the last of the Edinburgh-based papers did not appear in print until 1963. These papers firmly placed the young Edwards at the forefront of studies on the genetic manipulation of development and started to attract attention.

It was also in Edinburgh that Edwards' interest in ethics was first sparked by the interdisciplinary debates among scientists and theologians that Waddington organized, and, as a result, he went on what he describes as a "church crawl," trying the 10 or so variants of Christianity on offer in 1950s Edinburgh. He did not emerge from his consumer testing "God-intoxicated" (3), but convinced that man held his own future in his own hands. Edwards' humanist ethical sympathies and antipathy to the "revealed truths" of religion were to be developed further in all his later encounters (30).

AN AMERICAN DIVERSION

These 1950s studies in science and ethics were to form the platform on which Edwards' later IVF work was to be based, but before that his interests and life took a diversion to the California Institute of Technology for the year 1957–1958. He describes his year at Caltech as being "a bit of a holiday," but it was a holiday which with hindsight had both distracting and significant consequences. He went there to work with Albert Tyler [1906–1968; (33)], an influential elder statesman of American reproductive science, working on spermatozoon–egg interactions. Caltech was then a hot bed of developmental biology, and Tyler had clustered around him an exciting group of young scientists, which included that year a visit by the English doyen of fertilization, Lord Victor Rothschild FRS [1910–1990; (34)]. Rothschild was later to clash scientifically with Edwards over his IVF work (35), a clash in which the younger man triumphed again (36),

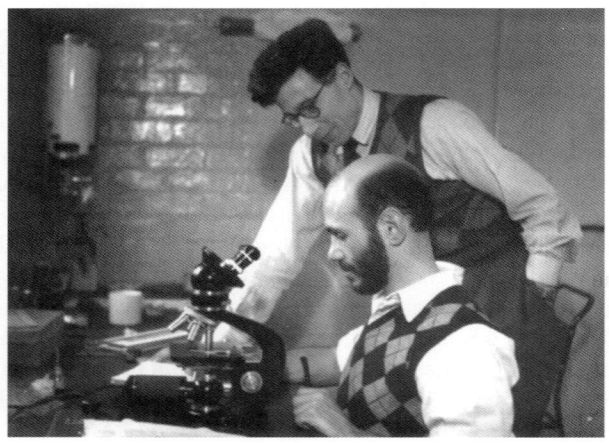

Figure 4 Julio Sirlin with Edwards in the 1950s. *Source*: Courtesy of Julio Sirlin.

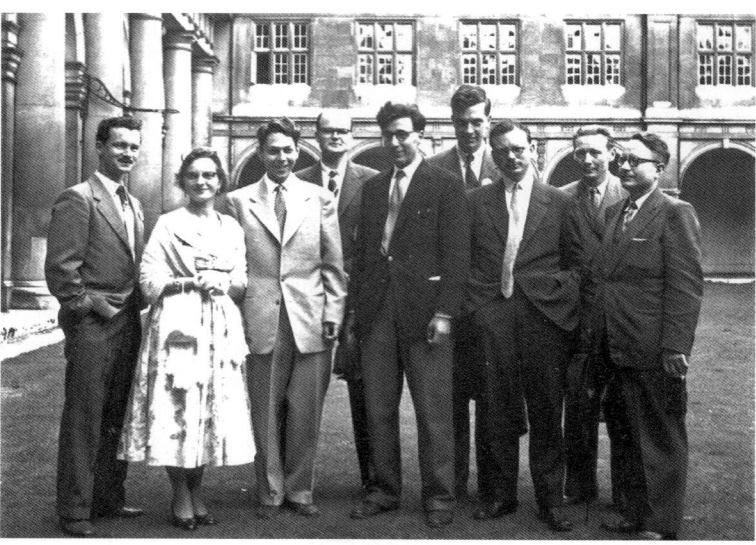

Figure 5 Edwards as "a very recent PhD student" (*centre*) and Alan Gates (*extreme left*) at a meeting in Trinity College Cambridge in the late 1950s. *Source*: Courtesy of Ruth Edwards.

just as he had with Pincus. Tyler was exploring the molecular specificity of egg–spermatozoon interactions and had turned for a model to immunology. Immunology was then at an exciting phase in its development, with the engaging Sir Peter Medawar FRS [1915–1987, Nobel Laureate in Physiology or Medicine, 1960; (37)], influentially for Bob, extending his ideas on immunological tolerance to the paradox of the "fetus as an allograft": a semi-paternal graft nonetheless somehow protected from maternal immune attack inside the mother's uterus (38). This confluence of reproduction and immunology excited Edwards' restless curiosity and hence the choice of Tyler. Significantly, the subject also offered funding possibilities via the Ford and Rockefeller Foundations and the Population Council, which were increasingly concerned about world population growth and the need for better methods to control fertility (39–41). Immunocontraception then seemed to offer tantalizingly specific possibilities, alas not much closer to being realized today (42).

So when Edwards returned to the United Kingdom from CalTech in 1958 at Alan Parkes' invitation to join him at the Medical Research Council (MRC) National Institute for Medical Research (NIMR) at Mill Hill in north London, it was to work on the science of immunocontraception (5). This period in the United States initiated a series of 23 papers on the immunology of reproduction between 1960 and 1976 (30). It also prompted Edwards' first involvement in founding an international society in 1967 in Varna Bulgaria, (Fig. 6) when the International Coordinating Committee for the Immunology of Reproduction was created (43). Immunoreproduction was, in retrospect, to prove a distracting diversion from what was to become Edwards' main work, albeit one that continued to enthuse and stimulate his imagination for many years. Indeed, it was his research into immunoreproduction that led serendipitously to his first meeting with Patrick Steptoe (see later). The period at Mill Hill, between 1958 and 1962, seems to have been a period of increasing intellectual conflict for him. While being enthusiastic about the science underlying immunocontraception, his old interests in eggs, fertilization and, in particular, the genetics of development were gradually reasserting themselves. His day job was therefore increasingly supplemented by evening and weekend flirtations with egg maturation.

THE CRUCIAL EGG-MATURATION STUDIES

The stimulus that re-awakened Edwards' interest in eggs was provided by the then recent consensus about the number of human chromosomes and, more particularly the descriptions in 1959 of the pathologies in man that resulted from chromosomal anomalies. Thus, his 1962 *Nature* paper begins: "Many of the chromosomal anomalies in man and animals arise through non-disjunction or lagging chromosomes during meiosis in the oocyte. Investigation of the origin and primary incidence of such anomalies would be greatly facilitated if meiotic stages etc., were easily available" (44).

The idea that these aneuploidies in humans might result from errors in the complex chromosomal dance that he and Gates had observed in maturing mouse eggs drove his thinking. The possible clinical relevance of his work on egg maturation and aneuploidy in the mouse was becoming significant.

So Edwards resumed his experimenting with mice, trying to mimic in vitro the in-vivo maturation of eggs, one rationale being that this route would open the possibility of similar studies in humans, in which not even induced ovulation had then been described (45). He tried releasing the immature eggs from their ovarian follicles into culture medium containing the ovulatory hormone human chorionic gonadotropin, to explore whether he could simulate their in-vivo development.

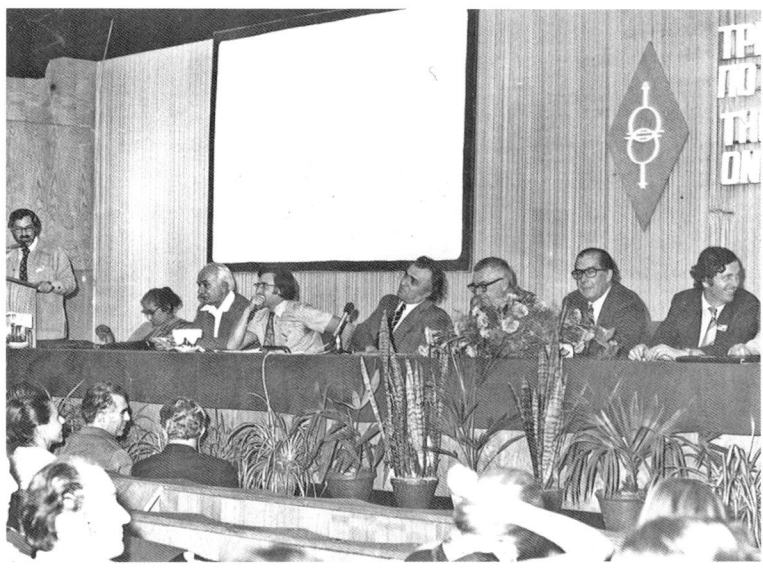

Figure 6 Edwards at one of the Varna meetings on Immunoreproduction; Schulman is speaking and to Edwards' left is Bratanov, and seated two to his right is Shanta Rao. *Source*: Courtesy Barbara Rankin.

Amazingly he found it worked first time; the eggs seemed to mature at the same rate as they had in vivo. However, they did so whether or not the hormone had been added. The eggs evidently were maturing spontaneously when released from their follicles. The same happened in rats and hamsters. If this also were to happen in humans, then the study of the chromosomal dance during human egg maturation was a realistic practical possibility, as was IVF and thereby studies on the genetics of early human development. Edwards' excitement at seeing eggs spontaneously maturing was temporarily blunted by his library discovery that Pincus in the 1930s (46,47) and M C Chang [1908–1991; (48,49)] earlier in the 1950s had been there before him, using both rabbit and, Pincus claimed, human eggs.

In order to pursue his cytogenetic studies on maturation, he needed a reliable supply of human ovarian tissue from which to retrieve and mature eggs. This requirement posed difficulties for a scientist with no medical qualification, given the elitist attitudes and lack of scientific awareness then prevalent amongst most of the U.K. gynecological profession (2,50,51). His first breakthrough came with Molly Rose, who was a gynecologist at the Edgeware General Hospital, northwest London, near Mill Hill. Edwards was introduced to her through John Humphrey FRS [1915–1997; (52)], who was the medically qualified Head of Immunology at Mill Hill. Humphrey, notwithstanding his more privileged social background, was a kindred spirit for Edwards, sharing his passion for science, its social application and utility, as well as his left-wing politics; indeed he had been a Marxist until 1940 and was for many years denied entry to the United States as a result. Edwards asked Humphrey if he knew anyone who might be helpful, and he not only suggested Rose, but also offered to arrange an introduction. Rose was to provide biopsied ovarian samples intermittently for the next 10 years.

Between 1960 and 1962, Edwards used human ovarian biopsies provided by Rose to try to repeat and extend Pincus' observations from the 1930s. Given the sporadic supply of human material, he also tried dog, monkey and baboon ovarian eggs, but in all cases with limited success compared with smaller rodents. In the 1962 Nature paper (44), he cautiously interprets the few maturing human (3/67), monkey (10/56) and baboon (13/90) eggs that he had observed as most likely arising from in-vivo stimulation and thus partially matured at the time of their recovery from the biopsy. He suggests that Pincus' observations on human eggs are also likely to be artifactual, the source of his Venice spat with Pincus some 4 years later (vide supra). This 1962 paper ends with the report of an ingenious experimental approach to try and persuade the reluctant human eggs to mature. Thus, the ovarian arteries of patients undergoing ovarian removal were cannulated and perfused with hormones post-removal, perhaps unsurprisingly in retrospect, without success.

However, by this time, his quest for human eggs, and his dreams of IVF and studying the genetics and development of early human embryos, had reached the ears of the then Director of the Institute, Sir Charles Harington FRS [1897–1972; (53)], who banned any work on human IVF at NIMR (3). Alan Parkes was no longer able to defend Edwards, having left in 1961 to take up his chair in Cambridge and, although he had asked Edwards to join him there, funding was not available until 1963. So by the time Edwards left Mill Hill in 1962 for a year in Glasgow, he had encountered a taste of the opposition to come.

GLASGOW AND STEM CELLS

Edwards had accepted an invitation from John Paul to spend a year in the biochemistry department at Glasgow University. Paul was then the acknowledged master of tissue culture in the United Kingdom and had got wind of some experiments that Edwards had been doing on the side at NIMR attempting to generate stem cells from rabbit embryo cultures (14). The objective of this strategy was to use these stem cells to study early developmental mechanisms, either in vitro, or in vivo after their incorporation into embryos. Paul had proposed that they work together, with fellow Glasgow biochemist Robin Cole, to see what progress might be made. This must have been an attractive invitation, not simply because the challenge was scientifically interesting, but also because Edwards could learn more about culture media for his eggs and hopefully later embryos, then an uncertain prospect, successful mouse embryo culture only recently having been described (54). However, by this time, the Edwards family was growing, so Ruth remained in north London with their young daughters, while her husband commuted to Glasgow for the working week.

The collaboration was to result in two papers (55,56) remarkable for their prescience. They described the production of embryonic stem cells from both rabbit blastocysts and the inner cell masses dissected from them. The cells were capable of proliferating through over 100 generations and of differentiating into various cell types. These experiments were initiated some 20 years before Evans and Kaufman (57) described the derivation of embryonic stem cells from mice. That this work has largely been ignored by those in the stem cell field is probably mainly attributable to its being too far ahead of its time (58). Thus, reliable molecular markers for different types of cells were not available then, nor were appropriate techniques with which to critically test the developmental potential of the cultured cells.

THE MOVE TO CAMBRIDGE

Edwards arrived in Cambridge from Glasgow in 1963 as a Ford Foundation Research Fellow. He had previously visited Cambridge at least once, as "a recently graduated PhD" in the late 1950s for a conference on Reproduction held in Trinity College (Fig. 5), where he recalls meeting some of the big names in the subject, including John Hammond, Alan Parkes, MC Chang, Thaddeus Mann, Rene Moricard, Bunny Austin, and Charles Thibault (14). Although Edwards was to remain in Cambridge for the rest of his career, in 1963 his reactions to the place were mixed. He describes how he immediately reacted against the then extant "misogynist public-school traditions; the exclusivity," "the privileges given to the already privileged." But he set against that the "sheer beauty of the place," the concern with the truth and high seriousness," the ambience of scientific excellence... I was surrounded by so many talented young men and women" (3). He, Ruth, and his five daughters settled in a house in Gough Way, off the Barton Road.

Edwards worked in a cluster of seven smallish rooms at the top of the Physiological Laboratory backing onto Downing Place (Fig. 7). These were collectively known as the "Marshall laboratory" and were to be shared eventually with two other groups. One group was led initially by Sir Alan Parkes, the first Mary Marshall and Arthur Walton Professor of Reproductive Physiology at the University (10), who had arrived in 1961. His group included scientists with mainly zoological or comparative interests, such as his wife Ruth Deansley, Bunny Austin, and Dick Laws FRS, who with Parkes was often away "in the field" collecting material, especially in Uganda at the Nuffield Unit of Tropical Animal Ecology (10). Much of this material was examined histologically under the skilled eye of Frank Lemon, the senior technician. Research students included Martin Richards, CJ Dominic, Margaret Mitchell, and Barbara Weir (59). Parkes was also much involved at this time in writing and committee work, especially with the World Health Organization which was then becoming concerned about world population growth and ways to curb it (10). Parkes was also acting as an unpaid company secretary to the then fledgling *Journal of Reproduction and Fertility* [called *Reproduction* since 2001; (59–61)].

In 1967, Parkes retired. Edwards applied for his chair on January 6, 1966 (62), but was unsuccessful, the chair passing to Thaddeus Mann FRS [1908–1993; (63)], who worked on the biochemistry of semen. Mann decided not to relocate to the Physiology Laboratory from his Cambridge base at the Agricultural Research Council Unit of Reproductive Physiology and Biochemistry at Huntingdon Road, where he was Director. Neither was the leadership of the Marshall laboratory to pass to Edwards, as the University appointed as its head his more senior colleague and friend Colin "Bunny" Austin [1914–2004; (64)], who had been in Cambridge intermittently since 1962 (Figs. 8 and 9). Austin was elected the first Charles Darwin Professor of Animal Embryology (1967–1981) and began attracting several upcoming reproductive biologists to the Marshall Laboratory, including John Marston, David Whittingham, and Matthew Kaufmann. In addition, a new group was formed in 1967, with the arrival from the Strangeways laboratory of Denis New (1929–2010), as university lecturer in histology (65). New built a group comprising initially research assistant Pat Coppola (to be followed later by Stephanie Ellington) and PhD students Chris Steele and David Cockroft, later joined by postdoc Frank Webb, and visiting scientists such as Joe Daniels Jr, on leave from the University of Colorado.

It was against this varied scientific background that Edwards, who was already 38 when he arrived in Cambridge, began for the first time to assemble his own group. Initially,

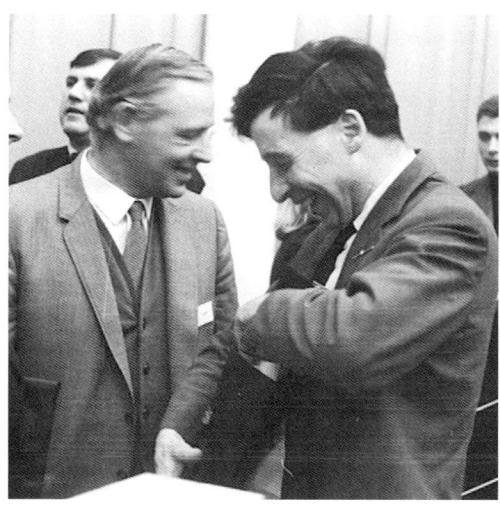

Figure 8 Edwards with "Bunny" Austin (1960s). *Source*: Courtesy of Ruth Edwards.

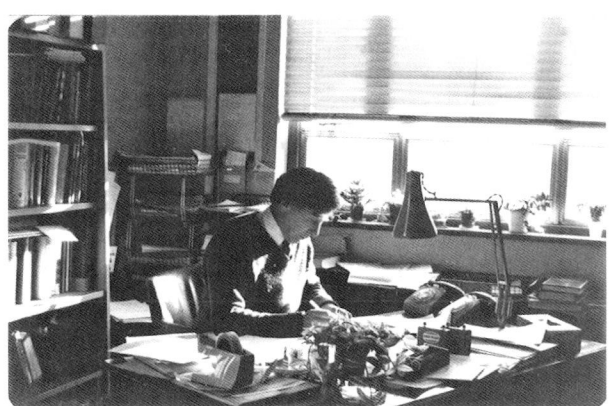

Figure 7 Edwards in his office backing onto Downing Place in the Marshall laboratory (1970s). *Source*: Courtesy of Barbara Rankin.

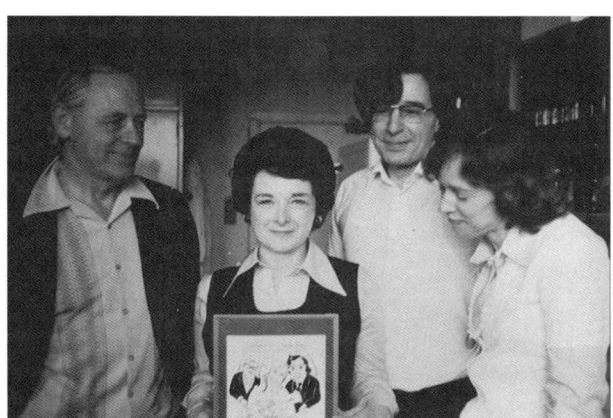

Figure 9 Barbara Rankin holding a cartoon of Edwards, Steptoe, and Purdy holding Lousie Brown drawn by Alan Handyside who also took the photograph. With Austin are (*left*) Edwards and Purdy (*right*) after the return of the latter two from Oldham and the birth of Louise Brown in 1978. *Source*: Courtesy of Barbara Rankin.

his technical assistance was provided by Clare Jackson and then Valerie Hunn, after whom he recruited Jean Purdy (Fig. 10) in 1968, one of her attractions being her nursing qualification, a sign of the increasing importance that his forays into use of clinical material was assuming. Purdy was to stay with him until her early death at age 39 in 1985 (66). Also joining him as a part-time secretary in 1969, Barbara Rankin (b. 1933; Fig. 9) was to remain with him until 1987. He also began recruiting his first graduate students. Initially, he helped co-supervise (with Alan Parkes) Anne Vickers (67), who sexed fixed whole-mouse blastocysts by karyotyping. This work led directly to his collaboration on preimplantation genetic diagnosis (PGD) (see later) with Richard Gardner, one half of his first pair of graduate students, the other being this author. The two students started PhD training with Edwards in 1966 (68,69). Gardner studied early mouse embryology from 1966 to 1971 and until 1973 as a postdoctoral worker, before moving to Zoology in Oxford. This author worked on immunoreproduction from 1966 to 1969, returning as a postdoc between 1971 and 1974 after two years in the United States before moving to the Anatomy Department in Cambridge.

From 1969 onwards, Edwards' group increased in size substantially as more accommodation was made available to the Marshall laboratory. David Griffin (now retired from the World Health Organization) was to join as Head Technician between 1970 and 1975, with junior technicians including Sheila Barton, Sally Fawcitt, Sylvia Jackson, Vinitha Dharawardena, and Brenda Dickstein, in addition to Jean Purdy. Early graduate students recruited included Roger Gosden (1970–1974), Carol Readhead (1972–1976), and Rob Gore-Langton (1973–1978), all working on follicle growth, Craig Howe (1971–1974) working on immunoreproduction, and Azim Surani (1975–1979) on implantation. A "third generation" of graduate students also arrived; for example, Janet Rossant (from 1972) studied with Gardner and Alan Handyside (from 1974) studied with Johnson. Postdoctoral workers also arrived, including Ginny Papaioannou (1971–1974), Hester Pratt (1972–1974), and Frank Webb (1976–1977). Ruth Fowler-Edwards also resumed working in the laboratory, developing hormonal assays and studying the endocrine aspects of follicle development and early pregnancy. Thus, slowly until 1969, and more rapidly thereafter, Edwards built a lively group, its members working in diverse areas of reproductive science that reflected his own broad interests and knowledge. Moreover, Edwards encouraged a spirit of open communication and egalitarianism, which extended across all three groups, with sharing of resources, space, equipment, knowledge, and ideas, as well as social activities.

Through the 1960s, Edwards was funded by the Ford Foundation via grants first to Parkes and then to Austin to continue work on basic reproductive mechanisms, with an eye to developing new methods of fertility control. So he continued to pursue both the immunology of reproduction and egg maturation, for the latter collecting pig, cow, sheep, the odd monkey, and some human eggs. He showed that eggs of all these species would indeed mature in vitro, but that the eggs of larger animals simply needed a longer time than those of smaller ones, human eggs taking up to 36 hours rather than the 12 hours or less erroneously reported by Pincus. These cytogenetic studies were reported in two seminal papers in 1965 (70,71), both of which are primarily concerned with understanding the kinetics of the meiotic chromosomal events during egg maturation. In its discussion, the Lancet paper displays a breathtaking clarity of vision as Edwards sets out a program of research that predicted the events of the next 20 years and beyond (Table 1). Significantly, if not surprisingly given his research interests, the early study and detection of genetic disease is afforded a heavy focus compared with the slight emphasis on infertility alleviation.

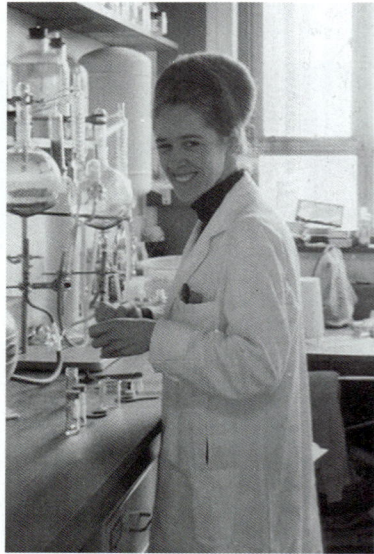

Figure 10 Jean Purdy (1946–1985). Source: Courtesy of Barbara Rankin.

Table 1 Key Points in the Program of Research Laid Out in the Discussion to Edwards' 1965 Lancet Paper

1. Studies on non-disjunction of meiotic chromosomes as a cause of aneuploidy in humans[a]
2. Studies on the effect of maternal age on non-disjunction in relation to the origins of trisomy 21[a]
3. Use of human eggs in IVF to study fertilization
4. Study of culture methods for human eggs fertilized in vitro
5. Use of priming hormones to increase the number of eggs per woman available for study/use
6. Study of early IVF embryos for evidence of ([ab]) normality – especially aneuploidies arising prior to or at fertilization[a]
7. Control of some of the genetic diseases in man[a]
8. Control of sex-linked disorders by sex detection at blastocyst stage and transfer of only female embryos[a]
9. Intracervical transfer of IVF embryos into the uterus
10. Use of IVF embryos to circumvent blocked tubes[b]
11. Avoidance of a multiple pregnancy (as observed after hormonal priming and in vivo insemination) by transfer of a single IVF embryo

[a]Five aims relating specifically to genetic disease.
[b]One aim relating specifically to infertility relief.

This genetic focus continues in his research papers over the next four years. Thus, within three years, working with a graduate student called Gardner, he provided proof of principle for PGD, in a paper on rabbit embryo sexing published in 1968 (72), a paper that was to anticipate the development of PGD clinically by some 22 years (73). Likewise, working with the Cambridge geneticist Alan Henderson, Edwards was to develop his "production line theory" of egg production to explain the origins of maternal aneuploidy in older women. Thus, the earliest eggs to enter meiosis in the fetal ovary were shown to have more chiasmata and to be ovulated earlier in adult life than those entering meiosis later in fetal life (Fig. 11) (74,75).

THE PROBLEM OF FERTILIZATION OF THE HUMAN EGG

Notwithstanding his broad range of scientific interests, Edwards' ambitions to achieve IVF in humans remained undiminished. In 1966, this was no trivial task, having been accomplished convincingly only in rabbit and hamster (76,77). In trying to achieve this aim, he was engaging in two struggles: the first being simply but critically the continuing practical difficulty in obtaining a regular supply of human ovarian tissue. Local Cambridge sources proved unreliable and Rose was now two to three hours' drive away in London; so, during the summer of 1965, Edwards turned to the United States for help and approached Victor McKusick, a leading American cytogeneticist at The Johns Hopkins University. There he initiated his longstanding contact with Howard and Georgeanna Jones in Obstetrics and Gynecology (78). The supply of American eggs they generated during his six-week stay allowed him to confirm the maturation timings that were published in 1965.

However, it was the second scientific struggle that was then occupying most of his attention, namely that in order to fertilize these in-vitro matured eggs, he had to "capacitate" the spermatozoa, a final maturation process which spermatozoa undergo physiologically in the uterus and that is essential for the acquisition of fertilizing competence. Failing to achieve this convincingly at Johns Hopkins, he made a second transatlantic summer journey in 1966 to visit Luther Talbot and his colleagues at Chapel Hill. He tried a variety of ways (79) to overcome the problem of "sperm capacitation," one of the most ingenious of which was to construct a 2.5 cm-long chamber from a nylon tube, plugged at each end, and with holes drilled in the walls which were encased in panels made of Millipore membrane (80). The chamber, which had a short thread attached to it, fitted snugly inside the inserter tube of an intrauterine device and so could be placed into the volunteer woman's uterus intracervically at mid-cycle, where it sat for up to 11 hours before being recovered by gently pulling on the thread, exactly as was being done routinely for insertion and removal of intrauterine devices. By placing spermatozoa within the chamber, the membrane of which permitted equilibration of its contents with uterine fluid, he hoped to expose them to a capacitating environment. However, this ingenious approach, like the many others, failed in this case most probably because the chamber itself induced an inflammatory response or a local bleed. For all the ingenuity of his various experimental approaches to achieve capacitation, and despite the occasional evidence of early stages of fertilization using such spermatozoa, no reliable evidence for the completion of the process was forthcoming. Then in 1968 both struggles began to resolve.

THE MEETING WITH PATRICK STEPTOE

Patrick Steptoe (1913–1988; Fig. 12) had been a consultant obstetrician at Oldham General Hospital since 1951 (81), where for several years he had been pioneering the development and use of the laparoscope in gynecological surgery (81,82). Much to his frustration, his progress had fallen on the largely deaf ears of the conservative gynecological hierarchy, and indeed incited considerable

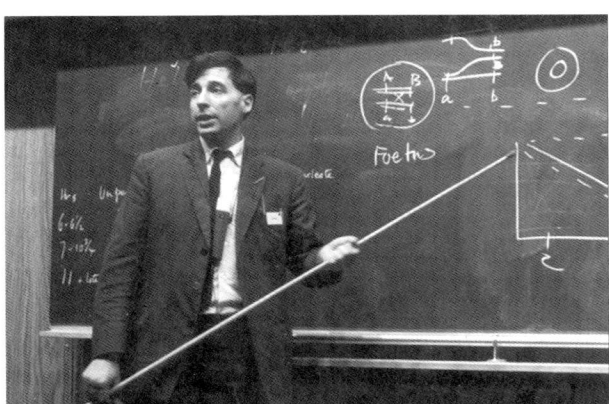

Figure 11 Edwards talks about his "production line" hypothesis (late 1960s). *Source*: Courtesy of Ruth Edwards.

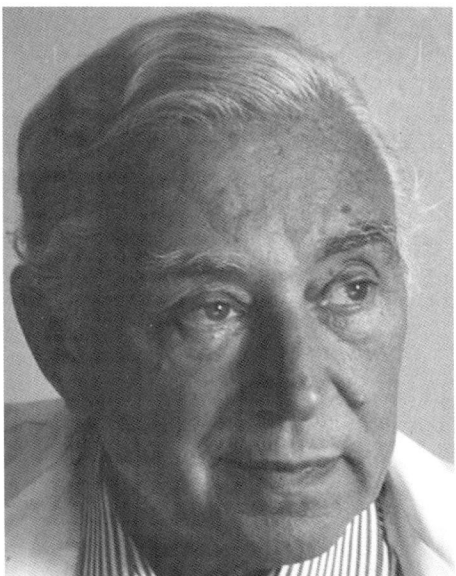

Figure 12 Patrick Steptoe (1913–1988). Source: Courtesy of Andrew Steptoe.

Table 2 Edited Record from the RSM Endocrinology Section: General Minutes, 1946–1975 (ref: RSM/J/19/4/1) p.365 (with permission)

A joint meeting of the SECTION OF ENDOCRINOLOGY of the Royal Society of Medicine with the SOCIETY FOR THE STUDY OF FERTILITY was held at 1 Wimpole Street, W.1., Wednesday, February 28, 1968, at 10.00 am.
The meeting was attended by approximately 127 Fellows, members, and guests and the program was as follows:

"FERTILITY AND INFERTILITY"

10.00: Chairman's opening remarks
10.10: Sperm capacitation. C.R. Austin, Department of Embryology, Cambridge
10.35: Immunological aspects of infertility. R.G. Edwards, Department of Physiology, Cambridge
11.00: Coffee
11.30: The rating of semen quality by chemical methods. Dr T Mann, Department of Physiology of Reproduction, Cambridge
11.55: Endocrine studies in women with secondary amenorrhea. Prof. Ivor H Mills and RJ Wilson, Department of Investigative Medicine, Cambridge
12.20: Some investigation in male hypogonadism. Prof. FTG Prunty, Department of Chemical Pathology, St Thomas's Hospital Medical School, London
12.45: Lunch
2.15: A gonadotropin stimulation test for ovarian responsiveness. GIM Sawyer, University College Hospital Medical School, London
2.40: Factors affecting the response to clomiphene therapy. D Ferriman, AW Purdie, and M Corns, North Middlesex Hospital, London
3.05: Comparison of clomiphene and FSH for treatment of anovulation. AD Tsapoulis and AC Crooke, Department of Clinical Endocrinology, Birmingham
3.30: Tea
4.00: Time cause of urinary oestrogen excretion after various schemes of Pergonal therapy. JK Butler, GD Searle and Co., High Wycombe, Bucks
4.25: Recent developments in the control of fertility. Sir Alan S Parkes, Cambridge
4.50: General discussion
[signed] CL Cope 26/6/1968 [pasted in] 26th June 1968

opposition and some outright hostility (83). Edwards' claim was that he was scanning the medical and scientific journals in the library and came across a paper by Steptoe describing his experiences with laparoscopy (3,81,84). Edwards goes on to describe how he rang Steptoe to discuss a possible collaboration, but was "warned off" Steptoe by London gynecological colleagues (85). This warning and the daunting prospect of collaboration in far-away Oldham, deterred him from following through. Finally, Edwards reported actually meeting Steptoe later at a meeting at the Royal Society of Medicine, at which, ironically, Edwards was talking about his work on immunoreproduction, not his attempts at IVF.

The Steptoe paper that Edwards found that day in the library was cited in his tributes to the then-deceased Steptoe (81,84) as being a Lancet paper entitled "Laparoscopy and ovulation" (86). However, these later recollections do not withstand scrutiny. Thus, the Lancet paper cited was published in October 1968, but their first meeting was in fact earlier that year, on Wednesday February 28, 1968 at a joint meeting of the Section of Endocrinology of the Royal Society of Medicine with the Society for the Study of Fertility held at 1 Wimpole Street (Table 2) (87). Moreover, according to Steptoe (88), they had already commenced collaborating prior to October 1968; indeed their first paper together was submitted for publication later that year in December 1968 (see next section). Clearly, the paper read by Edwards must have been another, earlier than October 1968, one that proceeded February 1968 by several months. Indeed, in an earlier account, Edwards describes the library "Eureka" moment as occurring in "one autumn day in 1967" (3). So which was the paper by Steptoe that Edwards saw and what about it attracted his attention? Looking at Steptoe's possible publications in journals, there is none listed for 1967, but there are two 1967 conference reports and Steptoe's book on gynecological laparoscopy (82,89,90). Of the few journal papers, only two concern laparoscopy, one from January 1966 in the British Medical Journal (BMJ), and one from August 1965 in the Journal of Obstetrics and Gynaecology of the British Commonwealth (JOGBrC). Which of these five publications (Table 3) did Edwards read? The 1966 BMJ publication (91) is a letter entitled "The fifth freedom." It responds to a paper by Sir Dugald Baird on the "problem of excessive fertility in women." Steptoe concurs that there is a problem, but disagrees with the proposed contraceptive solution, advising laparoscopic sterilization for women as safer and more effective. He also discusses how laparoscopy can be used postoperatively to confirm that tubes were indeed blocked. The JOGBrC paper (92) is entitled "Gynaecological endoscopy – laparoscopy and culdoscopy" and reviews the history of endoscopy and Steptoe's experiences with it. It is in essence a very abbreviated version of his book (82), which was to be published in the following year. The two reports of the conference proceedings (89,90) are slightly more detailed accounts than the BMJ letter and are much abbreviated versions of the JOGBrC paper.

Of these five publications, the Sydney conference proceedings (90) can probably be dismissed as they only arrived in the Cambridge library in May 1968. The proceedings from Stockholm (89) are now no longer available in Cambridge, but evidence of their presence in the Physiology library in 1967 has been uncovered in an old catalog record, and so they would have been newly available to Edwards from November 1967 at the earliest. The BMJ letter (91) seems unlikely.

Table 3 Steptoe's Papers from 1967 and Earlier

Publication	Title	Type of publication	Location in Cambridge; date of arrival
Steptoe (82)	Laparoscopy in gynaecology	Book	University library; March 1967
Steptoe (89)	A new method of tubal sterilisation	Conference proceedings (Stockholm)	Physiology library; arrival date unknown, published in November 1967
Steptoe (90)	Laparoscopic studies of ovulation, its suppression and induction, and of ovarian dysfunction	Conference proceedings (Sydney)	University library; May 1968
Steptoe (91)	The fifth freedom	BMJ letter (22 January), 234	Physiology library; January 1966
Steptoe (92)	Gynaecological endoscopy – laparoscopy and culdoscopy	Paper in J Obstet Gynaecol Br Commonw 72, 535–543	University library; August 1965 (moved to Clinical School library after 1973)

Although Edwards was involved in contraceptive studies over this period through his work on immunoreproduction and was a member of the Royal Society Population Study Group at the time (10), and so may well have read this correspondence, it seems unlikely that the BMJ letter would have caught his eye to such dramatic effect and so long after its publication in January 1966, being readily available each week in the Physiology Library. The JOGBrC paper from 1965 was located in the University library, which was physically more remote from Physiology and not so immediately available to Edwards. However, it was in exactly the sort of clinical journal that he might then have been trawling retrospectively in his attempts to solve the problem of sperm capacitation. Thus, although in the more recent accounts of these events, Edwards (84,81) records his motivation for contacting Steptoe as being the potential value of the laparoscopic approach for egg collection, in 1967 eggs was not the foremost subject on his mind. Indeed in two earlier accounts, one written (3) and one spoken ((85); Supplementary video), Edwards claims he saw laparoscopy as a way of recovering capacitated spermatozoa from the oviduct by flushing with a small volume of medium: "a practical way ... of letting spermatozoa be in contact with the secretions of the female tract" (3). He says he actually rang Steptoe to ask whether this really was possible and was reassured by him that this was the case.

However, the only publication by Steptoe that explicitly lays out this possibility is his book (82). Thus, on page 27 he reports "By means of laparoscopy, Sjovall (1964) has carried out extended post-coital tests and has recovered spermatozoa from the fimbriated end of the tubes ..."; and on page 70, he writes "An extended post-coital test can be done by aspirating fluid from the tubal ostium ...". Moreover, Steptoe's book arrived in the University library in March 1967. However, against this conclusion sits Steptoe's recollection that Edwards had rung him just before his book was published, that is before March 1967 (3). This memory conflicts with both his and Edwards' memories elsewhere of the phone conversation being in the autumn of 1967, so the matter remains one for conjecture, but the book seems the most likely source. It is possible that Edwards' attention was drawn to the book by a review of it in the BMJ on November 11, 1967 (93).

THE FERTILIZATION OF THE HUMAN EGG RESOLVED

Despite the initiation of the collaboration with Steptoe, the actual solution to the capacitation problem existed nearer to home than Oldham, in the laboratories shared with Austin. In the early 1950s, Austin, and independently MC Chang, had discovered the requirement for sperm capacitation (94,95). After his appointment to the Cambridge chair, Austin's first graduate student (1967–1972) was Barry Bavister, who set to work to try and resolve the factors influencing the capacitation of hamster spermatozoa in vitro. In 1968, Bavister discovered a key role for pH, showing how higher rates of fertilization could be obtained by simply increasing the alkalinity of the medium (96). Edwards seized on this observation and co-opted Bavister to his project. That proved to do the trick, and in December 1968 Edwards, together with Bavister and Steptoe, submitted the paper to *Nature*, in which IVF in humans was described convincingly for the first time (97).

The 1969 *Nature* paper makes modest claims. Only 18 of 56 eggs assigned to the experimental group showed evidence of "fertilization in progress"; of which only two were described as having the two pronuclei to be expected if fertilization was occurring normally (Table 4). However, like Edwards' other papers, this one is a model of clarity, describing well-controlled experiments, cautiously interpreted. Despite the relatively small numbers, this paper convinced where previous claims had failed (98–103), precisely because the skilled hands and creative intellect that were behind it are so evident from its text.

The provenance of the eggs described in the 1969 paper is not immediately clear from the paper itself. All were obtained by in-vitro maturation after ovarian biopsy. In addition to Steptoe's coauthorship, four other gynecologists are thanked in the Acknowledgements section of the paper: Molly Rose, Norman Morris [1920–2008; Professor of Obstetrics and Gynecology at Charing Cross Hospital, London from 1958 to 1985; (104)], Janet Bottomley (1915–1995; Consultant Obstetrician and Gynecologist at Addenbrooke's Hospital, Cambridge from 1958 to 1976) and Sanford Markham (b. 1934; Chief of the Section of Obstetrics and Gynecology at the U.S.

Table 4 Summary of Data from Ref. 97

Egg characteristic	Experimental group	Control group
Assigned	56	17
Surviving	54/56	17/17
Matured to metaphase II	34/54	7/17
Some evidence of sperm penetration	18/34	
Spermatozoon within the zona pellucida	6/18	
Spermatozoon inside zona pellucida (c.7 hr post insemination)	5/18	
Evidence of pronuclei (c.11 hr post insemination)	7/18	0/7
No. with two pronuclei	2/18	

Air Force Hospital, South Ruislip, to the north west of London from 1967 to 1972). Markham, now Professor of Obstetrics and Gynecology at Florida International University, Miami, writes:

"I believe that I met Bob by introduction from Dr. Roger Short at a Royal College of Medicine conference in London ... probably in early 1968 [possibly the Royal Society of Medicine's 28 February meeting at which Steptoe and Edwards first met?]. Bob mentioned that he was in need of ovarian tissue from reproductive aged women ... I offered to obtain tissue if we could work out a scheme to transport the tissue ... to Cambridge ... He provided the media and container and a driver that came to our hospital ... I remember three samples, however, there may have been others. In each case the whole wedge ... or ... ovary was sent (after sampling for pathology). In all cases the patients provided their consent for utilization of their tissue for research. They were not told what the research work involved. These samples were most likely sent in mid to late 1968 and possibly in early 1969. ... These ... were planned surgeries which were accomplished at specific times in their menstrual cycle. Unfortunately, I do not know if the tissues supplied were indeed the tissues used in data for his 1969 paper published in *Nature*."

It is possible that they were used, but unsuccessfully, not contributing to the 18 eggs showing fertilization. Thus, according to Edwards (3), Jean Purdy drove to Edgeware General Hospital to collect:

"the last piece of ovarian tissue that I was to obtain from the Edgware General Hospital. It yielded me 12 human eggs. Those eggs were soon ripening in mixtures of culture medium I had used over many years to which some of Barry [Bavister]'s fluid had been added. Thirty-six hours later we judged that they were ready for fertilization."

Nine of these were inseminated, leaving three as controls. Ten hours later, when Edwards and Bavister returned to the laboratory late at night:

"a spermatozoon was just passing into the first egg ... An hour later we looked at the second egg. Yes, there it was, the earliest stages of fertilization. A spermatozoon had entered the egg without any doubt – we had done it ... We examined other eggs and found more and more evidence. Some ova were in the early stages of fertilization with the sperm tails following the sperm heads into the depths of the egg; others were even more advanced with two nuclei – one from the sperm and one from the egg – as each gamete donated its genetic component to the embryo."

This (unverified) account suggests that Rose provided the first group of eggs to be fertilized in "Bavister's medium." Moreover, since only 18 of the eggs in the paper showed evidence of fertilization (Table 4), nine of those seem to have come from Rose, including presumptively the two described as having two pronuclei. Rose was invited to be a co-author, but she declined for reasons unknown. The source of the remaining nine eggs is unknown, but may have come from Oldham General Hospital. The Acknowledgements section thanks Drs C Abberley, G Garrett, and L Davies "for their help," all from Oldham General. John Webster, a later gynecological colleague of Steptoe, having consulted his colleague John Battie, writes of these:

"Cyril Adderley, not Abberley, was the Group Pathologist in Oldham. Geoff Garrett ... was also a pathologist there ... there was no L. Davies there but a John Davies, a haematologist, and a Vincent John Davies, a histologist ... and my money would go on V. J. as I think a histologist rather than a haematologist would have been of more help to him ...?"

The first two of these have elsewhere been described as helpful in setting up the embryology laboratory in Oldham, largely through the provision or loan of equipment required locally for egg maturation and fertilization, so their involvement in direct provision of eggs seems unlikely.

The *Nature* paper also supports Oldham as the source of the remaining eggs: "Some eggs were transported from Oldham to Cambridge" (97), and in his retrospective 1980 account of the events, Edwards says that at Oldham they began to repeat the experiment:

"Twelve women whose ovaries had to be removed [presumably laparoscopically] for serious medical conditions provided us with the necessary eggs over the next few months. We fertilized many more eggs and were able to make detailed examinations of the successive stages of fertilization (3)."

So it seems reasonable to conclude that those eggs described in the paper as "undergoing fertilization" were provided in roughly equal numbers by Rose and Steptoe.

However, with Steptoe on board, Rose no longer featured as a supplier of eggs (3). While the initial attraction of laparoscopy for Edwards had been the recovery of capacitated spermatozoa from the oviduct, once working with Steptoe he rapidly saw the wider possibilities for recovery of in-vivo matured eggs from the ovary (86). Indeed, the 1969 paper includes the following statement:

"Problems of embryonic development are likely to accompany the use of human oocytes matured and fertilized in vitro. When oocytes of the rabbit and other species were matured in vitro and fertilized in vivo, the pronuclear stages appeared normal but many of the resulting embryos had subnuclei in their blastomeres, and almost all of them died during the early cleavage stages ... When maturation of rabbit oocytes was started in vivo by injecting gonadotropins into the mother, and completed in the oviduct or in vitro, full term rabbit fetuses were obtained (97)."

The paper goes onto discuss how the use of hormonal priming to stimulate intrafollicular egg maturation might be achieved and reports: "Preliminary work using laparoscopy has shown that oocytes can be recovered from ovaries by puncturing ripening follicles in vivo. ..."

Through these preliminary collaborative studies, Edwards and Steptoe were already building a research partnership. Although both were very different personalities, and brought very different skills to the project, they shared energy, commitment, and vision. Each was also marginalized by his professional peers, a marginalization that also perhaps helped to cement their partnership (2).

With the paper's publication, announced to the media on St Valentine's day (105), all hell was let loose. The impossible tangle of TV cables and pushy reporters trying to force their way up the stairs to the fourth floor laboratories proved a major disruption to the Physiological laboratory in general and to the members of the Marshall laboratory in particular. It was something that was to recur episodically over the next 10 years.

THE BATTLES BEGIN

However, 1969 seemed to be a good year for Edwards. Not only did IVF succeed at long last, and his partnership with Steptoe seemed set to flourish, but also so impressed were the Ford Foundation with his work that in late 1968 they had established, at Austin's prompting (106), an endowment fund with the University of Cambridge to cover the salary cost of a Ford Foundation Readership [a half-way step to a professorship; (107)]. Elated by his promotion and their achievement, Edwards and Steptoe pressed on, the latter's laparoscopic skills coming to the fore, first in 1970 with the collection of in-vivo matured eggs from follicles after mild hormonal stimulation (108), and then achieving regular fertilization of these eggs and their early development through cleavage to the blastocyst stage (109,110). So well was the work going that in late 1970 and early 1971 they confidently applied to the U.K. Medical Research Council for funding.

However, any illusions that Edwards may have had that their achievements would prove a turning point in his fortunes were soon shattered. The hostility of much of the media coverage to his work in 1969 heralded the dominant pattern of scientific and medical responses for the next 10–15 years and resulted just two months later in the MRC rejecting the grant application (2). The practical consequences of this rejection were profound – both psychologically and physically – not least that for the next seven years, Edwards and Purdy shuttled on the 12-hour round trip between Cambridge and Oldham, Greater Manchester, paradoxically just north of his schoolboy haunts of Gorton, where Steptoe and he set up a small laboratory and clinic in Dr Kershaw's cottage hospital, all the while leaving Ruth and his five daughters in Cambridge.

The professional attacks on Edwards and his work took a number of forms (2), and one must try to make a mental time trip back to the 1960s and 1970s to understand their basis. Despite the nature of the political and religious battles to come, his scientific and medical colleagues did not focus on the special status of the human embryo as an ethical issue. Ethical issues were raised professionally, but took quite a different form. It is perhaps difficult now to comprehend the complete absence of infertility from the consciousness of most gynecologists in the United Kingdom at the time, of whom Steptoe was a remarkable exception (81). Indeed, even Edwards' strong commitment to treating infertility came to the fore only after he had teamed up with Steptoe, his previous priority being the study and prevention of genetic and chromosomal disorders.

In the several reports from the Royal College of Obstetricians and Gynaecologists and the MRC during the 1960s examining the areas of gynecological ignorance that needed academic attention, infertility simply did not feature (50,51). Overpopulation and family planning were seen as dominant concerns and the infertile were ignored as, at best, a tiny and irrelevant minority and at worst as a positive contribution to population control. This was a values system that Edwards did not accept (111), and the many encouraging letters he received from infertile couples spurred him on and provided a major stimulus to his continued work later, despite so much professional and press antagonism. For his professional colleagues, however, the fact that infertility was not seen as a significant clinical issue meant that any research designed to alleviate it was viewed not as experimental treatment, but as using humans in experiments. Given the sensitivity to the relatively recent Nazi "medical experiments," the formal acceptance of the Helsinki Declaration (112,113) and the public reaction and disquiet surrounding the recent publication of "Human guinea-pigs" (114), this distinction was critical. The MRC, in rejecting the grant application, took the position that what was being proposed was human experimentation, and so were very cautious, emphasizing risks rather than benefits, of which they saw few if any (2).

Edwards and Steptoe were also attacked for their willingness to talk with the media. It is difficult nowadays, when the public communication of science is embedded institutionally, to understand how damaging to them this was. The massive press interest of the late 1960s was unabated in the ensuing years, and so Edwards was faced with a choice: either he could keep his head down and allow press fantasies and speculations to go unanswered and unchallenged, or he could engage, educate, and debate. For him this was no choice, regardless of the consequences professionally (30). His egalitarian spirit demanded that he trust common people's common sense. His radical political views demanded that he fought the corner of the infertile: the underdog with no voice. The Yorkshireman in him relished engagement in the debate and argument. In Edwards and Sharpe (111), he sets out his reasons for public engagement and acknowledges the risk to his own interests:

> "Scientists may have to make disclosures of their work and its consequences that run against their immediate interests; they may have to stir up public opinion, even lobby for laws before legislatures."

And risk it was. One of the scientific referees on their MRC grant application started his referee's report declaring the media exposure distasteful:

> "Dr. Edwards feels the need to publicise his work on radio and television, and in the press, so that he can change public attitudes. I do not feel that an ill-informed general public is capable of evaluating the work and seeing it in its proper perspective. This publicity has antagonised a large number of Dr. Edwards' scientific colleagues, of whom I am one (2)."

Edwards' pioneering role in the public communication of science proved to be disadvantageous to his work.

The Edwards and Sharpe (111) paper is a tour de force in its survey of the scientific benefits and risks of the science of IVF, in the legal and ethical issues raised by IVF, and in the pros and cons of the various regulatory responses to them. It sets out the issues succinctly and anticipates social responses that were some 13–19 years into the future. Edwards built on his strong commitment to social justice based on a social ethic in subsequent years, as he engaged at every opportunity with ethicists, lawyers and theologians, arguing, playing "devil's advocate" (literally, in the eyes of some), and engaging in what would now be called practical ethics as he hammered out his position and felt able to fully justify his instincts intellectually.

However, the establishment was, with few exceptions, unwilling to engage seriously in ethical debates (115,116) in advance of the final validation of IVF that was to come in 1978 with the birth of Louise Brown (Fig. 13) (117). Only then did the UK social, scientific, and medical hierarchies, such as the MRC, the British Medical Association, the Royal Society, and Government move gradually from their almost visceral reactions against IVF and its possibilities to serious engagement with the issues (118). Then, to their credit, both the MRC and the Thatcher Government of the time came on board, but it was not until 1989, 24 years after Bob's 1965 visionary paper in the Lancet, that the UK Parliament finally gave its stamp of approval to his vision, and then only after a fierce battle lasting some 11 years (118,119).

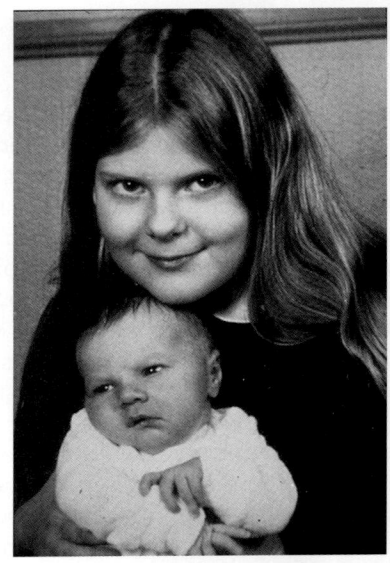

Figure 13 Louise Brown holding the 1000th Bourn Hall baby, 1987. *Source*: Courtesy of Bourn Hall Clinic.

DISCUSSION

This paper describes some of the early years of Edwards' life and work, in order to provide a context for the events leading up to the 1969 *Nature* paper describing IVF and the final validation of the claims made in that paper with the birth of Louise Brown in 1978. It is evident even from the earliest stages of his late entry into research that Edwards is a man of extraordinary energy and drive, qualities sustained throughout his long career, witnessing his prodigious output of papers between 1954 and 2008 (30). Indeed, several of the referees on the unsuccessful MRC grant application specifically criticized his "overenthusiasm," doubting that he could achieve the program he sets out therein as "too ambitious" (2). Tenacity of purpose comes through clearly in Edwards' work, a trait he is inclined to attribute to his Yorkshire origins, but which may also be fuelled by his working-class determination to show himself as good as the next (wo)man.

The influence of Waddington's Edinburgh Institute, of Waddington himself, and of his supervisor, Alan Beatty, on Edwards' interests and values is also clear from the dominant role that developmental genetics played in his thinking, especially until the time he met Steptoe. Indeed, from examination of Edwards' papers and interests, his passionate conversion to the cause of the infertile seems directly attributable to Steptoe's influence. Admittedly, Edwards' forays into immunoreproduction did involve consideration of immunological causes of infertility, but these were more usually of interest to him as models for developing new contraceptive agents. Indeed, Edwards was as captured as most reproductive biologists of the time by the 1960s' consensus on the need for better methods of world population control. This position was understandable given the reality of those concerns, as is demonstrated now in the problem of global warming that is attributable at least in part to a failure to control population growth. It is a measure of his imagination and empathy that he could grasp so rapidly Steptoe's understanding of the plight of the infertile and so flexibly incorporate this understanding into his plans. That empathy clearly reflects his underprivileged origins, his espousal of the cause of the junior, the disadvantaged, the ill-informed, and the underdog being a thread running through his career. Edwards can be very critical, but I have found no one who can remember him ever being nasty or vindictive. Even when he disagrees with someone passionately, he never loses his respect for them as people. That Steptoe tapped into this sentiment is clear.

The way in which Edwards met Steptoe has been absorbed into folklore, but an examination of the evidence seems to warrant some revision to commonly held later reminiscences. It remains uncertain exactly which publication(s) by Steptoe it was that Edwards read in 1967, but seems likely that he did read Steptoe's book. Thus, it was spermatozoa, not eggs, that were exercising Edwards in 1967, and it was the problem of sperm capacitation, not egg retrieval, to which Steptoe and his laparoscope seemed to offer a solution. The book is the only place that this issue is specifically addressed. Their actual meeting at the Royal Society of Medicine is also re-evaluated: Edwards was an invited speaker lecturing about his work on immunoreproduction; so paradoxically, what has been seen as a side track to his main work was, albeit serendipitously, the reason for their actual meeting.

The early collaboration between them involved the recovery of ovarian biopsies, just like those Rose and others had been providing. However, the attractions of preovulatory follicular egg recovery were already clear to them both by the end of 1968, and became, with embryo replacement, the central planks of their partnership. Steptoe and Edwards were in many ways an unlikely partnership. Their personal styles were very different, and there are clear hints in his writings that Edwards found their early days together difficult. But like most successful partnerships, their differences were sunk in a mutual respect for the other's pioneering skills and willingness to take on the established conventions. In Jean Purdy, they also had a partner who smoothed the bumps on the path of their work together (Fig. 14).

However, it remains Edwards' extraordinary foresight that marks him out so distinctively. His combination of vision and intellectual rigor is evident not just in his work on stem cells, PGD and, with Steptoe, infertility, but also in his pioneering work in the public communication of science, in how ethical discourse about reproduction is conducted, and in consideration of regulatory issues. The epithet "the father of Assisted Reproductive Technique" is surely deservedly appropriate.

ACKNOWLEDGMENTS

I thank the Edwards' family for their help in writing this account, for which, however, I take full responsibility. I also thank Sandy Markham and John Webster for allowing me to quote our correspondence, Margaret Wilson

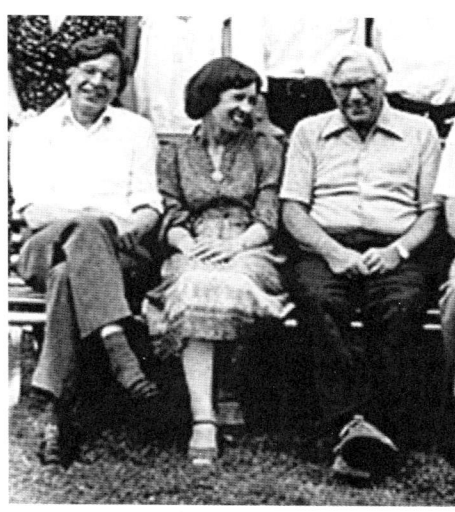

Figure 14 Edwards, Purdy, and Steptoe at Bourn Hall, 1981. *Source*: Courtesy of Bourn Hall Clinic.

for her help with locating books and periodicals, and Kay Elder, Ralph Robinson, and Sarah Franklin for their unfailing wisdom and help. I also thank Barry Bavister, Richard Gardner, Roger Gosden, David Griffin, Ginny Papaioannou, Barbara Rankin, Carol Readhead, Martin Richards, Janet Rossant, Pat Tate, and Frank Webb for contributing their own memories from their own papers and for correcting mine. I thank Ruth Edwards for permission to reproduce Figures 1–3, 5, 8, and 11, Barbara Rankin for permission to reproduce Figures 6, 7, 9, and 10, Andrew Steptoe for permission to reproduce Figure 12, Bourn Hall Clinic for permission to reproduce Figures 13 and 14, and Peter Williams for permission to include the movie clip in the Supplementary material. The research was supported by a grant from the Wellcome Trust (088708), which otherwise had no involvement in the research or its publication.

REFERENCES

1. Nobel, 2010. [Available from: http://nobelprize.org/nobel_prizes/medicine/laureates/2010/announcement.html].
2. Johnson MH, Franklin SB, Cottingham M, Hopwood N. Why the medical research council refused Robert Edwards and Patrick Steptoe support for research on human conception in 1971. Hum Reprod 2010; 25: 2157–74.
3. Edwards RG, Steptoe PC. A Matter of Life: The Story of a Medical Breakthrough. London, UK: Hutchinson, 1980.
4. Massey H, Feather N. James Chadwick. 20 October 1891–24 July. Biogr Mems Fell R Soc 1974; 22: 10–70.
5. Ashwood-Smith M. Robert Edwards at 55. Reprod BioMed Online 2002; 4(Suppl 1): 2–3.
6. Ingle DJ. Gregory Goodwin Pincus. April 9, 1903-August 22, 1967. Biogr Mems Natl Acad Sci USA 1971: 229–270. [Available from: http://www.nap.edu/readingroom.php?book=biomemsandpage=ggpincus.html].
7. Slee J. RGE at 25 – personal reminiscences. Reprod BioMed Online 2002; 4(Suppl 1): 1.

8. Oakley CL. Francis William Rogers Brambell. 1901–1970. Biogr Mems Fell R Soc 1973; 19: 129–171.
9. Parkes AS. Francis Hugh Adam Marshall. 1878–1949. Biogr Mems Fell R Soc 1950; 7: 238–251.
10. Polge C. Sir Alan Sterling Parkes. 10 September 1900–17 July. Biogr Mems Fell R Soc 2006; 52, 263–283.
11. Robertson A. Conrad Hal Waddington. 8 November 1905–26 September. Biogr Mems Fell R Soc 1977; 23: 575–622.
12. Milne EA. Ralph Howard Fowler. 1889–1944. Biogr Mems Fell R Soc 1945; 5: 60–78.
13. Eve AS, Chadwick J. Lord Rutherford. 1871–1937. Biogr Mems Fell R Soc 1938; 2: 394–423.
14. Edwards RG. An astonishing journey into reproductive genetics since the 1950's. Reprod Nutr Dev 2005; 45: 299–306.
15. Watson JD, Crick FH. Genetical implications of the structure of deoxyribonucleic acid. Nature 1953a; 171: 964–7.
16. Watson JD, Crick FH. Molecular structure of nucleic acids: a structure for deoxyribose nucleic acid. Nature 1953b; 171: 737–8.
17. Franklin R, Gosling R. Molecular configuration in sodium thymonucleate. Nature 1953; 171: 740–1.
18. Wilkins MHF, Stokes AR, Wilson HR. Molecular structure of deoxypentose nucleic acids. Nature 1953; 171: 738–40.
19. Gurdon JB. The developmental capacity of nuclei taken from intestinal epithelium cells of feeding tadpoles. Development 1962a; 10: 622–40.
20. Gurdon JB. Adult frogs derived from the nuclei of single somatic cells. Dev Biol 1962b; 4: 256–73.
21. Gurdon JB, Elsdale TR, Fischberg M. Sexually mature individuals of Xenopus laevis from the transplantation of single somatic nuclei. Nature 1958; 182; 64–5.
22. Weinberg AM. Messenger RNA: origins of a discovery. Nature 2001; 414: 485.
23. Ford CE, Hamerton JL. The chromosomes of man. Nature 1956; 178: 1020–23.
24. Tjio JH, Levan A. The chromosome number of man. Hereditas 1956; 42: 1–6.
25. Conference, Denver. A proposed standard system of nomenclature of human mitotic chromosomes. Lancet 1960; 275: 1063–65.
26. Ford CE, Jones KW, Polani PE, De Almeida JC, Briggs JH. A sex-chromosome anomaly in a case of gonadal dysgenesis (Turner's syndrome). Lancet 1959a; 273: 711–13.
27. Ford CE, Polani PE, Briggs JH, Bishop PM. A presumptive human XXY/XX mosaic. Nature 1959b; 183: 1030–32.
28. Jacobs PA, Strong JA. A case of human intersexuality having a possible XXY sex-determining mechanism. Nature 1959; 183: 302–3.
29. Lejeune J, Gautier M, Turpin R. Etude des chromosomes somatiques de neuf enfants mongoliens. Comptes Rendus Hebd Seances Acad Sci 1959; 248: 1721–22.
30. Gardner RL, Johnson MH. Bob Edwards and the first decade of reproductive biomedicine. Online Reprod BioMed Online 2011; 22: 106–24.
31. Fowler RE, Edwards RG. Induction of superovulation and pregnancy in mature mice by gonadotrophins. J Endocr 1957; 15: 374–84.
32. Edwards RG, Gates AH. Timing of the stages of the maturation divisions, ovulation, fertilization and the first cleavage of eggs of adult mice treated with gonadotrophins. J Endocr 1959; 18: 292–304.
33. Horowitz NH, Metz CB, Piatigorsky J, Piko L, Spikes JD, Ycas M. Albert Tyler. Science 1969; 163: 424.
34. Reeve S. Nathaniel Mayer Victor Rothschild, G.B.E., G.M. Third Baron Rothschild. 31 October 1910–20 March. Biogr Mems Fell R Soc 1994; 39: 364–80.
35. Rothschild. Did fertilization occur? Nature 1969; 221: 981.
36. Edwards RG, Bavister BD, Steptoe PC. Early stages of fertilization in vitro of human oocytes matured in vitro. Nature 1969b; 221: 632–5.
37. Mitchison NA. Peter Brian Medawar. February 1915–2 October. Biogr Mems Fell R Soc 1990; 35: 282–301.
38. Medawar PB. Some immunological and endocrinological problems raised by the evolution of viviparity in.vertebrates. Symp Soc Exp Biol 1953; 7: 320–38.
39. Clarke AE. Disciplining Reproduction: Modernity, American Life Sciences, and the Problems of Sex. Berkeley, California, USA: University of California Press, 1998.
40. Connelly M. Fatal Misconception: The Struggle to Control World Population. Cambridge, USA: Harvard University Press, 2008.
41. Marks LV. Sexual Chemistry: A History of the Contraceptive Pill. New Haven, USA: Yale University Press, 2001.
42. Naz RK, Gupta SK, Gupta JC, Vyas HK, Talwar GP. Recent advances in contraceptive vaccine development: a mini-review. Hum Reprod 2005; 20: 3271–83.
43. Rukavina D. The history of reproductive immunology: my personal view. Am J Reprod Immunol 2008; 59: 446–50.
44. Edwards RG. Meiosis in ovarian oocytes of adult mammals. Nature 1962; 196: 446–50.
45. Gemzell CA. The induction of ovulation with human pituitary gonadotrophins. Fertil Steril 1962; 13: 153–68.
46. Pincus G, Enzmann EV. The comparative behavior of mammalian eggs in vivo and in vitro I. the activation of ovarian eggs. J Exp Med 1935; 62: 665–75.
47. Pincus G, Saunders B. The comparative behavior of mammalian eggs in vivo and in vitro VI. The maturation of human ovarian ova. Anat Rec 1939; 75: 537–45.
48. Greep RO. Min Chueh Chang. October 10, 1908–June 5, 1991. Biogr Mems Natl Acad Sci USA. 2010. [Available from: http://www.nap.edu/readingroom.php?book=biomemsandpage=mchang.html].
49. Chang MC. The maturation of rabbit oocytes in culture and their maturation, activation, fertilization and subsequent development in the Fallopian tubes. J Exp Zool 1955; 128: 379–405.
50. MRC. 1969. Research in Obstetrics and Gynaecology: Report to the Secretary of the Council by Section A1, General Clinical Medicine. National Archives, FD 7/912.
51. RCOG. Macafee Report. The Training of Obstetricians and Gynaecologists in Britain, and Matters Related Thereto: The Report of a Select Committee to the Council of the Royal College of Obstetricians and Gynaecologists. London, UK: RCOG, 1967.
52. Askonas BA. John Herbert Humphrey. 16 December 1915–25 December. Biogr Mems Fell R Soc 1990; 36: 274–300.

53. Himsworth H, Pitt-Rivers R. Charles Robert Harington. 1897–1972. Biogr Mems Fell R Soc 1972; 18, 266–308.
54. McLaren A, Biggers JD. Successful development and birth of mice cultivated in vitro as early embryos. Nature 1958; 182: 877–8.
55. Cole RJ, Edwards RG, Paul J. Cytodifferentiation in cell colonies and cell strains derived from cleaving ova and blastocysts of the rabbit. Exp Cell Res 1965; 37: 501–4.
56. Cole RJ, Edwards RG, Paul J. Cytodifferentiation and embryogenesis in cell colonies and tissue cultures derived from ova and blastocysts of the rabbit. Dev Biol 1966; 13: 385–407.
57. Evans MJ, Kaufman MH. Establishment in culture of pluripotential cells from mouse embryos. Nature 1981; 292: 154–6.
58. Edwards RG. IVF and the history of stem cells. Nature 2001; 413: 349–51.
59. Parkes AS. Off-beat Biologist. Cambridge, UK: The Galton Foundation, 1985.
60. Cook B. JRF – the first 100 volumes. Reproduction 1994; 100: 2–4.
61. Clarke J. The history of three scientific societies: the Society for the Study of Fertility (now the Society for Reproduction and Fertility) (Britain), the Societe 'Francaise pour l'Etude de la Fertilite', and the Society for the Study of Reproduction (USA). Stud Hist Phil Biol Biomed Sci 2007; 38: 340–57.
62. Edwards RG. Letter to Cambridge University Registrary, plus supporting documents, applying for the Mary Marshall and Arthur Walton Professorship of the Physiology of Reproduction. Edwards' papers, 6 Jan 1966. Uncatalogued, Churchill College Archive. 1966.
63. Polge C. 1993. Obituary: Professor Thaddeus Mann. The Independent, 9 December.
64. Short R. Colin Austin. Aust Acad Sci Newslett 2004; 60: 11.
65. Arechaga J. Technique as the basis of experiment in developmental biology: An interview with Denis A.T. New Int J Dev Biol 1997; 41: 139–52.
66. Edwards RG, Steptoe PC. Preface. In: Edwards RG, Purdy JM, Steptoe PC, eds. Implantation of the Human Embryo. London, UK: Academic Press, 1985: vii–viii.
67. Vickers AD. A direct measurement of the sex-ratio in mouse blastocysts. Reproduction 1967; 13: 375–6.
68. Gardner RL. Bob Edwards – 2010 nobel laureate in physiology or medicine. Physiology News 2011; 82: 18–22.
69. Gardner RL, Johnson MH. Robert Edwards. Hum Reprod 1991; 6: iii–iv.
70. Edwards RG. Maturation in vitro of human ovarian oocytes. Lancet 1965a; 286: 926–929.
71. Edwards RG. Maturation in vitro of mouse, sheep, cow, pig, rhesus monkey and human ovarian oocytes. Nature 1965b; 208: 349–51.
72. Gardner RL, Edwards RG. Control of the sex ratio at full term in the rabbit by transferring sexed blastocysts. Nature 1968; 218: 346–9.
73. Theodosiou AA, Johnson MH. The politics of human embryo research and the motivation to achieve PGD. Reprod BioMed Online 2011; 22: 457–71.
74. Edwards RG. Are oocytes formed and used sequentially in the mammalian ovary? Phil Trans R Soc B 1970; 259: 103–5.
75. Henderson SA, Edwards RG. Chiasma frequency and maternal age in mammals. Nature 1968; 218: 22–8.
76. Chang MC. Fertilization of rabbit ova in vitro. Nature 1959; 184: 466–7.
77. Yanagimachi R, Chang M.C. Fertilization of hamster eggs in vitro. Nature 1963; 200: 281–2.
78. Jones Jr HW. From reproductive immunology to Louise Brown. Reprod BioMed Online 2002; 4(Suppl 1): 6–7.
79. Edwards RG, Donahue RP, Baramki TA, Jones Jr HW. Preliminary attempts to fertlilize human oocytes matured in vitro. Am J Obstet Gynecol 1966; 96: 192–200.
80. Edwards RG, Talbert L, Israelstam D, Nino HN, Johnson MH. Diffusion chamber for exposing spermatozoa to human uterine secretions. Am J Obstet Gynecol 1968; 102: 388–396.
81. Edwards RG. Patrick Christopher Steptoe, C. B. E. 9 June 1913–22 March 1988. Biogr Mems Fell R Soc 1996; 42: 435–52.
82. Steptoe PC. Laparoscopy in Gynaecology. Edinburgh, UK: E and S Livingstone, 1967a.
83. Philipp E. Obituary: P C Steptoe CBE, FRCSED, FRCOG, FRS. Br Med J 1988; 296: 1135.
84. Edwards RG. Tribute to Patrick Steptoe: beginnings of laparoscopy. Hum Reprod 1989; 4(Suppl): 1–9.
85. Edwards RG. Interviewed in: To Mrs. Brown a daughter. Peter Williams TV: The Studio, Boughton. Faversham, UK (see Supplementary Material), 1978.
86. Steptoe PC. Laparoscopy and ovulation. Lancet 1968; 292: 913.
87. Hunting P. The history of the royal society of medicine. London, UK: The Royal Society of Medicine Press Ltd, 2002.
88. Steptoe PC. Laparoscopy: diagnostic and therapeutic uses. Proc Roy Soc Med 1969; 62: 439–441.
89. Steptoe PC. A new method of tubal sterilisation. In: Westin B, Wiqvist N, eds. Amsterdam: Fertility and Sterility: Proc 5th World Congress June 16–22, 1966. Stockholm: International Congress Series no. 133, Excerpta Medica Foundation, 1967b: 1183–1184.
90. Steptoe PC. Laparoscopic studies of ovulation, its suppression and induction, and of ovarian dysfunction. In: Wood C, Walters WAW, eds. Fifth World Congress of Gynaecology and Obstetrics, held in Sydney, Australia, September, 1967. Butterworths, Sydney, Australia, 1967c: 364.
91. Steptoe PC. The fifth freedom. Br Med J 1966; 1: 234.
92. Steptoe PC. Gynaecological endoscopy–laparoscopy and culdoscopy. J Obstet Gynaecol Br Commonwealth 1965; 72: 535–43.
93. Morrison DL. Laparoscopy. BMJ 1967; 4: 34.
94. Austin CR. Observations of the penetration of sperm into the mammalian egg. Aust J Sci Res B 1951; 4: 581–96.
95. Chang MC. Fertilizing capacity of spermatozoa deposited into the fallopian tubes. Nature 1951; 168: 697–8.
96. Bavister BD. Environmental factors important for in vitro fertilization in the hamster. Reprod 1969; 18: 544–545.
97. Edwards RG, Bavister BD, Steptoe PC. Did fertilization occur? Nature 1969a; 221: 981–2.
98. Hayashi M. Fertilization in vitro using human ova. In: Proceedings of the 7th International Planned Parenthood Federation, Singapore. Excerpta Medica International Congress Series No. 72. Amsterdam, Netherlands, 1963.

99. Petrov GN. Fertilization and first stages of cleavage of human egg in vitro. Arkhiv Anatomii Gistologii i Embriologii 1958; 35: 88–91.
100. Petrucci D. Producing transplantable human tissue in the laboratory. Discovery 1961; 22: 278–83.
101. Rock J, Menkin M. In vitro fertilization and cleavage of human ovarian eggs. Science 1944; 100: 105–7.
102. Shettles LB. A morula stage of human ovum developed in vitro. Fertil Steril 1955; 9: 287–9.
103. Yang WH. The nature of human follicular ova and fertilization in vitro. J Jpn Obstet Gynecol Soc 1963; 15: 121–130.
104. Anon, 2008. Morris, Prof. Norman Frederick. In: Who Was Who 1920–1980. A & C Black and Oxford University Press. [Available from: http://www.ukwhoswho.com/view/article/oupww/whowaswho/U28190].
105. Anon, 1969. New step towards test-tube babies. Nature-Times News Service; The Times 14 February, 1.
106. Holmes RF. Letter to D Kellaway, (Sec Fac Board Biol. B), dated 21 May. University of Cambridge Archives, 1968; 731.020.
107. Hankinson GS. Letter (G.B.6812.534) from the General Board of the Faculties, the Old Schools, Cambridge to RG Edwards detailing some aspects of the Ford Foundation endowment fund, 20 December 1968. Edwards papers uncatalogued, Churchill College Archive.1968.
108. Steptoe PC, Edwards RG. Laparoscopic recovery of preovulatory human oocytes after priming of ovaries with gonadotrophins. Lancet 1970; 295: 683–9.
109. Edwards RG, Steptoe PC, Purdy JM. Fertilization and cleavage in vitro of preovulatory human oocytes. Nature 1970; 227: 1307–9.
110. Steptoe PC, Edwards RG, Purdy JM. Human blastocysts grown in culture. Nature 1971; 229: 132–3.
111. Edwards RG, Sharpe DJ. Social values and research in human embryology. Nature 1971; 231: 87–91.
112. Helsinki Declaration, Human Experimentation: Code of Ethics of World Medical Association. Br Med J 1964; 2: 177.
113. Hazelgrove J. The old faith and the new science. the Nuremberg Code and human experimentation ethics in Britain 1946–73. Soc Hist Med 2002; 15: 109–135.
114. Pappworth MH. Human Guinea-Pigs. London, UK: Routledge and Keegan Paul, 1967.
115. Edwards RG. Fertilization of human eggs in vitro: morals, ethics and the law. Q Rev Biol 1974; 49: 3–26.
116. Jones A, Bodmer WF. Our Future Inheritance: Choice or Chance? London, UK: Oxford University Press, 1974.
117. Edwards RG, Steptoe PC. Birth after the reimplantation of a human embryo. Lancet 1978; 312: 366.
118. Johnson MH, Theodosiou AA. PGD and the making of the genetic embryo as a political tool. In: McLean S, ed. Regulating PGD: A Comparative and Theoretical Analysis. London, UK: Routledge, 2011.
119. Mulkay M. The embryo research debate: science and the politics of reproduction. Cambridge, UK: Cambridge University Press, 1997.

Setting up an ART laboratory

Jacques Cohen, Mina Alikani, Antonia Gilligan, and Tim Schimmel

There are a number of ways to set up and operate a successful assisted reproductive technique (ART) laboratory; one set-up may have little in common with another but may prove to be equally successful. It is important that one remembers this before venturing into establishing a new clinic. Facilities for ART range from a makeshift in vitro fertilization (IVF) laboratory with a minimum of equipment to a fully equipped laboratory specifically designed for ART and additional space dedicated to clinical care and research. This chapter does not cover makeshift laboratories, which may incorporate retrieval and transport of gametes and embryos from other locations. While such models can be successful under some circumstances, compelling evidence showing that they produce optimal results is still lacking (1,2). Both IVF and intracytoplasmic sperm injection (ICSI) can be applied to transported oocytes, and in certain situations "transport IVF" is a welcome alternative for those patients whose reproductive options have been limited by restrictive governmental regulations (3,4). This chapter discusses the more typical purpose-built all-inclusive laboratories that are adjacent or in close proximity to oocyte retrieval and embryo transfer facilities, with emphasis on the special problems of construction. For choices of culture system, culture medium, supplementation, viability assays, and handling and processing of gametes and embryos including freezing and vitrification, the reader is referred to other relevant chapters in this textbook.

PERSONNEL AND EXPERIENCE

While the environment, physical plant, and equipment require special consideration in the design of an integrated gamete and embryo culture facility, it is the staff members who will carry out the procedures and are essential for the success of the entire operation. Successful clinical practice in general and ART in particular are almost entirely dependent on the experience level of medical and laboratory personnel. For the laboratory staff, enthusiasm is another key factor to success, especially because there are still few formal teaching and skills examination programs in place for a specialty in ART. Good clinical outcome requires a cautious and rational assessment of individual abilities, so laboratory staff, directors, and embryologists must consider their experience in the context of what will be required of them. This chapter aims to provide information necessary for experienced practitioners to set up a new laboratory. Setting up a new laboratory or thoroughly renovating an existing facility is very much an art as is the practice of ART itself.

Programs should develop a strong (though friendly) system of tracking individual performances for crucial clinical and laboratory procedures such as embryo transfer efficiency, ICSI and biopsy proficiency, etc. Certain regulatory bodies such as the College of American Pathology and the Human Fertilization and Embryology Authority in the United Kingdom provide guidelines and licensing for embryologists, sometimes even for subspecialties such as the performance of ICSI, the practice of embryo biopsy, and directing IVF and andrology laboratories. So far, such licensing has done little more than provoke debate, because licensing does not necessarily guarantee skill (or success) and the licenses are not valid across borders from one country to another.

Tradition also plays its role. For example, in some Asian countries embryology directors are usually medical professionals. Thus academic titles are often seen as being more important than actual qualifications. What then qualifies someone to be a laboratory director or an embryologist? The answer is not a simple one. In general, current licensing authorities including the American Board of Bioanalysis consider individuals trained in general pathology or reproductive medicine and holding an MD degree as well as individuals holding a PhD degree qualified to be laboratory director if they meet some other requirements. However, pathologists do not necessarily have experience in gamete and embryo cell culture, and some reproductive medicine specialists, such as urologists and immunologists, may have never worked with gametes and embryos. It is possible for a medical practitioner to direct a laboratory in certain countries without ever having practiced gamete and embryo handling! As Galileo said, "*Eppur si muove*" ("and yet it moves") when condemned by the Roman inquisition for heresy of accepting Copernican astronomy, once there are rules, even silly ones, it may be hard to change them.

EMPIRICAL AND STATISTICAL REQUIREMENTS FOR STAFF

There is considerable disagreement about what should be the required experience for embryologists. Hands-on experience in all facets of clinical embryology is an absolute requirement when starting a new program. Even highly experienced experimental embryologists and animal scientists should be directly supervised by experienced clinical personnel. The period during which a detailed supervision must continue depends on the types of skills required, the daily caseload, and time spent performing procedures. Clearly, performing 100 cases over a one-year period is a very different circumstance than performing the same number over six weeks; the period of supervision then should be adjusted accordingly.

The optimal ratio of laboratory staff to the expected number of procedures is debatable, and unfortunately, economics plays an all-too important role here. Nevertheless, it is safe to say that the ratio should be low so that embryologists can spend a reasonable portion of their time on quality control, training, and procedural details to ensure the high standards required for success. In practice, however, the staff to procedure ratio is often suboptimal for economic reasons or as a consequence of national health systems or insurance mandates that must provide a wide range of services on a minimal budget. Needless to say, patients usually do not benefit from these constraints; this is most obvious when comparing outcomes between the various health service systems in Western countries.

The job description for the embryologist ideally includes all embryology and andrology tasks, except for medical and surgical procedures. Embryologists are often involved in other important tasks as well, including patient management, follicular monitoring, genetic counseling, marketing, and administration. However, it should be realized that these tasks seriously detract them from their main responsibilities. First and foremost, the embryologist's duty is to perform gamete and embryo handling and culture procedures. Secondly, but equally important, the embryologist should maintain quality control standards, both by performing routine checks and tests and by maintaining detailed logs of incidents, changes, unexpected events, and corrective measures. Across all these duties, the following seven positions can be clearly defined: director, supervisor, senior embryologist, embryologist, trainee, assistant, and technician, their actual numbers varying according to the number of procedures performed annually. There may also be positions for others to do pre-implantation genetic diagnosis, research, or secretarial work. Obviously, not all of these positions are necessary for smaller centers.

Although a seemingly unimportant detail, one of the most important jobs in the IVF laboratory at Bourn Hall Clinic in Cambridge, United Kingdom, during the first few years of operation was that of a professional witness and embryology assistant. This position was the brainchild of Jean Purdy, the third person who was involved in the work that led to the birth of Louise Brown. The embryology assistant effectively enforced and oversaw the integrity of the chain of custody of gametes and embryos during handling, particularly when large numbers of patients were being treated simultaneously. The "witness" also ensured that embryologists performed only those procedures for which they were qualified. In general, embryologists should concentrate on only gamete and embryo handling, and any laboratory with a relatively high number of annual procedures should have additional embryology technicians and assistants who can order and maintain equipment, and record laboratory data. In short, skimping on staff can be self-defeating in the IVF laboratory.

FACILITY, DESIGN, AND BUDGET

In the early days of IVF some clinics were built in remote areas, based on the premise that environmental factors such as stress could affect the patient and thereby the outcome of treatment. Today's laboratories are commonly placed in city centers and large metropolitan areas in order to service large populations. It is important that patients understand that there have been millions of others like them before and that in general IVF is a routine, though complex, medical procedure. It is clear that the choice of a laboratory site is of great importance for a new program. The recent development of better assays for determining the baseline quality of the environment facilitates site selection. There is now awareness that some buildings or building sites could be intrinsically harmful to cell tissue culture (5–7).

A laboratory design should be based on the anticipated caseload and any subspecialty. Local building and practice permits must be assessed prior to engaging and completing a design. There are five basic types of design:

1. Laboratories using only transport IVF
2. Laboratories adjacent to clinical outpatient facilities that are only used part of the time
3. Full-time clinics with intra-facility egg transport using portable warming chambers
4. Fully integrated laboratories with clinical areas
5. Moveable temporary laboratories

Before developing the basic design for a new laboratory, environmental factors must be considered. While the air quality in modern laboratories can be controlled to a degree, it can never be fully protected from the exterior environment and adjoining building spaces. Designers should first determine whether the building or the surrounding site is scheduled to undergo renovations, demolition, or major changes of any kind in the foreseeable future. City planning should also be reviewed. Historical environmental data and trends, future construction, and the ability of maintenance staff to maintain and service the IVF laboratory need to be determined. Activity related to any type of construction can have a significant negative impact on any proposed laboratory. Prevalent wind direction, industrial hazards, and general pollution reports such as ozone measurements should also be determined. Even when these factors are all deemed acceptable, basic air sampling and determination of volatile organic compound (VOC) concentrations is necessary inside and outside the proposed building area. The outcome of these tests will determine which design requirements are needed to remove VOCs from the laboratory area. In most cases an over-pressured laboratory (at least 0.10–0.20 inches of water) that uses a high number (7–15) of fresh air changes per hour (FACH) is the best solution, because it also provides for proper medical hygiene. The laboratory walls and ceiling should have the absolute minimum number of penetrations. This generally requires a solid ceiling, sealed lighting, and airtight utility connections. Contrary to many vendors' representations, commercial suspended ceilings using double-sided tape and clips are not ideal. Doors will require seals and sweeps, and should be lockable. Ducts and equipment must be laid out in such a way that routine and emergency maintenance and repair work can be performed outside the laboratory with minimal disruption to the laboratory. Air handling must not use an open plenum design. In the ideal case, 100% outside air with chemical and physical filtration will be used with sealed supply and return ducts. While providing cleaner air, 100% outside air sourcing will maximize the life of a chemical filter and will provide a lower concentration of VOC in the IVF laboratory's air. In climates where temperatures routinely exceed 32°C with 85% plus relative humidity, 100% outside air could result in an unacceptable level of humidity (>60%), which could allow mold growth. In these cases the use of limited return air from the lab is acceptable. A 50% outside air system with 15–30 total air changes per hour does work well and the relative humidity becomes very controllable. To place this in perspective, traditional medical operating room design calls for 10–15% outside air. The air supply equipment may supplement outside air with recirculated air, with processing to control the known levels of VOCs. On rare occasions, laboratories will require full-time air recirculation while most may actually find the outside air to be perfectly clean at least most of the time. Outside air is often erroneously judged to be polluted without proper chemical analysis, while inside air is usually considered "cleaner" because it may "smell" better (5). In most laboratory locations, conditions are actually the reverse, and designers should not "follow their instincts" in these matters. Humidity must also be completely controlled according to climate and seasonal variation. The system must be capable of supplying the space with air with a temperature as high as 30–35°C at less than 40% relative humidity. Air inlets and outlets should be carefully spaced to avoid drafts that can change local "spot" temperatures, or expose certain equipment to relatively poor air or changes in air quality. Laminar flow hoods and micromanipulation workstations should not be located too close to air supply fixtures to avoid disruption of the sterile field and to minimize cooling on the microscope stage. A detailed layout and assessment of all laboratory furniture and equipment is therefore essential prior to construction and has many other benefits.

Selection of an experienced and subspecialized (and flexible) architect and a mechanical engineer for the project is essential. Confirm what their past experience has been in building biologically clean rooms. The use of "environmentally friendly" or "green" products has been suggested by some designers. The reliance on "natural" products does not ensure a clean laboratory. In one case, wood casework with a green label was found to be a major source of formaldehyde. Floor coverings using recycled vinyl and rubber were selected for their low environmental impact, without considering the significant release of trapped gasses by the material.

Supervision of the construction is also critical. Skilled tradesmen using past training and experience may not follow all of the architect's instructions. The general contractor and the builders must be briefed on why these novel construction techniques are being used. They must understand that the use of untested methods and products can compromise the project (and the payment of their fees!). Contractual agreement is recommended. Just as the organization and flow of traffic in a world-class restaurant results in a special ambience where more than just the food is the attraction, appropriate modular placement of equipment ensures safety and comfort in the IVF laboratory. Placement of stacks of incubators, gamete handling areas (laminar flow units or isolettes), and micromanipulation stations should minimize distances that dishes and tubes need be moved. Ideally, an embryologist should be able to finish one complete procedure without moving more than three meters in any direction; not only is this efficient but also it minimizes accidents in a busy laboratory. The number of modules can easily be determined by the expected number of cases and procedure types, the average number of eggs collected, and the number of embryologists expected to work simultaneously. Each person should be provided with sufficient workspace to perform all procedures without delay. Additional areas can contain simple gamete-handling stations or areas for concentrating incubators. Cryopreservation and storage facilities are often located in a separate space, although this is not strictly necessary; if separated, these areas should always be adjacent to the main laboratory. Another separate laboratory or module may contain an area for culture medium preparation, sterilization, and water treatment; however, the need for such an area is diminishing now that commercial manufacturers provide all the basic needs of an IVF laboratory. Administration should be performed in separate offices.

Last but not least, it is preferable to prepare semen in a separate laboratory altogether, adjacent to a collection room. The semen laboratory should have ample space for microscopes, freezing, and sterile zoning. Proper separation of patient samples during processing is essential and some elemental design features may be considered before the first procedures are carried out. Some thought should go into planning the semen collection area. This room should be at the end of a hallway, preferably with its own exit; it should be soundproofed, not too large, with a sink. Clear instructions of how to collect semen for ART should be provided in the room. The room should also be adjacent to the semen preparation laboratory, preferably with a double-door pass-through for samples. This pass-through should have a signaling device so the patient can inform the embryologist that the sample is ready; it also permits male patients to leave the area without having to carry a specimen container.

EQUIPMENT AND STORAGE

A detailed list of equipment should be prepared and checked against the planned location of each item; it can later be used as the basis of maintenance logs. It is important to consider the inclusion of extra crucial equipment and spare tools in the laboratory design, to allow for unexpected malfunction. It is particularly important to have redundant elements of the cryopreservation system—including cryopreservation and storage equipment. Similarly, two or more spare incubators should not be seen as excessive; at least one spare follicle aspiration pump and micromanipulation station should also be included. There are many other instruments and equipment pieces, the malfunction of which would jeopardize patient care, although some spares need not be kept on hand as manufacturers may have them available; however, such details need to be repeatedly checked as suppliers' stock continues to change. It may also be useful to team up with other programs or an embryology research laboratory locally so that a crucial piece of equipment can be exchanged in case of unexpected failure.

Some serious thought is needed when contemplating the number of incubators and incubator spaces. The ratio of cases per incubator depends on incubator size and capacity but it varies considerably from program to program. It is clear that the number and type of incubator, as well as the length and number of incubator door openings affect results. In principle, the number of cases per incubator should be kept to a minimum; we prefer a limit of four cases per large standard incubator. The smaller incubators should not handle more than two to three cases. In bench-top incubators, the use of one dish slot per patient is not recommended. Several other incubators can be used for general purpose during micromanipulation and for other generic uses to limit further the number of incubator openings. Strict guidelines must be implemented and adhered to when maintaining distinct spaces for separating culture dishes or tubes of different patients. Tracking of incubators and even shelves within each incubator is recommended so their performance can be evaluated on an ongoing basis. Separate compartments within an incubator may be helpful and can be supplied by certain manufacturers. Servicing and cleaning of equipment such as incubators may have to be done when the laboratory is not performing procedures. Placement of incubators and other pieces of equipment on large castors may be helpful in programs where downtime is rare. Pieces of equipment can then be serviced outside the laboratory. New incubators and equipment pieces that come in contact with gametes and embryos must be "burned-in" or "off-gassed." Protocols vary per equipment type and manufacturer.

When there are several options available to the laboratory designer, supply and evacuation routes should be planned in advance. One of the most susceptible aspects of ART is cryopreservation. In case of an emergency such as fire or power failure, it may be necessary to relocate the liquid nitrogen–filled dewars without using an elevator, or to relocate the frozen samples using a temporary container. This may seem an extreme consideration, especially in the larger laboratories that stockpile thousands of samples, but plans should be made. It may be possible to keep a separate storage closet or space near the building exit, where long-term samples, which usually provide the bulk of the storage, can be kept; this would require a repeated checking of a facility that is not part of the laboratory. Liquid nitrogen tank alarms with remote notification capability should be installed on all dewars holding gametes and embryos. The route of delivery of liquid nitrogen and other gas cylinders must be made relatively easy, without stairways between the laboratory and the delivery truck, and should be sensibly planned in advance. Note that the flooring of this route is usually destroyed within months because of liquid nitrogen spills and wear caused by delivery containers, so the possibility of an alternative delivery corridor should be considered for these units.

Liquid nitrogen containers and medical gas cylinders are preferentially placed immediately adjacent to the laboratory in a closet or a small, ventilated room with outside access. Pipes and tubes enter the laboratory from this room, and cylinders can be delivered to this room without compromising the laboratory area in any way. Providing liquid nitrogen and even liquid oxygen vapor to triple gas incubators is nowadays a preferred option since vapor is cleaner than compressed gas. This allows liquid nitrogen vapor to be pumped into the cryopreservation laboratory using a manifold system and minimal lining. Lines should be properly installed and insulated to ensure that they do not leak or allow condensation and conserve energy at the same time. Medical gases can be directed into the laboratory using pre-washed vinyl/Teflon-lined tubing such as fluorinated ethylene propylene or FEP, which has high humidity, temperature, and UV radiation stability. Lines should be properly marked every meter indicating the incubators supplied in order to facilitate later maintenance. Alternatively, solid manifolds made from stainless steel with suitable compression fittings can be used. Avoid soldered or brazed copper lines used in domestic plumbing applications wherever possible; copper lining can be used but should be cleaned and purged for a prolonged period prior to use in the laboratory. Copper line connections should not be soldered as this could cause continuous contamination. This recommendation may conflict with existing building codes, but noncontaminating alternatives can be found. A number of spare lines hidden behind walls and ceilings should be installed as well, in case of later renovation or facility expansion.

Large programs should consider the use of exterior bulk tanks for carbon dioxide and liquid nitrogen. This removes the issues of tanks for incubators or cryopreservation. These tanks are located where delivery trucks can hook onto and deliver directly to the tank. Pressurized gas lines or cryogenic lines then run the carbon dioxide or liquid nitrogen to the IVF laboratory for use.

Placement of bulky and difficult pieces of equipment should be considered when designing doorways and electrical panels. Architects should be fully informed of all equipment specifications to avoid the truly classic door-width mistake. Emergency generators should always be installed, even where power supplies are usually reliable. The requirements can be determined by an electrical engineer. Thankfully, these units can be well removed from the laboratory, but must be placed in well-ventilated areas that are not prone to flooding. Additional battery "uninterruptible power systems" may be considered as well but are of very limited capability. Buildings should also be checked for placement of the main power inlets and distribution centers, especially because sharing power lines with other departments or companies may not be advisable. Circuit breakers should be easily accessible to embryologists or building maintenance staff. General knowledge of mechanical and electrical engineering of the building and the laboratory specifically will always be advantageous. Leaving all the building mechanics and facilities to other individuals is often counterproductive. Embryologists need to be involved with facilities management and be updated with construction decisions in and outside the building in a timely manner.

Ample storage spaces should always be planned for IVF laboratories. In the absence of dedicated storage space, laboratory space ends up being used instead, filling all cabinets and negating any advantages of the original design. This storage area should be used to stock all materials in sufficient quantity to maintain a steady supply. A further reason to include storage areas in laboratory design, sufficient on its own to justify the space, is that new supplies, including sterile disposable items, release multiple compounds for prolonged periods. This "out-gassing" has been determined to be a major cause of air pollution in a number of laboratories in which supplies are stored inside the lab. Separate storage space therefore provides the best chance of good air quality, especially when it is supplied by a separate air handling system. It should be large enough to handle bulky items as well as mobile shelving for boxes. One should be careful to avoid the natural inclination to save extra trips by bringing too many items into the laboratory, or the purpose of a careful design may be lost.

MICROSCOPES AND VISUALIZATION OF CELLS

Although dissecting microscopes are crucial for the general handling of gametes and embryos, many people still consider inverted microscopes to be a luxury even though they are in regular use with micromanipulation systems. Proper visualization of embryos is key to successful embryo selection for transfer or freezing; if the equipment is first class, the visualization can be done quickly and accurately (8). Even so, an appropriately detailed assessment is still dependent on the use of an oil overlay system to prevent damage by prolonged exposure. Each workstation and microscope should be equipped with a still camera and/or video camera and monitor. Still photos can be placed in the patient file and the video footage permits a speedy review of embryonic features with colleagues after the gametes are safely returned to the incubator; this is also helpful for training of new embryologists. Interference optics such as Hoffman and Nomarski are preferable because they permit the best measure of detail and depth. Novel visualization of internal elements such as spindles using polarized microscopy requires more complicated equipment, but can still be part of a routine operation (9). Ideally, the captured photos should be digitally stored for recall in the clinic's medical database.

CONSTRUCTION, RENOVATION, AND BUILDING MATERIALS

Construction and renovation can introduce a variety of compounds into the environment of the ART laboratory, either temporarily or permanently. Both can have major adverse effects on the outcome of operations (5–7,10,11). The impact of the exterior environment on IVF success has been demonstrated. Pollutants can have a significant negative effect on success in an IVF laboratory. These effects can range from delayed or abnormal embryonic development, reduced or failed fertilization, and reduced implantation rates to failure of a treatment cycle. Many of the damaging materials are organic chemicals that are released or out-gassed by paint, adhesives from flooring, cabinets, and general building materials, as well as from laboratory equipment and procedures. It is important to realize that the actual construction phase of the laboratory can cause permanent problems. Furthermore, any subsequent adjacent renovation can also cause similar, or even greater, problems. Neighboring tenants can be informed of the sensitivity of gametes and embryos in culture. At the very least, changes undertaken in adjacent areas should be supervised by IVF laboratory personnel to minimize potential damage. However, new construction immediately outside the building is considerably more problematic. City works such as street construction are very hard to predict and nearly impossible to control. A good relationship with the neighbors should be maintained and a working relationship with building owners and city planners should be established so that the IVF laboratory is kept informed of upcoming changes.

For construction of a new laboratory or if changes are to be made to areas adjacent to the IVF facility, the following guidelines should be followed. First, the area to be demolished and reconstructed needs to be physically isolated from the IVF laboratory (if this is not the new IVF laboratory itself). The degree of isolation should be equivalent to an asbestos or lead abatement project. The isolation should be done through (*i*) physical barriers, consisting of polysheeting supported by studding where needed; (*ii*) limited access to the construction area and the use of an access passageway with two doors in series; (*iii*) removal of all construction waste via an exterior opening or proper containment of waste before using an interior exit; (*iv*) negative air pressure in the construction area, exhausting to the exterior, far removed from the laboratory's air intake, and properly located with regard to the prevailing winds and exterior airflow; (*v*) extra interior fans during any painting or the use of adhesives to maximize removal of noxious fumes; (*vi*) compiling and logging of material safety data sheets for all paints, solvents, and adhesives in use.

Follow-up investigations with manufacturers and their representatives may be helpful because specifications of equipment may be changed without notice. The negative pressurization of the laboratory space requires continuous visual confirmation via a ball and tube pressure indicator or simply paper strips. Periodic sampling for particulates, aldehydes, and organics could be done outside the demolition and construction site, provided this is economically feasible. Alternatively, tracer gas studies can be done to verify containment. The general contractor of the demolition and construction should be briefed in detail on the need to protect the IVF facility and techniques to accomplish this. When possible, the actual members of the construction crew should be selected and briefed in detail. Large filter units using filter pellets of carbon and permanganate can be placed strategically. Uptake of organics can be assayed, but the frequency of routine filter changes should be increased during periods of construction activity.

SELECTION OF BUILDING MATERIALS

Many materials release significant amounts of VOCs and a typical list includes paints, adhesives, glues, sealants, and caulking materials, which release alkanes, aromatics, alcohols, aldehydes, ketones, and other classes of organic materials. This section outlines steps to be taken in order to reduce these out-gassing chemicals. Any and all interior painting throughout the facility should only be done on prepared surfaces with water-based paint formulated for low VOC potential. During any painting, auxiliary ventilation should be provided using large industrial construction fans, with exhaust vented to the exterior. Paints that can significantly influence air quality should be emission tested (some suppliers already have these test results available). Material safety data sheets are generally available for construction materials. Suppliers should be encouraged to conduct product testing for the emission potential. The variety of materials and applications complicates the testing process, but several procedures have been developed to identify and quantify the compounds released by building materials and furnishings. Interior paints must be water-based, low-volatile paints with acrylic, vinyl acrylic, alkyd, or acrylic latex polymers. Paints meeting this specification can also contain certain inorganic materials. Paints with low volatiles may still contain low concentrations of certain organics. No interior paint should contain formaldehyde, acetaldehyde, isocyanates, reactive amines, phenols, and other water-soluble volatile organics. Adhesive glues, sealants, and caulking materials present some of the same problems as paints. None of these materials used in the interior should contain formaldehyde, benzaldehyde, phenol, and like substances. Although water-based versions of these are generally not available, their composition varies widely. Silicone materials are preferred whenever possible, particularly for sealant and caulking works. A complete list of guidelines for material use during construction of a tissue culture laboratory is available elsewhere (12).

"BURNING-IN" OF THE FINISHED FACILITY

New IVF laboratories and new facilities around existing laboratories have often been plagued by complaints of occupants who experience discomfort from the chemicals released by new construction and furnishings. The ambient levels of many of these materials can be reduced by "burning-in" the facility. A typical burn-in consists of increasing the temperature of the new area by 10–20°C and increasing the ventilation rate; even higher temperatures are acceptable. The combination of elevated temperature and higher air exchange aids in the removal of the volatile organics. Upon completion of the construction, the air handling system should be properly configured for the burn-in of the newly constructed area. As previously stated, the system must be capable of supplying the space with air with a temperature of 30–35°C, at less than 40% relative humidity. The burn-in period can range from 10 to 28 days, and the IVF laboratory should be kept closed during this time. If these temperatures cannot be reached by the base system, use auxiliary electrical heating to reach the minimum temperature. During a burn-in, all lighting and some auxiliary equipment should be turned on and left running the whole time. Naturally, ventilation is critical if redistribution of irritants is to be avoided; the whole purpose is to purge the air repeatedly. Auxiliary equipment should of course be monitored during the burn-in.

The same burn-in principle applies to newly purchased incubators. Removal of volatile organics is especially important in the critical microenvironment of the incubator. Whenever possible, it is advantageous to purchase incubators months in advance of their intended initial use and to operate them at an elevated temperature in a clean, protected location. An existing embryology laboratory is not a good space for burn-in of a new incubator.

After the burn-in is complete, a commissioning of the IVF suite should be conducted to verify that the laboratory meets the design specifications. The ventilation and isolation of the laboratory should be verified by a series of tests using basic airflow measurements and tracer gas studies. The particulate levels should be determined to verify that the high-efficiency particulate air (HEPA) system is functional. Particulate sampling can be performed using U.S. Federal Standard 209E. Microbial sampling for aerobic bacteria and fungi is often done in new facilities using an Andersen sampler followed by microbiological culturing and identification. The levels of VOC contamination should be determined. Possible methods are included in the U.S. Environmental Protection Agency protocols using gas chromatography/mass spectroscopy and high-performance liquid chromatography sensitive at the microgram per cubic meter level (13–15).

MAINTENANCE PLANNING AND STERILIZATION

Even the best systems and designs will eventually fail unless they are carefully maintained. The heating, ventilation, and air conditioning (HVAC) will require filter changes, coil cleaning, replacement of drive belts, and chemical purification media. The most prevalent failure concerns the initial particulate filter. These are inexpensive filters designed to keep out large dust particles, plant debris, insects, etc. If such filters are not replaced promptly and regularly, they will fail, allowing the HVAC unit to become contaminated. The HEPA filters and chemical media also require inspection and periodic replacement. Maintenance staff should report their findings to the IVF laboratory.

The IVF laboratory must have a cleaning facility for surgical instruments. Ongoing use of an autoclave is not a problem as long as the released steam is rapidly exhausted to the outside. This keeps the relative humidity in the facility to controllable limits. Autoclaves should not be placed on the IVF laboratory's HVAC system, but rather in a room that is built using tight construction and is exhausted directly outside of the building. The use of cold sterilizing agents is not advised. Aldehydes such as glutaraldehyde and *ortho*-phthalaldehyde from the autoclave can be transported inside the IVF laboratory.

INSURANCE ISSUES

Assisted reproductive techniques have become common practice worldwide and are regulated by a combination of legislation, regulations, or committee-generated practice standards. The rapid evolution and progress of ARTs reveal new legal issues that require consideration. Even the patients themselves are changing, as it becomes more acceptable for single women and homosexual couples to seek and receive treatment. Donation of gametes, embryos, and gamete components, enforcement of age limits for treatment, selective fetal reduction, preimplantation genetic diagnosis, surrogacy, and many other practices in ARTs present practitioners and the society at large with challenges, which are often defined by social norms, religion, and law and are specific to each country.

Furthermore, financial and emotional stresses often burden patients seeking treatment in countries where medicine is not socialized and infertility treatment is not covered by insurance. This translates into an increasing number of ART lawsuits related to failed treatments in spite of generally improved success rates. Laboratory personnel and the laboratory owner should therefore obtain an insurance policy of sufficiently high level and quality commencing prior to the first day of operations.

Litigation-prone issues need special consideration and include the following:

- Cancellation of a treatment cycle prior to egg retrieval
- Failure to become pregnant
- Patient identification errors
- Cryostorage mishaps

These issues occur even if experienced practitioners consider themselves at low risk of exposure. Prior to engaging in the practice of ART, protocols must be established to identify potential problem areas and establish countermeasures.

CONCLUSIONS

It may be surprising how many professionals continue to pursue the establishment of new ART clinics at a time when competition is fierce, financial benefits are small, and existing ART services may appear to be approaching saturation in many areas and countries. Appearances can be misleading, however, and ART centers of excellence that deserve the trust and confidence of patients and serve as models for other practices are always needed.

This chapter provides some guidance for those who aspire to establish such outstanding, well thought out and planned ART practices. Although it cannot safeguard practitioners against adverse events, it introduces concepts in proper design, construction, and operation of ART facilities that are of fundamental importance to treatment success; these guidelines have been painstakingly compiled through decades of practical experience and research. The approach is best adopted as a whole rather than dissected into its components and adopted in part or selectively. Keep in mind that resisting the urge to cut corners in the wrong places avoids future headaches and positions you and your patients on the path to success.

REFERENCES

1. Jansen CA, van Beek JJ, Verhoeff A, Alberda AT, Zeilmaker GH. In vitro fertilisation and embryo transfer with transport of oocytes. Lancet 1986; 22: 676.
2. Verhoeff A, Huisman GJ, Leerentveld RA, Zeilmaker GH. Transport in vitro fertilization. Fertil Steril 1993; 60: 187–8.
3. Coetsier T, Verhoeff A, De Sutter P, Roest J, Dhont M. Transport in vitro fertilization/intracellular sperm injection: a prospective randomized study. Hum Reprod 1997; 12: 1654–6.
4. De Sutter P, Dozortsev D, Verhoeff A, et al. Transport intracytoplasmic sperm injection (ICSI): a cost-effective alternative. J Assist Reprod Genet 1996; 13: 234–7.
5. Cohen J, Gilligan A, Esposito W, Schimmel T, Dale B. Ambient air and its potential effects on conception in vitro. Hum Reprod 1997; 12: 1742–9.
6. Cohen J, Gilligan A, Willadsen S. Culture and quality control of embryos. Hum Reprod 1998; 13(Suppl 3): 137–44.
7. Merton JS, Vermeulen ZL, Otter T, et al. Carbon-activated gas filtration during in vitro culture increased pregnancy

rate following transfer of in vitro-produced bovine embryos. Theriogenology 2007; 67: 1233–8.
8. Alikani M, Cohen J, Tomkin G, et al. Human embryo fragmentation in vitro and its implications for pregnancy and implantation. Fertil Steril 1999; 7: 836–42.
9. Navarro PA, Liu L, Trimarchi JR, et al. Noninvasive imaging of spindle dynamics during mammalian oocyte activation. Fertil Steril 2005; 83(Suppl 1): 1197–205.
10. Hall J, Gilligan A, Schimmel T, Cecchi M, Cohen J. The origin, effects and control of air pollution in laboratories used for human embryo culture. Hum Reprod 1998; 13(Suppl 4): 146–55.
11. Boone WR, Johnson JE, Locke AJ, Crane MM 4th, Price TM. Control of air quality in an assisted reproductive technology laboratory. Fertil Steril 1999; 71: 150–4.
12. Gilligan A. Guidelines for Material Use in the USA During Construction of a Tissue Culture Laboratory. New Jersey: Alpha Environmental, 2006.
13. Sarigiannis DA, Karakitsios SP, Gotti A, et al. Exposure to major volatile organic compounds and carbonyls in European indoor environments and associated health risk. Environ Int 2011; 37: 743–65.
14. Federal Standard 209E. Washington, DC: General Services Administration, US Federal Government, 1992.
15. Compendium of Methods for the Determination of Toxic Organic Compounds in Ambient Air, US EPA 600/4-84-041, April 1984/1988. [Available from the US EPA through the Superintendent of Government Documents, Washington, DC.]

2

Quality control: Maintaining stability in the laboratory

David H. McCulloh

INTRODUCTION

The field of assisted reproductive techniques (ARTs), primarily involving in vitro fertilization, embryo culture, and embryo transfer (collectively known as IVF), has matured significantly in its development. Since the birth of Louise Brown in 1978, the field has grown immensely, and its success has improved steadily and impressively (as measured by the incidence of live births per cycle initiated) from less than 1% to a remarkable incidence of over 41% in under 35 years. Equally remarkable is the observation that, throughout the field, the majority of attempts are followed by failure. Hence, despite the improvements of the past third of a century, there remains a need to optimize procedures.

Let us concentrate on the steady improvement in success that has been documented over this period. To what can we attribute the improved success, from nearly nonexistent to success exceeding 60% in some programs? There are at least three general areas in which changes have impacted on outcome.

New Products

New products have revolutionized patient treatment. There have been steady improvements in many areas, including the generalized use of gonadotropin-releasing hormone analogs to control the pituitary's release of gonadotropins (follicle-stimulating hormone and luteinizing hormone). There have been significant improvements in culture media, both through mass production leading to more uniform and repeatable production of media and through developments in new media leading to stepwise media changes that are currently the standard of care. Newer formulations propose the use of a single medium that can be used throughout the entire in vitro culture period. Production of media for gamete and embryo culture has become a competitive and complicated business. Now it is unusual for laboratories to fabricate their own medium since individual production is prone to error. The introduction of soft catheters has also become extremely competitive, with many manufacturers vying for our programs' business. The introduction of recombinant gonadotropins has led to much more uniform and stable formulations that yield more reproducible responses in patients. The use of drugs designed to treat type II diabetes (metformin and rosiglitazone) has begun as an adjunct to treatment of patients with polycystic ovaries. Many of these improvements have benefited from the use of more uniform products, manufactured to more stringent standards requiring quality control measures to assure lack of toxicity.

New Procedures

New procedures have resulted in such a dramatic improvement in success that our field is experiencing a shift in the type of patients treated. The introduction of the laboratory technique of intracytoplasmic sperm injection (ICSI) revolutionized the field so that our most optimistic cases are now couples for whom the only diagnosis is a male factor that precludes fertilization. Prior to the inception of ICSI around 1993, these patients were unlikely to achieve fertilization without the use of donor sperm. Micro tools fabricated previously in the laboratory are now commercially available. In addition, the improved sensitivity of Kruger's strict criteria for scoring sperm morphology has resulted in improved detection of men with poor prognosis. The use of ICSI has also advanced the field so that azoospermic men can now be the source of sperm, which result in live births, since sperm obtained by surgical techniques are quite effective for use in ARTs.

A second procedural advancement that is revolutionizing the field is the extended culture of embryos to the fifth or sixth day after oocyte retrieval. This advancement is founded on the research determining that embryos' metabolic needs vary during the first few days of development. Extended culture has permitted more critical assessment and selection of embryos. The ability to select the most rapidly developing embryos has focused attention on replacing fewer embryos and thereby eliminating the dangerous occurrence of triplet and higher-order multiple pregnancies. A recent trend has been to transfer only one single embryo to avoid the occurrence of twins. The more sensitive assessment of embryos possible through extended culture has, no doubt, affected many aspects of IVF treatment, including embryo culture and even improvements in ovulation induction.

A third procedural improvement is the institution of novel techniques of embryo selection. Foremost among these is embryo biopsy in conjunction with genetic screening or genetic testing. Implementation of biopsy plus genetic screening is implicated in improving success to high levels, with incidences of live birth approaching 80% in several programs, some employing transfer of only single embryos. The identification of euploid embryos and embryos not affected by genetic diseases is an exciting new application of ART. Further procedures, including less invasive techniques that involve assessment of the medium surrounding cultured embryos, also promise to yield improved outcomes. Evaluation of the medium is important in performing proteomic and metabolomic analyses to select embryos. Such procedures have been used and are presently becoming more widespread.

Women too have benefited from improved protocols for controlled ovarian hyperstimulation and through the development of more critical tests of ovarian reserve prior to treatment.

New Legislation

New legislation has both directly and indirectly assisted with the improved outcome of ART. In 1988, a legislation was enacted in the United States (1) that defined standards for all clinical laboratories. In particular, it stated that laboratories performing quantitative semen analysis (andrology laboratories) must comply. Standards included qualifications for personnel and specific requirements for a quality assurance program involving frequent quality control measurements. Although the Clinical Laboratory Improvement Amendments of 1988 (CLIA '88) did not specifically dictate standards for embryology laboratories, they strongly influenced many programs to adopt CLIA '88 as standards for their embryology laboratories also. The College of American Pathologists in association with the American Fertility Society (now the American Society for Reproductive Medicine, ASRM) formed its Reproductive Laboratory Accreditation Program and adopted specific standards for accreditation (the first agency achieving deemed status with a specific program for andrology/embryology laboratories). Updated recommendations were published by the ASRM (2,3) and included personnel qualifications as well as standards for quality assurance, including quality control. Standards were also defined for personnel involved in direct clinical patient care during ART.

The passage of the Fertility Clinic Success Rate and Certification Act of 1992 (4) mandated that all ART programs report their ART success and undergo certification, additionally challenging programs to improve, undergo certification, or face extinction.

More recently, in 1998, the "Obstetric and Gynecologic devices; Reclassification and Classification of medical devices used for in vitro fertilization and related assisted reproduction procedures" (5) legislated that the Food and Drug Administration (FDA) must regulate the devices used in ART. Their regulation was largely responsible for causing manufacturers to alter their production practices and to require more stringent quality control measures to assure that the products are not toxic.

In addition, the adoption of the legislation entitled "Human Cellular and Tissue-Based Products or HCT/Ps" (6) effective from March 25, 2005, has changed the complexion of donor gamete use in ART. This legislation was designed to improve the safety of donor gametes (oocytes and sperm) by regulating the screening and testing of donors for infectious diseases prior to obtaining gametes. In addition, several laboratory functions, including labeling of gamete containers and housekeeping, are also regulated.

During this same period, facilities have worked feverishly to improve their success through application of stringent standards of practice. It is difficult to determine just what has led to the consistent improvement in IVF success over the years. Has it been federal regulation of the assisted reproduction industry or has it been patient selection? However, a large portion of the improvements, including new products and practices, are founded on more careful quality control practices in the highly regulated pharmaceutical and medical device industry. A careful quality control system can lead to much more stable products with less variability and less likelihood of toxicity. Maintenance of stable conditions from these industries has benefited the practice of ART, and its implementation in our own programs is the focus of this chapter. Quality control is also crucial for the clinical ART program where stability is also advantageous. The stability afforded by careful quality control may effectively confirm that any patient-related success or failure is really specific to the patient or the patient's treatment rather than an inconsistency in the program.

Introductory Comments

This chapter is an extension of three previously published reviews on this subject (7–9). An update to the article on quality control and quality assurance that previously appeared (7) summarizes the new legislation that has occurred since the article was written, including the ASRM's revised guidelines and the FDA legislation. In addition, there is a section devoted to staffing norms that was available only in the previous two editions (9,10). This edition includes the addition of humidity as an important quality control parameter, some questions about the optimal temperature, CO_2, and humidity for use in gamete and embryo culture, and an expanded review of the bioassays used to maintain quality in many IVF programs. Other additions include brief discussions of embryo biopsy and the institution of the use of witnesses to confirm unique embryo identification.

This chapter begins with a definition of quality control, and continues by describing several features of quality control: record keeping, quality control of personnel, procedures, equipment, computers, and that of materials and supplies. Descriptions of process testing, including sperm survival assays (SSAs) and mouse embryo testing, and mention of quality control of the entire process by consideration of patient treatment data, are discussed as overall quality control checks that should be performed by the program. Although written from a U.S. perspective, the contents of this chapter are adaptable and applicable to all IVF laboratories.

DEFINITION OF QUALITY CONTROL

Although ART success has improved remarkably since its inception, the field of human-assisted reproduction overall remains relatively poor in providing patients with demonstrably high levels of success. As practitioners in the field, we must constantly attempt to improve our success. Until we can offer nearly 100% success throughout the field, we must strive to maintain a stable level of success so that we may provide our patients with honest, realistic estimates of their chances of achieving their goal of bearing a healthy child.

Quality control is the process whereby all aspects of the program are monitored and confirmed to be functioning within limits previously determined to be tolerable. The program must remain within these limits to ensure that the program operates in a stable, repeatable fashion. *The goal of quality control is to confirm and document that the program maintains stable conditions.* This stability provides a constant backdrop against which all patient treatment is performed. Without this stability, it is impossible to know whether an unusual outcome for a particular patient is associated with a patient-specific issue or a programmatic failure.

Quality assurance is the overall process (that includes quality control as a subset) by which the program undergoes improvements and corrective actions to maintain or improve its processes. The goal of quality assurance is to improve the outcome. Quality control is a necessary portion of the quality assurance program. It is the quality control assessment of personnel, procedures, equipment, and materials that provides most of the data used in performing quality assurance/improvement activities.

FEATURES OF QUALITY CONTROL

Quality control records should be maintained to demonstrate that quality control was performed and so that data may be analyzed at a later time to detect the source of problems and determine ways to rectify problems. Data should be accumulated in several different categories, as described next.

Record Keeping

While performing quality control, the monitored parameters should be recorded and maintained so that they will be available for review in the future. When a problem arises or improvements are desired, the assembled data will be useful in determining the necessary corrective actions that should be taken (quality assurance/improvement task). The natural variability in quality control data is a source of variation that can be analyzed to assess trends for improvement (7,11). Records of quality control tasks must be maintained for several years in many localities. In instances of use of donor gametes, you may be required to maintain the records for up to 21 years. Check with your local regulations.

Quality control data may be maintained in one of at least two forms, either paper records or electronic records. Paper records have been used for years as the major method of data recording. When an analysis of data is required, the data must be transferred from the paper records into a form for analysis. This often involves conversion of data from paper records to electronic records. Electronic records (maintenance in a computer spreadsheet or database) are quickly replacing paper records as the preferred method of data recording, since the data recorded electronically are ready for analysis nearly immediately, much more quickly than those in paper records. This will require off-site backup of all data.

Quality Control of Laboratory Personnel

Employees in ART laboratories must adhere to predetermined standards. They must have appropriate training and must be able to demonstrate competence with the procedures that they will perform. Standards have been provided within CLIA '88 (1) describing the educational requirements for personnel in different positions within laboratories performing high-complexity testing. Personnel in andrology laboratories (any laboratory performing semen analysis) must adhere to these standards, because laboratories performing semen analysis are specifically designated as laboratories performing high-complexity testing. The qualifications for personnel in laboratories performing high-complexity testing (specifically andrology laboratories) are summarized in Table 2.1. Each laboratory must have a laboratory director, a technical supervisor, a general supervisor, a clinical consultant, and testing personnel. One individual may share multiple positions.

While legally defined standards exist for andrology laboratories, similar standards do not exist for embryology laboratories in the United States. Embryology laboratories are neither specifically included in the CLIA '88 documents defining high-complexity testing, nor are they excluded as waived testing. Moreover, the U.S. congress has not defined embryology procedures as high-complexity testing, opting rather to consider embryology procedures as medical procedures. However, the ASRM has provided guidelines for staffing (2). These guidelines are summarized in Table 2.2 and are applicable globally.

Personnel hired to perform an andrology and/or embryology procedure, once they satisfy the educational requirements for the position, are also required to demonstrate competency to perform the procedure. CLIA requirements do not indicate a particular mechanism for this other than the requirement to participate in routine, periodic proficiency testing, thereby demonstrating a

Table 2.1 Personnel Qualifications Required for High-Complexity Testing in Andrology Laboratories as Specified by the Clinical Laboratory Improvement Amendments of 1988 (1)

Laboratory Director[a] (or Clinical Consultant) must possess Laboratory Director License in the state (if available) and satisfy one complete row

Degree[a]	Certification	Experience[b]	Supervision[c]
MD or DO, and licensed to practice medicine anatomic pathology, or clinical pathology in the state or both	Certified by ABP or AOBP		
MD, DO, or DPM and licensed to practice medicine, osteopathy, or podiatric medicine in the state	None	≥2 yr	≥2 yr
Doctoral degree[d]	Certified by ABMM, ABCC, ABB, or ABMLI	2 yr[e]	2 yr[e]
No doctoral degree	Certification prior to 2/28/1992	2 yr	2 yr

Technical Supervisor: must possess Technical Supervisor License in state (if available) and satisfy one complete row[f]

Degree[a]	Certification	Experience[g]
MD, DO, or DPM and licensed to practice medicine, osteopathy, or podiatric medicine in the state	Certified in both anatomic and clinical pathology by ABP, AOBP, or equivalent	
Doctoral degree[d]	None	1 yr
Master's degree[d]	None	2 yr
Bachelor's degree[d]	None	4 yr

General Supervisor: must possess General Supervisor License in state (if available) and satisfy one complete row

Education	Qualification as:	Experience[b]
(See above)	Laboratory Director	1 yr
(See above)	Technical Supervisor	1 yr
(See below)	Testing Personnel	2 yr
Independent of education	Qualified as General Supervisor prior to 2/28/92	None
Graduate of MLT/CLT program[a]	Qualified as General Supervisor prior to 9/1/92	None
High School Graduate (or GED)	Qualified as General Supervisor prior to 9/1/92	None

Testing Personnel: must possess Testing Personnel License in state (if available) and satisfy one complete row

Education[a]	Experience[b]	Further Qualifications
MD, DO, DPM, licensed to practice in the state	None	None
Doctoral degree[d], master's degree[d], bachelor's degree[d], or in medical technology	None	None
Associate Degree[h]	None	None
Education equivalent to an Associate Degree	None	24 semester hr of MLT courses
Education equivalent to an Associate Degree	Completion of CLT program[i]	24 semester hr of science, specifically 6 hr chemistry, 6 hr biology, 12 hr chemistry, biology, or MLT
Education equivalent to an associate degree	3 months of laboratory training in each specialty	24 semester hr of science, specifically 6 hr chemistry, 6 hr biology, 12 hr chemistry, biology, or MLT
Education equivalent to an associate degree	None	Prior qualification as a technologist before 2/28/1992
High school graduate or equivalent	Completion of CLT program[i,j]	None

[a] Degree must be from an accredited institution.
[b] Training or experience must be gained in clinical laboratory.
[c] Experience as a director or supervisor of high complexity testing.
[d] The degree must be in chemical, physical, biological, or clinical laboratory science.
[e] Effective from 4/24/2003.
[f] Other than state licensure, no specific qualifications for Technical Supervisors are listed in the field of andrology. If andrology is considered a discipline in hematology, these qualifications apply.
[g] Experience must be in the specific field to be supervised (hematology/andrology).
[h] Associate degree in a laboratory science or medical laboratory technology.
[i] Completion of a clinical laboratory training program accredited or approved by the Accreditation Bureau of Health Education Schools (ABHES), the Committee on Allied Health Education and Accreditation (CAHEA), or other program approved by HHS.
[j] Successful completion of an official U.S. military medical laboratory procedures training course and hold the enlisted occupational specialty of Medical Laboratory Specialist.

Abbreviations: ABB, American Board of Bioanalysis; ABCC, American Board of Clinical Chemistry; ABMLI, American Board of Medical Laboratory Immunology; ABMM, American Board of Medical Microbiology; ABP, American Board of Pathology; AOBP, American Osteopathic Board of Pathology; CLT, clinical laboratory training; DO, doctor of osteopathy; DPM, doctor of podiatric medicine; GED, high school equivalency demonstrated by examination; MD, doctor of medicine; MLT, medical laboratory training.

Table 2.2 Personnel Qualifications Recommended for Embryology Programs by ASRM (2)

Laboratory Director: must satisfy one complete row

Degree[a]	Certification	Experience[b]	ART procedures[c]
PhD[d,e], MD[e], or DO[e]	In embryology	2 yr	60 ART procedures
No doctoral degree	In embryology, qualification prior to January 1992	2 yr	60 ART procedures

Supervisor[f]: must satisfy one complete row

Degree[a]	Experience[b]	ART procedures[c]
Master's or Bachelor's degree[d]	6 months	60 ART procedures

Technologist: must satisfy the complete row

Degree[a]	ART procedures[c]
Bachelor's Degree[d]	30 ART procedures, under supervision

[a]Degree should be from an accredited institution.
[b]Documented pertinent experience in a program performing IVF-related procedures, including quality control, detailed knowledge of cell culture, ART, and andrology procedures.
[c]Number of ART procedures completed (each procedure including examination of follicular aspirates, insemination, documentation of fertilization, and preparation for embryo transfer) in a program performing at least 100 IVF procedures per year with a minimum annual 10% IVF live birth rate per retrieval.
[d]Degree should be from an accredited institution, in a chemical, physical, or biological science as the major subject.
[e]Education should include expertise and/or special training in biochemistry, cell biology, and physiology of reproduction with experience in experimental design, statistics, and problem solving/trouble shooting.
[f]If the laboratory director is also the medical director, there should be a qualified designated supervisor.
Abbreviations: ART, assisted reproductive technique; ASRM, American Society for Reproductive Medicine; DO, DO, doctor of osteopathy; MD, doctor of medicine.

competence to perform the procedure. The ASRM guidelines suggest that personnel should perform a minimum of 30 complete procedures in order to qualify as a technologist, or 60 complete procedures to qualify as a laboratory director or a supervisor. This competency should be documented in the quality control records.

At the present time, there are very few academic programs in the United States offering training for individuals in the fields of andrology and/or embryology. Therefore, it is difficult to receive formal training in these fields. Most training occurs "on the job" at facilities where the procedures are performed. Good practices should be in place to assure that trainees are overseen throughout their training process and that the training is documented. It is wise for staff members to keep track of the number of procedures that they have personally performed.

Further demonstration of competency should be achieved by each staff member's participation in proficiency testing exercises. A rotation should be instituted that assures that each laboratory staff member performs the proficiency testing, thereby demonstrating competency using an unknown analyte at least periodically.

Laboratory Staffing Norms

In addition to covering all the functions required by law/guidelines, sufficient personnel should be available to perform all the andrology/embryology work without subjecting either the personnel or the patients to undue risk. Staffing norms are not widely available. However, it is clearly a quality control issue to be certain that enough staff members are available to provide the desired volume of laboratory services safely and efficiently. Reference and hospital laboratories provide many broadly distributed laboratory services (especially for stat testing) seven days per week. To do this they have large numbers of staff who are broadly cross trained. However, ART laboratories are generally staffed with fewer individuals, often with a repertoire limited specifically to the field of gamete testing and manipulation, and yet the staff members are expected to provide services seven days per week for extended periods of weeks. The effect of fatigue in this environment has not been evaluated, despite the possibly severe consequences of an error such as specimen misidentification.

For many years, staffing norms were circulated by word of mouth throughout the field, without any published standards. The circulated norm suggested that one embryologist is necessary for each 100 IVF procedures performed per year. This number emerged prior to the introduction of widespread micromanipulation techniques that require a longer time to perform. Despite the widespread addition of this time-consuming activity, no changes in staffing norms occurred. During the Survey of 1999 Compensation conducted in 2000 (12), staffing norms were estimated although they were not published. The average workload of laboratory personnel in ART laboratories was calculated to be 77.2 cases per laboratory person (average of 286.9 IVF cases per program with an average of 3.72 personnel in each of 110 laboratories in the year 1999). However, this simple ratio is probably not a fair representation of the staffing needs of a program.

It is clear that more procedures per employee can be performed in a large program than in a smaller program. There is a fixed volume of work (largely the quality control functions) that must be performed in order to maintain an ART laboratory, even with no performance of ART cases. Likewise, ART laboratories generally operate seven days per week. It is unreasonable and unethical, if not illegal, to expect a technologist to work seven days per week. For these reasons, it is more reasonable to consider that a fixed number of personnel are required to perform the fixed volume of work. Additional personnel are required to perform the ART cases. Two examples follow.

Example 1

The number of laboratory personnel was determined using linear regression of the data from the 110 programs represented in the above Survey of 1999 Compensation (12). The relationship between IVF cases and personnel (Table 2.3) indicates that roughly 0.5 staff is required without the performance of any IVF procedures. One additional staff person is required for each additional 88.5 embryo transfers. The number of embryo transfers is used as an estimate of the number of IVF treatments performed per year. This estimate could misrepresent the number of IVF treatments performed due to inclusion of embryo transfers from frozen–thawed embryo treatments and due to IVF treatments resulting in no embryo transfer. However, this analysis estimates that the average program will have 1.6 laboratory staff to perform 100 embryo transfers per year. Five laboratory staff persons are employed to perform 400 embryo transfers per year.

Example 2

Similar analysis has been applied more recently and more directly by counting individual procedures (oocyte retrieval, insemination, ICSI, fertilization check, embryo transfer, and embryo cryopreservation) (13) instead of counting embryo transfers only. The relationship (Table 2.3) from the preliminary work derived by averaging 47 laboratories in the United States is that staffing requires 2.92 personnel prior to the performance of any andrology or IVF treatments. One additional staff member is required for every 500 procedures (where a procedure is defined to be much less than a complete IVF treatment). In Table 2.3, a minimum of roughly seven procedures is performed in one IVF treatment. When seven procedures are involved with an ART treatment, a staff of roughly 4.3 laboratory personnel is needed to perform the first 100 IVF cases (700 procedures), assuming that no other andrology activities occur.

Discrepancies between these two examples of staffing norms could be due to differences in the surveyed year (1999 (12) *vs* 2001(13)), differences in the programs that

Table 2.3 Staffing Norms for ART Facilities in the United States

	Number of laboratory staff		
Number of IVFs	McCulloh[a]	Boone and Higdon[b]	ASRM[c]
0	0.47	2.92	Not provided
150	2.2	5.0	2
300	3.9	7.1	3
600	7.2	11.3	4
1000	11.7	16.9	6

[a]Data assembled in conjunction with McCulloh (12). Average number of laboratory staff in 110 programs responding to the 2000 Survey of 1999 Compensation. Values were determined according to the linear regression equation:

$$\#Staff = 0.47 + ([Number\ of\ IVFs]/88.5)$$

where (Number of IVFs) was estimated by the number of embryo transfers. The correlation coefficient was 0.697 for the data in this analysis.
[b]Data from Boone and Higdon (13). Average number of laboratory staff in 47 programs responding to their 2002 survey. Values were determined according to the linear regression equation:

$$\#Staff = 2.92 + (Number\ of\ procedures)\ 0.002$$

where (Number of procedures) was estimated by multiplying the (Number of IVFs) by seven procedures per IVF. (Note that one IVF involves the sum of at least seven procedures: (1) a prior semen analysis, (2) identification of oocytes from follicular aspirates, (3) sperm preparation, (4) in vitro insemination, (5) fertilization scoring, (6) embryo scoring, and (7) preparation of embryos for transfer. The estimates in this table neglect the staffing needs of procedures unrelated to IVF such as sperm preparation for intrauterine inseminations and other diagnostic testing).
[c]Data assembled from guidelines published by the Practice Committees of ASRM and SART[w] with the number of personnel indicating the minimum number to provide up to the number of IVF's indicated. The guidelines indicate that the additional number of personnel (over 4) required when over 600 cases per year are performed is equal to (the number of cases – 600)/200.
Abbreviations: ART, assisted reproductive technique; ASRM, American Society for Reproductive Medicine.

responded, and/or major differences in the emphasis of the surveys. The Survey of Compensation (12) was directed at determining an individual's compensation, whereas the Boone and Higdon survey (13) was directed at assessing all of the tasks performed by personnel in programs, and focused on procedures. The equivalency of all procedures is not clear (e.g., is one determination of sperm count and motility equivalent to the performance of ICSI on all of one patient's oocytes?). The analysis in conjunction with the Survey of Compensation (12) focused on embryo transfers performed, neglecting all the ART procedures that failed to result in embryo transfer and totally neglecting the variability of andrology activities from program to program. Despite these discrepancies, the two examples provide a range of values that are now available for discussion and consideration (Table 2.3).

More recently, the ASRM has provided staffing guidelines (3) that estimate the minimum number of staff required to perform various numbers of procedures. It is not clear how the ASRM arrived at these guidelines and it

Table 2.4 Preparing a Protocol: When Preparing a Written Protocol, Include the Following Information

Principle and/or purpose of the test	Provide a general outline of the point of the procedure and how the procedure is performed
Specimen required for the test	Describe any instructions necessary to be certain that the specimen is collected in a way that will assure correct processing and testing
Reagents, standards, controls, media	List any materials needed to perform the procedure
Instrumentation	List any instruments to be used and any quality control procedures needed to assure that the instrument is functioning correctly
Step-by-step instruction	Carefully describe in narrative form exactly how the procedure is to be performed
Calculations	Describe how to perform any necessary calculations
Frequency and tolerance of controls	Describe any controls that should be run to assure quality of the performance of the procedure
Expected values	List expected values for the results so that the performer will know whether the values are within a reasonable range
Limitations	Describe any limitations on the interpretation of the results or on the utility of the procedure
References	List sources of information that the user may wish to consult if questions arise
Effective date and schedule for review	Indicate the date that the procedure will become effective, and date(s) that it is scheduled for review
Distribution	List all persons/locations to which the procedure has been sent
Author	List the person who wrote the procedure

Source: From Ref. 14.

seems rather arbitrary that only one additional staff member is required for the additional 300 cases performed for a program increasing from 300 to 600 IVF's per year, whereas increases above 600 cases per year require a greater staffing increment of one per every 200 additional cases. Keep in mind that the ASRM guidelines are intended to be minimum standards (3), while the staffing norms presented by McCulloh (12) and by Boone and Higdon (13) utilized regression analysis to achieve average staffing employed in practices in the United States. Also realize that publication of these three estimates pre-dates widespread performance of embryo biopsy for genetic screening and diagnosis. Hence, these published norms/guidelines underestimate the staff needed with the increased requirements placed on laboratory personnel due to additional highly technically complex laboratory procedures.

QUALITY CONTROL OF PROCEDURES

Uniformity of procedures and enforcement of uniform performance will aid in confirming that every procedure is performed consistently. A written protocol for each procedure performed in the facility must be available near the site of performance. Each protocol should be written in a way whereby anyone reading it could perform the procedure. Standards for written laboratory protocols have been assembled by the National Committee for Clinical Laboratory Standards (NCCLS) (14). These guidelines are summarized in Table 2.4. The protocol should include a clearly understandable, step-by-step description of exactly how to perform the procedure. Since stability is the goal of quality control, consistency of performance is the goal to be achieved by clearly describing the procedure. Procedures will probably be repeated more consistently by different individuals, when the written protocol describes precisely how to perform the procedure.

In addition, all materials and equipment that are necessary should be clearly listed in the protocol. Any calculations required should be described simply and directly. Any specific limitations of the technique should be listed. References that have been used in creating the procedure should be listed.

It is generally agreed that the laboratory director is responsible for creating and approving all laboratory protocols. The maintenance of a protocol that describes how to write a protocol is often overlooked. It is a simple solution to maintain a copy of NCCLS GP2–A3 (14) or its equivalent Table 2.4 in the laboratory.

All protocols must be reviewed at least annually (and approved by the laboratory director) in order to comply with the guidelines of the College of American Pathologists. Any improvements in methodology should be instituted during this review. This may include any changes brought about following intensive quality assurance/improvement investigations.

Each person responsible for performance of the procedure must be familiar with the procedure. If any changes in the procedure are made during review, then the procedure must be reviewed in turn by the testing personnel. This important step assures that all personnel know how the procedure is to be performed. This is often accomplished by requiring staff members to sign a form indicating that they have read the procedure and are aware of any changes.

QUALITY CONTROL OF EQUIPMENT

We must be certain that all equipment operate within tolerable limits. This requires periodic testing to confirm proper operation. Tolerable limits should be set prior to use of the equipment, with knowledge of what values are biologically optimal for the specimens and with knowledge of the variability of the instrument. Biologically optimal conditions have yet to be demonstrated for human gametes/embryos (see the section, "Periodic Review of Daily Quality Control Records). Laboratories generally have many pieces of equipment, including but not necessarily limited to incubators, microscopes, heating surfaces, heating blocks, water baths, refrigerators, freezers, controlled rate freezers, and storage dewars. The single task in the ART laboratory that is often not recognized or acknowledged and that takes the most time is the performance of daily quality control monitoring for equipment. The final publication of CLIA '88 (1) has amended the requirement for performance of quality control monitoring for equipment. The new standard defers to the manufacturer to define the frequency of quality control monitoring. Although the standard has changed, it is wise to perform equipment quality control monitoring at least daily (some manufacturers will suggest with each shift or with each run, which could be more frequently or less frequently). This means that each piece of equipment should be checked for proper function on at least each day of use. Table 2.5 lists some commonly used equipment and the types of testing that should be performed. Any equipment with an "out-of-tolerance" quality control value should have corrective actions performed to rectify the problem.

Daily Temperature Quality Control

Gamete/embryo temperature is one of the most important determinants of IVF success that is controlled by the laboratory. Equipment designed to maintain a particular temperature should be monitored daily using a thermometer (external to the unit) that can be traced to a standard thermometer approved by the National Institutes of Standards and Technology (NIST) or some other reliable source. It is standard practice to perform quality control monitoring as the first event in the morning. This time is chosen because most equipment have stabilized overnight. Incubator doors and refrigerator/freezer doors have not been opened; new objects have not been placed on heating surfaces or in heating blocks or water baths. Temperatures should be determined and recorded. Comparison of the value to the tolerable limits should be made.

The use of a reference thermometer of demonstrable accuracy cannot be emphasized enough, especially when calibrating the temperature of incubators. In the United States, the line voltage is generally well regulated, providing a constant source of power to the incubator. However,

Table 2.5 List of Equipment, Parameters for QC, and Frequency of QC

Equipment	Parameter for QC	Frequency of QC	Comments
Incubator	Temperature	Daily	Annual preventive maintenance
	CO_2	Daily	
	Humidity	Daily	
Heating surfaces	Temperature	Daily	
Heating bath	Temperature	Daily	
	Water level	Daily	
Heating block	Temperature	Daily	
Microscope	Image quality	Daily	Annual preventive maintenance
Laser (for zona ablation)	Alignment of beam	Each use	Annual preventive maintenance
	Power/pulse duration	Each use	
CASA	Sperm count	Daily	Annual preventive maintenance
	Motility (%)	Daily	
	Motility (velocities)	Daily	
	Morphology (%)	Daily	
Controlled rate freezer	Sufficient refrigerant	Each use	Annual preventive maintenance
	Start temperature	Each use	
	Seeding temperature	Each use	
	Final temperature	Each use	
Storage dewars	Liquid N_2 level	Daily	
Refrigerator	Temperature	Daily	
Freezer	Temperature	Daily	
Heating, ventilation, and air conditioning systems	Room temperature	Daily	Clean filters/humidifiers periodically
	Room humidity	Daily	
QC Equipment			
Thermometers	Temperature (accuracy/precision)	Periodically	
pH meters	pH (accuracy/precision)	Each use (daily)	Annual preventive maintenance
Osmometers	Osmolality (accuracy/precision)	Each use (daily)	Annual preventive maintenance
Hygrometers	Humidity (accuracy/precision)	Periodically	
Timers	Time (Accuracy/precision)	Periodically	
CO_2 monitor	$\%CO_2$ (accuracy/precision)		Fyrite should be changed every 300 determinations

Abbreviations: CASA, computerized semen analyzer; QC, quality control.

I have observed incubators under less stable conditions with dire consequences. "Backup" power may not be identical to the power that is typically provided to the incubator. On one occasion, during a sustained, overnight power failure, incubators powered by "backup" power continued to function, indicating the same temperature with their digitally displayed temperatures. However, independent, external thermometers indicated a drop of chamber temperature by more than 1°C to values less than 36.0°C. Embryos inside the incubators maintained overnight at these low temperatures failed to undergo cell division, despite the presence of multiple nuclei in cells. This observation suggests that cytokinesis is more temperature sensitive than mitosis is. On another occasion, a new laboratory had set up a new incubator. The new incubator's temperature was calibrated using an inaccurate thermometer (the only thermometer available). Several days later, it was discovered that this reference thermometer indicated a temperature of 37°C when the actual temperature inside the incubator was 41°C. This difference of 4°C was extremely detrimental to embryogenesis. On the mornings following ICSI, the incidence of normal fertilization was very low (3/26) and the incidence of oocytes with more than two pronuclei was very high (5/26). Expectations based on prior experience in my laboratory are 71.4% (normal fertilization) and 4.4% (more than two pronuclei). Further culture at this elevated temperature resulted in no cell divisions (no cytokinesis) for embryos with either two pronuclei or more than two pronuclei. Immediately after correction of the incubator temperature, normal fertilization and cell divisions occurred as expected for subsequent patients. Therefore, I must conclude that embryos display exquisite temperature sensitivity. Hence, we must calibrate the incubator temperature and maintain it at a value verified by an independent and accurate thermometer. It is important that embryos be cultured at demonstrably permissive temperatures. (It is important to distinguish between long-term developmental exposure to temperatures diverging from body temperature (~37°C) and brief departures of temperature during cryopreservation where development is hoped to be halted and then resumed upon warming. The brief exposure (a few minutes during cryopreservation and a few minutes during warming after cryopreservation) may avoid temperature-sensitive periods that could be critically affected by prolonged developmental exposure.)

Daily Quality Control of CO_2 Levels

The pH of the medium is another determinant of IVF success that is controlled by the laboratory. The pH of bicarbonate-buffered medium is regulated through a complex equilibrium driven by the CO_2 content of the atmosphere above the medium. Equipment that controls gas concentrations (incubator with elevated CO_2 levels) should be monitored daily using a method that is sensitive to CO_2 levels in the range to be maintained. Several methods exist. The Fyrite (Bacharach, Inc., New Kensington, PA 15068) device uses Bacharach solution (potassium hydroxide solution) that absorbs CO_2. The partial volume of gas removed by absorption/dissolution of CO_2 is measured, indicating the percentage of the gaseous volume occupied by CO_2.

An alternative to the Fyrite device is the use of a CO_2 monitor that is typically used to monitor CO_2 in exhaled gases. Both of these devices should undergo periodic quality control monitoring also, to confirm their accuracy prior to use as quality control monitoring devices. In some laboratories a supply of 5% CO_2 mixed gas is available and may serve as a calibrator for CO_2 monitors.

A third method of monitoring CO_2 levels in the incubator is the determination of pH in culture medium maintained in the incubator. Since most culture media for embryo culture are prepared with bicarbonate as a pH buffer, the pH of the medium is controlled by the equilibrium of atmospheric CO_2, dissolved CO_2, bicarbonate, and hydrogen ions in solution. The major purpose for maintenance of CO_2 levels in the incubator is the maintenance of medium pH. Therefore it is sensible to monitor the pH of a small amount of medium that can be maintained in the incubator. This medium should be discarded after its use as a determinant of whether the CO_2 levels are appropriate. The pH meter must be calibrated immediately prior to use, and pH measurements must be made rapidly to avoid off-gassing of CO_2 after opening the incubator door to insert the pH probe in the medium.

Among these three methods, which method is best to achieve our goals? Generally, the partial pressure of CO_2 in the incubator atmosphere is maintained near 38 mmHg (5% of standard atmospheric pressure, 1 atm = 760 mmHg) in order to maintain the pH of the culture medium. There are difficulties with each method of performing quality control. The use of a Fyrite analyzer with Bacharach solution (that measures the percentage of the gas that comprises CO_2) is generally accepted to have an error of roughly 0.25–0.50%. Care must be taken to avoid saturation of the Bacharach solution with CO_2 (the solution should be replaced after ~300 determinations). Saturation will lead to underestimates of the actual %CO_2.

Anesthesia equipment designed to measure the CO_2 in exhaled air is expensive and requires calibration. Such an instrument may not permit the display of %CO_2 (the value displayed on the incubator display). Rather it may display the partial pressure of CO_2 in mmHg. The partial pressure of CO_2 in the atmosphere is actually the parameter that determines the dissolved CO_2 in the aqueous phase. (Note that in order to maintain a partial pressure of 38 mmHg for CO_2, it may be necessary to raise the %CO_2 to values exceeding 5%, especially in laboratories at high altitudes, where the atmospheric pressure is reduced.)

If the goal of this quality control exercise is to control the pH of the medium, then it may seem logical to perform this exercise by monitoring the pH of the medium maintained in the incubator. However, this can be fraught with problems since pH meters require daily calibration. Calibration must be performed at the incubator temperature (the difference between room temperature and incubator temperature leads to a 5% change in the slope of the voltage *vs* pH relationship [Nernst equation]). Secondly, an incubator door must be opened to insert the pH probe into a medium that has equilibrated with the incubator's gas mixture. The door opening will affect the very gas mixture that controls the pH of the solution. Although this pH measurement attempts to monitor the endpoint of the CO_2 control, it is tricky to perform. In addition, the sensitivity of the medium's pH to the %CO_2 in the atmosphere surrounding the medium is rather weak. Near the desired value of roughly 5% CO_2, medium pH changes only 0.1 pH unit for each 1% change of the CO_2 in the atmosphere. So, given the typical precision of pH measurement (0.1 pH unit) and the difficulty of performing these measurements in a closed incubator, one can only hope to achieve a precision of 1% in the CO_2 control. Therefore, once a pH measurement demonstrates a pH near the level desired, and assuming no changes in medium composition, it is more practical and precise to control the pH by controlling the %CO_2 using methods that yield more precise levels of CO_2 (Fyrite or calibrated anesthesia monitor), thereby controlling the pH to within roughly 0.025–0.05 pH units.

Daily Quality Control of Humidity

The humidity of the incubator environment can be a determinant in IVF success. Low levels of humidity can lead to desiccation of a medium thereby resulting in increases in the colloid osmolality of the medium. Increased osmolality, while integral in the dehydration of embryos for cryopreservation, is generally considered less than optimal for embryo culture. Each day, the relative humidity of the incubator's gas phase should be ascertained. A large pan of water is maintained within the incubator to maintain high humidity, near saturation. Humidity may be determined by the use of a hygrometer; however, this is unwieldy. Inexpensive, modern digital devices can be placed within the incubator to monitor the relative humidity. Humidity should be maintained high, in the range of 90–100% relative humidity.

One pertinent issue is that some of the incubators that assess the CO_2 level using a thermal conductivity sensor are quite sensitive to relative humidity. Failure to maintain a consistent high humidity rate can lead to inaccuracy in the level of CO_2 controlled by the incubator. Resultant changes in CO_2 levels can result in changes of the pH for culture medium as discussed in the previous section.

Daily Quality Control of Computerized Semen Analyzers

Computerized semen analyzers can be used to determine sperm concentration (sperm count), motility (percentage motile), sperm velocities, and sperm morphology (percentage normal morphology). Proper functioning for these tests should be confirmed on each day of use. Methods of performing quality control can include using a known concentration of latex beads (probably only valuable as quality control material for concentration). Unfortunately, latex spheres are neither the same size nor the same shape as sperm. Therefore, although the spheres can be counted, they are not a test of the algorithm that distinguishes sperm from nonsperm objects in semen. In addition, spherical beads do not exhibit reproducible motility. Therefore, some other mechanism must be used to perform quality control of motility.

Videotaped sequences of motile and nonmotile sperm, for which the concentration is known, can be used as standards for quality control checks of concentration and motility. The tapes should be created using the computerized semen analyzer to generate the images to be stored on videotape. An additional possible source would be the production of digital video recordings on digital videodisks. Primary calibration of the material used to create these recorded sequences should be performed prior to their use as quality control standards.

Likewise, video records can be generated (with videotape, DVD, or digital still images) using sperm stained for morphology determinations. Such images can be used as quality control images for the computerized semen analyzer. These images should be evaluated as primary standards prior to use as quality control standards. Prestained sperm smear slides are available commercially, which are created from samples evaluated by well-known authorities on morphology. These can serve as primary sources for calibration of computerized semen analyzers, or as controls for periodic quality control of personnel who perform sperm morphology determinations.

Daily Quality Control of Microscopes

Microscopes are used daily during diagnostic testing in the andrology laboratory and daily during therapeutic procedures in both the andrology and embryology laboratories. Clarity of images should be confirmed at least daily and should be documented. Procedures for alignment of the optical path and for alignment of any apertures and analyzers should be available near the microscope laboratory bench. Any lack of clarity should be noted and rectified, to be certain that consistency in specimen analysis and procedure performance is maintained. This is generally noticed easily by microscope users.

Quality Control of Lasers with Each Use

Use of a laser mounted on the embryology microscope has become routine to create a breech in the zona pellucida by disintegration of zona pellucida material. This procedure is used for assisted zona pellucida hatching and in conjunction with embryo biopsy. In addition, use of the laser to help in obtaining biopsies of trophectoderm cells for genetic screening/diagnosis is becoming more widespread. With each use, the laser's alignment should be confirmed by demonstrating that the beam is directed to a known position within the microscope's field of view. Frequent confirmation of alignment is extremely important since lasers are often mounted so that the position of the microscope's objective lens affects the alignment. In addition, it is important to confirm that the laser's power is set (by adjustment of the intensity of the beam and/or the duration of the light pulse) so that the desired power is delivered when desired. Documentation of the alignment and power test is useful in demonstrating that the laser has not damaged embryos during the procedures due to preventable misalignment or maladjustment of power.

Periodic Review of Daily Quality Control Records

Daily quality control records should be reviewed periodically by supervisory personnel to confirm that first, data were collected; secondly, corrective actions were taken when needed; and thirdly, corrective actions rectified any problem(s).

In addition to the periodic review of the quality control records to ensure that equipment are functioning as intended, it is valuable to review the daily quality control records to determine whether the values maintained are associated with patient outcomes. It is rather universally accepted that core body temperature is 37.0°C, CO_2 levels in arteriolar blood approximate levels are associated with a blood gas level of 5%, and osmolality is controlled by homeostatic mechanisms. Despite this acceptance, it has been demonstrated for some time that core body temperature undergoes a daily circadian fluctuation of 0.6°C (15) to 1.0°C (16) with warming during daytime hours of greater activity and cooling during the night time periods of decreased activity and sleep. Women undergo a monthly rhythm with slightly elevated temperatures during the luteal phase (17–19) that corresponds to the period of embryo culture. In fact, the optimal temperature, CO_2 level, and humidity for culture of gametes and embryos are really not well substantiated.

Over the period of time between 2003 and 2009, my previous laboratory maintained electronic (database) records of all daily quality control information. In addition, many parameters of patient IVF treatments were maintained in another database. Information from the two databases could be merged to associate patient outcome with incubator and room conditions. Since quality control data were collected daily, values were associated with each day of IVF treatment between day 0 (the day of oocyte retrieval), day 3 (the most common day of embryo transfers), and day 5 (the day of blastocyst transfers). Over 1300 IVF treatments were investigated to see whether any information about IVF outcome might be associated with incubator or room quality control values for days 0 through 3. Nearly 300 cases were examined on days 4 and 5 because blastocyst transfers were performed. Female patient age (36.0 ± 4.6 years) at the initiation of the cycle and live birth outcome (1 for live birth of any number of infants and 0 for no live born infants) were assembled for each cycle. Quality control parameters were assembled for incubator temperature (37.08° ± 0.14°C; mean ± standard deviation), CO_2 level (5.37% ± 0.31%) and relative humidity (88.1% ± 6.6%), for room temperature (21.7°C ± 1.2°C) and relative humidity (35.5% ± 14.5%) and for the surface temperature of the dissecting microscope (36.7°C ± 0.39°C) used for oocyte retrievals and transfers, the surface temperature of the inverted compound microscope (36.8°C ± 0.4°C) used for ICSI and daily embryo scoring, the surface temperature of a warming surface (37.00°C ± 0.11°C) in a chamber where oocytes were maintained for a period of 15–45 minutes during oocyte retrievals (FIV). The atmosphere inside this chamber was flushed with 5% CO_2: 20% O_2: 75% N_2 humidified by bubbling through a self-contained water bath. All quality control values were recorded in the morning prior to opening incubators and prior to the performance of any procedures. Hence, the quality control data are indicative of the stable levels maintained throughout the night preceding any procedures performed.

Data were assembled for the roughly six and one-half year-period and records with clear erroneous mis-entries were removed for each day of IVF treatment. Multiple linear regression analysis was performed to examine which (if any) parameters (including patient age) had significant linear regressions associated with live birth outcome. For each day of culture, there was a significant negative regression slope relating live birth to female patient age (negative slope means that younger patients were more successful). Most of the quality control temperature and CO_2 parameters were not significantly associated with live birth. This affirms that most of the quality control parameters did not affect live birth outcome and that the ranges of values were acceptable or that linear regression did not capture the essence of a non-linear relationship. However, there were a few examples of significant relationships between quality control parameters and incidence of live birth. These include a significant positive slope relating live birth to incubator humidity (positive slope means that a higher humidity value was beneficial), on days 1 and 3. In addition, a significant positive slope associated live birth with room temperature on day 2 (positive slope means that a higher room temperature was beneficial). A significant negative slope related live birth with surface temperature of the FIV unit on day 1, the day following oocyte retrieval (cooler temperature was beneficial). There were no significant relationships between live birth and quality control values for days 0, 4, or 5.

The observation of a significant relationship between incubator humidity and live birth outcome underscores the importance of maintaining high humidity, either to maintain osmolality or incubator CO_2. The significant relationship between live birth and room temperature on day 2 suggests that day 2 is a period during the embryo's development when it is most susceptible to temperature fluctuations associated with exposure of culture dishes to room temperature during day 2 examinations. Day 2 is also the period of development when the embryonic genome is activated (4–8 cell stage) and has been suggested as a period of hypersensitivity (20). The insensitivity of live birth to quality control values on day 0 (when oocytes/embryos have not yet been exposed to overnight incubator conditions) is not surprising. It is not clear whether the insensitivity of embryos on days 4 and 5 is due to low numbers of patients examined or actual decreased sensitivity of embryos during these later periods when the embryo begins to establish and control its own internal blastocele environment.

The evidence of embryo sensitivity to conditions in vitro (20,21) provides evidence that we should make efforts to determine the optimal temperature, CO_2 levels and humidity for human embryos, so that we can strive to optimize the conditions for each patient's embryos. Further, the changes in sensitivity over the period of culture suggest that conditions for optimal culture may change with time, thereby requiring different conditions for different stages of development to achieve optimal outcomes.

In addition to daily quality control, equipment should be serviced at regular intervals to prolong its useful lifetime and to prevent any calamitous equipment failures. Records of this preventive maintenance must be kept to demonstrate the performance of these crucial functions. This can be done with the annual preventive maintenance. Automated equipment should be serviced routinely to make sure that it is functioning to manufacturers' standards. Microscopes should be cleaned routinely to eliminate any distortion-producing imperfections within the optical path. There are requirements that the electrical integrity and polarity of electrical equipment be checked at least annually (Occupational Safety and Health Administration).

An additional method to confirm that equipment are functioning properly is the performance of proficiency testing two or three times per year. Enrolment in a proficiency testing program is available for many commonly performed tests and is a means of performing testing on unknown samples. In the United States, proficiency testing samples are available for sperm count, sperm motility (%), sperm morphology, sperm viability, antisperm antibody detection, culture media toxicity testing, and pH and osmolality determinations. Samples should be treated as they would be for standard patient testing. Results are submitted to the proficiency testing agency and are compared with the results of other laboratories. Proficiency testing exercises provide an opportunity to detect equipment malfunction; but these events are designed to test more than the equipment alone. A comparison of your laboratory's results should be made with the published outcome of other laboratories. This comparison permits you to assess how well your laboratory is performing relative to the other participating laboratories using the same methodology. Documentation of this review is necessary for compliance with accreditation authorities.

Quality Control of Computers

As we move forward and adopt the use of electronic records for patient data and quality control data, we are obliged to perform quality control monitoring on the computers and computer systems used for data entry and storage. Prior to use for data storage, the computer system must be assessed for its ability to handle the task(s) it is planned to perform. Does the system have enough data storage capability? Will it be sufficient to support growth of the practice? Can it function rapidly enough to meet the needs of the personnel using it? Mechanisms for keeping records of problems encountered, maintenance, and upgrades must be implemented. There should be a mechanism to demonstrate that data will not be corrupted through long-term use.

Prior to the use of the computer system for generation of patient reports using stored data, the ability of the report to present the correct information must be verified and documented. Records of personnel entering data and making changes to any report should be maintained. Any calculations performed must be verified as accurate and must be documented. The accuracy of reports generated from remote locations must be verified and documented. If there are any changes in reported values or with reference ranges, it must be verified that any report should be printed with the reference range used at the time that the test was performed.

Patient confidentiality must be protected (22). Access to computer data must be restricted so that no unauthorized user may inspect any patient data. This is most readily accomplished by the implementation of restricted access requiring authorized users to enter passwords to gain access to computer operating systems. Further levels of security may be implemented by requiring further password-protected log-ins to sensitive data. Passwords should be changed periodically. Monitors displaying data should be situated in such a way that unauthorized persons cannot inspect the displayed data. In addition, displays that go unused for a brief period of time should be logged off or locked out (requiring password use to re-enter), preventing casual, unauthorized users from gaining access to privileged information.

Imagine the person-hours required to enter all the data in your system. Data entry is of such great value that it is clearly reasonable to create back-up copies of the already-entered data at regular intervals so that in the inevitable event that the data are lost or corrupted, they may be restored. Upon restoration, the data will return to their state at the time of backup. You will need to enter (again) any data that had been entered since the back-up operation. Clearly, less re-entry is necessary when the calamity occurs close in time to the back-up event. Therefore, it is wise to perform back-up operations frequently. Frequent backup assures that data loss occurs shortly after the most recent backup.

Data backup varies with the type of computer system. A small laboratory database may fit on one floppy disk. Larger practice databases may require more space for storage and backup such as streaming tape or compact disks. Some systems perform automatic back-up procedures daily, making copies to several internal magnetic disks and to removable media. Removable media should be removed following each back-up operation and stored in a remote, safe place where the data will not be corrupted by any event that might corrupt the original copy of the data. An additional alternative is to hire a company to perform remote data backup. These companies can back up your data automatically over telephone lines or via internet connections that are rapid and secure, but may require encryption of data to assure privacy. Since the companies are not located at your site, they provide added safety of remote storage that is not likely to be affected by a local event that could destroy data. Data restoration times may vary with these different back-up techniques; however, the convenience of having back-up copies may far outweigh the inconvenience of a longer wait prior to data restoration.

QUALITY CONTROL OF MATERIALS AND SUPPLIES

It should be confirmed that gametes and embryos are never exposed to a substance that will deleteriously impact their development. Exposure can occur during gamete acquisition, via culture in media, or via plastic ware with which the medium has come in contact, or via any airborne volatile or nonvolatile agent that may affect the culture material either directly or indirectly. The effects of electromagnetic radiation are not clearly defined. The purpose of performing quality control for materials and supplies is to determine whether these materials bring some "toxic" substance into the laboratory or into the culture milieu. Any material introduced into the laboratory or culture system that is associated with diminished development should probably be removed from use during human gamete preparation or embryo culture.

Gametes and embryos are maintained in a culture medium throughout their duration in the ART laboratory. The medium must sustain gametes and support optimal development of embryos. This may be tested using an embryo development assay (usually using mouse embryos, see "Process testing"). The manufacturer tests commercially available IVF media and provides the results of their testing with the shipment of media. It may be advisable to test media upon arrival to confirm that nothing occurred during shipping that affected the medium.

Most maintenance and culture of human gametes and embryos is performed in a plastic ware. Great variability exists between different manufacturers of certain plastic ware as well as between different lots of the same item (23). However, rinsing the plastic ware with medium prior to use can greatly diminish any toxic effects (23). It is now possible to purchase plastic ware products that have already tested non-toxic using a mouse embryo assay (MEA). Manufacturers are testing more and more contact materials prior to distribution to assure that they are not toxic Table 2.6. The results of toxicity testing are generally included with the shipment.

Gametes and embryos are maintained in plastic containers within incubators during most of their time in the laboratory. The incubator environment is controlled by maintenance of temperature and gas concentrations. Many incubators regulate the partial pressure of CO_2 inside the incubator. The gas tanks used to supply gases for use in incubators may have high levels of toxicants, of which the suppliers may be unaware (24,25). Although 4–7% of the incubator environment is CO_2, the remaining 93–96% is ambient air from within the laboratory

Table 2.6 Contact Materials and Availability of Prior Mouse Embryo Testing

Item	Whether available with prior mouse embryo assay
Culture medium	Yes
Culture dishes	Yes
Embryo transfer catheters	Yes
Pipettes, serological	No, requires testing
Pipettes, micropipettes for moving embryos	Yes
Pipettes, Pasteur	Yes
Micropipettes for ICSI, AZH, biopsy and holding	Yes
Centrifuge tubes	No, requires testing
Culture tubes	No, requires testing
Pipette tips	Yes
Gases for maintenance of CO_2 levels	No, requires testing
Filters for gases or medium	No, requires testing

Abbreviations: ICSI, intracytoplasmic sperm injection; AZH, assisted zona hatching.

that is circulated into the incubator by a fan. The quality of the ambient air can vary from laboratory to laboratory and within the same laboratory from time to time. There have even been suggestions that success can vary from shelf to shelf within the same incubator and from position to position within the same controlled-rate freezer (Boone, pers. comm.).

The field of airborne toxicants is beginning to grow. Airborne toxic agents fall into several classes: volatile compounds dissolved in the atmosphere and particulate agents that are suspended in the atmosphere. Paint applied to ceilings or walls in the embryology area or even in a distant location may expose gametes/embryos to toxic fumes. The same is true for construction adhesives (24). Particulate agents can be filtered from the atmosphere; however, volatile agents dissolved in the atmosphere are much more difficult to remove. Carbon filters are capable of absorbing some dissolved agents. Gametes and embryos do not have purification systems such as lungs and livers to detoxify their environments, so we must be very careful what we expose gametes and embryos to. Maintenance of a low content of particulates (26) and low concentration of volatile organic compounds (24,25) is associated with improved incidence of pregnancy.

The use of an oil overlay, covering the medium used for ART procedures, may be an effective way of detoxifying the drops of medium that the oil overlays. Any toxicants with a high oil–water partition coefficient will be more concentrated in the oil overlay phase than in the water (culture medium) phase. This can help to remove lipid-soluble toxicants from the aqueous medium. In addition, the presence of an oil overlay creates an oil barrier between the atmosphere and the aqueous medium phase, thereby decreasing the likelihood that water-soluble or particulate toxicants will ever achieve high concentrations in the aqueous (medium) phase. In addition to the presumed advantage of decreased gas diffusion (decreased loss of CO_2), the oil overlay may also be advantageous in slowing toxic agent accumulation in the medium. Although it may be considered a barrier to penetration, the oil overlay may really act only to slow the approach of equilibrium of toxicant between the ambient atmosphere and the culture medium.

In the past several years, more and more products for human IVF and embryo culture have become available that have been manufactured to more exacting standards, as required by the FDA (5). Most of the contact materials for the IVF/embryology laboratory can be purchased having already undergone toxicity testing Table 2.6 (usually by an MEA). This may simplify our lives; however, one always wonders if the manufacturers are using as stringent conditions for the assay as we would in our own laboratories. We also question whether there could be exposure or accumulation of toxic substances during shipping (do Styrofoam packing peanuts impart styrene to previously packaged and tested materials?).

PROCESS TESTING

Once we are certain that all personnel are sufficiently educated and trained, all procedures are intact, all equipment are functioning according to predetermined standards, and all contact materials are confirmed to be nontoxic, we still will like to be able to confirm that the entire process of gamete handling and embryo culture can be performed in a way that does not harm the gametes/embryos. Although there are no perfect tests of the conditions for culture of human gametes and embryos, various survival/development assays have been used for just this purpose. The three major tests are the hamster sperm motility assay (SMA), the human sperm survival assay (SSA) and the mouse embryo assay (MEA). All of these assays challenge the ensemble of personnel, procedures, equipment, and materials in order to assess the ability of the program to sustain sperm or achieve highly developed embryos. It is assumed that the optimal conditions for these assays mimic the conditions that are optimal for maintenance of human gametes and culture of human embryos. Unfortunately, there is very little standardization of these assays, and results in one laboratory may not be the same as results in another laboratory for a variety of reasons.

Many things influence the outcome of ART procedures, including patient selection, patient preparation, gamete handling, and gamete/embryo culture conditions. It is not clear which of these is the factor that affects outcome for any particular patient.

The purpose of strict quality control of culture conditions is to assure that the gamete/embryo culture conditions in the laboratory are uniform and, in theory, optimal so that they are not a negative influence on patients' outcome.

In order to provide control over the quality of culture for gametes/embryos, bioassays utilize similar gametes/embryos, cultured under conditions that simulate human gamete/embryo culture system. Quality control procedures compare different factors (media, plastic ware, culture conditions, etc.) versus control conditions. Control conditions generally employ medium, plastic ware, and incubation conditions that were previously demonstrated to provide adequate culture of gametes/embryos. If a particular aspect of medium, plastic ware, or incubation conditions is found to be significantly detrimental in the bioassay, that particular component is avoided or eliminated from use in culturing human gametes/embryos.

Bioassays must be capable of detecting any and all agents that are detrimental to gametes/embryo, a daunting task in light of our lack of knowledge of everything that affects embryos. At the same time, bioassays should be specific for agents that affect human embryos and not specifically the nonhuman gametes used for testing. The intersection of these two qualities is most probably not achievable using nonhuman gametes/embryos. But alas, we have no better option, at present. Indeed, such quality control exercises have been used in labs that achieve extremely high success with human gametes/embryos. It is possible that some facilities with poorer human outcomes might improve through implementation of better quality control procedures in their facilities.

In subsequent paragraphs, I will describe the three most commonly employed bioassay methods used for quality control of culture conditions: the hamster SMA, the human SSA and the MEA.

Hamster SMA

General Description of the Hamster SMA

Hamster sperm are obtained by allowing them to swim out through several lacerations of the epididymis while the epididymis is maintained in medium. The original solution used for testing is Tyrode's Solution modified by the addition of bovine serum albumin, lactate, and pyruvate (27). All media for testing are supplemented with polyvinyl alcohol, penicillamine, and hypotaurine and an adrenergic agent (epinephrine or isoproterenol). Sperm are introduced to the prepared medium and cultured at a concentration of 1–2 million per ml in 2 ml of medium under oil in an incubator at 37°C with 5% CO_2. Sperm are examined using a dissecting stereomicroscope after four hours of exposure (a time when sperm tend to exhibit their maximal hyperactivation) and scored for both percent motile and quality of motion. Both percent motility and the quality of motion are "estimated" by an overview of the specimen and scoring the "average vigor" of the specimen. A motility score is obtained by multiplying these two values (27). The assay relies upon the timely appearance of hyperactivated sperm in high quantities to achieve adequate motility scores. Determination of two factors in the motility score and particularly the quality of motion value are not well defined and require that personnel performing the scoring have a sufficient level of competency.

Control cultures are prepared using a medium that had previously been demonstrated to perform well in the assay. Sperm motility scores are compared between test and control conditions by performing statistical comparisons between three or four replicates.

Improvements in Sensitivity

Motility scores are affected by albumin. Albumin can obscure the effects of the factors in the media that were considered detrimental to sperm hyperactivation (27). Therefore, the assay's sensitivity is improved by using solutions without albumin.

Significant Conditions that have been Detected

Hamster SMA has been demonstrated to detect differences between media prepared with different water sources (tap water vs clinical laboratory water even after purification by reverse osmosis, Milli-Q filtration, and double distillation) (27–29) and between water passed through unrinsed sterilization filters (27).

Advantages/Disadvantages

The primary advantage of the hamster SMA is that it is brief, requiring only four to 6 hours to arrive at results. Disadvantages of the assay include the need for hamsters (not typically maintained in IVF laboratories) and that it focuses on only the hyperactivation of sperm, only one of the functions that sperm must perform during IVF. Unfortunately, the use of hamster sperm may not represent the sensitivity of human sperm or human embryos to culture conditions. In addition, it requires that nonculture constituents be added to the medium that all the media used in the assay.

Human SSA

General Description of the Human SSA

Human sperm are obtained either from patient samples donated for research (30–36), or frozen sperm samples (37). Since human material is used, there is increasing consideration of whether informed consent is required for use of specimens that would otherwise be discarded. Sperm are prepared for culture by techniques that isolate sperm from seminal plasma and/or cryoprotectants, typically by centrifugation of semen layered over density sedimentation media or a discontinuous sedimentation gradient (30,32–34,38,39).

Control solutions for sperm culture are selected because they previously supported acceptable prolonged culture of sperm. Separate vessels (typically culture tubes) of media are prepared so that test solutions (either new medium or media that have been exposed to test conditions) are compared with control solutions. Sperm harvested following sperm preparation are aliquoted into the control and test solutions at equal concentrations. Sperm cultures are maintained for periods of several minutes (36) to several days (30,34,36–39). Uniform, constant temperatures for culture were maintained, most commonly at room temperature (31,32) or at 37°C (32–34,39). Sperm survival declines over time.

At specified times, sperm survivals for specimens cultured under both the test and control conditions are assessed. The assessment of survival is most commonly made by determination of the percent motile (31,38,37) or the percent of sperm with progressive motility (30,33,36) although other measures of survival have been used such as the percent viable (31) (by use of a vital stain exclusion or by hypo-osmotic swelling), morphology (31) or mitochondrial function (31).

Survival values for replicate specimens from each test group are determined and compared with the values determined for the control specimens. The assay relies on the ability of sperm to sustain their survival; however, it is assessed in different conditions. Statistical comparisons reveal if any test conditions are significantly different from the control conditions. It is common to require that control solutions support motility of 70–85% of the initial motility (30,38) after 48–96 hours for the assay to be considered valid. Rather than relying totally on statistical criteria, it is common to use a defined survival level 75% of the control as a threshold. For the test condition to be considered sufficient to be used in human culture, sperm in the test solution must not decline below this threshold (36).

Improvements in Sensitivity

Early versions of the assay relied upon culture durations of 48 and/or 96 hours at room temperature (40,38). Prolonged survival is observed when sperm culture is performed at room temperature (31,32) or 4°C (32) when compared with culture that was performed at 37°C (32,34,39). More prolonged survival may increase the difference of survival observed at any particular culture time (38). While differences in survival are seldom detectable during the first minutes of culture, significant differences are more easily detected around 48 or 96 hours of culture at room temperature (30–32,38). The duration of exposure and the duration of culture have been useful in improving the sensitivity of the assay. Culture at 37°C, rather than room temperature, leads to a more rapid demise of sperm and earlier detection of effects on sperm survival, thereby improving the sensitivity of the assay at shorter time periods (33,38,39).

The desire to improve the sensitivity and reliability of the human SSA has led to several improvements over the years. Use of replicates (38) is helpful in comparing two treatments at the same point in time. Other statistical methods have been employed to improve the sensitivity, including the use of the rate of decline in motility (slope of the motility as a function of time) or the use of an index relating the rate of decline to the rate of decline for sperm in the control conditions (37).

Additional improvements in sensitivity have been achieved through the use of qualitative assessments of sperm motility (30,33,36,39) that distinguish between tails barely shaking on sperm that are not progressive, sperm that swim slowly in straight lines and hyperactivated sperm that swim in ways that might be personified as feverish and frantic. By implementing qualitative assessment of motility, the assay may be equally sensitive with less time (39) for some toxicants, but it still continues to have increased sensitivity with longer durations. Attempts at implementation of other measures of survival (viability using vital stain or hypo-osmotic swelling, morphology, or mitochondrial function (31)) have not led to improvements in sensitivity.

Other methods to improve the sensitivity of the human SSA include omission of protein or albumin from the medium, and decreasing the concentration of sperm cultured (38).

Significant Conditions that have been Detected

Conditions found to be detrimental to human sperm survival are those to which the human SSA is sensitive. These include overlay oil that had been demonstrated to affect development of nonhuman primate embryos (34) or proved spermicidal for nonhuman primate sperm (34), contact materials used for IVF (ultrasound probe covers, transfer catheters, gloves for personal protection) (30), cumene hydroperoxide (34), gloves for IVF use (36), and proficiency testing samples (37) for which the toxicant is not defined. Addition of glucose to a simple medium (with daily replacement of the medium) has been shown to prolong the survival of sperm (32).

Advantages/Disadvantages

Advantages of the human SSA include that it uses human sperm, material that is commonly available in the IVF laboratory, and that the sperm used are of the same species that is used in performance of human IVF, a distinct improvement of relevance over the hamster SMA. Disadvantages include that human sperm samples vary substantially from male to male. It is not clear whether this male-to-male variability also impacts the sensitivity of sperm to culture conditions. Survival of sperm for days is certainly not the only function of sperm during human IVF. Use of qualitative scoring of motility to improve the sensitivity is somewhat arbitrary and requires trained personnel for reproducible performance. Sensitivity of the assay generally is improved by increased duration of the culture duration. However, during human IVF, sperm generally enter oocytes within the first few hours after insemination. Is survival for two to five days relevant? In addition, other functions of sperm (ability to capacitate, hyperactivate, fertilize, and activate oocytes) may not be well discriminated by the assay.

Mouse Embryo Assay

General Description of the Assay

Mouse embryos are obtained either by super ovulation, mating, and harvesting fresh embryos (28,36,41) or by thawing frozen embryos (34,35). The typical starting stage for embryos is either the one-cell (zygote) stage (20,34,36,41) or the two-cell stage (34,35). Solutions (at least one Control medium and one Test medium) are prepared and maintained at 37°C. Embryos at the starting stage are introduced into the control or test media and cultured in incubator-like conditions with a gas environment appropriate for the medium used, either 5% CO_2 in air (41,42) or a higher percentage of the air replaced by CO_2 (34–36). Development of the embryos to a particular advanced stage is assessed at a predetermined time. Typically, the advanced stage is the blastocyst stage (20,28,36,41,43) or the expanded blastocyst stage (34,35) on the fourth day of embryonic development. Embryos containing a blastocele are considered blastocysts. Blastocysts with a blastocele that has enlarged and has stretched the zona pellucida to a diameter larger than the zona pellucida of a zygote or two-cell embryo are considered expanding blastocysts. Other stages used have been the compacted morula stage (28,42) on the third day of embryonic development or the hatching or hatched blastocyst stage on the fifth day of embryonic development (28,34,35,43). Hatching blastocysts have a portion of the blastocyst spilling outside of the zona pellucida. A hatched blastocyst is one that has escaped from its zona pellucida. The blastocyst or hatching blastocyst stage is scored on the fourth day following introduction of one-cell zygotes into culture (fourth day of embryonic development) or on the third day after introduction of two-cell embryos into culture (also the fourth day of embryonic development). The number or percentage of embryos attaining the desired advanced stage is compared between embryos cultured in test medium and embryos cultured in control medium. Some labs are now determining the number of cells in the blastocyst (30,34,44). If the percentage of embryos achieving the advanced stage is significantly lower in the test conditions than in the control conditions, then the test conditions are considered insufficient to support human embryos and those conditions are avoided or not permitted for use with humans.

Improvements in Sensitivity

The sensitivity of the assay is associated with a number of factors. First, the strain of mouse generating the gametes determines the sensitivity of the assay (reviewed in (20)). Inbred mice (28) are less sensitive to conditions than are F1 hybrids of inbred mice (36,41) and these in turn are less sensitive to conditions than outbred mice (20,44). Second, the starting stage of the embryos determines the sensitivity of the assay. Embryos introduced to culture conditions as zygotes are more sensitive to conditions than are those introduced to culture conditions as two-cell embryos (20,34). The two-cell block in mice corresponds to the time of onset of expression of the embryonic genome (analogous to the four- to eight-cell stage in humans). Embryos placed in culture prior to the onset of expression of the embryonic genome are more sensitive to their conditions (20). Third, the stage that must be attained affects the sensitivity. The general rule is that reliance upon more advanced stages increases the sensitivity of the assay to culture conditions. This was shown by Rinehart et al. (28) when they demonstrated that sensitivity to culture conditions (presence vs absence of protein) was evident at the blastocyst and hatching blastocyst stages when it was not evident at the morula stage using two-cell mouse embryos as the starting point. Others have extended the assay to use expanded, hatching and/or hatched blastocysts as the endpoint of the assay (34,35,42). The use of cell numbers as the endpoint of the assay, further increases the sensitivity of the assay (20,34,44) as may the use of gene expression (20), apoptotic index (20,34), and/or fetal development (20). Suggestions have been made that results from multiple stages should be considered together to improve the sensitivity of the assay (44).

Other procedural differences used to improve sensitivity that have been explored are culture of embryos singly, each embryo in a separate drop of culture medium (34) and/or culture of zona-free embryos (36,44,45). In many respects, the sensitivity can be improved by formulating substandard conditions that barely support embryo development so that effects of any further detrimental condition will be accentuated. Culturing embryos in a medium that is not covered by oil makes the medium more susceptible to changes in environment and may improve the sensitivity to lipid-soluble agents (46). Culture in a medium lacking amino acids, protein, albumin, or serum is commonly used to increase the sensitivity of the assay (44,47). Further refinement may include culture for 24 hours with albumin (to permit development beyond the two-cell block) and then transfer to a medium lacking albumin for extended culture (44). An additional suggestion is to culture the mouse embryos under an atmosphere containing 20% oxygen rather than a lower level (44).

Further improvements in the testing paradigm include increasing the number of embryos cultured and improving the statistical design so that equal numbers of embryos from each mated pair of mice are allotted to control and test conditions and are compared in a stratified test (akin to paired comparisons)(41). In this method, mated pairs of mice with too few or too many embryos were excluded from use in the testing. In this method, a minimum of 69 embryos is required for each group tested (69 embryos in the control group, and 69 in each test group, using equal numbers of embryos from each mated pair of mice (41). The need for such large numbers of embryos and mated pairs of mice results in very high power but at a high cost in terms of animals and personnel time and leads to the question, "How many mice must die for one human to be born?"

Significant Conditions that have been Detected

The MEA has been demonstrated to detect the presence or absence of pyruvate in the culture medium (20), the presence or absence of protein supplementation in the medium (20), the quality of maternal serum used for supplementation (48), serum from women who smoked cocaine paste up to two months prior to collection of the serum, the presence of cumene hydroperoxide a lipid-soluble compound in overlay oil (34), endotoxin (49), or ammonium (a metabolite of amino acids in the medium) (20), exposure of medium to material from sterile gloves used for personnel during IVF procedures (36) or to the sterilizing agents Cidex (Civco Medical Solutions, Kalona, IA 52247) and ethylene oxide (50). MEAs detected a detrimental effect of culture on Matrigel (BD Biosciences, San Jose, CA 95131) (51), a cell surface-like agent used for somatic cell culture. MEAs have detected differences in media or products that had previously been found to be associated with poor development or outcomes with patient gametes/embryos (28) or in oils for overlay found to be detrimental to live birth outcomes in mice or spermicidal for non-human primate sperm (34,35). Further, the assay has led to the observation that glucose and inorganic phosphate are detrimental to embryonic development (52) and that the inclusion of glutamine (an amino acid) and/or EDTA (a divalent/heavy metal chelator) is beneficial for embryonic development (52). Further, it has been instrumental, during the formulation of KSOM (a potassium enhanced version of the simplex optimized medium devised in the laboratory of John Biggers) (53).

Advantages/Disadvantages

Advantages of the MEA are that it tests the ability of embryos to undergo sustained development through the early stages and to result in embryos of a particular quality. The conditions are quite similar to those used for culture of human embryos. Disadvantages are that mouse embryos may not be sensitive to the same array of culture conditions that may affect human embryo development. The MEA requires a lengthy duration of culture and yet does not generally assess the ability of the conditions to support implantation, fetal growth, and delivery (although this rather impractical feat has been implemented by some and has demonstrated that some early exposures can result in poor fetal development even when there are no recognized effects during culture (20)).

Comparison of Sensitivities

Sensitivities of these assays vary and some assays may be sensitive to detrimental conditions when others are not. The hamster SMA detected differences in media prepared using tap water versus Milli-Q water, whereas the MEA (albeit using an inbred strain of mice) did not detect any difference (28). The human SSA detected the exposure of media to the material from several different types of gloves that were not detected as toxic when using the standard MEA (36). After increasing the sensitivity of the MEA by using frozen zona-free embryos, the media deemed toxic by the human SSA were found to be inadequate to support mouse embryos. However, most commonly, (although it may not be appropriate) the MEA is accepted to be more sensitive to detrimental conditions than are the other two assays. In direct comparison, the MEA, using frozen zygotes, was able to detect lower concentrations of cumene hydroperoxide in the overlay oil than the human SSA (34). Direct comparisons resulted in the observation that mouse zygotes cultured individually in 10 µl drops of medium detected cumene hydroperoxide in the oil overlay at half the concentration detected by mouse zygotes cultured in groups of 10 in 10 μl drops of medium. Zygotes cultured in groups detected cumene hydroperoxide at roughly half the concentration detected by two-cell embryos cultured in groups. Two-cell mouse embryos cultured in groups detected cumene hydroperoxide in oil overlay at a concentration that was one-tenth the concentration detected by the human SSA (including qualitative assessment of sperm motility)(34). Similarly, the MEA detected the effects of overlay by a particular oil that was not detected by the human SSA (35). This particular oil previously had been selected for its bad effects on live birth of mouse embryos in a transgenic facility. An obvious conclusion is that some detrimental conditions are detected more sensitively by sperm and some are detected more sensitively by embryos. Knowledge of these diverse spectra of sensitivities has led some to conclude that more than one assay should be used to assess the acceptability of culture conditions ((34–36,54,55), reviewed in (44)).

In most human IVF facilities, we would avoid any conditions that are known to be detrimental to sperm or to embryos. It would make sense to use one assay for sperm sensitivity and another assay for embryo sensitivity to make sure that no toxic substance "squeaks by." It is reasonable to suspect that a sperm assay would detect conditions that affect sperm but that it would not detect all conditions that might be detrimental to embryos. Likewise, it is reasonable to suspect that an embryo assay would detect conditions that affect embryos but that it would not detect all conditions that might be detrimental to sperm or to the steps of fertilization, for that matter. Perhaps it would make sense to include an assay for conditions that affect sperm–egg interactions and fertilization. I have found few reports of a mouse IVF assay involving fertilization in the medium, which should, in theory, test for effects on sperm, oocytes, and embryos (28,53). Although this assay has been the crux of development of a very successful medium for human embryo culture (53), one early version of the assay failed to detect the differences in media that had been formulated using tap water, HPLC grade water, or ultrapure Milli-Q water (28). In contrast, these authors found that the hamster SMA could discriminate the three sources of water tested (that were not detected by use of mouse embryos); however, there was no direct demonstration of the causal factor (contaminant or omission from the medium) that led to their observed differences in human IVF outcome. While laboratory conditions should always be scrutinized, this author believes that it remains possible that clinical parameters other than age and number of oocytes may have influenced the human IVF outcome that led to the investigations summarized in the publication (28). Therefore, it may be fruitful to reinvestigate the use of an IVF assay (involving culture of sperm, culture of oocytes, fertilization of oocytes, and culture of embryos) for future scrutiny of conditions that may affect human IVF outcome. The applicability of such an assay may be questioned, however, in light of the increasingly common use of ICSI as the insemination method of choice in many facilities.

The use of somatic cell lines or embryonic stem cells for quality control has been reviewed elsewhere (44,56) and since it does not include sensitivity to gamete/embryo-specific conditions, these are not considered in this chapter.

Sensitivity vs Sensibility

Great advancements have been made toward improving the sensitivity for the human sperm survival and mouse embryo assays. These include use of a greater number of gametes/embryos and a stratified approach to analysis (41), a high ratio of gamete or embryo to medium (lower sperm concentration (38) or culture of single embryos (35)) and removal of any protective layers surrounding the embryo (36). However, as the sensitivity of the bioassay improves, one wonders whether the bioassay becomes more specific for the particular gamete/species used and less sensitive for factors that affect human gametes and embryos. Some investigators have indicated that the results of the MEA do not correlate with the outcome of human embryo culture (57), but may be indicative of the ability to support oocyte fertilization without any predictive value for pregnancy (58). Others have expressed concern that none of the assays that we use may detect some conditions that may be detrimental specifically to human embryos (47,52). Most improvements in sensitivity result in increased costs for the bioassay through more personnel time, more animals, or bioassay material used or more supplies. Costs can become prohibitive especially in laboratories with decreasing revenue in difficult economic times with declining patient numbers and insurance reimbursements.

Improvements in sensitivity have generally been made by tailoring the bioassay to a particular detrimental factor. Such improvements improve the sensitivity for that particular factor; but, this does not assure that the assay's sensitivity has been improved for all detrimental factors. As we improve the sensitivity of a bioassay to detect one toxicant, we may actually obscure other sources of toxicants. For example, the use of smaller drops of medium in the singly cultured MEA (34) improved the sensitivity of the assay when the lipid soluble toxicant, cumene hydroperoxide, originated in the oil phase. However, when the toxicant originates in the water phase and is lipid soluble, a large oil overlay will provide protective benefits (46) as the lipid-soluble toxicant partitions into the overwhelmingly voluminous oil phase. Creating smaller culture drops in this situation would be expected only to dilute the toxicant even further, thereby reducing sensitivity.

Issues about specificity for bioassay materials raise the question of just how sensitive our assays should be for various functions. If we use a very sensitive test for all contact materials, then more contact material will be rejected. Use of some bioassays has led to the rejection of roughly 25% of the materials purchased for use in the laboratory (30) and 80% of the gloves for use as personal protective equipment (36). Rejection of these materials was made using human SSA alone (30) and together with the MEA (36) but there was no confirmation of toxicity using human embryos. Just how stringent should a bioassay be when used to reject supplies, especially if there is an increase of costs? And how much do we believe that human sperm and mouse embryos behave exactly like human embryos? Unfortunately, ethical considerations preclude us from using human embryos in a widespread manner to screen for toxicity of supplies in the IVF laboratory. While there are clear limitations to the bioassays available, these bioassays are the best that we have, at present, to assess the quality of our culture conditions. Reliance upon these procedures has been crucial to achieving the improvements with human embryos that have led to excellent success in excellent programs. While rejection of supplies can be costly, it is difficult, indeed, to determine the marginal cost of rejecting supplies per additional healthy baby born. The approach that you use should be tailored to your laboratory's individual stringency versus cost relationship and should be widely shared with the clinicians who will be using the laboratory's services.

QUALITY CONTROL OF THE ART

Despite demonstration of all aspects of the ART process, by performance of quality control for every employee, every procedure, every piece of equipment, and all materials and supplies, and following the use of survival/development assays, it is necessary to confirm that the clinical treatment procedures as they are applied to patients are resulting in an acceptable incidence of pregnancy for the treated patients. A target for the incidence of pregnancy should be determined prior to the onset of treatment. Treatment of patients should continue only as long as the incidence of pregnancy continues to remain at or above the predetermined target. Any failure to maintain success above the predetermined level requires the institution of quality assurance procedures.

It may be considered questionable ethically to use patient material as testing material for quality control exercises; however, it would be equally questionable not to cease treatments when success drops below a predetermined level of success. Further, it is difficult to determine what will result in an improvement without performing patient treatments.

Similar standards for several outcome parameters should be monitored to determine that all procedures are succeeding. Among these could be the recovery of sperm during sperm processing for insemination, incidence of fertilization following standard in vitro insemination, incidence of fertilization following ICSI, incidence of embryo development to an acceptable stage on day 3 or day 5, incidence of survival following cryopreservation, or incidence of implantation (per embryo transferred). Some newer techniques also should be monitored to control the quality of performance. These include confirmation that embryo biopsy yields embryos that are capable of further development (unharmed) in addition to the demonstration that the biopsied material can yield a genetic screening result or genetic diagnosis with a high degree of repeatability. Once data for success as well as all quality control parameters have been entered as data, quality assurance/improvement analysis of any trends can be conducted (7,11,59).

Quality Control of Embryo and Specimen Identification: Witnesses

In the earlier days of ART, laboratory personnel were quite intent on assuring that sperm, eggs, and embryos were accurately labeled and associated with the patient couple for whom they were intended. However, now, with the increasing prevalence of embryo testing used to aid in the selection of individual embryos for transfer, it has become necessary to maintain unique identifiability of each embryo throughout embryo culture, catheter loading, and embryo transfer. Emphasis on each embryo's identity, rather than just the patients' identities, has made the task of identification more difficult by an order of magnitude (typically 10–20 embryos per couple). Embryo biopsies must be performed using methods that provide errorless association of the results of embryo testing (results of genetic diagnosis and/or screening and/or testing of the medium surrounding each embryo) with the embryo that was tested. Thus far, this has required that embryos be cultured individually in separate and uniquely identified drops of medium or wells of a culture plate. Whenever embryos or samples are removed from these separate drops/wells, there is a risk of losing the identity of the embryo through misidentification of test materials or by moving embryos to culture locations that are not the appropriate locations for the identity of the embryo. Busy, overworked staff members are particularly at risk of such misidentifications. One method that has been applied widely to avoid misidentification is the use of a witness to confirm that all steps involving possible misidentification. The witness confirms that the person performing the step (biopsy, pipetting of biopsied material into the reaction tube, the replacement of the embryo into its culture drop, and any transfer of embryos from one culture drop to another) maintains the correct identification of the material. Similar witnessing steps have been put in place to assure that the correct sperm are used for insemination/ICSI of oocytes. Use of witnesses not only decreases the probability of misidentification but it also is an effective sales point that addresses patients' concerns over the possibility of misidentification in the laboratory. The avoidance of misidentification is well worth the added personnel cost. This author believes that the use of a witness familiar with identification techniques should be part of every risky step in every IVF cycle performed in every ART laboratory. The personnel performing the witness function may be laboratory personnel, medical assistants, nurses, physicians, or anyone else familiar with the methods involved in unique patient identification.

SUMMARY

Quality control procedures are performed in order to confirm that all aspects of the program are operating as expected. By careful performance of quality control, the program will continue to operate under stable conditions that should help to result in stable, repeatable results for patients. Critical features that should be performed are listed in this chapter.

Experienced practitioners realize that the achievement of fertilization and transfer of attractive embryos will not guarantee pregnancy. There are many biological processes in the establishment of pregnancy that remain poorly understood. While improvements of our treatment paradigms fall into the domain of quality assurance or quality improvement, monitoring success is a quality control task. Monitoring success is necessary to have the data available to attempt improvements. Each quality control parameter measured should be recorded so that it is documented for use when unexpected events occur. The maintenance of this data is necessary to simplify the analytical process that can be used to institute improvements in the program.

I believe that quality control will continue to evolve in the future, including more widespread use of quality control monitoring for all tests and procedures, even those that are not considered laboratory procedures, such as ultrasound measurements. More and more programs will store their quality control data electronically, thereby simplifying the analysis process. The recent FDA regulations have led to more widespread availability of materials and supplies that can be purchased after testing for gamete and embryo toxicity. I also expect that in the near future daily quality control will become more automated. Temperatures can be monitored digitally by sensors and be logged into a database remotely. This could also be designed to monitor quality control parameters more frequently, perhaps hourly or every 10 minutes, to assure that quality control values are more verifiably constant. I believe that proficiency testing will improve to the point that it will be available for all tests performed in the andrology/embryology laboratory. In addition, the use of proficiency testing will be more clearly matched to test the appropriate process to be monitored, whether it is a test of the personnel or a test of the conditions, and will be designed to provide proficiency testing for the clinical components in addition to the laboratory component.

As the success of assisted reproduction procedures improves, the methods of performing quality control will also evolve. Within the next decade, ART programs will become more uniform in their ability to provide a high incidence of success (pregnancy or delivery). When most programs can offer a high incidence of pregnancy, issues of patient satisfaction other than simple measures of pregnancy outcomes will become much more important in affecting patients' decisions about which program to choose for treatment. As this evolves, patient satisfaction surveys will become more important in our assessment of the quality of the services that we provide.

Until the time when all treated patients can be promised a viable pregnancy, we must continue to perform quality control activities and a careful recording of the data so that we may concentrate on improving the outcome of our procedures.

ACKNOWLEDGMENTS

I acknowledge gratefully the assistance that I received from two students who helped me assemble the references during the preparation of this chapter. Thanks to Katherine E. McCulloh and Patrick S. McCulloh who had access to literature that was not accessible to me at the time of writing.

REFERENCES

1. Medicare, Medicaid and CLIA Programs; Laboratory requirements relating to quality systems and certain personnel qualifications; Final rule. 42 CFR Part 493, 2003.
2. American Society for Reproductive Medicine. Revised minimum standards for in vitro fertilization, gamete intrafallopian transfer, and related procedures. Fertil Steril 1998; 53: 225–6.
3. American Society for Reproductive Medicine. Revised guidelines for human embryology and andrology laboratories. Fertil Steril 2008; 90: S45–59.
4. The Fertility Clinic Success Rate and Certification Act of 1992. 42 U.S.C. 263a-1, 1992.
5. Obstetric and gynecologic devices; Reclassification and classification of medical devices used for in vitro fertilization and related assisted reproduction procedures. 21 CFR Part 884, 1998.
6. Human Cellular and Tissue-Based Products or HCT/Ps. 21 CFR Part 1271, 2001.
7. McCulloh DH. Quality control and quality assurance: record keeping and impact on ART performance and outcome. Infertil Reprod Med Clin North Am 1998; 9: 285–309.
8. Weimer KE, Anderson A, Weikert L. Quality control in the IVF laboratory. In: Gardner DK, Weissman A, Howles CM, Shoham Z, eds. Textbook of Assisted Reproductive Techniques: Laboratory and Clinical Perspectives. London: Taylor & Francis, 2001: 27–33.
9. McCulloh DH. Quality control: maintaining stability in the laboratory. In: Gardner DK, Weissman A, Howles CM, Shoham Z, eds. Textbook of Assisted Reproductive Techniques: Laboratory and Clinical Perspectives, 3rd edn. London: Informa Healthcare, 2009: 9–24.
10. McCulloh DH. Quality control: maintaining stability in the laboratory. In: Gardner DK, Weissman A, Howles CM, Shoham Z, eds. Textbook of Assisted Reproductive Techniques: Laboratory and Clinical Perspectives, 2nd edn. London: Taylor & Francis, 2004: 25–39.
11. McCulloh DH. Quality assurance in the ART program: can we learn anything from it? Presented at In Vitro Fertilization and Embryo Transfer: A Comprehensive Update – 2001: Minisymposium on the IVF Laboratory. Santa Barbara, UCLA School of Medicine, 2001.
12. McCulloh DH. 2000 Survey of 1999 Compensation. Birmingham: Reproductive Laboratory Technology

Professional Group and Reproductive Biology Professional Group of the American Society for Reproductive Medicine, 2000.
13. Boone WR, Higdon HL. Time and staffing issues as they relate to assisted reproductive technology (ART) laboratories in the US. Bull Am Assoc Bioanalysts 2003; 47: 1–7.
14. NCCLS. Clinical Laboratory Technical Procedure Manuals. 3rd edn. 1996; Approved guideline GP2-A3.
15. Squire W. Observations on the temperature of the body in health and disease. Br Med J 1871; 1: 32.
16. Bardswell ND, Chapman JE. Some observations upon the deep temperature of the human body at rest and after muscular exertion. Br Med J 1911; 1: 106–1110.
17. Nakayama K, Nakagawa T, Hiyama T, et al. Circadian changes in body temperature during the menstrual cycle of healthy adult females and patients suffering from premenstrual syndrome. Int J Clin Pharmacol Res 1997; 17: 155–64.
18. Cagnacci A, Volpe A, Paoletti AM, Melis GB. Regulation of the 24-hour rhythm of body temperature in menstrual cycles with spontaneous and gonadotropin-induced ovulation. Fertil Steril 1997; 68: 421–5.
19. Coyne MD, Kesick CM, Doherty TJ, et al. Circadian rhythm changes in core temperature over the menstrual cycle: method for noninvasive monitoring. Am J Physiol Regul Integr Comp Physiol 2000; 279: R1316–20.
20. Lane M, Mitchell M, Cashman KS, Feil D. To QC or not to QC: the key to a consistent laboratory? Reprod Fertil Dev 2008; 20: 23–32.
21. Johnson MT, Gardner DK. Embryo culture in the twenty-first century. In: Gardner DK, Rizk BRMB, Falcone T, eds. Human Assisted Reproductive Technology: Future Trends in Laboratory and Clinical Practice. Cambridge: Cambridge University Press, 2011.
22. United States Department of Health and Human Services. OCR Privacy Brief: Summary of the HIPAA Privacy Rule,revised May 2003. [Available from: http://www.hhs.gov/ocr/hipaa]
23. Boone WR, Shapiro SS. Quality control in the in vitro fertilization laboratory. Theriogenology 1990; 33: 23–50.
24. Cohen J, Gilligan A, Willadsen S. Culture and quality control of embryos. Hum Reprod 1998; 13(Suppl 3): 137–44.
25. Hall J, Gilligan A, Schimmel T, Cecchi M, Cohen J. The origin, effects and control of air pollution in laboratories used for human embryo culture. Hum Reprod 1998; 13(Suppl 4): 146–55.
26. Boone WR, Johnson JE, Locke AJ, Crane MM, Price TM. Control of air quality in an assisted reproductive technology laboratory. Fertil Steril 1999; 71: 150–4.
27. Bavister BD, Andrews JC. A rapid sperm motility bioassay procedure for quality-control testing of water and culture media. J In Vitro Fert Embryo Transf 1988; 5: 67–75.
28. Rinehart JS, Bavister BD, Gerrity M. Quality control in the in vitro fertilization laboratory: comparison of bioassay systems for water quality. J In Vitro Fert Embryo Transf 1988; 5: 335–42.
29. Gorrill MJ, Rinehart JS, Tamhane AC, Gerrity M. Comparison of the hamster sperm motility assay to the mouse one-cell and two-cell embryo bioassays as quality control tests for in vitro fertilization. Fertil Steril 1991; 55: 345–54.
30. Nijs M, Franssen K, Cox A, et al. Reprotoxicity of intrauterine insemination and in vitro fertilization-embryo transfer disposables and products: a 4-year study. Fertil Steril 2009; 92: 527–35.
31. Hossain AM, Osuamkpe CO, Magamani M. Extended culture of human spermatozoa in the laboratory may have practical value in the assisted reproductive procedures. Fertil Steril 2008; 89: 237–9.
32. Amaral A, Paiva C, Baptista M, et al. Exogenous glucose improves long-standing human sperm motility, viability, and mitochondrial function. Fertil Steril 2011; [Epub ahead of print].
33. Vargas J, Crausaz M, Senn A, Germond M. Sperm toxicity of "nonspermicidal" lubricant and ultrasound gels used in reproductive medicine. Fertil Steril 2011; 95: 835–6.
34. Hughes PM, Morbeck DE, Hudson SBA, et al. Peroxides in mineral oil used for in vitro fertilization: defining limits of standard quality control assays. J Assist Reprod Genet 2010; 27: 87–93.
35. Morbeck DE, Khan Z, Barnidge DR, Walker DL. Washing mineral oil reduces contaminants and embryotoxicity. Fertil Steril 2010; 94: 2747–52.
36. Lierman S, DeSutter P, Dhont M, Van der Elst J. Double-quality control reveals high-level toxicity in gloves used for operator protection in assisted reproductive technology. Fertil Steril 2007; 88(Suppl 2): 1266–72.
37. DeJonge CJ, Centola GM, Reed ML, et al. Human sperm survival assay as a bioassay for the assisted reproductive technologies laboratory. J Androl 2003; 24: 16–18.
38. Claassens OE, Wehr JB, Harrison KL. Optimizing sensitivity of the human sperm motility assay for embryo toxicity testing. Hum Reprod 2000; 15: 1586–91.
39. Hossain A, Subbhash A, Osuampke C, Phelps J. Human sperm bioassay for reprotoxicity testing in embryo culture media: Some practical considerations in reducing the assay time. Adv Urol 2010; [Epub ahead of print].
40. Critchlow JD, Matson PL, Newman MC, et al. Quality control in an in vitro fertilization laboratory: use of human sperm survival studies. Hum Reprod 1989; 4: 545–9.
41. Punt van der Zalm JPEM, Hendriks JCM, Westphal JR, et al. Toxicity testing of human assisted reproduction devices using the mouse embryo assay. Reprod Biomed Online 2009; 18: 529–35.
42. Del Valle LJ, Pella R, Mercedes A, et al. Embryotoxicity of serum from women smoking cocaine paste (CBP). Eur J Obstet Gyn Reprod Med 2008; 139: 28–31.
43. Svalander P, Anderson E, Hyllner J, et al. Quality assurance methods for production of culture media and equipment essential for high success rate. In: Maximizing the Potential of Every Embryo to Minimize Multiple Embryo Transfer, Textbook for the Postgraduate Course at the Meeting of the American Society for Reproductive Medicine. American Society for Reproductive Medicine. San Francisco, October 1998: 1–15.
44. Gardner DK, Reed L, Linck D, et al. Quality control in human in vitro fertilization. Semin Reprod Med 2005; 23: 319–24.
45. Fleetham JA, Pattinson HA, Mortimer D. The mouse embryo culture system: improving the sensitivity for use as a quality control assay for human in vitro fertilization. Fertil Steril 1993; 59: 192–6.
46. Quinn PJ. AAB embryology proficiency testing (PT) surveys as a tool to distinguish variables affecting

outcomes. Presented at the AAB College of Reproductive Biology Seventh Annual Symposium. Broomfield, CO, June 2003.
47. Taft RA. Virtues and limitations of the preimplantation embryo as a model system. Theriogen 2008; 69: 10–16.
48. Deaton JL, Dempsey RA, Miller KA. Serum from women with polycystic ovary syndrome inhibits fertilization and embryonic development in the murine in vitro fertilization model. Fertil Steril 1996; 65: 1224–8.
49. Dubin NH, Bornstein DR, Gong Y. Use of endotoxin as a positive (toxic) control in the mouse embryo assay. J Assist Reprod Genet 1995; 12: 147–52.
50. Ackerman SB, Stokes GL, Swanson RJ, Taylor SP, Fenwick L. Toxicity testing for human in vitro fertilization programs. J In Vitro Fert Embryo Transf 1985; 2: 132–7.
51. Dawson KM, Baltz JM, Claman P. Culture with Matrigel inhibits development of mouse zygotes. J Assist Reprod Genet 1997; 14: 543–8.
52. Quinn P, Horstman FC. Is the mouse a good model for the human with respect to the development of the preimplantation embryo in vitro? Hum Reprod 1998; 13(Suppl 4): 173–83.
53. Summers MC, Bhatnagar PR, Lawitts JA, Biggers JD. Fertilization in vitro of mouse ova from inbred and outbred strains: complete preimplantation embryo development in glucose-supplemented KSOM. Biol Reprod 1995; 53: 431–7.
54. Muller CH. The andrology laboratory in an assisted reproductive technologies program. Quality assurance and laboratory methodology. J Androl 1992; 13: 349–60.
55. Scott L, Smith S. Mouse in vitro fertilization, embryo development and viability, human sperm motility in substances used for human sperm preparation for assisted reproduction. Fertil Steril 1997; 67: 372–81.
56. Castilla JA, Ruiz de Assin R, Gonzalvo MC, et al. External quality control for embryology laboratories. Reprod Biomed Online 2010; 20: 68–74.
57. Clarke RN, Griffin PM, Biggers JD. Screening of maternal sera using a mouse embryo culture assay is not predictive of human embryo development or IVF outcome. J Assist Reprod Genet 1995; 12: 20–5.
58. van den Bergh M, Baszo I, Diramane J, et al. Quality control in IVF with mouse bioassays: a four years' experience. J Assist Reprod Genet 1996; 13: 733–8.
59. McCulloh DH. Quality control and quality assurance: a means of improving and stabilizing IVF results. Presented at In Vitro Fertilization and Embryo Transfer: A Comprehensive Update – 2003: Minisymposium on the IVF Laboratory. Santa Barbara, UCLA School of Medicine, July 2003.

3

The ART laboratory: Current standards

Cecilia Sjöblom

INTRODUCTION

Quality assurance (QA), quality control (QC), and accreditation are concepts that seem to touch on a wide range of functions in our society. QC system and standardization is especially needed in units for assisted reproductive techniques (ART) to assure reproducibility of all methods and that all members of staff are competent to perform their duties. The necessity of a QC system becomes even clearer when considering the possible risks of ART.

Over the years that ARTs have been practiced, extensive knowledge has been gained on how to run an ART laboratory and what methods to use in order to achieve ultimate success. Facing the future, we encounter other variables such as the safety and efficiency of the laboratory and quality and standardization become key features. Professional, national and international guidelines on how ART should be performed have been established over the years, and many countries have legislation concerning how ART should be practiced (1–3). Among others, England, Australia, and the United States have instituted a system whereby the ART clinics have to be licensed to practice these techniques and the clinic as well as the laboratory are audited by a third-party authority in order to assure correct practice (4–7). However, with the increased knowledge of the importance of implementing quality systems most clinics choose to conform to any of a range of available standards.

This chapter first covers an overview of the most common laboratory standards together with some regional/national guidelines and regulation. Then it provides a simple "how to" guide for laboratories seeking to conform to internationally recognized standardization. Then most importantly, goes beyond the standards to establish some key determinants to success, which are interdependent on maintaining high quality standards, safety, and improved results in the IVF laboratory.

STANDARDS

International Standards and Regulatory Frameworks

International Organization for Standardization (ISO) 9001 (8) is the most widely used standard in ART clinics and involves the quality system of the whole organization. This standard covers the need for quality management and the provision of resources (both personnel and equipment), and a substantial section involves customer satisfaction and how to improve service. A more detailed overview of ISO 9001:2008 is presented in chapter 32 (9).

ISO 17025:2005, specifying general requirements for the competence of testing and calibration laboratories (10), is the main international standard for laboratory accreditation. It is based on the European norm (EN) 45001 (11), and was originally modeled on the corresponding ISO/International Electrotechnical Commission (IEC) guide (12). The scope of this standard is specialized and is aimed toward assurance of methods and includes both the quality system and the technical part of the activities such as validations of methods, QA, QC, and calibration of equipment. In 1997, Fertility Centre Scandinavia became the first IVF laboratory to be accredited according to this international standard (13).

With an increase in laboratory accreditation it was evident that ISO 17025, aiming to standardize testing and calibration laboratories could not fully accommodate and cover the complexities of a medical testing laboratory. The ISO 15189, on medical laboratories, particular requirements for quality and competence, was issued to aid the accreditation of methods used in medical testing. It was first issued in 2003 with the current second edition issued in 2007 (14). It is used for the accreditation of medical laboratories and brings together the quality system requirements of ISO 9001 and the competency requirements of ISO 17025, and addresses the specific needs of medical laboratories.

Most medical laboratories in Europe are accredited according to ISO 15189:2007 or ISO 17025:2005. There are differences between the two laboratory standards with the ISO 15189 focusing on patient outcome without downgrading the need for accuracy, and emphasizes not only the quality of the measurement, but the total service provided by a medical lab. The language and terms are familiar to the medical profession, and it highlights important features of pre- and post-investigational issues while addressing ethics and the information needs of the medical laboratory. ISO 15189:2007 addresses the need for equivalency of quality management systems and competency requirements between laboratories. The need for this becomes more obvious at a time when potential and actual patients are increasingly mobile—the systems to collect medical data on these patients must be standardized independently from their location.

IVF laboratories located in the EU are required to adhere to the Directive on setting standards of quality and safety for the donation, procurement, testing, processing, preservation, storage, and distribution of human tissues and cells, usually called the European Union Tissue and Cells Directive (EUTCD) (15). European Society of Human Reproduction and Embryology (ESHRE) have issued a position paper on the EUTCD (16), and it is important to underline that regardless of ESHRE's recommendations, each EU country interprets the directive differently. However, one part of the EUTCD is very clear; the demand for a quality system. The directive states that "Tissue establishments shall take all necessary measures to ensure that the quality system includes at least the following documentation; standard operating procedures (SOPs), guidelines training and reference manuals." Certainly, by achieving accreditation to either ISO 15189 or ISO 17025 this demand will be fulfilled along with several other demands of the directive.

Joint Commission (JC, USA) and Joint Commission International (JCI) accredit and certify hospitals and health care organizations worldwide. It is a non-profit organization with the main focus on improving patient safety. JCI have a range of standards including Accreditation Standards for Clinical Laboratories (17). The World Health Organization (WHO) in collaboration with JC and JCI has developed a core program for patient safety solutions. It brings attention to patient safety and practices, which can help reduce risks involved with medical procedures. The most recent advice builds on "nine patient safety solutions" including patient identification, and recommend actions in four basic categories: (*i*) Risk Management and Quality Management Systems; (*ii*) Policies, Protocols, and Systems; (*iii*) Staff Training and Competence; and (*iv*) Patient Involvement (18).

The Clinical and Laboratory Standards Institute (CLSI) is another global not-for-profit standards development organization, and while mostly applicable to the United States, the CLSI standards are of great help for improving laboratory quality and safety (for further information, see chap. 2 (19,20)).

Other standards that might be less suitable for the IVF laboratory are the Good Manufacturing Practice/Good Laboratory Practice guides (GMP/GLP). These standards apply to research laboratories and the pharmaceutical production industry. They include demands on the laboratory facilities that will be difficult to meet with the limited resources that many IVF clinics face (21,22).

In addition to these quality system–driven standards, there are many IVF-specific standards and guidelines including WHO laboratory manual for the examination and processing of human sperm (23) and the Alpha/ESHRE consensus on embryo assessment (24). The Alpha/ESHRE consensus group is currently working on a consensus for cryopreservation establishing key performance indices (KPIs) for both slow freezing and vitrification. These will be published in due time by Human Reproduction and Alpha.

National/Regional Standards

While the ISO standards cover the fundamental needs for quality systems in the IVF laboratory, many regions and countries have specific guidelines, laws, and regulations. It is important to note that while some of these regulatory frameworks are standards and others are license requirements or law, when it comes to inspections and audits the laboratory is expected to conform.

Europe

With the EUTCD in place all IVF laboratories handling gametes and embryos are required to have a quality system and fulfill the demands of the directive and the national interpretation of it. This has led to most of the IVF laboratories in the EU holding or working toward formal accreditation to ISO 15189 or ISO 17025. In the United Kingdom, where all IVF clinics are required to be licensed by the Human Fertilization and Embryology Authority (HFEA) (25), there are further guidelines regulating the IVF laboratory as detailed in the HFEA code of practice (HFEA CoP) (26). Specifically the CoP contains demands for risk management, sample identification, and embryology staffing as described later in this chapter.

Australia and New Zealand

In Australia, the Reproductive Technology Accreditation Committee (RTAC) undertakes the licensing of IVF clinics. While the RTAC code of practice (7) is far less comprehensive than its U.K. counterpart, it contains critical criteria with focus on risk management, staffing, and sample identification and further guidelines covering the requirement of a quality management system. In addition to the code, Fertility Society Australia issues technical bulletins, which act as educational communication to all units and certifying bodies, offering advice and guidance. It is not enforceable (27). In New Zealand RTAC licensing is optional, but most clinics hold an RTAC licence. While the majority of IVF clinics hold an ISO 9001 certification, most are also accredited by NATA to ISO 15189 for some of the crucial methods such as semen analysis. However, very few laboratories hold ISO 15189 accreditation for the overall IVF laboratory processes.

Asia

At the time of publication, there were few, if any IVF laboratories in Asia, accredited according to ISO 15189 or similar standards and the laboratory accreditation was not widespread. However, there is an increased interest and need for standardization. Many private IVF centers throughout the region have ISO 9001 certification.

Memorial Hospital in Istanbul, Turkey was recently the first IVF laboratory in the region to achieve ISO 15189 accreditation (acknowledging that Turkey is a transcontinental country at the junction of Europe and Asia).

China has implemented rather strict guidelines for IVF clinics as set by the Ministry of Health in 2001. Up until

2008/2009 all clinics had to be approved by the Ministry of Health before starting; however, now the Ministry of Health entrusts their offices at the provincial level to do the audit and registration. For the embryologist training there are specific rules; however, there are no specific demands for standards in the laboratory itself.

In 2005, India introduced National Guidelines for Accreditation, Supervision, and Regulation of ART Clinics; however, these are yet to be legislated (28). The guidelines cover issues such as staff qualifications and laboratory procedures, but have no formal demand for quality systems. The PNDT Act (Prenatal Diagnostic Techniques) prohibits sex selection pre- and post conception. ISO certification is not widespread for individual IVF clinics but larger hospitals that have IVF departments are commonly ISO certified.

In Japan the Japanese Gynaecology Society has guidelines for IVF clinics, but they don't comprehensively cover the laboratory or the need for quality systems.

In Singapore the Ministry of Health has recently introduced stringent licensing requirements for assisted re production services in private hospitals and clinics. It covers demands for QC, facilities, embryology training, and sample identification (29).

Middle East

ART in many of the Muslim countries is covered by a number of fatwas (religious opinion concerning an Islamic law issued by an Islamic scholar) (30). The first fatwa relating to ART was issued in 1980 by His Excellency Gad El Hak Ali Gad El Hak, the Grand Sheikh of Egypt's Al-Azhar University. The core requirement is that the couple is married and the use of donor sperm or oocytes is prohibited (31).

Apart from the fatwas, there are very little regulations and standards for IVF laboratories in the Middle East and few laboratories are formally accredited to international standards, but many larger hospitals hold JCI and ISO accreditations.

Saudi Arabia has a comprehensive fatwa containing demands for documented SOPs, safeguarding of sample ID and prevention of mix-ups etc. The Ministry of Health has started setting standards and some centers have had their first audit by the authorities (30).

The United Arab Emirates (UAE) has recently introduced laws regulating IVF and the laboratories have recently gone through a first round of audits by the UAE health authority. The law includes demands on the embryology staff degrees and training, laboratory facilities, documented protocols and procedures and QC. For a brief period the regulations prohibited cryopreservation of embryos; however, this prohibition has now been partially lifted (32).

Latin America

The Latin American Network of Assisted Reproduction (RED) covers most of the Latin American clinics. While membership in the organization is voluntary, over 90% of clinics participate in the data collection, accreditation, and continuous professional development training programs. The accreditation includes external audits and follows the Standard Rules for the Accreditation of the ART center and it's laboratories of Embryology and Andrology (33) involving among other QC, KPIs, staff requirements, equipment, and materials.

Russia

There are no IVF laboratories in Russia accredited to ISO 15189. However, with the growing interest in IVF tourism and with the prospect of attracting patients from Europe, many clinics in Russia are working toward implementing European standards. So far only the AVA PETER clinic in St Petersburg holds an ISO 9001:2008 certification. Russia has limited standards and regulations for IVF and separates between state and private clinics. The state clinics are required to report data to the Ministry of Health, but there are no formal audits and so implementation of the rules is not widespread.

North America

In 2004, the Canadian Federal Government passed the Assisted Human Reproduction Act and created the Federal agency Assisted Reproduction Canada (34,35). The Act is divided into prohibited activities, including cloning, non-medically-indicated sex selection, and the payment of donors, and controlled activities, covering the performance of all procedures involved in IVF. The Act was challenged by the province of Quebec leading to a lengthy complicated legal battle ending with the Supreme Court of Canada ruling that much of the AHR Act was unconstitutional (36). In the meantime, Quebec had passed an Act of its own, and is also so far the only province or territory to provide full public funding for IVF. The Canadian Fertility and Andrology Society has recently ratified comprehensive professional standards concerning the laboratory activities involved in IVF prepared by its ART Lab Special Interest Group, as well as training and competency requirements that include continuing professional development of all ART laboratory scientists (37).

In the United States, the practice committee of the American Society for Reproductive Medicine and the practice committee of the society for assisted reproductive technology have issued guidelines for human embryology and andrology laboratories (38,39). A comprehensive overview of the U.S. standards and regulations for IVF laboratories can be found in chapter 2 (20).

HOW TO ACHIEVE LABORATORY ACCREDITATION

It is important to underline that in no way are all the quality standards independent of each other. ISO 17025:2005 is basically the same standard as ISO 15189:2007 with the major difference being the medical laboratory terminology used in 15189. The quality system requirements of the both are based on ISO 9001:2000. As a result of this, laboratories within ISO 9001 certified clinics seeking accreditation will have major parts of the system requirements of the two laboratory standards already in place. It could be recommended that the first step toward accreditation is to get the clinic certified to ISO 9001; further details on this subject are found in chapter 30 (9). The requirements discussed throughout the continuation of this part of the chapter will be for laboratory accreditation to ISO 15189 or ISO 17025 on top of (over and above) what is already required for certification to ISO 9001. For example, scope, organization and document control are found in all the standards and many of the demands are the same, but the requirements discussed in these sections below will be what ISO 15189 has (hereinafter referred to as the standard) in addition to what has already been implemented through ISO 9001 certification. Correlation tables for ISO 9001, 17025, and 15189 can be found in the standards themselves.

GETTING STARTED

The first step toward an accreditation is to make sure that everyone in the organization wants to achieve the same goal. The full understanding of how everyone benefits from an accreditation will make the process easier. A good way to ensure this is to have staff meetings throughout the process and involve all staff from the very beginning The most frequent mistake organizations make when trying to implement a QC system is not to involve everyone. Divide the project into smaller sections and give out personal responsibilities enabling all staff to be included in the preparation work. This will also make the implementation easier. A suggestion of how to divide the project and put together a "task force" is given in Appendix 1.

A good way to make sure that all demands in the standard are covered is to make up a table of contents—using the ISO 15189:2007 standard table of contents as a template (Table 3.1). An assessment can then be made of what needs to be added to the quality manual and other documentation. It is important to note while the standards have demands for management structure, internal audit, or document control, the laboratory standards have some more specified demands not found in ISO 9001 and these need to be added to the specific procedures.

METHODS AND SOPs

Examination Procedures (ISO 15189:2007; 5.5)

The methods and procedures we use in the embryology laboratory and their efficacy have a direct impact on the pregnancy results of the clinic. It is therefore hugely important that we standardize these methods and make sure that they are reproducible. In simple words, an ICSI should be done in the same way using the same disposals and equipment by all embryologists in the lab, assuring that an ICSI done by embryologist A on a Monday is performed in

Table 3.1 Table of Contents ISO 15189:2007

1 Scope
2 Normative references
3 Terms and definitions
4 Management requirement
   4.1 Organization and management
   4.2 Quality management system
   4.3 Document control
   4.4 Review of contracts
   4.5 Examination by referral laboratories
   4.6 External services and supplies
   4.7 Advisory services
   4.8 Resolution of complaints
   4.9 Identification and control of nonconformities
   4.10 Corrective action
   4.11 Preventive action
   4.12 Continual improvement
   4.13 Quality and technical records
   4.14 Internal audits
   4.15 Management review
5 Technical requirements
   5.1 Personnel
   5.2 Accommodation and environmental conditions
   5.3 Laboratory equipment
   5.4 Pre-examination procedures
   5.5 Examination procedures
   5.6 Assuring quality of examination procedures
   5.7 Post-examination procedures
   5.8 Reporting of results

exactly the same way and with the same level of skill as the ICSI done by embryologist B on a Friday. Assuring the correct methods is done through several steps. First we need to make sure that the processes and methods we use are correct and up to date with the latest developments in ART. Hence, a clear starting point should be a literature search, together with the knowledge gained from workshops, external training, and visits to other clinics. Once the details of the methods have been agreed between the embryology team members they need to be documented. A document describing a method or process used in a laboratory is commonly called SOP. A good SOP should follow a set format and ISO 15189: 2007; 5.5.3 contains a very good guide for SOP's layouts. The SOP title should be followed by a short clinical description of the method. The analytic principles need to include a theoretical description of the method and review of current literature. The SOP should outline the competence demands on embryologists performing the process. Collection and handling of gametes and embryos should include the sampling procedures and the physical environmental issues such as temperature. Remember that all variables in the SOP, such as those referring to the measurement of temperature, have to give a precise range, followed by a description of how the temperature is measured, the accuracy of the thermometer, and how often and how it is calibrated. There should be clear descriptions of how the sample is labeled and, considering the risks associated with the work in an IVF laboratory (40), the marking should be logical and clear, to eliminate completely the risk of mixing of samples (for further details refer to the section, "Sample Identification, Witnessing, and Prevention of Misidentification"). The description of the procedural steps should be written in an uncomplicated way so that they can be easily followed by any new member of staff under supervision.

All equipment used for the method should be listed with references to handling instructions and calibration protocols. Any safety routines and occupational hazards involved should be discussed and clearly known by the embryologists. References to any textbooks or publications concerning the method should be included last.

The standard demands that the procedures used should meet the requirements of the users of the laboratory service, preferably using methods that have been published in established/authoritative textbooks, peer-reviewed texts, or journals. If in-house methods are used, these need to be appropriately validated for the intended use and fully documented by the laboratory.

When the SOP is written it needs to e-communicated to all members of the embryology team, and it is important to allow them to comment, give feedback, and suggest changes before the document is formally issued and implemented. The way to check that all embryologists follow the new SOP is to undertake audits and it is suggested to audit all processes three months after the issue of the SOP. If the audit findings include discrepancies between the written SOP and the embryologists' hands-on-working procedure, then either the SOP needs to be changed to reflect the actual hands on procedure, or the member of staff needs to be re-trained and reminded of the importance of following the agreed SOP. No embryologists can insist on doing things "their own way" in a standardized high quality IVF laboratory.

Once the SOPs are fully implemented and the audits show that we have achieved the required reproducibility, then we need to ask: is it working? Is the method we agreed upon successful? The standard calls this validation and it is the process, which confirms that the techniques and methods used in the IVF laboratory are suitable for the production of good embryos, viable pregnancies, and live birth. All methods have to be validated regularly, and the SOP should include information on how often and how validations are done. The EUCTD includes demands for validation and in the United Kingdom HFEA CoP (26) requires that all processes in the IVF laboratory should be validated. Some methods and techniques used in the laboratory can be difficult to validate, and it is acceptable to use retrospective analysis of fertilization, damage, and pregnancy rates to validate ICSI and IVF. Appropriate validation of new techniques can become very difficult when considering the sample size needed to prove a null hypothesis or small increase in pregnancy rates. An accurate validation of a new culture medium will need hundreds of patients in each study group. Adding to the complexity of validation practice is the fine line between validation and research and questions are raised regarding the need for ethical approval to undertake validations (41). However, it is highly recommended to regularly validate other practices in the lab such as changes of osmolarity during preparation of dishes, temperature fluctuation during denudation, and temperature distribution in incubators. Validation of temperature in a culture medium in different types of dishes on all heated stages in the laboratory should confirm the appropriate range of surface temperature of the heated stage.

HANDLING OF GAMETES AND EMBRYOS

Pre- and Post-Examination Procedures (ISO 15189:2007; 5.4, 5.7)

The standard has specific demands on how the sample, that is, gametes and embryos should be collected and stored. The samples have to be correctly and safely identified and any laws regulating the identification of patient samples have to be taken into account (see further in the section "Identification, Witnessing, and Prevention of Misidentification"). The sample should be accompanied with a written, standardized request of what procedure the sample should be used for. It is a common occurrence that the requests for treatment are unclear and that couples who could have had normal IVF end up having ICSI due to poor communication. Senior embryologists with considerable experience in assessing sperm samples are more suitable to make the final decision on IVF or ICSI in conjunction with the couple on the day of treatment when the sample has been washed, then the referring doctor who takes the decision of whether IVF or ICSI based solely on a semen analysis report. Other procedures where clear requests are crucial are frozen embryo transfer cycles to assure that the embryo is thawed on the correct day. For collection of sperm, the date and time of collection should be noted by the patient and date and time of receipt should be recorded by the laboratory.

Usually the procedures for collecting samples, pre- and post-examination procedures are documented in the applicable laboratory SOPs for sperm processing and oocyte collection. However, it is important to include the specific demands of the standards for these procedures and the documentation of them.

LABORATORY SHEETS AND REPORTS

Reporting Results (ISO 15189:2007; 5.8)

The details from assessments of gametes and embryos we document in the laboratory on lab sheets are referred to in the standard as reports. The reporting of results should always be accurate, clear, unambiguous, and objective. This requires that the lab sheets be standardized and follow a set format. They should be filled out in a neat manner, no scribbling allowed. All entries and comments on a lab sheet should be accompanied by a date and signature. For sperm assessment, sources of errors and uncertainty of measurements should be stated and properly calculated for each method. Formal reports, such as seminal fluid analysis reports should also be checked and signed off by the senior andrologist/embryologist before being issued.

Many laboratories have computerized databases and enter the information from the lab sheets to the database. It is important to understand that the handwritten lab sheet is considered source data and therefore needs to be archived correctly, not destroyed after computer entry. If the laboratory wants to go paper free it has to indeed be paper free and allow for direct data entry on to the computer without an in-between paper sheet. When considering the need for signatures and witnessing, a complete paperless IVF laboratory could be difficult to create.

THE EMBRYOLOGY LABORATORY

Facilities (ISO 15189:2007; 5.2)

A laboratory needs to ensure that the environmental conditions of the laboratory are suitable for the safe handling of gametes and embryos and do not invalidate the results or adversely affect the quality of any procedure. In simple words, this means that the IVF laboratory has to be designed in such a way that the outcome of any procedure is optimal and not affected by environmental parameters.

Live birth results following IVF treatment vary from country to country, clinic to clinic, and often within a clinic from month to month. It is a general consensus that it is the patient demographics, such as age and cause of infertility are the main factors affecting the outcome. Considering a varying population of patients, it is of great importance that parameters in the laboratory are stable. Defining the environment and setting limits for acceptable working conditions will help in reducing variables and result in the patient being the only factor that varies. Exactly what this encompasses will always be down to interpretation and international, national or regional regulations; however, the standard has some clear demands and some environmental factors cannot be ignored.

General Laboratory Layout

Theater for oocyte retrieval and embryo transfer should be in close vicinity to the laboratory. The laboratory layout should further make sure safe handling of gametes and embryos; small crowded laboratories impose a significant risk for accidents resulting in loss of gametes and embryos.

The laboratory should never double as an embryologist office. There needs to be a minimal allowance of paper in the laboratory as this can increase the amount of particles in the air. Therefore, only patient records necessary for ongoing treatment should be kept in the laboratory. Also, laboratory is not the place for cardboards as these involve a high risk of fungus infections. Furthermore, the laboratory is not a storage room for disposables; only a weekly stock of disposables should be kept inside the lab, further storage can be managed elsewhere. The equipment held in the laboratory should be limited to the absolute necessary; again the laboratory is not a storage room for old lab equipment.

Access Rules

The laboratory should have limited access ensured by use of locks, swipe card, or other access control. It should also hold documentation verifying who has access to the laboratory. There should be documented and implemented rules for what is required for access to the laboratory including demands for change of clothes and shoes, the use of hair cover and masks and washing of hands. While some embryologists insist that changing clothes and covering hair are of no importance, it is important to understand that embryology and handling of gametes and embryos are sterile processes with a need to protect the samples from microbes and contaminants. The correct degree of cleanliness is impossible to reach if the embryologists are using their own clothes or only minimal cover such as laboratory coats. Best practice is to change clothes and preferably use scrubs, which are made of low-lint, no shedding material; cotton is high lint and not advisable. Many embryologists complain that these types of scrubs are uncomfortable and that they will not use them as cotton is comfortable, but it is important to understand that we are not embryologists to be comfortable, we need to do what is best for gametes and embryos. Further all hair should be covered, and again some might see the cap as a fashion item looking much better if hair is allowed outside but they need to be reminded to tuck in all hair before entering the laboratory. Changing into clean room shoes comes without saying. Best practice is to have all-white shoes with white soles in the laboratory. This makes it easy to spot any spillage on them. Also, the rack for these shoes should be designed so that the shoes are hung up with soles facing out, allowing for daily inspection of the cleanliness of the shoes. If colored shoes are used outside the laboratory it will be easy to spot anyone who has forgotten to change shoes. Hands should be washed using a proper disinfectant soap before entering the laboratory. Furthermore, jewelry, nail polish, long fingernails, and perfumes should not be worn in the laboratory.

Health and Safety

The laboratory is required to ensure the safety of its entire staff. This includes providing an environment that minimizes the risk of transfer of any contagious contaminants through the use of class II bio-safety cabinets when handling unscreened patient materials.

Temperature

The optimal IVF laboratory temperature is a matter of great debate; however, it has to be defined to a limited range. Some embryologists argue that an elevated laboratory temperature benefits the embryos through reduced risk of cooling during transport from the incubator to the heated stage. However, high laboratory temperatures will provide a perfect environment for microbes and contaminants. All laboratory equipment is designed to operate in room temperature, usually defined as $22 \pm 2°C$ and unless the laboratory can show process verification at a different temperature this range will be the one demanded by the standard. A laboratory without temperature control cannot be accredited.

Light

The embryo is extremely sensitive to light exposure; however, there is a wide range of opinions on whether light in the laboratory or from microscopes will harm embryos or not. It has been very elegantly demonstrated in a large study on hamster and mouse embryos that cool fluorescent light increases the reactive oxygen species production and apoptosis in blastocysts and reduces the development of live-term fetuses (42). The embryos were handled under minimal light conditions and the test groups were exposed to 5–30 minutes of cool white, warm white, or midday sunlight. A 44% of blastocysts exposed to cool white light and transferred to recipients developed to term of pregnancy (day 19), compared with 73% in the control; 58% of blastocysts exposed to warm white light developed to term (day 19). When embryos were exposed to only one minute of sunlight only 25% of embryos developed to term with 35% resorbed. In the light of these findings best practice should be to have a dim light in the laboratory and close out any daylight.

Air Quality

Another area of great debate is the demands of clean air in the laboratory and this has also been affected by regional interpretation of the EUCTD. The standard requires that attention is paid to sterility and presence of dust and it is highly recommended that laboratories periodically monitor the particle count and presence of volatile organic compounds (VOCs) in the air together with microbial monitoring using blood agar settle plates to detect bacteria and Sabouraud dextrose agar (SAB) plates for detection of fungus. The plates should be exposed in key positions in the laboratory, theater, and treatment rooms for four hours. Acceptable limits are zero colonies inside the flow hoods or handling chambers and <10 colonies outside the hoods in the laboratory.

General Cleanliness

An IVF laboratory should always be clean and the laboratory standards demand that documented frequent cleaning procedures are implemented and that cleaning is confirmed by active signatures. The use of harsh detergents is not recommended and cleaning should be undertaken using 70% alcohol and sterile water or other products tested for embryology use such as Oosafe® (SparMED, Stenløse, Denmark) (43). Steam cleaners are suitable for the cleaning of floors.

CULTURE MEDIUM, DEVICES, AND DISPOSABLES

(ISO 15189:2007 4.6)

All devices used in ART, such as culture media and consumables, will affect the outcome of the treatment. First, the laboratory needs to decide what their own requirements for culture medium, oocyte collection needles, culture dishes etc. This includes limits in toxicity and results from mouse embryo assays for culture media, oocyte pickup needles, or plasticware. There is solid evidence that many of the devices and disposables we use in the embryology laboratory are indeed reprotoxic and it is our duty to make sure that we don't use items which will expose the embryos to stress (44). It is important to take into account any national, regional, or local regulation which applies. EUTCD stipulates that all devices which come in to contact with cells, gametes, or embryos need to be tested according to the EU devices directives (45,46) and be CE (Conformité Européenne) marked. The laboratory also has to define requirements for the safe transport of devices from supplier to the laboratory, and how they will be inspected when they arrive to ensure they meet the limits specified. For example there has to be a system to assure that the box containing the culture medium is still cold when it arrives. This can easily be done by inserting a temperature probe into the box upon arrival, or request that the medium provider pack a temperature data logger with the medium, which you can attach to your computer when the medium arrives and ascertain that the temperature inside has been constant and correct throughout the transport. Moreover, consumables then have to be verified before taken into use. Some laboratories choose to culture excess embryos or undertake sperm survival assays in new batches of culture medium; however, this type of verification is not demanded by the standard and could be argued if it is really necessary (for testing methods, see chap. 2) (20). If all the devices conform to the EU devices regulation they should already have been stringently tested. ISO 15189 only demands that the laboratory actively checks the test reports issued by the manufacturer and confirm that the report complies with their own limits for use.

When the devices have been accepted for use it is crucial that they are stored correctly to ensure their continued suitability for use. The laboratory has to safeguard correct storage by defining the exact storage environment. Limits for temperature in refrigerators and freezers are crucial and culture medium should be stored in a pharmaceutical refrigerator which assures constant temperature throughout, whereas a normal kitchen refrigerator is not acceptable (chap. 2). The environment in general storage rooms is also important as plasticware stored at high temperatures will not be suitable for use.

All purchased supplies, reagents, and consumables should be included in the laboratory inventory. Information in the inventory shall include LOT number (batch number), date of reception, and date taken into use. The inventory for equipment should include unique identification, date of arrival, date placed in service, last calibration or service, and periodicity of service and calibration. The laboratory is required to keep a list of approved suppliers and critically evaluate all suppliers on an annual basis.

The batch or LOT number of any device that comes into contact with a given patient's gametes or embryos needs to be recorded on that individual patient's records.

It is not appropriate to have a list of batches currently used in the lab and draw conclusions from this using date and make a guesswork of what device was used for what patient.

It is of great advantage to have a computerized case file system whereby each cycle has a batch record page attached. This page includes a full list of culture media and laboratory-ware and the batches in use, and with a simple mouse-click, marks what materials were used in every step of the cycle, from culture media down to pipette tips.

EQUIPMENT

(ISO 15189:2007; 5.3)

A laboratory should have all the equipment needed to assure the best service. The standards require a documented program for preventive maintenance and it is the responsibility of the laboratory manager to regularly monitor and ensure appropriate service, calibration, and function of all equipment. All equipment used in an accredited laboratory have to be clearly labeled with a unique identifier, date of last calibration or service, and date or expiration criteria as to when re-calibration/service is due. Together with this, all equipment used should be included in an equipment record containing information listed in ISO 15189:2007; 5.3.4. There should be clearly documented processes for validation of equipment function before it is taken into use. The standard of equipment used in IVF laboratories is generally very high, but even the best equipment can fail and not function optimally if it is not appropriately maintained. All embryologists should have solid knowledge of how to operate all equipment and there should be written implemented procedures in place for action taken if there happens to be an equipment failure. Crucial equipment such as incubators should always be connected to auto-dialers enabling staff to promptly respond to any faults out of hours.

Equipment should be verified by test runs; for example, before a new centrifuge is taken into use in the laboratory, a series of mock sperm preparations have to be undertaken and documented.

MONITORING AND TRACEABILITY

(ISO 15189:2007; 5.2, 5.3, 5.5)

Chapter 2 presents a detailed report of monitoring of equipment and laboratory parameters and traceability of reference equipment (20).

Monitoring of KPIs

Most of the clinics have a quality system in place to monitor KPIs. Similar to the monitoring of laboratory environmental parameters, each clinic has to agree on documented limits of performance. Usually, when monitoring parameters such as live birth, clinical pregnancy, and fertilization, there is no upper limit; however, a lower limit is necessary as well as documented plans for immediate action whenever a KPI falls under the agreed limit.

The KPIs essential for monitoring in connection with the laboratory include, but are not limited to, fertilization rates for IVF and ICSI, damage rates for ICSI, survival of embryos after thawing, and pregnancy results from embryo transfer. These KPIs should be monitored for the whole laboratory and for each embryologist and doctor. It is important to underline the importance of confidentiality when monitoring individual performance, taking into account the need for training of any embryologist falling under the given limit, but not ignoring the stress and decrease in self-confidence this can lead to. All members of staff need to understand that the monitoring is not a way of punishing people, but to assure that all embryologists perform to the same high standard, minimizing variables. Another important outcome of individual performance monitoring is to identify persons with exceptionally high results so that others can learn more and thereby increase the overall success.

QUALITY ASSURANCE

Assuring Quality (ISO 15189:2007; 5.6)

Quality assurance makes sure that you are doing the right thing in the right way and QC makes sure that what you have done is what you expected. In short, quality assurance is process oriented and QC is product oriented. When discussing QA/QC it is easy to get confused; however the terminology is not important, what is important is that the laboratory has control mechanisms in place to assure that they perform according to the SOPs and to the highest standard. ISO 15189:2007 demands that the laboratory has QC and QA systems in place for monitoring of the validity of the methods used. This includes the demand of internal and external controls and inter/intra laboratory comparisons and validations. The laboratory is required to determine the uncertainty of results. This can be difficult with a subjective parameter such as embryo scoring; however, it can easily be done for the assessment of sperm. Through assessment of a series of sperm samples by all laboratory staff involved in the preparation of sperm, a coefficient of variance (CV%) can be calculated, usually resulting in a 10–15% variance.

The standard also demands that all embryologists/andrologists assess sperm samples and photos or movies of embryos on a regular basis, usually at least every three months. It is the responsibility of the laboratory manager to document the results from these comparisons and calculate variations and address any deviance. To collect samples and photos and arrange these types of intra-laboratory comparisons takes time and over and above this, the standards also demand that the laboratory participates in interlaboratory comparisons. A laboratory can share photos of embryos and samples of sperm with other centers and set up an interlaboratory comparison scheme, although the standard clearly states that self-developed programs like this should not be used when organized external schemes are available. In the United Kingdom, most laboratories participate in the U.K.National External Quality Assessment Service (UKNEQAS) andrology scheme, which uses the DVD/video of sperm for motility assessment (47).

A web based interlaboratory comparison scheme is run by Dr James Stanger and includes schemes for assessment of all stages of human pre-implantation embryos, sperm morphology and concentration, and ultrasound measurement of follicles (www.fertaid.com). The scheme provides monthly assessments of embryos and sperm and allows the laboratory manager to use the information for intra-laboratory comparison. As each of the different schemes has some 200–300 participants around the world the intra-laboratory comparison scheme provides a solid reference for the laboratory management to implement corrective actions when deviations are found (48). This comparison program is in substantial agreement with the ISO/IEC guide 43–1 which is a requirement by the standard (49).

PATIENT CONTACT

Advisory Services (15189:2007 4.7)

In most IVF clinics the embryologists have none or very little contact with the patient and also very little input in the exact treatment options. In an accredited laboratory the standard demands that the laboratory actively provides advice on choice of treatment and clarification of any laboratory outcomes. As discussed previously, some decisions such as fertilizing oocytes using IVF or ICSI should be taken by a senior embryologist rather than a doctor. The ultimate approach is to have the couple/patient sit down with the embryologist after oocyte and sperm collection for a "post-OPU chat." This gives the opportunity for the embryologist to discuss with the couple issues such as the quality and numbers of sperm and oocytes, and advise them on the best procedure ahead. This short chat should also include reminding the patient of risk and success; that is, there is always a risk for failed fertilization, failed cleavage, or failed blastocyst development. If the couple has been reminded of these risks it makes it somewhat less stressful to make a call to them to report a failed fertilization. ISO 15189 even demands that the embryologist should take part in the clinical rounds (i.e., meeting with the patients) enabling advice and guidance on embryology in general and in individual cases.

AUDITS

(ISO 15189:2007 4.14)

Audits can be internal or external, vertical or horizontal, or process oriented or system oriented. Therefore, it is easy to get confused and caught up in terminology, and to miss out on the great opportunity as audits are to improve the system and our service to patients. To find nonconformities at an audit is not bad, it is proof that the system is working and we are capable of recognizing our weaknesses and faults and ready to learn and improve on them. For general internal audit principles, see chap. 32 (9).

Internal Audits

The laboratory standards are more precise in what exactly should come out of an audit and what is needed for a correct audit process. When preparing, writing, and implementing internal audit procedures ISO 15189 is very precise and elaborate on what exactly is needed. In relation to ISO 9001 internal audit demands, the laboratory standards are more stringent with how often internal audits need to be undertaken and requires all accredited methods and procedures to be audited on an annual basis.

External Audits

If the laboratory aims to seek formal accreditation to ISO 15189, the National Authority for Conformity Assessment performs the external audits. A formal accreditation is always advantageous, but in many countries this option is not available and as it is a rather pricey process, some laboratories choose to state that they adhere to the standard without formal accreditation.

When a laboratory is ready to be formally accredited they need to apply for accreditation and the national authority will assess whether they have the appropriate expertise to perform the audit. If not, they can seek help from other members of the European Cooperation for Accreditation who has the appropriate experienced auditors. Together with the application, the laboratory has to supply evidence of a fully compliant quality system and it is essential that all methods, for which accreditation is sought, have gone through a series of internal audits. Result documentation from these audits is supplement to the application. The accreditation body then arranges a preaudit to assess the readiness of the laboratory and pending the outcome of this pre-audit an accreditation audit will be arranged. When the accreditation audit has been done, the lead auditor or any technical experts can only recommend that the laboratory be awarded accreditation. This recommendation is then passed on to the board of the accreditation body, which will decide if the laboratory is to be awarded accreditation.

BEYOND THE STANDARDS

While the embryology laboratory could be seen as any other clinical medical laboratory, there are some major differences to do with the delicacy of the samples it handles. While a mistake in the day-to-day pathology laboratory mostly can be rectified by re-sampling, a mistake in the embryology laboratory can lead to major irreparable trauma for the patients (40). Therefore, it is of great importance that we acknowledge these differences and implement processes which help safeguard us from incidents. While some national and regional guidelines acknowledge these differences, IVF laboratories worldwide need to understand and address this. There are three major areas concerning the safeguarding of the patients' gametes and embryos, but also aiming to protect the embryologists working in the laboratory: (*i*) training of embryologists to make sure that the staff handling these delicate samples and undertaking the complex IVF processes are properly trained; (*ii*) appropriate sample identification processes, and (*iii*) implementation of risk management processes.

Training and Accreditation of Embryologists

Personnel (ISO 15189:2007; 5.1)

Clinical embryology is a highly skilled profession and the main contributor to IVF success is the skills and knowledge of the embryologists. When considering the impact the training of embryologists has on results it is evident that there is a need for formalized training programs in every clinical IVF laboratory.

When looking at the international ISO standards, the requirement for personnel is not clearly defined. They state that the laboratories need to define all personnel groups within the laboratory in respect of education and experience and the areas of responsibility should be clearly outlined together with duties in the documented job descriptions. The quality manual should include documentation on how proof of competence is issued and how introduction of new personnel is performed, and the management of the laboratory should formulate goals for each member of staff with respect to further education and training. These goals should be assessed and discussed at annual appraisals, which should be documented but kept confidential. There should be clearly documented procedures in place for the introduction and training of new staff and the re-introduction of staff after long periods of absence or leave.

In recent years there has been an increased focus on the training and accreditation/certification of clinical embryologists. In the United Kingdom, there has been a formal training program in place for embryologists since 1995 through Association of Clinical Embryologists (ACE) (50). The original program included a minimum of two years and has both practical and theoretical components. The current ACE certificate has to be completed within two to four years and involves a training log, which lists all the practical elements and a training manual, which involves written work. There are 15 modules and they comprise short answer questions and case reports. Apart from the essential IVF components such as sperm, oocytes, fertilization, and embryos the modules also include regulation, health and safety, equipment, and quality management (50). Trainees have to submit their work on a six-monthly basis and then they have a two to three hour viva at the end by an external assessor. If the certificate is not awarded within four years then the candidate essentially fails. After attaining the ACE certificate, embryologists follow a clear career pathway including gaining certification from the Association of Clinical Sciences (ACS; state registration and membership of the Royal Collage of Pathologists). ACE also provides an online Continual Professional Development scheme. In October 2011, ACE issued a consultation paper on the future workforce of the embryology laboratory (51), which outlines the future career pathway in embryology. In the future the embryologists training will include a Master of Science in Clinical Sciences, where embryology will follow the cellular sciences pathway. Students will combine theoretical university-based teaching at the University of Nottingham with 10–25 work-based placements over three years.

In 2008, ESHRE introduced a certification for embryologists with the aim to certify competence of clinical embryologists working in IVF and to develop a formal recognition for embryologists (52). It provides three different pathways to certification: a fast-track where senior embryologists with experience at laboratory director level for at least 10 years are given certification through a grandfathering process, a regular track for senior level clinical embryologists, and a regular track for clinical embryologists. The trainee has to have a minimum of Bachelor of Science in Natural Sciences and be a member of ESHRE. The assessment includes a logbook outlining the procedures included in the training and the minimum cases done, and passing a multiple-choice examination. The steering group is also in the process of introducing a Continuous Embryology Education Credit system with the credits needed for three-yearly renewal of the certificate.

Canadian Fertility and Andrology Society recently issued guidelines for an applied training program and evaluation and development of competencies for ART laboratory professionals and will in the near future implement a formal certification/accreditation (37).

For a comprehensive overview of embryologist requirements in the United States see chapter 2 (20).

In Australia, the Scientists in Reproductive Technologies (SIRT) is in the process of formalizing embryology training with the aim for a future certification and continuous professional development system.

With the U.K. career development pathway being available for U.K. embryologists only and the ESHRE certification at the time of publication available only for European embryologists, there is still a need for clinics to find ways of formalizing training for their embryologists. Every clinic should have documented training procedures clearly stating the minimum of supervised procedures a trainee has to undertake before being signed off for independent work. For the ESHRE certification this includes 50 procedures of each of OPU, Semen analysis and preparation, insemination, ICSI, zygote and embryo evaluation, ET, cryopreservation of oocytes/embryos, and thawing of oocytes/embryos. Obviously the outcome of those procedures needs to be evaluated too and the trainees have to meet the set KPIs of the clinic to be approved. To assure the theoretical component, that the trainee knows why, and not only how, it is suggested that essays set on subjects such as preimplantation genetic diagnosis and embryo development are included along with a small examination. It is also crucial to fulfill the need for continued professional development, allowing embryologists to attend conferences and workshops and to participate in research.

Sample Identification, Witnessing, and Prevention of Misidentification

One of the most crucial tasks in the IVF lab is to assure the correct identity (ID) of gametes and embryos. Over the years there have been numerous reports of misidentification resulting at best in a cancelled cycle if the mistake is identified before embryo transfer, in tragedy if realized after the embryo transfer or indeed birth. These errors are generally the result of trained personnel not following the known procedure for reasons such as distraction, tiredness, or being rushed (53,54). Alternatively, it is caused by poorly written or nonexisting policies and protocols (Active Failure vs Latent Condition). The solution to misidentification is the development of robust identification procedures, which are risk assessed (see further "Risk Management").

The EU tissue directive includes demands for appropriate sample identification with the core being a unique identifier for each sample. However, the most stringent guidelines involving safe sample identification procedures are provided by the HFEA CoP (26). In the United Kingdom it is a licensing requirement to have robust ID systems (Mandatory Requirement T71, HFEA CoP) and all IVF laboratories have to put in place processes to ensure that no mismatches of gametes or embryos or identification errors occur. With this comes a demand for double witnessing of the identification at all critical pints of the IVF laboratory process. The witnessing has to be signed at the time of the checked step and records must be kept in each patient's case file. Together with this license requirement the guidelines stipulate that all samples of gametes and embryos be labeled with at least the patient's name and a unique identifier. Most clinics interpret this as using the surname and a clinic or cycle-specific couple identifying a number such as couple number. It is important to note that a patient's name or date of birth is not a unique identifier. The witnessing is mandatory and required every time gametes or embryos changes vessel (dish or tube) and the person checking should have full understanding of the process they are witnessing, allowing only clinic staff named on the HFEA license to undertake the check. At semen sample hand-over, oocyte retrieval and embryo transfer the patient is required as an active participant in the identification. Identification checks can also be electronic with several witnessing systems available for embryology purposes. The most commonly used are based on bar codes (Matcher; fertqms.com, Trusty; optimalivf.com.au, Ferti Proof™; mtg-de.com) or using radio frequency technology (RI Witness™, research-instruments.com). The advantages of automated systems are that their accuracy is not affected by lack of concentration or poor protocols (54), and they have a significantly lower error rate than human error (0.001% compared with 1–3%) (55). So by introducing electronic witnessing we can possibly reduce errors in misidentification and potentially add an extra level of patient safety (55,56). But at the same time it is important to underline that all the current electronic witnessing systems are based on some type of sticker being attached to the tubes and dishes and mistakes can certainly occur in printing and labeling. Moreover, while the systems are not fail proof, they are expensive and some are bulky taking up a substantial space. The development of electronic witnessing systems for IVF is only at its infancy and the technology will more than likely be refined in the future.

In addition to the HFEA CoP, which is IVF specific, there are several standards and recommendations on the subject of patient and sample identification. The CLSI guideline on Accuracy in Patient and Sample Identification (56) describes the essential components of processes and systems, which needs to be implemented for accurate patient and sample identification. It covers the whole process from the pre-examination phase to the reporting of results underlining the importance of staff training, risk assessment, and the use of unique identifiers and relates to both manual and electronic systems. The previously mentioned "Nine patient safety solutions" from WHO/JCI have patient identification at its core (18). The ISO standards also have demands of correct simple labeling; however, they offer little information on safe solutions.

There are certainly huge advantages with the use of manual double witnessing, but there is always a slight risk that a procedure like this can cause mistakes, as we cannot double the embryologist workforce. One major source of incidents in the IVF laboratory is insufficient staffing, and to be interrupted while working with embryos can have disastrous consequences. In a busy IVF lab setting, scientists need to switch repeatedly between the patients' material they are working on to the patients' material they are being asked to check (57,58). In practice, the principle operator interrupts their workflow to locate a "witness" and the "witness" is interrupted from their own task to carry out the double check. Daniel Brison (59) estimated that, in a well-staffed IVF lab, each embryologist was witnessing 15–20 other procedures in a morning on top of their own workload. Many laboratories today have very few embryologists, and with a witnessing routine in place this will not only increase the workload, it will also add a heightened risk of distraction when an embryologist has to interrupt others' work to get them to witness a certain step in the procedure. Moreover, human beings and systems under stress will underperform in rushed situations and stress is known to affect human performance in many sectors including the IVF laboratory. Most clinics have periods when patient throughput is increased without compensation in relation to staffing levels. Systematic overtime, overloaded work schedules, high cognitive loads, and chronic staff shortages contribute to error-inducing environments (60–62). But also other forms of stress such as inadequate training and lack of guidance have been identified as sources of identification errors (63).

When introducing a robust safe ID system in the laboratory, the best way of starting is to avoid re-inventing the wheel. Even if your laboratory is located outside the United Kingdom, the HFEA CoP section 18 provides a great guide of how to ensure that the correct gametes are mixed and right embryos transferred (26). To make it simple, the IVF laboratory has to have written protocols for witnessing and each step involved has to be risk assessed (documented). As a part of the standardization introduced in a laboratory there will be written SOPs and flow chart and it is easy to identify each step where a gamete or embryo changes tubes or dishes. Simply add a witnessing signature to the laboratory sheet to each of those steps (the procedure itself should already have a signature on the sheet). An exception to the witnessing requirements is the so-called "Forced Functions," for example when a clinic receives only one sperm sample on a given day, and so there will be a forced function when the sample is transferred from one tube to another. If the clinic takes use of this it has to be risk assessed.

With the first step in the process being reception of gametes, semen sample, or oocytes and the last step being embryo transfer, the HFEA CoP underlines the need for the patient to be involved in this crucial identification step. Here it is important to implement a process which involves positive patient identification, which is the foundation for error prevention (64). In simple words the embryologist will ask the patient to audibly read out his/her name and any other identifier you have chosen such as date of birth, and at the same time have a witness, the doctor or nurse, to confirm this positive identification step being done.

The witnessing action itself also needs to be done correctly. It should include three major components: (*i*) the ID labeled vessel which holds the gametes or embryos, (*ii*) the new vessel which the sample is being moved in to, labeled with the same ID, and (*iii*) the patient documentation, i.e. the laboratory sheet containing the full identification of the patient. In addition to these three components, the embryologist performing the "move" (principle operator) reads the name aloud and unique identifier loud from the sample vessel, the new vessel, and the laboratory sheet, followed by the witness reading aloud the same.

Other hugely important factors are the strength and quality of the identifier itself. The need for a strong unique identifier together with the name is paramount. With the date of birth being too weak and not considered unique, the clinic or laboratory needs to create a couple-specific identifying number such as a unit number or couple number. A patient-specific number such as medical records number is not advisable as the embryo mostly belongs to the couple, not one patient only. This identification, name, and couple number then need to be affixed to the vessel in a clear safe manner. The most widely used labeling is handwriting with a nontoxic pen. Usually the ID is written on the side of tubes and bottom of dishes (mirrored from the outside) to allow easy noticing. Printed stickers are also being used, however, it should be made clear that stickers contain glue and when placed in a humidified incubator this results in an increase of VOCs which in turn can be embryo toxic. Another way of labeling is etching the ID into the plastic using a small syringe, but scratching of plastic will also increase VOCs and can be embryo toxic. Moreover, the etched details appear very faint and cannot be considered safe from a clear witnessing point of view. Finally, the ID should always be affixed to the part of the vessel actually carrying the sample. Labeling the lid of a dish or a tube is not acceptable.

If a process involving gametes or embryos changing vessel several times during a short time period, such as sperm preparation or embryo freezing/thawing, then it can be acceptable to witness the whole area. For example, a laboratory preparing sperm can have multiple biosafety cabinets with one designated centrifuge and other equipment assigned to a specific defined work area. Note that each work area has to have a designated centrifuge and two samples cannot be centrifuged together if this approach is adapted. When a sample is being brought in to this area all tubes involved can be witnessed at the same time with the prospect that only one sample will be handled through the whole process from start to finish (Fig. 3.1). Obviously this process needs to be risk assessed if adapted.

Correct labeling together with witnessing procedures will help minimizing the risk of misidentification, but it is also absolutely imperative that only one couple's samples

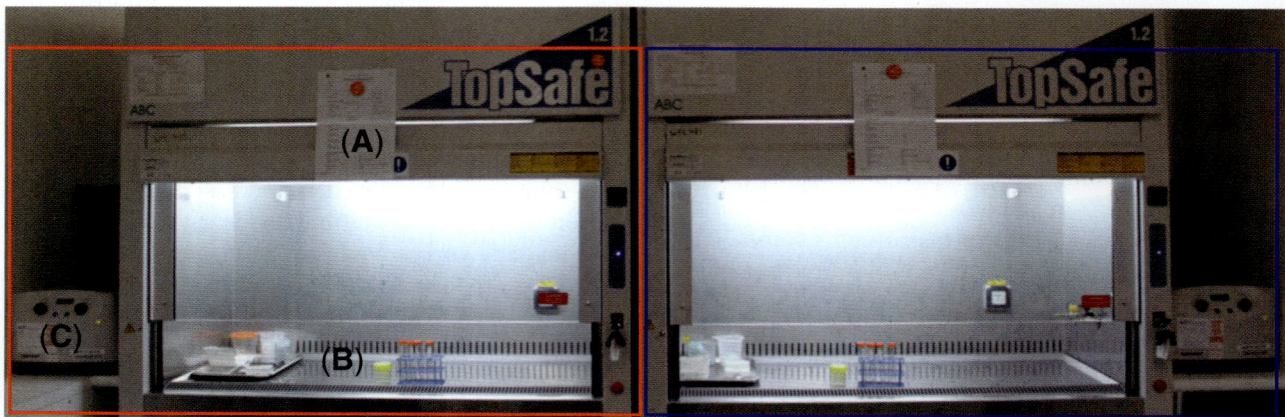

Figure 3.1 Sperm preparation area RED and BLUE each containing all equipment needed for a complete sperm preparation. (**A**) Documentation for the patient assigning work area RED to this patient. (**B**) Labeled sample pot and preparation tubes are double witnessed when brought into the area. (**C**) Only the sample currently being prepared in area RED is centrifuged in the area designated centrifuge. When the preparation is complete, the area is sterilized before being assigned to the next patient.

are handled at any one time. Preparation of a number of sperm samples, or cryopreservation or thawing of multiple patients' embryos at the same time poses a huge risk for mix-ups and should never be done.

Risk Identification, Management, and Prevention

According to the WHO one in six couples experience difficulties in conceiving and would need some form of assisted reproduction method (65). Worldwide over 3.75 million children have been born as a result of an ART treatment and it is approximated that over 800,000 treatment cycles are undertaken annually (66–68). With the increase in IVF cycle number worldwide it has become evident that just like in other areas of medicine and health care, errors are inherent. But it is important to remember that these errors are most often resulting from a complex interplay of multiple factors; only rarely are they due to the carelessness or misconduct of single individuals. Historically, rather than addressing the source of errors, prevention strategies have relied almost exclusively on enhancing the carefulness of the caregiver. (69). A culture of blame and finding a scapegoat has commonly been the response to adverse events and this is an approach, which can never improve the system and prevent the incident form reoccurring. The portioning of blame to an individual usually comes with a promise that it "will never happen again" (70). The crucial changes in the approach to risk management in IVF clinics are presented in Table 3.2.

In order to prevent errors and identify risks IVF laboratories must introduce robust risk management including an analysis of systems and structures in advance of those risks actually materializing, so embedding a risk management into the daily routine for embryologists. The international standard, ISO 31000:2009 Risk Management – Principles and guidelines (71), is the most widely acknowledged tool for addressing, managing, and preventing risk. Implementing this standard will vastly decrease the risk of adverse events and near misses, but also provide tools for how to learn from incidences when they happen and prevent them from happening again. ISO 31000 will provide a clear guide of how to set up a risk management policy and clearly outlines what needs to be included.

Errors and incidents result from failures and these can be categorized as active failures or latent conditions (72,73). Active failures result from violation of the agreed protocols, lapses, or mistakes. Latent conditions or errors include error-provoking conditions such as workload, fatigue, knowledge, supervision, and equipment and weaknesses in defence including unworkable procedures or switching off a malfunctioning alarm. Latent conditions are embedded in all systems as it is not possible to foresee all error-producing situations. However as they pre-exist, the active failures they may be able to be identified prior to adverse events occurring. Therefore, these conditions tend to be the targets of risk management systems.

The first step toward risk management in the laboratory is to have a clear overview of the protocols and procedures undertaken by the embryologists. This should be

Table 3.2 Shift in Approaches to Risk Management in IVF Clinics

Outdated approach	Modern approach
Main Goal	
To protect the IVF clinic's reputation	To improve patient safety; minimize risk of harm to and misidentification of embryos and gametes through better understanding of systemic factors that affect the risk for incidents
Reporting	
Acknowledge only reports submitted in writing	Variety of methods to report: paper form, electronic form, telephone call, anonymous reporting, person to person reporting
Investigation	
Investigate only the serious occurrences	Encourage reporting of "near misses" and investigate and discuss the potential
Interview staff one on one when there is an adverse incident	Have root cause analysis meetings with the entire team
Corrective/Preventive Action	
Blame and train (or dismissal)	Perform a criticality analysis chart and determine the root cause of the "near miss" or the adverse occurrence
Work with department involved to develop corrective action	Work with the team to develop a safety improvement plan
Information from investigation kept confidential	Develop corrective action, share with the whole IVF team
Communication	
Talk to the patients only if necessary and be vague about incident/findings	Advise clinic director to speak directly with the patients and discuss any unexpected outcome and error; keep them appraised of steps taken to make environment safe for the next patient
Long-Term Follow-up	
Assume that action is taken to correct the problem that occurred, notice only when it happens again that no action is taken	Monitor and audit to determine whether changes have been initiated and whether or not they have made a difference

Source: Adapted from Ref. 69.

provided already as a part of the quality system and demand for SOPs. With the use of process maps and flow charts for the procedures it will be easy to identify areas and procedures which could be high risk, but total risk management has to include all processes and procedures. Mortimer and Mortimer (74) provide a simple summary of risk management by asking and answering three basic questions: What can go wrong? What will we do? If something happens, how will we resolve it? There are three core tools for helping us address risk and answer those questions: Failure Mode and Effects Analysis (FMEA), Root Cause Analysis, and Audit.

A comprehensive way of proactively addressing risk is to make use of an FMEA. Like many approaches that improve quality and safety, FMEA has its origins in the army, space, and aviation industry, but is now used as a tool for error prevention in a wide range of industries including heath care. The aim of an FMEA is to try to think of every possible way a process can go wrong, how serious it would be, and how the process can be improved to avoid failure. It is important that all embryologists in the team are involved in assessing each process using FMEA. A simple format for FMEA is illustrated in Table 3.3. The first step is to identify the process to be assessed, using the example insemination, mixing of oocytes, and sperm for IVF. They identify what could go wrong (Potential Failure Mode) for example, an embryologist forgets to inseminate, mixing the wrong oocytes and sperm, losing oocytes, bumping a dish etc. Then ask "what could be the result of this failure?" It could be failed fertilization, creation of an embryo or indeed child with the "wrong parents," and decreasing the chances of pregnancy. Then assess the seriousness of the suggested failures using a 1–10 scale with 1 being no effect and 10 being critical. For failed fertilization one could argue a seriousness of 8 but the creation of a mixed-up embryo having a severity of 10. Once severity has been established, address the different causes for the failure, in this case being rushed, low staffing levels, poor processes, lack of checklists, and no witnessing system. The rate how often this would happen, occurrence and rate from 1 being no known occurrences, has never happened in any IVF clinic and 10 being very high risk with this happening regularly. Forgetting to inseminate happens in all clinics but one could argue that it is very rare, so an occurrence of 2 or 3 would be appropriate. Then discuss and list the current controls, for example use of daily work sheets or reminders followed by assessing what chance there is that we detect the failure. With forgetting to inseminate, this will be evident the morning after when the oocytes are found without sperm and unfertilized and we can assign this a 1 with detection every time it happens. However, with the case of a mix-up, this could go completely undetected and should be assigned a 9–10; the fault will be passed to the customer undetected or in IVF terms, the resulting embryo will be transferred leaving the patient or child to detect the failure. Then calculate the risk priority number (RPN) by multiplying the severity, occurrence, and detection, for forgetting to inseminate $8 \times 3 \times 1 = 24$. Now the initial analysis is done and the embryology team has the task of lowering the RPN. There needs to be an active discussion on how we can change the procedure, allowing everyone in the team to come with suggestions. Remember that we can some time get accustomed to our own best practices, should consider the suggestions from trainees, whom after all provide us with a fresh pair of eyes. Preventing failure in insemination could include the introduction of daily worksheets and checklists together with witnessing and improved ID checks. For example, Westmead Fertility Centre in Sydney has a system where each insemination is noted on the database and if one patient's oocytes have not been inseminated by 4 pm an automated text message will be sent to the senior embryologists and scientific director. When these suggested changes have been discussed, documented, and implemented, a new value for severity, occurrence, and detection is assigned and the new RPN should hopefully be significantly lower than the original.

The FMEA exercise is not only a mathematical exercise resulting in reduced risk through the actions taken, it is also a great way of making all embryologists aware of what risks are involved in each step of the IVF process and this awareness itself can help reducing risks.

Even the best risk management systems have incidents and near misses. So what can be done when the incident occurs? The answer is root cause analysis, which is the reactive component in a risk management system. A root cause analysis is simply an analysis of the very reason for the incident occurring. A simple example is when recently trialing a new incubator, the lid accidentally fell over the hand of the embryologist while placing dishes inside, resulting in the spill of the medium and loss of

Table 3.3 FMEA Work Sheet

Item/Function	Potential Failure Mode	Potential Effects of Failure	S Rating 1–10	Potential Cause(s)	O Rating 1–10	Current Controls	D Rating 1–10	RPN	Recommendations Action	Action Taken	New S 1–10	New O 1–10	New D 1–10	New RPN

Abbreviations: D, Detection; FMEA, Failure Mode and Effects Analysis; O, Occurrence; RPN, Risk Priority Number; S, Severity.

one out of 23 oocytes. The root cause analysis included discussing the incident at the lab meeting. Had it happened before? Were there any near misses previously where the lid had been falling without incident? But also we discussed how we place dishes in the incubators. Are we sometimes carrying more than one dish? We further contacted the supplier to see whether it was a fault of the incubator itself. It was concluded that the lid of our trial incubator did not recline and was a risk if left open without holding on to it. We implemented a procedure where only one dish could be carried and placed in the incubator at any one time, always allowing one hand to be free to hold up the lid. At no time is it appropriate to revert to the old outdated way of thinking where we portion blame; this can never result in improvement. More complex root cause analysis could involve the failure to inseminate as used for the FMEA, but instead of looking at it proactively doing a root cause analysis after the fact. Mortimer and Mortimer (74) provide an interesting example of root cause analysis of poor fertilization results and with the outcome being a complete re-formulation of the fertilization medium.

Many root cause analyses I had been involved in had concluded that the level of staffing was inappropriate. It is important to underline that staffing issues, such as overworking and poor training are main contributors to incidents. There is also the issue with staff who are not accepting professional responsibility and do not take enough care to undertake their duties or following protocols, they should not continue to work in the laboratory (74).

Finally the very effective tool in addressing and analyzing risk is audits. All incidents, followed by a root cause analysis will include suggestion for change and continuous improvement. To assure these have been implemented and are indeed effective is to undertake internal audits (see the Audits section).

Another side to safe practice is to have robust contingency plans. There should always be a documented agreed plan B. This will include having a backup for all equipment, such as a minimum of two microscopes, heated stages, centrifuges etc. For more expensive equipment such as ICSI rigs, oocyte aspiration pumps, and controlled freezers where sometimes the clinic cannot afford to have two sets, there needs to be a written agreement with another IVF clinic to utilize their equipment.

CONCLUDING REMARKS AND FUTURE ASPECTS

Throughout completing the long and work-intensive process of applying standardized systems in an embryology laboratory, one might ask what it has meant for the embryologists and the results of the clinic. There is no doubt that introducing and fully implementing a quality system standardizes methods and the way in which embryologists perform their work. The troubleshooting, maintenance of equipment, and the milieu are improved and standardized. This guarantees optimal handling of a couple's gametes, and embryos and inevitably will lead to improved outcome.

The number of ART treatment cycles undertaken worldwide is increasing every year and with the improvement of the techniques we use, more babies are born as a result of IVF. With the outcome improving we are aiming toward a future where more focus will be on the safety of treatment and indeed the long-term health of children resulting from ART. With this comes a demand for standardization and improvement of quality. The introduction of quality management systems will assure reproducibility and traceability, which will be crucial for future follow-up of these children.

To face the future we need to improve our understanding of the long-term effects of our laboratory procedures on the embryo health, acknowledging that some of our methods might deliver in numbers but might be detrimental when considering the long-term epigenetic outcome. A review of follow-up of children born from IVF over 25 years in Sweden has revealed that in contrast to cleavage stage transfer, children born after blastocyst transfer exhibited a higher risk of preterm birth and congenital malformations (75). This report clearly underlines that suboptimal culturing and handling of embryos have long reaching effects far beyond blastocyst development, successful pregnancy, and live birth. It indicates that what we do in the clinical embryology laboratory is closely connected to the adult health of children born from IVF. This further highlights the importance of standardization, but also implementing processes which goes beyond the standards; working toward improved risk management, robust and thorough training of clinical embryologists and processes to assure correct identification and preventing mix-ups.

Finally, it is important to acknowledge that quality management together with a never-ending commitment to improve our service, beyond standards, is the only way forward toward a future where we can guarantee safe efficient IVF treatment for all patients and the birth of children, who go on to live a healthy life.

ACKNOWLEDGMENTS

Thanks to Dr Diego Ezcurra for commenting on the layout of this chapter. Deep gratitude goes to the friends who have helped with the information on national and regional regulations in no specific order; David Mortimer, Ann-Sofie Forsberg, Lyndsay Devlin, Meishan Jin, Marcus Hedenskog, CT Yeong, Ahmad Suleiman, Rosemary Cullinan, Nader Abdelmonheim, Semra Kahraman, Andrey Kovtyushenko, and Amal Atared.

REFERENCES

1. ISO/IEC Guide 2:2004 Standardization and related activities – General vocabulary. 2004 International Organization for standardization. Geneva, Switzerland. [Available from: www.ISO.org]
2. Hazekamp JT. Current differences and consequences of legislation on practice of assisted reproductive technology in the Nordic countries. The Nordic Committee on Assisted Reproduction of the Scandinavian Federation

of Societies of Obstetrics and Gynecology. Acta Obstet Gynecol Scand 1996; 75: 198–200.
3. Clinical and laboratory guidelines for assisted reproductive technologies in the Nordic Countries: NFOG bulletin supplement. NFOG 1997; 3.
4. Dawson KJ. Quality control and quality assurance in IVF laboratories in the UK. Hum Reprod 1997; 12: 2590–1.
5. Pool TB. Practices contributing to quality performance in the embryo laboratory and the status of laboratory regulation in the US. Hum Reprod 1997; 12: 2591–3.
6. Lieberman BA, Matson PL, Hamer F. The UK human fertilisation and embryology Act 1990. How well is it functioning? Hum Reprod 1994; 9: 1779–82.
7. Code of Practice for Assisted Reproductive Technology Units. Fertility Society of Australia Reproductive Technology Accreditation Committee (RTAC) revised October 2010. [Available from: www.fertilitysociety.com.au/wp.../201011201-final-rtac-cop.pdf]
8. ISO 9001: 2008. Quality Management Systems, Requirements. 4th edn. Geneva, Switzerland: International Organization for standardization, 2008.
9. Keck C, Sjoblom C, Fischer R, Baukloh V, Alper M. Quality management in reproductive medicine. In: Gardner D, ed. Textbook of Assisted Reproductive Techniques (Ch. 32). 4th edn. London: Informa, 2012.
10. ISO 17025:2005. General Requirements for the Competence of Testing and Calibration Laboratories. Geneva, Switzerland: International Organization for standardization, 2005.
11. EN 45001. General Criteria for the Operation of Testing Laboratories. Geneva, Switzerland: International Organization for standardization, 1989.
12. ISO/IEC Guide 25. General Requirements for the Competence of Calibration and Testing Laboratories. 3rd edn. Geneva, Switzerland: International Organization for standardization, 1990.
13. Wikland M, Sjoblom C. The application of quality systems in ART programs. Mol Cell Endocrinol 2000; 166: 3–7.
14. ISO 15189:2007. Medical laboratories—Particular Requirements for Quality and Competence. 2nd edn. Geneva, Switzerland: International Organization for standardization, 2007.
15. Directive 2003/23/EC of the European Parliament and of the Council of 31 March 2004 on setting standards of quality and safety for the donation, procurement, testing, processing, preservation, storage and distribution of human tissues and cells. Official J Eur Union 2004; 102: 48–58. [Available from: http://europa.eu.int/eur-lex/en/oj/]
16. ESHRE position paper on the EU Tissues and Cells Directive EC/2004/23, November, 2007. [Available from: www.eshre.com/file.asp?filetype=doc/04/010/eshre_position_paper_on_the_eu_tissues_and_cells_directive_ec_final.pdf]
17. Joint Commission International Accreditation Standards for Clinical Laboratories. Joint Commission International. 2 edn, 2010.[Available from: www.jointcommissioninternational.org]
18. WHO Collaborating Centre for Patient Safety Solutions. Patient Safety Solutions. [Available from: http://www.ccforpatientsafety.org/Patient-Safety-Solutions/]
19. Clinical and Laboratory Standards Institute. [Available from: http://www.clsi.org/]
20. McCulloh D. Quality control: Maintaining stability in the laboratory. In: Gardner D. ed. Textbook of Assisted Reproductive Techniques (Ch. 2). 4th edn. London: Informa, 2012.
21. The Commission of the European Communities. Commission Directive 2003/94/EC, Laying down the principles and guidelines of good manufacturing practice in respect of medicinal products for human use and investigational medicinal products for human use. Off J Eur Union 2003; 14: L262/22–6.
22. European Commission. EC Guide to Good Manufacturing Practice, Revision to Annex 1. Manufacture of Sterile Medicinal Products. Brussels: Enterprise Directorate-General, 2003.
23. WHO laboratory manual for the Examination and processing of human sperm. 5th edn, 2010. [Available from: t:whqlibdoc.who.int/publications/2010/9789241547789_eng.pdf]
24. Balaban B, Brison D, Calderon G, et al. The Istanbul consensus workshop on embryo assessment; proceedings of an expert meeting. Hum Reprod 2011; 26: 1270–83.
25. Human Fertilisation and Embryology Authority (HFEA). [Available from: www.HFEA.gov.uk]
26. Human Fertilisation and Embryology Authority (HFEA) Code of Practice, 8th Edition published 2009, revised 2011. [Available from: http://www.hfea.gov.uk/code.html]
27. Reproductive Technology Accreditation Committee RTAC Technical Bulletins. [Available from: http://www.fertilitysociety.com.au/rtac/technical-bulletins/]
28. National Guidelines for Accreditation, Supervision & Regulation of ART Clinics in India. Indian Council of Medical Research National Academy of Medical Sciences (India), 2005. [Available from: http://icmr.nic.in/art/art_clinics.htm]
29. Licensing terms and conditions on assisted reproduction services. Section 6(5) of the private hospitals and medical clinics act (CAP248). [Available from: https://www.moh-ela.gov.sg/ela/]
30. Inhorn MC. Making Muslim babies: IVF and gamete donation in Sunni v. Shi'a Islam. Cult Med Psychiatry 2006; 30: 427–50.
31. Ali A. The Conditional Permissibility of In Vitro Fertilisation under Islamic Jurisprudence. Al-Ghazzali awareness paper, Al-Ghazzali centre for Islamic sciences and human development 2004. [Available from: http://alghazzali.org/]
32. Cabinet decision (36) of 2009 Issuing the implementing regulation of federal law No. (11) of concerning licensing of fertilisation centres in the State. Health Authority Abu-Dhabi (HAAD) 2008. [Available from: http://www.haad.ae/haad/tabid/852/Default.aspx]
33. Normas para la acreditacion de centros de reproduccion asistida y sus laboratorios de embriologia y andrologia. Version 12, 2007. [Available from: http://redlara.com/aa_ingles/default.asp]
34. Department of Justice Canada. Assisted Human Reproduction Act. S.C. c.2 2004. [Available from: http://laws-lois.justice.gc.ca/eng/acts/A-13.4/]
35. Federal agency Assisted Reproduction Canada (AHRC). [Available from: http://www.ahrc-pac.gc.ca]
36. Supreme Court of Canada Citation: Reference re Assisted Human Reproduction Act. BETWEEN:

Attorney General of Canada Appellant and Attorney General of Quebec. [Available from: scc.lexum.org/en/2010/2010scc61/2010scc61.html]
37. Canadian Fertility and Andrology Society (CFAS), ART Lab Special Interest Group. [Available from: http://www.cfas.ca/index.php?option=com_content&view=article&id=742&Itemid=522]
38. American Society for Reproductive Medicine. Revised minimum standards for in vitro fertilization, gamete intrafallopian transfer, and related procedures. Fertil Steril 1998; 70(4 Suppl 2): 1S–5S.
39. American Society for Reproductive Medicine. Revised guidelines for human embryology and andrology laboratories. Fertil Steril 2008; 90: S45–59.
40. Van Kooij JR, Peeters MF, Te Velde ER. Twins of mixed races: consequences for Dutch IVF laboratories. Hum Reprod 1997; 12: 2585–7.
41. Hartshorne GM, Baker H. Fads and foibles in ART; where is the evidence? Hum Fertil (Camb) 2006; 9: 27–35.
42. Takenaka M, Horiuchi T, Yanagimachi R. Effects of light on development of mammalian zygotes. Proc Natl Acad Sci USA 2007; 104: 14289–93.
43. Oosafe MEA tested IVF laboratory disinfectants. Denmark, Sparmed, Stenlose. [Available from: http://www.sparmed.dk/en/product.asp?cid=122&pid=129]
44. Nijs M, Franssen K, Cox A, et al. Reprotoxicity of intrauterine insemination and in vitro fertilization-embryo transfer disposables and products: a 4-year study. Fertil Steril 2009; 92: 527–35.
45. Council Directive 93/42/EEC of 14 June 1993 concerning medical devices, OJ L 169, 12.7.1993. Directive last amended by Regulation (EC) No 1882/2003 of the European Parliament and of the Council (OJ L 284, 31.10.2003).
46. Directive 98/79/EC of the European Parliament and of the Council of 27 October 1998 on in vitro diagnostic medical devices. OJ L 331, 7.12.1998, Directive as amended by Regulation (EC) No 1882/2003.
47. United Kingdom National External Quality Assessment Service (NEQUAS). [Available from: www.ukneqas.org.uk]
48. QAP online FertAid. [Available from: www.fertaid.com]
49. ISO/IEC guide 43-1 1997: International Organization for standardization, Geneva, Switzerland.
50. The Association of Clinical Embryologists (ACE). [Available from: https://www.embryologists.org.uk/]
51. Paget J, Blower J. The future workforce of the embryology laboratory. Consultation paper, 2011 The Association of Clinical Embryologists.
52. European Society of Human Reproduction and Embryology (ESHRE) Certification for Embryologists. [Available from: http://www.eshre.eu/ESHRE/English/Accreditation-and-Certification/Certification-for-embryologists/page.aspx/109]
53. Australian Commission on Safety and Quality in Health Care (ACSQHC). Technology Solutions to Patient Misidentification - Report of Review ACSQHC (2008).
54. Lusky K. Patient ID Systems Offer Smart Start. Collage of American Pathologists Periodical, CAP Today, 2005.
55. Aller R. Positive patient identification. More than a double check (positive patient identification systems and products). Collage of American Pathologists Periodical, CAP Today, 2005: 26–34.
56. Clinical and Laboratory Standards Institute (CLSI). Accuracy in Patient and Sample Identification. Approved Guideline (GP33-A). Pennsylvania: CLSI, 2010.
57. Adams S, Carthey J. IVF Witnessing and electronic systems. HFEA commissioned report comparing the relative risks of witnessing systems. [Available from: www.hfea.gov.uk/docs/Witnessing_samples_id_report.pdf]
58. Kerr A. A problem shared...? Teamwork, autonomy and error in assisted conception. Soc Sci Med 2009; 69: 1741–9.
59. Brison D. Reducing risk in the IVF laboratory: implementation of a double witnessing system. Clinical Risk 2004; 10: 176–80.
60. Amalberti R, Auroy Y, Berwick D, et al. Five system barriers to achieving ultrasafe health care. Ann Intern Med 2005; 142: 756–64.
61. Leape LL, Berwick DM. Safe health care: are we up to it? BMJ 2000; 320: 7256.
62. Toft B, Mascie-Taylor H. Involuntary automaticity: a work-system induced risk to safe health care. Health Serv Manage Res 2005; 18: 211–16.
63. Kennedy CR, Mortimer D. Risk management in IVF. Best Pract Res Clin Obstet Gynaecol 2007; 21: 691–712.
64. Lippi G, Blanckaert N, Bonini P, et al. Causes, consequences, detection, and prevention of identification errors in laboratory diagnostics. Clin Chem Lab Med 2009; 47: 143–53.
65. Edi-Osagie E, Hooper L, Seif MW. The impact of assisted hatching on live birth rates and outcomes of assisted conception: a systematic review. Hum Reprod 2003; 18: 1828–35.
66. Zegers-Hochschild F, Adamson GD, de Mouzon J. International Committee for Monitoring Assisted Reproductive Technology (ICMART) and the World Health Organization (WHO) revised glossary of ART terminology. Fertil Steril 2009; 92: 1520–4.
67. Capri Workshop Group for the European Society of Human Reproduction and Embryology (ESHRE). Intrauterine insemination. Hum Reprod Update 2009; 1: 1–13.
68. Connolly M, Hoorens S, Chambers GM. The costs and consequences of assisted reproductive technology: an economic perspective. Hum Reprod Update 2010; 16: 603–13.
69. Kuhn AM, Youngberg BJ. The need for risk management to evolve to assure a culture of safety. Qual Saf Health Care 2002; 11: 158–62.
70. Wu AW. Medical error: the second victim. The doctor who makes the mistake needs help too. BMJ 2000; 320: 726–7.
71. ISO 31000:2009. Risk management – Principles and guidelines. Geneva, Switzerland: International Organization for standardization, 2009.
72. Reason J. The contribution of latent human failures to the breakdown of complex systems. Philos Trans R Soc Lond B Biol Sci 1990; 327: 475–84.
73. Reason J. Human Error: models and management. BMJ 2000; 320: 768–7074.
74. Mortimer D, Mortimer ST. Quality and Risk Management in the IVF Laboratory. Cambridge: Cambridge University Press, 2005.
75. Finnström O, Källén B, Lindam A, et al. Maternal and child outcome after in vitro fertilization–a review of 25 years of population-based data from Sweden. Acta Obstet Gynecol Scand 2011; 90: 494–500.

4

Evaluation of sperm

Kaylen M. Silverberg and Tom Turner

INTRODUCTION

Abnormalities in sperm production or function, alone or in combination with other factors, account for 35–50% of all cases of infertility. Although a battery of tests and treatments have been described and continue to be used in the evaluation of female infertility, the male has been essentially neglected. It would appear that the majority of programs offering advanced reproductive technologies (ARTs) employ only a cursory evaluation of the male—rarely extending beyond semen analysis and antisperm antibody detection. Several factors certainly account for this disparity. First, most practitioners of ARTs are gynecologists or gynecologic subspecialists who have little formal training in the evaluation of the infertile or subfertile men. Second, the urologists, who perhaps theoretically should have taken the lead in this area, have devoted little of their literature or research budgets to the evaluation of the infertile male. Third, and perhaps the most important, is the inescapable fact that sperm function testing remains a very controversial area of research. Many tests have been described, yet few have been extensively evaluated in a proper scientific manner. Those that have continue to be criticized for poor sensitivity or specificity, a lack of standardization of methodology, suboptimal study design, problems with outcome assessment, and the lack of long-term follow-up. Although many of these same criticisms could also be leveled against most diagnostic algorithms for female infertility, in that arena, the tests continue to prevail over their critics. Fourth, like female infertility, male infertility is certainly multifactorial. It is improbable that one sperm function test will prove to be a panacea, owing to the multiple steps involved in fertilization. In addition to arriving at the site of fertilization, sperm must undergo capacitation and the acrosome must allow for penetration of the cumulus cells and the zona pellucida, so the sperm head can fuse with the oolemma, activate the oocyte, undergo nuclear decondensation, form the male pronucleus, and then fuse with the female pronucleus. Finally, with the advent and rapid continued development of micro-assisted fertilization, sperm function testing has assumed a role of even lesser importance. As fertilization and pregnancy rates improve with procedures such as intracytoplasmic sperm injection (ICSI), more and more logical questions are being asked about the proper role for sperm function testing. This chapter reviews the most commonly employed techniques for sperm evaluation, and examines the issues surrounding their utilization in the modern ART program.

PATIENT HISTORY

A thorough history of the infertile couple at the time of the initial consultation will frequently reveal conditions that could affect semen quality. Some of the important factors to consider are as follows:

1. Reproductive history, including previous pregnancies with this and other partners
2. Sexual interaction of the couple, including frequency and timing of intercourse as well as the duration of their infertility
3. Past medical and surgical history: Specific attention should be paid to sexually transmitted diseases, prostatitis, or epididymitis, as well as scrotal trauma or surgery—including varicocele repair, vasectomy, inguinal herniorrhaphy, and vasovasostomy
4. Exposure to medication, drugs, toxins, and adverse environmental conditions such as temperature extremes in occupational and leisure activities, either in the past or in the present

SEMEN ANALYSIS

The hallmark of the evaluation of the male remains the semen analysis. It is well known that the intrapatient variability of semen specimens from fertile men can vary significantly over time (1). This variability decreases the diagnostic information that can be obtained from a single analysis, often necessitating additional analyses. What is also apparent from literature that analyzes samples from "infertile" patients is that the deficiencies revealed may not be sufficient to prevent pregnancy from occurring: rather, they may simply lower the probability of pregnancy, resulting in so-called "subfertility." Clearly, the overall prognosis for a successful pregnancy is dependent on the complex combination of variables in semen quality coupled with the multiple factors inherent in the female reproductive system that must each function

Table 4.1 WHO 4th and 5th Edition Reference Values for Semen Analysis (1,2)

Parameter	Reference values	
	(4th edn)	(5th edn)
Volume	>2.0 mL	1.5 (1.4–1.7)
Sperm concentration	20 × 10	15 (12–16) × 10^6
Total sperm count	40 × 10	39 (33–46) × 10^6
Total motility	50%	40% (38–42)
Progressive motility	25%	32% (31–34)
Vitality	50%	58% (55–63)
pH	7.2	7.2
Morphology	15%	4% (3.0–4.0)

Liquefaction: Complete within 60 minutes at room temperature.
Appearance: Homogeneous, gray, and opalescent.
Consistency: Leaves pipette as discrete droplets.
Leukocytes: Fewer than 1 million/mL.

flawlessly to enable a pregnancy to occur. The commonly accepted standard for defining the normal semen analysis is the criteria defined by the World Health Organization (WHO). These parameters for both the fourth and the fifth edition are listed in Table 4.1.

The normal or reference values for semen analyses have been altered with each new edition of the WHO. The values from the current edition (fifth edition) have been derived from a retrospective look at the semen parameters of men with two to seven days of abstinence whose partner conceived within 12 months after the cessation of the use of contraception. (2,3). There are significant changes in the parameters listed in the current edition compared with past editions. Some of these changes are due to observations made of the semen samples from the patients mentioned above. These real differences in declining sperm concentrations and normal morphology are thought to be due to environmental influences. However, the drastic changes in the morphology reference values are primarily due to the suggested use of the Kruger strict morphology method in the fifth edition. Many labs prefer to continue using the fourth edition because of the suggested use of the Kruger Strict morphology. The value of this method will be discussed in the sperm morphology section of this chapter.

COLLECTION OF THE SPECIMEN

When the semen analysis is scheduled, instructions should be given to the couple to ensure collection of an optimum semen sample. Written instructions are useful, especially if the patient is collecting the specimen outside of the clinical setting. During the initial infertility evaluation, a semen specimen should be obtained following a two to seven day abstinence from sexual activity (1). A shorter period of time may adversely affect the semen volume and sperm concentration, although it may enhance sperm motility. A longer period of abstinence may reduce the sperm motility. In light of the natural variability in semen quality that all men exhibit, the initial semen collection may not accurately reflect a typical ejaculate for that patient. A second collection, with a two to seven-day abstinence period, can eliminate the tension associated with the initial semen collection, as well as provide a second specimen from which a typical set of semen parameters can be determined. This second collection may also be used to determine the optimal abstinence period for this particular patient. Masturbation is the preferred method of collection. The use of lubricants is discouraged since most are spermicidal. However, some mineral oils and a few water-based lubricants are acceptable. Since masturbation may present significant difficulty for some men, either in the clinic or at home, an alternative method of collection must be available. The use of certain silastic condoms (seminal collection devices) during intercourse may be an acceptable second choice. Interrupted intercourse should not be considered, as this method tends to lose the sperm-rich initial few drops of semen while transferring many bacteria to the specimen container (1,4).

CARE OF THE SPECIMEN

Appropriate care of the ejaculate between collection and examination is important. Specimens should be collected only in approved, sterile, plastic, disposable cups. Many other plastic containers are toxic to sperm, especially if the sperm is allowed to remain in the containers for the duration of time that it takes to deliver the specimen from offsite. Washed containers may contain soap or residue from previous contents, which can kill or contaminate the sperm. Delivery of the semen to the laboratory should occur within 60 minutes of collection, and the specimen should be kept at room temperature during transport. These recommendations are designed to maintain optimal sperm viability until the time of analysis.

CONTAINER LABELING

The information recorded on the specimen container label should include the husband's name as well as a unique identifying number. Typically, a social-security number, birth date, or a clinic-assigned patient number is used. Other helpful information recorded on the label should include the date and time of collection and the number of days since the last ejaculation. When the specimen is received from the patient, it is important to confirm that the information provided on the label is complete and accurate.

EXAMINATION OF THE SPECIMEN

Liquefaction and Viscosity

When the semen sample arrives in the laboratory, it is checked for liquefaction and viscosity. Although similar, these factors are distinct from each other (5,6). Liquefaction is a natural change in the consistency of semen from a semi-liquid to a liquid. Before this process is completed, sperm are contained in a gel-like matrix that prevents their homogeneous distribution. Aliquots taken from this uneven distribution of sperm for the purpose of determining concentration, motility, or morphology may not be truly representative of the specimen as a whole. As liquefaction occurs over 15–30 minutes, sperm are released and distributed throughout the semen. Incomplete liquefaction may adversely affect the semen analysis by preventing this even distribution. The coagulum that characterizes freshly ejaculated semen results from secretions from the seminal vesicles. The liquefaction of this coagulum is the result of enzymatic secretions from the prostate. Watery semen, in the absence of a coagulum, may indicate the absence of the ejaculatory duct or nonfunctional seminal vesicles. Inadequate liquefaction, in the presence of a coagulum, may indicate a deficiency of prostatic enzymes (7,8).

Viscosity refers to the liquefied specimen's tendency to form drops from the tip of a pipette. If drops form and fall freely, the specimen has a normal viscosity. If drops will not form or the semen cannot be easily drawn up into a pipette, viscosity is high. Highly viscous semen may also prevent the homogeneous distribution of sperm. Treatment with an enzyme, such as chymotrypsin, (9) or aspiration of semen through an 18-gauge needle, may reduce the viscosity and improve the distribution of sperm before an aliquot is removed for counting. Any addition of medium-containing enzymes should be recorded, as this affects the actual sperm concentration. The new volume must be factored in when calculating the total sperm count.

Semen Volume

Semen volume is best measured with a serological pipette that is graduated to 0.1 mL. This volume is recorded and later multiplied by the sperm concentration in order to obtain the total count. A normal seminal volume before dilution is considered to be >1.4 mL (2).

Sperm Concentration

A variety of counting chambers are available for determining sperm concentration. Those more commonly used include the hemocytometer, the Makler counting chamber, and the MicroCell. Regardless of the type of chamber used, an aliquot from a homogeneous, mixed semen sample is placed onto a room temperature chamber. The chamber is covered with a glass coverslip, which allows the sperm to distribute evenly in a very thin layer. Sperm within a grid are counted, and a calculation is made according to the formula for the type of chamber used. Accuracy is improved by including a greater number of rows, squares, or fields in the count. Sperm counts should be performed immediately after loading semen onto the chamber. Waiting until the heat from the microscope light increases the speed of the sperm may inaccurately enhance the count. As indicated earlier, a particular patient's sperm count may vary significantly from one ejaculate to another. This observation holds true for both fertile and infertile males, further complicating the definition of a normal range for sperm concentration. Demographic studies employing historic controls were used to define a sperm concentration of <15 million/mL as abnormal (fifth edn) (2). Several investigators had observed that significantly fewer pregnancies occurred when men had sperm counts <15 million/mL; however, the prognosis for pregnancy did not increase proportionately to sperm concentrations above this threshold.

Sperm Motility

Sperm motility may be affected by many factors:

- Patient's age and general health
- Length of time since the last ejaculation
- Patient's exposure to outside influences such as excessive heat or toxins
- Method of collection
- Length of time and adequacy of handling from collection to analysis

When the aliquot of semen is placed on the room temperature counting chamber, the count and motility should be determined immediately. As previously stated, this will prevent the effect of the heat from the microscope light source from influencing the results. If a chamber with a grid is used to count the sperm, the motility can be determined at the same time as the concentration by using a multiple-click cell counter to tally motile and nonmotile sperm and then totaling these numbers to arrive at the true sperm concentration. The accuracy improves as more sperm are counted. If a wet-mount slide is used to determine motility, more than one area of the slide should be used, and each count should include at least 200 sperm. Prior to examining the specimen for motility, the slide or counting chamber should be examined for signs of sperm clumping. Sperm clumping to other sperm, head to head, head to tail, or tail to tail, may indicate the presence of sperm antibodies in the semen. This should not be confused with clumping of sperm to other cellular debris in the semen, which is not associated with the presence of antibodies. In either case, sperm clumping may affect the accuracy of both the sperm count and the motility (1,4).

Motility is one of the most important prerequisites for achieving fertilization and pregnancy. The head of the sperm must be delivered a great distance in vivo through the barriers of the reproductive tract to the site of the egg. Sperm must have sufficient motility in order to penetrate both the layers of coronal cells and the zona pellucida before fusing with the egg's cell membrane (oolemma). An exact threshold level of motility that is required to accomplish fertilization and pregnancy, however, has never been described (10). This may be due to variables in the equipment and techniques used in assessing motility.

Progression

While sperm motility represents the quantitative parameter of sperm movement expressed as a percentage, sperm progression represents the quality of sperm movement expressed on a subjective scale. A typical scale, such as the one below, attempts to depict the type of movement exhibited by most of the sperm visualized on a chamber grid. Progression of sperm may also be calculated with sperm motility as a percentage of sperm exhibiting "progressive motility." With the advent of successful microassisted fertilization, progression has assumed more limited utility. Nevertheless, for those laboratories that quantify progression of motility separately, a score of 0 means no motility; 1 means motility with vibratory motion without forward progression; 2 means motility with slow, erratic forward progression; 3 means motility with relatively straightforward motion; and 4 is motility with rapid forward progression (4).

Sperm Vitality

When a motility evaluation yields a low proportion of moving sperm (less than 50%), a vitality stain may be beneficial. This is a method used to distinguish nonmotile sperm that are living from those that are dead. This technique will be discussed later in the sperm function section.

Additional Cell Types

While observing sperm in a counting chamber or on a slide, additional cell types may also be seen. These include endothelial cells from the urethra, epithelial cells from the skin, immature sperm cells, and white blood cells. The most common and significant of these cell types is referred to collectively as "round cells." These include immature sperm cells and white blood cells. In order to distinguish between them, an aliquot of semen can be placed in a thin layer on a slide and air-dried. The cells are fixed to the slide and stained using a Wright–Giemsa or Bryan–Leishman stain. When viewed under 400× or 1000× power, cell types may be differentiated primarily by their nuclear morphology. Immature sperm have one to three round nuclei within a common cytoplasm. Polymorphonuclear leukocytes may also be multinucleate, but the staining method will typically reveal characteristic nuclear bridges between their irregularly shaped nuclei (1). A peroxidase stain may be used to identify granulocytes and to differentiate them from the immature sperm. The presence of greater than 1 million white blood cells per one milliliter of semen may indicate an infection in the urethra or accessory glands, which provide the majority of the seminal plasma. Such infections could contribute to infertility (1,11). As such, these samples must be cultured so that the offending organism can be identified and appropriate treatment can be instituted. Besides bacteria, white blood cells on their own, can contribute to infertility. They can especially be a detrimental factor in the in vitro fertilization (IVF) process. Even though the white blood cells can be removed by centrifugation of the semen sample through a layer of silica beads, the toxins produced by the cells, called leukokines, may pass through the layer and concentrate in the medium below containing the sperm. If this sperm is to be used in insemination of oocytes, the concentrated toxins will be in contact with the oocytes for several hours. These toxins may cause detrimental effects to the oocytes and to the embryos that develop from fertilization.

Sperm Morphology

Sperm morphology can be assessed in several ways. The most common classification systems are the fourth and fifth edition WHO standard that incorporate Kruger strict criteria (Fig. 4.1). Two easy methods of preparing slides for assessing normal morphology include the following; first, a 5–10 µl drop of semen is placed on a slide and a second slide is used to smear the sample in a very thin, smoothly distributed layer. The slide is air-dried and then a 5–10 µl drop of stain is placed on the dried sample and a coverslip is placed over the specimen. After placing a coverslip over the specimen, morphology may be determined at 400× using a phase contrast microscopy. Alternatively, the drop of semen may be mixed with an equal volume of fixative plus stain (typically Papanicolaou or a Diff-Quik kit) prior to placing it on the slide. With either method, at least 200 sperm must be counted at 400× or 1000× with phase contrast or bright field microscopy. WHO fourth edition criteria for assessing normal forms include the following:

- Head: Oval and smooth heads are normal; round, pyriform, pin, double, and amorphous heads are all abnormal.
- Mid-piece: A normal mid-piece is straight and slightly thicker than the tail.
- Tail: Single, unbroken, straight tails, without kinks or coils are normal.

A normal semen analysis should contain at least 15% normal sperm using WHO fourth edition criteria. In order to employ Kruger strict criteria, sperm morphology is evaluated by placing 5 µl of liquefied semen on a slide, making a thin smear, and air-drying it at room temperature. The slide is then fixed and stained (typically with a Papanicolaou stain or a Diff-Quik kit). Slides are read using bright field microscopy under 1000× or a higher magnification. At least 200 sperm should be counted for an accurate evaluation. The Kruger criteria for assessing normal forms include the following (Fig. 4.2): (13,14).

- Head: Smooth; oval configuration; length, 5–6 µm, diameter 2.5–3.5 µm; acrosome, must constitute 40–70% of the sperm head.
- Mid-piece: Slender, axially attached; <1 µm in width and approximately 1.5 µm in head length; no cytoplasmic droplets, >50% of the size of the sperm head.
- Tail: Single, unbroken, straight, without kinks or coils approximately 45 µm in length.

As described by Kruger et al., sperm forms that are not clearly normal should be considered abnormal. The presence of ≥15% normal sperm morphology should be interpreted as a normal result. Normal morphology of 4–14% should be considered to be borderline, and

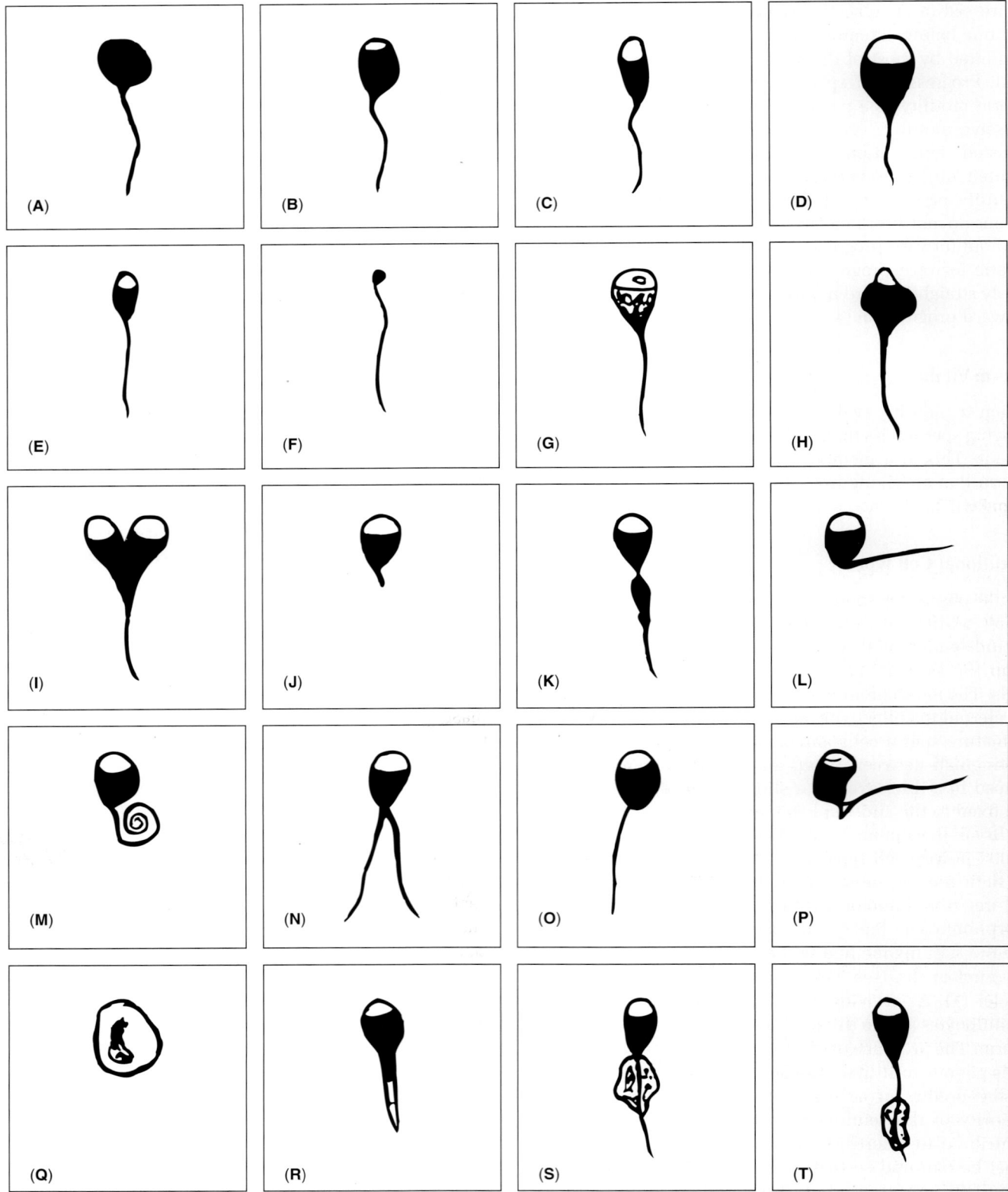

Figure 4.1 Different types of sperm malformations. (**A**) Round head/no acrosome; (**B**) small acrosome; (**C**) elongated head; (**D**) megalo head; (**E**) small head; (**F**) pinhead; (**G**) vacuolated head; (**H**) amorphous head; (**I**) bicephalic; (**J**) loose head; (**K**) amorphous head; (**L**) broken neck; (**M**) coiled tail; (**N**) double tail; (**O**) abaxial tail attachment; (**P**) multiple defects; (**Q**) immature germ cell; (**R**) elongated spermatid; (**S**) proximal cytoplasmic droplet; (**T**) distal cytoplasmic droplet. *Source*: Reproduced from Ref. 12.

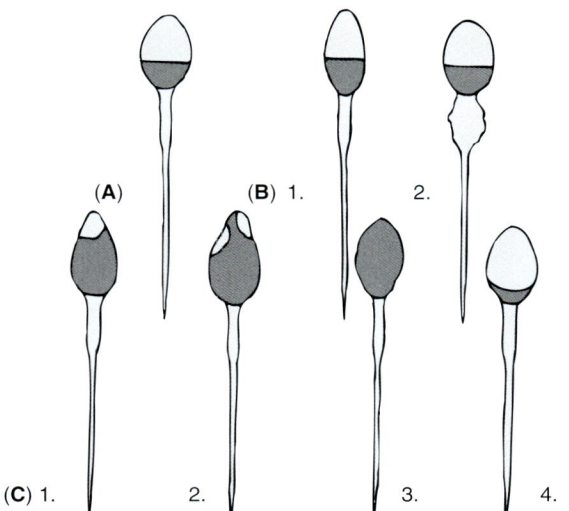

Figure 4.2 A diagrammatic representation of quick-stained spermatozoa. (**A**) Normal form; (**B.1**) slightly amorphous head; (**B.2**) neck defect; (**C.1** and **2**) abnormally small acrosome; (**C.3**) no acrosome; (**C.4**) acrosome 70% of sperm head. *Source*: Reproduced from Ref. 12.

normal morphology <4% is abnormal (13,14). Normal sperm morphology has been reported to be directly related to fertilization potential. This may be due to the abnormal sperm's inability to deliver normal genetic material to the cytoplasm of the egg. From video recordings, it appears that abnormal sperm are more likely to have diminished, aberrant, or absent motility. This reduced or unusual motility may result from hydrodynamic inefficiency due to the head shape, abnormalities in the tail structure which prevent normal motion, and/or deficiencies in energy production necessary for motility (15,16). In addition to compromised motility, abnormal sperm do not appear to bind to the zona of the egg as well as normal sperm. This has been demonstrated in studies employing the hemizona binding assay (17). IVF has helped further to elucidate the role that normal sperm morphology plays in the fertilization process and in pregnancy. Both the fourth edition WHO method and the Kruger strict method of determining normal sperm morphology have been used to predict a patient's fertility.

Several studies have concluded that the Kruger method of strict morphology determination shows the most consistent prediction of fertilization in vitro following conventional insemination (11,18,19). This method of assessing normal sperm morphology, because of its precise, nonsubjective nature, establishes a threshold below which abnormal morphology becomes a contributing factor in infertility. While Kruger strict morphology provides a repeatable, objective method of analyzing sperm morphology based on precise measurements, some IVF labs prefer to use the WHO fourth edition of sperm morphology (15%) as a cut-off point below which ICSI is used and above which, insemination may be used. The opinion in those labs is that the 15% level, while not as accurate as the Kruger method, is more realistic in determining patients who will do well with insemination. Setting the bar higher for patients who are considered "normal" ensures that ICSI will be employed on potential borderline normal patients who might not do well by using insemination.

COMPUTER-ASSISTED SEMEN ANALYSIS

Computer-assisted semen analysis (CASA) was initially developed to improve the accuracy of manual semen analysis. Its goal is to establish a standardized, objective, reproducible test for sperm concentration, motility, and morphology. The technique also attempts, for the first time, to actually characterize sperm movement. The automated sperm movement measurements—known as kinematics—include straight-line velocity, curvilinear velocity, and mean angular displacement (Table 4.2). The use of CASA requires specialized equipment, including a phase contrast microscope, video camera, video recorder, video monitor, computer, and printer.

To perform CASA, sperm are placed on either a Makler or a MicroCell chamber and they are then viewed under a microscope. The video camera records the moving images of the sperm cells and the computer digitizes them. The digitized images consist of pixels whose changing locations are recorded frame by frame. Thirty to 200 frames per minute are produced. The changing locations of each sperm are recorded and their trajectories are computed (Fig. 4.3) (20). In this manner, hyperactive motion can also be detected and recorded. Hyperactive sperm exhibit a whip-like, thrashing movement, which is thought to be associated with sperm that are removed from seminal plasma and ready to fertilize the oocytes (20,21). Persistent questions about the validity and reproducibility of results have kept CASA from becoming a standard procedure in the andrology laboratory. The accuracy of sperm concentration appears to be diminished in the presence of either severe oligospermia or excessive numbers of sperm. In cases of oligospermia, counts may be overestimated due to the machine counting debris as sperm. High concentrations of sperm may be underestimated in the presence of clumping. High sperm concentrations can also cause overestimations in counting due to the manner in which the software handles collisions between motile sperm and nonmotile sperm. In these cases, diluting the sample may improve the accuracy of the count (21,22). Sperm concentration also appears to be closely related with the type of counting chamber employed. Similar to the challenges reported with manual counting, sperm counts may vary whether it is a Makler or MicroCell.

Sperm motion parameters identified by CASA have been assessed by several investigators for their ability to predict fertilization potential. Certain types of motion have been determined to be important in achieving specific actions related to fertilization, such as cervical mucus penetration and zona binding. However, the overall potential of CASA in predicting pregnancy is still a subject of much debate. In summary, persistent questions about results and their interpretation continue to limit the routine use of CASA. As reproducibility improves overall ranges of sperm concentration, CASA may become the standard for semen analysis.

Table 4.2 Kinematic Measurements in CASA

Symbol	Name	Definition
VSL	Straight-line velocity	Time average velocity of the sperm head along a straight line from its first position to its last position
VCL	Curvilinear velocity	Time average velocity of the sperm head along its actual trajectory
VAP	Average path velocity	Time average velocity of the sperm head along its average trajectory
LIN	Linearity	Linearity of the curvilinear trajectory (VSL/VCL)
WOB	Wobble	Degree of oscillation of the actual sperm-head trajectory around its average path (VAP/VCL)
STR	Straightness	Straightness of the average path (VSL/VAP)
ALH	Amplitude of lateral head	Amplitude of variations of the actual sperm-head trajectory about its average trajectory displacement (the average trajectory is computed using a rectangular running average
RIS	Riser displacement	Point-to-point distance of the actual sperm-head trajectory to its average path (the average path is computed using an adaptive smoothing algorithm)
BCF	Beat-cross frequency	Time average rate at which the actual sperm trajectory crosses the average path trajectory
HAR	Frequency of the fundamental	Fundamental frequency of the oscillation of the curvilinear trajectory around its average harmonic path (HAR is computed using the Fourier transformation)
MAG	Magnitude of the Amplitude	Squared height of the HAR spectral peak (MAG is a measure of the peak to fundamental harmonic peak dispersion of the raw trajectory about its average path at the fundamental frequency)
VOL	Area of fundamental harmonic	Area under the fundamental harmonic peak in the magnitude spectrum (VOL is a harmonic measure of the power-bandwidth of the signal)
CON	Specimen concentration	Concentration of sperm cells in a sample in millions of sperm per mL of plasma or medium
MOT	Percentage motility	Percentage of sperm cells in a suspension that are motile (in manual analysis, motility is defined by a moving flagellum; in computer-assisted semen analysis (CASA), motility is defined by a minimum VSL for each sperm)

Source: Reproduced from Ref. 19.

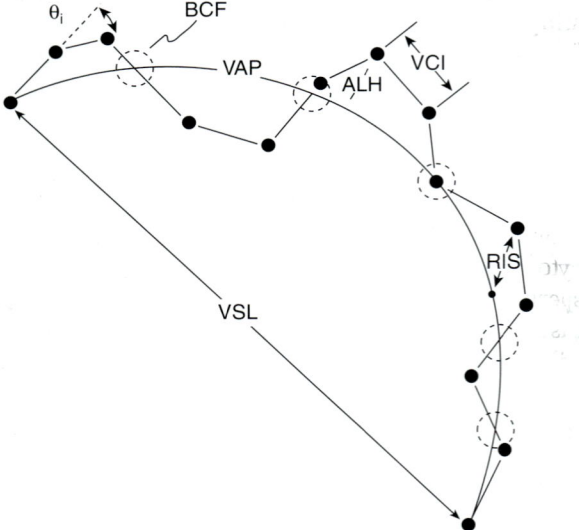

Figure 4.3 Examples of kinematic measurements involved in a single-sperm tracing. *Abbreviations*: ALH, amplitude of lateral head; BCF, beat-cross frequency; RIS, Riser displacement; VAP, average path velocity; VCL, curvilinear velocity; VSL, straight-line velocity. *Source*: Reproduced from Ref. 19.

The use of fluorescent DNA staining with CASA may also improve its reliability. In addition, as the kinematics of sperm motion becomes better understood, CASA may play an integral role in determining the optimal method of assisted reproductive technique that should be utilized for specific types of male factor patients.

SPERM ANTIBODIES

Because mature spermatozoa are formed after puberty, they can be recognized as foreign protein by the male immune system. In the testicle, the sperm are protected from circulating immunoglobulins by the tight junctions of the Sertoli cells. As long as the sperm are contained within the lumen of the male reproductive tract, they are sequestered from the immune system, and no antibodies form to their surface antigens. If there is a breach in this so-called "blood–testis barrier," an immune response may be initiated. The most common causes of a breach in the reproductive tract, which could initiate antibody formation, include vasectomy, varicocele repair, testicular biopsy, torsion, trauma, and infection (23,24). Once formed, antibodies are secreted into the fluids of the accessory glands, specifically the prostate and seminal vesicles. At the time of ejaculation, the fluids from these glands contribute most of the volume to the seminal plasma. These antibodies can then come into contact with the sperm and may cause them to clump. In women, the atraumatic introduction of sperm into the reproductive tract as a result of intercourse or artificial insemination does not appear to be a factor in the production of sperm antibodies. However, events that induce trauma, or introduce sperm to the mucous membranes outside of the reproductive tract, can induce antibody formation. Proposed examples of such events include trauma to the vaginal mucosa during intercourse or the deposition of sperm into the gastrointestinal tract by way of oral or anal intercourse (24). There are several tests currently employed for detecting the presence of sperm antibodies. The two most common are the mixed agglutination reaction (MAR) and the immunobead binding test.

The Mixed Agglutination Reaction

This test is performed by mixing semen, immunoglobulin G (IgG)- or IgA-coated latex beads or red blood cells, and IgG or IgA antiserum on a microscope slide. The slides are incubated and observed at 400× magnification. At least 200 sperm are counted. If antibodies are present, the sperm will form clumps with the coated latex beads or coated red blood cells. If antibodies are absent, the sperm will swim freely. The level of antibody concentration considered to be clinically relevant must be established by each center conducting the test. The WHO considers a level of binding of ≥50% to be clinically significant. This test is used only for detection of direct antibodies in men, and is not specific for the location of bead attachment to the sperm.

The Immunobead Binding Test

This test is performed by combining IgG- or IgA-coated latex beads and washed sperm on a slide. The sperm must be removed from the seminal plasma by washing the sample with media plus bovine serum albumin (BSA). The presence of human protein on the surface of the sperm interferes with the binding of the immunobeads to the sperm, and thus may mask a positive result. After washing, the sperm are placed on a slide with IgG- or IgA-coated latex beads and read at 200× or 400× magnification. If antibodies are present, the small beads will attach directly to the sperm. This test provides potentially greater information than the mixed agglutination reaction, as results consider the number of sperm bound by beads, the type of antigen involved in binding, and the specific location where the bead is bound to the sperm.

If antibodies are absent, the beads will not attach. This test can be used for the detection of direct antibodies in men. However, unlike the MAR test, it may also be used to detect antibodies produced in a woman's serum, follicular fluid, or cervical mucus by incubating these bodily fluids with washed sperm that have previously tested negative for antibodies. To perform an indirect test, known direct antibody negative sperm are washed free of seminal plasma and resuspended in a small volume of media plus BSA. They are incubated for one hour at 37°C with the bodily fluid to be tested. The sperm are then washed free of the bodily fluid, resuspended in media plus BSA, and mixed on a slide with IgG- or IgA-coated latex beads. The test is interpreted by noting the percentage and location of the bead attachment. Third edition WHO standard considers the level of binding of ≥20% as representing a positive test, whereas the fourth edition WHO standard considers the level of ≥50% to be a positive test. The level of binding of ≥50% is commonly considered to be clinically significant (10,25). The clinical value of antisperm antibody testing is predicated on the observation that the presence of a significant concentration of antibodies may impair fertilization. It has been reported that antibody-positive sperm may have difficulty penetrating cervical mucus. Although, in these cases, intrauterine insemination or IVF may improve the prognosis for fertilization, antibody levels >80%, coupled with subpar concentration, motility, or morphology, may necessitate the addition of ICSI in order to achieve the highest percentage of fertilization (26). As suggested by the literature, andrology laboratories may do a significantly better job of preparing sperm if they are aware of the presence of antibodies. Specifically, it has been demonstrated that the use of increased concentrations of protein in the media used for sperm preparation will reduce the adverse effect of antisperm antibodies on sperm motility. In summary, antisperm antibodies have been demonstrated to be a contributing factor in infertility. While their presence alone may not be sufficient to prevent pregnancy, their detection should encourage the andrologist to pursue additional appropriate action.

SPERM VITALITY

An intact plasma membrane is an integral component of, and possibly a biologic/diagnostic indicator for, sperm viability. The underlying principle is that viable sperm may contain intact plasma membranes that prevent the passage of certain stains, whereas nonviable sperm have defects within their membranes that allow for staining of the sperm. Several so-called vital stains have been employed for this purpose. They include eosin Y, trypan blue, and/or nigrosin (27). When viewed with either bright field or phase contrast microscopy, these stains allow for the differentiation of viable, nonmotile sperm from dead sperm. This procedure may, therefore, play a significant role in determining the percentage of immotile sperm that are viable and available for ICSI. Unfortunately, dyes such as eosin Y are specific DNA probes that may have toxic effects if they enter a viable sperm or oocyte, which precludes the use of these sperm that have been exposed to the dyes for ICSI or insemination. Flow cytometry has also been utilized for the determination of sperm viability. Like vital staining, flow cytometry is based on the principle that an intact plasma membrane will prevent the passage of nucleic acid-specific stains. Some techniques, such as the one described by Noiles et al., employ dual staining, which can differentiate between an intact membrane and a damaged membrane (28). There are no studies that prospectively evaluate sperm viability staining as a predictor of ART outcome.

HYPO-OSMOTIC SWELLING TEST

Another means of assessing the sperm plasma membrane is the hypo-osmotic swelling test (HOST). This assay is predicated upon the observation that all living cells are permeable to water, although in different degrees. The human sperm membrane has one of the highest hydraulic conductivity coefficients (2.4 µL/min/atm at 22°C) of any mammalian cell (29).

As originally described, the HOST involves placing a sperm specimen into hypotonic conditions of approximately 150 mosmol (30). This environment, while not sufficiently hypotonic to cause cell lysis, will cause swelling of the sperm cells. As the tail swells, the fibers curl, and this change can be detected by phase contrast microscopy, differential interference contrast, or Hoffman optics. The normal range for a positive test is typically considered to be a score ≥60%, that is, at least 60% of the cells demonstrate curling of the tails. A negative test is defined as <50% curling (31). This test generated a significant amount of initial interest, and several investigators compared it to the sperm penetration assay (SPA) as an in vitro surrogate for fertilization, reporting good correlation (32,33). In the 1990s, several investigators reported using the test as a predictor of ART outcome, with conflicting results. Although one group reported a favorable correlation, another found no predictive value for the test (34,35). It has also been suggested that, owing to sperm morphology changes in response to the test, the HOST may facilitate an embryologist's ability to select sperm appropriate for injection. Regardless, as evidenced by the fact that there have been essentially no new human studies on the HOST in the past 10 years, it is likely that the use of the HOST is not increasing significantly. In our program at the Texas Fertility Center, we use the HOST to identify sperm suitable for use in ICSI cases where all sperm are nonmotile. In summary, the HOST currently lacks sufficient critical evaluation to determine its true role in the assessment and/or treatment of the infertile male.

ASSAYS OF THE SPERM ACROSOME

The acrosome is an intracellular organelle, similar to a lysosome, which forms a cap-like structure over the apical portion of the sperm nucleus (36). The acrosome contains multiple hydrolytic enzymes, including hyaluronidase, neuraminidase, proacrosin, phospholipase, and acid phosphatase, which, when released, are thought to facilitate sperm passage through the cumulus mass, and possibly the zona pellucida as well (Fig. 4.4). Once sperm undergo capacitation, they are capable of an acrosome reaction. This reaction is apparently triggered by fusion of the sperm plasma membrane with the outer acrosomal membrane at multiple sites, leading to diffusion of the acrosomal enzymes into the extracellular space. This leads to the dissolution of the plasma membrane and acrosome, leaving the inner acrosomal membrane exposed over the head of the sperm (Fig. 4.5). Although electron microscopy has produced many elegant pictures of acrosome-intact and acrosome reacted sperm, it is not always possible to know whether sperm that fail to exhibit an acrosome have truly acrosome reacted, or could possibly be dead. In addition, electron microscopy is not a technique available to all andrologists.

This has led to the necessity for the development of biochemical markers for the acrosome reaction. Throughout the 1970s and 1980s, multiple biochemical tests were described using a variety of lectins, antibodies, and stains. Although they apparently correlated well with electron microscopy, the tests were still time consuming and difficult to perform (37,38). Contemporary assays for the determination of acrosomal status employ fluorescent plant lectins or monoclonal antibodies, which can be detected much more easily with fluorescence microscopy (39,40). These assays may prove to be of value if they can truly identify males who manifest deficiencies in their ability to undergo the acrosome reaction. Hypothetically, such patients may need to have their sperm specially preincubated—such as with follicular fluid or calcium ionophore—prior to insemination if they fail to acrosome-react on their own. Conversely, this test may help to identify

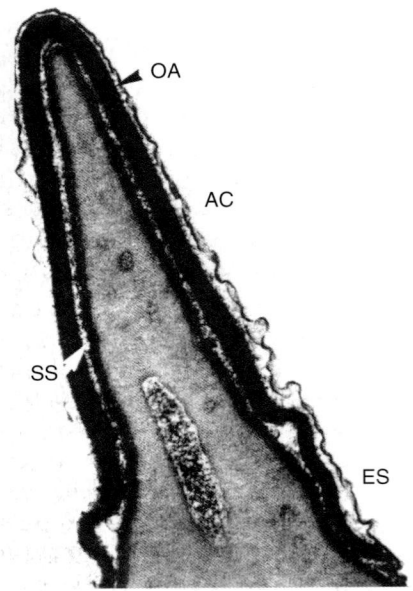

Figure 4.4 Sperm head with intact acrosome. *Abbreviations*: AC, acrosomal cap; ES equatorial segment; OA, outer acrosomal membrane; SS, subacrosomal space. *Source*: Reproduced from Ref. 12.

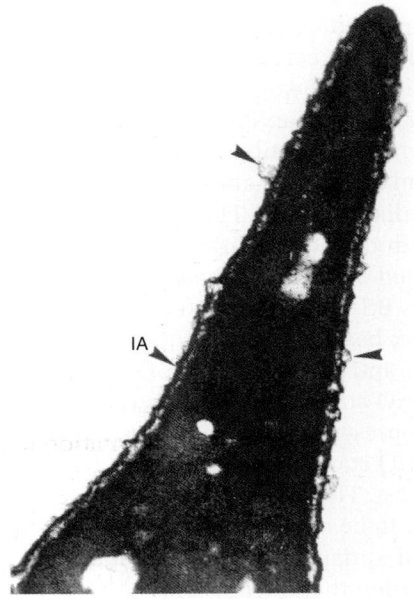

Figure 4.5 Acrosome-reacted sperm. *Abbreviation*: IA, inner acrosomal membrane. *Source*: Reproduced from Ref. 12.

a small subpopulation of males who prematurely acrosome-react. Several studies have reported an association between ejaculated sperm with low percentages of acrosome-intact sperm and poor subsequent fertilization (41). These areas certainly await additional study.

OTHER BIOCHEMICAL TESTS

As noted above, one of the predominant enzymes present in the acrosome is proacrosin. The enzymatic action of acrosin is not necessarily correlated to the presence of an intact acrosome; therefore, assays for the presence of acrosin have been described (42). Acrosin activity has been reported to be greater in fertile men than in infertile men; (43) however, there are no prospective evaluations correlating acrosin activity to fertilization rates in ART patients. Like all other tissues that require energy synthesis and transport, spermatozoa contain measurable levels of creatinine phosphokinase (CPK). Two isomers, CK-M and CK-B, have been described, and differences have been noted in these levels in semen specimens from fertile and infertile men. Specifically, CK-M levels exceed CK-B levels in normospermic males, while CK-B levels are greater in spermatozoa from oligospermic males (44).In this same study, researchers found that semen samples in which CK-M/CK-B ratios exceeded 10% exhibited higher fertilization rates in IVF than specimens with lower ratios. Few other studies have addressed this topic.

SPERM PENETRATION ASSAY

The SPA or hamster egg penetration assay (HEPA) was initially described by Yanagimachi et al. in 1976 (45). It measures the ability of sperm to undergo capacitation and the acrosome reaction, penetrate the oolemma, and then decondense. In this test, oocytes from the golden hamster are first treated in order to remove the zona pellucida. As one of the functions of the zona is to confer species specificity, its presence would preclude performance of this test. However, zona removal obviously prohibits the SPA from being able to assess sperm for the presence of zona receptors. Following zona removal, human sperm are incubated for 48 hours with the hamster oocytes, and the number of penetrations with nuclear decondensation is calculated. As originally described, it was hoped that the test would correlate with the ability of human sperm to fertilize human oocytes in vitro. Although the test was designed to assess the ability of sperm to fuse to the oolemma, it also indirectly assesses sperm capacitation, the acrosome reaction, and the ability of the sperm to be incorporated into the ooplasm. Unfortunately, however, intrinsic in the design of the test is its inability to assess the sperm's ability to bind to—and penetrate through—the zona pellucida. This factor continues to be one of the major criticisms that plague this test. Throughout the 1980s, multiple modifications of the SPA were published. These included modifications of the techniques for sperm preparation prior to the performance of the assay, such as inducing the acrosome reaction or incubation with TEST yolk buffer (Irvine Scientific, Irvine, California, USA), changes in the protocol methodology itself, and modifications of the scoring system (46,47). Published reports demonstrated widely varying conclusions, such as the finding that the SPA could identify anywhere from 0 to 78% of men whose sperm would fail to fertilize oocytes in ART procedures (48). Most criticisms of the SPA literature center on poor standardization of the assay, poor reproducibility of the test, and lack of a standard normal range.

Although some reports suggest a correlation between the SPA and fertility, neither a large literature review (48) nor a prospective long-term (five-year) follow-up study demonstrates such a correlation (49). In fact, a meta-analysis of 2906 subjects from 34 prospective, controlled studies suggested that the SPA is a poor predictor of fertilization (50). In light of these considerations, support for this test has gradually waned.

HEMIZONA ASSAY

Over the past several years, a growing body of research has demonstrated a significant correlation between tests of sperm–zona pellucida binding and subsequent fertilization in ART. This led the European Society for Human Reproduction and Embryology (ESHRE) Andrology Special Interest Group to recommend inclusion of such tests in the advanced evaluation of the male (51). Like the SPA, the hemizona assay (HZA) employs sperm and non-viable oocytes in an in vitro assessment of fertilization (52). In this test, however, both gametes are human in origin. As described, the HZA assesses the ability of sperm to undergo capacitation, acrosome react, and bind tightly to the zona. Classically, oocytes that failed to fertilize during an ART procedure are bisected, and then sperm from a proven fertile donor (500,000/mL) are added to one hemizona, while sperm from the subject male are added to the other hemizona. Following four-hour incubation, each hemizona is removed and pipetted in order to dislodge loosely attached sperm. A comparison or hemizona index (HZI) is then calculated by dividing the number of test sperm tightly bound to the hemizona by the number of control (fertile) sperm bound to the other hemizona:

$$HZI = \text{Number of test sperm bound/Number of control sperm bound} \times 100$$

This test assesses the ability of sperm to bind to the zona itself. Although HZA being expensive, labor-intensive, and difficult to perform, there are some data that suggest that the HZA may help to identify individuals with a poor prognosis for success with ART (53,54) (Fig. 4.6). A more recent prospective study employing receiver operating characteristic curve analysis has also suggested that HZA results may be used to predict subsequent fertilization in ART procedures with both high sensitivity and specificity (55).

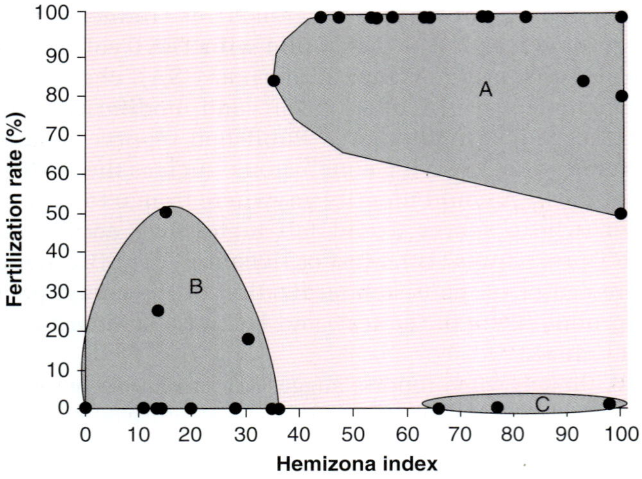

Figure 4.6 Cluster analysis of hemizona assay index and fertilization rate. (**A**), good fertilization; (**B**), poor fertilization; (**C**), false-positive hemizona assay index. *Source*: From Ref. 52.

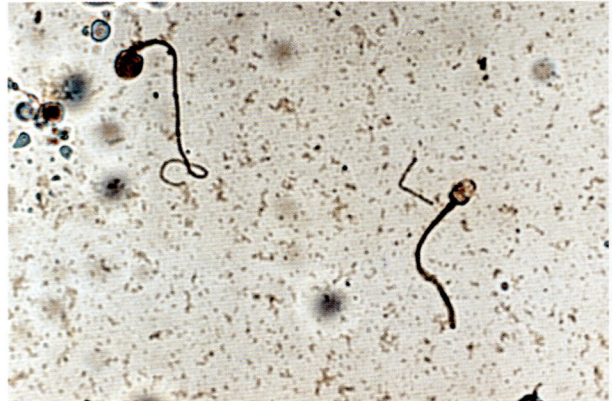

Figure 4.7 Mannose-positive (brown) and mannose-negative (clear) sperm. *Source*: Courtesy of Tammy Dey, Kaylen Silverberg.

MANNOSE BINDING ASSAY

Another test has been developed in order to assess the ability of sperm to bind to the zona. This in vitro procedure is based on a series of observations that suggest that sperm–oocyte interaction involves the recognition by a sperm surface receptor of a specific complementary receptor on the surface of the zona pellucida. This zona receptor appears to be a glycoprotein, the predominant sugar moiety of which is mannose (56). In an elegant series of experiments, Mori et al. determined that sperm–zona binding could be curtailed by the addition of a series of sugars to the incubating media. Although many sugars impaired binding, the addition of mannose totally inhibited sperm–oocyte interaction (57). In vitro assays in which labeled probes of mannose conjugated to albumin are co-incubated with semen specimens allow for the differential staining of sperm (Fig. 4.7). Those that bind the probe are thought to possess the sperm surface receptor for the mannose-rich zona glycoprotein. Several investigators, including our group, have subsequently demonstrated that sperm from fertile populations exhibit greater mannose binding than do sperm from infertile males (58–60). This new area shows promise in the area of sperm function testing, but also invites further study.

ASSAYS OF SPERM DNA INTEGRITY

The most current area of investigation into sperm function involves the assessment of sperm DNA integrity. Sperm chromatin has been demonstrated to be packaged very differently from chromatin in somatic cells. Specifically, the DNA is organized in such a manner that it remains very compact and stable (61). As there are many ways in which this DNA organization or the sperm chromatin itself can be damaged, several assays of sperm chromatin assessment have been developed. There are two basic types of assays: direct assays, such as the "Comet" and "TUNEL" assays, and indirect assays such as the sperm chromatin structure assay or acridine orange assay (62). The direct assays detect actual breakages in the DNA, while the indirect assays measure the relative proportions of single (abnormal) and double (normal) stranded DNA within the sperm following acid treatment. Data from several studies suggest that infertile men have significantly a greater amount of DNA damage than fertile men (61,63,64). There is also a suggestion that this finding is similarly present in the male partner of couples experiencing recurrent miscarriage. Despite these reports, at the present time, there is no conclusive correlation between the results of sperm DNA integrity testing and pregnancy rates achieved either naturally or with the ARTs. As such, the Practice Committee of the American Society for Reproductive Medicine recommended that the routine testing of sperm DNA integrity should not be included in the evaluation of the infertile couple (65).

CONCLUSION

In summary, there have been many recent advances in the diagnostic evaluation of sperm and sperm function. Although many tests of sperm function have been described, there remains a lack of consensus as to the role of testing and the identification of the appropriate test(s) to perform. Owing to the complicated nature of sperm function, it is improbable that a single test will emerge with sufficient sensitivity, specificity, and positive and negative predictive values required of a first-line diagnostic tool for all affected men. A more likely scenario will be similar to that in female infertility, where a battery of tests—each evaluating a specific function—are employed as needed. In light of profound recent advances in gamete micromanipulation, a more germane issue might be the overall relevance of sperm function testing in the contemporary andrology laboratory. Although this issue is quite controversial, it is likely that sperm function testing will continue to play a role in the evaluation of the infertile male. Just as ART is not the treatment of choice for all infertile women, it is not likely that micromanipulation will be the standard treatment for all infertile men. The gold standard of sperm function remains the ability to fertilize an oocyte in vitro. Therefore, in order to continue to address the above questions, it is incumbent upon investigators to design appropriate prospective trials to assess these tests thoroughly. Those tests that demonstrate a statistically significant correlation with fertilization in vitro must then undergo additional evaluation in order to assess clinical significance if we hope to develop an appropriate diagnostic algorithm.

REFERENCES

1. World Health Organization. WHO Laboratory Manual for the Examination of Human Semen and Sperm–Cervical Mucus Interaction. 4th edn. New York: Cambridge University Press, 1999; 4–33: 60–1.
2. World Health Organization. WHO Laboratory Manual for the Examination of Human Semen. 5th edn. Geneva, Switzerland: WHO Press, 2010: 223–5.
3. Cooper TG, Noonan E, von Eckardstein S, et al. World Health Organization reference values for human semen characteristics. Hum Reprod Update 2010; 16: 231–45.
4. Alexander NJ. Male evaluation and semen analysis. Clin Obstet Gynecol 1982; 25: 463–82.
5. Overstreet JW, Katz DF, Hanson FW, Foseca JR. A simple inexpensive method for objective assessment of human sperm movement characteristics. Fertil Steril 1979; 31: 162–72.
6. Overstreet JW, Davis RO, Katz DF, Overstreet JW, eds. Infertility and Reproductive Medicine. Clinics of North America. Philadelphia: WB Saunders, 1992: 329–40.
7. Koren E, Lukac J. Mechanism of liquefaction of the human ejaculate: I. Changes of the ejaculate proteins. J Reprod Fertil 1979; 56: 493–500.
8. Lukac J, Koren E. Mechanism of liquefaction of the human ejaculate: II. Role of collagenase like peptidase and seminal proteinase. J Reprod Fertil 1979; 56: 501–10.
9. Cohen J, Aafjes JH. Proteolytic enzymes stimulate human spermatozoal motility and in vitro hamster egg penetration. Life Sci 1982; 30: 899–904.
10. Van Voorhis BJ, Sparks A. Semen analysis: what tests are clinically useful? Clin Obstet Gynecol 1999; 42: 957–71.
11. Gangi CR, Nagler HM. Clinical evaluation of the subfertile man. In: Diamond MP, DeCherney AH, Overstreet JW, eds. Infertility and Reproductive Medicine. Clinics of North America. Philadelphia: WB Saunders, 1992; 3: 299–318.
12. Sathananthan AH, ed. Visual Atlas of Human Sperm Structure and Function for Assisted Reproductive Technique. Melbourne: La Trobe and Monash Universities, Singapore: National University, 1996.
13. Kruger TF, Acosta AA, Simmons KF, et al. Predictive value of abnormal sperm morphology in in vitro fertilization. Fertil Steril 1988; 49: 112–17.
14. Kruger TF, Menkveld R, Stander FS, et al. Sperm morphologic features as a prognostic factor in in vitro fertilization. Fertil Steril 1986; 46: 1118–23.
15. Katz DF, Overstreet JW. Sperm motility assessment by videomicrography. Fertil Steril 1981; 35: 188–93.
16. Katz DF, Diel L, Overstreet JW. Differences in the movements of morphologically normal and abnormal human seminal spermatozoa. Biol Reprod 1982; 26: 566–70.
17. Franken DR, Oehninger S, Burkman LJ, et al. The hemizona assay (HZA): a prediction of human sperm fertilizing potential in in vitro fertilization (IVF) treatment. J In Vitro Fert Embryo Transfer 1989; 6: 44–50.
18. Coetzee K, Kruger TF, Lombard CJ. Predictive value of normal sperm morphology: a structured literature review. Hum Reprod Update 1988; 4: 73–82.
19. Enginsu MF, Pieters MGEC, Dumoulin JCM, Evers JLH, Geruedts JPM. Male factor as determinant of in vitro fertilization outcome. Hum Reprod 1992; 7: 1136–40.
20. Davis R. The promise and pitfalls of computer aided sperm analysis. In: Diamond MP, DeCherney AH, Overstreet JW, eds. Infertility and Reproductive Medicine. Clinics of North America, Philadelphia: WB Saunders, 1992: 93: 341–52.
21. Irvine DS. The computer assisted semen analysis systems: sperm motility assessment. Hum Reprod 1995; 10(Suppl 1): 53–9.
22. Krause W. Computer assisted semen analysis systems: comparison with routine evaluation and prognostic value in male fertility and assisted reproduction. Hum Reprod 1995; 10(Suppl 4): 60–6.
23. Marshburn PB, Kutteh WH. The role of antisperm antibodies in infertility. Fertil Steril 1994; 61: 799–811.
24. Golumb J, Vardinon N, Hommonnai ZT, et al. Demonstration of antispermotozoal antibodies in varicocele-related infertility with an enzyme-linked immunosorbent assay (ELISA). Fertil Steril 1986; 45: 397–405.
25. Helmerhost FM, Finken MJJ, Erwich JJ. Detection assays for antisperm antibodies: what do they test? Hum Reprod 1999; 14: 1669–71.
26. Bronson R. Detection of antisperm antibodies: An argument against therapeutic nihilism. Hum Reprod 1999; 14: 1671–3.
27. World Health Organization. Manual for Examination of Human Semen and Semen–Cervical Mucus. Cambridge: Cambridge University Press, 1987: 1–12.
28. Noiles EE, Ruffing NA, Kleinhans FW, et al. Critical tonicity determination of sperm using dual fluorescent staining and flow cytometry. In: Johnson LA, Rath D, eds. Reproduction in Domestic Animals. (Suppl 1) Boar Semen Preservation II. Procedings of the Second International Conference on Boar Semen Presentation. Beltsville, MD: 1991. 359–64.
29. Noiles EE, Mazur. P, Watson PF, et al. Determination of water permeability coefficient for human spermatozoa and its activation energy. Biol Reprod 1993; 48: 99–109.
30. Jeyendran RS, Van der Ven JJ, Perez-Pelaez M. Development of an assay to assess the functional integrity of the human sperm membrane and its relationship to other semen characteristics. J Reprod Fertil 1984; 70: 219–28.
31. Zaneveld LJD, Jeyendran RS. Modern assessment of semen for diagnostic purposes. Semin Reprod Endocrinol 1988; 4: 323–37.
32. Chan SYW, Fox EJ, Chan MMC. The relationship between the human sperm hypoosmotic swelling test, routine semen analysis, and the human sperm zona free hamster ovum penetration test. Fertil Steril 1985; 44: 688–92.
33. Jeyendran RS, Zaneveld LJD. Human sperm hypoosmotic swelling test. Fertil Steril 1986; 46: 151–4.
34. Mladenovic I, Micic S, Genbacev O, et al. The hypoosmotic swelling test for quality control of sperm prepared for assisted reproduction. Arch Androl 1995; 34: 163–9.
35. Joshi N, Kodwany G, Balaiah D, et al. The importance of CASA and sperm function testing in a in vitro

fertilization program. Int J Fertil Menopausal Stud 1996; 41: 46–52.
36. Critser JK, Noiles EE. Bioassays of sperm function. Semin Reprod Endocrinol 1993; 11: 1–16.
37. Talbot P, Chacon RS. A triple stain technique for evaluating acrosome reaction of human sperm. J Exp Zool 1981; 215: 201–8.
38. Wolf DP, Boldt J, Byrd W, et al. Acrosomal status evaluation in human ejaculated sperm with monoclonal antibodies. Biol Reprod 1985; 32: 1157–62.
39. Cross NL, Morales P, Overstreet JW, et al. Two simple methods for detecting acrosome-reacted sperm. Gamete Res 1986; 15: 213–16.
40. Holden CA, Hyne RV, Sathananthan AH, et al. Assessment of the human sperm acrosome reaction using concanavalin A lectin. Mol Reprod Dev 1990; 25: 247–57.
41. Chan PJ, Corselli JU, Jacobson JD, et al. Spermac stain analysis of human sperm acrosomes. Fertil Steril 1999; 72: 124–8.
42. Kennedy WP, Kaminski JM, Van der Ven HH, et al. A simple clinical assay to evaluate the acrosin activity of human spermatozoa. J Androl 1989; 10: 221–31.
43. Mohsenian M, Syner FN, Moghissi KS. A study of sperm acrosin in patients with unexplained infertility. Fertil Steril 1982; 37: 223–9.
44. Huszar G, Vigue L, Morshedi M. Sperm creatinine phosphokinaseM-isoform ratios and fertilizing potential of men: a blinded study of 84 couples treated with in vitro fertilization. Fertil Steril 1992; 57: 882–8.
45. Yanagimachi R, Yanagimachi H, Rogers BJ. The use of zona-free animal ova as a free system for the assessment of their fertilizing capacity of human spermatozoa. Biol Reprod 1976; 15: 471–6.
46. Aitken RJ, Thatcher S, Glasier AF, et al. Relative ability of modified versions of the hamster oocyte penetration test, incorporating hyperosmotic medium of the ionophore A23187 to predict IVF outcome. Hum Reprod 1987; 2: 227–31.
47. Jacobs BR, Caulfield J, Boldt J. Analysis of TEST (TES and tris) yolk buffer effects on human sperm. Fertil Steril 1995; 63: 1064–70.
48. Mao C, Grimes DA. The sperm penetration assay: can it discriminate between fertile and infertile men? Am J Obstet Gynecol 1988; 159: 279–86.
49. O'Shea DL, Odem RR, Cholewa C, et al. Long-term follow-up of couples after hamster egg penetration testing. Fertil Steril 1993; 60: 1040–5.
50. Oehninger S, Franken DR, Sayed E, Barroso G, Kolm P. Sperm function assays and their predictive value for fertilization outcome in IVF therapy: A meta-analysis. Hum Reprod Update 2000; 6: 160–8.
51. ESHRE Andrology Special Interest Group. Consensus Workshop on Advanced Diagnostic Andrology Techniques. Hum Reprod 1996; 11: 1463–79.
52. Burkman LJ, Coddington CC, Franken DR, et al. The hemizona assay (HZA): development of a diagnostic test for the binding of human spermatozoa to the human hemizona pellucida to predict fertilization potential. Fertil Steril 1988; 49: 688–97.
53. Oehninger S, Acosta AA, Marshedi M, et al. Corrective measures and pregnancy outcome in in vitro fertilization in patients with severe sperm morphology abnormalities. Fertil Steril 1989; 50: 283–7.
54. Oehninger S, Toner J, Muasher S, et al. Prediction of fertilization in vitro with human gametes; is there a litmus test? Am J Obstet Gynecol 1992; 166: 1760–7.
55. Coddington CC, Oehninger SC, Olive DL, et al. Hemizona index (HZI) demonstrates excellent predictability when evaluating sperm fertilizing capacity in in vitro fertilization patients. J Androl 1994; 15: 250–4.
56. Mori K, Daitoh T, Irahara M, et al. Significance of D-mannose as a sperm receptor site on the zona pellucida in human fertilization. Am J Obstet Gynecol 1989; 161: 207–11.
57. Mori K, Daitoh T, Kamada M, et al. Blocking of human fertilization by carbohydrates. Hum Reprod 1993; 8: 1729–32.
58. Tesarik J, Mendoza C, Carreras R. Expression of D-mannose binding sites on human spermatozoa: comparison of fertile donors and infertile patients. Fertil Steril 1991; 56: 113–18.
59. Benoff S, Cooper GW, Hurley I, et al. Human sperm fertilizing potential in vitro is correlated with differential expression of a head-specific mannose ligand receptor. Fertil Steril 1993; 59: 854–62.
60. Silverberg K, Dey T, Witz C, et al. D-Mannose binding provides a more objective assessment of male fertility than routine semen analysis: correlation with in vitro fertilization. Presented at the 49th Annual Meeting of the American Fertility Society, 1993.
61. Agarwal A, Said T. Role of sperm chromatin abnormalities and DNA damage in male infertility. Hum Reprod Update 2003; 9: 331–45.
62. Evenson DP, Wixon R. Clinical aspects of sperm DNA fragmentation detection and male infertility. Theriogenology 2006; 65: 979–91.
63. Zini A, Bielecki R, Phang D, et al. Correlations between two markers of sperm DNA integrity, DNA denaturation and DNA fragmentation in fertile and infertile men. Fertil Steril 2001; 75: 674–7.
64. Evenson DP, Jost LK, Marshall D, et al. Utility of the sperm chromatin assay as a diagnostic and prognostic tool in the human fertility clinic. Hum Reprod 1999; 14: 1039–49.
65. The Practice Committee of the American Society for Reproductive Medicine. The clinical utility of sperm DNA integrity testing. Fertil Steril 2006; 86(Suppl 4): S35–7.

5

Sperm preparation techniques

Harold Bourne, Janell Archer, David H. Edgar, and H. W. Gordon Baker

OVERVIEW

The aim of sperm preparation for assisted reproductive techniques (ARTs) is to maximize the chances of fertilization to provide as many normally fertilized oocytes as possible for transfer to the uterus or cryopreservation (1). With normal semen it is easy to obtain motile sperm by a variety of techniques. Abnormal semen, which will not yield adequate sperm for standard in vitro fertilization (IVF), needs to be recognized so that intracytoplasmic sperm injection (ICSI) can be used. Refinements of the preparation procedures are required to obtain spermatozoa or elongated spermatids with the highest potential for normal fertilization from grossly abnormal semen samples or from samples obtained directly from the male genital tract. Sperm characteristics important for fertilization with standard IVF include normal morphology, normal intact acrosomes, straight line velocity (VSL) and linearity (LIN) and ability to bind to the zona pellucida, penetrate the zona pellucida, fuse with the oolemma, activate the oocyte, and form a male pronucleus (1). For ICSI, live sperm with an ability to activate the oocyte and form a pronucleus are necessary but morphology, motility, and acrosome status are generally not important (1–5). It is probably important to remove seminal plasma as it contains decapacitation factors and extraneous cells and degenerating sperm that may produce agents capable of damaging the sperm (6–8). For IVF or gamete intrafallopian transfer (GIFT), the medium should contain protein and buffers which promote sperm capacitation (1). While serum or high molecular weight fractions from serum appear to be important for sperm motility, more recently relatively pure preparations of human serum albumin, pasteurized to reduce the risk of transmitting infections, have been found to be adequate for sperm preparation for standard IVF and ICSI (9,10). Purified and appropriately tested human serum albumin preparations are now routinely available from the major IVF media suppliers. The inclusion of protein in the culture medium is required to prevent sperm from adhering to surfaces. Although the concentration of albumin in human periovulatory oviductal fluid is reported to be of the order of 30 mg/mL, concentrations of around 4 mg/mL will support normal sperm function in IVF. Bicarbonate ions are required for capacitation of sperm and are normally present at a concentration of about 25 mmol/L in the medium. Although glucose is utilized as a metabolic substrate by sperm it is not clear whether it is essential for normal function in vitro. It has been suggested that more recent media formulations, which do not contain glucose, may not be appropriate for fertilization stages of ART procedures.

Damage to the sperm from dilution, temperature change, centrifugation, and exposure to potentially toxic material must be minimized. Dilution should be performed slowly, especially with cryopreserved sperm. Temperature changes should be gradual. Preparation of the insemination suspension should be performed at or as close as practicable to 37°C. Centrifugal force should be the lowest possible required to bring down the most motile sperm. Minimizing centrifugation, particularly in the absence of seminal plasma, and separating the live motile sperm from the dead sperm and debris early in the procedure should limit oxidative damage caused by free oxygen radicals released from leukocytes or abnormal sperm (6,7,11).

Modifications of sperm preparation may be necessary for the various types of ART. For example, for GIFT or intratubal insemination, suspensions of spermatozoa are to be introduced into the fallopian tubes so debris and bacteria must be removed and no particulate material added which might damage the female genital tract. If cryopreserved donor sperm are to be used, matching and extra care in preparation of the sample is usually required. If the semen is severely abnormal, sperm are prepared for ICSI.

Combinations of gradient centrifugation and swim-up methods may produce higher yields of good quality sperm (12). In the era of ICSI, the need for special preparation techniques has receded as simple procedures with swim up, washing or allowing sperm to swim to the medium–oil interface from a centrifuged pellet placed in droplets of medium under oil, produce fertilization and pregnancy rates as good as those with sperm obtained by more careful and laborious preparation techniques (13). The use of gradient centrifugation may also provide additional safeguards in preparing sperm from men with a chronic viral illness (14,15).

The optimal number of sperm for insemination is poorly defined but several reviews of results of IVF suggest that there is an increase in fertilization rate with insemination of sperm at between 2000 and 500,000/mL (1). There may be some increase in risks of polyspermy with the higher sperm concentrations thus most groups inseminate oocytes with approximately 100,000 sperm/mL for standard IVF or GIFT. This is more than surround the oocyte in vivo and, if better selection of high quality sperm could be achieved, insemination with lower numbers could be as or more successful. It has been suggested that reduced exposure of the oocyte to sperm may result in improvement in embryo quality and higher implantation rates (16,17). The total volume of sperm suspension added should be minimized to restrict dilution of the oocyte medium.

METHODS

Procedures for preparation of the culture media and sperm isolation are given in appendices 1–8 and shown schematically in Figures 5.1–5.4.

Collection of Semen or Sperm

While semen is usually collected by masturbation for ART, sperm may be collected by a variety of methods from several sites in the male genital tract (Fig. 5.1). The man should collect semen into a sterile disposable plastic jar in a room adjacent to the IVF laboratory. The sperm should be prepared soon after liquefaction of the seminal plasma. If liquefaction is delayed or the specimen is particularly viscous, syringing the sample through a 21-gauge needle or mixing the specimen 1:1 with the medium followed by vigorous shaking may help. If the semen sample is unexpectedly poor, a second sample may provide sufficient sperm. Cryopreserved sperm can also be used, for example, as backup for ICSI for patients with motile sperm present in the semen only intermittently. The timing of semen collection and preparation does not appear to be critical especially with good semen samples. In general, the oocytes are inseminated four to six hours after collection and the sperm can be prepared during this time. The semen should be placed in a clean area of the laboratory or in a laminar flow hood. The sample must be mixed thoroughly because ejaculation does not result in a homogeneous suspension of sperm in the seminal plasma. The semen sample is examined, any particulate material is allowed to settle, and the supernatant is transferred to another tube if necessary. Following mixing, a small portion (~10 µL) of the sample is taken to check the sperm concentration and motility. With normal semen samples, usually 1 mL of sample is sufficient for preparation of adequate numbers of motile sperm. If the semen sample is mildly to moderately abnormal but judged adequate for standard IVF, then the whole semen volume should be distributed to several tubes for preparation of as many sperm as possible.

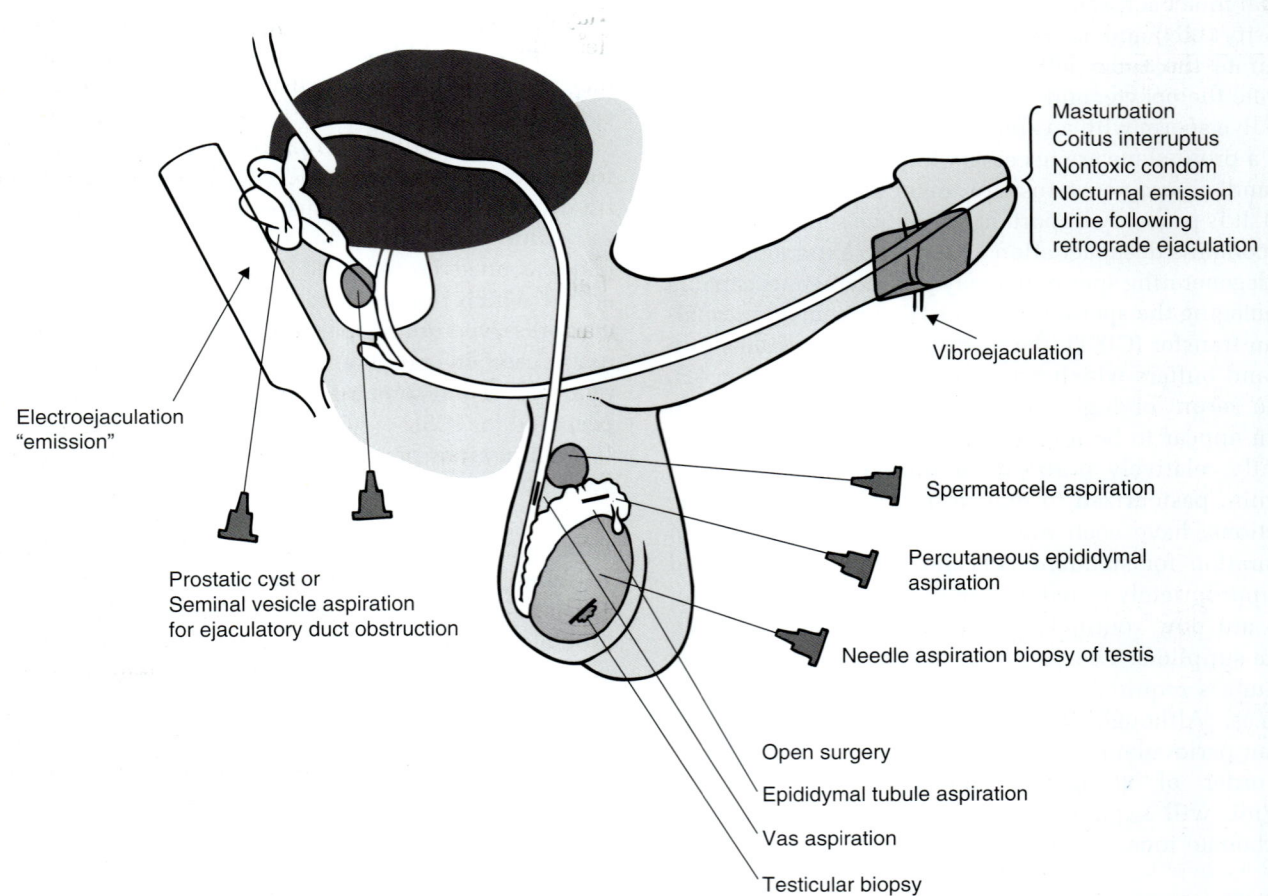

Figure 5.1 Possible sites of collection of sperm or elongated spermatids from the male genital tract for assisted reproduction.

Sperm Preparation

Initially, IVF involved repeated "washing" of the spermatozoa by dilution of the semen with culture medium supplemented with protein, followed by centrifugation and resuspension of the pellet. This technique has been criticized as it may result in oxidative damage of the sperm by free oxygen radicals (6,7,11,18,19). Sperm for ICSI may be harvested from the oil–medium interface after the sperm-containing material is placed in a drop of culture medium under oil (Fig. 5.3). Some prepare channels to outlaying smaller droplets for this purpose.

All plastic, glassware, and media should be checked for toxicity to sperm or embryos. Sperm may be immobilized by contact with rubber. A variety of media are suitable for sperm preparation for IVF. The medium chosen should be equilibrated with the gas mixture and the temperature maintained constant at 37°C. If not using a commercially available protein source suitable for human ART but preparing a protein source in-house from serum, then this needs to be checked for sperm antibodies and, if pools are used, the donors must be tested for viral illnesses including HIV and hepatitis. However the use of pooled serum samples is to be discouraged because of the risk of transmitting both known and unknown diseases. Heat inactivation of the serum should not be relied upon to overcome the risk of transmitting infections.

Swim Up

Several variations of the swim-up procedure are possible. The seminal plasma can be overlaid directly with culture medium and the sperm allowed to swim from the seminal plasma into the culture medium. Following this the sperm suspension should be washed to ensure adequate removal of seminal plasma constituents. Alternatively, the semen sample may be diluted and centrifuged and the pellet loosened and overlaid or the semen sample may be centrifuged without prior dilution of the seminal plasma and the pellet loosened and overlaid with medium for the swim-up procedure. The latter technique may be particularly useful for oligozoospermia as the sperm may be damaged by the dilution procedure. If cryopreserved semen is to be used, dilution of the semen sample should be slow with a drop-wise addition of culture medium to the thawed sample. If the thawed semen is overlaid directly, the need for slow dilution is eliminated.

After centrifugation the supernatant is aspirated off the pellet and the pellet is gently resuspended in a small volume of liquid. The overlay medium is then gently pipetted onto the surface of the pellet and the tube is incubated for 45–60 minutes. Prolonged incubation times may result in a reduced yield of motile sperm from gravitational effects. The use of a conical tube for centrifugation may help maximize yield as the pellet is easier to see and less likely to be disturbed during manipulation. Some recommend that the tubes be placed in the incubator at an angle to increase the surface area of the interface. Following incubation, the upper half to two-thirds of the overlay is aspirated and mixed and the sperm concentration is determined.

Density Gradients

Various gradient separation procedures have been introduced. The advantage is that the gradient separation techniques are rapid, requiring 20-minute centrifugation compared with an average of one-hour incubation for swim up. They are also relatively simple to perform under sterile conditions. The most popular of these is colloidal silica density gradient (CSDG) centrifugation but other agents have also been used (1,12,20). The colloidal silica particles are coated with polyvinylpyrrolidone for example, Percoll™ (Pharmacia AB, Uppsula, Sweden). However, concerns regarding the levels of endotoxins have resulted in the withdrawal of Percoll from use in ART. Other media containing silane-coated silica have become available for clinical use from the major IVF media companies and other specialist suppliers, including Isolate™ (Irvine Scientific, Santa Ana, California, USA), PureSperm™ (Nidacon Laboratories, AB, Gothenburg, Sweden), SpermGrad™ (Vitrolife, Englewood, Colorado, USA), SupraSperm™ (Medicult, Jyllinge, Denmark), PureCeption™ (Sage Biopharma,

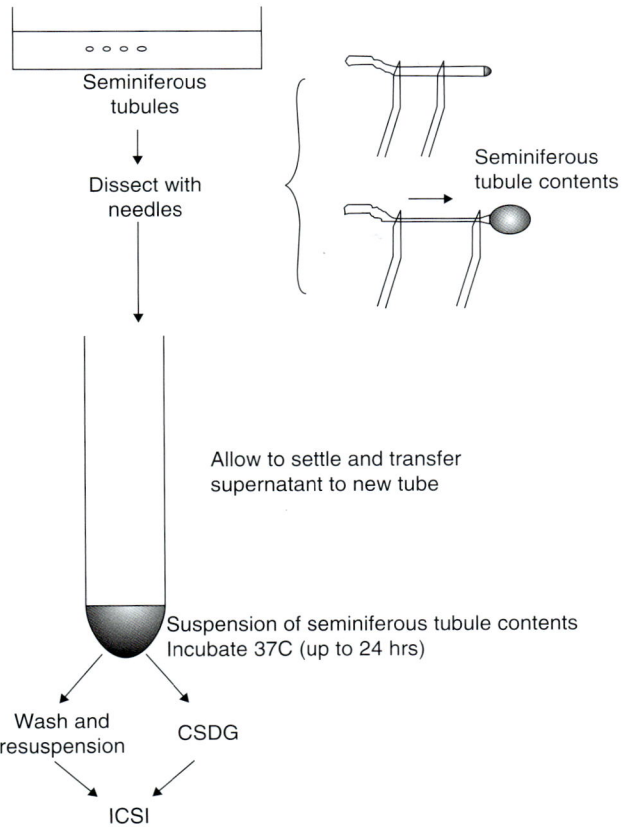

Figure 5.2 Procedure for seminiferous tubules obtained by fine needle tissue aspiration or open biopsy. *Abbreviations*: CSDG, colloidal silica density gradient; ICSI, intracytoplasmic sperm injection.

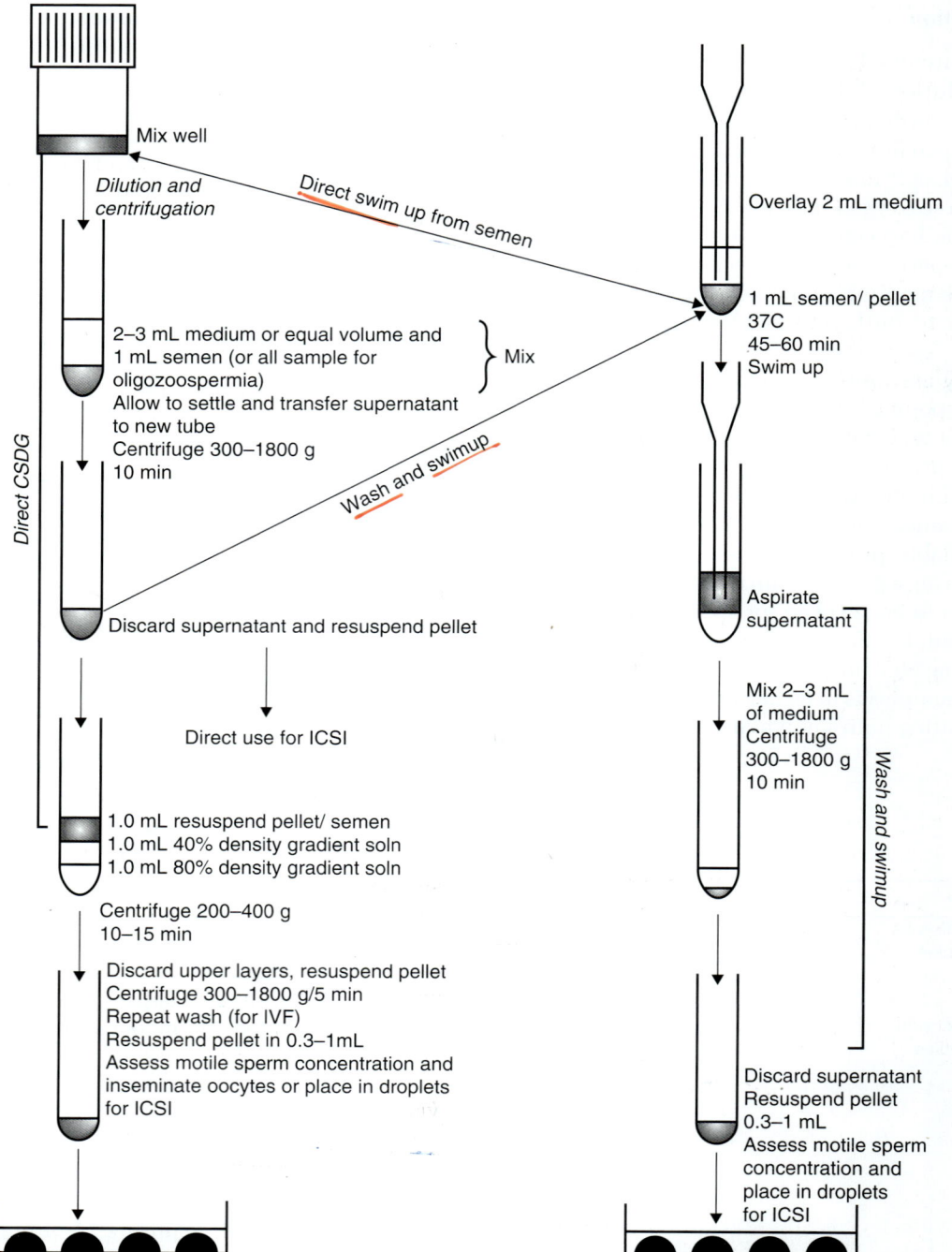

Figure 5.3 Methods of sperm preparation for assisted reproduction. *Abbreviations*: ICSI, intracytoplasmic sperm injection; IVF, in vitro fertilization.

Bedminster, New Jersey, USA), Sil-Select™ (FertiPro, Beeman, Belgium), and Sydney IVF density gradient media (William A. COOK, Brisbane, Queensland, Australia).

Discontinuous gradients of two or more steps are used. Sperm and other material form distinct bands at the interfaces on the CSDG (Fig. 5.4). It has been claimed that abnormal sperm as well as immotile sperm and debris are largely eliminated and a rapid and efficient isolation of motile human sperm, free from contamination with other seminal constituents, is possible. A number of studies have compared CSDG centrifugation with the swim-up and occasionally other sperm preparation techniques. The end points of the studies have been recovery of motile sperm, morphology, chromatin structure assessed by the various techniques, and ultrastructure. Generally the recovery of motile sperm is greater with the gradient techniques but the percentage of sperm with progressive motility is usually lower and the proportion of sperm with good morphology is lower with gradient centrifugation than with swim up (1,8,12,21–23). Some studies suggest that the gradient materials may damage the sperm (24,25). Others indicate gradient preparations produce sperm with less mitochondrial and DNA

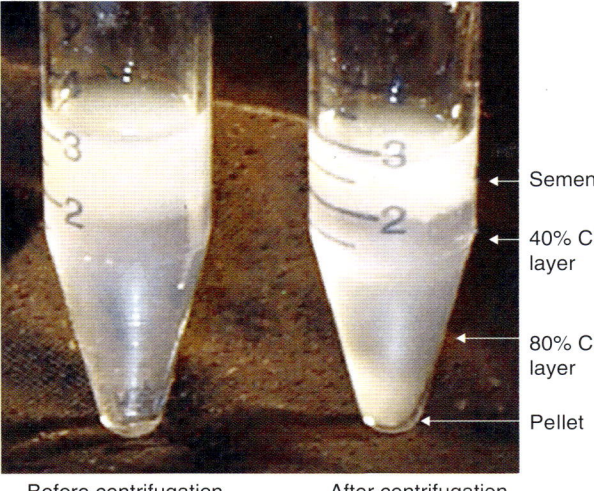

Figure 5.4 Appearance of gradient tubes with overlaid semen prior to and after centrifugation. *Abbreviations*: CSDG, colloidal silica density gradient.

damage than other procedures (26–29). However, while there are some reports of higher fertilization and pregnancy rates, improved results of IVF and ICSI are not consistently found (26,27). CSDG in combination with swim up has also been reported to reduce the viral load from samples carrying an infectious agent such as HIV (30–34) However, CSDG on its own, or in combination with swim up, should not be relied upon to minimize the risk of infection to the woman or any resulting pregnancy (31,35–39) although modifications to the procedure may further reduce the chance for viral contamination of the final preparation (39–41).

Sperm Preparation from Surgical Aspirates or Tissue Samples

Spermatozoa or elongated spermatids may be obtained for ICSI from the male genital tract by microsurgical epididymal sperm aspiration (MESA), percutaneous epididymal sperm aspiration (PESA), testicular open biopsy or fine needle aspiration biopsy, or other techniques (Fig. 5.1). Preparing tissue from a fine needle biopsy can be managed using fine gauge needles. Processing of large amounts of tissue may be expedited by using bigger implements (e.g., scalpel blades) and/or a sterile mortar and pestle homogenizer in the style of a small conical tube and insert. Methods for preparation are outlined in appendices 7 and 8.

Sperm Selection from Immotile Samples

ICSI with immotile sperm is often associated with low fertilization rates; thus, every attempt should be made to ensure that live sperm are injected (1–4,42). A variety of agents have been reported to enhance sperm motility (1). Pentoxifylline (POF) has been used for ART. The maximally effective dose of POF is between 0.3 and 0.6 mmol/L and many groups use 3.6 mmol/L (1 mg/mL). POF has been reported to provide greater stimulation of motility and velocity than caffeine or 2-deoxyadenosine. Exposure of sperm to hypo-osmotic medium is also used to identify potentially viable sperm by detecting membrane integrity. This method may reveal a higher proportion of viable sperm than when utilizing motility stimulants alone; however, it can be technically more difficult in cases where sperm density is high, or large amounts of debris or extraneous material are present. The use of a laser pulse, applied to the tail tip of an immotile sperm (43) and a mechanical touch technique (44) have also been suggested as useful tools to identify viable sperm for injection although both these approaches await verification in a wider setting. In practical terms, the generation of sperm movement from the use of motility stimulants has the added advantage of making live sperm more conspicuous and therefore may be the preferred first choice in identifying viable sperm from an immotile population. Appendices 10 and 11 give methods for stimulating sperm motility with POF and the use of hypo-osmotic media.

Preparation of Semen from HIV-Infected Men

The use of combination antiretroviral therapies has markedly improved the prognosis and life expectancy for men infected with HIV. A population of these men in a discordant relationship (i.e., where the man is seropositive and the women is uninfected) desire parenthood from their own gametes. With appropriate medical care and use of ART techniques, safe and effective treatment can now be offered for achieving a pregnancy while minimizing the risk of transmission to either the partner or the resulting baby. (14,15,45–52) Most protocols recommend the use of antiretroviral therapies to reduce viral load, subsequent testing of sperm samples for residual viral HIV RNA and DNA using sensitive PCR techniques and the preparation of cleared samples for clinical use via density gradient centrifugation. Normally, cryopreservation of the sperm is required to allow adequate time for the testing regimens to be completed. Samples with undetectable or sufficiently low viral loads are cleared for use and, depending on the quality of the sperm post thaw, an attempt at pregnancy is undertaken using intrauterine insemination, IVF, or ICSI. A flow diagram for the treatment of discordant couples where the male is seropositive is presented in Figure 5.5.

Sperm Selection Techniques

A variety of techniques have been reported for the selection of sperm with characteristics which may improve outcome. The quality of sperm DNA packaging, described in terms of DNA damage or fragmentation, has been implicated in poor embryo development and pregnancy loss. Methods to select sperm with reduced levels of damage have been sought in an attempt to improve clinical outcomes following ART.

The use of membrane-based electrophoretic filtration to potentially select sperm with reduced DNA damage has been reported (53). Clinical pregnancies have been achieved; however, sperm recovery, functional parameters, and clinical outcomes were comparable to sperm prepared by CSDG centrifugation and its benefit may be limited to the simplicity of use (54). Other methods utilizing magnetic activated cell sorting to remove apoptotic sperm, based on the externalization of phosphatidylserine residues, may prove to be more effective in selecting sperm with reduced DNA damage (55,56).

The selection of sperm defined as normal following evaluation under high magnification has been reported useful in improving outcomes with ICSI (57,58). The approach utilizes live examination of sperm under high power optics with further virtual magnification via

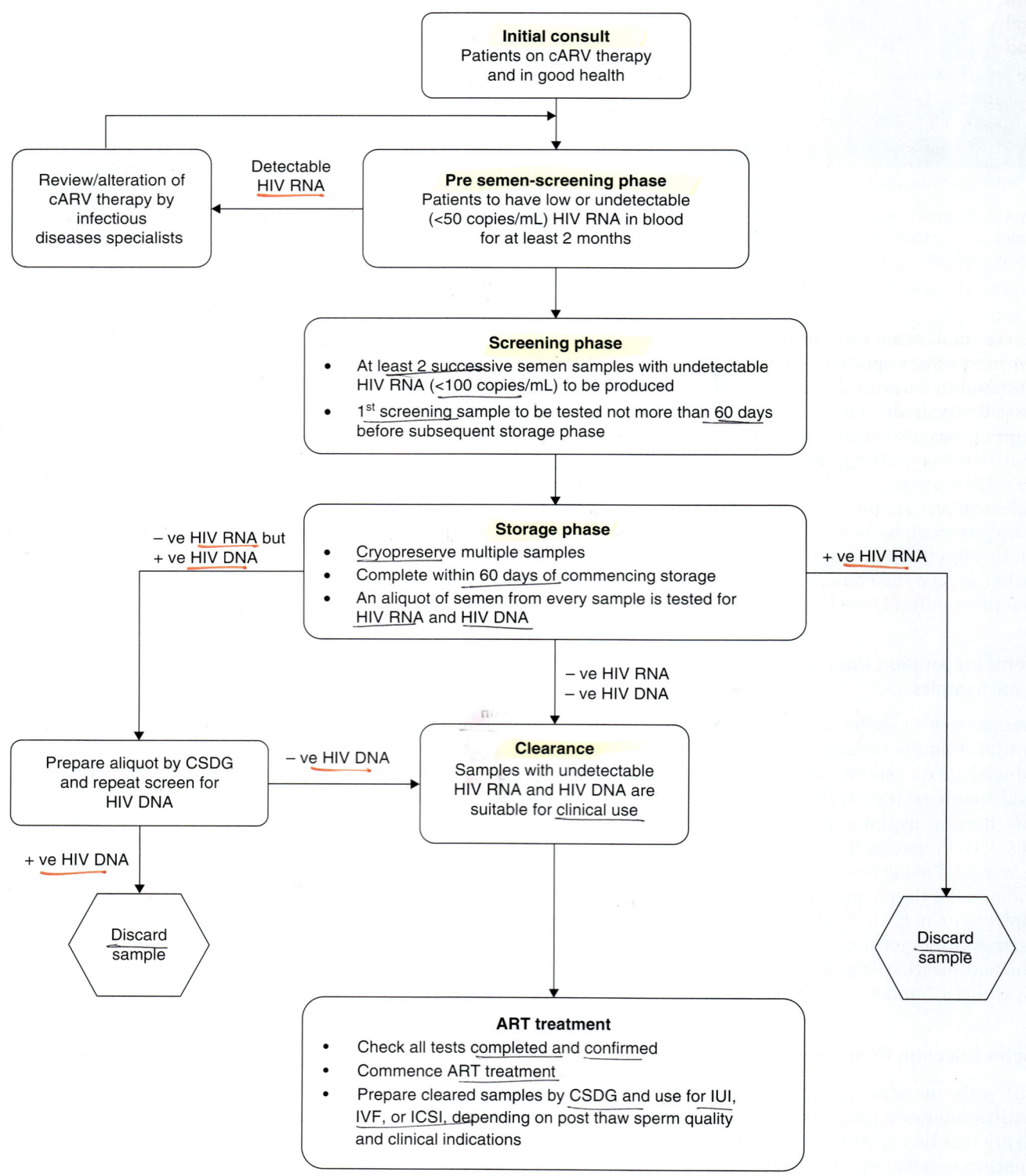

Figure 5.5 Flow chart for the treatment of HIV discordant couples; (male seropositive and female uninfected), using assisted reproduction to minimize the risk of HIV transmission. *Abbreviations*: cARV, combination antiretroviral; CSDG, colloidal silica density gradient; ICSI, intracytoplasmic sperm injection; IUI, intrauterine insemination; IVF, in vitro fertilization.

digital imaging. Those motile sperm exhibiting a normal nuclear profile based on shape and absence of vacuolization, and lacking neck and tail abnormalities, are preferentially selected for injection (59). Improvements in fertilization rate and early embryo development are generally not seen but significant improvements in implantation rate and reduced pregnancy loss have been reported (57,58). However, the technique is time consuming and requires some specialized equipment, and further prospective randomized controlled trials are still warranted to confirm the efficacy of this approach.

Sperm binding to hyaluronic acid has also been described as a sperm selection tool for ICSI and commercial products are available for clinical use. The ability of sperm to bind to hyaluronic acid is reported as related to normal morphology, maturity, and DNA integrity (60,61). Sperm are exposed to hyaluronic acid on a coated slide or Petri dish and those that bind are then preferentially used for ICSI (62). However, the ability of hyaluronic binding to identify functional sperm of better quality than by routine techniques may be limited. An alternative sperm binding method is to utilize human zonae. The ability of the human zona pellucida to selectively bind sperm with normal morphology and having an intact acrosome is well described (63–65). In this approach, immature eggs from the same cohort are incubated for two hours with prepared sperm. Sperm which bind are then removed by aspiration through a fine glass pipette and set aside for ICSI. Preliminary reports show improvements in embryo quality and implantation rate (66–68). However, further trials using sibling oocytes are needed to validate any benefits.

RESULTS

A comparison of normal fertilization and embryo utilization rates for swim up and CSDG, categorized according to male indication, is presented in Table 5.1. Apart from the improvement in the normal fertilization rate with CSDG for IVF with oligozoospermic samples, the results are similar. Results with sperm or elongated spermatids obtained from the genital tract, cryopreserved samples and those following the use of hypo-osmotic swelling have been published (4,69–71).

Fertilization results and incidence of poor outcome for different culture conditions and sperm preparation methods are presented in Table 5.2. The normal fertilization rate improved steadily following the introduction of closed, mini incubators (William A COOK) and the change from a single-stage medium (Human Tubal Fluid, HTF, Irvine Scientific; supplemented with 4 mg/mL human serum albumin, Albumex-20, CSL Ltd, Melbourne, Australia) to a sequential medium formulation containing a different albumin (Quinn's Advantage containing 4 mg/mL human albumin, Sage BioPharma). These results were matched by an overall decrease in the incidence of cycles with poor fertilization, indicating that increased fertilization was also achieved in patients with a poor prognosis.

Following the routine introduction of density gradient centrifugation, improvement in fertilization rate and a decrease in the incidence of poor fertilization cycles were found for standard IVF inseminations, probably due to a reduced chance for carry-over of inhibitory

Table 5.1 Comparison of Results Obtained with Swim Up and CSDG[a]

	IVF				ICSI			
	Oocytes collected	IVF	Normal fertilization	Embryo utilization	Oocytes collected	ICSI	Normal fertilization	Embryo utilization
Normal Semen								
Swim up	21255	21031	12286	10520	1396	1113	665	545
		99	58	49		80	48	39
CSDG	3319	3298	1833[b]	1577[b]	905	685	394	322
		99	55	48		76	44	36
Abnormal Semen								
Swim up	8826	8733	4236	3513	5718	4664	2804	2367
		99	48	40		82	49	41
CSDG	6126	5943	2720[b]	2338[b]	6387	5221	3054	2567
		97	44	38		82	48	40
Oligoasthenoteratozoospermia								
Swim up	360	354	97	93	1328	1072	610	514
		98	27	26		81	46	39
CSDG	1183	1158	416[b]	358	2436	2016	1142	941
		98	35	30		83	47	39

[a]Preparation of sperm from semen for IVF or ICSI from men with normal semen (sperm concentration $\geq 20 \times 10^6$/mL, progressive motility $\geq 40\%$, and abnormal morphology $\leq 85\%$); abnormal semen (sperm concentration $1–19 \times 10^6$/mL or progressive motility 1–39% or abnormal morphology 86–100%) or oligoasthenoteratozoospermia (sperm concentration $1–19 \times 10^6$/mL, progressive motility 1–39% and abnormal morphology 86–100%) from 1990 to 1999. Men with sperm autoimmunity were excluded. Embryo utilization is the sum of embryos transferred fresh and those frozen for later transfer. Percentages using oocytes collected as the denominator are shown in italics.
[b]Significant differences between results for swim up and CSDG; ($P < 0.05$, χ^2 test).
Abbreviations: CSDG, colloidal silica density gradient; ICSI, intracytoplasmic sperm injection; IVF, in vitro fertilization;

Table 5.2 Comparison of Fertilization Rate and Incidence of Cycles with Poor Fertilization (<20% of Eggs Fertilized Normally) for Different Culture Conditions and Sperm Preparation Methods, Introduced Sequentially Over a 3 Year Period

Period	Culture conditions	Sperm preparation	ICSI					Standard IVF		
			No. of cycles	Cycles with <20% Fert	Eggs injected	Fertilized normally	No of cycles	Cycles with <20% Fert	Eggs inseminated	Fertilized normally
1999–2000	HTF medium/open incubators	Swim up	1327	106 (8.0%^{a,b})	10188	6605 (64.8%^{e,f})	1372	254 (18.5%^{g,h})	12174	6455 (53.0%^{k})
2001	Sequential medium/open incubators	Swim up	330	32 (9.7%^{c,d})	2915	1977 (67.8%^{e})	324	59 (18.2%^{i,j})	3187	1699 (53.3%^{l})
		CSDG	465	24 (5.2%^{a,c})	3829	2597 (67.8%^{f})	392	45 (11.5%^{g,i})	3689	2152 (58.3%^{k,l})
2003	Sequential medium/mini incubators	CSDG	456	17 (3.7%^{b,d})	3921	2848 (72.6%^{e,f})	477	53 (11.1%^{h,j})	4473	2861 (64.0%^{k,l})

Results with the same superscripts are significantly different by χ^2.
Abbreviations: CSDG, colloidal silica density gradient; ICSI, intracytoplasmic sperm injection; IVF, in vitro fertilization; Fert, fertilization; HTF, Human Tubal Fluid.

components from seminal plasma following CSDG preparation. No difference in fertilization rate was observed between swim up and CSDG prepared sperm for ICSI.

Thus, improvements in fertilization results can be achieved by optimizing culture conditions. In preparing sperm for ART, CSDG centrifugation appears a more reliable method for standard IVF while swim-up provides a simple alternative approach for intracytoplasmic injection.

Results from the treatment of HIV discordant couples have been published (51,52). Pregnancy rates following the use of ART with washed sperm are similar to noninfected couples. Overall, the screening and storage of sperm prior to treatment appears an effective fertility treatment for couples where the male is HIV positive with no seroconversions reported in any women or delivered babies to date.

COMPLICATIONS

Although there is potential for semen or sperm-dependent complications of ART such as infections or allergic reactions these are very rare. Patients should be tested for serious transmissible infections such as HIV and hepatitis, and standard precautions for handling biological material must be practiced in the embryology laboratory. Transmission of genetic conditions to offspring is possible: suitable counseling and, where possible, screening should be part of the clinical work-up of the couple. Strict laboratory quality control should minimize the risks of loss or errors of identity of gametes or embryos.

With ICSI for primary spermatogenic disorders an increased frequency of sex chromosomal aneuploidies has been noted in the conceptuses (72). In some clinics there appears to be a higher rate of abnormal fertilization with ICSI using testicular sperm (70).

FUTURE DIRECTIONS AND CONTROVERSIES

The main problems to be solved in the future are the accurate identification of patients who are likely to have problems with fertilization and require ICSI, effective treatment of defective sperm production or function and improved implantation and pregnancy rates with ART. Improved prediction of results will come from the development of new methods of semen analysis such as automated sperm morphology and simple tests for assessing the ability of sperm to interact with oocytes (1). Effective treatment of most forms of male infertility is only a remote possibility, especially as the pathogenesis remains obscure (73). Further studies should resolve questions about the involvement of free oxygen species in the pathogenesis of sperm defects and whether this may affect the health of the offspring (6,11,18,19,74). New technology may improve the procedures for activation of the oocyte to allow direct injection of a sperm head or nucleus from spermatids or spermatocytes although there is rarely a need for this clinically (75). The contribution of the sperm to abnormal embryonic development, failure of implantation, and pregnancy wastage will probably become clear as preimplantation genetic diagnosis and other tests of embryos are more widely used. However, advances in sperm selection methods offer some prospect for improved clinical outcomes (76). Practical methods for selection of sperm with normal chromosomes or a desired sex chromosome are also likely to be developed (77).

CONCLUSION

The principles of sperm preparation for IVF and ICSI are outlined and practical methods are given.

APPENDICES

Appendix 1: Preparation of Media

- Suitable culture media are available from a variety of commercial suppliers. The methods in the following have been described using Quinn's Advantage (QA) sequential culture media (fertilization medium), QA medium with hydroxyethane propoxy ethane sulfonate buffer (QA/HEPES) and human albumin from Sage BioPharma and PureSperm™ CSDG from Nidacon Laboratories (Gothenburg Sweden). However, the methods can be followed using other products substituted where required, while taking note of the requirement for equilibration with CO_2 or room atmosphere as appropriate.
- As required, human albumin (ALB) solution (100 mg/mL, Sage BioPharma, pharmaceutical grade) is added (one part in 25), to give a final concentration of 4 mg/mL.
- QA fertilization medium with both albumin (QA fert/ALB) and QA/HEPES/ALB is prepared and refrigerated until required (maximum storage time according to the manufacturer's expiry date: about 6 weeks).
- Bicarbonate buffered media requiring CO_2 to attain physiological pH are equilibrated prior to use under a CO_2 atmosphere according to the manufacturer's recommendations

Appendix 2: Choice of Method

- Patient and sample identity should be checked with another person and recorded as a quality assurance measure.
- Examine a drop of undiluted semen (hemocytometer or Makler chamber):
- *For standard in vitro fertilization (IVF):*
    - Prepare sperm by density gradient centrifugation.
    - If the sample is unexpectedly poor on the day (e.g., concentration $<10 \times 10^6$/mL, <40% motility, and/or poor forward progression), ICSI should be considered.
- *For ICSI:*
    - Prepare sperm by density gradient centrifugation or swim up.
    - Even samples with severe oligozoospermia (down to ~10,000/mL) can be prepared using swim up as long as there are some sperm with good forward progression.

- Alternatively, samples may be concentrated by wash and resuspension and used directly or prepared further by density gradient centrifugation or swim up.
- Samples with large amounts of debris, extreme oligozoospermia, or severely compromised motility are better prepared by CSDG.
- Surgical samples obtained from the testis or epididymis and those collected by electroejaculation typically have a low motile sperm concentration and are more suited to CSDG separation to maximize the yield and remove tissue debris. Alternatively surgical samples can be used directly if there is little extraneous cellular material and sufficient progressive motility to allow sperm to migrate to the edge of the drop.

Appendix 3: Density Gradient

CSDG Stock Solutions

- "PureSperm" (to make 50 mL of solution)
  - Forty percent stock solution: 20 mL "PureSperm," 28 mL QA/HEPES, 2 mL of 100 mg/mL human albumin (pharmaceutical grade)
  - Eighty percent stock solution: 40 mL "PureSperm," 8 mL QA/HEPES, 2 mL of 100 mg/mL human albumin (pharmaceutical grade)

Preparation and Use of Gradients

- Prepare sufficient tubes for each patient
  - Dispense 1.0 mL of 40% gradient stock solution into a 15 mL conical tube (Falcon 2095, Becton Dickinson, NJ, USA)
  - With a clean Pasteur pipette, underlay 1.0 mL of 80% gradient stock solution
- Carefully overlay ~1 mL of semen (fresh or thawed) or sperm suspension directly on top of the gradient
  - Ensure gradients are at room temperature before overlaying
- Prepare multiple gradients if the sperm concentration is low
- To maximize the yield (for example, for severe oligozoospermia or testicular biopsy samples)
  - Samples may be concentrated by wash and resuspension prior to placing onto gradient
  - Centrifugation speed and time may be increased, as described below:
  - Additional sperm can also be obtained by wash and resuspension of the upper gradient layers/supernatant normally discarded after removal of the bottom gradient layer and pellet
- Centrifuge at 200–300 g for 10 minutes (braking may be used during deceleration)
  - Increase centrifugation to 400 g for 15 minutes to improve the yield of poor ICSI samples
- Gently remove all but the bottom 0.3–0.5 mL and place in a discard tube
- With a clean Pasteur pipette gently aspirate the remaining solution and pellet and transfer to a fresh conical tube containing ~8 mL of medium, in preparation for a single wash
  - Avoid contact with the sides of the tube to minimize carry-over of seminal plasma and debris
  - For IVF, the single large volume wash may be replaced by 2 smaller volume washes (~3 to 4 mL) each if there are concerns for carry-over of seminal components into the final preparation
- Centrifuge at 300 g for 5 minutes
  - Use increased centrifugation (up to 1800 g) to maximize the yield of poor ICSI samples
  - Remove supernatant and resuspend in 0.3–1.0 mL of QA/fert medium (for IVF) or QA/HEPES/ALB (for ICSI)
  - Assess sperm quality in the final sample (count, motility, and progression), and calculate volume required for insemination as follows:
  - Place ~5 μL of prepared sperm onto a counting chamber (hemocytometer or Makler chamber) and allow to settle for >3 minutes
  - Grade forward progression (FP) as follows: FP0: no movement, FP1: movement but minimal progression, FP2: slow progression FP3: moderate to rapid progression
  - Count the number of motile sperm in a minimum of 5 squares from the central 25 squares (hemocytometer), or a minimum of 10 squares (Makler chamber), to estimate the motile concentration (to improve accuracy, aim to count at least 50 sperm).
  - *For IVF*: Calculate volume of final sperm suspension required for insemination (ideally 10–50 μL) to give a total of 100,000–200,000 FP3 sperm/mL in the medium containing the oocytes.
- Incubate at 37°C under 5% CO_2 (IVF) or room atmosphere (ICSI) until required

Appendix 4: Swim Up

- After the semen has liquefied (usually 30 minutes at 37°C), 1 mL aliquots of semen are placed in 5 mL labeled tubes (Falcon 2003) and gently overlaid with 2 mL of medium (QA/HEPES/ALB)
  - For samples with poor mucolysis, dilute semen with 2 to 3 volumes of appropriate medium and mix vigorously; allow any particulate matter to settle, transfer supernatant to another test tube, and use as described for liquefied semen
  - Alternatively, samples may be prepared as described for wash and resuspension, or the semen may be centrifuged directly and the seminal plasma removed, prior to overlaying the resulting pellet with medium for swim up
- Incubate tubes at 37°C for 45–60 minutes to allow progressively motile sperm to swim into the overlaid medium
- Taking care not to disrupt the interface or collect any seminal plasma, collect the overlaid medium, mix with 2–3 mL of medium and centrifuge at 300 g for 5–10 minutes; (increase centrifugation up to 1800 g to maximize the yield of poor ICSI samples)

- Remove the resulting supernatant and resuspend the pellet in 0.3–1.0 mL of fresh medium
- Assess sperm quality (count, motility, and velocity) and incubate at 37°C until required, as previously described

Appendix 5: Wash and Resuspension

- Allow semen to liquefy at 37°C for 30 minutes.
- Mix 1 mL of semen with 2–3 mL of appropriate medium; alternatively, to maximise motility in poorer samples, centrifuge the neat semen and remove the seminal plasma prior to diluting with medium.
- Centrifuge for 10 minutes at 300 g, (increase centrifugation up to 1800 g to maximize the yield of poor ICSI samples)
- Aspirate supernatant and resuspend pellet in 0.3–1.0 mL of appropriate medium.
- Assess sperm quality in the final sample (count, motility and progression) and incubate at 37°C until required, as previously described.

Appendix 6: Preparation of Slow Frozen Sperm

- Double check straw/vial code and patient identity
- *For straws*:
  - Thaw straw in air for 10–20 minutes; check integrity of the straw and discard if damaged.
  - Soak straw in hypochlorite solution prepared fresh daily (~0.5% available chlorine; e.g., 1:1 dilution of Milton antibacterial solution, Proctor and Gamble, Australia) for at least 2 minutes to disinfect outside of straw and reduce chance for cross-infection; rinse in fresh water and wipe excess solution from the straw after soaking.
- Cut one end and aspirate contents.
- *For vials*:
  - Loosen cap (to prevent the build-up of pressure during thawing) and thaw at 37°C.
- Assess sperm concentration, motility, and progression.
- Prepare sample by density gradient centrifugation as previously described.
  - Alternatively, samples for ICSI may be prepared by swim up, if sufficient motile sperm are present, or wash and resuspension if there is minimal extraneous cellular material or debris.
- Assess sperm count, motility, and progression in the final suspension. For IVF samples, calculate the volume required for insemination.
- Incubate at 37°C under 5% CO_2 (IVF) or room atmosphere (ICSI) until required.

Appendix 7: MESA/PESA

- Epididymal sperm are obtained either by microsurgery, (microsurgical epididymal sperm aspiration, MESA), or by percutaneous, fine needle aspiration (percutaneous epididymal sperm aspiration, PESA).
- Expel aspirates into a small Petri dish of warm QA/HEPES/ALB.
- Pool samples and concentrate if necessary.
- Depending on concentration, motility and amount of debris, either use directly, prepare by wash and resuspension or separate on a density gradient.
- Leave to incubate to allow sperm to gain motility
  - Up to 24 hours in QA Fert/ALB at 37°C under 5% CO_2
  - For same day use, prepare plate for ICSI and leave at 37°C in QA/HEPES/ALB (room atmosphere)
- If extra sperm are available, consider freezing the excess. Samples with >5000 motile sperm/mL should have a sufficient yield of live sperm post thaw for subsequent ICSI treatments. A method for cryopreservation of such samples is given in appendix 9.

Appendix 8: Testicular Biopsy

- Testicular tissue is obtained either by open biopsy (TEsticular Sperm Extraction (TESE)) or percutaneous fine needle aspiration (TEsticular Sperm Aspiration (TESA)).
- Place tissue into a small Petri dish of warm QA/HEPES/ALB.
- Dissect tubules using fine gauge needles (Fig. 5.2), sterile scalpel blades, and/or macerate using a sterile mortar and pestle style homogenizer.
- Transfer raw suspension to a test tube.
- Depending on the concentration, motility, and amount of debris, either use directly, prepare by wash and resuspension or separate on a density gradient.
- Leave to incubate to allow sperm to gain motility.
  - Keep in QA fert/ALB at 37°C under 5% CO_2 for up to 24 hours.
  - For same day use, prepare plate for ICSI and leave at 37°C in QA/HEPES/ALB (room atmosphere).
- If extra sperm are available, consider freezing the excess (Appendix 9).

Appendix 9: Freezing Protocol for Oligozoospermia and Washed Sperm

- Semen containing only a few motile sperm and sperm suspensions obtained from the genital tract can be stored for subsequent ICSI.
- Epididymal, testicular, and oligozoospermic sperm suspensions are routinely processed by density gradient centrifugation or wash and resuspension.
- Sperm excess to that required for treatment can be cryopreserved with glucose-citrate-glycine (GCG)-glycerol cryoprotectant supplemented with human albumin.
- *GCG-glycerol cryoprotectant*:
  - Dissolve glucose (1.0 gm) and sodium citrate (1.0 gm) in 40 mL of sterile deionized water.
  - Add glycine (1.0 g), (pH ~7.5, and osmolality ~500 mOsm/kg).
  - Add 10 mL of glycerol, mix and filter (0.2 µm).
  - Store in 2 mL volumes at −70°C.
- *Albumin stock solution*:
  - Dilute albumin (Sage BioPharma, 100 mg/mL) 1:1 with Tyrode buffer to make albumin stock solution (50 mg/mL); filter (0.45 µm) and store at −70°C.

- As required, thaw a vial of GCG-glycerol.
- Add equal volume of albumin stock solution to the sperm sample and mix well.
- Add GCG-glycerol solution to sperm/albumin suspension 1:2; (1 volume of GCG-glycerol to 2 volumes of sperm/albumin) gradually over ~10 minutes with mixing.
- Package in cryovials (Nunc A/S, Denmark) and freeze.
  - Freeze gradually by suspending in liquid nitrogen vapor and store similarly.
- Alternatively, samples can be frozen using commercially available freezing media; (e.g., QA Sperm Freeze, Sage BioPharma).
  - Add 1 volume of freezing medium, drop by drop, to an equal volume of sperm suspension; (add slowly over ~5 minutes and mix well between additions).
  - Place the final sperm/cryoprotectant mixture into cryovial (~1.5 mL per vial).
  - Freeze and store over liquid nitrogen vapor as described above.

Appendix 10: Use of Pentoxifylline

- Prepare a 10× concentrated solution of pentoxifylline (POF, Sigma) in protein-free QA/HEPES (POF MW = 278.3; 10× concentrate = 10 mg/mL).
- Sterilize through a 0.2 μm filter and store at 4°C.
- Dilute 1:9 with sperm suspension to expose sperm to a final concentration of 1 mg/mL POF (3.6 mM).
- Spread the treated sperm suspension adjacent to the holding drops in the injection plate.
- Functional sperm should show motility within 10 minutes of exposure to the stimulant.
- Move the motile sperm to clean, stimulant-free medium.
- Expel the treated medium from the injection pipette and rinse with the untreated, clean medium in the holding drop; repeat rinsing of sperm and injection pipette.
- Immobilize the selected sperm and perform ICSI as usual.
- Aim to collect the motile sperm without excessive delay (within ~3 hours) as the treated sperm may lose motility with time.

Appendix 11: Use of a Hypo-osmotic Medium

- Prepare a 100–150 mOsm/kg solution by diluting QA/HEPES/ALB 1:1 or 1:2 with purified water.
- Filter and store at 4°C.
- Add a drop of hypo-osmotic medium adjacent to the holding drops in the injection plate.
- Transfer sperm using the injection pipette to the hypo-osmotic medium.
- Immotile sperm with an intact plasma membrane should coil their tails shortly after contacting the hypo-osmotic medium.
- Move the presumptive live sperm to the normo-osmotic oocyte holding drop and leave briefly to equilibrate.
- Expel the hypo-osmotic medium from the injection pipette and rinse with normo-osmotic medium; repeat rinsing of sperm and injection pipette.
- Immobilize the selected sperm and perform ICSI as usual.

ACKNOWLEDGMENTS

The authors thank Associate Professor GN Clarke for the advice about cryopreservation procedures; Dr M Giles, Dr A Mijch, Dr P Foster, Professor S Garland, and Associate Professor Sepehr Tabrizi for their assistance with the management and testing of HIV discordant couples, and Dr C Garrett and Ms P Sourivong for their assisting with the figures.

REFERENCES

1. Baker G, Liu DY, Bourne H. Assessment of the male and preparation of sperm for ARTs. In: Trounson AO, Gardner DK, eds. Handbook of in Vitro Fertilization. Boca Raton: CRC Press, 1999: 99–126.
2. Nagy Z, Liu J, Cecile J, et al. Using ejaculated, fresh, and frozen-thawed epididymal and testicular spermatozoa gives rise to comparable results after intracytoplasmic sperm injection. Fertil Steril 1995; 63: 808–15.
3. Nagy ZP, Verheyen G, Tournaye H, et al. Special applications of intracytoplasmic sperm injection: the influence of sperm count, motility, morphology, source and sperm antibody on the outcome of ICSI. Hum Reprod 1998; 13(Suppl 1): 143–54.
4. Bourne H, Richings N, Liu DY, et al. Sperm preparation for intracytoplasmic injection: methods and relationship to fertilization results. Reprod Fertil Dev 1995; 7: 177–83.
5. Dozortsev D, Rybouchkin A, De Sutter P, et al. Human oocyte activation following intracytoplasmic injection: the role of the sperm cell. Hum Reprod 1995; 10: 403–7.
6. Aitken RJ, Gordon E, Harkiss D, et al. Relative impact of oxidative stress on the functional competence and genomic integrity of human spermatozoa. Biol Reprod 1998; 59: 1037–46.
7. Mortimer D. Sperm preparation techniques and iatrogenic failures of in-vitro fertilization. Hum Reprod 1991; 6: 173–6.
8. Mortimer D. Sperm recovery techniques to maximize fertilizing capacity. Reprod Fertil Dev 1994; 6: 25–31.
9. Adler A, Reing AM, Bedford JM, et al. Plasmanate as a medium supplement for in vitro fertilization. J Assist Reprod Genet 1993; 10: 67–71.
10. Laverge H, De Sutter P, Desmet R, et al. Prospective randomized study comparing human serum albumin with fetal cord serum as protein supplement in culture medium for in-vitro fertilization. Hum Reprod 1997; 12: 2263–6.
11. Aitken RJ, Sawyer D. The human spermatozoon—not waving but drowning. Adv Exp Med Biol 2003; 518: 85–98.
12. Ng FL, Liu DY, Baker HW. Comparison of Percoll, mini-Percoll and swim-up methods for sperm preparation from abnormal semen samples. Hum Reprod 1992; 7: 261–6.
13. De Vos A, Nagy ZP, Van de Velde H, et al. Percoll gradient centrifugation can be omitted in sperm preparation

for intracytoplasmic sperm injection. Hum Reprod 1997; 12: 1980–4.
14. Savasi V, Ferrazzi E, Lanzani C, et al. Safety of sperm washing and ART outcome in 741 HIV-1-serodiscordant couples. Hum Reprod 2007; 22: 772–7.
15. Bujan L, Sergerie M, Kiffer N, et al. Good efficiency of intrauterine insemination programme for serodiscordant couples with HIV-1 infected male partner: A retrospective comparative study. Eur J Obstet Gynecol Reprod Biol 2007.
16. Gianaroli L, Cristina Magli M, Ferraretti AP, et al. Reducing the time of sperm-oocyte interaction in human in-vitro fertilization improves the implantation rate. Hum Reprod 1996; 11: 166–71.
17. Gianaroli L, Fiorentino A, Magli MC, et al. Prolonged sperm-oocyte exposure and high sperm concentration affect human embryo viability and pregnancy rate. Hum Reprod 1996; 11: 2507–11.
18. Twigg J, Irvine DS, Houston P, et al. Iatrogenic DNA damage induced in human spermatozoa during sperm preparation: protective significance of seminal plasma. Mol Hum Reprod 1998; 4: 439–45.
19. Twigg JP, Irvine DS, Aitken RJ. Oxidative damage to DNA in human spermatozoa does not preclude pronucleus formation at intracytoplasmic sperm injection. Hum Reprod 1998; 13: 1864–71.
20. Ord T, Patrizio P, Marello E, et al. Mini-Percoll: a new method of semen preparation for IVF in severe male factor infertility. Hum Reprod 1990; 5: 987–9.
21. Claassens OE, Menkveld R, Harrison KL. Evaluation of three substitutes for Percoll in sperm isolation by density gradient centrifugation. Hum Reprod 1998; 13: 3139–43.
22. Carrell DT, Kuneck PH, Peterson CM, et al. A randomized, prospective analysis of five sperm preparation techniques before intrauterine insemination of husband sperm. Fertil Steril 1998; 69: 122–6.
23. Centola GM, Herko R, Andolina E, et al. Comparison of sperm separation methods: effect on recovery, motility, motion parameters, and hyperactivation. Fertil Steril 1998; 70: 1173–5.
24. Grab D, Thierauf S, Rosenbusch B, et al. Scanning electron microscopy of human sperms after preparation of semen for in-vitro fertilization. Arch Gynecol Obstet 1993; 252: 137–41.
25. Sterzik K, De Santo M, Uhlich S, et al. Glass wool filtration leads to a higher percentage of spermatozoa with intact acrosomes: an ultrastructural analysis. Hum Reprod 1998; 13: 2506–11.
26. Hammadeh ME, Kuhnen A, Amer AS, et al. Comparison of sperm preparation methods: effect on chromatin and morphology recovery rates and their consequences on the clinical outcome after in vitro fertilization embryo transfer. Int J Androl 2001; 24: 360–8.
27. Tomlinson MJ, Moffatt O, Manicardi GC, et al. Interrelationships between seminal parameters and sperm nuclear DNA damage before and after density gradient centrifugation: implications for assisted conception. Hum Reprod 2001; 16: 2160–5.
28. Marchetti C, Obert G, Deffosez A, et al. Study of mitochondrial membrane potential, reactive oxygen species, DNA fragmentation and cell viability by flow cytometry in human sperm. Hum Reprod 2002; 17: 1257–65.
29. O'Connell M, McClure N, Powell LA, et al. Differences in mitochondrial and nuclear DNA status of high-density and low-density sperm fractions after density centrifugation preparation. Fertil Steril 2003; 79(Suppl 1): 754–62.
30. Semprini AE, Levi-Setti P, Bozzo M, et al. Insemination of HIV-negative women with processed semen of HIV-positive partners. Lancet 1992; 340: 1317–19.
31. Marina S, Marina F, Alcolea R, et al. Human immunodeficiency virus type 1–serodiscordant couples can bear healthy children after undergoing intrauterine insemination. Fertil Steril 1998; 70: 35–9.
32. Kim LU, Johnson MR, Barton S, et al. Evaluation of sperm washing as a potential method of reducing HIV transmission in HIV-discordant couples wishing to have children. Aids 1999; 13: 645–51.
33. Hanabusa H, Kuji N, Kato S, et al. An evaluation of semen processing methods for eliminating HIV-1. Aids 2000; 14: 1611–16.
34. Pasquier C, Daudin M, Righi L, et al. Sperm washing and virus nucleic acid detection to reduce HIV and hepatitis C virus transmission in serodiscordant couples wishing to have children. Aids 2000; 14: 2093–9.
35. Chrystie IL, Mullen JE, Braude PR, et al. Assisted conception in HIV discordant couples: evaluation of semen processing techniques in reducing HIV viral load. J Reprod Immunol 1998; 41: 301–6.
36. Leruez-Ville M, de Almeida M, Tachet A, et al. Assisted reproduction in HIV-1-serodifferent couples: the need for viral validation of processed semen. Aids 2002; 16: 2267–73.
37. Fiore JR, Lorusso F, Vacca M, et al. The efficiency of sperm washing in removing human immunodeficiency virus type 1 varies according to the seminal viral load. Fertil Steril 2005; 84: 232–4.
38. Garrido N, Meseguer M, Bellver J, et al. Report of the results of a 2 year programme of sperm wash and ICSI treatment for human immunodeficiency virus and hepatitis C virus serodiscordant couples. Hum Reprod 2004; 19: 2581–6.
39. Politch JA, Xu C, Tucker L, et al. Separation of human immunodeficiency virus type 1 from motile sperm by the double tube gradient method versus other methods. Fertil Steril 2004; 81: 440–7.
40. Kato S, Hanabusa H, Kaneko S, et al. Complete removal of HIV-1 RNA and proviral DNA from semen by the swim-up method: assisted reproduction technique using spermatozoa free from HIV-1. Aids 2006; 20: 967–73.
41. Loskutoff NM, Huyser C, Singh R, et al. Use of a novel washing method combining multiple density gradients and trypsin for removing human immunodeficiency virus-1 and hepatitis C virus from semen. Fertil Steril 2005; 84: 1001–10.
42. Casper RF, Meriano JS, Jarvi KA, et al. The hypo-osmotic swelling test for selection of viable sperm for intracytoplasmic sperm injection in men with complete asthenozoospermia. Fertil Steril 1996; 65: 972–6.
43. Aktan TM, Montag M, Duman S, et al. Use of a laser to detect viable but immotile spermatozoa. Andrologia 2004; 36: 366–9.
44. de Oliveira NM, Vaca Sanchez R, Rodriguez Fiesta S, et al. Pregnancy with frozen-thawed and fresh testicular biopsy after motile and immotile sperm microinjection, using the mechanical touch technique to assess viability. Hum Reprod 2004; 19: 262–5.
45. Manigart Y, Rozenberg S, Barlow P, et al. ART outcome in HIV-infected patients. Hum Reprod 2006; 21: 2935–40.

46. Gilling-Smith C, Nicopoullos JD, Semprini AE, et al. HIV and reproductive care–a review of current practice. Bjog 2006; 113: 869–78.
47. Terriou P, Auquier P, Chabert-Orsini V, et al. Outcome of ICSI in HIV-1-infected women. Hum Reprod 2005; 20: 2838–43.
48. Semprini AE, Fiore S. HIV and reproduction. Curr Opin Obstet Gynecol 2004; 16: 257–62.
49. Ohl J, Partisani M, Wittemer C, et al. Assisted reproduction techniques for HIV serodiscordant couples: 18 months of experience. Hum Reprod 2003; 18: 1244–9.
50. Pena JE, Thornton MH, Sauer MV. Assessing the clinical utility of in vitro fertilization with intracytoplasmic sperm injection in human immunodeficiency virus type 1 serodiscordant couples: report of 113 consecutive cycles. Fertil Steril 2003; 80: 356–62.
51. van Leeuwen E, Repping S, Prins JM, et al. Assisted reproductive technologies to establish pregnancies in couples with an HIV-1-infected man. Neth J Med 2009; 67: 322–7.
52. Vitorino RL, Grinsztejn BG, de Andrade CA, et al. Systematic review of the effectiveness and safety of assisted reproduction techniques in couples serodiscordant for human immunodeficiency virus where the man is positive. Fertil Steril 2011; 95: 1684–90.
53. Ainsworth C, Nixon B, Jansen RP, et al. First recorded pregnancy and normal birth after ICSI using electrophoretically isolated spermatozoa. Hum Reprod 2007; 27: 197–200.
54. Fleming SD, Ilad RS, Griffin AM, et al. Prospective controlled trial of an electrophoretic method of sperm preparation for assisted reproduction: comparison with density gradient centrifugation. Hum Reprod 2008; 23: 2646–51.
55. Dirican EK, Ozgun OD, Akarsu S, et al. Clinical outcome of magnetic activated cell sorting of non-apoptotic spermatozoa before density gradient centrifugation for assisted reproduction. J Assist Reprod Genet 2008; 25: 375–81.
56. Said TM, Agarwal A, Zborowski M, et al. Utility of magnetic cell separation as a molecular sperm preparation technique. J Androl 2008; 29: 134–42.
57. Nadalini M, Tarozzi N, Distratis V, et al. Impact of intracytoplasmic morphologically selected sperm injection on assisted reproduction outcome: a review. Reprod Biomed Online 2009; 19(Suppl 3): 45–55.
58. Souza Setti A, Ferreira RC, Paes de Almeida Ferreira Braga D, et al. Intracytoplasmic sperm injection outcome versus intracytoplasmic morphologically selected sperm injection outcome: a meta-analysis. Reprod Biomed Online 2010; 21: 450–5.
59. Bartoov B, Berkovitz A, Eltes F. Selection of spermatozoa with normal nuclei to improve the pregnancy rate with intracytoplasmic sperm injection. N Engl J Med 2001; 345: 1067–8.
60. Huszar G, Jakab A, Sakkas D, et al. Fertility testing and ICSI sperm selection by hyaluronic acid binding: clinical and genetic aspects. Reprod Biomed Online 2007; 14: 650–63.
61. Nasr-Esfahani MH, Razavi S, Vahdati AA, et al. Evaluation of sperm selection procedure based on hyaluronic acid binding ability on ICSI outcome. J Assist Reprod Genet 2008; 25: 197–203.
62. Huszar G, Ozkavukcu S, Jakab A, et al. Hyaluronic acid binding ability of human sperm reflects cellular maturity and fertilizing potential: selection of sperm for intracytoplasmic sperm injection. Curr Opin Obstet Gynecol 2006; 18: 260–7.
63. Menkveld R, Franken DR, Kruger TF, et al. Sperm selection capacity of the human zona pellucida. Mol Reprod Dev 1991; 30: 346–52.
64. Liu DY, Baker HW. Acrosome status and morphology of human spermatozoa bound to the zona pellucida and oolemma determined using oocytes that failed to fertilize in vitro. Hum Reprod 1994; 9: 673–9.
65. Liu DY, Baker HW. Human sperm bound to the zona pellucida have normal nuclear chromatin as assessed by acridine orange fluorescence. Hum Reprod 2007; 22: 1597–602.
66. Paes Almeida Ferreira de Braga D, Iaconelli A Jr, Cassia Savio de Figueira R, et al. Outcome of ICSI using zona pellucida-bound spermatozoa and conventionally selected spermatozoa. Reprod Biomed Online 2009; 19: 802–7.
67. Black M, Liu de Y, Bourne H, et al. Comparison of outcomes of conventional intracytoplasmic sperm injection and intracytoplasmic sperm injection using sperm bound to the zona pellucida of immature oocytes. Fertil Steril 2010; 93: 672–4.
68. Liu F, Qiu Y, Zou Y, et al. Use of zona pellucida-bound sperm for intracytoplasmic sperm injection produces higher embryo quality and implantation than conventional intracytoplasmic sperm injection. Fertil Steril 2011; 95: 815–18.
69. Harari O, Bourne H, McDonald M, et al. Intracytoplasmic sperm injection: a major advance in the management of severe male subfertility. Fertil Steril 1995; 64: 360–8.
70. Watkins W, Nieto F, Bourne H, et al. Testicular and epididymal sperm in a microinjection program: methods of retrieval and results. Fertil Steril 1997; 67: 527–35.
71. Sallam HN, Farrag A, Agameya AF, et al. The use of the modified hypo-osmotic swelling test for the selection of immotile testicular spermatozoa in patients treated with ICSI: a randomized controlled study. Hum Reprod 2005; 20: 3435–40.
72. Bonduelle M, Wilikens A, Buysse A, et al. A follow-up study of children born after intracytoplasmic sperm injection ICSI with epididymal and testicular spermatozoa and after replacement of cryopreserved embryos obtained after ICSI. Hum Reprod 1998; 13(Suppl 1): 196–207.
73. De Kretser DM, Baker HW. Infertility in men: recent advances and continuing controversies. J Clin Endocrinol Metab 1999; 84: 3443–50.
74. Baker HWG. Marvellous ICSI: the viewpoint of a clinician. Int J Androl 1998; 21: 249–52.
75. Antinori S, Versaci C, Dani G, et al. Successful fertilization and pregnancy after injection of frozen-thawed round spermatids into human oocytes. Hum Reprod 1997; 12: 554–6.
76. Said TM, Land JA. Effects of advanced selection methods on sperm quality and ART outcome: a systematic review. Hum Reprod 2011; 17: 719–33.
77. Fugger EF, Black SH, Keyvanfar K, et al. Births of normal daughters after microsort sperm separation and intrauterine insemination, in-vitro fertilization, or intracytoplasmic sperm injection. Hum Reprod 1998; 13: 2367–70.

6

Sperm chromatin assessment

Ashok Agarwal, Igor Tsarev, Juris Erenpreiss, and Rakesh Sharma

INTRODUCTION

Semen analysis is used routinely to evaluate infertile men. Attempts to introduce quality control within and between laboratories have highlighted the subjectivity and variability of traditional semen parameters. A significant overlap in sperm concentration, motility, and morphology between fertile and infertile men has been demonstrated (1). In addition, standard measurements may not reveal subtle sperm defects such as DNA damage and can these defects affect fertility. New markers are needed to better discriminate infertile men from fertile ones, predict pregnancy outcome in the female partner, and calculate the risk of adverse reproductive events.

In this context, sperm chromatin abnormalities have been studied extensively in past decades as a cause of male infertility (2). Focus on the genomic integrity of the male gamete has been intensified by the growing concern about transmission of damaged DNA through assisted reproductive techniques (ARTs), especially intracytoplasmic sperm injection (ICSI). It is a particular concern if the amount of damage exceeds the DNA repair capacity of oocytes. There are concerns related to potential chromosomal abnormalities, congenital malformations, and developmental abnormalities in ICSI-born progeny (3–6).

Accumulating evidence suggests that a negative relationship exists between disturbances in the organization of the genomic material in sperm nuclei and the fertility potential of spermatozoa, whether in vivo or in vitro (2,7–14). Abnormalities in the male genome characterized by damaged sperm DNA may be indicative of male subfertility regardless of normal semen parameters (15,16). Sperm chromatin structure evaluation is an independent measure of sperm quality that provides good diagnostic and prognostic capabilities. Therefore, it may be considered a reliable predictor of a couple's inability to become pregnant (17). This may have an impact on the offspring, resulting in infertility (18).

Sperm DNA integrity correlates with pregnancy outcome in in vitro fertilization (IVF) (17,19–22). High sperm DNA fragmentation can compromise embryo quality and result in pregnancy loss (10). In addition, sperm DNA fragmentation may also compromise the progression of pregnancy and result in spontaneous miscarriage or biochemical pregnancy following ART.

Sperm DNA fragmentation seems to affect embryo post-implantation development in ICSI procedures (10). Therefore, it is recommended that sperm DNA fragmentation analysis should be included in the evaluation of the infertile male (22).

Many techniques have been described for evaluation of the chromatin status. In this chapter, we describe the normal sperm chromatin architecture and the causative factors leading to its aberrations. We also provide the rationale for sperm chromatin assessment and discuss the different methods used to analyze sperm DNA integrity.

HUMAN SPERM CHROMATIN STRUCTURE

In many mammals, spermatogenesis leads to the production of highly homogenous spermatozoa. For example, more than 95% of the nucleoprotein in mouse sperm nuclei is composed of protamines (23). This allows mature sperm nuclei to adopt a volume 40 times less than that of normal somatic nuclei (24). The final, highly compact packaging of the primary sperm DNA filament is produced by DNA–protamine complexes. Contrary to nucleosomal organization in somatic cells, which is provided by histones, these DNA–protamine complexes approach the physical limits of molecular compaction (25,26). Human sperm nuclei, on the other hand, contain considerably fewer protamines (around 85%) than sperm nuclei of the bull, stallion, hamster, and mouse (27,28). Mature human spermatozoa contain some levels of nucleosomes which are believed to be necessary for organizing higher-order genomic structure through interactions with the nuclear matrix. These regions are distributed nonrandomly throughout the sperm genome (29). Human sperm chromatin is therefore less regularly compacted and frequently contains DNA strand breaks (30,31).

To achieve this uniquely condensed state, sperm DNA must be organized in a specific manner that differs substantially from that of somatic cells (24). The fundamental packaging unit of mammalian sperm chromatin is a toroid containing 50–60 kilobases of DNA. Individual toroids represent the DNA loop-domains highly condensed by protamines and fixed at the nuclear matrix. Toroids are cross-linked by disulfide bonds formed by the oxidation of sulfhydryl groups of cysteine present in the protamines (25,32). Thus, each chromosome represents a garland of toroids, while all 23 chromosomes are clustered by centromeres into a compact chromocenter positioned well inside the nucleus; the telomere ends are united into dimers exposed to the nuclear periphery (33,34). This condensed, insoluble, and highly organized nature of sperm chromatin acts to protect the genetic integrity during transport of the paternal genome through the male and female reproductive tracts. It also ensures that the paternal DNA is delivered in the form that sterically allows the proper fusion of two gametic genomes and enables the developing embryo to correctly express the genetic information (34–36).

In comparison with other species (37), human sperm chromatin packaging is exceptionally variable both within and between men. This variability has been mostly attributed to its basic protein component. The retention of 15% histones, which are less basic than protamines, leads to the formation of a less-compact chromatin structure (28). Moreover, in contrast to the bull, cat, boar, and ram—whose spermatozoa contain only one type of protamine (P1)—human and mouse spermatozoa contain a second type of protamine called P2, which is deficient in cysteine residues (38). Consequently, the disulfide cross-linking responsible for more stable packaging is diminished in human sperm as compared with species containing P1 alone (39). It is interesting to note that altered P1/P2 ratios and the absence of P2 are associated with male fertility problems (40–44). P1/P2 ratio has been shown to correlate with sperm DNA fragmentation, and significant differences were detected between fertile and infertile men (45). The reference range reported for P1/P2 in a fertile, normozoospermic population ranges from 0.54 to 1.43. Such a wide range of P1/P2 shows that abnormal protamination can be an indicator of other disturbances during spermatogenesis than the mechanism to cause infertility (46).

ORIGIN OF SPERM CHROMATIN ABNORMALITIES

The susceptibility of male germ cells to DNA damage stems partly from the downregulation of DNA repair systems during late spermatogenesis. In addition, the cellular machinery that allows these cells to undergo complete apoptosis is progressively lost during spermatogenesis. As a result, the advanced stages of germ cell differentiation cannot be deleted even though they may have proceeded some way down the apoptotic pathway. As a consequence, the ejaculated gamete may exhibit genetic damage. Such DNA damage will be carried into the zygote by the fertilizing spermatozoon and must be then repaired, preferably prior to the first cleavage division. Several studies have shown that oocytes and early embryos can repair sperm DNA damage (47,48). Consequently, the biological effect of abnormal sperm chromatin structure depends on the combined effects of sperm chromatin damage and the capacity of the oocyte to repair it. Any errors that may occur during this postfertilization period of DNA repair have the potential to create mutations that can affect fetal development and, ultimately, the health of the child (18,49).

The exact mechanisms by which chromatin abnormalities/DNA damage arise in human spermatozoa are not completely understood. Three main theories have been proposed: defective sperm chromatin packaging, abortive apoptosis, and oxidative stress (OS). Deficiencies in recombination may also play a role.

Defective Sperm Chromatin Packaging

Stage-specific introduction of transient DNA strand breaks during spermiogenesis has been described (50–52). DNA breaks have been found in round and elongated spermatids. Such breaks are necessary for transient relief of torsional stress. During maturation, the nucleosome histone cores in elongating spermatids are cast off and replaced with transitional proteins and protamines (50,52–54). Thus, chromatin repackaging includes a sensitive step necessitating endogenous nuclease activity, which is evidently fulfilled by coordinated loosening of the chromatin by histone hyperacetylation and introduction of breaks by topoisomerase II that is able to create and ligate breaks (53,54). Although there is little evidence to suggest that spermatid maturation-associated DNA breaks are fully ligated, unrepaired DNA breaks are not allowed (55).

Ligation of DNA breaks is necessary not only to preserve the integrity of the primary DNA structure but also for reassembly of the important unit of genome expression—the DNA loop domain. However, if these temporary breaks are not repaired because of excessive topoisomerase II activity or a deficiency of topoisomerase II inhibitors (56,57), then DNA fragmentation in ejaculated spermatozoa may result. Similarly, if appropriate disulphide bridge formation does not occur because of inadequate oxidation of thiols during the epididymal transit, the DNA will be more vulnerable to damage caused by suboptimal compaction. Recent studies have postulated the hypothesis that large nuclear vacuoles could be an indicator of abnormal chromatin packaging (58,59).

Abortive Apoptosis

The incidence of apoptosis in ejaculated sperm is still a contentious issue. Until recently, the inability of a mature spermatozoon to synthesize new proteins was believed to make it impossible for such cells to respond to any of the signals that lead to the programmed death cascade. However, a number of recent observations have raised the possibility that abortive apoptosis may contribute to DNA damage in human spermatozoa: (*i*) the detection of Fas on ejaculated spermatozoa (60), (*ii*) the high proportion of spermatozoa with potentially apoptotic mitochondria (61), and (*iii*) the finding that potential mediators of apoptosis, including endonuclease activity, are present in spermatozoa (62). It has been postulated that OS can interfere with sperm chromatin remodeling. Cells with altered chromatin structure can enter apoptotic pathway, which is characterized by loss of motility, caspase activation, phosphatidylserine externalization, and the activation of reactive oxygen species (ROS) generation by the mitochondria. ROS causes lipid peroxidation and oxidative DNA damage, which, in turn, leads to DNA fragmentation and eventually cell death (63).

It has been suggested that an early apoptotic pathway, initiated in spermatogonia and spermatocytes, is mediated by Fas protein. Fas is a type I membrane protein that belongs to the tumor necrosis factor-nerve growth factor receptor family (64,65). It has been shown that Sertoli cells express Fas ligand, which by binding to Fas, leads to cell death via apoptosis (64,65). This in turn limits the size of the germ cell population to a number that Sertoli cells can support (66). Ligation of Fas ligand to Fas in the cellular membrane triggers the activation of caspases and therefore, this pathway is also characterized as a caspase-induced apoptosis (67).

Men exhibiting deficiencies in their semen profile often possess a large number of spermatozoa that bear Fas. This fact prompts the suggestion that these dysfunctional cells are the product of an incomplete apoptotic cascade (68). However, the contribution of aborted apoptosis in the DNA damage seen in the ejaculated spermatozoa is doubtful in cases where this process is initiated at the early stages of spermatogenesis. This is because at the stage of DNA fragmentation, apoptosis is an irreversible process (69), and these cells should be digested by Sertoli cells and removed from the pool of ejaculated sperm. Some studies have not found correlations between DNA damage and Fas expression (70), or, in contrast, have not revealed ultrastructural evidence for the association of apoptosis with DNA damage in sperm (71). Alternatively, if the apoptotic cascade is initiated at the round spermatid phase, where transcription (and mitochondria) is still active, abortive apoptosis might be an origin of the DNA breaks. A Bcl2 antiapoptotic family gene member called Bclw has been shown to suppress apoptosis in elongating spermatids (72).

Although many apoptotic biomarkers have been found in the mature male gamete, particularly in infertile men, their definitive association with DNA fragmentation remains elusive (73–82).

Oxidative Stress

ROS play an important physiological role, modulating gene and protein activities vital for sperm proliferation, differentiation, and function. In the semen of fertile men, the amount of ROS generation is controlled by seminal antioxidants. The pathogenic effects of ROS occur when they are produced in excess of the antioxidant capabilities of the male reproductive tract or seminal plasma (83). The human spermatozoon is highly susceptible to OS. This process induces peroxidative damage in the sperm plasma membrane and DNA fragmentation. Such stress may arise from a variety of sources. Morphologically abnormal spermatozoa (with residual cytoplasm, in particular) and leukocytes are the main sources of excessive ROS generation in semen (83). Also, a lack of antioxidant protection and the presence of redox cycling xenobiotics may be the cause of OS. Whenever levels of OS in the male germ line are high, the peroxidation of unsaturated fatty acids in the sperm plasma membrane leads to the depressed fertilization rates associated with DNA damage (18).

Deficiencies in Recombination

Meiotic crossing-over is associated with the genetically programmed introduction of DNA double-strand breaks (DSBs) by specific nucleases of the SPO11 family (84). These DNA DSBs should be ligated until the end of meiosis I. Normally, a recombination checkpoint in meiotic prophase does not allow meiotic division I to proceed until DNA is fully repaired or defective spermatocytes are ablated (84,85). However, a defective checkpoint may lead to persistent sperm DNA fragmentation in ejaculated spermatozoa. Direct data for this hypothesis in humans are lacking.

The processes leading to DNA damage in ejaculated sperm are inter-related. For example, a defective spermatid protamination and disulfide bridge formation caused by inadequate oxidation of thiols during epididymal transit, resulting in diminished sperm chromatin packaging, makes sperm cells more vulnerable to ROS-induced DNA fragmentation. A two-step hypothesis has been proposed, suggesting that OS acts on poorly protaminated cells, that are generated as a result of defective spermiogenesis (86).

CONTRIBUTING FACTORS

Advancing age has been associated with an increased percentage of ejaculated spermatozoa with DNA damage (11,87,88). Young men with cancer typically have poor semen quality and sperm DNA damage even before starting therapy. Further damage from radiation or chemotherapy is dependent on both the duration and dose of radiation (89,90).

Spermatogenesis may not occur months to years after therapy, but evidence of sperm DNA damage often persists beyond that period (91,92). A recent study on men with testicular cancer showed that radiation therapy induced transient sperm DNA damage and that this damage was present three to five years later, but three or more cycles of chemotherapy, in turn, decreased the percentage of sperm with DNA damage (92).

Cigarette smoking is associated with a decrease in sperm count and motility and an increase in abnormal sperm forms and sperm DNA damage (93). It is suggested that smoking increases production of leukocyte-derived ROS; the OS may be the underlying reason why sperm DNA from smokers contain more strand breaks than that from nonsmokers (93,94). Also, genital tract infections and inflammation result in leukocytospermia and have been associated with OS and subsequent sperm DNA damage (95). Exposure to pesticides (organophosphates), persistent organochlorine pollutants, and air pollution have also been associated with sperm DNA damage (11,96-98). Varicoceles have been associated with seminal OS and sperm DNA damage (99–101). Sperm DNA integrity has been shown to improve after varicocele repair (102,103).

A deficiency in gonadotropic hormones such as follicle stimulating hormone (FSH) can cause sperm chromatin defects. FSH-receptor knock-out mice have been found to have higher levels of sperm DNA damage (104). A febrile illness has been shown to cause an increase in the histone/protamine ratio and DNA damage in ejaculated sperm (105). Direct testicular hyperthermia has also been shown to cause these effects (106,107). Finally, sperm preparation techniques involving repeated high-speed centrifugation and the isolation of spermatozoa from the seminal plasma, which is a protective antioxidant environment, may contribute to increased sperm DNA damage via mechanisms that are mediated by the enhanced generation of ROS (14,108).

INDICATIONS FOR SPERM CHROMATIN ASSESSMENT

Evaluating sperm chromatin can be challenging for several reasons: it can be difficult to link the results of chromatin integrity tests to known physiological mechanisms; the role that sperm chromatin structure assessment plays in clinical practice (especially in ART) is still controversial; and there is no one standardized method for measuring sperm chromatin integrity. On the other hand, sperm chromatin structure is complex, and several methods may be necessary to assess it. In addition, a number of confounding factors can complicate the interpretation of the results including heterogeneity in the sperm population and the fact that not all DNA damage is lethal (most DNA contains non-coding regions or introns, and oocytes can repair sperm DNA damage). Nevertheless, at the present time, it is clear that sperm chromatin assessment provides good diagnostic and prognostic capabilities for fertility/infertility.

It must be stressed that among all methods employed for sperm chromatin assessment, clinical thresholds so far have been demonstrated only for the sperm chromatin structure assay (SCSA) and terminal deoxynucleotidyl transferase (TdT)-mediated deoxyuridine triphosphate (dUTP) nick end labeling assay (TUNEL), and these thresholds have been confirmed by different laboratories for SCSA only. Also, the reported biological variability of sperm DNA damage within men over time should be considered, although it is more stable than standard semen parameters (109–111).

Diagnosis of Male Infertility

Sperm DNA damage has a significant impact on in vivo fertilization. Many studies have shown, using a variety of techniques, significant differences in sperm DNA damage levels between fertile and infertile men (112–117). Moreover, spermatozoa from infertile patients are generally more susceptible to the effects of DNA-damaging agents such as H_2O_2 and radiation (118). The probability of fertilization in vivo seems to be close to zero if the proportion of sperm cells with DNA damage exceeds 30% as detected by the SCSA (17,112) or 20% as detected by TUNEL (119). Thus, sperm DNA integrity may be considered an objective marker of sperm function that serves as a significant prognostic factor for male infertility (7). Also, a significant increase in SCSA-defined DNA damage in sperm from infertile men with normal sperm parameters has been demonstrated (117), indicating that the analysis of sperm DNA damage may reveal a hidden sperm abnormality in infertile men classified with idiopathic infertility based on apparently normal standard semen parameters.

Assisted Reproductive Techniques

The probability of fertilization by intrauterine insemination (IUI) also seems to be close to zero if the proportion of sperm cells with DNA damage exceeds 30% by means of SCSA (12,19,120,121), or 12% by TUNEL (19). Whether sperm DNA damage negatively affects the results of IVF and ICSI is controversial. Although no association between sperm DNA damage and IVF/ICSI outcome has been demonstrated in some studies (122) most of the studies show a significant negative correlation between sperm DNA damage and embryo quality in IVF cycles (123), blastocyst development following IVF (124), and fertilization rates following IVF (125) and ICSI (126), even though sperm DNA damage may not necessarily preclude fertilization and pronucleus formation during ICSI (127). Two recent meta-analyses concluded that sperm DNA damage is predictive for reduced pregnancy success using routine IVF but has no significant effect on ICSI outcome (9,128). Thus, assessment of sperm chromatin may help predict the success rates of IUI and IVF. It has been also suggested that in patients with a high proportion of DNA-damaged sperm who are seeking ART, ICSI should be the method of choice (12).

Embryonal Loss

Data on miscarriages as a possible consequence of sperm DNA damage is rather scarce. It has been shown that the proportion of sperm with DNA damage is significantly higher in men from couples with recurrent pregnancy loss than in the general population or fertile donors (129). It has also been reported that 39% of miscarriages could be predicted using a combination of selected cut-off values for percentage spermatozoa with denatured (likely fragmented) DNA and/or abnormal chromatin packaging as assessed by SCSA (17). An increased trend of spontaneous abortions following IVF/ICSI was also demonstrated when sperm from men with a large amount of damaged DNA were used (130,131). Thus, it is possible that the assessment of sperm DNA damage could be a good predictor of possible miscarriage. However, the above mentioned findings need to be supported by additional studies.

Cancer Patients

Patients with cancer are often referred to sperm banks before chemotherapy, radiation therapy, or surgery is initiated. Although pregnancies and births have been reported using cryopreserved sperm from patients with cancer, these semen samples have decreased fertilization potential. The extent of DNA damage may help to determine how semen should be cryopreserved before therapy begins. Specimens with high sperm concentration and motility and low levels of DNA damage should be preserved in relatively large aliquots that are suitable for IUI. If a single specimen of good quality is available, then it should be preserved in multiple small aliquots suitable for IVF or ICSI (132).

EVALUATION OF SPERM NUCLEAR DNA DAMAGE

Different methods may be used to evaluate the status of the sperm chromatin for the presence of abnormalities or simply immaturity Table 6.1. These assays include simple staining techniques such as the acidic aniline blue (AAB) and basic toluidine blue (TB) stains, fluorescent staining techniques such as the sperm chromatin dispersion (SCD) test, chromomycin A_3 (CMA_3), DNA breakage detection- fluorescent in situ hybridization assay (DBD-FISH), in situ nick translation (NT), and flow cytometric based SCSA. Some assays employ more than one method for the analysis of their results. Examples of these assays include the acridine orange (AO) and TUNEL assays. Other methods less frequently used include measurement of 8-hydroxy-2-deoxyguanosine by high-performance liquid chromatography (HPLC).

AAB Stain

Principle

The AAB stain discriminates between lysine-rich histones and arginine/cysteine-rich protamines. This technique provides a specific positive reaction for lysine and reveals differences in the basic nuclear protein composition of ejaculated human spermatozoa. Histone-rich nuclei of immature spermatozoa are rich in lysine and will consequently take up the blue stain. On the other hand, protamine-rich nuclei of mature spermatozoa are rich in arginine and cysteine and contain relatively low levels of lysine, which means they will not take up the stain (143).

Technique

Slides are prepared by smearing 5 µL of either raw or washed semen sample. The slides are air-dried and fixed for 30 minutes in 3% glutaraldehyde in phosphate-buffered saline (PBS). The smear is dried and stained for five minutes in 5% aqueous aniline blue solution (pH 3.5). Sperm heads containing immature nuclear chromatin stain blue and those with mature nuclei do not. The percentage of spermatozoa stained with aniline blue is determined by counting 200 spermatozoa per slide under bright field microscopy (133).

Modification of the AAB Assay with Eosin

Visualization of unstained sperm cells can be difficult under ordinary light microscopy when using AAB staining. Counterstaining technique using eosin-Y stain can be adopted to overcome this limitation. Glass slides are prepared by fixing the sperm smears in 4% formalin solution for five minutes and rinsing in water. Slides are stained in 5% aniline blue prepared in 4% acetic acid (pH 3.5) solution for five minutes. After five minutes, the slides are rinsed in water and stained in 0.5% eosin for 1 minute. This is followed by rinsing and air drying of the slides (144).

Table 6.1 Various Methods for Assessing Sperm Chromatin Abnormalities

Assay	Parameter	Method of analysis
Acidic aniline blue (133)	Nuclear maturity (DNA protein composition)	Optical microscopy
Toluidine blue staining (134)	Nuclear maturity (DNA protein composition)	Optical microscopy
Chromomycin A_3 (135)	Nuclear maturity (DNA protein composition)	Fluorescent microscopy
DNA breakage detection-fluorescent in situ hybridization (136)	DNA fragmentation (ssDNA)	Fluorescent microscopy
In situ nick translation (137)	DNA fragmentation (ssDNA)	Fluorescent microscopy, Flow cytometry
Acridine orange (138)	DNA denaturation (acid)	Fluorescent microscopy, Flow cytometry
Sperm chromatin dispersion (139)	DNA fragmentation	Fluorescent microscopy
Comet (neutral) (140)	DNA fragmentation (dsDNA)	Fluorescent microscopy
(alkaline) (141)	DNA fragmentation (ssDNA/dsDNA)	
TUNEL (71)	DNA fragmentation	Fluorescent microscopy, Flow cytometry
Sperm chromatin structure assay (17)	DNA denaturation (acid/heat)	Flow cytometry
8-OHdG measurement (142)	8-OHdG	High-performance lipid chromatography

Abbreviations: 8-OHdG, 8-hydroxy-2-deoxyguanosine; dsDNA, double-stranded DNA; ssDNA, single-stranded DNA.

Clinical Significance

Results of AAB staining have shown a clear association between abnormal sperm chromatin and male infertility (145). However, the correlation between the percentage of aniline blue-stained spermatozoa and other sperm parameters remains controversial. Immature sperm chromatin may or may not correlate with asthenozoospermic samples and abnormal morphology patterns (142,143). Most important is the finding that chromatin condensation as visualized by aniline blue staining is a good predictor for IVF outcome, although it cannot determine the fertilization potential and the cleavage and pregnancy rates following ICSI (144,146). Evaluation of the sperm chromatin quality using AAB staining could be considered as one of the complementary tests of semen analysis for assessment of male factor infertility (147,148). Counterstaining with Eosin can improve the assessment of sperm chromatin quality (144).

TB Stain

Principle

Toluidine blue is a basic planar nuclear dye used for metachromatic and orthochromatic staining of chromatin. The phosphate residues of sperm DNA in nuclei with loosely packed chromatin and/or impaired DNA become more liable to binding with basic TB, providing a metachromatic shift from light blue to purple-violet color (149). This stain is a sensitive structural probe for DNA structure and packaging.

Technique

The protocol of the TB stain includes four steps. The smears are air-dried, fixed in freshly made 96% ethanol–acetone (1:1) at 4°C for at least 30 minutes, hydrolyzed in 0.1 N HCl at 4°C for five minutes, and rinsed three times in distilled water for two minutes each. Smears are stained with 0.05% TB for five minutes. The staining buffer consists of 50% citrate phosphate (McIlvaine buffer, pH 3.5). Permanent preparations are dehydrated in tertiary butanol twice for three minutes each at 37°C, and in xylene twice for three minutes each and preparations are embedded in DPX. Sperm heads with good chromatin integrity stain light blue and those of diminished integrity stain violet (purple)(150). The results of the TB test are visualized using light microscope. Based on the different optical densities of cells stained by the TB, the image analysis cytometry test has been elaborated (Fig. 6.1A) (133).

Clinical Significance

TB staining may be considered a fairly reliable method for assessing sperm chromatin. Abnormal nuclei (purple-violet sperm heads) have been shown to be correlated with counts of red-orange sperm heads as revealed by the AO method (149). Significant correlations between the results of the TB, SCSA, and TUNEL tests have been demonstrated (150). Clinical applicability of the TB test for male fertility potential assessment also has been demonstrated, with specificity for infertility diagnosis as high as 92% and sensitivity reaching 42% when the threshold of 45% is used for sperm cells with abnormal nuclei (151). TB staining has been used in several studies for evaluating sperm chromatin quality (152–156), alone and in conjunction with other tests, proving it to be an effective tool for evaluation of the chromatin status.

Advantages and Limitations

In general, the AAB and TB methods are simple and inexpensive and have the advantage of providing permanent preparations for use on an ordinary microscope. The smears stained with the TB method can also be used for morphological assessment of the cells. Also, with the threshold for infertility diagnostics using TB staining having been established, TB staining method is more advantageous. However, these methods may have the inherent limitations of reproducibility dictated by the limited number of cells, which can be reasonably scored.

CMA_3 Assay

Principle

CMA_3 is a guanine–cytosine-specific fluorochrome that reveals chromatin that is poorly packaged in human spermatozoa via indirect visualization of protamine-deficient DNA. CMA_3 is specific for GC-rich sequences and is believed to compete with protamines for binding to the minor groove of DNA. Therefore, high CMA_3 fluorescence is a strong indicator of the low protamination state of spermatozoa (134).

Technique

For CMA_3 staining, semen smears are first fixed in methanol–glacial acetic acid 3:1 at 4°C for 20 minutes and are then allowed to air-dry at room temperature for 20 minutes. The slides are treated for 20 minutes with 100 μL CMA_3 solution. The CMA_3 solution consists of 0.25 mg/mL CMA_3 in McIlvaine buffer (pH 7.0) supplemented with 10 mmol/L $MgCl_2$. The slides are rinsed in buffer and mounted with 1:1 v/v PBS glycerol. The slides are then kept at 4°C overnight. Fluorescence is evaluated using a fluorescent microscope. A total of 200 spermatozoa are randomly evaluated on each slide. CMA_3 staining is evaluated by distinguishing spermatozoa that stain bright yellow (CMA_3 positive) from those that stain a dull yellow (CMA_3 negative) (138).

Clinical Significance

As a discriminator of IVF success (>50% oocytes fertilized), CMA_3 staining has a sensitivity of 73% and specificity of 75%. Therefore, it can distinguish between IVF success and failure (157). In cases of ICSI, Sakkas et al. (158) reported that the percentage of CMA_3 positivity does not indicate failure of fertilization entirely and

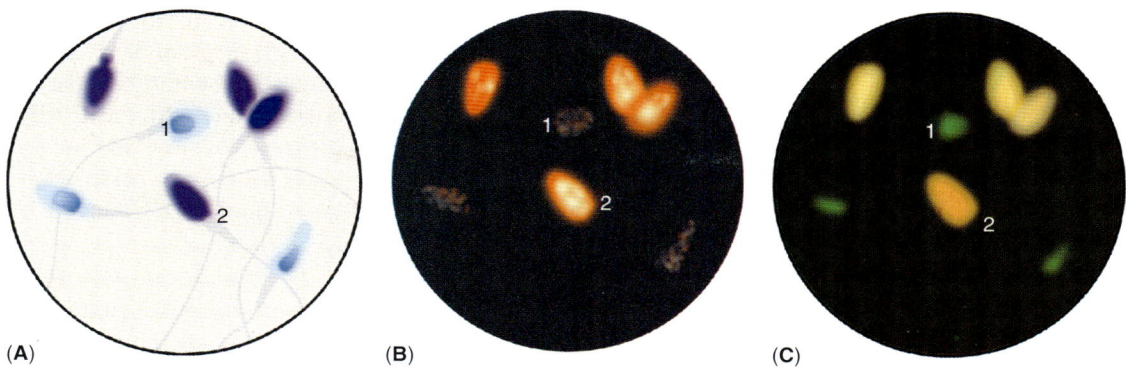

Figure 6.1 (**A**) Human ejaculate stained with toluidine blue: (1) sperm heads with normal chromatin conformation are light blue; (2) sperm heads with abnormal chromatin conformation are violet. (**B**) DNA breakage detection-fluorescence in situ hybridization (DBD-FISH) labeling with a whole genome probe (red fluorescence), demonstrating extensive DNA breakage in those nuclei that are intensely labeled. (**C**) Acridine orange (AO) stain to native DNA fluoresces green (1); whereas relaxed/denatured DNA fluoresces red (2).

suggested that poor chromatin packaging contributes to a failure in the decondensation process and probably reduced fertility. It appears that semen samples with high CMA_3 positivity (>30%) may have significantly lower fertilization rates if used for ICSI (159), but this observation is not seen in studies (160).

Advantages and Limitations

The CMA_3 assay yields reliable results as it is strongly correlated with other assays used in the evaluation of sperm chromatin (134,161) CMA_3 staining results have been reported to have strong negative correlation with sperm concentration, motility, and especially normal morphology. Men with low scores of morphologically normal spermatozoa tend to have a greater degree of protamine deficiency and DNA damage (158,161). In addition, the sensitivity and specificity of the CMA_3 stain are comparable with those of the AAB stain (75% and 82%, 60% and 91%, respectively) if used to evaluate the chromatin status in infertile men (135). However, the CMA_3 assay is limited by observer subjectivity.

DBD-FISH Assay

Principle

Cells embedded within an agarose matrix on a slide are exposed to an alkaline unwinding solution, which transforms DNA-strand breaks into ssDNA motifs. After neutralization and protein removal, ssDNA is accessible to hybridization with whole genome or specific DNA probes. The probe highlights the chromatin area to be analyzed. As DNA breaks increase, the more ssDNA is produced by the alkaline solution and the probe hybridizes more, resulting in an increase in the fluorescence intensity and surface area of the FISH signal. Abnormal chromatin packaging in sperm cells greatly increases the accessibility of DNA ligands and the sensitivity of DNA to denaturation by alkali, and this relates to the presence of intense labeling (red fluorescence) by DBD-FISH. Therefore, DBD-FISH allows in situ detection and quantification of DNA breaks and reveals structural features in the sperm chromatin (135,162).

Technique

To perform this assay, sperm cells are mixed with low-melting-point agarose to a final concentration of 0.7% at 37°C. A volume of 300 µL of the mixture is pipetted onto polystyrene slides and allowed to solidify at 4°C. The slides are immersed into a freshly prepared alkaline denaturation solution (0.03 mol/L NaOH, 1 mol/L NaCl) for five minutes at 22°C in the dark to generate ssDNA from DNA breaks. The denaturation is then stopped, and proteins are removed by transferring the slides to a tray with neutralizing and lysing solution 1 [0.4 mol/L Tris, 0.8 mol/L dithiothreitol (DTT), 1% sodium dodecylsulfate (SDS), and 50 mmol/L ethylenediaminetetraacetic acid (EDTA), pH 7.5] for 10 minutes at room temperature, which is followed by incubation in a neutralizing and lysing solution 2 (0.4 mol/L Tris, 2 mol/L NaCl, and 1% SDS, pH 7.5) for 20 minutes at room temperature. The slides are thoroughly washed in Tris-borate-EDTA buffer (0.09 mol/L Tris-borate and 0.002 mol/L EDTA, pH 7.5) for 15 minutes, dehydrated in sequential 70%, 90%, and 100% ethanol baths (two minutes each), and air-dried. A human whole-genome probe is hybridized overnight [4.3 ng/µL in 50% formamide/2× standard saline citrate (SSC), 10% dextran sulfate, and 100 mmol/L calcium phosphate, pH 7.0] (1× SSC is 0.015 mol/L sodium citrate and 0.15 mol/L sodium chloride, pH 7.0). It is then washed twice in 50% formamide/2× SSC, pH 7.0, for five minutes, and twice in 2× SSC (pH 7.0) for three minutes at room temperature. The hybridized probe is detected with streptavidin and indocarbocyanine (1:200; Sigma Chemical Co., St Louis, Missouri, USA) and cells are counterstained with 4′,6-diamidino-2-phenylindole (DAPI; 1 µg/mL) and visualized using fluorescent microscopy (Fig. 6.1B) (135).

Advantages and Limitations

Although the assay reveals chromatin structural features, it is expensive and time consuming and involves sophisticated procedures. Its major advantage is the possibility to simultaneously detect and discriminate single-stranded and double-stranded DNA breaks (163). The assay is of less clinical value because the results are not superior to those of other, less cumbersome assays.

In Situ NT Assay

Principle

The NT assay is a modified version of TUNEL assay; it quantifies the incorporation of biotinylated dUTP at ssDNA breaks in a reaction that is catalyzed by the template-dependent (unlike TUNEL) enzyme DNA polymerase I. It specifically stains spermatozoa that contain appreciable and variable levels of endogenous DNA damage. The NT assay indicates anomalies that have occurred during remodeling of the nuclear DNA in spermatozoa. In doing so, it is more likely to detect sperm anomalies that are not indicated by morphology.

Technique

To perform the assay, smears containing 500 sperm each should be prepared. The fluorescent staining solution is prepared by mixing 10 μL streptavidin-fluorescein-isothiocyanate, 90 μL Tris buffer, and 900 μL double distilled water. One hundred microliters of this solution is added to the slides. The slides are incubated in a moist chamber at 37°C for 30 minutes. After incubation, the slides are rinsed in PBS twice, washed with distilled water, and finally mounted with a 1:1 mixture of PBS and glycerol. The slides are examined using fluorescent microscopy. A total of 100–200 spermatozoa should be counted, and those fluorescing and hence incorporating the dye are classified as having endogenous nicks (136).

Clinical Significance

Sperm nuclear integrity as assessed by the NT assay demonstrates a very clear relationship with sperm motility and morphology and, to a lesser extent, sperm concentration (164-166). Results of the assay are supported by the strong positive correlations detected with the sensitivity of CMA_3 and TUNEL assays ($r = 0.86$; $p < 0.05$ and $r = 0.87$; $p < 0.05$, respectively) (134). The NT assay can also indicate whether there is damage arising from factors such as heat exposure (167) or the generation of ROS following exposure to leukocytes within the male reproductive tract (168).

Advantages and Limitations

The advantage of the NT assay is that the reaction is based on direct labeling of the termini of DNA breaks. Thus, the lesions that are measured are identifiable at the molecular level. In addition, if flow cytometry is used to analyze the results, it may be performed on fixed cells, as the time of cell storage in ethanol may vary (136) NT assay has lower sensitivity when compared with other assays, and does not correlate with fertilization in in vivo studies.

AO Assay

Principle

The AO assay measures the susceptibility of sperm nuclear DNA to acid-induced denaturation in situ by quantifying the metachromatic shift of AO fluorescence from green (native DNA) to red (denatured DNA). The fluorochrome AO intercalates into double-stranded DNA (dsDNA) as a monomer and binds to ssDNA as an aggregate. The monomeric AO bound to native DNA fluoresces green, whereas the aggregated AO on relaxed or denatured DNA fluoresces red (Fig. 6.1C) (169).

Technique

The AO assay may be used for either fluorescence or flow cytometry. To perform this assay for fluorescent microscopy, thick smears are fixed in Carnoy's fixative (methanol:acetic acid, 1:3) for at least two hours. The slides are stained for five minutes and gently rinsed with deionized water. At least 200 cells should be counted so that the estimate of the numbers of sperm with green and red fluorescence is accurate.

For flow cytometry, aliquots of semen (about 25–100 μL, containing 1 million spermatozoa) are suspended in 1 mL of ice-cold PBS (pH 7.4) and centrifuged at 600 g for five minutes. The pellet is resuspended in ice-cold TNE (0.01 mol/L Tris-HCl, 0.15 mol/L NaCl, and 1 mmol/L EDTA, pH 7.4) and again centrifuged at 600 g for five minutes. The pellet is then resuspended in 200 μL of ice-cold TNE with 10% glycerol and immediately fixed in 70% ethanol for 30 minutes. The fixed samples are treated for 30 seconds with 400 μL of a solution of 0.1% Triton X-100, 0.15 mol/L NaCl, and 0.08N HCl, pH 1.2. After 30 seconds, 1.2 mL of staining buffer (6 μg/mL AO, 37 mmol/L citric acid, 126 mmol/L Na_2HPO_4, 1 mmol/L disodium EDTA, and 0.15 mol/L NaCl, pH 6.0) is added to the test tube and analyzed by flow cytometry. After excitation by a 488-nm wavelength light source, AO bound to dsDNA fluoresces green (515–530 nm) and AO bound to ssDNA fluoresces red (630 nm or greater). A minimum of 5000 cells are analyzed by fluorescent activated cell sorting (FACS) (137).

Clinical Significance

Staining with AO shows a significant difference between fertile men and those who are infertile with different andrologic pathologies like varicocele (155). AO-positive cells are likely to have more structural abnormalities (like sperm nucleus with vacuoles) than AO-negative cells (170). Negative correlation has been shown between AO test results and conventional sperm parameters (171). The "cut-off" value set to differentiate between fertile and infertile men varies between 20% and 50% (17,172,173). Studies show that ssDNA that is detected by a low incidence (<50%) of green AO fluorescence negatively affects the fertilization process in a classical IVF program, resulting in lower fertilization and pregnancy rates and lower proportion of grade A embryos (169,174–177). However, no correlation was found with pregnancy rate and live births achieved by ICSI, except in patients having 0% of spermatozoa with ssDNA, in whom the pregnancy rate was significantly high (174,177).

Advantages and Limitations

The AO assay is a biologically stable measure of sperm quality. The interassay variability is less than 5%, rendering the technique highly reproducible (178). A strong positive correlation exists between the AO assay and other techniques used to evaluate ssDNA, for example, the TUNEL assay (179). The AO assay still requires expensive instrumentation if flow cytometry is used to interpret the results. Also, observer subjectivity may hinder the results if fluorescent microscopy is used.

SCD Test (Halo Sperm Assay)

Principle

If spermatozoa with nonfragmented DNA are immersed in an agarose matrix and directly exposed to lysing solutions, the resulting deproteinized nuclei (nucleoids) show extended halos of DNA dispersion as monitored by fluorescent microscopy. The presence of DNA breaks promotes the expansion of the halo of the nucleoid (138,180–184). The SCD test is based on the principle that when sperm are treated with an acid solution prior to lysis buffer, the DNA dispersion halos that are observed in sperm nuclei with nonfragmented DNA after the removal of nuclear proteins are either minimally present or not produced at all in sperm nuclei with fragmented DNA.

Technique

Aliquots of either raw or washed semen samples should be adjusted to concentrations ranging between 5 and 10 million/mL. The suspensions are mixed with 1% low-melting-point aqueous agarose (to obtain a 0.7% final agarose concentration) at 37°C. Aliquots of 50 μL of the mixture should be pipetted onto a glass slide precoated with 0.65% standard agarose dried at 80°C, covered with a coverslip, and left to solidify at 4°C for four minutes. The coverslips are then carefully removed, and the slides are immediately immersed horizontally in a tray of freshly prepared acid denaturation solution (0.08N HCl) for seven minutes at 22°C in the dark, which generates restricted ssDNA motifs from DNA breaks. Denaturation is then stopped, and the proteins are removed by transferring the slides to a tray with neutralizing and lysing solution 1 (0.4 mol/L Tris, 0.8 mol/L DTT, 1% SDS, and 50 mmol/L EDTA pH 7.5) for 10 minutes at room temperature. The slides are then incubated in neutralizing and lysing solution 2 (0.4 mol/L Tris, 2 mol/L NaCl, and 1% SDS, pH 7.5) for five minutes at room temperature. The slides are thoroughly washed in Tris-borate EDTA buffer (0.09 mol/L Tris-borate and 0.002 mol/L EDTA, pH 7.5) for two minutes, dehydrated in sequential 70%, 90%, and 100% ethanol baths (two minutes each), and air-dried. Cells are stained with DAPI (2 μg/mL) for fluorescence microscopy (Fig. 6.2A) (138).

Advantages and Limitations

The major advantage of the SCD test is that it does not require the determination of color or fluorescence intensity. Rather, the percentage of spermatozoa with nondispersed (very small halos or none at all) or dispersed nuclei is determined, which can be easily and reliably accomplished by the naked eye. Furthermore, the test is simple, fast, and reproducible, and its results are comparable to those of the SCSA (181,184) and TUNEL (185). SCD test is successfully used in clinical studies for sperm DNA damage detection (186). If required, SCD test can be simultaneously combined with FISH (SCD-FISH) assay for detection of aneuploidy in sperm cells (187). Oxidative DNA damage also can be simultaneously determined in the same sperm cell by combining SCD test and incubation with an 8-oxoguanine DNA probe (188). Commercially available Halosperm® kit (Halotech DNA SL, Madrid, Spain; Conception Technologies, San Diego,

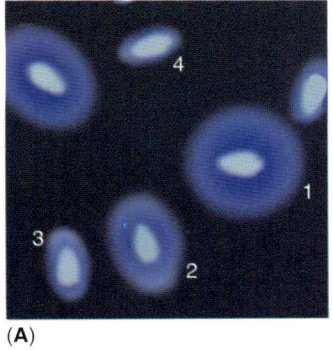
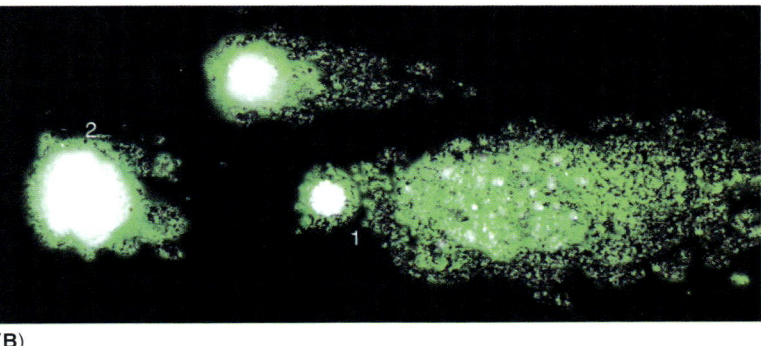

(A)   (B)

Figure 6.2 (**A**) Spermatozoa embedded in an agarose microgel stained with 4′,6-diamidino-2-phenylindole (DAPI) staining (blue fluorescence) and showing spermatozoa with different patterns of DNA dispersion: big-sized halo (1); medium-sized halo (2); very small-sized halo (3); no halo (4). (**B**) Comet images showing damaged (1) and undamaged DNA (2).

USA) has been recently developed (189). Reports suggest that sperm DNA fragmentation as reported by the SCD test are negatively correlated with fertilization rate and embryo quality in IVF/ICSI, but not with clinical pregnancy rates or births (182,190).

Comet Assay

Principle

The comet assay, also known as single-cell gel electrophoresis for analysis of DNA damage in an individual cell, was first introduced by Ostling and Johanson in 1984 (191). Neutral electrophoresis buffer conditions were used to show that the migration of dsDNA loops from a damaged cell in the form of a tail unwinding from the relaxed supercoiled nucleus was proportional to the extent of damage inflicted on the cell. This finding took on the appearance of a comet with a tail when viewed using the fluorescent microscope and DNA stains. Singh et al. modified the comet assay in 1988 (140) by using alkaline electrophoresis buffers to expose alkali-labile sites on the DNA; this modification increased the sensitivity of the assay to detect both single- and dsDNA breaks (140). Comet assay is unable to differentiate between ssDNA breaks and dsDNA breaks in the same sperm cell. To overcome this limitation, the two-tailed comet assay (2T-Comet)—a modification of the original comet assay developed for the simultaneous evaluation of DNA SSB and DSB—was introduced (192). Chromosome-comet assay was designed, which can be used to generate comets in subnuclear units, such as chromosome, based on the chromosome isolation protocols currently used for whole chromosome mounting in electron microscopy, to detect DNA damage and link it to specific chromosomes. However, it is not evaluated on sperm cells so far (193).

The damage is quantified by measuring the displacement between the genetic material of the nucleus "comet head" and the resulting tail. The tail lengths are used as an index for the damage. Also, the tail moment—the product of the tail length and intensity (fraction of total DNA in the tails)—has been used as a measuring parameter. The tail moment can be more precisely defined as being equivalent to the torsional moment of the tail (194).

Technique

In this assay, sperm cells are cast into miniature agarose gels on microscope slides and lysed in situ to remove DNA-associated proteins and to allow the compacted DNA in the sperm to relax. The lysis buffer (Tris 10 mmol/L, 0.5 mol/L EDTA, and 2.5 mol/L NaCl, pH 10) contains 1% Triton X-100, 40 mmol/L DTT, and 100 µg/mL proteinase K. Slides immersion time in alkaline lysis solution ranges between one and 20 minutes and does not affect assay results (195). Micro-gels are then electrophoresed (20 minutes at 25 V/0.01 A) in neutral buffer (Tris 10 mmol/L containing 0.08 mol/L boric acid and 0.5 mol/L EDTA, pH 8.2), during which the damaged DNA migrates from the nucleus toward the anode. The DNA is visualized by staining the slides with the fluorescent DNA binding dye SYBR Green I. Comet measurements are performed using fluorescent microscopy. These measurements can be done either manually or with computerized image analysis (Fig. 6.2B) (139).

2T-Comet: Technique

Sperm cells should be diluted in PBS to a concentration of 10×10^6 spermatozoa/mL; 25 µl of the cell dilution was mixed with 50 µl of 1% low-melting-point agarose in distilled water at 37°C. Then 15 µl of the mixture was placed on a slide, covered with a coverslip, and transferred to an ice-cold plate. As soon as the gel solidified, coverslips were removed, the slides were rinsed in two lysing solutions: lysing solution 1 (0.4 mol/L Tris–HCl, 0.8 mol/L DTT, 1% SDS, pH 7.5) for 30 minutes, followed by lysing solution 2 (0.4 mol/L Tris–HCl, 2 mol/L NaCl, 1% SDS, 0.05 mol/L EDTA, pH 7.5) for 30 minutes. Then, slides were rinsed in TBE buffer (0.09 mol/L Tris–borate, 0.002 mol/L EDTA, pH 7.5) for 10 minutes, transferred to an electrophoresis tank and immersed in fresh TBE electrophoresis buffer. Electrophoresis was performed at 20 V (1 V/cm), 12 mA for 12.5 minutes. After washing in 0.9% NaCl, nucleoids were unwound in an alkaline solution (0.03 mol/L NaOH, NaCl 1 mol/L) for 2.5 minutes, transferred to an electrophoresis chamber, and oriented 90° to the first electrophoresis.

The second electrophoresis is performed at 20 V (1 V/cm) 12 mA for 4 minutes in 0.03 mol/L NaOH. Then, slides are rinsed in a neutralization buffer (0.4 mol/L Tris-HCl, pH 7.5) for 5 minutes, briefly washed in TBE buffer, dehydrated in increasing concentrations of ethanol, and air-dried DNA are stained with SYBR Green I at a 1:3000 dilution in Vectashield (Vector Laboratories, Burlingame, California, USA). Samples are assessed by visual scoring or digitalization and image processing. The frequency of sperm cells with fragmented DNA is established by measuring at least 500 sperm cells per slide. Cells are classified as undamaged (no DNA migration) or damaged (migrated DNA) cells and the types are assessed; sperm cells were classified as containing SSB (up-down migration), DSB (right-left migration) or both (192).

Clinical Significance

The assay has been successfully used to evaluate DNA damage after cryopreservation (196). It may also predict embryo development after IVF and ICSI, especially in couples with unexplained infertility (197,198), and some clinical thresholds were set for infertility diagnostics and IVF outcome prediction (199–202), although some studies fail to demonstrate such an association (203). Modified version of comet assay protocol is capable for detection of different mutagen impact on sperm DNA integrity (204).

Advantages and Limitations

The comet assay is a well-standardized assay that correlates significantly with the TUNEL and SCSA assays (205).

It is simple to perform, has a low intra-assay coefficient of variation, and is inexpensive. 2T comet is capable of discriminating between SNA SSBs and DSBs, for example resistance of sperm DNA to oxidative damage can be specifically assessed (206). Because it is based on fluorescent microscopy, the assay requires an experienced observer to analyze the slides and interpret the results.

TUNEL Assay

Principle

The TUNEL assay quantifies the incorporation of dUTP at double-strand DNA breaks in a reaction catalyzed by the template-independent enzyme TdT. This enzyme incorporates biotinlyated deoxyuridine to 3'-OH of DNA to create a signal, which increases with the number of DNA breaks. Sperm with normal DNA, therefore, have only background staining/fluorescence, while those with fragmented DNA (multiple chromatin 3'-OH ends) stain/fluoresce brightly (136).

Technique

Identification of strand breaks can be quantified by flow cytometry or fluorescent microscopy in which DNA-damaged sperm fluoresce intensely (15). To assess the DNA fragmentation by TUNEL, about 2×10^6 sperm are fixed with 1% formaldehyde for 10 minutes at room temperature. The sample is centrifuged at $10,000g$ for four minutes. After the sperm are washed in PBS (pH 7.4), they are resuspended in 100 μL prewash buffer containing single-strength One-Phor-All® (GE Healthcare Biosciences, Pittsburg, PA) buffer (100 mmol/L Tris-acetate, 100 mmol/L magnesium acetate, 500 mmol/L potassium acetate, and 0.1% Triton X-100) for 10 minutes at room temperature. Fixed sperm are spun out of the buffer and resuspended in 50 μL of TdT buffer containing 3 μmol/L biotin-16-dUTP, 12 μmol/L deoxyadenosine triphosphate, 0.1% Triton X-100, and 10 U of TdT enzyme and incubated at 37°C for 60 minutes. After two washes in PBS, the fixed permeabilized sperm are resuspended in 100 μL of staining buffer consisting of 0.1% Triton X-100 and 1% streptavidin/Texas red antibiotin and incubated at 4°C in the dark for 30 minutes. The stained cells are washed in PBS/0.1% Triton X-100. To create negative controls, the enzyme terminal transferase may be omitted from the reaction mixture. To create positive controls, the samples are pretreated with 0.1 IU DNAase I for 30 minutes at room temperature and then labeled. Results may be interpreted by assessing 100–500 sperm cells under fluorescent microscopy or by using FACS flow cytometry (Fig. 6.3A and B) (71).

Standard TUNEL assay could be improved to become more sensitive to DNA damage if sperm cells are incubated in 2 mm DTT solution for 45 minutes prior to fixation with formaldehyde. This modified version of the TUNEL assay significantly enhanced its sensitivity. Study by Mitchell et al. refined the TUNEL methodology by incorporating a vital staining of sperm cells by spermatozoa incubating for 30 minutes at 37°C with LIVE /DEAD Fixable Dead Cell Stain (far red; Molecular Probes, Eugene, Oregon, USA). After this the cells were washed three times with Biggers-Whitten-Whittingham medium (BWW) before incubation with DTT, so both DNA integrity and vitality could be simultaneously assessed (207).

Clinical Significance

The TUNEL assay has been widely used in male infertility research related to sperm chromatin/DNA abnormalities. It provides useful information in many cases of male infertility. A negative correlation was found between the percentage of DNA-fragmented sperm and the motility, morphology, and concentration in the ejaculate. It also appears to be potentially useful as a predictor for IUI pregnancy rate, IVF embryo cleavage rate, and ICSI fertilization rate. In addition, it provides an explanation for recurrent pregnancy loss (18,19,129,205). Recently a predictive threshold of 19.2% has been shown that could differentiate between fertile and infertile men with a sensitivity of 64.9% and specificity of 100% (205,208). This is higher than that demonstrated for IUI procedures (12%) (19).

Advantages and Limitations

TUNEL assay is relatively expensive and labor consuming. It has been demonstrated that the measures of sperm DNA fragmentation are significantly affected by fixative and its concentration, the time of storage of fixed samples, the fluorochrome used to label DNA breaks, and the method used to analyze flow cytometric data (209). Flow cytometric method of assessment is generally more accurate and reliable than fluorescent microscopy, but it is also more sophisticated and expensive, and it presents limitations in the accuracy and reproducibility of the measures of sperm DNA fragmentation (210). Fairly good quality control parameters have been demonstrated for the fluorescent TUNEL assay (the intraobserver variability was found to be <8% and the interobserver variability was <7%) (71,211), although other authors mention high intra-assay and interlab variability (212).

Sperm Chromatin Structure Assay

Principle

The SCSA measures in-situ DNA susceptibility to the acid-induced conformational helix-coil transition by AO fluorescence staining. The extent of conformational transition in situ following acid or heat treatment is determined by measuring the metachromatic shift of AO fluorescence from green (native DNA) to red (denatured or relaxed DNA). This protocol has been divided into $SCSA_{acid}$ and $SCSA_{heat}$ to distinguish the physical means of inducing conformational transition. The two methods give essentially the same results, but the $SCSA_{acid}$ method is much easier to use. DNA damage that is SCSA-defined is manifested by the DNA Fragmentation Index (DFI) (17).

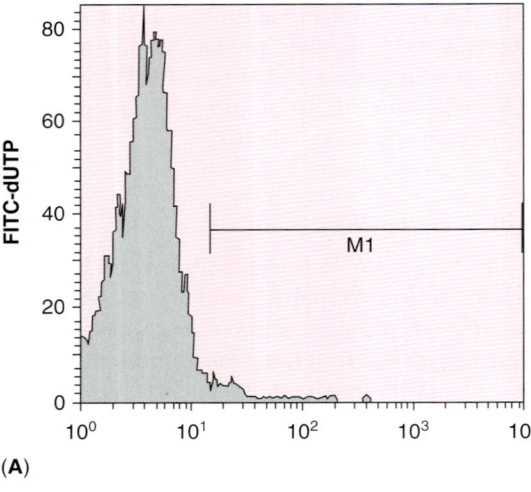 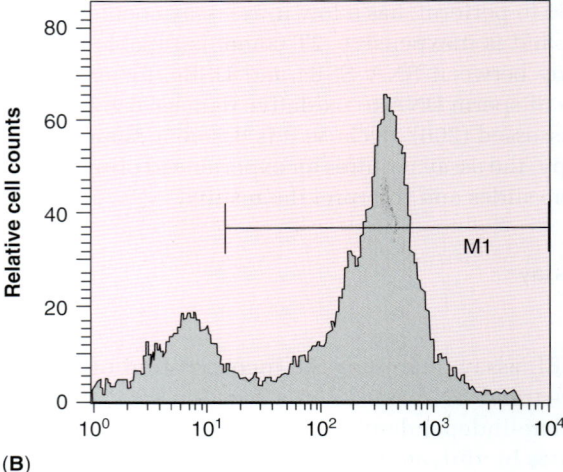

Figure 6.3 (**A**) Terminal deoxynucleotidyl transferase-mediated fluorescin-deoxyuridine triphosphate-nick end labeling (TUNEL) assay fluorescent activated cell sorting (FACS) histograms with markers (M1) for detection of fluorescence set at 650 nm semen sample with low percentage of sperm DNA fragmentation; (**B**) TUNEL assay FACS histograms with markers (M1) for a semen sample with high percentage of sperm DNA fragmentation. *Abbreviations*: dUTP, deoxyuridine triphosphate; FITC, fluorescein isothiocyanate.

Technique

To perform SCSA, an aliquot of unprocessed semen (about 13–70 µL) is diluted to a concentration of $1-2 \times 10^6$ sperm/mL with TNE buffer (0.01 M Tris-HCl, 0.15 M NaCl, and 1 mM EDTA, pH 7.4). This cell suspension is treated with an acid detergent solution (pH = 1.2) containing 0.1% Triton X-100, 0.15 mol/L NaCl, and 0.08 N HCl for 30 seconds, and then stained with 6 mg/L purified AO in a phosphate-citrate buffer, pH 6.0. The stained sample is placed into the flow cytometer sample chamber (17).

Clinical Significance

Because the SCSA is more constant over prolonged periods of time than routine World Health Organization (WHO) semen parameters, it may be used effectively in epidemiological studies of male infertility (213). No significant male age-related increase in DFI was demonstrated (214). Currently, SCSA is the only assay that has clearly established clinical thresholds for utility in the human infertility clinic (215). In clinical applications, the SCSA parameters not only distinguish fertile and infertile men but also are able to classify men according to the level of in vivo fertility: high fertility (pregnancy initiated in less than three months) moderate fertility (pregnancy initiated within 4–12 months) and no proven fertility (no pregnancy by 12 months). In addition, a DFI threshold was established that identifies samples compatible with in vivo pregnancy (<30%) (12,216–219). To the best of our knowledge, SCSA is the most successful assay in predicting the various outcomes of ART; however, this is true only for neat semen (220) including the fertilization and implantation rates (9,12,128,221,222), but this is not supported by some studies, where only increased abortion rate in the high DFI (>27%) group was found (223). Recent reports suggest that DFI can be used as an independent predictor of fertility in couples undergoing IUI (221), but so far association between SCSA results and IVF and ICSI outcomes is not strong enough (224). It is also proposed that all infertile men should be tested with SCSA as a supplement to the standard semen analysis (225). Recent data suggest that ICSI should be the method of choice when DFI exceeds 30% (12).

Advantages and Limitations

The SCSA accurately estimates the percentage of DNA-damaged sperm and has a cut-off point (30% DFI) to differentiate between fertile and infertile samples (216,221). However, it requires the presence of expensive instrumentation (flow cytometer) and highly skilled technicians. SCSA DFI showed significant association with TUNEL assay results when Spearman's rank correlation was used; however, regression and concordance correlation results have shown that these methods are not comparable. SCSA rather measures DNA damage in terms of susceptibility to DNA denaturation, while TUNEL measures "real" DNA damage (226).

Measurement of 8-OHDG

Principle

This assay measures levels of 8-hydroxy-2-deoxyguanosine (8-OHdG), which is a byproduct of oxidative DNA damage, in the spermatozoa. It is the most commonly studied biomarker for oxidative DNA damage. Among various oxidative DNA adducts, 8-OHdG has been selected as a representative of oxidative DNA damage owing to its high specificity, potent mutagenicity, and relative abundance in DNA (227).

Technique

Step I DNA extraction is performed with chloroform–isoamyl alcohol (12:1 v/v) after the sperm cells are washed with sperm wash buffer (10 mmol/L Tris-HCl, 10 mmol/L EDTA, 1 mol/L NaCl, pH 7.0) and lysed at 55°C for 1 hour with 0.9% SDS, 0.5 mg/mL proteinase K, and 0.04 mol/L DTT. After being treated with ribonuclease A to remove RNA residue, the extracted DNA is dissolved in 10 mmol/L Tris-HCl (pH 7.0) for DNA digestion.

Step II Enzymatic DNA digestion is performed with three enzymes: DNAase I, nuclease P1, and alkaline phosphatase. The final solution is dried under reduced temperature and pressure and is redissolved in distilled and deionized water for HPLC.

Step III The third step is HPLC analysis. The HPLC system used for 8-OHdG measurements consists of a pump, a partisphere 5 C18 column, an electrochemical detector, an ultraviolet detector, an autosampler, and an integrator. The mobile phase consists of 20 mmol/L $NH_4H_2PO_4$, 1 mmol/L EDTA, and 4% methanol (pH 4.7). The calibration curves for 8-OHdG are established with standard 8-OHdG, and the results are expressed as 8-OHdG/10^4 dG (141).

Clinical Significance

The assay provides the most direct evidence suggesting that oxidative sperm DNA damage is involved in male infertility, based on the finding that levels of 8-OHdG in sperm are significantly higher in infertile patients than in fertile controls and have an inverse relationship with sperm concentration (141). DNA fragmentation and 8-OHdG formation assessed by TUNEL are highly correlated with each other (228). The 8-OHdG levels also are highly correlated with the disruption of chromatin remodeling (86). Levels of 8-OHdG in sperm DNA have been reported to be increased in smokers, and they inversely correlate with the intake and seminal plasma concentration of vitamin C—the most important antioxidant in sperm. It is demonstrated that infertile patients with varicocele have increased 8-OHdG expression in the testes which is associated with deficient spermatogenesis (229). If not repaired, 8-OHdG modifications in DNA are mutagenic and may cause embryo loss, fetal malformations, or childhood cancer. Moreover, this modification could be a marker of OS in sperm, which may have negative effects on sperm function (230,231).

Advantages and Limitations

Although 8-OHdG is a potential marker for oxidative DNA damage, artificial oxidation of dG can occur during the analysis, which can lead to inaccurate results. A fixed number of sperm cells should be analyzed as a precaution. However, the DNA yield cannot be excluded as a potential confounder.

STRATEGIES TO REDUCE SPERM DNA DAMAGE

In view of the impact sperm DNA fragmentation has on reproductive outcomes, it is important to develop and implement appropriate treatment methods and strategies to minimize DNA damage in spermatozoa used in assisted reproduction. Some of the strategies are discussed next.

Appropriate Sperm Preparation Methods

Most of the commonly used methods such as density gradient centrifugation, swim-up, and glass wool filtration yield sperm with better DNA integrity than native semen (14). Sperm preparation should be aimed at minimizing damage to the spermatozoa. This may be accomplished by exercising some simple precautions such as (*i*) slow dilution of the samples, especially when using cryopreserved spermatozoa, (*ii*) a gradual change in temperature and tests performed at 37°C, (*iii*) a minimal use of centrifugation, and when necessary, this should be carried out at the lowest possible speeds, and (*iv*) controlled exposure to potentially toxic materials. Plastic glassware and media should be checked for potential toxicity to spermatozoa and contact with gloves as it may immobilize the spermatozoa. In patients who are unable to create a sperm sample by masturbation, use of nontoxic condoms is important, and when necessary, a second sample should be collected a few hours after the first.

Electrophoretic Separation of Sperm

This is based on the principle that high-quality spermatozoa tend to be viable and morphologically normal and have a low degree of DNA fragmentation as measured by TUNEL assay (232).

Antioxidant Treatments

One of the causes of sperm DNA damage is OS. Studies have investigated the ability of antioxidant treatments to manage male subfertility, both in vivo and in vitro. It is generally accepted that antioxidants may be beneficial in reducing sperm DNA damage, but their exact mechanism of action still not established, and some studies along with positive effect of antioxidants demonstrated possible adverse events of such treatment like increase in sperm chromatin decondensation (233,234). Significant improvement in clinical pregnancy and implantation rates have been shown in patients with high sperm DNA damage as assessed by TUNEL assay when treated with antioxidants before assisted reproduction (235,236). Therefore, in patients in whom OS is the cause of sperm DNA damage, adequate oral antioxidant treatment appears to be a simple strategy to enhance sperm genome integrity and the reproductive outcome. Designing standard and reliable oral antioxidant treatment protocols and alternative treatment strategies for nonresponders is needed (237).

Magnetic Cell Separation

Magnetic cell separation is a useful technique to separate apoptotic and nonapoptotic spermatozoa (238). All of these strategies are designed to help select vital, nonapoptotic spermatozoa with minimal DNA damage and positively affect the success rate and safety of ART.

High Magnification ICSI for Patients with Sperm DNA Fragmentation

Using inverted microscopes with Nomarski differential interference contrast optics combined with digitally enhanced secondary magnification (239,240) allows the observation of spermatozoa with apparently normal morphology and shows intranuclear vacuoles that appear to be associated with chromatin packaging.

CONCLUSION

In summary, we emphasize the importance of assessing sperm for chromatin abnormalities as it may provide useful information in cases of male idiopathic infertility and in couples pursuing assisted reproduction. Pathologically increased sperm DNA fragmentation is one other main paternal-derived cause of repeated assisted reproduction failures in the ICSI era. Several studies have demonstrated that sperm DNA integrity correlates with pregnancy outcome in in vitro fertilization. Therefore, sperm DNA fragmentation should be included in the evaluation of the infertile male. Assessment of sperm DNA damage appears to be a potential tool for evaluating semen samples prior to their use in assisted reproduction. It allows the selection of spermatozoa with intact DNA or with the least amount of DNA damage for use in assisted conception. It provides better diagnostic and prognostic capabilities than standard sperm parameters for male fertility potential.

There are multiple assays that may be used to evaluate sperm chromatin. Most of these assays have many advantages as well as limitations. Choosing the right assay depends on many factors such as the expense, the available laboratory facilities, and the presence of experienced technicians. The establishment of a cut-off point between normal levels in the average fertile population and the minimal levels of sperm DNA integrity required for achieving pregnancy still remains to be investigated. Such an average range or value confirmed by different laboratories is still lacking for most of these assays except for the SCSA. Given the importance of sperm DNA integrity, it is important to determine the real cause of DNA damage and provide proper therapeutic treatment. Furthermore, methods for selecting sperm with undamaged DNA should be designed, especially in cases where ICSI is strongly recommended.

REFERENCES

1. Guzick DS, Overstreet JW, Factor-Litvak P, et al. National Cooperative Reproductive Medicine Network. Sperm morphology, motility, and concentration in fertile and infertile men. N Engl J Med 2001; 45: 388–93.
2. Agarwal A, Said TM. Role of sperm chromatin abnormalities and DNA damage in male infertility. Hum Reprod Update 2003; 9: 31–45.
3. Hansen M, Kurinczuk JJ, Bower C, et al. The risk of major birth defects after intracytoplasmic sperm injection and in vitro fertilization. N Engl J Med 2002; 346: 25–30.
4. Schieve LA, Meikle SF, Ferre C, et al. Low and very low birth weight in infants conceived with use of assisted reproductive technique. N Engl J Med 2002; 346: 731–7.
5. Moll AC, Imhof SM, Cruysberg JR, et al. Incidence of retinoblastoma in children born after in-vitro fertilisation. Lancet 2003; 361: 309–10.
6. Orstavik KH, Eiklid K, van der Hagen CB, et al. Another case of imprinting defect in a girl with Angelman syndrome who was conceived by intracytoplasmic semen injection. Am J Hum Genet 2003; 72: 218–19.
7. Agarwal A, Allamaneni SS. Sperm DNA damage assessment: a test whose time has come. Fertil Steril 2005; 84: 850–3.
8. Erenpreiss J, Spano M, Erenpreisa J, et al. Sperm chromatin structure and male fertility: biological and clinical aspects. Asian J Androl 2006; 8: 11–29.
9. Evenson D, Wixon R. Meta-analysis of sperm DNA fragmentation using the sperm chromatin structure assay. Reprod Biomed Online 2006; 12: 466–72.
10. Borini A, Tarozzi N, Bizzaro D, et al. Sperm DNA fragmentation: paternal effect on early post-implantation embryo development in ART. Hum Reprod 2006; 21: 2876–81.
11. Aitken RJ, De Iuliis GN. Origins and consequences of DNA damage in male germ cells. Reprod Biomed Online 2007; 14: 72–33.
12. Bungum M, Humaidan P, Axmon A, et al. Sperm DNA integrity assessment in prediction of assisted reproductive technique outcome. Hum Reprod 2007; 22: 174–9.
13. Ozmen B, Koutlaki N, Youssry M, et al. DNA damage of human spermatozoa in assisted reproduction: origins, diagnosis, impacts and safety. Reprod Biomed Online 2007; 14: 384–95.
14. Tarozzi N, Bizzaro D, Flamigni C, et al. Clinical relevance of sperm DNA damage in assisted reproduction. Reprod Biomed Online 2007; 14: 746–57.
15. Lopes S, Jurisicova A, Sun JG, et al. Reactive oxygen species: potential cause for DNA fragmentation in human spermatozoa. Hum Reprod 1998; 13: 896–900.
16. Sakkas D, Tomlinson M. Assessment of sperm competence. Semin Reprod Med 2000; 18: 133–9.
17. Evenson DP, Jost LK, Marshall D, et al. Utility of the sperm chromatin structure assay as a diagnostic and prognostic tool in the human fertility clinic. Hum Reprod 1999; 14: 1039–49.
18. Aitken RJ. The Amoroso Lecture. The human spermatozoon-a cell in crisis? J Reprod Fertil 1999; 115: 1–7.
19. Sun JG, Jurisicova A, Casper RF. Detection of deoxyribonucleic acid fragmentation in human sperm: correlation with fertilization in vitro. Biol Reprod 1997; 56: 602–7.
20. Duran EH, Morshedi M, Taylor S, et al. Sperm DNA quality predicts intrauterine insemination outcome: a

prospective cohort study. Hum Reprod 2002; 17: 3122–8.
21. Larson KL, DeJonge CJ, Barnes AM, et al. Sperm chromatin structure assay parameters as predictors of failed pregnancy following assisted reproductive techniques. Hum Reprod 2000; 15: 1717–22.
22. DeJonge C. The clinical value of sperm nuclear DNA assessment. Hum Fertil 2002; 5: 51–3.
23. Bellve AR, McKay DJ, Renaux BS, et al. Purification and characterization of mouse protamines P1 and P2. Amino acid sequence of P2. Biochem 1988; 27: 2890–7.
24. Ward WS, Coffey DS. DNA packaging and organization in mammalian spermatozoa: comparison with somatic cells. Biol Reprod 1991; 44: 569–74.
25. Fuentes-Mascorro G, Serrano H, Rosado A. Sperm chromatin. Arch Androl 2000; 45: 215–25.
26. Oliva R, Castillo J. Proteomics and the genetics of sperm chromatin condensation. Asian J Androl 2011; 13: 24–30.
27. Gatewood JM, Cook GR, Balhorn R, et al. Sequence-specific packaging of DNA in human sperm chromatin. Science 1987; 236: 962–4.
28. Bench GS, Friz AM, Corzett MH, et al. DNA and total protamine masses in individual sperm from fertile mammalian subjects. Cytometry 1996; 23: 263–71.
29. Johnson GD, Lalancette C, Linnemann AK, et al. The sperm nucleus: chromatin, RNA, and the nuclear matrix. Reproduction 2011; 141: 21–36.
30. Sakkas D, Mariethoz E, Manicardi G, et al. Origin of DNA damage in ejaculated human spermatozoa. Rev Reprod 1999; 4: 31–7.
31. Irvine DS, Twigg JP, Gordon EL, et al. DNA integrity in human spermatozoa: relationships with semen quality. J Androl 2000; 21: 33–44.
32. Ward WS. Deoxyribonucleic acid loop domain tertiary structure in mammalian spermatozoa. Biol Reprod 1993; 48: 1193–201.
33. Zalensky AO, Allen MJ, Kobayashi A, et al. Well-defined genome architecture in the human sperm nucleus. Chromosoma 1995; 103: 577–90.
34. Solov'eva L, Svetlova M, Bodinski D, et al. Nature of telomere dimers and chromosome looping in human spermatozoa. Chromosome Res 2004; 12: 817–23.
35. Ward WS, Zalensky AO. The unique, complex organization of the transcriptionally silent sperm chromatin. Crit Rev Eukaryot Gene Expr 1996; 6: 139–47.
36. De Jonge CJ. Paternal contributions to embryogenesis. Reprod Med Rev 2000; 8: 203–14.
37. Lewis JD, Song Y, de Jong ME, et al. A walk through vertebrate and invertebrate protamines. Chromosoma 1999; 111: 473–82.
38. Corzett M, Mazrimas J, Balhorn R. Protamine 1 : Protamine 2 stoichiometry in the sperm of eutherian mammals. Mol Reprod Dev 2002; 61: 519–27.
39. Jager S. Sperm nuclear stability and male infertility. Arch Androl 1990; 25: 253–9.
40. Balhorn R, Reed S, Tanphaichitr N. Aberrant protamine 1/protamine 2 ratio in sperm of infertile human males. Experientia 1988; 44: 52–5.
41. Bench G, Corzett MH, De Yebra L, et al. Protein and DNA contents in sperm from an infertile human male possessing protamine defects that vary over time. Mol Reprod Dev 1998; 50: 345–53.
42. de Yebra L, Ballesca JL, Vanrell JA, et al. Detection of P2 precursors in the sperm cells of infertile patients who have reduced protamine P2 levels. Fertil Steril 1998; 69: 755–9.
43. Nasr-Esfahani MH, Salehi M, Razavi S, et al. Effect of protamine-2 deficiency on ICSI outcome. Reprod Biomed Online 2004; 9: 652–8.
44. Aoki VW, Liu L, Carrell DT. Identification and evaluation of a novel sperm protamine abnormality in a population of infertile males. Hum Reprod 2005; 20: 1298–106.
45. García-Peiró A, Martínez-Heredia J, Oliver-Bonet M, et al. Protamine 1 to protamine 2 ratio correlates with dynamic aspects of DNA fragmentation in human sperm. Fertil Steril 2011; 95: 105–9.
46. Nanassy L, Liu L, Griffin J, Carrell DT. The clinical utility of the protamine 1/protamine 2 ratio in sperm. Protein Pept Lett 2011; 18: 772–7. Review.
47. Matsuda Y, Tobari I. Chromosomal analysis in mouse eggs fertilized in vitro with sperm exposed to ultraviolet light (UV) and methyl and ethyl methanesulfonate (MMS and EMS). Mutat Res 1988; 198: 131–44.
48. Genesca A, Caballin MR, Miro R, et al. Repair of human sperm chromosome aberrations in the hamster egg. Hum Genet 1992; 89: 181–6.
49. Aitken RJ, Krausz C. Oxidative stress, DNA damage and the Y chromosome. Reproduction 2001; 122: 497–506.
50. McPherson SM, Longo FJ. Nicking of rat spermatid and spermatozoa DNA: possible involvement of DNA topoisomerase II. Dev Biol 1993; 158: 122–30.
51. Sakkas D, Manicardi G, Bianchi PG, et al. Relationship between the presence of endogenous nicks and sperm chromatin packaging in maturing and fertilizing mouse spermatozoa. Biol Reprod 1995; 52: 1149–55.
52. Marcon L, Boissonneault G. Transient DNA strand breaks during mouse and human spermiogenesis: new insights in stage specificity and link to chromatin remodeling. Biol Reprod 2004; 70: 910–18.
53. McPherson SM, Longo FJ. Localization of DNase I-hypersensitive regions during rat spermatogenesis: stage-dependent patterns and unique sensitivity of elongating spermatids. Mol Reprod Dev 1992; 31: 268–79.
54. Laberge RM, Boissonneault G. On the nature and origin of DNA strand breaks in elongating spermatids. Biol Reprod 2005; 73: 289–96.
55. Kierszenbaum AL. Transition nuclear proteins during spermiogenesis: unrepaired DNA breaks not allowed. Mol Reprod Dev 2001; 58: 357–8.
56. Morse-Gaudio M, Risley MS. Topoisomerase II expression and VM-26 induction of DNA breaks during spermatogenesis in Xenopus laevis. J Cell Sci 1994; 107: 2887–98.
57. Bizzaro D, Manicardi G, Bianchi PG, et al. Sperm decondensation during fertilisation in the mouse: presence of DNase I hypersensitive sites in situ and a putative role for topoisomerase II. Zygote 2000; 8: 197–202.
58. Franco Jr JG, Mauri AL, Petersen CG, et al. Large nuclear vacuoles are indicative of abnormal chromatin packaging in human spermatozoa. Int J Androl 2012; 35: 46–51.
59. Boitrelle F, Ferfouri F, Petit JM, et al. Large human sperm vacuoles observed in motile spermatozoa

under high magnification: nuclear thumbprints linked to failure of chromatin condensation. Hum Reprod 2011; 26: 1650–8.
60. Sakkas D, Mariethoz E, St John JC. Abnormal sperm parameters in humans are indicative of an abortive apoptotic mechanism linked to the Fas-mediated pathway. Exp Cell Res 1999; 251: 350–5.
61. Donnelly ET, O'Connell M, McClure N, et al. Differences in nuclear DNA fragmentation and mitochondrial integrity of semen and prepared human spermatozoa. Hum Reprod 2000; 15: 1552–61.
62. Spadafora C. Sperm cells and foreign DNA: a controversial relation. Bioessays 1998; 20: 955–64.
63. Aitken RJ, Koppers AJ. Apoptosis and DNA damage in human spermatozoa. Asian Journal of Andrology 2011; 13: 36–42.
64. Suda T, Takahashi T, Golstein P, et al. Molecular cloning and expression of the Fas ligand, a novel member of the tumor necrosis factor family. Cell 1993; 75: 1169–78.
65. Krammer PH, Behrmann I, Daniel P, et al. Regulation of apoptosis in the immune system. Curr Opin Immunol 1994; 6: 279–89.
66. Rodriguez I, Ody C, Araki K, et al. An early and massive wave of germinal cell apoptosis is required for the development of functional spermatogenesis. Embo J 1997; 16: 2262–70.
67. Said TM, Paasch U, Glander HJ, et al. Role of caspases in male infertility. Hum Reprod Update 2004; 10: 39–51.
68. Sakkas D, Mariethoz E, Manicardi G, et al. Origin of DNA damage in ejaculated human spermatozoa. Rev Reprod 1999; 4: 31–7.
69. Zhivotovsky B, Kroemer G. Apoptosis and genomic instability. Nat Rev Mol Cell Biol 2004; 5: 752–62.
70. Muratori M, Piomboni P, Baldi E, et al. Functional and ultrastructural features of DNA-fragmented human sperm. J Androl 2000; 21: 903–12.
71. Barroso G, Morshedi M, Oehninger S. Analysis of DNA fragmentation, plasma membrane translocation of phosphatidylserine and oxidative stress in human spermatozoa. Hum Reprod 2000; 15: 1338–44.
72. Ross AJ, Waymire KG, Moss JE, et al. Testicular degeneration in Bclw-deficient mice. Nat Genet 1998; 18: 251–6.
73. Sakkas D, Moffatt O, Manicardi GC, et al. Nature of DNA damage in ejaculated human spermatozoa and the possible involvement of apoptosis. Biol Reprod 2002; 66: 1061–7.
74. Sutovsky P, Neuber E, Schatten G. Ubiquitin-dependent sperm quality control mechanism recognizes spermatozoa with DNA defects as revealed by dual ubiquitin-TUNEL assay. Mol Reprod Dev 2002; 61: 406–13.
75. Muratori M, Maggi M, Spinelli S, et al. Spontaneous DNA fragmentation in swim-up selected human spermatozoa during long term incubation. J Androl 2003; 24: 253–62.
76. Sakkas D, Seli E, Bizzaro D, et al. Abnormal spermatozoa in the ejaculate: abortive apoptosis and faulty nuclear remodelling during spermatogenesis. Reprod Biomed Online 2003; 7: 428–32.
77. Cayli S, Sakkas D, Vigue L, et al. Cellular maturity and apoptosis in human sperm: creatin kinase, caspase-3 and Bcl-XL levels in mature and diminished maturity sperm. Mol Hum Reprod 2004; 10: 365–72.
78. Henkel R, Hajimohammad M, Stalf T, et al. Influence of deoxyribonucleic acid damage on fertilization and pregnancy. Fertil Steril 2004; 81: 965–72.
79. Lachaud C, Tesarik J, Canadas ML, et al. Apoptosis and necrosis in human ejaculated spermatozoa. Hum Reprod 2004; 19: 607–10.
80. Moustafa MH, Sharma RK, Thornton J, et al. Relationship between ROS production, apoptosis, and DNA denaturation in spermatozoa from patients examined for infertility. Hum Reprod 2004; 19: 129–38.
81. Paasch U, Sharma RK, Gupta AK, et al. Cryopreservation and thawing is associated with varying extent of activation of apoptotic machinery in subsets of ejaculated human spermatozoa. Biol Reprod 2004; 71: 1828–37.
82. Sutovsky P, Hauser R, Sutovsky M. Increased levels of sperm ubiquitin correlate with semen quality in men from an andrology clinic population. Hum Reprod 2004; 19: 628–35.
83. Aitken RJ, Buckingham D, West K, et al. Differential contribution of leucocytes and spermatozoa to the generation of reactive oxygen species in the ejaculates of oligozoospermic patients and fertile donors. J Reprod Fertil 1992; 94: 451–62.
84. Bannister LA, Schimenti JC. Homologous recombinational repair proteins in mouse meiosis. Cytogenet Genome Res 2004; 107: 191–200.
85. Page AW, Orr-Weaver TL. Stopping and starting the meiotic cell cycle. Curr Opin Genet Dev 1997; 7: 23–31.
86. De Iuliis GN, Thomson LK, Mitchell LA, et al. DNA damage in human spermatozoa is highly correlated with the efficiency of chromatin remodeling and the formation of 8-hydroxy-2'-deoxyguanosine, a marker of oxidative stress. Biol Reprod 2009; 81: 517–24.
87. Singh NP, Muller CH, Berger RE. Effects of age on DNA double-strand breaks and apoptosis in human sperm. Fertil Steril 2003; 80: 1420–30.
88. Schmid TE, Eskenazi B, Baumgartner A, et al. The effects of male age on sperm DNA damage in healthy non-smokers. Hum Reprod 2007; 22; 180–7.
89. Morris ID. Sperm DNA damage and cancer treatment. Int J Androl 2002; 25: 255–61.
90. Sailer BL, Jost LK, Erickson KR, et al. Effects of X-irradiation on mouse testicular cells and sperm chromatin structure. Environ Mol Mutagen 1995; 25: 23–30.
91. Fossa SD, De Angelis P, Kraggerud SM, et al. Prediction of posttreatment spermatogenesis in patients with testicular cancer by flow cytometric sperm chromatin structure assay. Cytometry 1997; 30: 192–6.
92. Stahl O, Eberhard J, Jepson K, et al. Sperm DNA integrity in testicular cancer patients. Hum Reprod 2006; 21: 3199–205.
93. Potts RJ, Newbury CJ, Smith G, et al. Sperm chromatin damage associated with male smoking. Mutat Res 1999; 423: 103–11.
94. Saleh RA, Agarwal A, Sharma RK, et al. Effect of cigarette smoking on levels of seminal oxidative stress in infertile men: a prospective study. Fertil Steril 2002; 78: 491–9.
95. Erenpreiss J, Hlevicka S, Zalkalns J, et al. Effect of leukocytospermia on sperm DNA integrity: a negative effect in abnormal semen samples. J Androl 2002; 23: 717–23.

96. Stronati A, Manicardi GC, Cecati M, et al. Relationships between sperm DNA fragmentation, sperm apoptotic markers and serum levels of CB-153 and p,p'-DDE in European and Inuit populations. Reproduction 2006; 132: 949–58.
97. Rubes J, Selevan SG, Evenson DP, et al. Episodic air pollution is associated with increased DNA fragmentation in human sperm without other changes in semen quality. Hum Reprod 2005; 20: 2776–83.
98. Sanchez-Pena LC, Reyes BE, Lopez-Carrillo L, et al. Organophosphorous pesticide exposure alters sperm chromatin structure in Mexican agricultural workers. Toxicol Appl Pharmacol 2004; 196: 108–13.
99. Saleh RA, Agarwal A, Sharma RK, et al. Evaluation of nuclear DNA damage in spermatozoa from infertile men with varicocele. Fertil Steril 2003; 80: 1431–6.
100. Fischer MA, Willis J, Zini A. Human sperm DNA integrity: correlation with sperm cytoplasmic droplets. Urology 2003; 61: 207–11.
101. Zini A, Defreitas G, Freeman M, et al. Varicocele is associated with abnormal retention of cytoplasmic droplets by human spermatozoa. Fertil Steril 2000; 74: 461–4.
102. Zini A, Blumenfeld A, Libman J, et al. Beneficial effect of microsurgical varicocelectomy on human sperm DNA integrity. Hum Reprod 2005; 20: 1018–21.
103. Werthman P, Wixon R, Kasperson K, et al. Significant decrease in sperm deoxyribonucleic acid fragmentation after varicocelectomy. Fertil Steril 2008; 90: 1800–4.
104. Xing W, Krishnamurthy H, Sairam MR. Role of follitropin receptor signaling in nuclear protein transitions and chromatin condensation during spermatogenesis. Biochem Biophys Res Commun 2003; 312: 697–701.
105. Evenson DP, Jost LK, Corzett M, et al. Characteristics of human sperm chromatin structure following an episode of influenza and high fever: a case study. J Androl 2000; 21: 739–46.
106. Sailer BL, Sarkar LJ, Bjordahl JA, et al. Effects of heat stress on mouse testicular cells and sperm chromatin structure. J Androl 1997; 18: 294–301.
107. Banks S, King SA, Irvine DS, et al. Impact of a mild scrotal heat stress on DNA integrity in murine spermatozoa. Reproduction 2005; 129: 505–14.
108. Zalata A, Hafez T, Comhaire F. Evaluation of the role of reactive oxygen species in male infertility. Hum Reprod 1995; 10: 1444–51.
109. Sergerie M, Laforest G, Boulanger K, et al. Longitudinal study of sperm DNA fragmentation as measured by terminal uridine nick end-labelling assay. Hum Reprod 2005; 20: 1921–7.
110. Erenpreiss J, Bungum M, Spano M, et al. Intra-individual variation in sperm chromatin structure assay parameters in men from infertile couples: clinical implications. Hum Reprod 2006; 21: 2061–4.
111. Smit M, Dohle GR, Hop WC, et al. Clinical correlates of the biological variation of sperm DNA fragmentation in infertile men attending an andrology outpatient clinic. Int J Androl 2007; 30: 48–55.
112. Spano M, Bonde JP, Hjollund HI, et al. Sperm chromatin damage impairs human fertility. The Danish First Pregnancy Planner Study Team. Fertil Steril 2000; 73: 43–50.
113. Larson-Cook KL, Brannian JD, Hansen KA, et al. Relationship between the outcomes of assisted reproductive techniques and sperm DNA fragmentation as measured by the sperm chromatin structure assay. Fertil Steril 2003; 80: 895–902.
114. Host E, Lindenberg S, Kahn JA, et al. DNA strand breaks in human sperm cells: a comparison between men with normal and oligozoospermic sperm samples. Acta Obstet Gynecol Scand 1999; 78: 336–9.
115. Gandini L, Lombardo F, Paoli D, et al. Study of apoptotic DNA fragmentation in human spermatozoa. Hum Reprod 2000; 15: 830–9.
116. Zini A, Bielecki R, Phang D, et al. Correlations between two markers of sperm DNA integrity, DNA denaturation and DNA fragmentation, in fertile and infertile men. Fertil Steril 2001; 75: 674–7.
117. Saleh RA, Agarwal A, Nelson DR, et al. Increased sperm nuclear DNA damage in normozoospermic infertile men: a prospective study. Fertil Steril 2002; 78: 313–18.
118. McKelvey-Martin V, Melia N, Walsh I, et al. Two potential clinical applications of the alkaline single-cell gel electrophoresis assay: (1). Human bladder washings and transitional cell carcinoma of the bladder; and (2). Human sperm and male infertility. Mutat Res 1997; 375: 93–104.
119. Sergerie M, Laforest G, Bujan L, et al. Sperm DNA fragmentation: threshold value in male fertility. Hum Reprod 2005; 20: 3446–51.
120. Saleh RA, Agarwal A, Nada ES, et al. Negative effects of increased sperm DNA damge in relation to seminal oxidative stress in men with idiopathic and male factor infertility. Fertil Steril 2003; 79: 1597–605.
121. Bungum M, Humaidan P, Spano M, et al. The predictive value of sperm chromatin structure assay (SCSA) parameters for the outcome of intrauterine insemination, IVF and ICSI. Hum Reprod 2004; 19: 1401–8.
122. Payne JF, Raburn DJ, Couchman GM, et al. Redefining the relationship between sperm deoxyribonucleic acid fragmentation as measured by the sperm chromatin structure assay and outcomes of assisted reproductive techniques. Fertil Steril 2005; 84: 356–64.
123. Tomlinson MJ, Moffatt O, Manicardi GC, et al. Interrelationships between seminal parameters and sperm nuclear DNA damage before and after density gradient centrifugation: implications for assisted conception. Hum Reprod 2001; 16: 2160–5.
124. Seli E, Gardner DK, Schoolcraft WB, et al. Extent of nuclear DNA damage in ejaculated spermatozoa impacts on blastocyst development after in vitro fertilization. Fertil Steril 2004; 82: 378–83.
125. Hammadeh ME, Stieber M, Haidl G, et al. Association between sperm cell chromatin condensation, morphology based on strict criteria, and fertilization, cleavage and pregnancy rates in an IVF program. Andrologia 1998; 30: 29–35.
126. Lopes S, Sun JG, Jurisicova A, et al. Sperm deoxyribonucleic acid fragmentation is increased in poor-quality semen samples and correlates with failed fertilization in intracytoplasmic sperm injection. Fertil Steril 1998; 69: 528–32.
127. Twigg JP, Irvine DS, Aitken RJ. Oxidative damage to DNA in human spermatozoa does not preclude

pronucleus formation at intracytoplasmic sperm injection. Hum Reprod 1998; 13: 1864–71.
128. Li Z, Wang L, Cai J, et al. Correlation of sperm DNA damage with IVF and ICSI outcomes: a systematic review and meta-analysis. J Assist Reprod Genetics 2006; 23: 367–76.
129. Carrell DT, Liu L, Peterson CM, et al. Sperm DNA fragmentation is increased in couples with unexplained recurrent pregnancy loss. Arch Androl 2003; 49: 49–55.
130. Virro MR, Larson-Cook KL, Evenson DP. Sperm chromatin structure assay (SCSA) parameters are related to fertilization, blastocyst development, and ongoing pregnancy in in vitro fertilization and intracytoplasmic sperm injection cycles. Fertil Steril 2004; 81: 1289–95.
131. Check JH, Graziano V, Cohen R, et al. Effect of an abnormal sperm chromatin structural assay (SCSA) on pregnancy outcome following (IVF) with ICSI in previous IVF failures. Arch Androl 2005; 51: 121–4.
132. Kobayashi H, Larson K, Sharma R, et al. DNA damage in cancer patients before treatment as measured by the sperm chromatin structure assay. Fertil Steril 2001; 75: 469–75.
133. 133. Baker H, Liu D. Assessment of nuclear maturity. In: Acosta A, Kruger T, eds. Human Spermatozoa in Assissted Reproduction. London: CRC Press, 1996: 193–203.
134. Erenpreisa J, Erenpreiss J, Freivalds T, et al. Toluidine blue test for sperm DNA integrity and elaboration of image cytometry algorithm. Cytometry 2003; 52: 19–27.
135. Manicardi GC, Bianchi PG, Pantano S, et al. Presence of endogenous nicks in DNA of ejaculated human spermatozoa and its relationship to chromomycin A3 accessibility. Biol Reprod 1995; 52: 864–7.
136. Fernandez JL, Vazquez-Gundin F, Delgado A, et al. DNA breakage detection-FISH (DBD-FISH) in human spermatozoa: technical variants evidence different structural features. Mutat Res 2000; 453: 77–82.
137. Gorczyca W, Gong J, Darzynkiewicz Z. Detection of DNA strand breaks in individual apoptotic cells by the in situ terminal deoxynucleotidyl transferase and nick translation assays. Cancer Res 1993; 53: 1945–51.
138. Zini A, Fischer MA, Sharir S, et al. Prevalence of abnormal sperm DNA denaturation in fertile and infertile men. Urology 2002; 60: 1069–72.
139. Fernandez JL, Muriel L, Rivero MT, et al. The sperm chromatin dispersion test: a simple method for the determination of sperm DNA fragmentation. J Androl 2003; 24: 59–66.
140. Singh NP, McCoy MT, Tice RR, et al. A simple technique for quantitation of low levels of DNA damage in individual cells. Exp Cell Res 1988; 175: 184–91.
141. Singh NP, Danner DB, Tice RR, et al. Abundant alkali-sensitive sites in DNA of human and mouse sperm. Exp Cell Res 1989; 184: 461–70.
142. Kodama H, Yamaguchi R, Fukuda J, et al. Increased oxidative deoxyribonucleic acid damage in the spermatozoa of infertile male patients. Fertil Steril 1997; 68: 519–24.
143. Hammadeh ME, Zeginiadov T, Rosenbaum P, et al. Predictive value of sperm chromatin condensation (aniline blue staining) in the assessment of male fertility. Arch Androl 2001; 46: 99–104.
144. Wong A, Chuan SS, Patton WC, et al. Addition of eosin to the aniline blue assay to enhance detection of immature sperm histones. Fertil Steril 2008; 90: 1999–2002.
145. Foresta C, Zorzi M, Rossato M, et al. Sperm nuclear instability and staining with aniline blue: abnormal persistence of histones in spermatozoa in infertile men. Int J Androl 1992; 15: 330–7.
146. Hammadeh ME, Stieber M, Haidl G, et al. Association between sperm cell chromatin condensation, morphology based on strict criteria, and fertilization, cleavage and pregnancy rates in an IVF program. Andrologia 1998; 30: 29–35.
147. Kazerooni T, Asadi N, Jadid L, et al. Evaluation of sperm's chromatin quality with acridine orange test, chromomycin A3 and aniline blue staining in couples with unexplained recurrent abortion. J Assist Reprod Genet 2009; 26: 591–6.
148. de Jager C, Aneck-Hahn NH, Bornman MS, et al. Sperm chromatin integrity in DDT-exposed young men living in a malaria area in the Limpopo Province, South Africa. Hum Reprod 2009; 24: 2429–38.
149. Erenpreiss J, Bars J, Lipatnikova V, et al. Comparative study of cytochemical tests for sperm chromatin integrity. J Androl 2001; 22: 45–53.
150. Erenpreiss J, Jepson K, Giwercman A, et al. Toluidine blue cytometry test for sperm DNA conformation: comparison with the flow cytometric sperm chromatin structure and TUNEL assays. Hum Reprod 2004; 19: 2277–82.
151. Tsarev I, Bungum M, Giwercman A, et al. Evaluation of male fertility potential by Toluidine Blue test for sperm chromatin structure assessment. Hum Reprod 2009; 24: 1569–74.
152. Sadeghi MR, Lakpour N, Heidari-Vala H, et al. Relationship between sperm chromatin status and ICSI outcome in men with obstructive azoospermia and unexplained infertile normozoospermia. Rom J Morphol Embryol 2011; 52: 645–51.
153. Carretero MI, Giuliano SM, Casaretto CI, Gambarotta MC, Neild DM. Evaluation of the effect of cooling and of the addition of collagenase on llamasperm DNA using toluidine blue. Andrologia. Published Online 8 June 2011.
154. Rybar R, Kopecka V, Prinosilova P, Markova P, Rubes J. Male obesity and age in relationship to semen parameters and sperm chromatin integrity. Andrologia 2001; 43: 286–91.
155. Talebi AR, Moein MR, Tabibnejad N, Ghasemzadeh J. Effect of varicocele on chromatin condensation and DNA integrity of ejaculated spermatozoa using cytochemical tests. Andrologia 2008; 40: 245–51.
156. Mahfouz RZ, Sharma RK, Said TM, Erenpreiss J, Agarwal A. Association of sperm apoptosis and DNA ploidy with sperm chromatin quality in human spermatozoa. Fertil Steril 2009; 91: 1110–18.
157. Esterhuizen AD, Franken DR, Lourens JG, et al. Sperm chromatin packaging as an indicator of in-vitro fertilization rates. Hum Reprod 2000; 15: 657–61.
158. Sakkas D, Urner F, Bianchi PG, et al. Sperm chromatin anomalies can influence decondensation after intracytoplasmic sperm injection. Hum Reprod 1996; 11: 837–43.
159. Sakkas D, Urner F, Bizzaro D, et al. Sperm nuclear DNA damage and altered chromatin structure: effect

on fertilization and embryo development. Hum Reprod 1998; 13: 11–19.
160. Nijs M, Creemers E, Cox A, et al. Chromomycin A3 staining, sperm chromatin structure assay and hyaluronic acid binding assay as predictors for assisted reproductive outcome. Reprod Biomed Online 2009; 19: 671–84.
161. Manochantr S, Chiamchanya C, Sobhon P. Relationship between chromatin condensation, DNA integrity and quality of ejaculated spermatozoa from infertile men. Andrologia 2012; 44: 187–99.
162. Fernandez JL, Goyanes VJ, Ramiro-Diaz J, et al. Application of FISH for in situ detection and quantification of DNA breakage. Cytogenet Cell Genet 1998; 82: 251–6.
163. Fernández JL, Cajigal D, Gosálvez J. Simultaneous labeling of single- and double-strand DNA breaks by DNA breakage detection-FISH (DBD-FISH). Methods Mol Biol 2011; 682: 133–47.
164. Irvine DS, Twigg JP, Gordon EL, et al. DNA integrity in human spermatozoa: relationships with semen quality. J Androl 2000; 21: 33–44.
165. Tomlinson MJ, Moffatt O, Manicardi GC, et al. Interrelationships between seminal parameters and sperm nuclear DNA damage before and after density gradient centrifugation: implications for assisted conception. Hum Reprod 2001; 16: 2160–5.
166. Shamsi MB, Kumar R, Dada R. Evaluation of nuclear DNA damage in human spermatozoa in men opting for assisted reproduction. Indian J Med R 2008; 127: 115–23.
167. Setchell BP, Ekpe G, Zupp JL, et al. Transient retardation in embryo growth in normal female mice made pregnant by males whose testes had been heated. Hum Reprod 1998; 13: 342–7.
168. Aitken RJ, Irvine DS, Wu FC. Prospective analysis of sperm-oocyte fusion and reactive oxygen species generation as criteria for the diagnosis of infertility. Am J Obstet Gynecol 1991; 164: 542–51.
169. Hoshi K, Katayose H, Yanagida K, et al. Kimura Y, Sato A. The relationship between acridine orange fluorescence of sperm nuclei and the fertilizing ability of human sperm. Fertil Steril 1996; 66: 634–9.
170. Skowronek F, Casanova G, Alciaturi J, et al. DNA sperm damage correlates with nuclear ultrastructural sperm defects in teratozoospermic men. Andrologia 2012 Feb; 44(1): 59–65.
171. Varghese AC, Bragais FM, Mukhopadhyay D, et al. Human sperm DNA integrity in normal and abnormal semen samples and its correlation with sperm characteristics. Andrologia 2009; 41: 207–15.
172. Zini A, Fischer MA, Sharir S, et al. Prevalence of abnormal sperm DNA denaturation in fertile and infertile men. Urology 2002; 60: 1069–72.
173. Gopalkrishnan K, Hurkadli K, Padwal V, et al. Use of acridine orange to evaluate chromatin integrity of human spermatozoa in different groups of infertile men. Andrologia 1999; 31: 277–82.
174. Virant-Klun I, Tomazevic T, Meden-Vrtovec H. Sperm single-stranded DNA, detected by acridine orange staining, reduces fertilization and quality of ICSI-derived embryos. J Assist Reprod Genet 2002; 19: 319–28.
175. Katayose H, Yanagida K, Hashimoto S, et al. Use of diamide-acridine orange fluorescence staining to detect aberrant protamination of human-ejaculated sperm nuclei. Fertil Steril 2003; 79: 670–6.
176. Lazaros LA, Vartholomatos GA, Hatzi EG, et al. Assessment of sperm chromatin condensation and ploidy status using flow cytometry correlates to fertilization, embryo quality and pregnancy following in vitro fertilization. J Assist Reprod Genet 2011; 28: 885–91.
177. Zhang Y, Wang H, Wang L, et al. The clinical significance of sperm DNA damage detection combined with routine semen testing in assisted reproduction. Mol Med Report 2008; 1: 617–24.
178. Zini A, Kamal K, Phang D, et al. Biologic variability of sperm DNA denaturation in infertile men. Urology 2001; 58: 258–61.
179. Zini A, Bielecki R, Phang D, et al. Correlations between two markers of sperm DNA integrity, DNA denaturation and DNA fragmentation, in fertile and infertile men. Fertil Steril 2001; 75: 674–7.
180. Ankem MK, Mayer E, Ward WS, et al. Novel assay for determining DNA organization in human spermatozoa: implications for male factor infertility. Urology 2002; 59: 575–8.
181. Muriel L, Meseguer M, Fernandez JL, et al. Value of the sperm chromatin dispersion test in predicting pregnancy outcome in intrauterine insemination: a blind prospective study. Hum Reprod 2006; 21: 738–44.
182. Muriel L, Garrido N, Fernandez JL, et al. Value of the sperm deoxyribonucleic acid fragmentation level, as measured by the sperm chromatin dispersion test, in the outcome of in vitro fertilization and intracytoplasmic sperm injection. Fertil Steril 2006; 85: 371–83.
183. Muriel L, Goyanes V, Segrelles E, et al. Increased aneuploidy rate in sperm with fragmented DNA as determined by the sperm chromatin dispersion (SCD) test and FISH analysis. J Androl 2007; 28: 38–49.
184. Fernandez JL, Muriel L, Goyanes V, et al. Halosperm is an easy, available, and cost-effective alternative for determining sperm DNA fragmentation. Fertil Steril 2005; 84: 860.
185. Zhang LH, Qiu Y, Wang KH, et al. Measurement of sperm DNA fragmentation using bright-field microscopy: comparison between sperm chromatin dispersion test and terminal uridine nick-end labeling assay. Fertil Steril 2010; 94: 1027–32.
186. Meseguer M, Santiso R, Garrido N, et al. Sperm DNA fragmentation levels in testicular sperm samples from azoospermic males as assessed by the sperm chromatin dispersion (SCD) test. Fertil Steril 2009; 92: 1638–45.
187. Balasuriya A, Speyer B, Serhal P, Doshi A, Harper JC. Sperm chromatin dispersion test in the assessment of DNA fragmentation and aneuploidy in human spermatozoa. Reprod Biomed Online 2011; 22: 428–436.
188. Santiso R, Tamayo M, Gosálvez J, et al. Simultaneous determination in situ of DNA fragmentation and 8-oxoguanine in human sperm. Fertil Steril 2010; 93: 314–18.
189. Fernández JL, Cajigal D, López-Fernández C, Gosálvez J. Assessing sperm DNA fragmentation with the sperm chromatin dispersion test. Methods Mol Biol 2011; 682: 291–301.
190. Velez de la Calle JF, Muller A, Walschaerts M, et al. Sperm deoxyribonucleic acid fragmentation as

190. assessed by the sperm chromatin dispersion test in assisted reproductive technique programs: results of a large prospective multicenter study. Fertil Steril 2008; 90: 1792–9.
191. Ostling O, Johanson KJ. Microelectrophoretic study of radiation-induced DNA damages in individual mammalian cells. Biochem Biophys Res Commun 1984; 123: 291–8.
192. Enciso M, Sarasa J, Agarwal A, Fernández JL, Gosálvez J. A two-tailed Comet assay for assessing DNA damage in spermatozoa. Reprod Biomed Online 2009; 18: 609–16.
193. Cortés-Gutiérrez EI, Dávila-Rodríguez MI, Fernández JL, et al. New application of the comet assay: chromosome-comet assay. J Histochem Cytochem 2011; 59: 655–60.
194. Hellman B, Vaghef H, Bostrom B. The concepts of tail moment and tail inertia in the single cell gel electrophoresis assay. Mutat Res 1995; 336: 123–31.
195. Kusakabe H, Tateno H. Shortening of alkaline DNA unwinding time does not interfere with detecting DNA damage to mouse and human spermatozoa in the comet assay. Asian J Androl 2011; 13: 172–4.
196. Duty SM, Singh NP, Ryan L, et al. Reliability of the comet assay in cryopreserved human sperm. Hum Reprod 2002; 17: 1274–80.
197. Morris ID, Ilott S, Dixon L, et al. The spectrum of DNA damage in human sperm assessed by single cell gel electrophoresis (Comet assay) and its relationship to fertilization and embryo development. Hum Reprod 2002; 17: 990–8.
198. Tomsu M, Sharma V, Miller D. Embryo quality and IVF treatment outcomes may correlate with different sperm comet assay parameters. Hum Reprod 2002; 17: 1856–62.
199. Lewis SE, Agbaje IM. Using the alkaline comet assay in prognostic tests for male infertility and assisted reproductive technique outcomes. Mutagenesis 2008; 23: 163–70.
200. Shamsi MB, Venkatesh S, Tanwar M, et al. Comet assay: a prognostic tool for DNA integrity assessment in infertile men opting for assisted reproduction. Indian J Med Res 2010; 131: 675–81.
201. Simon L, Lutton D, McManus J, Lewis SE. Sperm DNA damage measured by the alkaline Comet assay as an independent predictor of male infertility and in vitro fertilization success. Fertil Steril 2011; 95: 652–7.
202. Lewis SE, Simon L. Clinical implications of sperm DNA damage. Hum Fertil (Camb) 2010; 13: 201–7.
203. Abu-Hassan D, Koester F, Shoepper B, et al. Comet assay of cumulus cells and spermatozoa DNA status, and the relationship to oocyte fertilization and embryo quality following ICSI. Reprod Biomed Online 2006; 12: 447–52.
204. Villani P, Spanò M, Pacchierotti F, Weimer M, Cordelli E. Evaluation of a modified comet assay to detect DNA damage in mammalian sperm exposed in vitro to different mutagenic compounds. Reprod Toxicol 2010; 30: 44–9.
205. Benchaib M, Braun V, Lornage J, et al. Sperm DNA fragmentation decreases the pregnancy rate in an assisted reproductive technique. Hum Reprod 2003; 18: 1023–8.
206. Enciso M, Johnston SD, Gosálvez J. Differential resistance of mammalian sperm chromatin to oxidative stress as assessed by a two-tailed comet assay. these cells from the genotoxic effects of adverse environments. Reprod Fertil Dev 2011; 23: 633–7.
207. Mitchell LA, De Iuliis GN, Aitken RJ. The TUNEL assay consistently underestimates DNA damage in human spermatozoa and is influenced by DNA compaction and cell vitality: development of an improved methodology. Int J Androl 2011; 34: 2–13.
208. Sergerie M, Laforest G, Bujan L, et al. Sperm DNA fragmentation: threshold value in male fertility. Hum Reprod 2005; 20: 3446–51.
209. Muratori M, Tamburrino L, Tocci V, et al. Small variations in crucial steps of TUNEL assay coupled to flow cytometry greatly affect measures of sperm DNA fragmentation. J Androl 2010; 31: 336–45.
210. Muratori M, Tamburrino L, Marchiani S, et al. Critical aspects of detection of sperm DNA fragmentation by TUNEL/flow cytometry. Syst Biol Reprod Med 2010; 56: 277–85.
211. Sharma RK, Sabanegh E, Mahfouz R, et al. TUNEL as a test for sperm DNA damage in the evaluation of male infertility. Urology 2010; 76: 1380–6.
212. Erenpreiss J, Spano M, Erenpreisa J, et al. Sperm chromatin structure and male fertility: biological and clinical aspects. Asian J Androl 2006; 8: 11–29.
213. Spano M, Kolstad AH, Larsen SB, et al. The applicability of the flow cytometric sperm chromatin structure assay in epidemiological studies. Hum Reprod 1998; 13: 2495–505.
214. Nijs M, De Jonge C, Cox A, et al. Correlation between male age, WHO sperm parameters, DNA fragmentation, chromatin packaging and outcome in assisted reproductive technique. Andrologia 2011; 43: 174–9.
215. Evenson DP, Kasperson K, Wixon RL. Analysis of sperm DNA fragmentation using flow cytometry and other techniques. Soc Reprod Fertil 2007; 65: 93–113.
216. Evenson DP, Larson KL, Jost LK. Sperm chromatin structure assay: its clinical use for detecting sperm DNA fragmentation in male infertility and comparisons with other techniques. J Androl 2002; 23: 25–43.
217. Bungum M, Bungum L, Giwercman A. Sperm chromatin structure assay (SCSA): a tool in diagnosis and treatment of infertility. Asian J Androl 2011; 13: 69–75.
218. Castilla JA, Zamora S, Gonzalvo MC, et al. Sperm chromatin structure assay and classical semen parameters: systematic review. Reprod Biomed Online 2010; 20: 114–24.
219. Giwercman A, Lindstedt L, Larsson M, et al. Sperm chromatin structure assay as an independent predictor of fertility in vivo: a case-control study. Int J Androl 2010; 33: e221–7.
220. Bungum M, Spanò M, Humaidan P, et al. Sperm chromatin structure assay parameters measured after density gradient centrifugation are not predictive for the outcome of ART. Hum Reprod 2008; 23: 4–10.
221. Evenson D, Wixon R. Meta-analysis of sperm DNA fragmentation using the sperm chromatin structure assay. Reprod Biomed Online 2006; 12: 466–72.
222. Miciński P, Pawlicki K, Wielgus E, Bochenek M, Tworkowska I. The sperm chromatin structure assay (SCSA) as prognostic factor in IVF/ICSI program. Reprod Biol 2009; 9: 65–70.
223. Lin MH, Kuo-Kuang Lee R, Li SH, et al. Sperm chromatin structure assay parameters are not related to fertilization rates, embryo quality, and pregnancy

rates in in vitro fertilization and intracytoplasmic sperm injection, but might be related to spontaneous abortion rates. Fertil Steril 2008; 90: 352–9.
224. Collins JA, Barnhart KT, Schlegel PN. Do sperm DNA integrity tests predict pregnancy with in vitro fertilization? Fertil Steril 2008; 89: 823–31.
225. Lewis SE, Agbaje I, Alvarez J. Sperm DNA tests as useful adjuncts to semen analysis. Syst Biol Reprod Med 2008; 54: 111–25.
226. Henkel R, Hoogendijk CF, Bouic PJ, Kruger TF. TUNEL assay and SCSA determine different aspects of sperm DNA damage. Andrologia 2010; 42: 305–13.
227. Shen H, Ong C. Detection of oxidative DNA damage in human sperm and its association with sperm function and male infertility. Free Radic Biol Med 2000; 28: 529–36.
228. Aitken RJ, De Iuliis GN, Finnie JM, Hedges A, McLachlan RI. Analysis of the relationships between oxidative stress, DNA damage and sperm vitality in a patient population: development of diagnostic criteria. Hum Reprod 2010; 25: 2415–26.
229. Ishikawa T, Fujioka H, Ishimura T, Takenaka A, Fujisawa M. Increased testicular 8-hydroxy-2'-deoxyguanosine in patients with varicocele. BJU Int 2007; 100: 863–6.
230. Loft S, Kold-Jensen T, Hjollund NH, et al. Oxidative DNA damage in human sperm influences time to pregnancy. Hum Reprod 2003; 18: 1265–72.
231. Agarwal A, Varghese AC, Sharma RK. Markers of oxidative stress and sperm chromatin integrity. Methods Mol Biol 2009; 590: 377–402.
232. Ainsworth C, Nixon B, Aitken RJ. Development of a novel electrophoretic system for the isolation of human spermatozoa. Hum Reprod 2005; 20: 2261–70.
233. Zini A, San Gabriel M, Baazeem A. Antioxidants and sperm DNA damage: a clinical perspective. J Assist Reprod Genet 2009; 26: 427–32.
234. Ménézo YJ, Hazout A, Panteix G, et al. Antioxidants to reduce sperm DNA fragmentation: an unexpected adverse effect. Reprod Biomed Online 2007; 14: 418–21.
235. Agarwal A, Nallella KP, Allamaneni SS, et al. Role of antioxidants in treatment of male infertility: an overview of the literature. Reprod Biomed Online 2004; 8: 616–27.
236. Greco E, Romano S, Iacobelli M, et al. ICSI in cases of sperm DNA damage: beneficial effect of oral antioxidant treatment. Hum Reprod 2005; 20: 2590–4.
237. Rolf C, Cooper TG, Yeung CH, et al. Antioxidant treatment of patients with asthenozoospermia or moderate oligoasthenozoospermia with high-dose vitamin C and vitamin E: a randomized, placebo-controlled, double-blind study. Hum Reprod 1999; 14: 1028–33.
238. Said T, Agarwal A, Grunewald S, et al. Selection of nonapoptotic spermatozoa as a new tool for enhancing assisted reproduction outcomes: An in vitro model. Biol Reprod 2006; 74: 530–7.
239. Berkovitz A, Eltes F, Lederman H. et al. How to improve IVF-ICSI outcome by sperm selection. Reprod Biomed Online 2006; 12: 634–8.
240. Hazout A, Dumont-Hassan M, Junca AM, et al. High-magnification ICSI overcomes paternal effect resistant to conventional ICSI. Reprod Biomed Online 2006; 12: 19–25.

7

Oocyte retrieval and selection

Laura F. Rienzi and Filippo M. Ubaldi

INTRODUCTION

Of the several factors that affect oocyte quality, controlled ovarian stimulation protocols comprise one of the most important. To better understand the treatment strategies, their application, and their potential impact on oocyte quality, it is of utmost importance to know the physiology of the ovarian function.

The demise of corpus luteum at the end of the luteal phase of the menstrual cycle is responsible for the sudden fall of 17 beta estradiol (E2), inhibin A, and progesterone, which induces an increased frequency of pulsatile gonadotropin releasing hormone (GnRH) secretion and rising serum follicle-stimulating hormone (FSH) levels (1). When serum FSH concentration reaches a critical "threshold" level for ovarian stimulation, class 5 follicles departing from the resting pool are recruited and start a well-characterized growth trajectory (2,3). In the early follicular phase, the increased production of estrogens resulting from the FSH-dependent granulosa cell aromatase activity, together with the increase of inhibin B, is responsible for the falling circulating levels of FSH (4,5) which restricts the time when FSH levels remain above the "threshold" (6,7). As a result, one (dominant) follicle continues its growth, probably due to upregulation by intraovarian factors that may increase sensitivity for FSH stimulation (8,9), whereas other (nondominant) follicles (of the same cohort) enter atresia due to diminished sensitivity to FSH and estrogen biosynthesis (as well as elevated intrafollicular androgen levels) (9–11).

On the basis of these findings, the "FSH window" concept has been introduced, suggesting the importance of the duration of FSH elevation above the threshold level rather than the height of the elevation of FSH for single dominant follicle selection (6,7,12). The different stimulation protocols used for controlled ovarian hyperstimulation are based on the concept of widening the FSH window with the use of exogenous gonadotropins from the early follicular phase to the day of human chorionic gonadotropin (hCG) administration.

Over the last 25 years different stimulation protocols have been proposed. Easier stimulation regimens such as clomiphene citrate (CC) alone or in combination with human menopausal gonadotropin (hMG) and urinary FSH were gradually abandoned in favor of more complex protocols where GnRH agonists are used in combination with gonadotropins. These lengthy protocols, which are still the most widely used treatments for ovarian stimulation, allow us to manage the activity of in vitro fertilization (IVF) centers more easily, lower cancellation rates, and raise the number of preovulatory follicles, the number of oocytes retrieved, and the number of good quality embryos for transfer, thus leading to better pregnancy rates (13). However, these regimens are not free from complications and costs for the patients. The clinical introduction of GnRH antagonists in IVF (14–16), with their immediate suppression of the pituitary function, allows the administration of low doses of gonadotropins from mid follicular phase, resulting in more "patient friendly" stimulation protocols (17,18) with fewer days of stimulation, lower amounts of gonadotropins administered, and fewer oocytes retrieved.

However, if these milder protocols may improve patients" compliance, reducing the burden of IVF on the couple, the question that remains to be answered is whether the reduced number of oocytes obtained after mild protocols may impair the clinical outcome. Whatever stimulation regimen is used for controlled ovarian hyperstimulation, once the correct follicular and hormonal parameters are reached, a bolus of hCG is administered to trigger ovulation. The oocyte meiosis (blocked at the prophase of the first meiotic division) is then reinitiated, going through the germinal vesicle (GV) breakdown, the formation and extrusion of first polar body (IPB). After entering in the second meiotic division, a second arrest occurs at metaphase stage II (MII). Oocyte retrieval is performed 34–36 hours following hCG administration.

Once in the laboratory, the oocyte quality is evaluated. This assessment is based on the aspect of the cumulus–corona cells, and if denudation is performed, also on the basis of the morphology of the oocyte cytoplasm and on the aspect of the extracytoplasmic structures [such as zona pellucida (ZP), first polar body, and perivitelline space (PVS)]. Oocyte selection prior to insemination is potentially very important in IVF/ intracytoplasmic sperm injection (ICSI) programs because of the following:

- It gives important information with regard to the subsequent developmental ability of the deriving embryo.

- It helps to reduce the number of inseminated oocytes and thus the amount of supernumerary embryos.
- It helps to avoid inseminating "bad quality oocytes" potentially at risk of carrying chromosomal abnormalities.
- It helps to choose the appropriate number of oocytes in egg donation programs.

However, the current literature on oocyte assessment is controversial and the selection methods proposed are still largely ineffective. The presence of cumulus and corona cells makes the morphological oocyte evaluation difficult to perform prior to standard IVF. Moreover, the quality and the degree of expansion of these cells seem to be poor markers of oocyte maturity and mostly depend on the type of ovarian stimulation protocol used (19–22). The oocyte can be easily observed only after cumulus–corona cell removal. The presence of the first polar body is normally considered as a marker of oocyte nuclear maturity. However, recent studies using polarized light microscopy have shown that oocytes displaying an IPB may still be immature (23–25). Moreover, nuclear maturity alone is not enough to determine the quality of an oocyte. In fact, nuclear and cytoplasmic maturation should be completed in a coordinated manner to ensure optimal conditions for subsequent fertilization.

However, cytoplasmic maturation assessment is still unclear. It has been suggested that disturbances or asynchrony of these two maturation processes may result in a variety of oocyte morphological abnormalities (26–29). Abnormal ZP, large PVS, vacuoles, refractile bodies, increased cytoplasmic granularity, smooth endoplasmic reticulum clusters, and abnormal, fragmented or degenerated first polar body can be observed after oocyte denudation. The correlation between these abnormal morphotypes and oocyte developmental ability is discussed in this chapter.

OVARIAN STIMULATION PROTOCOLS

Although the first successful pregnancy after IVF and embryo transfer was performed in the natural unstimulated cycle of an infertile woman with a tubal factor (30), it was soon observed that pregnancy rates per IVF attempt increase when more than one embryo is transferred into the uterine cavity (31). Subsequently, natural cycle IVF was replaced by stimulated cycles, allowing significant clinical outcome improvement. Over the last 25 years different stimulation protocols have been proposed. More complex and more demanding protocols have gradually replaced easier stimulation regimens such as CC alone or in combination with hMG and urinary FSH.

At the beginning of the 1990s, short-term treatments with GnRH agonists and gonadotropins were abandoned in favor of long-term GnRH agonist stimulation protocols that allowed retrieval of more oocytes selection of one or more embryos for transfer, suggesting that the more oocytes obtained the higher the chance of conception (32,33). Recent evidence, however, suggests that excessive ovarian stimulation may have detrimental effects on oocyte quality (34–36) and that there might be an optimal range of oocyte retrieval, below and above which the clinical outcome might be compromised (37).

This observation suggests that among the cohort of recruited follicles only the most sensitive to stimulation are likely to give better-quality embryos, whereas all the additional oocytes resulting from maximal stimulation might be of impaired quality. Alternatively, the reduction of pregnancy rate observed after maximal stimulation might be due to a direct effect of high serum estradiol concentrations on oocytes, quality (18,38), or on endometrial receptivity (38–40).

About 10 years ago, GnRH antagonists were clinically introduced in IVF (14–16). These GnRH analogs induce an immediate suppression of the pituitary function, which allows the administration of low doses of gonadotropins from mid follicular phase, resulting in shorter and more "patient friendly" stimulation protocols (17,18). With these milder regimens the number of oocytes retrieved is lower, but a significantly higher proportion of high-quality embryos (according to their morphology) might be obtained, suggesting a better oocyte quality (probably because of less interference with natural follicle selection) (18). Although embryo morphology is commonly used to select the best embryo for transfer and is correlated with pregnancy rates (18), it gives limited information regarding the chromosomal constitution of the embryo (41). It has been suggested that ovarian stimulation protocols may affect embryo aneuploidy (42,43).

Reducing the duration and intensity of the pharmacological interventions might interfere less with natural follicle selection and result in better oocyte quality, with more physiological chromosome segregation behavior during meiosis and early embryo development (18). To investigate this hypothesis, very recently Baart et al. (36) designed a prospective, randomized study where the chromosomal constitution of the embryos obtained after mild or conventional stimulation was analyzed by preimplantation genetic screening (PGS) in patients younger than 38 years of age. The number of oocytes retrieved and of embryos obtained was higher in the conventional stimulation group but, as previously reported (18), the proportion of good morphology embryos was significantly higher in the mild stimulation group. Similarly, a significantly higher proportion of euploid embryos per patient and a lower proportion of mosaic embryos per patient were observed in the mild stimulation group.

Furthermore, the same authors reported a significant positive correlation between the number of oocytes retrieved and the proportion of abnormal embryos in patients stimulated with milder regimens. On the contrary, no correlation was observed in the conventional stimulation group. These findings suggest that the reduced number of oocytes retrieved in the mild stimulation group is the result of a more physiological oocyte selection, whereas in the conventional stimulation group a low ovarian response is a sign of ovarian aging (36). Although these results seem very interesting, further larger prospective studies are needed to confirm these data. Moreover, with mild protocols a significantly reduced number of oocytes can be retrieved and, unfortunately, so far, no data regarding the cumulative pregnancy rates obtained after mild or standard regimens are available.

Whatever stimulation protocol is used, the different pharmaceutical preparations of human gonadotropins that can induce the multiple follicular growth might also influence the oocyte quality. During the last 15 years, many studies have compared the efficacy and safety of different gonadotropin preparations (recombinant FSH vs. urinary FSH vs. highly purified FSH vs. hMG vs. highly purified hMG), reporting conflicting data (44–51). Most of these trials focus on clinical parameters such as number of oocytes, dosage, and duration of gonadotropin used, fertilization, pregnancy, and implantation rates. The reported conflicting results might be due to either different intrinsic factors, such as cause of infertility, age, ovarian reserve, individual FSH–FSH receptor interaction, and ethnic background, or extrinsic factors such as stimulation protocols, cigarette smoking, and sample size (52–55). The few studies that have examined the effect of different gonadotropin preparations on oocyte and embryo quality have reported conflicting results. Some (56), but not all authors, (57,58) reported a significantly higher proportion of metaphase II oocytes and fewer oocytes with dark cytoplasm in women receiving highly purified FSH when compared with those treated with hMG. The use of recombinant FSH may induce a better cytoplasmic maturation, which might be negatively influenced by the large amount of urinary proteins (cytokines, growth factors, transferrins, and other proteins) that are found in urinary FSH (51).

However, these results were not confirmed in previous (59) and in more recent studies (60). Several factors might explain these conflicting data: timing of hCG administration, interval between hCG and oocyte retrieval, and interval between oocyte retrieval and oocyte insemination. These aspects are further discussed in this chapter.

PERIFOLLICULAR VASCULARIZATION EVALUATION

Besides stimulation protocols and gonadotropin preparations, oocyte quality might be influenced by perifollicular vascularization. It has been suggested that an insufficient perifollicular vascularization measured using color Doppler ultrasonography correlates with intrafollicular hypoxia (61–63), inducing oocyte cytoplasmic defects, disorganized chromosomes, reduced fertilization, and embryos with multinucleated blastomeres (62,64,65). Embryos with high implantation potential originate from well-vascularized and oxygenated follicles (64). According to these data, several studies have also shown higher pregnancy and implantation rates when embryos resulting from the fertilization of oocytes from better-perfused follicles are transferred (66–70). Unfortunately, other studies were not able to confirm the clinical value of the association between perifollicular vascularization and oocyte competence to improve the reproductive outcomes in young infertile patients who undergo either intrauterine insemination cycles (71) or IVF cycles (72–75). Moreover, it is not technically easy to assess the perifollicular vascularity during the oocyte retrieval procedure and to perform the aspiration and flushing of the selected follicle until the oocytes are retrieved. For these reasons, further prospective randomized studies are needed to verify whether a relationship exists between the perifollicular vascularization of selected follicles measured using color Doppler ultrasonography and their reproductive competence.

SERUM AND FOLLICULAR ANTI-MÜLLERIAN HORMONE MEASUREMENTS

Very recent evidence indicates that anti-Müllerian hormone (AMH), a member of the transforming growth factor-beta superfamily produced by the granulosa cells of ovarian follicles, mainly from the primary to the preantral and early antral stages of folliculogenesis and independently from FSH (76), is a unique biomarker of ovarian follicular status (77–79). Serum day 3 AMH levels have been strongly correlated with ovarian reserve (80,81) and ovarian response to controlled ovarian hyperstimulation (82–84), showing a better cycle-to-cycle reproducibility than serum inhibin B and FSH levels (85). Furthermore, a positive correlation between serum AMH measured around the time of hCG administration and the number of oocytes retrieved, the fertilization rates, the embryo score, and the implantation rates was recently reported (86). Similarly, lower serum concentrations of AMH were correlated with reduced fertilization rates and increased miscarriage rates, suggesting serum AMH as a predictor of oocyte quality (87). On the contrary, other recent studies did not confirm these results (88). The observation in the animal model (77,89), and woman (79) that AMH is not expressed by the granulosa cells of atretic follicles suggests a more interesting role of this biomarker measured in the follicular fluid to predict the oocyte competence (89). In a very recent study the AMH levels in follicular fluid from women undergoing IVF with fertilized oocytes were statistically significantly higher than in the follicular fluid of patients with fertilization failure, suggesting that high follicular fluid AMH (FF AMH) levels positively correlate with oocyte quality (88). Similarly, FF AMH concentrations observed in natural IVF cycles were strongly and positively correlated with embryo implantation, suggesting FF AMH as a better predictor of oocyte quality than serum AMH (90). According to these results, it can be suggested that FF AMH concentrations may be used for oocyte selection in stimulated cycles. However, although these data are very interesting and promising, further prospective randomized studies are needed to draw any conclusion.

OOCYTE–CORONA–CUMULUS COMPLEX EVALUATION

Cumulus cells are Graafian follicular cells that surround and nourish the oocyte during its development in the ovary. The innermost layer of cumulus cells, immediately adjacent to the ZP, is called corona radiata. Cells of the corona radiata extend their cytoplasm toward the oocyte through the ZP. Communications (either paracrine interaction or gap junction) occur between the oocyte and the cumulus–corona cells. Such interactions allow oocyte nutrition and maturation during its preovulatory growth from the diplotene to the MII stage (91,92). Corona radiata and cumulus cells maintain their contact with the oocyte at the time of ovulation, during a normal menstrual cycle, or after withdrawal by aspiration, in hormonally stimulated assisted reproduction cycles. In mature oocytes, the cumulus–corona mass appears as an expanded and mucified layer, due to the active secretion of hyaluronic acid. This extracellular component interposes among the cells and separates them, conferring to the cumulus–corona mass a fluffy appearance.

During unstimulated cycles, the stage of oocyte nuclear maturation is coupled with an increased expansion and mucification of the cumulus layer (19). However, stimulated cycles may be characterized by an asynchrony of these two processes (20). This was suggested to be caused by a different sensitivity of the oocyte and the cumulus–corona mass to the stimulants (20,93).

Early studies from Rattanachaiyanont et al. (22), performed on oocytes scheduled for denudation and insemination by ICSI, reported no correlation between oocyte–corona–cumulus complex (OCCC) morphology and nuclear maturity, fertilization rate, and embryo cleavage. Ebner et al. (94) have performed similar grading and had a similar conclusion; however, they found that the presence of blood clots (but not that of amorphous clumps) were associated with dense central granulation of oocytes and had negative effect on fertilization and blastocyst rates. Both studies have found a correlation between very dense corona radiata layer and decreased maturity of oocytes. On the other hand, other authors reported that OCCC scoring was related with fertilization and pregnancy rates (95) as well as to blastocyst quality and development (96). Lin and colleagues (95) proposed a grading system of OCCCs based on the morphology of the oocyte cytoplasm, cumulus mass, corona cells, and membrana granulosa cells, for oocytes prior to insemination by conventional IVF.

Five grades (mature group, approximately mature, immature, postmature, and atretic) were described, as shown in Table 7.1 (96). The authors reported higher fertilization rates for the oocytes belonging to the mature group compared with those belonging to the other groups. Moreover, the immature group was characterized by a higher incidence of poor morphology day 3 embryos as compared with the mature group. In support of a positive effect of cumulus–corona cells on oocyte development, it was shown that the partial removal of this layer prior to ICSI improves embryo quality and development (97). It has been suggested that the presence of cumulus–corona cells may help embryonic metabolism, by either stimulating gene expression (98) or reducing oxidative stress (99). Although, cumulus–corona mass observation is not sufficient to evaluate oocyte maturity and competence, it is reasonable to hypothesize that ooplasm development is

Table 7.1 Oocyte–Corona–Cumulus Complex Evaluation Scheme

Groups	OCCC morphology
Mature	Expanded cumulus
	Radiant corona
	Distinct zona pellucida, clear ooplasm
	Expanded well-aggregated membrane granulosa cells
Approximately mature	Expanded cumulus mass
	Slightly compact corona radiata
	Expanded, well-aggregated membrana granulosa cells
Immature	Dense compact cumulus if present
	Adherent compact layer of corona cells
	Ooplasm if visible with the presence of germinal vesicle
	Compact and nonaggregated membrana granulosa cells
Postmature	Expanded cumulus with clumps
	Radiant corona radiata, yet often clumped, irregular, or incomplete
	Visible zona, slightly granular or dark ooplasm
	Small and relatively nonaggregated membrana granulosa cells
Atretic	Rarely with associated cumulus mass
	Clumped and very irregular corona radiata if present
	Visible zona, dark and frequently misshapen ooplasm
	Membrana granulosa cells with very small clumps of cells

Source: Adapted from Ref. 95.

influenced by the action of these cells. In accordance with this hypothesis, it has been suggested that cumulus–corona cells play an important role in the in vitro maturation of oocytes that were immature at the time of retrieval (100,101). Therefore, a careful observation of OCCC morphology may be a useful tool for oocyte selection in those circumstances where no direct evaluation of the oocyte is possible. In addition, in our laboratory, where a maximum of three oocytes can be inseminated according to the Italian law, we use OCCC evaluation prior to denudation for ICSI. In fact, as suggested by Canipari et al. (102), we hypothesize that there is a higher probability of obtaining a better-quality mature oocyte in a normally expanded cumulus than in a nonexpanded one.

OOCYTE NUCLEAR MATURITY EVALUATION

Direct observation of oocyte morphology, including the extracytoplasmic components, is possible only after the denudation of its cumulus and corona layers. The use of hyaluronidase enzyme and mechanical pipetting facilitates the breaking down of the cumulus–corona extracellular matrix. This method is normally used when insemination by ICSI is going to be performed. A meiotically mature

Table 7.2 Relationship Between the Presence of a Detectable MS in Fresh MII Oocytes and the ICSI Outcome

	Meiotic spindle presence							
	Yes				No			
	Wang et al. (121)	Moon et al. (123)	Rienzi et al. (124)	Cohen et al. (126)	Wang et al. (121)	Moon et al. (123)	Rienzi et al. (124)	Cohen et al. (126)
Injected oocytes (%)	1266 (82.0)	523 (83.5)	484 (91.0)	585 (76.0)	278 (18.0)	103 (16.5)	48 (9.0)	185 (24.0)
Fertilized oocytes (%)	879 (69.4)[a]	430 (82.2)	362 (74.8)[b]	412 (70.4)[c]	175 (62.9)[d]	79 (75.7)	16 (33.3)[e]	115 (62.2)[f]
Good quality embryos (%)	583 (46.0)[g]	276 (52.8)[h]	268 (55.4)[i]	169 (47.2)	97 (34.9)[j]	28 (27.2)[k]	9 (18.7)[l]	32 (35.6)

[a,d] $p < 0.05$; [b,e] $p < 0.01$; [c,f] $p < 0.035$; [g,j] $p < 0.01$; [h,k] $p < 0.01$; [i,l] $p < 0.01$.
Source: Adapted from Refs. 120,122,123,125.

oocyte is blocked at the MII stage. Completion of the meiotic maturation occurs only after sperm entry and consequent oocyte activation. Currently, oocyte nuclear maturity is determined by the presence of an extruded IPB in the perivitelline space and by the absence of a GV. Nonsynchronous oocyte maturation is often observed after ovarian hyperstimulation.

Approximately 85% of the denuded oocytes display the IPB and are classified as MII. In about 10% a GV is present in the oocyte cytoplasm; approximately 5% of the oocytes are in the metaphase of the first meiotic division (MI) with no visible GV and IPB (103). Immature oocytes (GV and MI) can potentially be matured in vitro (104–106). However, the fertilization rate of such oocytes after ICSI is significantly lower than that which can be obtained with in vivo matured oocytes (105). Although some successful pregnancies are reported with the use of these cells, a high incidence of genetical abnormalities has been observed in the embryos derived from in vitro matured oocytes (107). Therefore, immature oocytes obtained by ovarian hyperstimulation should not be selected for insemination.

At MII stage the oocyte chromosomes are aligned at the equatorial region of the *meiotic spindle* (MS). This structure plays a crucial role in the sequence of events leading to the correct completion of meiosis and fertilization and thus is a key determinant of oocyte developmental potential. However, the MS microtubules, which are responsible for proper chromosomal segregation, are highly sensitive to chemical and physical changes that may occur during oocyte retrieval and handling. It has been shown that the oocyte exposure to slight temperature fluctuations dramatically affects microtubular structure, with deleterious consequences on chromosomal organization (108–112). Other parameters, such as increased maternal age (113,114) and oocyte in-vitro aging (115) are also associated with the disruption of MS architecture. The most potentially dramatic consequences of MS alteration are the unbalanced disjunction and/or non-disjunction of chromatids, chromosome scattering, and the formation of aneuploid embryos (113,116,117).

The introduction of a novel orientation-independent polarized light microscopy system (Spindle View Pol-Scope system, CRI, Woburn, Massachusetts, USA), coupled with an image-processing software, allows the visualization of MS in living oocytes (118–120). Parallel-aligned MS microtubules are birefringent and able to shift the plane of polarized light, inducing retardance. These properties enable the system to generate contrast and image the MS structure. Moreover, digital processing enhances signal sensitivity. Unlike conventional methods of MS imaging, the Spindle View system does not require oocyte fixation and staining. In this way the MS can be visualized in a noninvasive way, preserving oocyte viability.

Using the Spindle View system, new information about human oocyte maturity and developmental potentiality has been recently produced. Several studies (121–128) indicate the importance of the presence of a detectable MS in the oocyte cytoplasm prior to ICSI. A clear positive correlation between MS visualization, fertilization rate, and/or embryo development and/or blastocyst progression was described in these studies (Table 7.2). The absence of a detectable MS and the consequent oocyte developmental impairment may be primarily ascribed to oocyte immaturity (117). It has been hypothesized that the lack of MS formation can be the result of aberrant signaling pathways or low energy supply during oocyte growth, resulting in both nuclear and cytoplasmic immaturity (12,117). Moreover, some oocytes were found to be clearly immature at the stage of telophase I (Fig. 7.1) when observed with the Spindle View system (23–25). At this stage there is continuity between the ooplasm and the cytoplasm of the forming IPB, and the MS is interposed between the two separating cells. These oocytes would have been classified as "mature" MII with light microscopy, based on the presence of an IPB (Fig. 7.1A). Therefore, the use of the Spindle View system allows an accurate determination of oocyte nuclear maturity and selection of fully mature eggs. However, it must be underlined that unfavorable culture conditions may also induce MS disassembly (11,121,122). In this case the

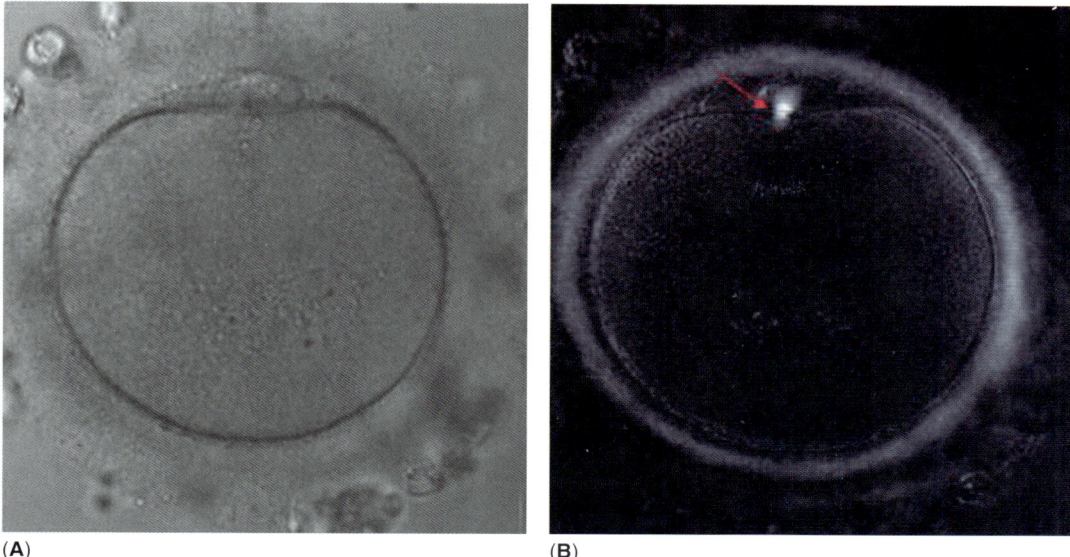

Figure 7.1 (**A**) Telophase I oocyte observed with light microscopy (Hoffman contrast) and (**B**) with polarized light microscopy (Spindle View system). Only with this latter system is it possible to observe the immature meiotic spindle (*arrow*) and to assess the maturation stage of this oocyte. (Magnification 400×).

lack of MS should be ascribed to environmental stress and not to oocyte incompetence to reach maturity.

The percentage of oocytes displaying a detectable MS varies between 60% and 90% in the different studies (Table 7.2) (121,123,124,126). This difference seems to be related to some important laboratory and clinical parameters: (*i*) the thermal control during oocytes handling (112,129); (*ii*) the technique of MS visualization (124,126,127); and (*iii*) the time elapsed from hCG administration (126). Because of the high sensitivity of the MS to temperature variations, thermal stability is necessary during oocyte observation and manipulation. In addition, oocyte rotation, by means of a micropipette, allows correct orientation of the MS structure, which therefore becomes more favorable to visualization under polarized light (124,125).

Finally, Cohen and coauthors (126) found that the percentage of oocytes with detectable MS was positively related with the time elapsed from hCG administration. For this reason it was suggested to postpone ICSI to 38–42 hours after hCG injection in order to allow complete oocyte maturation prior to insemination. Besides its role in chromosome segregation, the MS is also a key organelle in the creation of the IPB. Its position at the very periphery of the cell, attached to the oolemma cortex (130), dictates the orientation of the cleavage furrow and thus the IPB extrusion site. However, IPB has been found to be frequently dislocated from the MS location after the denudation procedure (123,124). Artifactual displacement of the IPB from its original extrusion place adjacent to the MS position is believed to be due to the manipulation required for cumulus–corona cell removal (124). No relationship between moderate degree of IPB/MS deviation and ICSI outcomes has been described in these studies. However, we (124) found that the mechanical stress that induces IPB dislocation more than 90 degrees from the MS position

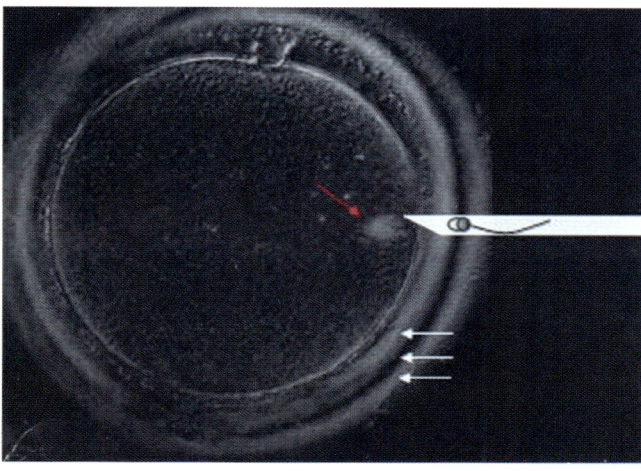

Figure 7.2 Metaphase II oocyte with a meiotic spindle located at 3 o'clock (*red arrow*) in the way of the injection pipette. The three different layers of the zona pellucida are clearly visible (*white arrows*). (Magnification 400×).

correlates with lower fertilization ability (124). In addition, MS dislocation is reported to affect embryo development since its position is involved in the correct orientation of the first cleavage plane (125). Another possible drawback of IPB displacement is the potential injury to the MS during microinsemination. In fact, the ICSI procedure is performed with the IPB at 90 degrees from the injection pipette entry site. Displaced IPB may thus expose the MS to the injection pipette passageway during oocyte microinsemination and therefore to mechanical damage (Fig. 7.2). The Spindle View system may thus be a useful tool to perform ICSI since it allows the correct orientation of the oocyte with the MS (and not the IPB) as far as possible from the injection needle.

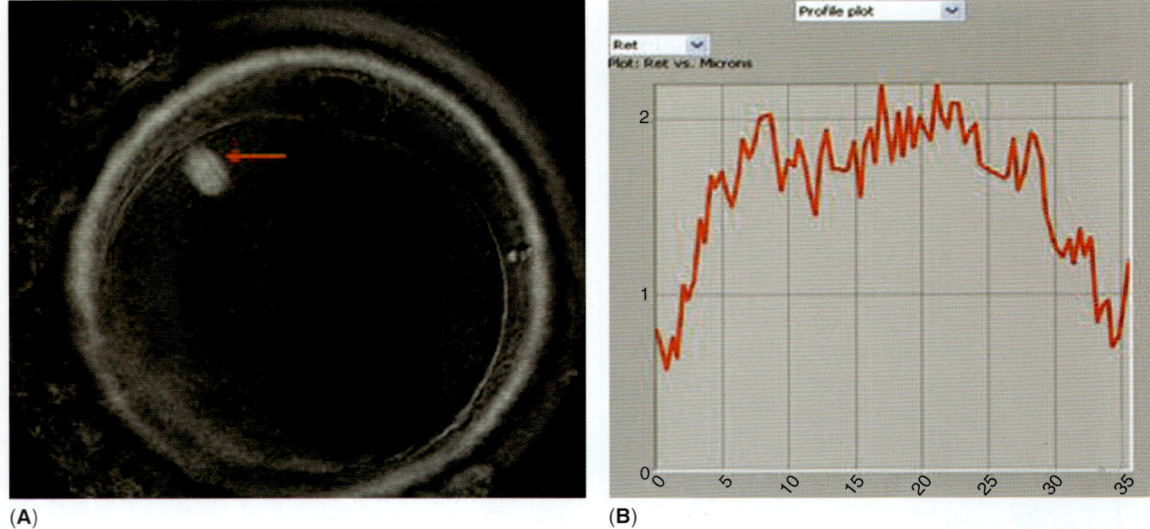

Figure 7.3 Metaphase II oocyte observed with the Spindle View system (**A**). Retardance profile of the meiotic spindle (**B**). (Magnification 400×).

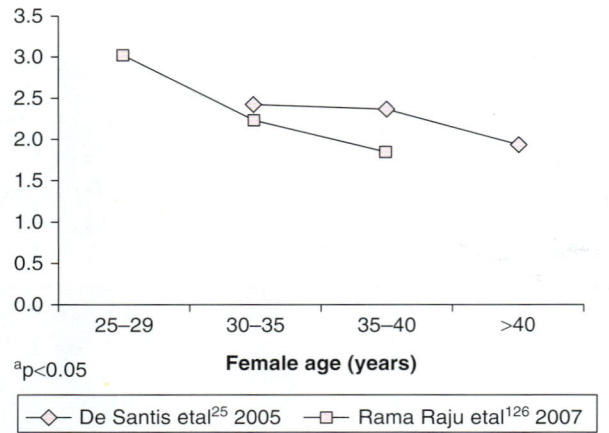

Figure 7.4 Relationship between MS retardance and female age. *Source*: Adapted from Refs. 25,127.

The Spindle View system can also produce quantitative information about the MS. The degree of birefringence is in fact directly proportional to the molecular organization of the structure (Fig. 7.3). It has been described that increased temperatures cause a decrease in spindle retardance, suggesting a partial loss of MS polymerization (131). A possible correlation between MS birefringence, oocyte quality, and embryo development has also been suggested (25,127,132). Moreover, a negative correlation between female age and MS retardance has been found (Fig. 7.4) (25,127). These data suggest that older women have a lower MS microtubular density, which could explain their higher risk of producing aneuploid embryos. These results are in agreement with observations by confocal microscopy that MS architecture is strictly related to female age (113).

METAPHASE II OOCYTE MORPHOLOGICAL EVALUATION

It is generally recognized that a "normal" human MII oocyte should have a round, clear ZP, a small PVS containing a single, not fragmented IPB and a pale, moderately granular cytoplasm with no inclusions (97,133–138). However, the majority of the oocytes retrieved after ovarian hyperstimulation exhibit one or more morphological abnormalities involving the cytoplasm aspect and/or the extracytoplasmic structures (97,134–139). The actual negative impact of the different oocyte "abnormalities" on IVF and ICSI outcome is unclear (reviewed in Ebner et al. (97), Balaban and Urman, (137) and Rienzi et al. (140)).

Some authors have suggested that all oocytes could be fertilized by ICSI independently from their morphological appearance (134,136). Furthermore, no impact on embryo quality has been associated with oocyte morphology. Similar clinical pregnancy and implantation rates were also obtained after transferring embryos derived from "abnormal" oocyte as compared with those obtained with embryos derived from "normal" appearing oocytes (22,25,134,136) (135,141–144). On the other hand, different authors have reported a correlation between oocyte morphology and embryo developmental potential. Regarding the *cumulative effect of multiple morphological features*, Xia (135) showed that oocyte grading based on IPB morphology, size of PVS, and cytoplasmic inclusions was correlated with its developmental potential after ICSI. In the study of Chamayou et al. (143) the cumulative effect of morphological features including cytoplasmic texture, inclusions, vacuoles, refractile bodies, and central granulation was found to be related with impaired embryo quality, but did not influence pregnancy rates. A completely different conclusion has been obtained by Serhal et al. (145) who found that similar features did not influence in vitro developmental parameters, but implantation and pregnancy rates were

Table 7.3 Morphological Features of Oocytes with ("Yes") or Without ("No") Predictive Value on In Vitro or In Vivo Outcome in Selected Publications

	COCs	Zona	Perivit	PBshape	Oshape	Darkdifg	Vac RB	Cgran	Spind	Multiple	Remark
Balaban et al. 1998 (136)	–	No	No	–	No	No	No	–	–	No	
Balakier et al. 2002 (165)	–	–	–	–	Yes	–	–	–	–	–	
Chamayou et al. 2006 (143)	–	–	Yes	Yes	No	+	+	+	No	Yes	Giant oocytes
Ciotti et al. 2004 (147)	–	–	–	No	–	–	–	–	Yes	–	Presence
Cohen et al. 2004 (126)	–	–	–	–	–	–	–	–	Yes	–	Presence
Cookeet et al. 2003 (125)	–	–	–	–	–	–	–	–	–	–	
De sutter et al. 1996 (134)	–	No	No	–	No	No	No	–	–	–	
Ebner et al. 2000 (138)	–	–	–	Yes	–	–	–	–	–	–	Blood clots in cum
Ebner et al. 2008 (94)	Yes	–	–	–	–	–	–	Yes	–	–	Fragmented better; Large impaired
Fancsovits et al. 2006 (151)	–	–	–	Yes	–	–	–	–	–	–	Thickness variation
Host et al. 2002 (158)	–	Yes	–	–	–	–	–	–	–	–	
Kahraman et al. 2000 (29)	–	–	–	–	–	–	–	Yes	–	–	
La Sala et al. 2009 (144)	+	+	+	+	–	+	+	–	–	No	
Lin et al. 2003 (95)	Yes	No	–	–	–	–	Yes	–	–	–	
Loutradis et al. 1999 (28)	–	–	–	–	–	Yes	–	–	–	–	Retardation
Madaschi et al. 2009 (128)	–	Yes	–	–	–	–	–	–	Yes	–	Presence
Moon et al. 2003 (123)	–	–	–	Yes	–	–	–	–	Yes	–	Presence+angle
Navarro et al. 2009 (150)	–	–	–	–	–	–	–	–	–	–	Large polar body
Ng et al. 1999 (95)	Yes	–	–	–	–	–	–	–	–	–	
Otsuki et al. 2004 (162)	–	–	–	–	–	Yes	Yes	–	–	–	Smoother cluster
Rama Raju et al. 2007 (127)	–	Yes	–	–	(m)Yes	No	–	–	Yes	–	Retardation, thickness
Rattana et al. 1999 (22)	No	–	–	–	–	–	–	–	–	–	
Rienzi et al. 2003 (124)	–	No	–	–	Yes	–	Yes	–	Yes	–	Presence, retard
Rienzi et al. 2008 (148)	–	–	Yes	Yes	No	Yes	Yes	Yes	–	Yes	Presence, position
Shen et al. 2006 (159)	–	–	–	–	–	–	–	–	Yes	–	Retardation
Ten et al. 2007 (152)	No	Yes	No	No	Yes	No	Yes	–	–	–	
Verlinsky et al. 2003 (142)	–	–	–	No	–	–	–	–	–	–	
Wang et al. 2001 (112)	–	–	–	–	–	–	–	–	Yes	–	Presence
Wilding et al. 2007 (164)	–	–	–	–	–	Yes	Yes	No	–	Yes	(M)membr.
Xia et al. 1997 (135)	–	–	+	+	–	–	Yes	–	–	Yes	Properties

Simplified version of the comprehensive table from Ref. 140.
Abbreviations: Cgran, central granulation; COC, cumulus–oocyte complex; Darkdifg, dark ooplasm or diffuse granulation; Multiple, multiple features evaluated together using a scoring system; Oshape, shape of the oocyte; PB shape, shape of the first polar body; Perivit, perivitelline space; Spind, meiotic spindle; VacRB, vacuoles, inclusions, refractile bodies; Zona, zona pellucida.

CONCLUSIONS

Useful, effective, and noninvasive grading tools are available for pronuclear, embryo, and blastocyst stage scoring (166–170). Combining several morphological criteria, each of which has been individually shown to be predictive for embryo competence, an accurate embryo selection is possible (23,145,171–173). In addition to morphological assessment, other features of the human embryo may be useful for a more accurate selection. Embryo physiology, evaluated by measurements of metabolic activity and normality, may help to determine embryonic "health" (174–179). Moreover, PGS of blastomeres' chromosomal constitution may give important information about embryonic developmental potential (180–182). With the current trend being toward limiting the number of embryos to be transferred, and thus the occurrence of multiple pregnancies, the ability of the embryologist to identify the embryo with the highest implantation potential is crucial. Nowadays, limited noninvasive tools exist to permit classification of human oocyte quality prior to fertilization.

As described above, the stimulation protocols, the different pharmacological preparations, and the perifollicular vascularization might influence human oocyte quality. Very recently, follicular fluid AMH has been positively correlated with oocyte quality, fertilization rate (88), and embryo implantation (90), suggesting that this biomarker is a very promising predictor of oocyte competence. In addition, oocyte observation under light microscopy provides assessments of several morphological characteristics. It seems, however, that slight deviations from the morphological normality should not be considered as abnormal phenotypes. Only some specific and evident oocyte morphological abnormalities, such as increased cytoplasmic granularity, vacuolization, presence of abnormal IPB, and ZP inner layer low retardance, have been linked to oocyte developmental potentiality. However, the limited predictive power and reliability of these parameters on implantation potential is generally reported. The reason may be ascribed to the subjectivity and inaccuracy in the evaluation.

The analysis of MS in living oocytes with the Spindle View system has shown that detectable MS are functionally superior to nondetectable ones (112,121,122,183). Furthermore, embryos derived from oocytes with functionally poor MS have impaired cell development (123,124,126). However, it must be underlined that more than 90% of the MII oocytes, not exposed to unfavorable laboratory conditions, display a detectable MS when observed with the Spindle View system. Therefore, while having ascertained that the absence of a signal is an important negative prognostic factor, the presence of MS, which involves the majority of the MII subjected to this evaluation, is of limited value for oocyte selection (25). In our opinion, MS qualitative analysis by measuring polarized light retardance, whose value is directly proportional to microtubule density, is a promising tool for oocyte quality assessment.

In addition to the above-mentioned evaluation criteria (such as serum and FF AMH measurements, and screening of intracellular and extracellular morphological features), other methods could be able to provide additional information on oocyte quality. Current research (reviewed in Wang and Sun (184)) is focusing on the following:

- Assessment of granulosa and cumulus cells' apoptosis status (185–187)
- Evaluation of oxidative stress in follicular fluid and granulosa cells (188–191)
- Follicular cells, gene expression profiles, by real-time polymerase chain reaction or DNA microarray (98,192)
- Measurement of follicular fluid leptin (192–195), growth factors and related binding proteins, that is insulin-like growth factor (IGF)/IGF binding protein / IGF-BP); members of the transforming growth factor (TGF-®) superfamily) (196–199)
- Quantitation of follicular steroids (such as estradiol, testosterone, progesterone, and prolactin) (195,200–205)
- Ultramicrofluorimetric quantitation of oocyte carbohydrate consumption and metabolite release in the culture medium (206).

Although potentially useful, further investigation is needed to ensure the consistency, reliability, and sensitivity of these methods. In addition, some of these methods are characterized by time-consuming protocols that imply in vitro oocyte aging.

On the basis of the above-mentioned potentialities of oocyte selection tools, future perspectives for the betterment of assisted reproductive techniques reside in creating a direct connection between IVF laboratories and research units.

To date, oocyte evaluation taking into account both clinical (ovarian stimulation protocols and follicular vascularization) and biological parameters (AMH measurements, aspect of the cumulus–corona cells, presence and position of the MS, morphology of the oocyte cytoplasm, and of the extracytoplasmic structures) gives some important information about the oocyte maturity stage and developmental fate of the deriving embryo. It is important that during laboratory evaluation procedures, the environmental conditions to which the oocytes are exposed should be as stable as possible. In this way these oocytes are preserved from stressful changes that could compromise their developmental potential. To this end, the use of chambers equipped with temperature/gas control is advisable during handling and observation.

From observing the egg with light microscopy and with polarized light, it is possible to identify "bad" quality oocytes. However, these evaluations are insufficient to select from normal-appearing oocytes the one with the higher developmental potential. Thus far, in order to gain reliable information about embryo implantation fate, pronuclear stage and embryo assessment are still essential in routine clinical applications. More efforts are needed to identify early markers of embryo quality, at the oocyte stage prior to fertilization. In the future, cellular/molecular approaches may help to provide such markers. The current trend is toward limiting the creation of supernumerary human embryos, and the identification of efficient parameters for oocyte competence assessment is a priority.

REFERENCES

1. Le Nestour E, Marraoui J, Lahlou N, et al. Role of estradiol in the rise in follicle stimulation hormone levels during the luteal-follicular transition. J Clin Endocrinol Metab 1993; 77: 439–42.
2. Hodgen GD. The dominant ovarian follicle. Fertil Steril 1982; 38: 281–300.
3. Goungeon A, Testart J. Influence of human menopausal gonadotropin on the recruitment of human ovarian follicles. Fertil Steril 1990; 54: 848–52.
4. Messinis IE, Templeton AA. The importance of follicle-stimulating hormone increase for folliculogenesis. Hum Reprod 1990; 5: 153–6.
5. Van Der Meer M, Hompes PGA, Scheele F, et al. Follicle stimulating hormone (FSH) dynamics of low dose step-up ovulation induction with FSH in patients with polycystic ovary syndrome. Hum Reprod 1994; 9: 1612–17.
6. Baird DT. A model for follicular selection and ovulation: lessons from superovulation. J Steroid Biochem 1987; 27: 15–23.
7. Brown JB. Pituitary control of ovarian function: concepts derived from gonadotropin therapy. Aust NZ J Obstet Gynaecol 1978; 18: 46–54.
8. Erickson GF, Danforth DR. Ovarian control of follicle development. Am J Obstet Gynecol 1995; 172: 736–47.
9. Fauser BC, Van Heusden AM. Manipulation of human ovarian function: physiological concepts and clinical consequences. Endocr Rev 1997; 18: 71–106.
10. Zelenzik AJ, Kubik CJ. Ovarian responses in macaques to pulsatile infusion of follicle-stimulating hormone (FSH) and luteinizing hormone: increased sensitivity of the maturing follicle to FSH. Endocrinology 1986; 119: 2025–32.
11. Van Santbrink EJ, Hop WC, Van Dessel TJ, de Jong FH, Fauser BC. Decremental follicle-stimulating hormone and dominant follicle development during the normal menstrual cycle. Fertil Steril 1995; 64: 37–43.
12. Fauser BC. Step-down follicle-stimulating hormone regimens in polycystic ovary syndrome. In: Filicori M, Flamigni C, eds. Ovulation Induction: Basic Science and Clinical Advances. Amsterdam: Elsevier, 1994: 153–62.
13. Hughes EG, Fedorkow DM, Daya S, et al. The routine use of gonadotropin-Releasing hormone agonists prior to in vitro fertilization and gamete intrafallopian transfer: a meta-analysis of randomized controlled trials. Fertil Steril 1992; 58: 888–96.
14. Albano C, Felberbaum RE, Smitz J, et al. Ovarian stimulation with HMG: results of a prospective randomized phase III European study comparing the luteinizing hormone-Releasing hormone (LHRH)-antagonist cetrorelix and the LHRH-agonist buserelin. Hum Reprod 2000; 15: 526–31.
15. Olivennes F, Belaisch-Allart J, Emperaire JC, et al. Prospective, randomized, controlled study of in vitro fertilization-embryo transfer with a single dose of a luteinizing hormone-releasing hormone (LH-RH) antagonist (cetrorelix) or a depot formula of an LH-RH antagonist (triptorelin). Fertil Steril 2000; 73: 314–20.
16. Fluker M, Grifo J, Leader A, et al. Efficacy and safety of ganirelix acetate versus leuprolide acetate in women undergoing controlled ovarian hyperstimulation. Fertil Steril 2001; 75: 38–45.
17. De Jong D, Macklon NS, Fauser BC. A pilot study involving minimal ovarian stimulation for in vitro fertilization: extending the "follicle-stimulating hormone window" combined with gonadotropinreleasing hormone antagonist cetrorelix. Fertil Steril 2000; 73: 1051–4.
18. Hohmann FP, Macklon NS, Fauser BC. A randomized comparison of two ovarian stimulation protocols with gonadotropin-releasing hormone (GnRH) antagonist cotreatment for in vitro fertilization commencing recombinant follicle-stimulating hormone on cycle day 2 or 5 with the standard long GnRH agonist protocol. J Clin Endocrinol Metab 2003; 88: 166–73.
19. Testart J, Lassalle B, Frydman R, Belaisch JC. A study of factors affecting the success of human fertilization in vitro. II. Influence of semen quality and oocyte maturity on fertilization and cleavage. Biol Reprod 1983; 28: 425–31.
20. Laufer N, Tarlatzis BC, DeCherney AH, et al. Asynchrony between human cumulus–corona cell complex and oocyte maturation after human menopausal gonadotropin treatment for in vitro fertilization. Fertil Steril 1984; 42: 366–72.
21. Khamsi F, Roberge S, Lacanna IC, Wong J, Yavas Y. Effects of granulosa cells, cumulus cells, and oocyte density on in vitro fertilization in women. Endocrine 1999; 10: 161–6.
22. Rattanachaiyanont M, Leader A, Leveille MC. Lack of correlation between oocyte–corona–cumulus complex morphology and nuclear maturity of oocytes collected in stimulated cycles for intracytoplasmic sperm injection. Fertil Steril 1999; 71: 937–40.
23. Rienzi L, Ubaldi F, Iacobelli M, et al. Significance of morphological attributes of the early embryo. Reprod Biomed Online 2005; 10: 669–81.
24. Montag M, Schimming T, van der Ven H. Spindle imaging in human oocytes: the impact of the meiotic cell cycle. Reprod Biomed Online 2006; 12: 442–6.
25. De Santis L, Cino I, Rabellotti E. Polar body morphology and spindle imaging as predictors of oocyte quality. Reprod Biomed Online 2005; 11: 36–42.
26. Hassan-Ali H, Hisham-Saleh A, El-Gezeiry D, et al. Perivitelline space granularity: a sign of human menopausal gonadotrophin overdose in intracytoplasmic sperm injection. Hum Reprod 1998; 13: 3425–30.
27. Eichenlaub-Ritter U, Schmiady H, Kentenich H, Soewarto D. Recurrent failure in polar body formation and premature chromosome condensation in oocytes from a human patient: indicators of asynchrony in nuclear and cytoplasmic maturation. Hum Reprod 1995; 10: 2343–9.
28. Loutradis D, Drakakis P, Kallianidis K, et al. Oocyte morphology correlates with embryo quality and pregnancy rate after intracytoplasmic sperm injection. Fertil Steril 1999; 72: 240–4.
29. Kahraman S, Yakin K, Donmez E, et al. Relationship between granular cytoplasm of oocytes and pregnancy

outcome following intracytoplasmic sperm injection. Hum Reprod 2000; 15: 2390–3.
30. Steptoe P, Edwards R. Birth after the reimplantation of a human embryo. Lancet 1978; 12: 366.
31. Laufer N, DeCherney AH, Haseltine FP, et al. The use of high-dose human menopausal gonadotropin in an in vitro fertilization program. Fertil Steril 1983; 40: 734–41.
32. Edwards RG, Lobo R, Bouchard P. Time to revolutionize ovarian stimulation. Hum Reprod 1996; 11: 917–19.
33. Fauser BC, Devroey P, Yen SS, et al. Minimal ovarian stimulation for IVF: appraisal of potential benefits and drawbacks. Hum Reprod 1999; 14: 2681–6.
34. Pena JE, Chang PL, Chan LK, et al. Supraphysiological estradiol levels do not affect oocyte and embryo quality in oocyte donation cycles. Hum Reprod 2002; 17: 83–7.
35. Greb RR, Behre HM, Simoni M. Pharmacogenetics in ovarian stimulation – current concepts and future options. Reprod Biomed Online 2005; 11: 589–600.
36. Baart EB, Martini E, Eijkemans MJ, et al. Milder ovarian stimulation for in-vitro fertlization reduces aneuploidy in the human preimplantation embryo: a randomized controlled trial. Hum Reprod 2007; 22: 980–8.
37. van der Gaast MH, Eijkemans MJ, van der Net JB, et al. Optimum number of oocytes for a successful first IVF treatment cycle. Reprod Biomed Online 2006; 13: 476–80.
38. Fauser BC, Devroey P, Macklon NS. Multiple birth resulting from ovarian stimulation for subfertility treatment. Lancet 2005; 365: 1807–16.
39. Simón C, Garcia Velasco JJ, Valbuena D, et al. Increasing uterine receptivity by decreasing estradiol levels during the preimplantation period in high responders with the use of a follicle-stimulating hormone stepdown regimen. Fertil Steril 1998; 70: 234–9.
40. Macklon NS, Fauser BC. Impact of ovarian hyperstimulation on the luteal phase. J Reprod Fertil 2000; 55: 101–8.
41. Munné S. Chromosome abnormalities and their relationship to morphology and development of human embryos. Reprod Biomed Online 2006; 12: 234–53.
42. Munné S, Magli MC, Adler A, et al. Treatmentrelated chromosome abnormalities in human embryos. Hum Reprod 1997; 12: 780–4.
43. Katze-Jaffe MG, Linck DW, Schoolcraft WB, Gardner DK. A proteomic analysis of mammalian preimplantation development. Reproduction 2005; 130: 899–905.
44. Recombinant Human FSH Study Group. Clinical assessment of recombinant human follicle-stimulating hormone in stimulating ovarian follicular development before in vitro fertilization. Fertil Steril 1995; 63: 77–86.
45. Out HJ, Mannaerts BM, Driessen SG, Bennink HJ. A prospective, randomized, assessor-blind, multicentre study comparing recombinant follicle-stimulating hormone (Puregon versus Metrodin) in in-vitro fertilization. Hum Reprod 1995; 10: 2534–40.
46. Bergh C, Howles C, Borg K, et al. Recombinant human follicle stimulating hormone (r-hFSH; Gonal-F) versus highly purified urinary FSH (Metrodin HP): results of a randomized comparative study in women undergoing assisted reproductive techniques. Hum Reprod 1997; 10: 2133–9.
47. Daya S, Gunby J, Hughes EG, Collins JA, Sagle MA. Follicle-stimulating hormone versus human menopausal gonadotrophin for in vitro fertilization cycles: a meta-analysis. Fertil Steril 1995; 64: 347–54.
48. Agarwal R, Holmes J, Jacobs HS, et al. Recombinant human follicle-stimulating hormone or human menopausal gonadotrophin for ovarian stimulation in in vitro fertilization cycles: a metaanalysis. Fertil Steril 2000; 73: 338–43.
49. Daya S. Updated meta-analysis of recombinant folliclestimulating hormone (FSH) versus urinary FSH for ovarian stimulation in assisted reproduction. Fertil Steril 2002; 77: 711–14.
50. Al-Inany H, Aboulghar M, Mansour R, Serour G. Meta-analysis of recombinant versus urinaryderived FSH: an update. Hum Reprod 2003; 18: 305–13.
51. Huang FJ, Lan KC, Kung FT, et al. Human cumulus-free oocyte maturational profile and in vitro developmental potential after stimulation with recombinant versus urinary FSH. Hum Reprod 2004; 19: 306–15.
52. Sherins RJ, Thorsell LP, Dorfmann A, et al. Intracytoplasmic sperm injection facilitates fertilization even in the most severe forms of male infertility: pregnancy outcome correlation with maternal age and number of eggs available. Fertil Steril 1995; 64: 369–75.
53. Garrido N, Navarro J, Remohí J, Simon C, Pellicer A. Follicular hormonal environment and embryo quality in women with endometriosis. Hum Reprod Update 2000; 6: 67–74.
54. Perez Mayorga M, Gromoll J, Behre HM, et al. Ovarian response to follicle-stimulating hormone (FSH) stimulation depends on the FSH receptor genotype. J Clin Endocrinol Metab 2000; 85: 3365–9.
55. Sudo S, Kudo M, Wada S, et al. Genetic and functional analyses of polymorphisms in the human FSH receptor gene. Mol Hum Reprod 2002; 8: 893–9.
56. Mercan R, Mayer JF, Walker D, et al. Improved oocyte quality is obtained with follicle stimulating hormone alone than with follicle stimulating hormone/human menopausal gonadotrophin combination. Hum Reprod 1997; 12: 1886–9.
57. Jacob S, Drudy L, Conroy R, Harrison RF. Outcome from consecutive in-vitro fertilization/intracytoplasmic sperm injection attempts in the final group treated with urinary gonadotrophins and the first group treated with recombinant follicle stimulating hormone. Hum Reprod 1998; 13: 1783–7.
58. Weissman A, Meriano J, Ward S, Gotlieb L, Casper RF. Intracytoplasmic sperm injection after follicle stimulation with highly purified human folliclestimulating hormone compared with human menopausal gonadotropin. J Assist Reprod Genet 1999; 16: 63–8.
59. Ng EH, Lau EY, Yeung WS, Ho PC. HMG is as good as recombinant human FSH in terms of oocyte and embryo quality: a prospective randomized trial. Hum Reprod 2001; 16: 319–25.
60. Smitz J, Andersen AN, Devroey P, Arce JC; MERIT Group. Endocrine profile in serum and follicular fluid differs after ovarian stimulation with HPhMG or recombinant FSH in IVF patients. Hum Reprod 2007; 22: 676–87.
61. Van Blerkom J. The influence of intrinsic and extrinsic factors on the developmental potential and chromosomal normality of the human oocyte. J Soc Gynecol Investig 1996; 3: 3–11.

62. Van Blerkom J, Antezak M, Schrader R. The developmental potential of human oocyte is related to the dissolved oxygen content of follicular fluid: association with vascular endothelial growth factor levels and perifollicular blood flow characteristics. Hum Reprod 1997; 12: 1047–55.
63. Battaglia C, Genazzani AD, Regnani G, et al. Perifollicular doppler flow and follicular fluid vascular endothelial growth factor concentrations in poor responders. Fertil Steril 2000; 74: 809–12.
64. Van Blerkom J. Epigenetic influences on oocyte developmental competence: perifollicular vascularity and intrafollicular oxygen. J Assist Reprod Genet 1998; 15: 226–34.
65. Coulam CB, Goodman C, Rinehart JS. Colour Doppler indices of follicular blood flow as predictors of pregnancy after in-vitro fertilization and embryo transfer. Hum Reprod 1999; 14: 1979–82.
66. Chui DK, Pugh ND, Walker SM, Gregory L, Shaw RW. Follicular vascularity-the predictive value of transvaginal power Doppler ultrasonography in an in-vitro fertilization programme: a preliminary study. Hum Reprod 1997; 12: 191–6; 67.
67. Bhal PS, Pugh ND, Chui DK, et al. The use of transvaginal power Doppler ultrasonography to evaluate the relationship between perifollicular vascularity and outcome in in-vitro fertilization treatment cycles. Hum Reprod 1999; 14: 939–45.
68. Bhal PS, Pugh ND, Gregory L, O'Brien S, Shaw RW. Perifollicular vascularity as a potential variable affecting outcome in stimulated intrauterine insemination treatment cycles: a study using transvaginal power doppler. Hum Reprod 2001; 16: 1682–9.
69. Borini A, Maccolini A, Tallarini A, et al. Perifollicular vascularity and its relationship with oocyte maturity and IVF outcome. Ann NY Acad Sci 2001; 943: 64–7.
70. Costello MF, Sjoblom P, Shrestha SM. Use of doppler ultrasound imaging of the ovary during IVF treatment as a predictor of success. In: Rao KA, Brinsdon PR, Sathananthan H, eds. The Infertility Manual. New Delhi: JAYPEE Brothers Medical, 2004: 344–9.
71. Ragni G, Anselmino M, Nicolosi AE, et al. Follicular vascularity is not predictive of pregnancy outcome in mild controlled ovarian stimulation and IUI cycles. Hum Reprod 2007; 22: 210–14.
72. Huey S, Abuhamad A, Barroso G, et al. Perifollicular blood flow Doppler indices, but not follicular pO2, pCO2, or pH, predict oocyte developmental competence in vitro fertilization. Fertil Steril 1999; 72: 707–12.
73. Kan A, Ng EH, Yeung WS, Ho PC. Perifollicular vascularity in poor ovarian responders during IVF. Hum Reprod 2006; 21: 1539–44.
74. Ng EH, Tang OS, Chan CC, Ho PC. Ovarian stromal vascularity is not predictive of ovarian response and pregnancy. Reprod Biomed Online 2006; 12: 43–9.
75. Palomba S, Russo T, Falbo A. Clinical use of the perifollicular vascularity assessment in IVF cycles: a pilot study. Hum Reprod 2006; 21: 1055–61.
76. Eldar-Geva T, Ben-Chetrit A, Spitz IM, et al. Dynamic assays of inhibin b, anti-Müllerian hormone and estradiol following FSH stimulation and ovarian ultrasonography as predictors of IVF outcome. Hum Reprod 2005; 20: 3178–83.
77. Baarends WW, Uilenbroek JT, Kramer P, et al. Anti-Müllerian hormone and anti-Müllerian hormone type II receptor messenger ribonucleic acid expression in rat ovaries during postnatal development, the estrous cycle, and gonadotropin-Induced follicle growth. Endocrinology 1995; 136: 4951–62.
78. Durlinger AL, Visser JA, Themmen AP. Regulation of ovarian function: the role of anti-Müllerian hormone. Reproduction 2002; 124: 601–9.
79. Weenen C, Laven JS, Von Bergh AR, et al. Anti-Müllerian hormone expression pattern in the human ovary: potential implications for initial and cyclic follicle recruitment. Mol Hum Reprod 2004; 10: 77–83.
80. De Vet A, Laven JS, de Jong FH, Themmen AP, Fauser BC. Antimüllerian hormone serum levels: a putative marker for ovarian aging. Fertil Steril 2002; 77: 357–62.
81. Fanchin R, Schonauer LM, Righini C, et al. Serum anti-Müllerian hormone is more strongly related to ovarian follicular status than serum inhibin B, estradiol, FSH and LH on day 3. Hum Reprod 2003; 18: 323–7.
82. Seifer DB, MacLaughlin DT, Christian BP, Feng B, Shelden RM. Early follicular serum Müllerian inhibiting substance levels are associated with ovarian response during assisted reproductive technique cycles. Fertil Steril 2002; 77: 468–71; 83.
83. van Rooij IA, Broekmans FJ, et al. Serum anti-Müllerian hormone levels: a novel measure of ovarian reserve. Hum Reprod 2002; 17: 3065–71.
84. Hazout A, Bouchard P, Seifer DB, et al. Serum antimüllerian hormone/Müllerian-inhibiting substance appears to be a more discriminatory marker of assisted reproductive technique outcome than follicle-stimulating hormone, inhibin B, or estradiol. Fertil Steril 2004; 82: 1323–9.
85. Fanchin R, Taieb J, Lozano DH, et al. High reproducibility of serum anti-Müllerian hormone measurements suggests a multi-staged follicular secretion and strengthens its role in the assessment of ovarian follicular status. Hum Reprod 2005; 20: 923–7.
86. Silberstein T, MacLaughlin DT, Shai I, et al. Müllerian inhibiting substance levels at the time of HCG administration in IVF cycles predict both ovarian reserve and embryo morphology. Hum Reprod 2006; 21: 159–63.
87. Lekamge DN, Barry M, Kolo M, et al. Anti-Müllerian hormone as a predictor of IVF outcome. Reprod Biomed Online 2007; 14: 602–10.
88. Takahashi C, Fujito A, Kazuka M, et al. Anti-Müllerian hormone substance from follicular fluid is positively associated with success in oocyte fertilization during in vitro fertilization. Fertil Steril 2008; 89: 586–91.
89. Fanchin R, Louafi N, Mendez Lozano DH, et al. Per follicle measurements indicate that anti-Müllerian hormone secretion is modulated by the extent of follicular development and luteinization and may reflect qualitatively the ovarian follicular status. Fertil Steril 2005; 84: 167–73.
90. Fanchin R, Mendez Lozano DH, Frydman N, et al. Anti-Müllerian hormone concentrations in the follicular fluid of the preovulatory follicle are predictive of the implantation potential of the ensuing embryo obtained by in vitro fertilization. J Clin Endocrinol Metab 2007; 92: 1796–802.

91. Dong J, Albertini DF, Nishimori K, et al. Growth differentiation factor-9 is required during early ovarian folliculogenesis. Nature 1996; 383: 531–5.
92. Albertini DF, Combelles CM, Benecchi E, Carabatsos MJ. Cellular basis for paracrine regulation of ovarian follicle development. Reproduction 2001; 121: 647–53.
93. Bar-Ami S, Gitay-Goren H, Brandes JM. Different morphological and steroidogenic patterns in oocyte/cumulus–corona cell complexes aspirated at in vitro fertilization. Biol Reprod 1989; 41: 761–70.
94. Ebner T, Moser M, Shebl O, et al. Blood clots in the cumulus-oocyte complex predict poor oocyte quality and post-fertilization development. Reprod Biomed Online 2008a; 16: 801–7.
95. Ng ST, Chang TH, Wu TC. Prediction of the rates of fertilization, cleavage, and pregnancy success by cumulus-coronal morphology in an in vitro fertilization program. Fertil Steril 1999; 72: 412–17.
96. Lin YC, Chang SY, Lan KC, et al. Human oocyte maturity in vivo determines the outcome of blastocyst development in vitro. J Assist Reprod Genet 2003; 20: 506–12.
97. Ebner T, Moser M, Tews G. Is oocyte morphology prognostic of embryo developmental potential after ICSI? Reprod Biomed Online 2006; 12: 507–12.
98. McKenzie LJ, Pangas SA, Carson SA, et al. Human cumulus granulosa cell gene expression: a predictor of fertilization and embryo selection in women undergoing IVF. Hum Reprod 2004; 19: 2869–74.
99. Fatehi AN, Roelen BA, Colenbrander B, et al. Presence of cumulus cells during in vitro fertilization protects the bovine oocyte against oxidative stress and improves first cleavage but does not affect further development. Zygote 2005; 13: 177–85.
100. Goud PT, Goud AP, Qian C, et al. In-vitromaturation of human germinal vesicle stage oocytes: role of cumulus cells and epidermal growth factor in the culture medium. Hum Reprod 1998; 13: 1638–44.
101. Yamazaki Y, Wakayama T, Yanagimachi R. Contribution of cumulus cells and serum to the maturation of oocyte cytoplasm as revealed by intracytoplasmic sperm injection (ICSI). Zygote 2001; 9: 277–82.
102. Canipari R, Camaioni A, Scarchilli L, Barberi M, Salustri A. Oocyte maturation and ovulation: mechanism of control. 2PN Attual Scient Biol Ripr 2004; 1: 62–8.
103. Ubaldi F, Rienzi L. Micromanipulation techniques in human infertility: PZD, SUZI, ICSI, MESA, PESA, FNA and TESE. In: Revelli A, Tur-Kaspa I, Holte JG, Massobrio M, eds. Biotechnology of Human Reproduction. Oxford: Parthenon Publishing, 2003: 315–36.
104. Nagy ZP, Cecile J, Liu J, et al. Pregnancy and birth after intracytoplasmic sperm injection of in vitro matured germinal-vesicle stage oocytes: case report. Fertil Steril 1996; 65: 1047–50.
105. De Vos A, Van de Velde H, Joris H, Van Steirteghem A. In-vitro matured metaphase-I oocytes have a lower fertilization rate but similar embryo quality as mature metaphase-II oocytes after intracytoplasmic sperm injection. Hum Reprod 1999; 14: 1859–63.
106. Edirisinghe WR, Junk SM, Matson PL, Yovich JL. Birth from cryopreserved embryos following in vitro maturation of oocytes and intracytoplasmic sperm injection. Hum Reprod 1997; 12: 1056–8.
107. Nogueira D, Staessen C, Van de Velde H, Van Steirteghem A. Nuclear status and cytogenetics of embryos derived from in vitro-matured oocytes. Fertil Steril 2000; 74: 295–8.
108. Sathananthan AH, Trounson A, Freemann L, Brady T. The effects of cooling human oocytes. Hum Reprod 1988; 3: 968–77.
109. Pickering SJ, Braude PR, Johnson MH, Cant A, Currie J. Transient cooling to room temperature can cause irreversible disruption of the meiotic spindle in the human oocyte. Fertil Steril 1990; 54: 102–8.
110. Almeida PA, Bolton VN. The effect of temperature fluctuations on the cytoskeletal organisation and chromosomal constitution of the human oocyte. Zygote 1995; 3: 357–65.
111. Zenzes MT, Bielecki R, Casper RF, Leibo SP. Effects of chilling to 0°C on the morphology of meiotic spindles in human metaphase II oocytes. Fertil Steril 2001; 75: 769–77.
112. Wang WH, Meng L, Hackett RJ, Odenbourg R, Keefe DL. Limited recovery of meiotic spindles in living human oocytes after cooling–rewarming observed using polarized light microscopy. Hum Reprod 2001; 16: 2374–8.
113. Battaglia DE, Goodwin P, Klein NA, Soules MR. Influence of maternal age on meiotic spindle assembly in oocytes from naturally cycling women. Hum Reprod 1996; 11: 2217–22.
114. Volarcik K, Sheean L, Goldfarb J, et al. The meiotic competence of in-vitro matured human oocytes is influenced by donor age: evidence that folliculogenesis is compromised in the reproductively aged ovary. Hum Reprod 1998; 13: 154–60.
115. Eichenlaub-Ritter U, Vogt E, Yin H, Gosden R. Spindles, mitochondria and redox potential in ageing oocytes. Reprod Biomed Online 2004; 8: 45–58.
116. Bernard A, Fuller BJ. Cryopreservation of human oocytes: a review of current problems and perspectives. Hum Reprod Update 1996; 2: 193–207.
117. Eichenlaub-Ritter U, Shen Y, Tinneberg HR. Manipulation of the oocyte: possible damage to the spindle apparatus. Reprod Biomed Online 2002; 5: 117–24.
118. Oldenbourg R, Mei G. New polarized light microscope with precision universal compensator. J Microsc 1995; 180: 140–7.
119. Oldenbourg R. Polarized light microscopy of spindles. Methods Cell Biol 1999; 61: 175–208.
120. Liu L, Trimarchi JR, Oldenbourg R, Keefe DL. Increased birefringence in the meiotic spindle provides a new marker for the onset of activation in living oocytes. Biol Reprod 2000; 63: 251–8.
121. Wang WH, Meng L, Hackett RJ, Keefe DL. Developmental ability of human oocytes with or without birefringent spindles imaged by Polscope before insemination. Hum Reprod 2001; 16: 1464–8.
122. Wang WH, Meng L, Hackett RJ, et al. The spindle observation and its relationship with fertilization after intracytoplasmicsperm injection in living human oocytes. Fertil Steril 2001; 75: 348–53.
123. Moon JH, Hyun CS, Lee SW, et al. Visualization of the metaphase II meiotic spindle in living human oocytes using the polscope enables the prediction of embryonic developmental competence after ICSI. Hum Reprod 2003; 18: 817–20.
124. Rienzi L, Ubaldi F, Martinez F, et al. Relationship between meiotic spindle location with regard to the polar body position and oocyte developmental potential after ICSI. Hum Reprod 2003; 18: 1289–93.

125. Cooke S, Tyler JP, Driscoll GL. Meiotic spindle location and identification and its effect on embryonic cleavage plane and early development. Hum Reprod 2003; 18: 2397–405.
126. Cohen Y, Malcov M, Schwartz T, et al. Spindle imaging: a new marker for optimal timing of ICSI? Hum Reprod 2004; 19: 649–54.
127. Rama Raju GA, Prakash GJ, Krishna KM, Madan K. Meiotic spindle and zona pellucida characteristics as predictors of embryonic development: a preliminary study using PolScope imaging. Reprod Biomed Online 2007; 14: 166–74.
128. Madaschi C, Aoki T, de Almeida Ferreira Braga DP, et al. Zona pellucida birefringence score and meiotic spindle visualization in relation to embryo development and ICSI outcomes. Reprod Biomed Online 2009; 18: 681–6.
129. Wang WH, Meng L, Hackett RJ, Oldenbourg R, Keefe DL. Rigorous thermal control during intracytoplasmic sperm injection stabilizes the meiotic spindle and improves fertilization and pregnancy rates. Fertil Steril 2002; 77: 1274–7.
130. Maro B, Verlhac MH. Polar body formation: new rules for asymmetric divisions. Nat Cell Biol 2002; 4: E281–3.
131. Sun XF, Wang WH, Keefe DL. Overheating is detrimental to meiotic spindles within in vitro matured human oocytes. Zygote 2004; 12: 65–70.
132. Trimarchi JR, Karin RA, Keefe DL. Average spindle retardance observed using the polscope predicts cell number in day 3 embryos. Fertil Steril 2004; 82: S268.
133. Alikani M, Palermo G, Adler A, et al. Intracytoplasmic sperm injection in dysmorphic human oocytes. Zygote 1995; 3: 283–8.
134. De Sutter P, Dozortsev D, Qian C, Dhont M. Oocyte morphology does not correlate with fertilization rate and embryo quality after intracytoplasmic sperm injection. Hum Reprod 1996; 11: 595–7.
135. Xia P. Intracytoplasmic sperm injection: correlation of oocyte grade based on polar body, perivitelline space and cytoplasmic inclusions with fertilization rate and embryo quality. Hum Reprod 1997; 12: 1750–5.
136. Balaban B, Urman B, Sertac A, et al. Oocyte morphology does not affect fertilization rate, embryo quality and implantation rate after intracytoplasmic sperm injection. Hum Reprod 1998; 13: 3431–3.
137. Balaban B, Urman B. Effect of oocyte morphology on embryo development and implantation. Reprod Biomed Online 2006; 12: 608–15.
138. Ebner T, Yaman C, Moser M, et al. Prognostic value of first polar body morphology on fertilization rate and embryo quality in intracytoplasmic sperm injection. Hum Reprod 2000; 15: 427–30.
139. Mikkelsen AL, Lindenberg S. Morphology of in-vitro matured oocytes: impact on fertility potential and embryo quality. Hum Reprod 2001; 16: 1714–18.
140. Rienzi L, Vajta G, Ubaldi F. Predictive value of oocyte morphology in human IVF: a systematic review of the literature. Hum Reprod Update 2011; 17: 34–45.
141. Esfandiari N, Burjaq H, Gotlieb L, et al. Brown oocytes: implications for assisted reproductive technique. Fertil Steril 2006; 86: 1522–5.
142. Verlinsky Y, Lerner S, Illkevitch N, et al. Is there any predictive value of first polar body morphology for embryo genotype or developmental potential? Reprod Biomed Online 2003; 7: 336–41.
143. Chamayou S, Ragolia C, Alecci C, et al. Meiotic spindle presence and oocyte morphology do not predict clinical ICSI outcomes: a study of 967 transferred embryos. Reprod Biomed Online 2006; 13: 661–7.
144. La Sala GB, Nicoli A, Villani MT, et al. The effect of selecting oocytes for insemination and transferring all resultant embryos without selection on outcomes of assisted. Fertil Steril 2009; 91: 96–100.
145. Serhal PF, Ranieri DM, Kinis A, et al. Oocyte morphology predicts outcome of intracytoplasmic sperm injection. Hum Reprod 1997; 12: 1267–70.
146. Ebner T, Moser M, Yaman C, et al. Elective transfer of embryos selected on the basis of first polar body morphology is associated with increased rates of implantation and pregnancy. Fertil Steril 1999; 72: 599–603.
147. Ciotti PM, Notarangelo L, Morselli-Labate AM, et al. First polar body morphology before ICSI is not related to embryo quality or pregnancy rate. Hum Reprod 2004; 19: 2334–9.
148. Rienzi L, Ubaldi FM, Iacobelli M, et al. Significance of metaphase II human oocyte morphology on ICSI outcome. Fertil Steril 2008; 90: 1692–700.
149. Ebner T, Moser M, Sommergruber M, et al. First polar body morphology and blastocyst formation rate in ICSI patients. Hum Reprod 2002; 17: 2415–18.
150. Navarro PA, de Araujo MM, de Araujo CM, et al. Relationship between first polar body morphology before intracytoplasmic sperm injection and fertilization rate, cleavage rate, and embryo quality. Int J Gynaecol Obstet 2009; 104: 226–9.
151. Fancsovits P, Tothne ZG, Murber A, et al. Correlation between first polar body morphology and further embryo development. Acta Biol Hung 2006; 57: 331–8.
152. Ten J, Mendiola J, Vioque J, et al. Donor oocyte dysmorphisms and their influence on fertilization and embryo quality. Reprod Biomed Online 2007; 14: 40–8.
153. Verlinsky Y, Lerner S, Illkevitch N, et al. Is there any predictive value of first polar body morphology for embryo genotype or developmental potential. Reprod Biomed Online 2003; 7: 336–41.
154. Verlhac MH, Lefebvre C, Guillaud P, Rassinier P, Maro B. Asymmetric division in mouse oocytes: with or without Mos. Curr Biol 2000; 10: 1303–6.
155. Ebner T, Yaman C, Moser M, et al. A prospective study on oocyte survival rate after ICSI: influence of injection technique and morphological features. J Assist Reprod Genet 2001; 18: 623–8.
156. Plachot M, Selva J, Wolf JP, Bastit P, de Mouzon J. Consequences of oocyte dysmorphy on the fertilization rate and embryo development after intracytoplasmic sperm injection. A prospective multicenter study. Gynecol Obstet Fertil 2002; 30: 772–9.
157. Balaban B, Urman B. Embryo culture as a diagnostic tool. Reprod Biomed Online 2003; 7: 671–82.
158. Høst E, Gabrielsen A, Lindenberg S, et al. Apoptosis in human cumulus cells in relation to zona pellucida thickness variation, maturation stage, and cleavage of the corresponding oocyte after intracytoplasmic sperm injection. Fertil Steril 2002; 77: 511–15.
159. Shen Y, Stalf T, Mehnert C, Eichenlaub-Ritter U, Tinneberg HR. High magnitude of light retardation by the zona pellucida is associated with conception cycles. Hum Reprod 2005; 20: 1596–606.

160. Serhal PF, Ranieri DM, Kinis A, et al. Oocyte morphology predicts outcome of intracytoplasmic sperm injection. Hum Reprod 1997; 12: 1267–70.
161. Meriano JS, Alexis J, Visram-Zaver S, Cruz M, Casper RF. Tracking of oocyte dysmorphisms for ICSI patients may prove relevant to the outcome in subsequent patient cycles. Hum Reprod 2001; 16: 2118–23.
162. Otsuki J, Okada A, Morimoto K, Nagai Y, Kubo H. The relationship between pregnancy outcome and smooth endoplasmic reticulum clusters in MII human oocytes. Hum Reprod 2004; 19: 1591–7.
163. Ebner T, Moser M, Sommergruber M, et al. Occurrence and developmental consequences of vacuoles throughout preimplantation development. Fertil Steril 2005; 83: 1635–40.
164. Wilding M, Di ML, D'Andretti S, et al. An oocyte score for use in assisted reproduction. J Assist Reprod Genet 2007; 24: 350–8.
165. Balakier H, Bouman D, Sojecki A, Librach C, Squire JA. Morphological and cytogenetic analysis of human giant oocytes and giant embryos. Hum Reprod 2002; 17: 2394–401.
166. Scott LA, Smith S. The successful use of pronuclear embryo transfers the day following oocyte retrieval. Hum Reprod 1998; 13: 1003–13.
167. Tesarik J, Greco E. The probability of abnormal preimplantation development can be predicted by a single static observation on pronuclear stage morphology. Hum Reprod 1999; 14: 1318–23.
168. Van Royen E, Mangelschots K, De Neubourg D. Characterization of a top quality embryo, a step towards single-embryo transfer. Hum Reprod 1999; 14: 2345–9.
169. Van Royen E, Mangelschots K, De Neubourg D, et al. Calculating the implantation potential of day 3 embryos in women younger than 38 years of age: a new model. Hum Reprod 2001; 16: 326–32.
170. Gerris J, De Neubourg D, Mangelschots K, et al. Prevention of twin pregnancy after in-vitro fertilization or intracytoplasmic sperm injection based on strict embryo criteria: a prospective randomized clinical trial. Hum Reprod 1999; 14: 2581–7.
171. Gerris J, De Neubourg D, Mangelschots K. Elective single day 3 embryo transfer halves the twinning rate without decrease in the ongoing pregnancy rate of an IVF/ICSI programme. Hum Reprod 2002; 17: 626–31.
172. Scott L. Pronuclear scoring as a predictor of embryo development. Reprod Biomed Online 2003; 6: 201–14.
173. Rienzi L, Ubaldi F, Iacobelli M, et al. Day 3 embryo transfer with combined evaluation at the pronuclear and cleavage stages compares favourably with day 5 blastocyst transfer. Hum Reprod 2002; 17: 1852–5.
174. Lane M, Gardner DK. Selection of viable mouse blastocysts prior to transfer using a metabolic criterion. Hum Reprod 1996; 11: 1975–8.
175. Gardner DK. Changes in requirements and utilization of nutrients during mammalian preimplantation embryo development and their significance in embryo culture. Theriogenology 1998; 49: 83–102.
176. Conaghan J, Hardy K, Handyside AH, Winston RM, Leese HJ. Selection criteria for human embryo transfer: a comparison of pyruvate uptake and morphology. J Assist Reprod Genet 1993; 10: 21–30.
177. Jones GM, Trounson AO, Vella PJ, et al. Glucose metabolism of human morula and blastocyst-stage embryos and its relationship to viability after transfer. Reprod Biomed Online 2001; 3: 124–32.
178. Houghton FD, Hawkhead JA, Humpherson PG, et al. Non-invasive amino acid turnover predicts human embryo developmental capacity. Hum Reprod 2002; 17: 999–1005.
179. Sakkas D, Gardner DK. Noninvasive methods to assess embryo quality. Curr Opin Obstet Gynecol 2005; 17: 283–8.
180. Gianaroli L, Magli MC, Ferraretti AP. The in vivo and in vitro efficiency and efficacy of PGD for aneuploidy. Mol Cell Endocrinol 2001; 22: 8–13.
181. Pehlivan T, Rubio C, Rodrigo L. Impact of preimplantation genetic diagnosis on IVF outcome in implantation failure patients. Reprod Biomed Online 2001; 6: 232–7.
182. Hardarson T, Caisander G, Sjögren A, et al. A morphological and chromosomal study of blastocysts developing from morphologically suboptimal human pre-embryos compared with control blastocysts. Hum Reprod 2003; 18: 399–407.
183. Wang WH, Keefe DL. Prediction of chromosome misalignment among in vitro matured human oocytes by spindle imaging with the PolScope. Fertil Steril 2002; 78: 1077–81.
184. Wang Q, Sun QY. Evaluation of oocyte quality: morphological, cellular and molecular predictors. Reprod Fertil Dev 2007; 19: 1–12.
185. Piquette GN, Tilly JL, Prichard LE, Simon C, Polan ML. Detection of apoptosis in human and rat ovarian follicles. J Soc Gynecol Investig 1994; 1: 297–301.
186. Nakahara K, Saito H, Saito T. The incidence of apoptotic bodies in membrana granulosa can predict prognosis of ova from patients participating in in vitro fertilization programs. Fertil Steril 1997; 68: 312–17.
187. Yuan YQ, Van Soom A, Leroy JL, et al. Apoptosis in cumulus cells, but not in oocytes, may influence bovine embryonic developmental competence. Theriogenology 2005; 63: 2147–63.
188. Seino T, Saito H, Kaneko T, et al. Eight-hydroxy-22-deoxyguanosine in granulosa cells is correlated with the quality of oocytes and embryos in an in vitro fertilization–embryo transfer program. Fertil Steril 2002; 77: 1184–90.
189. Bedaiwy MA, Falcone T, Mohamed MS, et al. Differential growth of human embryos in vitro: role of reactive oxygen species. Fertil Steril 2004; 82: 593–600.
190. Kim KH, Oh DS, Jeong JH, et al. Follicular blood flow is a better predictor of the outcome of in vitro fertilization–Embryo transfer than follicular fluid vascular endothelial growth factor and nitric oxide concentrations. Fertil Steril 2004; 82: 586–92.
191. Lee TH, Wu MY, Chen MJ, et al. Nitric oxide is associated with poor embryo quality and pregnancy outcome in in vitro fertilization cycles. Fertil Steril 2004; 82: 126–31.
192. Zhang X, Jafari N, Barnes RB, et al. Studies of gene expression in human cumulus cells indicate pentraxin 3 as a possible marker for oocyte quality. Fertil Steril 2005; 83: 1169–79.
193. Barroso G, Barrionuevo M, Rao P, et al. Vascular endothelial growth factor, nitric oxide, and leptin fol-

licular fluid levels correlate negatively with embryo quality in IVF patients. Fertil Steril 1999; 72: 1024–6.
194. Tsai EM, Yang CH, Chen SC. Leptin affects pregnancy outcome of in vitro fertilization and steroidogenesis of human granulosa cells. J Assist Reprod Genet 2002; 19: 169–76.
195. Anifandis G, Koutselini E, Louridas K, et al. Estradiol and leptin as conditional prognostic IVF markers. Reproduction 2005; 129: 531–4.
196. Kawano Y, Narahara H, Matsui N, et al. Insulinlike growth factor-binding protein-1 in human follicular fluid: a marker for oocyte maturation. Gynecol Obstet Invest 1997; 44: 145–8.
197. Oosterhuis GJ, Lambalk CB, Michgelsen HW, et al. Follicle-stimulating hormone measured in unextracted urine: a reliable tool for easy assessment of ovarian capacity. Fertil Steril 1998; 70: 544–8.
198. Fried G, Remaeus K, Harlin J, et al. Inhibin B predicts oocyte number and the ratio IGF-I/IGFBP-1 may indicate oocyte quality during ovarian hyperstimulation for in vitro fertilization. J Assist Reprod Genet 2003; 20: 167–76.
199. Chang CL, Wang TH, Horng SG, et al. The concentration of inhibin B in follicular fluid: relation to oocyte maturation and embryo development. Hum Reprod 2002; 17: 1724–8.
200. Xia P, Younglai EV. Relationship between steroid concentrations in ovarian follicular fluid and oocyte morphology in patients undergoing intracytoplasmic sperm injection (ICSI) treatment. J Reprod Fertil 2000; 118: 229–33.
201. Chiu TT, Rogers MS, Law EL, et al. Follicular fluid and serum concentrations of myo-inositol in patients undergoing IVF: relationship with oocyte quality. Hum Reprod 2002; 17: 1591–6.
202. Wunder DM, Mueller MD, Birkhauser MH, Bersinger NA. Steroids and protein markers in the follicular fluid as indicators of oocyte quality in patients with and without endometriosis. J Assist Reprod Genet 2005; 22: 257–64.
203. Wise T, Suss U, Maurer RR. The relationships of oocyte quality and follicular fluid prolactin and progesterone in superovulated beef heifers with and without norgestomet implants. Adv Exp Med Biol 1987; 219: 697–701.
204. Wiswedel K. Granulosa cell metabolism and the assessment of oocyte quality in IVF. Hum Reprod 1987; 2: 589–91.
205. Lindner C, Lichtenberg V, Westhof G, Braendle W, Bettendorf G. Endocrine parameters of human follicular fluid and fertilization capacity of oocytes. Horm Metab Res 1988; 20: 243–6.
206. Preis KA, Seidel G Jr, Gardner DK. Metabolic markers of developmental competence for in vitro-matured mouse oocytes. Reproduction 2005; 130: 475–83.

8

Preparation and evaluation of oocytes for ICSI

Irit Granot and Nava Dekel

INTRODUCTION

Resumption of meiosis in the oocyte is an essential prelude for successful fertilization. The meiotic division of the mammalian oocyte is initiated during fetal life, proceeds up to the diplotene stage of the first prophase, and arrests at birth. Meiotic arrest persists throughout childhood until the onset of puberty. In a sexually mature female, at each cycle one or more oocytes, according to the species, reinitiate the meiotic division. The chromatin in the meiotically arrested oocytes is encapsulated by a nuclear structure known as germinal vesicle (GV; Fig. 8.1A). The GV in oocytes resuming meiosis disappears (Fig. 8.1B), the condensed chromosomes align on the newly formed meiotic spindle, and the pairs of homologous chromosomes segregate between the oocyte and the first polar body (Fig. 8.1C). Emission of the first polar body, which represents the completion of the first round of meiotic division, is immediately followed by the formation of the second meiotic spindle with the remaining set of homologous chromosomes aligned on its equatorial plate. The whole series of events, initiated by GV breakdown (GVB) and completed at the metaphase of the second round of meiosis (MII), leads to the production of a mature fertilizable oocyte, also known as an egg. The egg is arrested at MII and will complete the meiotic division only after the penetration of the spermatozoon (1).

The physiological stimulus for reinitiation of meiosis is provided by the preovulatory surge of luteinizing hormone (LH) (2). Once oocyte maturation is completed, LH further induces ovulation, during which the follicle releases the mature oocyte that is picked up by the infundibular fimbria of the oviduct.

The egg released from the ovarian follicle is accompanied by the cumulus cells. Prior to ovulation, in concomitance with oocyte maturation, the cumulus undergoes characteristic transformations that are also stimulated by LH. In response to this gonadotropin the cumulus cells produce specific glycosaminoglycans, the secretion of which results in cumulus mucification and its expansion. The major component of the extracellular matrix secreted by the cumulus cells is hyaluronic acid (3–7).

The mucified cumulus mass that encapsulates the ovulated egg is penetrated by the spermatozoon that uses enzymes localized on its surface membrane to accomplish this mission. Sperm membrane protein PH-20, which is present on the plasma membrane of sperms of many species such as guinea pigs, mice, macaques, and humans exhibits hyaluronidase-like activity that facilitates this action (8–11). Furthermore, a later study has demonstrated that a plasma membrane–associated hyaluronidase is localized to the posterior acrosomal region of equine sperm (12).

Having traversed the cumulus, the spermatozoon undergoes acrosome reaction and binds to the zona pellucida. Sperm–zona pellucida binding is mediated by specific sperm surface receptors. The primary ligand on the zona pellucida, ZP3, specifically binds to the plasma membrane of the acrosomal cap of the intact sperm. The secondary zona ligand, ZP2, binds to the inner acrosomal membrane of the spermatozoon (13–15). One of the inner acrosomal membrane sperm receptors was identified as acrosin (16–18).

In order to penetrate the zona pellucida the spermatozoon utilizes enzymatic, as well as mechanical mechanisms. Specific enzymes that are released by the acrosome-reacted spermatozoon allow the invasion of the zona pellucida by local degradation of its components (19,20). This enzymatic action is assisted by mechanical force generated by vigorous tail beatings that facilitate the penetration of the sharp sperm head (18–22).

Having penetrated the zona pellucida the sperm crosses the perivitelline space and its head attaches to the egg's plasma membrane (oolemma). Sperm head attachment to the oolemma is followed by its incorporation into the egg cytoplasm (ooplasm). Sperm incorporation is initiated by phagocytosis of the anterior region of its head followed by fusion of the head's posterior region as well as the tail with the egg membrane (23–25).

The scientific efforts that have been invested by reproductive biologists in studying the process of gametogenesis and fertilization in animal models laid the groundwork for the design of in vitro procedures for assisted reproduction. These procedures that are successfully practiced at present in human patients, essentially attempted to mimic the biological processes in vivo. In vitro fertilization (IVF) regimens of treatment, which are continuously being improved, have allowed the birth of over a million babies all over the world.

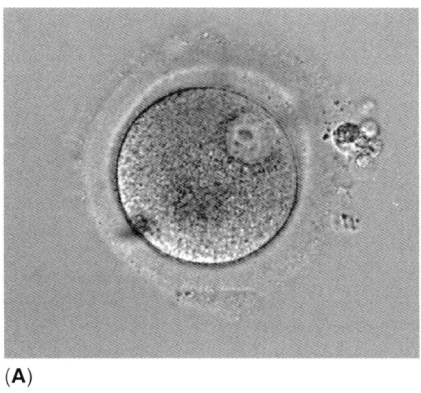 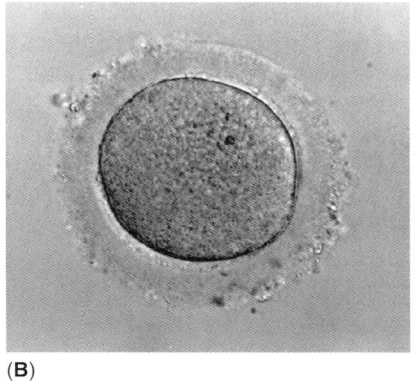 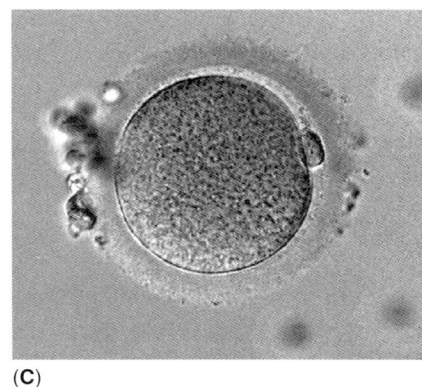

Figure 8.1 Morphological markers characterizing the meiotic status of oocytes. (**A**) Immature germinal vesicle (GV) oocyte: meiosis has not been reinitiated and the typical nuclear structure is visible. (**B**) Immature GV breakdown oocyte (metaphase I, MI): meiosis has been reinitiated, the GV has disappeared, but the first polar body is still absent. (**C**) Mature oocyte (MII): the GV has disappeared and the first polar body has been extruded.

One such improvement, which represents a major breakthrough in this area, is intracytoplasmic sperm injection (ICSI). Until 1992, most infertility failures originating from a severe male factor were untreatable. Micromanipulation techniques such as partial zona dissection (26–29) and subzonal sperm injection (28,30–34), designed to overcome the poor performance of sperm cells, did not result in a substantial improvement of the rate of success of in vivo fertilization. However, ICSI which was established by the team led by Professor Van Steirteghen at the Free University in Brussels, Belgium and initially reported by Palermo et al., (34) has generated dramatic progress (35–38).

The ICSI procedure involves the injection of a single sperm cell intracytoplasmically into an egg. Fertility failures associated with an extremely low sperm count were found to be successfully treated by this technique. Furthermore, as the sperm is microinjected into the ooplasma, it bypasses the passage through the zona pellucida and is not required to interact with the oolemma. Therefore, infertility problems that originate from faulty sperm–egg interaction may also be resolved by this IVF protocol of treatment.

HANDLING OF OOCYTES

Similar to conventional IVF, patients for ICSI undergo programmed induction of superovulation followed by scheduled oocyte retrieval (chap. 7). Under all protocols of treatment, identification of the cumulus–oocyte complexes and evaluation of their maturity are carried out immediately after follicle aspiration, as described in chapter 7. However, unlike conventional IVF, in which intact mature cumulus–oocyte complexes are inseminated, cumulus cells that surround the eggs are removed before microinjection.

Denudation of the mature oocytes is an essential prerequisite for ICSI. Cumulus cells may block the injecting needle, thus interfering with oocyte microinjection. Furthermore, in the presence of the cumulus, visualization of the egg is very limited. Since only mature oocytes that have reached MII are suitable for ICSI, optimal optical conditions that allow the assessment of the meiotic status of the oocytes are required. Oocyte maturation is determined morphologically, by the absence of the GV and the presence of the first polar body. Good optical conditions are also necessary for the positioning of the mature oocyte in the right orientation for injection (chap. 13).

Preparation of the retrieved mature oocytes for ICSI should be carried out under conditions of constant pH of 7.3 and a stable temperature of 37°C. In order to maintain the appropriate pH, 4-(2-hydroxyet4hyl)-1-piperazineethane sulfonic acid (HEPES)-buffered culture media are used. The correct temperature is maintained during egg handling by the use of a microscope equipped with a heated stage. Most of the procedures are performed under Earle's balanced salts solution-treated and CO_2-equilibrated paraffin/mineral oil that prevents evaporation of the medium and minimizes the fluctuations of both the pH and the temperature.

Temperature fluctuations, likely to accompany the handling of eggs have been shown to be specifically detrimental for the microtubular system. Changes in spindle organization were observed in human mature oocytes cooled to room temperature for only 10 minutes. These changes included a reduction in spindle size, disorganization of microtubules within the spindle, and, in some cases, even a complete absence of microtubules (39,40). The susceptibility of the microtubules to temperature variations has been also shown in mature mouse oocytes (41). Interference with spindle organization can disturb the faithful segregation of the chromosomes resulting in aneuploidy.

LABORATORY PROCEDURES

Removal of the surrounding cumulus cells is accomplished by a combined enzymatic and mechanical treatment carried out under a stereoscopic dissecting microscope. A preincubation period of at least three hours between oocyte retrieval and removal of the cumulus cells was recommended by one study (42). This recommendation was challenged by other studies, which did not demonstrate differences in ICSI outcomes that correlated with the time interval between egg aspiration and microinjection (43,44). On the other hand, preincubation time that exceeded nine hours resulted in embryos of lower quality (43). Since oocyte denudation cannot be carried out before some preliminary laboratory preparations that are described below are completed, a preincubation period of at least one hour is unavoidable. During this period, the retrieved mature cumulus–oocyte complexes are kept in the incubator at 37°C with 5–6% CO_2 according to the recommendations of the culture media manufacturer.

Preliminary Preparations for Oocyte Denudation

Injecting Dish

A special shallow Falcon dish (type 1006) is used for placing the denuded eggs. Nine small droplets of HEPES-buffered culture media, 5 µL each, are arranged in a square of 3 × 3 within this dish. An additional 10th droplet serves for orientation. The middle droplet, in which the sperm will be placed, contains 10% polyvinylpyrrolidone. The droplets are then covered with either paraffin or mineral oil, and the dish is placed on the heated area in the hood, to warm up before removal of the cumulus cells.

Enzymatic Solution

Since hyaluronic acid is a major component of the mucified cumulus mass that surrounds the mature oocyte, hyaluronidase is employed for enzymatic removal of these cells (80 IU/mL; Sage In-Vitro fertilization Inc., Trumbull, Connecticut, USA). The high concentration of 760 IU/mL of hyaluronidase that was used initially (1991) was found to induce parthenogenetic activation of the mature oocytes. A lower concentration of the enzyme, such as 80 IU/mL, which is being commonly used, significantly decreased the rate of parthenogenesis (45). According to our experience hyaluronidase at a concentration of 60 IU/mL effectively denudes the oocytes. Others have reported that a concentration as low as 10 IU/mL is also sufficient (46).

Denuding Dish

A drop of 100 µL of hyaluronidase solution and five drops of HEPES-buffered medium covered with oil are placed in a large culture dish and placed on the heated area in the hood to warm up for 10 minutes.

In order to maintain the drops at 37°C, the temperature in the working areas (hood and microscope) must be calibrated to a higher temperature (around 38°C).

Removal of the Cumulus Cells

Cumulus–oocyte complexes are transferred into the drop of hyaluronidase solution and repeatedly aspirated through a Pasteur pipette for up to 30–40 seconds. At this time dissociation of the cells is initially observed. Further mechanical denudation is carried out in the enzyme-free HEPES-buffered medium drops by repeated aspiration through commercially prepared stripper tips with decreasing inner diameters of 150 and 135 µM. The oocytes are then transferred through the drops of medium, until all coronal cells have been finally removed and all traces of enzyme have been washed off. This procedure is carried out very gently in order to avoid mechanical damage to the oocytes. Pricking of the oocyte has been shown to induce parthenogenetic activation (47,48). Finally, the denuded oocytes are placed in the droplets of the injecting dish and their morphology and meiotic status are evaluated. These procedures are performed on the heated area in the hood.

In cases of extremely low sperm count or testicular sperm injection, oocytes must be kept in the incubator in CO_2-equilibrated culture medium until a sufficient number of sperm cells have been collected.

Evaluation of Denuded Oocytes for ICSI

Oocytes are assessed for their maturation and for their morphology under an inverted microscope equipped with Nomarski differential interference contrast optics, at 200× magnification. It is commonly accepted that only mature oocytes that resume their first meiotic division, reaching MII, are appropriate for ICSI. Evaluation of the meiotic status of the oocyte is based on morphological markers. In mature oocytes, the GV has disappeared and the first polar body is present and localized in the perivitelline space (Fig. 8.1C).

Several studies have reported that 10–12% of the retrieved oocytes have not resumed their meiotic division (49–52). These oocytes can be divided into two categories: first, GV oocytes in which meiosis has not been reinitiated and the typical nuclear structure is visible (Fig. 8.1A), and second, GVB oocytes in which meiosis has been reinitiated but did not proceed beyond the first metaphase (MI). In these oocytes the GV has disappeared but the first polar body has not been extruded (Fig. 8.1B). Oocytes in both of these categories are separated from the MII oocytes. MI oocytes are further incubated and those that extrude the first polar body within two to four hours are inseminated by ICSI (53).

It has been reported that 74% of the MI oocytes completed meiosis in vitro within 20 hours after retrieval. This report did not find differences in the rates of fertilization and embryo development between these oocytes and other oocytes retrieved at MII. However, only sporadic pregnancies were achieved following the transfer of embryos obtained from fertilized MI oocytes that had matured in vitro (54,55). Another study demonstrated that 26.7% of MI oocytes extruded the first polar body in vitro within four hours. These oocytes were injected on the same day of follicle aspiration in parallel to the oocytes retrieved at MII. In this study, however, the MI oocytes that completed their maturation in vitro exhibited a lower fertilization rate, but again no differences were observed in embryo quality between oocytes that underwent maturation in vitro and those retrieved at MII. Similar to the previous study, only sporadic pregnancies were obtained following transfer of embryos developed from MI oocytes that had matured in vitro (55,56).

More recent studies support these observations showing that although in vitro-matured (IVM) MI oocytes can be normally fertilized, the embryos derived from these oocytes rarely provide pregnancies (57,58). This is compatible with the findings that these embryos exhibit low morphological quality and a high rate of chromosomal abnormalities (53). In patients with few MII oocytes, rescue of MI oocytes may increase the number of embryos for transfer; however, the chance to improve pregnancy rates by this procedure is minimal.

Oocytes with GV require an overnight (30 hours) incubation in order to reach the MII stage. Only sporadic pregnancies were reported from oocytes that were at the GV stage when retrieved during standard IVF treatment with controlled ovarian hyperstimulation (56,57,59). Because of the poor results, these GV oocytes are usually discarded. Only cases in which very few or no MII oocytes are retrieved, are the GV oocytes rescued for fertilization, provided they complete their maturation.

Immature GV oocytes can also be retrieved from the small (3–13 mm) ovarian follicles present in unstimulated patients (60–63). Although these oocytes were not exposed to LH in vivo, they are apparently meiotically competent and can be expected to mature spontaneously in vitro and produce normal eggs. In 1998, Goud et al. showed a fertilization rate of 46% by ICSI of such IVM GV oocytes, (63) resulting in a few pregnancies. However, as more experience is gained in handling immature oocytes, success rates are increasing worldwide (64,65). Recent studies demonstrated that human chorionic gonadotropin (hCG) administration before oocyte retrieval from the small follicles, accelerates their IVM resulting in better embryonic development and leading to higher pregnancy rates. It was further demonstrated that administration of low doses of FSH before hCG priming, enables the retrieval of in vivo-matured oocytes (MII) from the small follicles (<10 mm). Such oocytes have a higher potential to develop into good-quality embryos than IVM oocytes achieving even higher pregnancy rates (66).

In addition to the meiotic status, the morphology of the oocytes is also evaluated before ICSI. The various morphological defects may be manifested by an amorphic shape of the oocyte, enlargement of or granularity in the perivitelline space, inclusions, vacuolization, granularity and dark color of the cytoplasm, changes in the color and construction of the zona pellucida as well as in the shape and size of the polar body (Fig. 8.2). Most defective oocytes exhibit more than one of the above mentioned abnormalities. All these observations should be recorded and may help in later analysis of the fertilization rate, embryo development, and pregnancy outcomes after ICSI.

The correlation between egg morphology and the rates of fertilization, embryo quality, and pregnancy after ICSI has been extensively studied. Most of the studies reported that abnormal egg morphology of patients undergoing

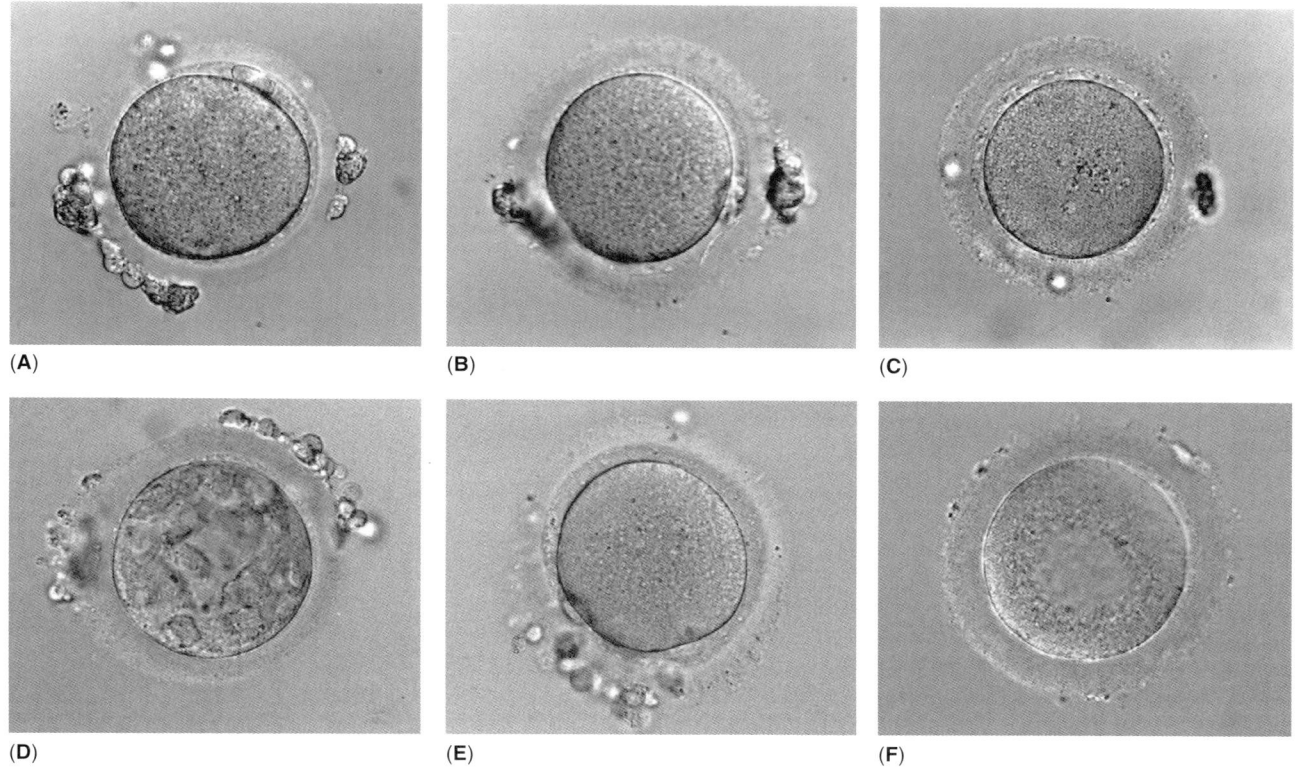

Figure 8.2 Various morphological abnormalities exhibited by oocytes. (**A**) Granulated perivitelline space; (**B**) a fragmented polar body; (**C**) thickened and dark-colored zona pellucida; (**D**) cytoplasmic inclusions; (**E**) enlarged and granulated perivitelline space; and (**F**) a large cytoplasmic vacuole.

ICSI, are associated with a lower rate of fertilization, embryos of poor quality, and, consequently, a lower success of pregnancy (67–69). Other studies demonstrated successful fertilization and normal early embryo development in microinjected eggs with defective morphology, such as large perivitelline space, cytoplasmic vacuoles, or a fragmented polar body (70–73). However, the transfer of these seemingly normal embryos resulted in a poor implantation rate (69) and a high incidence of early pregnancy loss (71). This controversy may be partially attributed to the absence of standard criteria for evaluation of oocyte morphology. To overcome this confusion, the use of triple markers namely polar body, size of the perivitelline space, and cytoplasmic inclusions has been suggested by Xia for human oocyte grading (68). This laboratory reported that the evaluation of oocyte quality based on these criteria correlated well with the rate of fertilization and with embryo quality after ICSI.

As mentioned previously in this chapter, the integrity of the meiotic spindle in MII oocytes is crucial for fertilization capacity and embryo development. Therefore, in addition to the above-mentioned features of the oocyte, the morphology of the spindle may serve as a reliable marker for predicting its potential for normal fertilization and embryonic development (74). A modification of the polarized light microscope, "Polscope" equipped with novel image-processing software (75) has emerged as a noninvasive tool to view the meiotic spindle in living oocytes and is being used in several IVF units worldwide (40,74,76,77). The image of the spindle is based on the highly birefringent characteristic of the microtubule filaments under a polarization microscope. The obvious advantage of the Polscope over conventional techniques such as immunocytochemistry and electron microscopy is that through a Polscope one can view the spindle in a living oocyte.

Use of the Polscope for examination of human oocytes has indeed demonstrated that the absence of, or abnormal morphology of the spindle is highly correlated with lower fertilization rates and impaired embryonic development (76–78). Furthermore, spindle assessment with the Polscope has been shown to facilitate the selection of embryos with high implantation potential for transfer (74). In most MII oocytes, the second meiotic spindle is adjacent to the first polar body (Fig. 8.3B), making the first polar body a marker for appropriate orientation of the ICSI micropipette to avoid interference with chromosome alignment. However, observations by Silva et al. (76) and ourselves that the meiotic spindle is not always adjacent to the polar body (Fig. 8.3C) has made use of the Polscope even more valuable. Furthermore, in those oocytes that have not yet completed the formation of the first polar body, the Polscope can detect the presence of microtubules in the midbody, suggesting that the second meiotic spindle has not yet been fully organized (Fig. 8.3A). These oocytes are considered suitable for ICSI, having high potential for developing into an embryo.

Appropriate ovarian stimulation protocols normally provide functional fertilizable mature oocytes, while oocytes of poor quality may represent a disturbed hormonal balance. For example, exposure to high dosage of human menopausal gonadotropin (hMG) has been shown to be associated with granularity of the perivitelline space (51). Moreover, an extended exposure to high doses of this hormone may lead to the senescence of the mature oocyte before retrieval. As previously mentioned, oocyte maturation and ovulation are both stimulated by LH. However, studies have shown that the ovulatory response is less sensitive to this gonadotropin, requiring higher concentrations of the hormone (79). Therefore, the relatively high concentration of LH in hMG effectively promotes oocyte maturation, but is insufficient to stimulate ovulation. Delayed administration of hCG in these patients entraps the mature oocytes in the follicle, leading to oocyte aging. One notable morphological marker in this case is the fragmentation of the first polar body (80). The presence of aged oocytes can also explain the decreased quality of oocytes and lower fertilization rate in polycystic ovarian syndrome patients (81) who exhibit relatively high serum concentrations of LH throughout their menstrual cycle (82). Nowadays pure FSH preparations (recombinant FSH) are widely used for

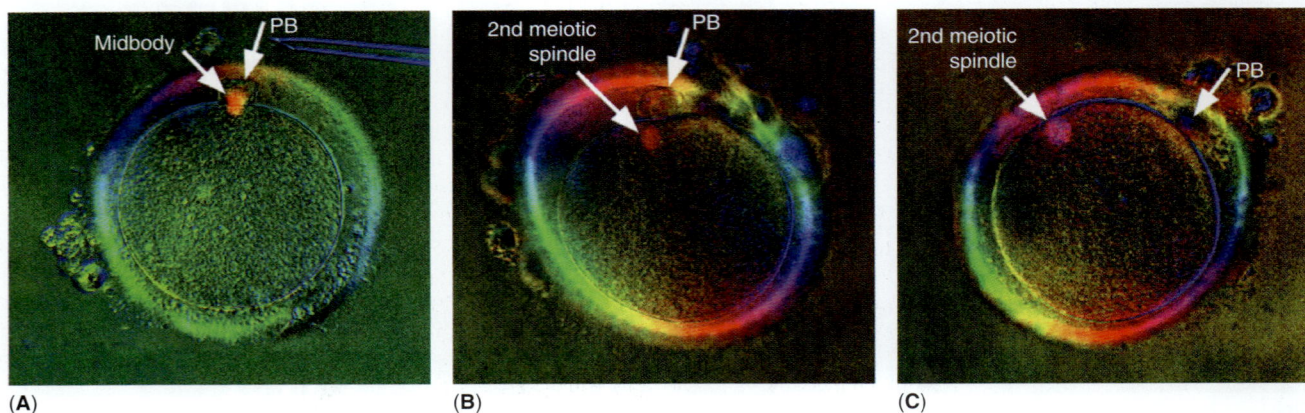

Figure 8.3 Microtubule images in metaphase II (MII) human oocytes. (**A**) Microtubules of the midbody extending from the cytoplasm into the first polar body (PB). (**B**) Microtubules of the second meiotic spindle located adjacent to the PB. (**C**) Microtubules of the second meiotic spindle at a distal location from the PB.

stimulation of follicular growth and development. However, it has been demonstrated that introducing low concentrations of LH (recombinant LH) in addition to FSH significantly improves IVF outcomes (82).

EPILOGUE

A baby girl is born with her ovaries containing about 2 million oocytes all of which arrested at the prophase of the first meiotic division. This pool of oocytes remains dormant throughout childhood until the onset of puberty. In sexually mature females, at each cycle, one such "sleeping beauty" is being kissed by the LH "prince" and awakened to continue its meiotic division. Once maturation has been completed the oocyte is released from the ovarian follicle into the fallopian tube, a site at which it will eventually meet the spermatozoon and undergo fertilization.

Hormonal stimulation protocols are designed to mimic the natural events that lead to the production of mature oocytes. In IVF patients, these oocytes are aspirated from the ovarian follicles prior to ovulation and allowed to meet the sperm cells in the Petri dish. A higher scale of assistance, designed to overcome the poor performance of spermatozoa, is offered by ICSI. The information regarding oocyte handling for this later modification of the classical IVF protocol has been summarized in this chapter.

APPENDIX

Laboratory Protocol

The following protocol is used in our laboratory:

Preliminary Preparations for Oocyte Denudation

1. Injecting dish: Place nine, 5 µL each, droplets of HEPES-buffered human tubal fluid medium containing 10% synthetic serum, arranged in a 3 × 3 square within a shallow Falcon dish (type 1006). Place one additional droplet for orientation. Cover with oil. Replace 4 µL of the middle droplet, with a solution of 10% polyvinylpyrrolidone where the sperm will be placed. Place the dish on the heated area in the hood to warm up. In cases of extremely low sperm counts, more than one droplet can be used for sperm.
2. Enzymatic solution: Dilute hyaluronidase solution of 80 IU/mL (Sage) with HEPES-buffered human tubal fluid medium containing 10% serum, to obtain a final concentration of 60 IU/mL and warm to 37°C.
3. Denuding dish: Place a drop of 100 µL of the above hyaluronidase solution and five drops of enzyme-free HEPES-buffered medium in a large culture dish. Cover with oil and place on the heated area in the hood to warm up.
4. Prepare two stripper tips with inner diameters of 150 and 135 µm.

Removal of the Cumulus Cells

1. Place the cumulus–oocyte complexes into the drop of the hyaluronidase solution (up to five complexes at a time) and aspirate repeatedly through a Pasteur pipette for up to 40 seconds.
2. Transfer the cumulus–oocyte complexes to a drop of enzyme-free HEPES-buffered medium and aspirate repeatedly through a 150 µµ diameter stripper tip. Continue aspirating with a 135 µm tip while passing the oocytes through the other four drops of the medium, until all coronal cells have been totally removed.
3. Transfer the denuded oocytes to the droplets of HEPES-buffered medium in the injecting dish, one in each droplet.

Microscopic Evaluation

1. Place the injecting dish containing the oocytes on the heated stage of an inverted microscope equipped with differential interference contrast.
2. Evaluate oocyte morphology and meiotic status at 200× magnification.

REFERENCES

1. Dekel N, Aberdam E, Goren S, Feldman B, Shalgi R. Mechanism of action of GnRH-induced oocyte maturation. J Reprod Fert 1989; 37: 319–27.
2. Lindner HR, Tsafriri A, Lieberman ME, et al. Gonadotropin action on cultured Graafian follicles: induction of maturation division of the mammalian oocyte and differentiation of the luteal cell. Recent Prog Horm Res 1974; 30: 79–138.
3. Dekel N. Hormonal control of ovulation. In: Litwack G, ed, Biochemical Action of Hormones. Orlando, Florida: Academic Press, 1986. 13: 57–90.
4. Buccione R, Vanderhyden BC, Caron PJ, Eppig JJ. FSH-induced expansion of the mouse cumulus oophorus in vitro is dependent upon a specific factor(s) secreted by the oocyte. Dev Biol 1990; 138: 16–25.
5. Salustri A, Yanagishita M, Hascall VC. Mouse oocytes regulate hyaluronic acid synthesis and mucification by FSH-stimulated cumulus cells. Dev Biol 1990; 138: 26–32.
6. Vanderhyden BC, Caron PJ, Buccione R, Eppig JJ. Developmental pattern of the secretion of cumulus expansion-enabling factor by mouse oocytes and the role of oocytes in promoting granulosa cell differentiation. Dev Biol 1990; 140: 307–17.
7. Vanderhyden BC. Species differences in the regulation of cumulus expansion by an oocyte secreted factor(s). J Reprod Fertil 1993; 98: 219–27.
8. Lin Y, Mahan K, Lathorp W, Myles D, Primakoff P. A hyaluronidase activity of the sperm plasma membrane protein PH-20 enables sperm to penetrate the cumulus cell layer surrounding the egg. J Cell Biol 1994; 125: 1157–63.
9. Cherr G, Meyers S, Yudin A, et al. The PH-20 protein in cynomolgus macaque spermatozoa: identification of two different forms exhibiting hyaluronidase activity. Dev Biol 1996; 175: 142–53.
10. Oversreet J, Lin Y, Yudin A, et al. Location of the PH-20 protein on acrosome-intact and acrosome-reacted spermatozoa of cynomolgus macaques. Biol Reprod 1995; 52: 105–14.

11. Sabeur K, Cherr G, Yudin A, et al. The PH-20 protein in human spermatozoa. J Androl 1997; 18: 151–8.
12. Meyers SA, Rosenberger AE. A plasma membrane-associated hyaluronidase is localized to the posterior acrosomal region of stallion sperm and is associated with spermatozoal function. Biol Reprod 1999; 61: 444–51.
13. Bleil JD, Wasserman PM. Autoradiographic visualization of the mouse egg's sperm receptor bound to sperm. J Cell Biol 1986; 102: 1363–71.
14. Beaver EL, Friend DS. Morphology of mammalian sperm membranes during differentiation, maturation, and capacitation. J Electr Microscop Tech 1990; 16: 281–97.
15. Mortillo S, Wasserman PM. Differential binding of gold-labeled zona pellucida glycoproteins mZP2 and mZP3 to mouse sperm membrane compartments. Development 1991; 113: 141–9.
16. Jones R. Interaction of zona pellucida glycoproteins, sulphated carbohydrates and synthetic polymers with proacrosin, the putative egg-binding protein from mammalian spermatozoa. Development 1991; 111: 1155–63.
17. Urch UA, Patel H. The interaction of boar sperm proacrosin with its natural substrate, the zona pellucida, and with polysulphated polysaccharides. Development 1991; 111: 1165–72.
18. Yanagimachi R. Fertilization and Embryonic Development in vitro. New York: Plenum Press, 1981.
19. Brown CR, Cheng WTK. Limited proteolysis of the porcine zona pellucida by homologous sperm acrosin. J Reprod Fertil 1985; 74: 257–60.
20. Dunbar BS, Prasad SV, Timmons TM. Comparative overview of mammalian fertilization. New York: Plenum Press, 1991.
21. Dunbar BS, Budkiewicz AB, Bundman DS. Proteolysis of specific porcine zona pellucida glycoproteins by boar acrosin. Biol Reprod 1985; 32: 619–30.
22. Yanagimachi R. Time and process of sperm penetration into hamster ova in vivo and in vitro. J Reprod Fertil 1966; 11: 359–70.
23. Phillips DM, Shalgi RM. Sperm penetration into rat ova fertilized in vivo. J Exp Zool 1982; 221: 373–8.
24. Shalgi R, Phillips D. Mechanics of sperm entry in cycling hamsters. J Ultrastruct Res 1980; 71: 154–61.
25. Shalgi R, Phillips DM, Jones R. Status of the rat acrosome during sperm-zona pellucida interactions. Gamete Res 1989; 22: 1–13.
26. Cohen J, Malter H, Fehilly C, et al. Implantation of embryos after partial opening of oocyte zonal pellucida to facilitate sperm penetration. Lancet 1988; 2: 162.
27. Cohen J, Malter H, Wright G, et al. Partial zona dissection of human oocytes when failure of zona pellucida is anticipated. Hum Reprod 1989; 4: 435–42.
28. Cohen J, Talanski BE, Malter HM, et al. Microsurgical fertilization and teratozoospermia. Hum Reprod 1991; 6: 118–23.
29. Tucker MJ, Bishop FM, Cohen J, et al. Routine application of partial zona dissection for male factor infertility. Hum Reprod 1991; 6: 676–81.
30. Laws-King A, Trounson A, Sathananthan H, et al. Fertilization of human oocytes by microinjection of single spermatozoon under zona pellucida. Fertil Steril 1987; 48: 637–42.
31. Ng SC, Bongso A, Ratnam SS, et al. Pregnancy after transfer sperm under zona. Lancet 1988; 2: 790.
32. Bongso TA, Sathananthan AH, Wong C, et al. Human fertilization by microinjection of immotile spermatozoa. Hum Reprod 1989; 4: 175–9.
33. Palermo G, Joris H, Devoroey P, et al. Induction of acrosome reaction in human spermatozoa used subzonal insemination. Hum Reprod 1992; 7: 248–54.
34. Palermo G, Joris H, Devoroey P, et al. Pregnancies after intracytoplasmic injection of a single spermatozoon into an oocyte. Lancet 1992; 340: 17–18.
35. Palermo G, Joris H, Devoroey P, et al. Sperm characteristics and outcome of human assisted fertilization by subzonal insemination and intracytoplasmic sperm injection. Fertil Steril 1993; 59: 826–35.
36. Van Steirteghem AC, Liu J, Nagy Z, et al. Use of assisted fertilization. Hum Reprod 1993; 8: 1784–5.
37. Van Steirteghem AC, Liu J, Joris H, et al. Higher success rate by intracytoplasmic sperm injection than by subzonal insemination. Reprod of second series of 300 consecutive treatment cycles. Hum Reprod 1993; 8: 1055–60.
38. Van Steirteghem AC, Nagy Z, Joris H, et al. High fertilization and implantation rates after intracytoplasmic sperm injection. Hum Reprod 1993; 8: 1061–6.
39. Pickering SJ, Braude PR, Johnson MH, Cant A, Currie J. Transient cooling to room temperature can cause irreversible disruption of the meiotic spindle in the human oocyte. Fertil Steril 1990; 54: 102–8.
40. Wang WH, Meng L, Hackett RJ, Odenbourg R, Keefe DL. Limited recovery of meiotic spindle in living human oocytes after cooling-rewarming observed using polarized microscopy. Hum Reprod 2001; 16: 2374–8.
41. Magistrini M, Szollosi D. Effects of cold and isopropyl-N-phenylcarbamate on the second meiotic spindle of mouse oocytes. Eur J Cell Biol 1980; 22: 699–707.
42. Rienzi L, Ubaldi F, Anniballo R, Cerulo G, Greco E. Preincubation of human oocytes may improve fertilization and embryo quality after intracytoplasmic sperm injection. Hum Reprod 1998; 13: 1014–19.
43. Yanagida K, Yazawa H, Katayose H, et al. Influence of preincubation time on fertilization after intracytoplasmic sperm injection. Hum Reprod 1998; 13: 2223–6.
44. Van de Velde H, De Vos A, Joris H, Nagy ZP, Van Steirteghem AC. Effect of timing of oocyte denudation and micro-injection on survival, fertilization and embryo quality after intracytoplasmic sperm injection. Hum Reprod 1998; 13: 3160–4.
45. Joris H, Nagy Z, Van de Velde H, De Vos A, Van Steirteghem A. Intracytoplasmic sperm injection: laboratory set-up and injection procedure. Hum Reprod 1998; 13(Suppl 1): 76–86.
46. Van de Velde H, Nagy ZP, Joris H, De Vos A, Van Steirteghem AC. Effects of different hyaluronidase concentrations and mechanical procedures for cumulus cell removal on the outcome of intracytoplasmic sperm injection. Hum Reprod 1997; 12: 2246–50.
47. Iritani A. Micromanipulation of gametes for in vitro assisted fertilization. Mol Reprod Dev 1991; 28: 199–207.
48. Flaherty SP, Payne D, Swann NG, et al. Aetiology of failed and abnormal fertilization after intracytoplasmic sperm injection. Hum Reprod 1995; 10: 2629–32.
49. Junca AM, Mandelbaum J, Belaisch-Allert J, et al. Oocyte maturity and quality: value of intracytoplasmic sperm injection. Fertility of microinjected oocytes after

in vitro maturation. Contracept Fertil Sex 1995; 23: 463–645.
50. Mandelbaum J, Junca AM, Balaisch-Allert J, et al. Oocyte maturation and intracytoplasmic sperm injection. Contracept Fertil Sex 1996; 24: 534–8.
51. Hassan-Ali H, Hisham-Saleh A, El-Gezeiry D, et al. Perivitelline space granularity: a sign of human menopausal gonadotropin overdose in intracytoplasmic sperm injection. Hum Reprod 1998; 13: 4325–30.
52. De Vos A, Van de Velde H, Joris H, Van Steirteghem A. In-vitro matured metaphase-I oocytes have a lower fertilization rate but similar embryo quality as mature metaphase-II oocytes after intracytoplasmic sperm injection. Hum Reprod 1999; 14: 1859–63.
53. Strassburger D, Goldstein A, Friedler S, et al. The cytogenetic constitution of embryos derived from immature (metaphase I) oocytes obtained after ovarian hyperstimulation. Fertil Steril 2010; 94: 971–8.
54. Coetzee K, Windt ML. Fertilization and pregnancy using metaphase I oocytes in an intracytoplasmic sperm injection program. J Assist Reprod Genet 1996; 13: 768–71.
55. Strassburger D, Friedler S, Raziel A, et al. The outcome of ICSI of immature MI oocytes and rescued in vitro matured MII oocytes. Hum Reprod 2004; 19: 1587–90.
56. Nagy ZP, Cecile J, Liu J, et al. Pregnancy and birth after intracytoplasmic sperm injection of in vitro matured germinal-vesicle stage oocytes: case report. Fertil Steril 1996; 65: 1047–50.
57. Jaroudi KA, Hollanders JMG, Sieck UV, et al. Pregnancy after transfer of embryos which were generated from in-vitro matured oocytes. Hum Reprod 1997; 12: 857–9.
58. Liu J, Katz E, Garcia JE, et al. Successful in vitro maturation of human oocytes not exposed to human chorionic gonadotropin during ovulation induction, resulting in pregnancy. Fertil Steril 1997; 67: 566–8.
59. Menezo YJ, Nicollet B, Rollet J, Hazout A. Pregnancy and delivery after in vitro maturation of naked ICSI-GV oocytes with GH and transfer of a frozen thawed blastocyst: case report. J Assist Reprod Genet 2006; 23: 47–9.
60. Edrishinghe WR, Junk SM, Matson PL, Yovich JL. Birth from cryopreserved embryos following in-vitro maturation of oocytes and intracytoplasmic sperm injection. Hum Reprod 1997; 12: 1056–8.
61. Trounson A, Anderiesz C, Jones GM, et al. Oocyte maturation. Hum Reprod 1998; 13(Suppl 3): 52–62; (discussion) 71–5.
62. Russel JB. Immature oocyte retrieval with in-vitro maturation. Curr Opin Obstet Gynecol 1999; 11: 289–96.
63. Goud PT, Goud AP, Qian C, et al. In-vitro maturation of human germinal vesicle stage oocytes: role of cumulus cells and epidermal growth factor in the culture medium. Hum Reprod 1998; 13: 1638–44.
64. Mikkelsen AL. Strategies in human in-vitro maturation and their clinical outcome. Reprod Biomed Online 2005; 10: 593–9.
65. Al-Sunaidi M, Tulandi T, Holzer H, et al. Repeated pregnancies and live births after in vitro maturation treatment. Fertil Steril 2007; 87: 1212. e9–12.
66. Weon-Young S, Seang LT. Laboratory and embryological aspect of hCG-primed in vitro maturation cycles for patients with polycystic ovaries. Hum Reprod 2010; 6: 675–89.
67. Sousa M, Tesarik J. Ultrastructural analysis of fertilization failure after intracytoplasmic sperm injection. Hum Reprod 1994; 9: 2374–80.
68. Xia P. Intracytoplasmic sperm injection: correlation of oocyte grade based on polar body, perivitelline space and cytoplasmic inclusions with fertilization rate and embryo quality. Hum Reprod 1997; 12: 1750–5.
69. Loutradis D, Drakakis P, Kallianidis K, et al. Oocyte morphology correlates with embryo quality and pregnancy rate after intracytoplasmic sperm injection. Fertil Steril 1999; 72: 240–4.
70. De Sutter P, Dozortsev D, Qian C, Dhont M. Oocyte morphology does not correlate with fertilization rate and embryo quality after intracytoplasmic sperm injection. Hum Reprod 1996; 11: 595–7.
71. Alikani M, Palermo G, Adler A, et al. Intracytoplasmic sperm injection in dismorphic human oocytes. Zygote 1995; 3: 283–8.
72. Serhal PF, Ranieri DM, Kinis A, et al. Oocyte morphology predicts outcome of intracytoplasmic sperm injection. Hum Reprod 1997; 12: 1267–70.
73. Balaban B, Urman B, Sertac A, et al. Oocyte morphology does not affect fertilization rate, embryo quality and implantation rate after intracytoplasmic sperm injection. Hum Reprod 1998; 13: 3431–3.
74. Kilani S, Cooke S, Tilia L, Chapman M. Does meiotic spindle normality predict improved blastocyst development, implantation and live birth rates? Fertil Steril 2011; 96: 389–93.
75. Oldenbourg R, Mei G. New polarized light microscope with precision universal compensator. J microsc 1995; 180: 140–7.
76. Silva CP, Kommineni K, Oldenbourg R, Keefe DL. The first polar body does not predict accurately the location of the metaphase II meiotic spindle in mammalian oocytes. Fertil Steril 1999; 71: 719–21.
77. Wang WH. Spindle observation and its relationship with fertilization after ICSI in living human oocytes. Fertil Steril 2001; 75: 348–53.
78. Moon JH, Hyun CS, Lee SW, et al. Visualization of the metaphase II meiotic spindle in living human oocytes using the Polscope enables the prediction of embryonic developmental competence after ICSI. Hum Reprod 2003; 18: 817–20.
79. Dekel N, Ayalon D, Lewysohn O, et al. Experimental extension of the time interval between oocyte maturation and ovulation: effect on fertilization and first cleavage. Fertil Steril 1995; 64: 1023–8.
80. Eichenlaub-Ritter U, Schmiady H, Kentenich H, et al. Recurrent failure in polar body formation and premature chromosome condensation in oocytes from a human patient: indicators of asynchrony in nuclear and cytoplasmic maturation. Hum Reprod 1995; 10: 2343–9.
81. Aboulghar MA, Mansour RT, Serour GI, Ramzy AM, Amin YM. Oocyte quality in patients with severe ovarian hyperstimulation syndrome. Fertil Steril 1997; 68: 1017–21.
82. Shoham Z, Jacobs HS, Insler V. Luteinizing hormone: its role, mechanism of action, and detrimental effects when hypersecreted during the follicular phase. Fertil Steril 1993; 59: 1153–61.
83. Franco JC Jr, Baruffi RLR, Oliveira JBA, et al. Effects of recombinant LH supplementation to recombinant FSH during induced ovarian stimulation in the GnRH-agonist protocol: a matched case-control study. Reprod Biol Endocrinol 2010; 94: 971–8.

9

Hyaluronic acid binding-mediated sperm selection for ICSI

Gabor Huszar

INTRODUCTION AND OVERVIEW

Intracytoplasmic sperm injection, or ICSI, was introduced in the mid 1990s, for treatment of male infertility patients with low sperm concentration and motility as a primary indication (1). ICSI can also be used in nonoligozoospermic men, either in those with unexplained male infertility, characterized by normal seminal sperm concentration and motility yet diminished fertilizing potential, or spermatozoa with diminished paternal contribution. Other patients, with normal or close-to-normal sperm concentration and motility, are treated with ICSI in order to increase fertilization rates and pregnancy success, particularly in couples that failed to achieve pregnancy in previous IVF cycles. As it will be discussed, a key issue of ICSI is sperm quality, which depends on the method of sperm selection. Sperm quality may be assessed by the objective sperm biomarkers that have been the primary focus of the Huszar laboratory in the past two decades (2).

Regarding ICSI sperm selection, it should be recognized that ideally, due to the historically known incidence of various adverse genetic events as a consequence of physiological fertilization, one will prefer to select and use for ICSI a sperm that exhibits properties of sperm normally binding to the zona pellucida of oocytes, and thus participate in physiological conception by intercourse or conventional in vitro fertilization (IVF). Hence, in sperm that participates in zona pellucida-interaction-based conception, the occurrence of genetic abnormalities and congenital adverse outcomes are already known.

SCIENTIFIC BASIS OF HYALURONIC ACID-MEDIATED SPERM SELECTION

The hyaluronic acid (HA) based sperm selection is based on the recognition of molecular and cellular aspects of sperm maturation, particularly the attributes of that are normally developed spermatozoa selected by nature for spontaneous fertilization. Conversely, it is now well established that the presence of some sperm attributes indicate failed development and so diminished fertilizing potential or deficient sperm paternal contribution (2).

Recognitions of such positive or negative sperm characteristics have evolved, biomarkers have been identified, and their role in sperm fertilizing potential, implantation, and success in causing pregnancy has been examined. In the first approach, sperm creatine kinase (CK) content and activity has been assessed, which reflects the presence of surplus cytoplasm, due to incomplete sperm cytoplasmic extrusion which is a key event of spermiogenesis (3–5). Indeed, it has been observed that normal spermatozoa which completed cytoplasmic extrusion are the only ones that are able to bind to the zona pellucida or to hemizonae (these are unfertilized human oocytes which were bisected in order to avoid inadvertent fertilization) (6). This experiment provided three novel conclusions of paramount importance: (*i*) sperm that failed to undergo cytoplasmic extrusion are unable to bind to the zona pellucida; (*ii*) sperm–oocyte interaction during fertilization is directed and regulated by the attributes of the spermatozoa. (*iii*) Another key element in the contemporary sperm research has been the recognition of the sperm plasma membrane remodeling, simultaneously with cytoplasmic extrusion in terminal spermiogenesis. This remodeling facilitates the formation of the zona pellucida-binding site(s) in spermatozoa. Thus, sperm that fail to undergo the plasma membrane remodeling process are unable to recognize the zona pellucida, and thus the fertilizing potential of such sperm is diminished. It has also been demonstrated that this failure of cytoplasmic extrusion and plasma membrane remodeling is linked to upstream higher spermatogenetic and spermiogenetic defects which adversely affect chromatin development, DNA integrity, and the frequency of chromosomal aneuploidies (2).

Another key biomarker identified in human sperm is the chaperone protein HspA2 (7,8). This protein is homologous to the HSP70 which has been found in the mouse system (9–11). Measurements of HspA2 levels in human sperm fractions has indicated that HspA2, which is part of the synaptonemal complex and also a key element of intracellular transport of DNA repair enzymes and other housekeeping elements in the developing spermatozoa, is a very important indicator of sperm fertilizing potential (12). HspA2 is also involved in the control of sperm DNA chain integrity and aneuploidy frequency. In the clinical arena, the markers of sperm CK and HspA2 levels were tested with respect to pregnancy success in blinded studies of intrauterine insemination (IUI) or IVF couples. The data indicated that the sperm CK content (a measure of excess cytoplasm in sperm) and HspA2 levels; provide an objective measure of sperm fertilizing potential. The first study was conducted on couples with oligozoospermic husbands who were treated with IUI. When sperm CK contents of couples with successful pregnancy and lack of pregnancy were compared, the data indicated that pregnancy success had no relationship with sperm concentrations, motility, or the amount of sperm inseminated. The important factor was sperm CK activity, which reflects sperm cytoplasmic content. The lower CK activity patients who had undergone cytoplasmic extrusion showed significantly higher pregnancy rates compared with those who had high CK activity and cytoplasmic retention. This indicates that the sperm biomarker CK reflecting extra cytoplasm is a negative factor with respect to fertility and pregnancy occurrence, whereas sperm concentration, motility, and total motile sperm are not contributing to the relationship between sperm developmental integrity and fertility, whether due to the fertilization process or to sperm paternal contribution (13).

The predictive value of sperm CK and HspA2 levels was also tested in the IVF setting. Similar to the IUI study, when the sperm CK activity was high in the samples, the IVF pregnancy success rate has declined in spite of comparable sperm concentration and motility in the semen samples with high CK and low HspA2 levels. In a blind collaborative study between Yale and Norfolk, we have analyzed IVF cycles in 82 couples and found that if the sperm CK activity in the husband's normozoospermic samples was high, the couples did not achieve pregnancy (14). In a similar study where sperm HspA2 was measured, we had a similar experience. With low HspA2 levels, there was a lack of pregnancies. In both of these studies, there were about 15% of men who were normozoospermic with good sperm concentration and motility, yet they did not achieve pregnancy either in the CK-focused or in the HspA2 chaperone protein-focused IVF groups (12). This is the basis for the idea of "unexplained male infertility" a concept (diminished fertility in spite of normal sperm concentration and motility) that we developed during the 1990s.

The discovery of the HspA2 chaperone in sperm has led our group to the developmental aspects of sperm genetic integrity. First, HspA2 is part of the synaptonemal complex of the developing sperm cell and, thus, the low levels of chaperone protein are leading to problems with respect to chromosomal aneuploidies, including disomies and diploidies. This phenomenon of the relationship between cytoplasmic retention and low HspA2 levels, as they are related to increase in chromosomal aneuploidies, was well demonstrated by the report of Kovanci et al. (15). When the spermatozoa were sorted by gradient centrifugation, sperm with cytoplasmic retention, which have decreased specific gravity due to the presence of cytoplasm, were compared with the developed spermatozoa following cytoplasmic extrusion. The sperm fraction with extra surplus cytoplasm exhibited a two and a half times higher incidence of chromosomal aneuploidies. Indeed, in the lighter sperm fraction, there was a close correlation ($r = 0.75$, $p < 0.002$) between residual cytoplasm and disomies of the 17 and Y chromosomes, as well as that of the XY sex chromosome.

The remodeling of sperm plasma membrane during spermiogenesis is extremely important. We have assessed in the same sperm fractions the amount of residual cytoplasm and also the presence of the enzyme galactosyltransferase, a unique sperm membrane marker signifying the normal development of the sperm plasma membrane. There was a very close inverse correlation ($r = >-0.9$) indicating that the spermatozoa which have surplus cytoplasm do also exhibit arrested sperm plasma membrane remodeling, Thus, sperm with the increased CK activity, indicating the failure of cytoplasmic extrusion, are unable to recognize and bind to the zona pellucida. These data are very important because they indicate that sperm plasma membrane remodeling is important in the formation of the zona pellucida-binding sites and development of sperm fertilizing potential (16).

SPERM PLASMA MEMBRANE REMODELING AND FORMATION OF THE ZONA PELLUCIDA RECEPTOR AND THE NEWLY RECOGNIZED HA RECEPTOR

HA or hyaluronan is a complex bioactive agent, which is well represented in the female reproductive tract. It is part of the cervical mucus spinnbarkeit during ovulation, and it is also a component of the cumulus oophorus which surrounds the oocytes. We recognized the sperm–HA interaction by observing that in the presence of HA, human sperm exhibited a substantially increased tail cross-beat frequency. Further, when we applied solid-state HA to a glass slide or a plastic surface, some of the sperm attached to it with head first: the sperm progress was diminished secondary to the head attachment, yet the tail-beating frequency increased and was maintained, sometimes even for days (17,18). During sperm plasma membrane remodeling in spermiogenesis, along with the formation of the zona pellucida receptors, receptors for HA are also formed. The common origin of the zona pellucida and HA receptors on sperm indicates that sperm binding to HA will also bind to the zona pellucida. Thus, the idea was conceived that we may select spermatozoa that would be participating in zona pellucida binding via a hyaluronan-mediated sperm selection (19).

The observations regarding the common origin of the zona pellucida and HA receptor lead to two important inventions:

1. For the first time in the history of andrology, there is now a 10 minutes laboratory semen test (in addition to assessment of sperm concentration, motility and

morphology), which predicts what percent of sperm in an ejaculate will have zona-binding properties (thus normally developed) and fertilizing potential. This is a very important advance and opportunity for physicians and patients (20).
2. The individual HA-bound spermatozoa are removable and may be used for intracytoplasmic sperm injection. This provides the opportunity for the embryologist to have ICSI fertilization with sperm which normally would have been fertilized in the zona pellucida–mediated physiological circumstances during intercourse or IVF. The shape and biochemical properties, as well as genetic attributes of HA-selected sperm are comparable to that of the zona pellucida-bound sperm that may perform the fertilization following physiological sperm–zona pellucida interaction. In the past few years, both HA-mediated devices, the sperm HA-binding assessment in the Andrology laboratory, and the ICSI sperm selection device, the so-called PICSI dish (an IVF Petri dish that carries an HA spot), has been increasingly accepted and used worldwide (21).

METHODS OF HA-MEDIATED ICSI SPERM SELECTION USING PICSI DISHES

The methods of PICSI dish mediated sperm selection, according to the manufacturer suggestions, maybe summarized as follows:

1. Sperm preparation is normally performed by using density gradient protocol (45% and 90% Isolate). A PICSI dish (a modified Petri dish) has orienting lines; each ending with a round HA-coated spot, in order to facilitate the approach to sperm selection. Washing media 5 to 10 µl (e.g., modified human tubal fluid with 10% human serum albumin) is added to each ring at 37°C, under sterile conditions, and covered up with oil.
2. Thereafter, 1–5 µl of sperm suspension prepared in fertilization media (the suspension is ready for ICSI) should be placed into the media drop around the PICSI HA spot. (The volume of the sperm suspension will depend on the motile sperm concentration in the suspension; the lower the motile sperm concentration, the more sperm suspension media is needed.)
3. The incubation with the PICSI dishes is carried out for 5–15 minutes at 34–36° C (The PICSI dish has some temperature filtering effect, thus alteration of the stage temperature should not be mandatory. During the observation time one can clearly distinguish between spermatozoa which are normally developed, have undergone the plasma membrane remodeling, and bind to the HA spot, as well as exhibit a higher tail cross-beat frequency and the dysmature spermatozoa that do not perceive the HA, and swims along.
4. Following the observation step, the PICSI dish is moved to the micromanipulation microscope. At this time Petri dishes should be ready to store the sperm collected from the PICSI dishes. Sperm should be collected using ICSI (microinjection) needle. In 5 to 15 minutes incubation time, there will be enough sperms attached to the HA spot. Using an ICSI needle 10–100 of attached sperm should be collected. The embryologist should prefer to pick up and collect sperm with the fastest sperm tail cross-beat frequency. This is important because of the sperm with a faster tail cross-beat frequency have a more enhanced HA receptor density, indicating that the sperm membrane remodeling has been more effective.
5. The sperm are collected from the PICSI HA spot with an ICSI needle and ejected into a sperm ICSI washing medium. This will be followed by the routine procedure of ICSI injection with the collected and washed sperm.

ATTRIBUTES OF HYALURONAN-BOUND SPERM

As discussed in the section on sperm biomarkers and sperm development, sperm with normal development and hyaluronan-binding properties (reflecting the completion of plasma membrane remodeling) show an inverse correlation with DNA degradation, diminished histone–protamine transition, or excess persistent histones and dark aniline blue staining (2). Further biomarkers are the presence or absence of caspase-3 and apoptotic changes, and the positive correlation between aneuploidy and abnormal sperm forms, as detailed in the paper on the relationship between sperm cytoplasmic retention, related abnormal morphology, and increased rates of chromosomal aneuploidies (22,23). However, it is also true that normal sperm morphology does not assure of low frequency of chromosomal aneuploidy. This was established in our studies demonstrating that the shape properties of sperm in the native or decondensed and denatured states necessary for fluorescence in situ hybridization have remained identical. Thus, we could study shape and aneuploidy in the same spermatozoa (23).

Regarding the features of arrested sperm development and biomarkers of sperm functional integrity, the work of Sati et al. provided a major insight into a very complex and intriguing feature (24). An inventive approach (aniline blue staining, recording of the sperm fields and destaining, followed by application of a second biomarker: see experiment design, Fig. 9.1) facilitated the study of double-stained spermatozoa, including aniline blue staining coupled with CK immunostaining (increased histone retention and cytoplasmic retention, Fig. 9.2), aniline blue staining and DNA fragmentation (histone retention and DNA fragmentation studied by in situ DNA nick translation, Fig. 9.3) and aniline blue staining and immunostaining with caspase-3 (increased histone retention and apoptotic process, Fig. 9.4), and the particularly relevant finding of the inverse correlation between persistent histones and normal Tygerberg Kruger sperm morphology, Fig. 9.5). When spermatozoa with these morphological or biochemical probes were studied in the double staining process, there was an approximately 80% agreement between the staining patterns, scored as light,

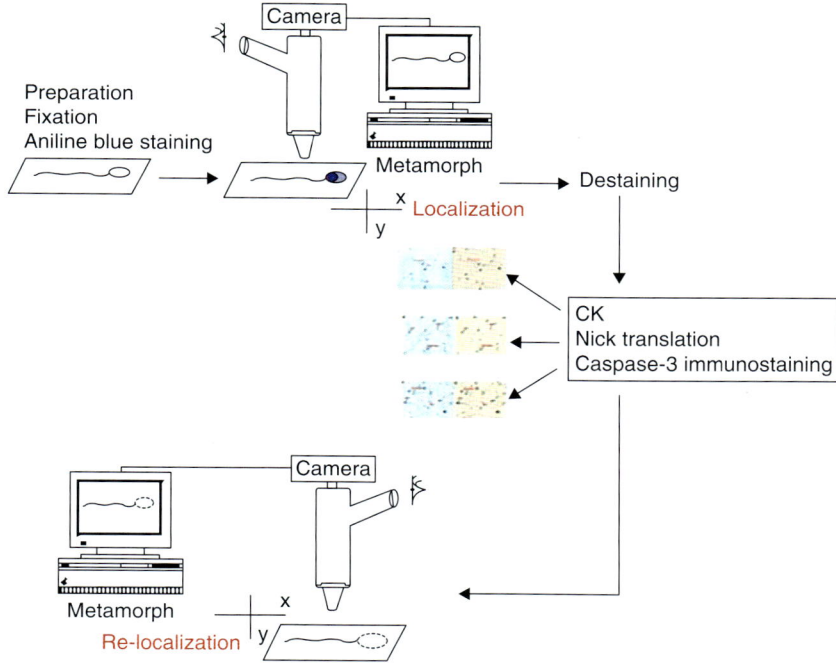

Figure 9.1 A flow chart of the experimental design. Aniline blue staining pattern recorded by Metamorph program, the slides are destained from aniline blue, and the slide (the same area is restained with a second probe), and the sperm field treated with the two probes are compared and the stainig is quantified as light, intermediate, and dark. *Abbreviation*: CK, creatine kinase. *Source*: From Ref. 9.

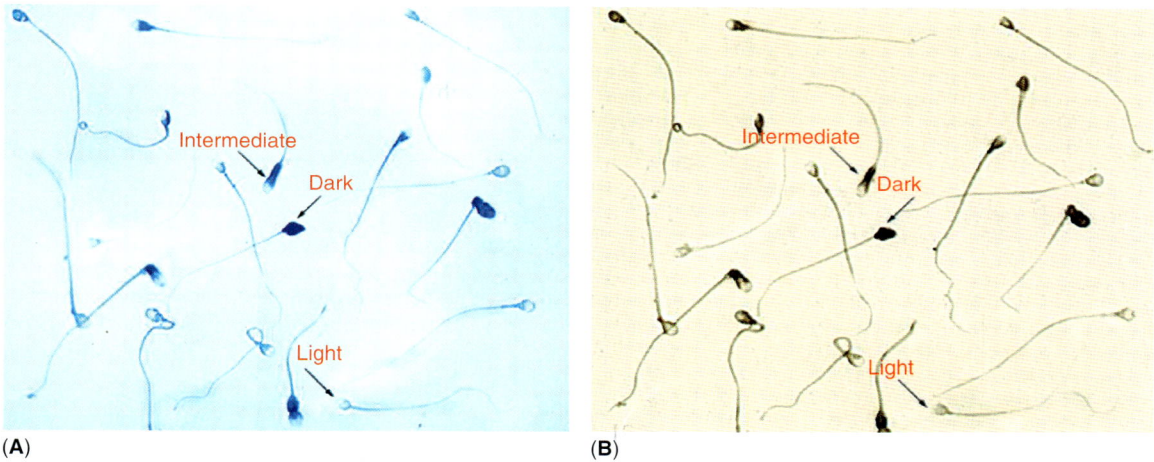

Figure 9.2 (**A**) Aniline blue staining and (**B**) creatine kinase (CK) immunostaining of the same spermatozoa. Note the substantial degree of similarity in the light-, intermediate- and dark-staining patterns with aniline blue and CK.

intermediate, and dark, with the various biochemical nuclear and cytoplasmic probes arising from early or late sperm development. Thus, abnormal sperm morphology and the underlying retention of cytoplasm and persistent histones, DNA chain fragmentation, aneuploidies, and the limited ability of the embryo for repair of the inborn deficiencies caused by the adverse sperm attributes mutually signal abnormal spermatozoa which is expected to provide lower fertilization rates, lesser embryonic development, lesser implantation, and higher rates of spontaneous abortion due to the arrested sperm development (2,24–34).

This is a potential point where the ICSI sperm selection via the HA-mediated process and by intracytoplasmic morphologically selected sperm injection (IMSI) sperm morphology selection may overlap. The issue needs to be studied, along with the potential inhibitory role of nuclear vacuoles, as well as the relationship between the biomarkers and vacuoles. The relationship between sperm shape and sperm development, due to the cytoplasmic retention, has been already demonstrated. Thus, once we understand the relationship between the already identified sperm biomarkers and perhaps the nuclear vacuoles in sperm, we may have a more extended and comprehensive global picture of how sperm shape or nuclear structure might support sperm selection to the same extent as hyaluronan-mediated or zona pellucida-mediated sperm selection.

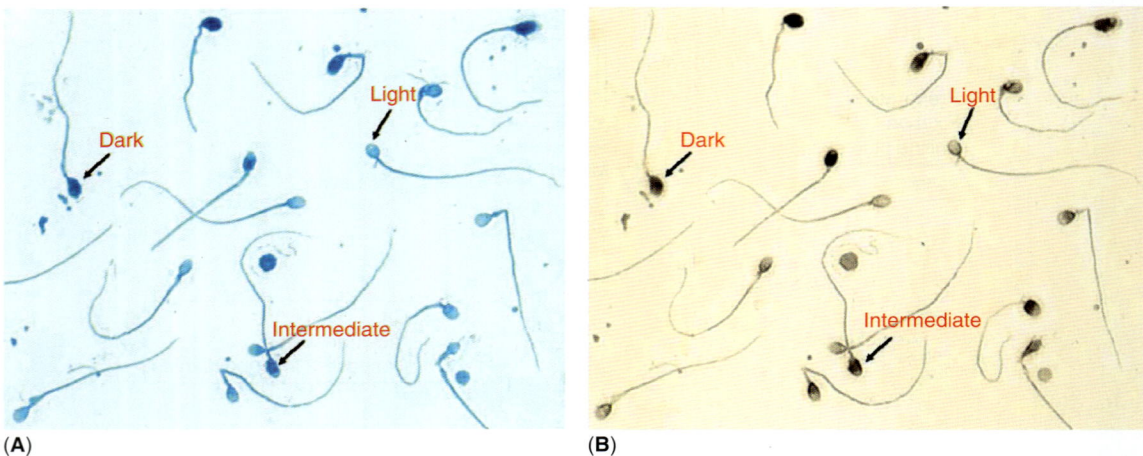

Figure 9.3 (**A**) Aniline blue staining and (**B**) DNA nick translation of the same spermatozoa. Note the substantial degree of similarity in the light-, intermediate- and dark-staining patterns with the two methods.

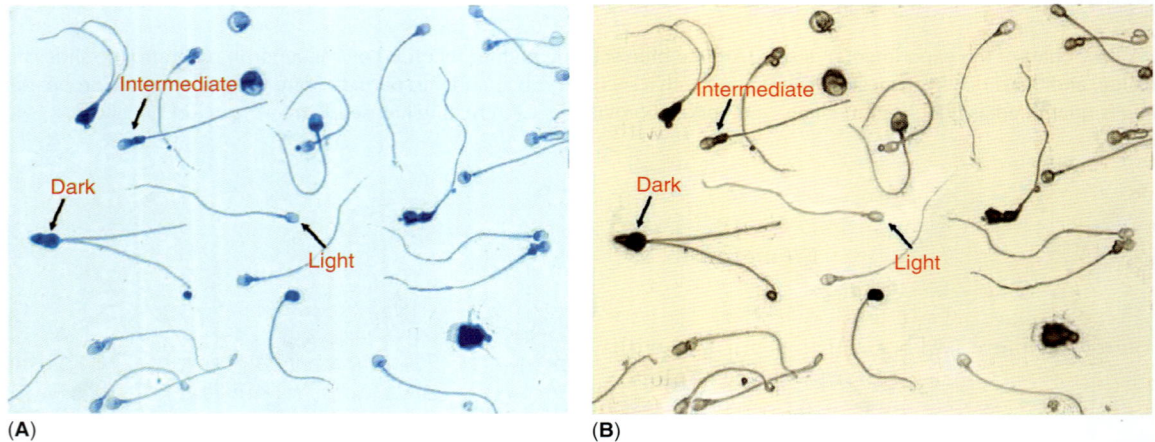

Figure 9.4 (**A**) Aniline blue staining and (**B**) caspase-3 immunostaining of the same spermatozoa. Note the similarity in the light-, intermediate- and dark-staining patterns of the aniline blue and caspase-3 panels. Also, caspase-3 immunostaining is present in the mid-piece of intermediate-type spermatozoa, whereas in dark spermatozoa with more extensive maturity arrest both the head and the mid-piece are stained (**A** and **B**).

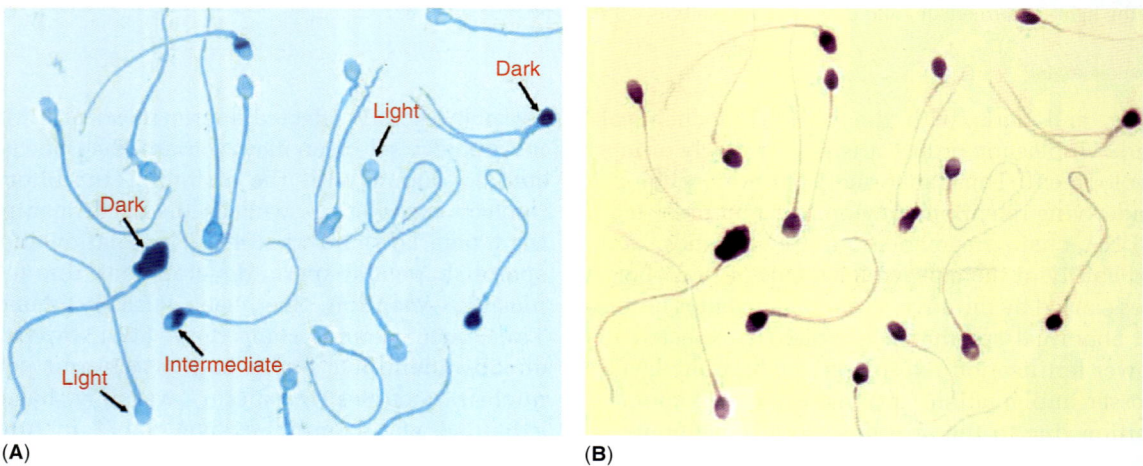

Figure 9.5 (**A**) Aniline blue staining and (**B**) creatine kinase immunocytochemistry staining of the same spermatozoa reveal inverse correlation between persistent histones and normal Tygerberg Kruger sperm morphology.

However, detection of normal sperm development with respect to the cytoplasmic extrusion and sperm plasma membrane remodeling is a more specific and powerful approach compared with the assessment of shape of the sperm head or nucleus. It is also important to appreciate that in spite of the efforts of comparing the high or lower magnification sperm morphology with various DNA and cytoplasmic attributes, this work was not yet initiated, and to date, none of the morphological attributes of IMSI are known to correlate to any of the sperm biomarkers.

Obviously, the discovery of the sperm plasma membrane remodeling and the formation of the zona pellucida and HA receptors, as well as the association between the lack of spermiogenetic development and sperm plasma membrane remodeling, along with the increased DNA fragmentation, chromosomal aneuploidies, that may affect the life time or cancer rate of the offspring, there are major concerns regarding the long-term public health effect of fertilization with spermatozoa that have never been selected by the sperm–oocyte interaction as a fertilizing sperm. One point which brings this concept home is the fact that the diminished HA binding, which is the related to the increased level of spermatozoa with arrested development, shows an inconsistency with sperm concentration and motility. More impressive evidence comes from the paper of Jakab et al. (27). In this report, the efficiency of HA binding in purifying sperm specimens with respect to sperm with chromosomal aneuploidies were demonstrated. Indeed, in 10 men who had a sperm concentration of over 100 million sperm/mL, and the sperm had been further purified with a density gradient, the sperm pellet has shown diploidy and sex and 17 disomy frequency of 0.9 (%), 0.2 (%), and 0.1 (%), whereas the chromosomal aneuploidy frequencies in the respective fractions of HA-bound spermatozoa were all in the range of 0.1–0.2% normal aneuploidy frequency rates.

Another supportive idea with respect to DNA fragmentation of spermatozoa is demonstrated most recently by Yagci et al. (34) in which sperm fractions were studied with acridine orange stain. The initial semen sperm fraction shows a close to 50–50% green and red fluorescence sperm pattern (high DNA chain integrity or fragmented DNA attributes, respectively). However, using the PICSI dish which facilitates the HA-mediated sperm selection for ICSI, the hundreds of selected HA-bound spermatozoa observed were all of acridine green fluorescence, indicating uncleaved high integrity DNA chains in those HA-bound spermatozoa (Fig. 9.6).

INTRACYTOPLASMIC MORPHOLOGICALLY SELECTED SPERM INJECTION (IMSI)

This alternative sperm selection approach is based on the shape or morphology of spermatozoa in which two sets of attributes may be considered: first, the shape of the sperm head and second, the shape of the nucleus evaluated by presence or absence or, if present, the size of nuclear vacuoles. In the classification of spermatozoa, regarding the sperm morphology for ICSI selection, the parameters evaluated are of the oval shape, having a low number of small vacuoles, larger or smaller vacuoles, and amorphous acrosomal head area with several vacuoles. (35). Some investigators have stated that in single sperm which had normal shape, the other physiological attributes, such as chromosomal aneuploidy, mitochondrial damage, and DNA fragmentation were lower than in sperm with vacuoles (36–38). Our experience does not agree with this finding (23).

IMSI is clearly a descriptive approach, whether it is used at low, high, or very high magnification, and is yet to be interpreted in light of the developmental sperm biomarkers discussed earlier that reflect the events of spermatogenesis and spermiogenesis, including cytoplasmic extrusion, chromatin maturation, DNA folding and DNA chain integrity, sperm plasma membrane remodeling, frequency of chromosomal aneuploidies, and apoptosis, all of which collectively affect the development of the embryo.

The IMSI selected for ICSI represents a very different approach from that of the HA-mediated ICSI sperm selection approach. Rather than an extensive work on sperm biomarkers and spermiogenetic events which has led to the discovery of the sperm plasma membrane remodeling in spermiogenesis, as well as the related formation of the zona pellucida and HA-binding sites which facilitate an "active" sperm selection with spermatozoa participation, IMSI is a descriptive and pragmatic approach in which the sperm is recovered as a "passive" participant. The fertilization outcome is described as "better," but there is an uncertainty regarding the sperm attributes, which may contribute to the "improved" outcome. This approach is an extension somewhat of the Tygerberg strict morphology approach

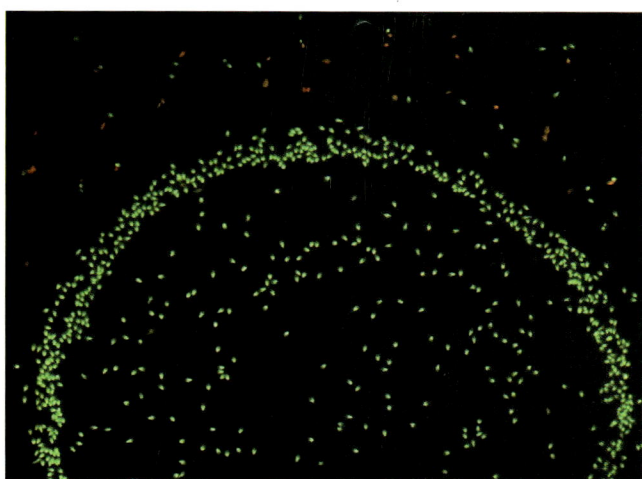

Figure 9.6 Acridine orange-stained spermatozoa in the outside and center of the hyaluronic acid (HA) spot of the HA-coated modified Petri dish (PICSI dish). The outside area with mixed orange (fragmented DNA) and green sperm (sperm with intact high integrity DNA) shows the DNA integrity in the initial semen sperm fraction. However, the hundreds of green sperm with intact DNA in the center of the dish, demonstrate the selection power of the HA spot with respect to sperm DNA integrity.

which had been invented in the mid-1980s by Dr Kruger who was looking for common shape elements in spermatozoa which could bind to the zona pellucida. The additional feature of IMSI is the focus upon the size, shape, and vacuole complement of the sperm nucleus.

It is also of interest that the sperm morphology features, according to the Tygerberg criteria, have little prognostic value with respect to the IMSI morphology and were not predictive with respect to ICSI outcome of embryo development, embryo morphology, or implantation rates (39,40). In similar matched studies (41,42) it was found that the implantation and pregnancy rates had increased two to three fold with IMSI compared with the conventional ICSI sperm selection by the embryologist.

CONSIDERATIONS REGARDING SPERM SELECTED BY PICSI AND IMSI

With respect to a morphologically defined normal nucleus without vacuoles with IMSI higher implantation and pregnancy rates were achieved in couples with previous ICSI failures (35,36,43). The improved IMSI outcome by the injection of spermatozoa without nuclear defects is related, perhaps, to improved chromatin status and reduced aneuploidy rates (37,44).

A negative feature of the IMSI sperm selection method is the fact that it is a time-consuming procedure which may require 90–120 minutes (35). It is also suspected that during this long period on the heated microscopic stage, the sperm cell and nucleus deterioration is enhanced along with a reactive oxygen species generation process, and will cause sperm DNA chain degradation, particularly in those sperm which are underdeveloped or damaged. In comparison, the HA selection of spermatozoa with the PICSI dish may take only a few minutes.

Further, the PICSI dish provides a spacious area for sperm selection. It is equipped with lines of orientation, and all spermatozoa are within the same level of microscopic focus range. Thus, the embryologist has a good opportunity to compare the available spermatozoa with respect to shape (morphology) and also HA binding, as well as the important specific response of the fully developed sperm to HA contact; two to four times increased cross-beat frequency. The motility arrest and the tail-beat response highlights the methodological advantage of HA-mediated sperm selection which is an efficient noninvasive process, and the fully completed sperm plasma membrane remodeling which also characterizes the biochemical attributes of "best" spermatozoa with respect to lack of cytoplasmic retention, lack of apoptotic process, high DNA chain integrity, high incidence of sperm with normal Tygerberg morphology, similar to the zona pellucida-bound sperm (45,46).

Regarding the various sperm attributes which are beneficial in the sperm selection process, whether by IMSI or PICSI, we have identified several biomarkers which may promote the sperm fertilization potential and paternal contribution of sperm. These biomarkers, including low CK content as a reflection of the completion of cytoplasmic extrusion, low levels of persistent histones, which reflect normal chromatin maturation with respect to progression from histones to intermediate proteins to protamine. The normal chromatin progression affects sperm function as well as normal DNA folding, and reduces the vulnerability to DNA degradation (45,46). We test for DNA integrity with the very highly accurate method of in situ DNA nick translation, and also with the sperm acridine orange fluorescence in situ. Further, we are testing for the presence of apoptotic agent caspase-3 which reflects the potential DNA degradation due to apoptosis (47).

The major biomarker which distinguishes the spermatozoa selected by HA-mediated binding compared with those used for eye-selected sperm in in vitro ICSI fertilization is the sperm binding, or lack of binding, to HA. This property represents the extent of sperm development or arrest of sperm development and the presence or absence of the zona pellucida and HA receptors, formation of which are simultaneously facilitated by the sperm membrane remodeling during terminal spermiogenesis.

On the contrary, sperm selected by IMSI are not characterized by the rigorous sperm biomarkers, and there are only occasional publication which indicate that the IMSI-selected sperm is superior compared with the sperm fractions in semen or with eye-selected sperm for conventional ICSI with respect to fertility, implantation, and pregnancy (or pregnancy loss) parameters. This is important, because in the case of HA-mediated ICSI sperm selection, the process is greatly supported by the sperm–hyaluronic acid-binding assay (HBA), a test which defines the proportion of motile sperm in a semen sample that will bind to HA, and, thus, will have completed the spermiogenetic membrane remodeling step. Accordingly, the HBA score, the proportion of sperm which are able to bind to HA, defines the improvement rates by HA-mediated sperm selection as the score provides a quantitative assessment. If the sperm-binding score is over 70–80%, it means that seven or eight of the 10 spermatozoa will be appropriate and fully developed. This almost gives comparable chance for pregnancy whether selecting sperm by eye or by the PICSI dish. However, in samples with low scores of 60%, 50%, or 25–40%, the chance for finding the appropriate sperm which is equivalent to the zona-binding sperm is 1:1 or 1;4 thus, the HA selection becomes an important factor. Indeed, in randomized studies in semen samples with low HA-binding scores, the HA-mediated selection gave improved 20–50% higher pregnancy rates than ICSI with eye-selected sperm, due to a combination of sperm quality and the substantial decline of miscarriage rates secondary to the improved DNA integrity in the sperm selected by the HA-mediated PICSI method.

In contrast, the IMSI method does not consider sperm function or sperm biomarkers. Sperm morphology or sperm nuclear morphology by IMSI provides a moderately higher level of fertilization or implantation, but it does lack two features: (*i*) There is no objective measure of comparison between ICSI candidates and the parameters used in morphology and nuclear morphology, the question of vacuoles and mid-piece attributes being not standardized. Further, there is a controversy among various IVF centers as to what morphological features are relevant, and how they may affect fertility and pregnancy outcome (48). All that is known is that the observation of morphological attributes at sperm selection improve fertilization, implantation rates, and somewhat diminish the spontaneous abortion rates. (*ii*) At the present time, as opposed to the HA mediated sperm ICSI selection, there are no well designed studies performed focusing upon DNA integrity, aneuploidy, or other sperm genetic studies in connection with the IMSI methods. Thus, it is unclear how IMSI provides any assurance for the future public health ICSI concerns with respect to the individual development and aneuploidy frequency of the offspring, as well as life span, and future cancer incidence in the post-IMSI offspring population (49,50).

Indeed, this is a challenge for the IMSI sperm selection investigators to develop the potential correlation between sperm morphological and nuclear morphology attributes, as well as biomarkers of cytoplasmic retention, aneuploidies, DNA fragmentation, DNA chain integrity, sperm paternal contribution for the HA sperm selection, and other aspects that have been already worked up for the HA-mediated sperm selection.

IMSI AND NUCLEAR ABNORMALITIES IN SPERM WITH LARGE VACUOLES

In the early 1990s, sperm shape evaluation was used for ICSI sperm selection as a potential enhancement. Bartoov et al. (51) developed a new method to assess morphology of the motile spermatozoa with high magnification, focusing on the sperm head shape and also the vacuoles in the nucleus. Regarding the vacuoles, 6.4% of the sperm nucleus area or under was considered to be normal and 13% area with nuclear vacuoles was considered severely abnormal. Perdrix et al. (48), in their study, examined additional sperm attributes related to vacuoles of normal spermatozoa with respect to sperm morphology (all 20 patients studied were teratozoospermic), acrosome morphology, and DNA fragmentation, via the TUNNEL assay. Chromatin, or persistent histones, was studied with aniline blue staining, and aneuploidies were assessed with FISH. The results indicate that the vacuoles were present in the anterior and medium sperm head, acrosome abnormalities were increased in sperm with large vacuoles (SLV) compared with the control. Microscopic observation showed the exclusively nuclear localization of vacuoles. Complete DNA fragmentation was higher in the native SLV sperm, whereas chromatin condensation was altered and aneuploidy frequencies were also increased in SLV. The problem with this study is that it was conducted on very few semen specimens.

It seems that the ICSI sperm selection by morphology creates internal controversy among the IMSI investigators. The main reason for this lack of consensus is because sperm morphology is not an objective science. There are variations between the sperm subpopulations selected, and it is difficult to evaluate what the shape differences mean in relation to sperm development and regarding the ability of spermatozoa for potential paternal contribution. Alternatively, the HA-mediated sperm selection, enhanced with the various sperm biomarkers, is based on objective measurable parameters of sperm development, fertilizing potential, and sperm paternal contribution toward the development of the embryo.

In a report supporting IMSI (43), a meta-analysis raised the fundamental question regarding the contrast between the conventional eye-selected sperm selection and IMSI sperm selection. The IMSI cycle data indicated a statistically significant improvement in implantation and pregnancy rates, and a significant reduction in miscarriage rates versus conventional ICSI. However, the authors seem to overlook the fact that no objective measures were used to compare the selected spermatozoa. Also, analysis of poorly correlated sperm shape attributes, which are known to be related to fertilization and paternal contribution of spermatozoa in these populations of hundreds of spermatozoa, may not be relevant, as only a few spermatozoa are selected for ICSI, and the attributes of these sperm seldom reflect the properties of all spermatozoa. It could be argued that it is not the question whether IMSI is better than ICSI; rather the focus should be on couples who, with the HA-mediated physiological sperm selection would achieve pregnancy, but are failing to succeed because of the arbitrary IMSI sperm morphology approach.

Another shortcoming of the IMSI studies is that no one can be sure that sperm shape or nuclear morphology are analyzed in comparable sperm cells. The reason is that there are no objective parameters for comparisons other than the sperm shape, which may be interpreted very differently from one IVF center to another (48).

Sperm selection by HA binding is based on the events related to sperm plasma membrane remodeling which is also related to the attributes of sperm biomarkers. The advantage of the HA-mediated selection of the best sperm, or the deselection of sperm with various negative attributes, such as abnormal morphology, apoptotic process, DNA fragmentation, increased aneuploidy frequency, cytoplasmic retention, and low concentration of the chaperone protein HspA2, are well studied of these markers were shown to adversely affect fertilization potential and paternal contribution of spermatozoa to the embryo and, thus, cause a decline in fertilization rates, embryo development, implantation rates, and pregnancy success (2,24,27–32,34).

Another controversy surrounds the origin and consequences of sperm head vacuoles. A large sperm head vacuole may originate in spermatogenetic or spermiogenetic impairment during the early stage of sperm development. The spermiogenetic events of acrosome formation, persistent histones, and increased DNA chain fragmentation are all related to the vacuoles, and it also has been reported by Sermondade et al. (55), that they were present in the anterior two-thirds of the sperm head; thus, the nucleus and the acrosomal area of sperm are the two main structures affected by the vacuoles. In general, the exclusive nuclear locations of vacuoles indicate some relationship to sperm development and functional quality. This idea is supported by the influence of sperm head vacuoles on late embryo development (56,38). However, the impact of vacuoles may also affect the paternal contribution of spermatozoa which indicate an association between DNA damage and the presence of nuclear vacuoles. In several studies, including (48), DNA fragmentation was not increased in spermatozoa with large vacuoles.

Further in the perdrix paper (46), with respect to patient-to-patient and laboratory-to-laboratory variations regarding a standardized sperm IMSI classification system. For instance, the large vacuoles may differ whether the vacuoles are present in the front of the nucleus or in other regions, and whether they are evaluated in an identical way because vacuoles may appear and be visible on one side, but not on the other aspect of the sperm cell. Also, regarding the proportion of vacuoles compared to the whole area of the nucleus, as the <6% or >13 or 14% parameters are not utilized uniformly in the various laboratories. Another issue is the head morphology which appears to be independent of the nuclear morphology; some investigators consider the acrosomal area morphology in the IMSI selection, which is part of the anterior sperm head.

A likely common feature between the spermatozoa with large vacuoles and also the HA-mediated ICSI selection of sperm for ICSI is the intensity or lack of aniline blue staining which represents the presence of persistent histones. It is higher in spermatozoa which are not selected by HA binding because persistent histones present in a higher proportion of spermatozoa which are not fully developed and failed to complete sperm plasma membrane remodeling (16). Also, it is of note that there is a high proportion of aniline blue stained sperm among vacuole-containing spermatozoa which are diminished in chromatin condensation (48). In both cases, this is obviously also related to erroneous DNA folding, diminished presence of protamine, and also vulnerability of DNA to chain fragmentation (25,28,30,31,57), (Simon et al., 2010a).

Further IMSI research and FISH analysis demonstrated that there was also an increase in chromosomal abnormalities (aneuploidy and diploidy) in the sperm which carried large nuclear vacuoles (48). However, the investigators only looked at about 1000 spermatozoa per sample which is not sufficient to provide statistical evaluation. In 1000 spermatozoa, assuming the normal disomy rate of 0.1–0.2% per chromosome, which is actually 1–2 sperm per 1000, the presence of disomies in three or four sperm, which is still a very low rate, would be a significant (33–100%) increase.

As opposed to IMSI, in the case of HA-mediated sperm selection, the semen may be evaluated with the sperm–HA-binding score, and the data indicate that the benefits of the HA-mediated sperm selection can be measured directly based on the HA-binding score (21,52). This is well coordinated with the fact that those spermatozoa which are able to bind to HA, thus, during spermatogenesis and spermiogenesis showed normal development all the way downstream to the key event of sperm plasma membrane remodeling and formation of the zona pellucida and HA-binding sites. In the poorly binding sperm samples, due to the lower frequency of the good spermatozoa which are greatly enhanced by HA-mediated selection of sperm without DNA fragmentation and aneuploidies, there is the expected improvement in higher pregnancy and lower miscarriage rates. Indeed this is well demonstrated by the multicenter study of Worrilow et al. which indicates a 10–30% improvement in pregnancy rates that are inversely correlated with the sperm–HA-binding score of the male partners (53).

With respect to "large" vacuoles, there is internal discrepancy. In the original publications of Bartoov et al. (51) and (54), large sperm vacuoles were those which had over 4% of the total head area. This was also true with Vanderzwalmen et al. (38). However, in more recent papers, for instance, Franco, et al. (36), large vacuoles were considered when >50% of the total head area was occupied. This is also true with Garolla et al. (37) where the large vacuoles were not specified with respect to their size. In the Perdrix study, a vacuole area occupying 13% was used to describe abnormal and large vacuoles (48). However, in a sperm fraction enhanced in teratozoospermic cells, the large vacuole-containing spermatozoa represented 38% of the nuclear surface area.

With respect to the comparison between the IMSI and the HA selection, it is a very important point that besides sperm abnormality and a high level of persistent histones described in some papers, a lack of chromatin condensation was also studied in the Huszar laboratory. Whereas a relationship which was tentative with the high morphology, in the paper by Sati et al. (24), the sperm were double labeled with chromatin condensation defect (aniline blue staining); subsequently, the sperm were destained from the aniline blue and were labeled with probes for DNA chain fragmentation, or with CK (demonstrating cytoplasmic retention which causes the abnormal sperm morphology), or with the apoptotic marker of caspase-3 for apoptosis and consequential DNA fragmentation. It is also of note that sperm were treated with double staining with aniline blue and with fluorescent in situ hybridization and also evaluated with aniline blue staining and Tygerberg strict morphology (24).

There were two remarkable set of data which appeared from the Sati study: First, it has become obvious that the aniline blue staining graded as light, intermediate or dark for persistent histones (which represents normal chromatin maturity, intermediate chromatin maturity, and diminished chromatin maturity). Second, the other biomarkers used were correlated with the absence or presence of cytoplasmic retention, absence or presence of DNA fragmentation, absence or presence of normal Kruger sperm morphology which is related to cytoplasmic retention, and finally to the absence or presence of chromosomal aneuploidies. For the most part, the light sperm did not show disomies; the intermediate sperm showed disomies. Most surprisingly, the dark aniline blue stained sperm, which have also shown diminished levels of protamine due to the lack of histone, transition protein to protamine conversion, and consequential improper DNA folding and extensive DNA fragmentation, did not show any FISH signal. Our explanation for this: Due to the extensive levels of DNA fragmentation and the broken DNA chain pieces, there were no adequate sites for the FISH probes to bind (58).

The relationship between sperm aneuploidy, sperm development, and morphology is controversial. It is relevant to refer again to the relationship between cytoplasmic retention and sperm aneuploidy frequency, which was well established by Kovanci et al. (15). The relationship between low HspA2 content in sperm (a chaperone protein which is present in the synaptonemal complex) and residual cytoplasm representing arrested spermiogenesis well explains the potential relationship. However, it is unclear how general this relationship is, because not all sperm with abnormal sperm morphology has shown to carry aneuploidies (23). Also, these studies were carried out based on the observation that spermatozoa in the native or decondensed\denatured state, steps that are necessary for performing FISH, maintain their original shape attributes, thus sperm shape and aneuploidy status may be examined in the same spermatozoa (59).

Indeed individual spermatozoa, which show perfect Tygerberg morphology and were evaluated with computerized morphometry for ideal shape, still have aneuploidies. This study was made possible by the novel demonstration that sperm maintain their initial shape after the steps of decondensation necessary for chromosome structure study by FISH. The data indicated with several representative pictures that the decondensed sperm maintain their morphology exactly as it was in the initial non-decondensed state (23,59). This technical invention made it possible for the first time to study sperm morphology and aneuploidy with FISH within the same spermatozoa. Although, there was some relationship between abnormal morphology and aneuploidies, the approach also demonstrated that aneuploidy may be found in perfectly normal spermatozoa. Finally, it should be pointed out that the double-stained sperm study by Sati et al. (24) indicated cytoplasmic retention, DNA fragmentation; thus, the sperm chromatin packaging or sperm morphology, or any other sperm attributes of arrested development would adversely affect embryo propagation, if such sperm is used for ICSI. Finally, due to the common origin of DNA fragmentation and arrested sperm maturation, no matter what sperm attributes the investigators may be looking at, it is most likely the DNA fragmentation which affects the paternal contribution to embryo development.

CLINICAL RESULTS: IMSI VS EYE-SELECTED CONVENTIONAL ICSI

In the paper of Antinori et al., a prospective randomized trial of IMSI and conventional ICSI was reported (35). The authors looked at the advantages of IMSI versus ICSI in couples with husbands of severe oligo-astheno-zoospermia.

The procedure of IMSI sperm selection was based on >6600 magnification. A total of 446 couples with three years of primary infertility and with a female age of <35 years were enrolled. ICSI was carried out on 219 patients, IMSI on 227 couples. The study considered pregnancy and miscarriage rates, as well as implantation rates. On the final analysis, IMSI versus ICSI resulted in higher clinical pregnancy rates (39.2 vs 26.5%, p = 0.004). In spite of the initial poor reproductive prognosis, patients with two or more previous failed IVF attempts, benefited most from IMSI versus ICSI in terms of pregnancy (29.8 vs 12.9, p = 0.02) and reduced miscarriage rates (17.4% vs 37.5%). At the time of the publication of this study there were only 35 babies born.

IVF–ICSI Data with HA-Mediated Sperm Selection

There are now several laboratories that have initiated HA-mediated sperm selection. It is important that none of the groups practicing the HA sperm selection reported any adverse effects regarding fertilization or embryo development. In one 2005 ESHRE presentation, preliminary data on 18 pregnancies were reported. Comparing ICSI results with those of visually selected ICSI sperm (N = 84) versus HA-selected ICSI sperm (N = 18), there were no differences in fertilization rates, proportion of good grade embryos, pregnancy and miscarriage rates, or take-home baby rates. Again, there were no adverse findings during the cycles (60).

A similar study was performed on 20 unselected couples treated with ICSI in which at least eight MII oocytes were recovered. The sibling oocytes were injected either with HA-selected or visually selected spermatozoa (N = 146 and 145). The fertilization rates (72.9% and 66.9%), oocyte degeneration rates (9.6% and 13.8%), rates of embryo cleavage, embryo quality, embryo transfer, and embryo cryopreservation rates were all similar (61). In a relevant publication, Park et al. (62) report improvements with HA-selected sperm in porcine IVF. Porcine embryos were produced by IVF, ICSI, and ICSI performed with HA-selected sperm. The HA-mediated sperm selection was superior to visual sperm selection in producing chromosomally normal embryos, and increasing ICSI efficiency by reducing the early embryonic mortality and thus enhancing ICSI success rates.

A related clinical aspect of the sperm biomarkers of sperm development and fertility is the enhancement of sperm with normal morphology in the HA-bound sperm fraction. Studies in the Huszar laboratory indicated that there was a two to threefold enrichment of Tygerberg normal sperm in the HA-bound fraction compared to the respective semen sperm fraction (63). This enhancement, interestingly, agreed with the finding of the Tygerberg group with respect to the enrichment of normal morphology sperm in the zona pellucida–bound versus semen sperm fraction (64). This is a further indication that sperm binding to the zona pellucida and to HA is not distinguishable from the point of view of the spermatozoa.

A number of recent studies have indicated that HA-bound sperm used in the ICSI procedure (the so-called physiological ICSI) may lead to increased fertilization and implantation rates (52,65,66). In the Parmegiani study, 293 couples were treated with HA-ICSI against 86 couples treated with conventional ICSI (historical control group). All outcome measures of fertilization, embryo quality, implantation, and pregnancy were the same or improved in the HA-mediated sperm selection group. The implantation rate was increased from 10.3% in conventional ICSI to 17.1% in the HA group. A smaller clinical trial assessing the same technology by Worillow et al. has also shown that clinical pregnancy rates are improved when using HA-selected sperm compared with conventional ICSI. Furthermore, the sperm HA-binding score (the proportion of sperm that underwent plasma membrane remodeling in spermatogenesis and binds to HA) is an important diagnostic indicator. Men with <55% binding score would particularly benefit, as their ICSI success rates were improved (15–30%) by using the HA-mediated sperm selection (53). Thus, it is important that in IVF programs, the andrology laboratory performs the sperm–HA-binding test for the husbands of IVF–ICSI couples. The HA-binding score provides the information on the proportion of sperm with attributes of incomplete development, such as DNA fragmentation, chromosomal aneuploidies, persistent histones, cytoplasmic retention, and lack of HA-binding ability. The IVF team should triage the couples according to their HA-binding score in order to perform IUI, IVF, or conventional ICSI or ICSI with HA-mediated sperm selection.

All these supporting data from various laboratories led to a recent multicenter trial. Among the couples enrolled, 802 men had an HA-binding score of <65% (approximately 200 eligible couples). These men were treated in two arms: one received conventional ICSI; the other group had HA-mediated ICSI sperm selection. However, the essential point is that the pairs matched with conventional or hyaluronan-mediated ICSI sperm selection had comparable HA-binding scores. The couples treated with the HA-mediated versus conventional ICSI sperm selection approach showed improved results: implantation rates: 37.4% versus 30.7%; clinical pregnancy rates: 50.8% versus 37.9%; pregnancy loss: 2% versus 16.8%, $P = 0.02$. This is an important study because of the strong points: (*i*) This is so far the largest patient population dealing with the benefits of the HA-mediated sperm selection; (*ii*) the multicenter participation and the double blinded design; (*iii*) the use of the sperm–hyaluronan-binding score-based matching of the randomized eye-selected and HA-selected sperm used for ICSI; (*iv*) confirmation of the increased pregnancy rates and statistically significant reduction in the spontaneous pregnancy loss in the group with HA-mediated sperm selection (21).

We can conclude that at the present stage of the ICSI sperm selection science, the data support a preference for the HA-mediated sperm selection. However, a more rigorous and valid comparison will be possible with studies in which the presence and size of the nuclear vacuoles in a sperm population, along with the HA-binding score, as well as the nuclear and cytoplasmic sperm biomarkers developed will be applied to spermatozoa selected by both HA binding and IMSI.

ACKNOWLEDGMENT

The editorial help by Dr Layla Sati in preparing this chapter is greatly appreciated.

REFERENCES

1. Palermo G, Joris H, Devroey P, Van Steirteghem AC. Pregnancies after intracytoplasmic injection of single spermatozoon into an oocyte. Lancet 1992; 340: 17–18.
2. Huszar G, Jakab A, Sakkas D, et al. Fertility testing and ICSI sperm selection by hyaluronic acid binding: clinical and genetic aspect. Reprod Biomed Online 2007; 14: 650–63.
3. Huszar G, Patrizio P, Vigue L, et al. Cytoplasmic extrusion and the switch from creatine kinase B to M isoform are completed by the commencement of epididymal transport in human and stallion spermatozoa. J Androl 1998; 19: 11–20.
4. Huszar G, Vigue L. Spermatogenesis-related change in the synthesis of the creatine kinase B-type and M-type isoforms in human spermatozoa. Mol Reprod Dev 1990; 25: 258–62.
5. Huszar G, Vigue L. Incomplete development of human spermatozoa is associated with increased creatine phosphokinase concentration and abnormal head morphology. Mol Reprod Dev 1993; 34: 292–8.
6. Huszar G, Vigue L, Oehninger S. Creatine kinase immunocytochemistry of human sperm-hemizona complexes: selective binding of sperm with mature creatine kinase-staining pattern. Fertil Steril 1994; 61: 136–42.
7. Huszar G, Stone K, Dix D, Vigue L. Putative creatine kinase M-isoform in human sperm is identifiedas the 70-kilodalton heat shock protein HspA2. Bio Reprod 2000; 63: 925–32.
8. Cayli S, Jakab A, Ovari L, et al. Biochemical markers of sperm function: male fertility and sperm selection for ICSI. Reprod Biomed Online 2003; 7: 462–8.
9. Allen JW, Dix DJ, Collins BW, et al. HSP70-2 is part of the synaptonemal complex in mouse and hamster spermatocytes. Chromosoma 1996; 104: 414–21.
10. Dix DJ, Allen JW, Collins BW, et al. Targeted gene disruption of Hsp70-2 results in failed meiosis, germ cell apoptosis, and male infertility. Proc Natl Acad Sci USA 1996; 93: 3264–8.
11. Eddy EM. Role of heat shock protein HSP70-2 in spermatogenesis. Reproduction 1999; 4: 23–30.
12. Ergur AR, Dokras A, Giraldo JL, et al. Sperm maturity and treatment choice of in vitro fertilization (IVF) or intracytoplasmic sperm injection: diminished sperm HspA2 chaperone levels predict IVF failure. Fertil Steril 2002; 77: 910–18.
13. Huszar G, Vigue L, Corrales M. Sperm creatine kinase activity in fertile and infertile oligospermic men. J Androl 1990; 11: 40–6.
14. Huszar G, Vigue L, Morshedi M. Sperm creatine phosphokinase M-isoform ratios and fertilizing potential of men: a blinded study of 84 couples treated with in vitro fertilization. Fertil Steril 1992; 57: 882–8.
15. Kovanci E, Kovacs T, Moretti E, et al. FISH assessment of aneuploidy frequencies in mature and immature human

spermatozoa classified by the absence or presence of cytoplasmic retention. Hum Reprod 2001; 16: 1209–17.
16. Huszar G, Sbracia M, Vigue L, Miller DJ, Shur BD. Sperm plasma membrane remodeling during spermiogenetic maturation in men: relationship among plasma membrane beta 1,4-galactosyltransferase, cytoplasmic creatine phosphokinase, and creatine phosphokinase isoform ratios. Biol Reprod 1997; 56: 1020–4.
17. Huszar G, Willetts M, Corrales M. Hyaluronic acid (sperm select) improves retention of sperm motility and velocity in normospermic and oligospermic specimens. Fertil Steril 1990; 54: 1127–34.
18. Sbracia M, Grasso J, Sayme N, Stronk J, Huszar G. Hyaluronic acid substantially increases the retention of motility in cryopreserved/thawed human spermatozoa. Hum Reprod 1997; 12: 1949–54.
19. Huszar G, Ozenci CC, Cayli S, et al. Hyaluronic acid binding by human sperm indicates cellular maturity, viability, and unreacted acrosomal status. Fertil Steril 2003; 79(Suppl 3): 1616–24.
20. Huszar G, Vigue L, Corrales M. Sperm creatine phosphokinase activity as a measure of sperm quality in normospermic, variablespermic, and oligospermic men. Biol Reprod 1988; 38: 1061–6.
21. Worrilow K, Eid S, Woodhouse J, et al. Prospective, multi-center, double-blind, randomized clinical trial evaluating the use of hyaluronan-bound sperm in ICSI: statistically significant improvement in clinical outcomes. Abstract, ASRM annual meeting. Florida: Orlando, 2011.
22. Gergely A, Kovanci E, Senturk L, et al. Morphometric assessment of mature and diminished-maturity human spermatozoa: sperm regions that reflect differences in maturity. Hum Reprod 1999; 14: 2007–14.
23. Celik-Ozenci C, Jakab A, Kovacs T, et al. Sperm selection for ICSI: shape properties do not predict the absence or presence of numerical chromosomal aberrations. Hum Reprod 2004; 19: 2052–9.
24. Sati L, Ovari L, Bennett D, et al. Double probing of human spermatozoa for persistent histones, surplus cytoplasm, apoptosis and DNA fragmentation. Reprod Biomed Online 2008; 16: 570–9.
25. Ebner T, Moser M, Sommergruber M, et al. Presence, but not type or degree of extension, of a cytoplasmic halo has a significant influence on preimplantation development and implantation behaviour. Hum Reprod 2003; 18: 2406–12.
26. Seli E, Sakkas D. Spermatozoal nuclear determinants of reproductive outcome: implications for ART. Hum Reprod Update 2005; 11: 337–49.
27. Jakab A, Sakkas D, Delpiano E, et al. Intracytoplasmic sperm injection: a novel selection method for sperm with normal frequency of chromosomal aneuploidies. Fertil Steril 2005; 84: 1665–73.
28. Zini A, Boman JM, Belzile E, Ciampi A. Sperm DNA damage is associated with an increased risk of pregnancy loss after IVF and ICSI: systematic review and meta-analysis. Hum Reprod 2008; 23: 2663–8.
29. Avendano C, Franchi A, Duran H, Oehninger S. DNA fragmentation of normal spermatozoa negatively impacts embryo quality and intracytoplasmic sperm injection outcome. Fertil Steril 2010; 94: 549–57.
30. Menezo Y, Dale B, Cohen M. DNA damage and repair in human oocytes and embryos: a review. Zygote 2010; 18: 357–65.
31. Sakkas D, Alvarez JG. Sperm DNA fragmentation: mechanisms of origin, impact on reproductive outcome, and analysis. Fertil Steril 2010; 93: 1027–36.
32. Simon L, Brunborg G, Stevenson M, et al. Clinical significance of sperm DNA damage in assisted reproduction outcome. Hum Reprod 2010; 25: 1594–608.
33. Simon L, Lutton D, McManus J, Lewis SE. Sperm DNA damage measured by the alkaline Comet assay as an independent predictor of male infertility and in vitro fertilization success. Fertil Steril 2010; 952: 652–7.
34. Yagci A, Murk W, Stronk J, Huszar G. Spermatozoa bound to solid state hyaluronic acid show chromatin structure with high DNA chain integrity: an acridine orange fluorescence study. J Androl 2010.
35. Antinori M, Licata E, Dani G, et al. Intracytoplasmic morphologically selected sperm injection: a prospective randomized trial. Reprod Biomed Online 2008; 16: 835–41.
36. Franco JG, Baruffi RL, Mauri AL, et al. Significance of large nuclear vacuoles in human spermatozoa: implications for ICSI. Reprod Biomed Online 2008; 17: 42–5.
37. Garolla A, Fortini D, Menegazzo M, et al. High-power microscopy for selecting spermatozoa for ICSI by physiological status. Reprod Biomed Online 2008; 17: 610–16.
38. Vanderzwalmen P, Hiemer A, Rubner P, et al. Blastocyst development after sperm selection at high magnification is associated with size and number of nuclear vacuoles. Reprod Biomed Online 2008; 17: 617–27.
39. Svalander P, Jakobsson AH, Forsberg AS, Bengtsson AC, Wikland M. The outcome of intracytoplasmic sperm injection is unrelated to 'strict criteria' sperm morphology. Hum Reprod 1996; 11: 1019–22.
40. French DB, Sabanegh ES Jr, Goldfarb J, Desai N. Does severe teratozoospermia affect blastocyst formation, live birth rate, and other clinical outcome parameters in ICSI cycles? Fertil Steril 2010; 93: 1097–103.
41. Bartoov B, Berkovitz A, Eltes F, et al. Pregnancy rates are higher with intracytoplasmic morphologically selected sperm injection than with conventional intracytoplasmic injection. Fertil Steril 2003; 80: 1413–19.
42. Berkovitz A, Eltes F, Yaari S, et al. The morphological normalcy of the sperm nucleus and pregnancy rate of intracytoplasmic injection with morphologically selected sperm. Hum Reprod 2005; 20: 185–90.
43. Souza Setti A, Ferreira RC, de Almeida Ferreira Braga DP, et al. Intracytoplasmic sperm injection outcome versus intracytoplasmic morphologically selected sperm injection outcome: a meta-analysis. Reprod Biomed Online 2010; 21: 450–5.
44. Boitrelle F, Ferfouri F, Petit JM, et al. Large human sperm vacuoles observed in motile spermatozoa under high magnification: nuclear thumbprints linked to failure of chromatin condensation. Hum Reprod 2011; 26: 1650–8.
45. Aoki VW, Carrell DT. Human protamines and the developing spermatid: their structure, function, expression and relationship with male infertility. Asian J Androl 2003; 5: 315–24.
46. Carrell DT, Emery BR, Hammoud S, et al. Altered protamine expression and diminished spermatogenesis: what is the link? Hum Reprod Update 2007; 13: 313–27.
47. Cayli S, Sakkas D, Vigue L, Demir R, Huszar G. Cellular maturity and apoptosis in human sperm: creatine

kinase, caspase-3 and Bcl-XL levels in mature and diminished maturity sperm. Mol Hum Reprod 2004; 10: 365–72.
48. Perdrix A, Travers A, Chelli MH, et al. Assessment of acrosome and nuclear abnormalities in human spermatozoa with large vacuoles. Hum Reprod 2011; 26: 47–58.
49. Simpson JL, Lamb DJ. Genetic effects of intracytoplasmic sperm injection. Semin Reprod Med 2001; 19: 239–49.
50. Bonduelle M, Liebaers I, Deketelaere V, et al. Neonatal data on a cohort of 2889 infants born after ICSI (1991-1999) and of 2995 infants born after IVF 1983-1999. Hum Reprod 2002; 17: 671–94.
51. Bartoov B, Berkovitz A, Eltes F. Selection of spermatozoa with normal nuclei to improve the pregnancy rate with intracytoplasmic sperm injection. N Engl J Med 2001; 345: 1067–8.
52. Parmegiani L, Cognigni GE, Ciampaglia W, et al. Efficiency of hyaluronic acid (HA) sperm selection. J Assist Reprod Genet 2010; 27: 13–16.
53. Worrilow K, Huynh H, Bower J, et al. The clinical impact associated with the use of PICSI derived embryos. Annual Meeting of ASRM. Atlanta, 2009.
54. Bartoov B, Berkovitz A, Eltes F, et al. Real-time fine morphology of motile human sperm cells is associated with IVF-ICSI outcome. J Androl 2002; 23: 1–8.
55. Sermondade N, Hafhouf E, Dupont C, et al. Successful childbirth after intracytoplasmic morphologically selected sperm injection without assisted oocyte activation in a patient with globozoospermia. Hum Reprod 2011; 26: 2944–9.
56. Berkovitz A, Eltes F, Ellenbogen A, et al. Does the presence of nuclear vacuoles in human sperm selected for ICSI affect pregnancy outcome? Hum Reprod 2006; 21: 1787–90.
57. Seli E, Gardner DK, Schoolcraft WB, Moffatt O, Sakkas D. Extent of nuclear DNA damage in ejaculated spermatozoa impacts on blastocyst development after in vitro fertilization. Fertil Steril 2004; 82: 378–83.
58. Ovari L, Sati L, Stronk J, et al. Double probing individual human spermatozoa: aniline blue staining for persistent histones and fluorescence in situ hybridization for aneuploidies. Fertil Steril 2010; 93: 2255–61.
59. Celik-Ozenci C, Catalanotti J, Jakab A, et al. Human sperm maintain their shape following decondensation and denaturation for fluorescent in situ hybridization: shape analysis and objective morphometry. Biol Reprod 2003; 69: 1347–55.
60. Sanchez M, Aran B, Blanco J, et al. Preliminary clinical and FISH results on hyaluronic acid sperm selection to improve ICSI. 21st Annual Meeting of European Society for Human Reproduction & Embryology (ESHRE), Copenhagen, Human Reproduction. Denmark 2005; 20(Suppl 1): 556.
61. Janssens R, Verheyen G, Bocken G, et al. Use of PICSI dishes for sperm selection in clinical ICSI practice: results of a pilot study. Annual Meeting of the Belgian Society Reproductive Medicine. 2006.
62. Park CY, Uhm SJ, Song SJ, et al. Increase of ICSI efficiency with hyaluronic acid binding sperm for low aneuploidy frequency in pig. Theriogenology 2005; 64: 1158–69.
63. Prinosilova P, Kruger T, Sati L, et al. Selectivity of hyaluronic acid binding for spermatozoa with normal Tygerberg strict morphology. Reprod Biomed Online 2009; 18: 177–83.
64. Menkveld R, Franken DR, Kruger TF, Oehninger S, Hodgen GD. Sperm selection capacity of the human zona pellucida. Mol Reprod Dev 1991; 30: 346–52.
65. Nasr-Esfahani MH, Razavi S, Vahdati AA, Fathi F, Tavalaee M. Evaluation of sperm selection procedure based on hyaluronic acid binding ability on ICSI outcome. J Assist Reprod Genet 2008; 25: 197–203.
66. Borini A, Tarozzi N, Bizzaro D, et al. Sperm DNA fragmentation: paternal effect on early post-implantation embryo development in ART. Hum Reprod 2006; 21: 2876–81.

10

Intracytoplasmic morphologically selected sperm injection

Monica Antinori

INTRODUCTION

Since its introduction, intracytoplasmic sperm injection (ICSI) has revolutionized the approach to male infertility by offering treatment to couples who were previously excluded from conventional in vitro fertilization (IVF).

Poor-quality samples with severe impairment of sperm count, motility, and morphology turned to be unexpectedly suitable to achieve pregnancy and deliver healthy babies (1). According to some authors, the only requirement of that approach is the presence of at least one motile spermatozoon, while its morphology does not seem to have any correlation with ICSI outcomes (2–5) given that fertilization can occur even in cases of total teratozoospermia (6), globozoospermia (7,8), and megalozoospermia (9). On the other hand, fertilization, pregnancy, implantation (9,10), embryo quality (11–13), and blastocyst formation (11,14) rates are negatively affected by severe morphological anomalies. Even if there is a tendency among embryologists to select for injection into the ooplasm only the most good-looking sperm and discard the most distorted ones (i.e., round, large, or tapered), visual assessment under 200–400× magnification can actually identify mostly rough alterations in sperm shape and size (15). However, it overlooks a variety of head defects (16–18), which could be indicative of impaired sperm function and DNA integrity, as is significantly frequent in cases of oligo-astheno-teratozoospermia (OAT) (19–25). Moreover, ICSI involves the use of a spermatozoon that would never be able to penetrate the zona pellucida because of structural defects whose severity seems to be related to the incidence of chromosome aneuploidies (26). Hence, its introduction into clinical practice has increased the likelihood that a genetically abnormal sperm may be selected for fertilization and participate in the embryo development. In this respect, several negative-impact factors, both genetic and epigenetic in origin, have been identified in embryos following an ICSI procedure (27–30), and there is considerable concern regarding the increased risk of chromosomal abnormalities in infants conceived through ICSI (31–33). Moreover, when considering that the European average "take-home baby" rates are essentially unchanged from a decade ago (34,35), and that, at present, the resulting pregnancy rates are only between 30% and 45% (36–38), it is reasonable to speculate that ICSI might have reached the highest success rate possible as against its technical limitations.

In 1999, seven sperm subcellular organelles (acrosome, postacrosomal lamina, nucleus, neck, axoneme, mitochondrial sheath, and outer dense fibers) were identified and "ultra-morphologically" analyzed by electron microscopy (namely scanning electron microscopy and transmission electron microscopy) (39). As a result, their highly predictive value for male fertility potential was demonstrated. However, analysis of the *sperm organellar morphological characteristics* involved high costs since it had to be carried out only on fixed and stained sperm cells from selected cases of unexplained infertility and repeated assisted reproductive technique (ART) failures. For that reason, a few years later *sperm functional morphology criteria* based on real-time observation of *individual* motile sperm cells under high magnification were developed. The new evaluation procedure, called motile sperm organellar morphology examination (MSOME), used an interference phase-contrast inverted microscope with Nomarski optics that combined objective magnification (100×), a magnification selector (1.5×), and a video monitor system (video camera plus monitor), which gave a final magnification of 6600× (40). On the basis of historical data, which demonstrated how proper sperm selection improves ICSI outcomes (10,14,41), MSOME, being able to detect subtle sperm morphological malformations, which might remain unnoticed during standard microinjection, and allow the identification of spermatozoa with the best morphology, was introduced to improve the ICSI success rates.

Out of the subcellular organelles examined, sperm nucleus turned out to be the most critical variable affecting the outcome of ICSI (40) particularly in the form of large nuclear vacuoles that were proposed to reflect damage in the nuclear DNA content and organization (42,43). Considering that, at present, we are not able to offer our patients a selection technique whereby spermatozoa used for fertilization are preventively tested for DNA integrity, the assumption that vacuolization of the sperm nucleus may reflect some underlying DNA defects, which could undermine male fertility potential, is a promising perspective.

Consequently, MSOME evaluation coupled with conventional ICSI gave rise to a new micromanipulation technique called intracytoplasmic morphologically selected sperm injection (IMSI), which is currently one of the most debated issues in the ART field.

The debate on the actual need to introduce such a new method into ART practice as an established treatment tool for infertile couples is lively, and it is not mitigated by the increasing data supporting its clinical effectiveness. Most opponents emphasize practical limitations arising from the technical peculiarities of the procedure including high-cost setting up of the necessary equipment, prolonged handling time of male gametes before fertilization, lack of standardized selection criteria, and problems in managing the ART laboratory. And some even go as far as negating any benefit from its application (44).

Despite those concerns, it is a fact that the implementation of this new method has rekindled interest in the role morphology would have to find functionally competent sperm with the highest fertility potentials. Nevertheless, only after extending its applications and adequate standardization will it be possible to clarify what the actual contribution of IMSI in defeating male infertility is.

EQUIPMENT

The apparatus used for sperm evaluation comprises an inverted microscope equipped with 20×, 40×, and 100× oil immersion objectives mounted preferably on a motorized revolver, and a Nomarski differential interference contrast (DIC) system. The images are captured by a three-charge-coupled device (CCD) video camera and visualized on a monitor screen (Fig. 10.1). Once assembled, the equipment is capable of high magnifications (over 6000×) required to achieve a detailed visualization of the sperm subcellular organelles. DIC is used for detecting optical gradients in the specimen and converting them into intensity differences; it produces monochromatic shadow-cast 3D images that provide information on the

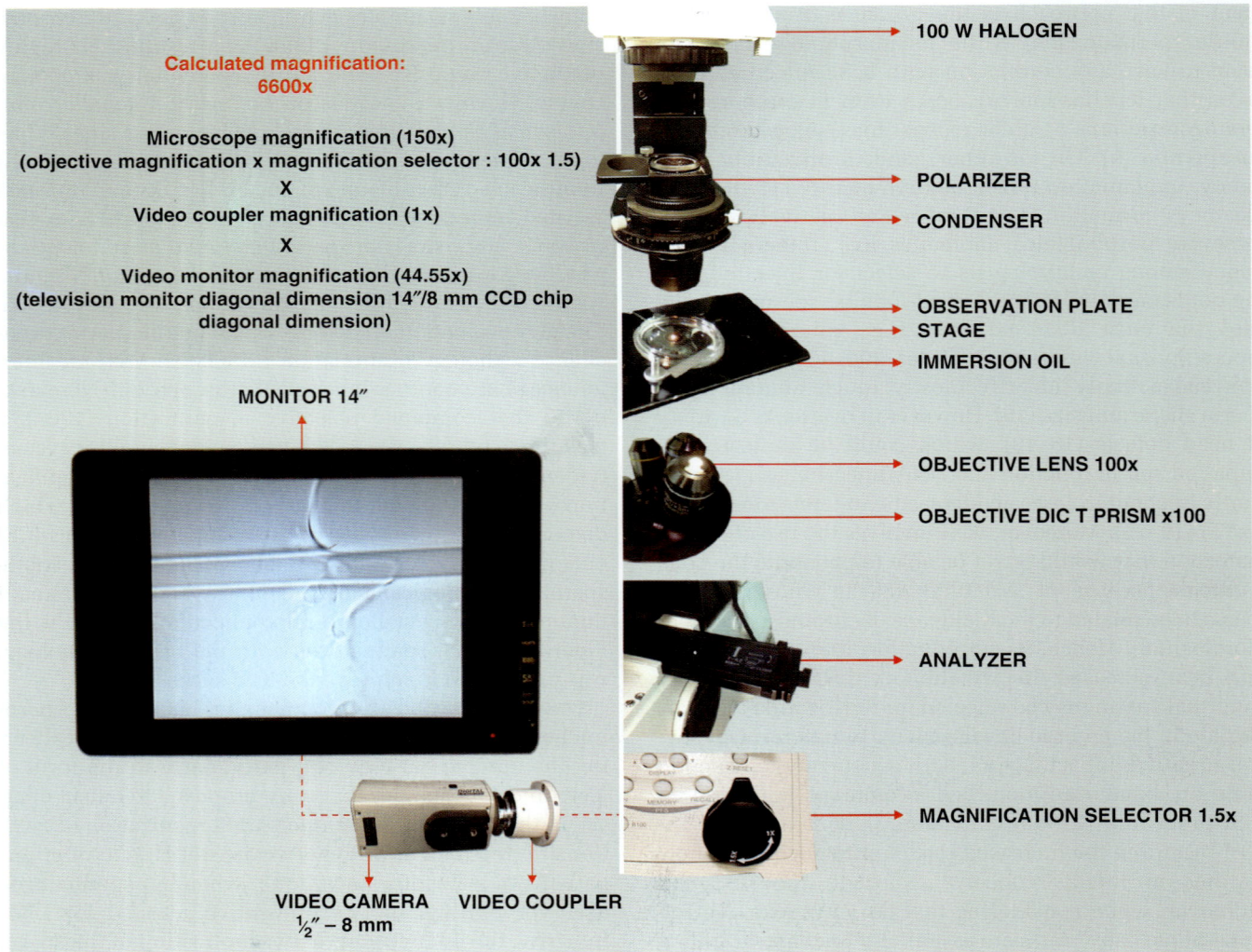

Figure 10.1 IMSI apparatus resulting in the corresponding calculated magnification. *Abbreviations*: DIC, differential interference contrast; CCD, charge-coupled device.

optical path length for both high and low spatial frequencies of the sample.

CALCULATION OF MAGNIFICATION

Calculation of the "total reached magnification" may vary depending upon the system components, but usually it is as follows (Fig. 10.1):

Microscope Magnification
(100 × objective magnification × 1.5 × magnification selector)
×
Video Coupler Magnification
(1 × when no other lenses are inserted)
×
Video Magnification [Monitor diagonal measurement (variable)/CCD chip diagonal measurement (variable)]

For example, to achieve a magnification of 6600×, a 14″ monitor (355.6 mm) and an 8 mm CCD (½-inch) are needed.

CHABLON CALCULATION AND DESIGN

The visualization varies with the technical features of the video camera and monitor, and the related magnification level achieved. The relation between the sperm sizes displayed on the monitor and the real ones has to be established. A chablon, that is a transparent celluloid form that can be superimposed on the monitor to determine whether the sperm under consideration fits the real regular shape and size required for selection (Fig. 10.2), can be calculated and designed using the following formula (see also www.microscopyu.com):

Specimen Real Size = Specimen Length Measured on Screen/Total Magnification

DISH PREPARATION

An IMSI dish could have a variety of designs; however, the basic idea should be to make it fit for the congenial way embryologists work in an IVF lab.

Due to the application of Nomarski optics, and in accordance with current literature, IMSI requires a sterile glass-bottomed dish featuring the following (Fig. 10.3):

- Observation droplets of sperm culture medium (with HEPES), each containing a different concentration (0–10%) of polyvinylpyrrolidone (PVP) solution and different quantities of sperm suspension according to the quality of the sample. Small bays extruding from the droplet rim are designed to capture the heads of motile spermatozoa. The PVP concentration has to be coordinated with the intensity of the sperm motility in order to slow down the sample and avoid total immobilization.
- Selection droplets of sperm culture medium, where selected, morphologically different sperm cells are positioned after MSOME evaluation. The number of droplets depends on the applied classification that differentiates sperm quality into choices/classes (best and second best (45); Class I–II–II (46)). Hence, every category has a corresponding selection droplet.
- Injection droplets of sperm culture medium that will host the oocytes to be injected in the following ICSI procedure, one for each oocyte available for microinjection. In some cases, embryologists prefer to move the selected sperm to a second plastic dish where the conventional ICSI procedure will take place. All microdroplets are placed under sterile liquid paraffin.

The choice of the glass dish is very important: the less hydrophilic, the more appropriate it is. Thanks to this feature the drop edge tends to remain well defined, which enables better focusing and retard drying of the drops.

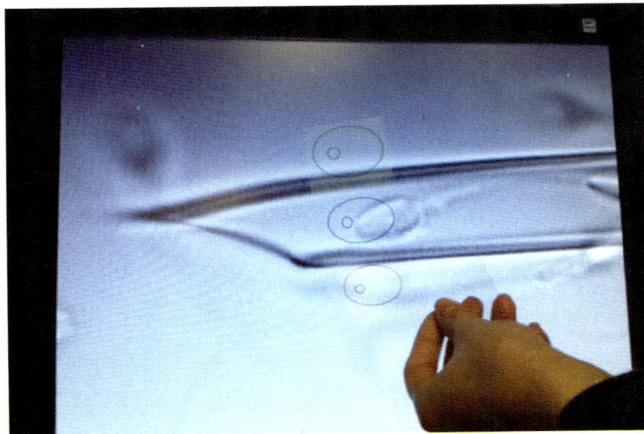

Figure 10.2 The chablon: a transparent celluloid form that can be superimposed on the monitor to verify sperm shape and size.

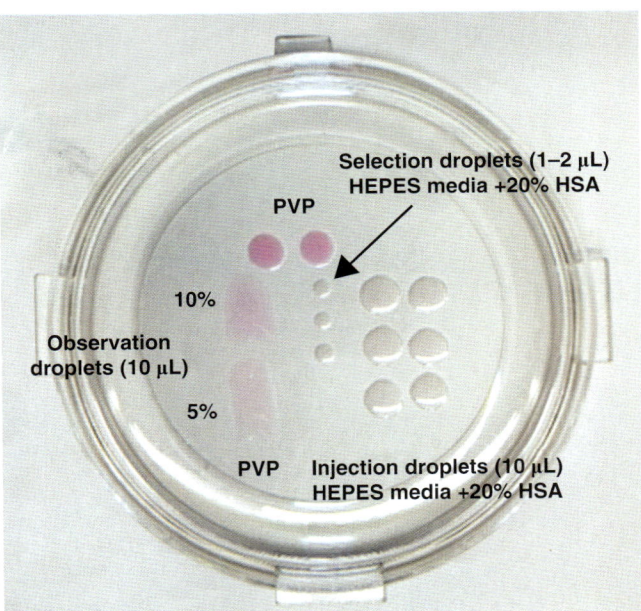

Figure 10.3 An example of a glass-bottomed dish prepared for IMSI (sperm selection and oocyte injection in the same dish). *Abbreviations*: HSA, human serum albumin; HEPES, N-(2-hydroxyethyl)piperazine-N′-ethanesulfonic acid; PVP, polyvinyl pyrrolidone.

SAMPLE PREPARATION

Freshly ejaculated semen is subjected to standard morphological selection of motile spermatozoa on the basis of a two-layer density gradient system: 1 mL of postejaculated liquefied semen is placed onto the gradient and centrifuged at 375 g for 15 minutes at 25°C. The sperm cell pellet is suspended by adding 3 mL of sperm culture medium, and then recentrifuged for 10 minutes. The supernatant is removed and replaced by sperm culture medium to bring the final concentration of motile sperm cells to about 4×10^6 spermatozoa per milliliter. In severe oligozoospermic cases with sperm density below 1×10^6 spermatozoa per ejaculate, liquefied semen are placed onto 1 mL of the low density layer only, and then centrifuged as described above. The final sperm cell pellet is resuspended in 0.1–0.2 mL of sperm culture medium.

MSOME Criteria and Evaluation Procedure

Based on data collected by scanning and transmission electron microscopy (39), the MSOME criteria for normally shaped nuclei are size (average length and width to be 4.75 ± 0.28 μm and 3.28 ± 0.20 μm, respectively), smoothness, symmetry, oval configuration (without extrusion or invagination of the nuclear mass also defined as a regional disorder), and homogeneity of the nuclear chromatin mass containing no more than one vacuole, which occupies less than 4% of the nuclear area (0.78 ± 0.18 μm) (Fig. 10.4). Spermatozoa with abnormal head size are excluded by using the transparent form called chablon (Fig. 10.2). Spermatozoa showing severe malformations, such as a pin, amorphous, tapered, round, or multinucleated head, which can be identified clearly even at low magnifications (200 to 400×), are not assessed by MSOME. Spermatozoa with an uncertain determination are excluded from selection. In order to perform an accurate sperm evaluation, embryologists follow each apparently suitable motile single sperm cell by moving the microscopic stage in the x, y, and z directions until the smallest details are also visualized. Some morphological defects, such as large vacuoles, are revealed only when sperm move. Therefore, motility can be beneficial to morphological observation. On the other hand, static sperm images only allow evaluation of the visible part, leaving some morphological alterations unveiled. Additionally, collaboration between two embryologists analyzing together the same sample at the same time is recommended in order to minimize the subjective nature of sperm evaluation. The amount of time needed to identify the best-looking spermatozoa in a particular sample depends on the quality.

Only motile spermatozoa with morphologically suitable nuclei are retrieved from the observation droplets and aspirated into a sterilized glass (angulated/nonangulated) pipette with a 9 μm inner diameter tip. Sperm cells are then placed into the corresponding selection droplets and finally injected into the oocytes for the traditional ICSI procedure (1) that is performed with a motorized micromanipulator system at room temperature, since prolonged manipulation at 37°C has demonstrated to be detrimental for preserving good sperm quality (47).

CLASSIFICATIONS

For those beginners, IMSI practice differs significantly from theory, being one of the issues that have often limited its wider introduction. The procedure might be perceived as a technically tricky method to learn, extremely complex as against the amount of morphological data to assess and classify. Thus, emerged the need to focus on specific aspects of the sperm morphology and to synthesize that information into classifications drawn from recent advances in the field of infertility and everyday use.

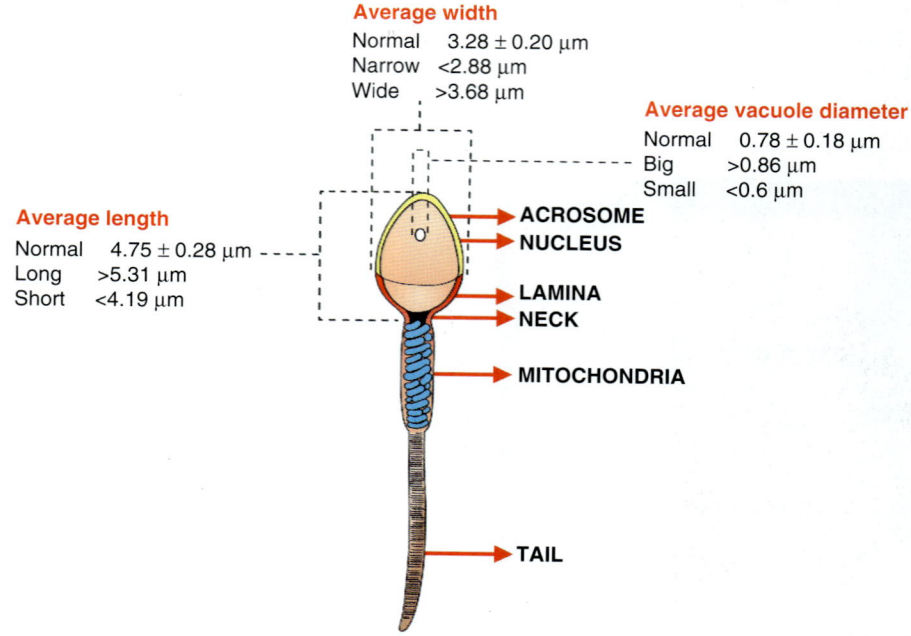

Figure 10.4 Six sperm subcellular organelles evaluated by MSOME criteria (40) and sperm standard dimensions.

Bartoov

Spermatozoa selected by MSOME criteria were evaluated as "best" and "second-best" based on the presence/absence of normal nuclei, respectively, in the test sample. In the second-best group, the following fixed levels of hierarchy were established to facilitate identification of the minimally impaired forms: large/small oval forms, narrow/wide forms, regional disorders, large vacuoles plus normal shape/size, and abnormal forms plus large vacuoles.

Fertilization, top embryo, implantation, pregnancy, and delivery rates per cycle were significantly higher within the "best" group, whereas the abortion rate was significantly lower among the "second-best" choices ($F = 10.5$, $P \leq 0.01$; $F = 4.6$, $P \leq 0.03$; $F = 23.4$, $P \leq 0.01$; $\chi^2 = 15.5$, $P \leq 0.05$; $\chi^2 = 19.6$, $P \leq 0.01$; and $\chi^2 = 5.5$, $P \leq 0.02$, respectively) (45).

Vanderzwalmen

Based on literature demonstrating the existence of a negative association between sperm nuclear vacuoles, natural fertility potential, (48,49) and pregnancy occurrence (43) Vanderzwalmen et al. (50) assume that, for specific morphological malformations, the presence of large vacuoles in the sperm nuclei indicates a more serious damage to the nuclear DNA content and organization than shape or size impairment. Hence, they classify spermatozoa into the following four groups based on the presence, size, and number of vacuoles (Figs. 10.5, 10.6): Grade I: normal shape and lack of vacuoles; Grade II: maximum two small vacuoles; Grade III: more than two small vacuoles or at least one large vacuole; Grade IV: large vacuoles and abnormal head shapes or other defects involving the sperm head base. In a group of 25 IMSI patients, the injection of a total of 442 oocytes with grade I (7%), II (60%), III (20%), and IV (13%) spermatozoa selected at 6600× did not determine any statistically significant difference among the four groups in the number of zygotes and embryo development to day 3. On the other hand, upon joint analysis and multiple comparisons (except for GI vs. GII and GIII vs. GIV), they differed significantly in their development into blastocysts and good-quality blastocysts. Being statistically acceptable to combine groups I and II ($n = 86$), and groups III and IV ($n = 78$), it was observed that, injection with grade I and grade II spermatozoa resulted in a higher rate of blastocyst and good quality blastocyst development compared with compromised spermatozoa (grade III and grade IV) (60.5% vs. 3.8%; $P < 0.001$ and 37.2% vs. 1.3%; $P < 0.001$). Hence, the size and number of nuclear vacuoles demonstrated a substantial negative effect on the embryo development into the blastocyst stage.

Cassuto and Barak

A scoring system was implemented to provide a friendly tool that will allow embryologists to rapidly classify

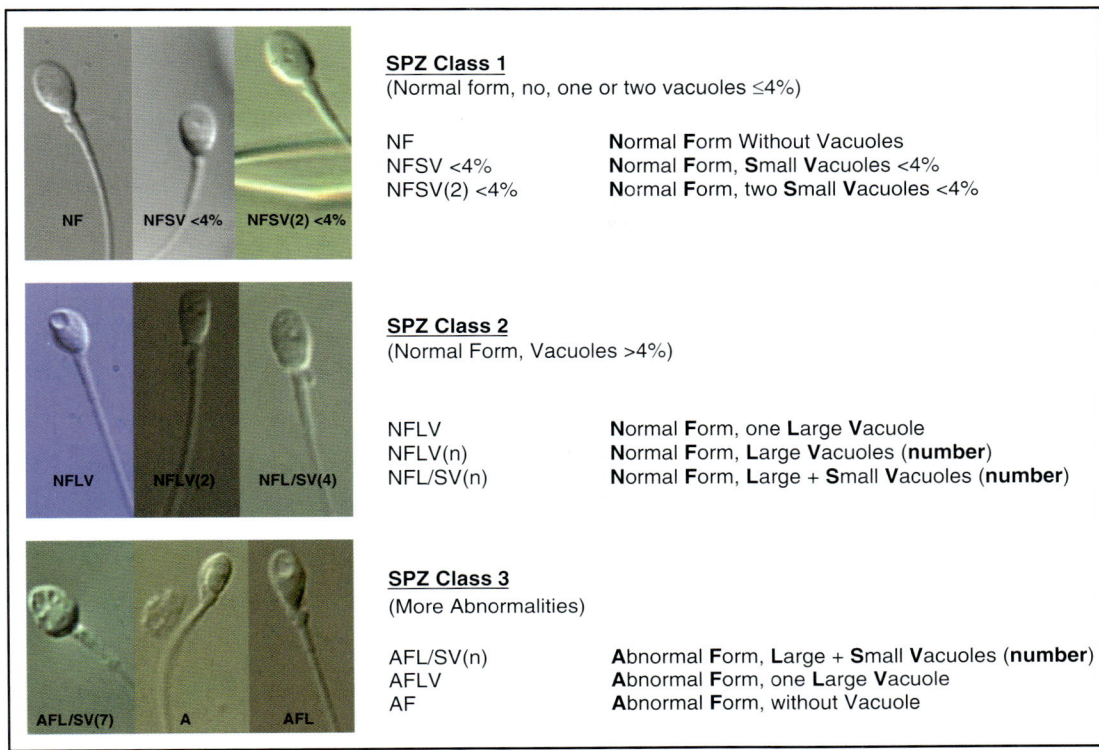

Figure 10.5 Morphological sperm classification at high magnification based on presence, size, and number of vacuoles (50). *Abbreviations*: SPZ, spermatozoa. *Source*: Courtesy of Pierre Vanderzwalmen.

sperm cells just prior ICSI, thus, shortening the prolonged time of the procedure (46). Based on the calculation of coefficients with area under the best ROC curve of 0.618, head shape, presence of vacuoles, and head base shape are identified as the major characteristics for sperm classification. As a result, a fixed total score of 6 points is assigned to sperm with morphologically normal head, vacuoles and base, distributed as follows: Head × 2 + Vacuole × 3 + Base 1. Conversely, 0 points are awarded to each morphologically abnormal sperm structure. Thus, the calculated total range of sperm scoring varies between 0 and 6. Based on the final score obtained, spermatozoa are categorized as follows: Class I (4–6 points) high-quality spermatozoa; Class II (1–3 points) medium-quality spermatozoa; Class III (0 points) poor-quality spermatozoa (Fig. 10.7). When the classification was applied to spermatozoa prior ICSI, following injection the three sperm classes exhibited a statistically significant difference in the fertilization potential: 79.2% for Class I, 63.2% for Class II, and 42.1% for Class III ($P < 0.04$; $\chi^2 = 6.25$). A trend toward a higher rate of development into blastocysts as a function of sperm classification was seen even if the small numbers prevented from reaching a statistical significance.

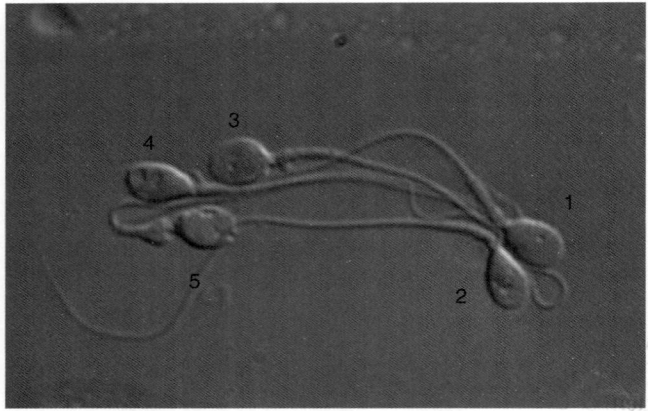

Figure 10.6 Examples of different sizes and numbers of vacuoles according to Ref. 50: 1. Normal shape, one small vacuole; 2. abnormal shape, one small and one large vacuole; 3. abnormal shape, one small vacuole; 4. abnormal shape, one small and one large vacuole; 5. abnormal shape, one small vacuole. Source: Courtesy of Pierre Vanderzwalmen.

IMSI REPRODUCTIVE OUTCOMES

Based on the assumption that morphologically severely impaired spermatozoa show reduced fertilization, pregnancy, and implantation rates (9,10), the impact of subtle morphological anomalies detected under high magnification (6600×) on ICSI outcome was investigated to identify the most relevant (40). A total of 10,000 spermatozoa (100 sperm samples, each including 100 spermatozoa) were evaluated. It was observed that in standard IVF-ICSI cycles patients who exhibited less than 20% spermatozoa with normal nucleus—according to MSOME criteria—did not achieve pregnancy. With respect to the ICSI fertilization rate, morphological normalcy of the entire sperm cell—according to MSOME criteria–showed a positive and significant correlation ($r = 0.52$, $P \leq 0.01$) and a very high predictive value (area under the ROC curve, 88%), whereas no association with pregnancy outcome was found. Normalcy of the sperm nucleus (shape + chromatin content), defined by MSOME, was significantly and positively correlated with both fertilization and pregnancy rates ($r = 0.42$, $P \leq 0.01$ and $r = 0.38$, $P \leq 0.01$, respectively). Else, the predictive value of normalcy of the sperm nucleus turned out to be significantly higher (areas under the ROC curve 72% and 74%, respectively). Hence, the authors could conclude that the sperm nucleus is the most important sperm parameter affecting ICSI outcome.

Later on MSOME criteria were applied to choose the morphologically best sperm cell to inject into the oocyte (51): Fifty IMSI couples were compared with 50 ICSI couples within a matched-control study (couples with a similar number of previous ICSI failures). Implantation and pregnancy rates following IMSI were significantly higher, whereas the abortion rate was significantly lower as against the present ICSI trial. In addition, the IMSI attempt produced a significantly higher top embryo percentage as against the present ICSI treatment. Moreover, 12 unmatched IMSI cases with an average of 9.1 ± 1.2 previous ICSI failures achieved a 50% pregnancy rate following their first IMSI trial. Overall, the results demonstrated a significant improvement in the IMSI success rate in couples with at least two previous ICSI failures. According to recent reports, these couples seem to have the worst reproductive prognosis with a dramatic reduction in pregnancy and implantation rates as compared with couples who underwent 0–1 previous IVF failed

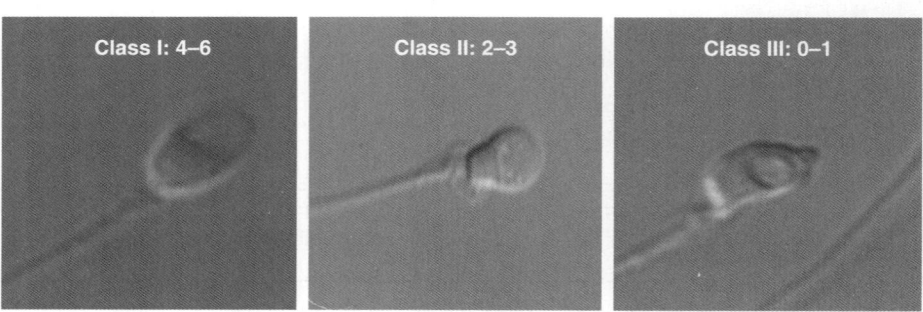

Figure 10.7 Cassuto and Barak score system. Source: Adapted from Ref. 46.

attempts (52,53). Antinori (54) designed a prospective, randomized, controlled protocol to assess the potential advantages offered by IMSI in the treatment of patients with severe OAT, regardless of previous ICSI failed attempts. The study participants were subsequently split into subgroups by the number of previous failed attempts (subgroup A: no previous attempts; sub-group B: 1 previous failed attempt; sub-group C: ≥2 previous failed attempts). The two different techniques were compared in terms of pregnancy, abortion, and implantation rates.

Pregnancy and implantation rates were statistically higher in the IMSI cycles than in the ICSI group (pregnancy rate: 39.2% vs. 26.5%; $P = 0.004$) (implantation rate: 17.3% vs. 11.3%; $P = 0.007$).

However, cases with two or more failed attempts benefited most from IMSI, with a significant doubling of pregnancy rates (12.9% vs. 29.8%; $P = 0.017$) and a remarkable 50% reduction in the abortion rate (17% vs. 35%). No statistical difference was observed in terms of abortions, but the clinical trend was clearly in favor of the IMSI method in cases with two or more previous failed attempts.

Based on the above results it can be speculated that, in those couples, the male factor could be featured by semen impairment, undetected by conventional diagnostic tools, thus reducing the effectiveness of previous ICSI treatments.

Those conclusions seem to be challenged by a prospective study on 200 couples with a history of at least two previous implantation failures due to mixed infertility factors enrolled by female age matching (≤39 years) in order to compare laboratory and clinical outcomes of IMSI ($n = 100$) and ICSI ($n = 100$) cycles (55). In spite of IMSI showing a positive clinical trend in terms of pregnancy (IMSI: 26% vs. ICSI: 19%), implantation (IMSI: 13.6% vs. ICSI: 9.8%), miscarriage (IMSI: 15.3% vs. ICSI: 31.7%), and live birth (IMSI: 21% vs. ICSI: 12%) rates, it did not produce a statistically significant improvement compared with ICSI. Similar results were obtained also by splitting the study population in subgroups, which could not prove statistically, male factor as a cause of infertility that could benefit the most from IMSI following repeated implantation failures after conventional ICSI.

The same issue was recently investigated by Balaban (56) who tested IMSI application within a prospective randomized study on an unselected infertile population (female age <35 years) to compare the clinical outcome of 87 IMSI and 81 ICSI cycles. Both groups were comparable in terms of fertilization rates and quantity and quality of embryos transferred. Implantation, pregnancy, and live birth rates showed a clinical trend in favor of the IMSI group over the ICSI group (28.9% vs. 19.5% and 54.0% vs. 44.4%, 43.7% vs. 38.3%, respectively; not significant), whereas the IMSI multiple pregnancy rate was significantly higher (34.0% vs. 16.7%; $P < 0.001$). Interestingly, when subgroup analyses on etiology of infertility were performed, male factor couples were seen to benefit more from the IMSI procedure, above all patients with sperm count under 1 million/mL in the basal ejaculate, as shown by significantly higher implantation rates (29.6% vs. 15.2%, $P = 0.01$).

A similar study population was investigated by Wilding (57) within a prospective randomized trial, which involved a heterogeneous population of 232 couples (1–3 years of infertility, sperm count 1×10^6/mL and 20×10^6/mL; female factor included, previous failures not mentioned) to be treated either by IMSI ($n = 122$) or ICSI ($n = 110$). Unlike Balaban's trial, this investigation was able to demonstrate the superior effectiveness of IMSI with respect to the number of good-quality embryos and pregnancy and implantation rates even when applied on an unselected infertile population.

The positive impact on embryo quality (57) and blastocyst development (50) previously reported in the literature, inspired Knez (58) to investigate the clinical role of IMSI on 57 randomized couples (37 IMSI vs. 20 ICSI) with poor semen quality and history of total cleavage arrest after day 5 culture in former ICSI attempts. Probably the lack of a preliminary power calculation, and the relating small size of the sample prevented the clinical outcomes from being significantly improved by IMSI with the exception of the cancellation rate/embryo transfer, which evidenced a significant reduction (IMSI 0% vs. ICSI 27%; $P \leq 0.05$).

The main possible reason for IMSI effectiveness might be the creation of genetically normal embryos with higher chances of implantation and birth, and a decreased abortion risk. To test this theory, Figueira (59) carried out an interesting randomized study on a total of 120 couples (60 IMSI, 60 ICSI) receiving preimplantation genetic screening [fluorescence in situ hybridization (FISH) analysis: x, y, 13, 16, 18, 21, 22] for advanced maternal age (severe OAT excluded). That was the first trial on the chromosomal status of IMSI-derived embryos, and showed the following statistically significant results: lower sex chromosome aneuploidies (IMSI 15% vs. ICSI 23.5%; $P = 0.0139$), lower chaotic chromosomal status with two or more chromosomal numerical abnormalities (IMSI 18.8% vs. ICSI 27.5%; $P = 0.0193$), higher incidence of XX euploid karyotype (IMSI 30% vs. ICSI 21.6%; $P = 0.0326$), and lower risk of transfer cancellation (IMSI 2.5% vs. ICSI 11.8%; $P = 0.0016$). Those outcomes confirm previous results regarding the role of IMSI as an indirect method for rescuing oocytes in patients aged 30 years and older, with impaired capability of repairing the DNA of the injected spermatozoon (46) and might provide a convincing explanation for IMSI effectiveness. However, even if in a recent methanolysis (60), involving a limited number of studies with variable designs, IMSI resulted more beneficial than ICSI in terms of top-quality embryo development, implantation, pregnancy rates and reduction of abortion, the number of RCTs is still too restricted to come to definitive conclusions (Table 10.1).

One of the conceivable expectations from the application of IMSI will be the reduction of congenital anomalies and genetic disorders due to the use of spermatozoa with a normal nucleus, which reduces the risk for DNA defects. That assumption was confirmed by Cassuto (62).

Table 10.1 IMSI Laboratory and Clinical Outcomes

	Study design	Population	Infertility factor/inclusion criteria	Female age (IMSI group)	Male age	Investigated variables	Main IMSI outcomes (Statistically significant)
Bartoov 2003 (53)	Comparative prospective study matched by previous ICSI failures	50 ICSI vs. 50 IMSI	Male/at least 2 ICSI failures	29.6 ± 3.5	31.7 ± 4.7	FR, Embryo quality, PR, IR, AR	Higher PR, Higher Embryo quality, Higher IR, Lower AR
Berkovitz 2006 (43)	Comparative prospective study matched by previous ICSI failures	80 ICSI vs. 80 IMSI	Male/at least 2 ICSI failures	32.3 ± 4.8	NP	FR, Embryo quality, PR, IR, AR	Higher PR, Higher embryo quality, Higher IR, Lower AR
Hazout 2006 (61)	Clinical observational	125 previous ICSI failures vs. 125 subsequent IMSI	Mixed/at least 2 ICSI failures	<38	NP	FR, Embryo quality, PR, IR	Higher PR, Higher IR
Antinori 2008 (54)	Randomized	219 ICSI vs. 227 IMSI	Male	31.65 ± 3.23	NP	FR, PR, IR, AR	Higher PR, Higher IR
Balaban 2011 (56)	Randomized	82 ICSI vs. 87 IMSI	Mixed	29.76 ± 4.03	33.97 ± 5.52	FR, PR, IR, LBR, MPR	Higher MPR, Higher IR, Only in male factor subgroup
Oliveira 2011 (55)	Comparative prospective study matched by female age	100 ICSI vs. 100 IMSI	Mixed	36.8 ± 3.9	39.8 ± 6.2	FR, Embryo quality, PR, IR, AR, LBR	None
Wilding 2011 (57)	Randomized	110 ICSI vs. 122 IMSI	Mixed	33.6 ± 4.5	NR	FR, Embryo quality, PR, IR, LBR	Higher PR, Higher embryo quality, Higher IR
Knez 2011 (58)	Randomized	37 ICSI vs. 20 IMSI	Mixed	35.8 ± 4.36	NR	FR, BDR, PR, IR	Lower total embryos arrest
Figueira 2011 (59)	Randomized	60 ICSI vs. 60 IMSI	Mixed/First ICSI attempt with PGS for Advanced maternal age	37.3 ± 3.2	43.6 ± 8.9	FR, Aneuploidies: X, Y, 13, 16, 18, 21, 22, Transfer cancellation rate	Lower sex chromosomal aneuploidies, Higher XX euploid embryos, Lower transfer cancellations

Abbreviations: AR, abortion rate; BDR, blastocyst development rate; FR, fertilization rate; ICSI, intracytoplasmic sperm injection; IMSI, intracytoplasmic morphologically selected sperm injection; IR, implantation rate; LBR, live birth rate; MPR, multiple pregnancy rate; NP, not present; NR, not rated; PGS, preimplantation genetic screening; PR, pregnancy rate.

He studied prospectively the follow-up of 1028 children conceived with IMSI (n = 450) and ICSI (n = 578), and compared their outcomes in terms of percentage of major malformations and genetic disorders. The results exhibited that IMSI is associated with significantly fewer birth defects than ICSI (1.77% vs. 4.15%, respectively). Additional evidence comes from the low prevalence (1.5%) of chromosomal abnormalities and birth defects observed by our group on a population of 443 children born after IMSI.

IMSI and DNA Integrity

When Kruger strict criteria were originally introduced (63), it was still not possible to associate poor sperm morphology with fragmented DNA (64,65), whereas following reports found that abnormal spermatozoa negatively correlate with DNA integrity (66,67), especially in case of head malformations (68–70). The potential relationship between sperm morphology and genetic integrity has become very relevant following the introduction of ICSI that gives a chance of fertilization even to those male gametes affected by severe malformations (13,67,71) but it is limited by its low magnification and low resolution of the sperm morphology assessment, which might miss some subtle defects. In both cases, there is considerable concern about the fact that morphologically abnormal spermatozoa with significantly elevated levels of numerical sperm chromosomal aberrations, reactive oxygen species (ROS) production, and DNA chain fragmentation (72,73) would contribute to impair fertilization, embryogenesis, or fetal development. The same considerable concern is still expressed on their contribution to the birth of infants with higher prevalence of chromosomal abnormalities and birth defects over natural conception (74).

Following the introduction of a new visual method applied on conventional ICSI technique called IMSI, sperm characteristics that were undetected by conventional microscopy can be clearly identified. This means that their association with the ICSI outcome can be investigated and can provide reliable evidence that a morphologically normal sperm nucleus is the most important sperm variable showing a close relation with both fertilization and pregnancy rates (40). Based on preliminary, unpublished data by Bartoov's group, which reported a significant negative correlation between the size of the nuclear vacuoles and chromatin stability assessed by sperm chromatin structure assay, and Lee (75), who demonstrated that no increase in chromosome aberrations was found in spermatozoa with large or small heads, it has been proposed that the existence of large sperm vacuoles in the sperm nuclei indicates more damage to nuclear DNA content and organization than nuclear shape or size impairment (43). Furthermore, large nuclear vacuole inoculation resulted in normal, early embryonic development (normal fertilization, development of top-quality embryos, and implantation) followed by impaired embryo survival (low pregnancy and high abortion rates) (43).

In order to prove that large nuclear vacuoles in the sperm cell may reflect some underlying chromosomal or DNA defect, the selection of sperm cells with and without large vacuoles from the same ejaculate and subsequent evaluation by different biochemical methods from an independent analytic system was recommended (43). Therefore, a report by Hazout (61) compared the outcomes of 125 couples with at least two previous ICSI failures and an undetected female infertility factor that received conventional and high-magnification ICSI in two sequential attempts. Following sperm injection into the oocytes without nuclear alterations, a double PR and a 50% decrease in the abortion rate were recorded as against similar cases treated by conventional ICSI. In 72 of 125 study patients, the degree of sperm DNA fragmentation was determined by terminal deoxynucleotidyl transferase dUTP nick end labeling (TUNEL) method, and the outcomes of high-magnification ICSI were compared in cases with different sperm DNA fragmentation degrees. However, that test was not performed directly with the ICSI-selected sperm samples. A marked rise in clinical implantation and birth rates was observed in patients with normal (<30%), moderately increased (30–40%), and highly (>40%) increased incidence of DNA fragmentation in the ejaculated spermatozoa.

In order to highlight the above assumptions, Franco (76) evaluated the extent of DNA fragmentation (TUNEL assay) and the presence of denatured single-stranded or normal double-stranded DNA (acridine orange fluorescence technique) in spermatozoa with large nuclear vacuoles selected under high magnification compared with those with normal nucleus. The percentage of positive DNA fragmentation was significantly higher ($P < 0.0001$) in large nuclear vacuole spermatozoa (29.1%) than in the normal nucleus group (15.9%). Similarly, the percentage of denatured single-stranded DNA was significantly higher ($P < 0.0001$) in the former (67.9%) than in the latter (33.1%).

So far, a direct relation to DNA quality has not been tested in single selected spermatozoa. With that in mind as a major goal, Garolla (77) evaluated 10 patients affected by severe testicular damage (severe oligozoospermia) by assaying the chromatin structure (sperm DNA integrity by acridine orange; DNA fragmentation by TUNEL assay) and sperm aneuploidies (FISH test) on single immotile sperm cells morphologically selected under high magnification (13,161×). Ten morphologically normal spermatozoa with no vacuoles (group A) and 10 morphologically normal spermatozoa with at least one large head vacuole (group B) were retrieved from each sample. Single cells from group A showed a more physiological status of DNA integrity and DNA fragmentation than cells from group B. Furthermore, no chromosomal alteration was detected by FISH analysis in group-A cells. Moreover, the authors reported that, when morphologically normal spermatozoa with or without large head vacuoles were considered as a single population, the mean results (data not shown) from all tests were significantly better than those obtained from unselected cells in the first part of the study (all $P < 0.001$).

As a result, a strong correlation between high-magnification morphology, sperm DNA status, and the chromatin origin of nuclear vacuoles visualized by MSOME was inferred, which could be indicative of molecular defects responsible for abnormal chromatin remodeling during sperm maturation, and sperm DNA damage (78), thus compromising ICSI outcomes.

Considering that DIC does may not allow intracellular evaluation (79–81) because of technical limitations, and that detection of chromatin vacuoles in the anterior part of the sperm head requires electron microscopy under a magnification factor of 20,000×, the acrosomal origin of the vacuoles was theorized (82). The first experiment of this study consisted of MSOME evaluation on immotile spermatozoa followed by assessment of the sperm acrosomal status using *Pisum sativum* agglutinin (PSA)-fluorescein isothiocyanate. In most cases (70.9%), the complete acrosome reaction corresponded to regularly shaped spermatozoa with no or minor vacuolization, whereas in sperm with incomplete or missing acrosome reaction the vacuole presence was 60.7%. The second experiment involved evaluation of immotile sperm by MSOME before and after inducing acrosome reaction by ionophore A23587. Vacuole-free spermatozoa increased from 41.2% to 63.8% ($P > 0.005$), so did acrosome-reacted gametes that rose from $17.4 + 7.8$ to $36.1 + 12.7$ ($P < 0.001$). The last part of the study was performed on motile acrosome-reacting spermatozoa that were analyzed by MSOME. Large protruding blebs, similar to vacuoles when seen upfront, as well as a sort of invagination looking like a vacuole, were seen in the following image. The author came to the conclusion that vacuole-free spermatozoa microinjected during IMSI are mostly acrosome-reacted spermatozoa.

Origin and significance of large nuclear vacuoles were also investigated by other groups. Almeida (83) evaluated 10,000 spermatozoa from 50 men (mean age: 31.4 ± 3.7 years; sperm count: 25.7×10^6 cells/mL; motility: 43.7%; Kruger normal forms: 5.5%) undergoing ICSI procedure by some MSOME criteria. A positive correlation was noted between the presence of large and small vacuoles, the level of fragmented DNA assessed by TUNEL test, and the patient's age, whereas no association was seen between chromosomal aneuploidies tested by FISH technique on chromosomes X, Y, 13, 18, 21 and the presence of nuclear vacuoles.

In a recent study (84), transmission electron microscopy was employed to determine the localization of spermatozoa with large vacuoles (defined as those occupying >13% of the head area) from three teratozoospermic, highly vacuolated samples (33%, 18%, and 40%). The result showed that their localization corresponded exactly to the nucleus. Then, confocal microscopy coupled with 4′,6-diamidino-2-phenylindole (DAPI) immunofluorescence was performed on the same samples and showed that mean DAPI fluorescence intensity has the same evolution in the nucleus and vacuoles, but it is significantly reduced in vacuoles as against the remaining nucleus (83.6 vs. 211.4; $P < 0.0001$).

As a second experiment, in the same trial, fresh samples from 20 teratozoospermic men were used to evaluate acrosome morphology (proacrosin immunolabeling), the level of DNA fragmentation (TUNEL test), and chromatin condensation (aniline blue staining), as well as the appearance of aneuploidies (fish) in both native and vacuolated spermatozoa selected by 6600× magnification. As shown by the results, vacuolated spermatozoa demonstrated a higher percentage of abnormal acrosome morphology (77.6% vs. 70.6%; $P = 0.014$), abnormal chromatin condensation (50.4% vs. 26.5%; $P < 0.0001$), and chromosome abnormalities (7.8% vs. 1.3%; $P < 0.0001$) than the native ones; however, no connection between vacuoles and DNA fragmentation was reported.

A further contribution to investigate the origin and structure of large vacuoles was given by Boitrelle (85). In her study, a population of 15 men with different quality of the sperm samples (five normospermic, five oligo-astheno-teratozoospermic, and five teratozoospermic) was enrolled to provide 30 top and vacuolated (>25%) spermatozoa. Each sperm cell was then compared with unselected sperm cells by using a triple probe procedure: aniline blue staining (condensation), TUNEL assay (DNA fragmentation), and FISH analysis (X,Y,18). The non-condensed chromatin rate resulted significantly higher in vacuolated spermatozoa than in "top" ($36.2\% + 1.9\%$ vs. $7.6\% + 1.3\%$, respectively; $P < 0.0001$) and unselected spermatozoa ($36.2\% + 1.9\%$ vs. $25.1\% + 3.7\%$, respectively; $P < 0.01$). DNA fragmentation rates were similarly low for both "top" and "vacuolated" spermatozoa ($0.7\% + 0.4\%$ vs. $1.3\% + 0.4\%$, respectively; $P = 0.25$). The "top" and "vacuolated" spermatozoa did not differ significantly in terms of aneuploidy rate ($1.1\% + 0.5\%$ vs. $2.2\% + 0.7\%$, respectively; $P = 0.25$). In the second study phase, atomic force microscopy was used to evaluate 10 "top" and 10 vacuolated sperm cells from two subjects (normozoospermic and oligo-astheno-teratozoospermic, respectively) in order to determine the mean cross-sectional area of the anterior and posterior portion of the head as well as large vacuoles. The vacuoles turned out to be a concavity in the intact structure of the plasma membrane (Fig. 10.8). That finding was further evaluated by 3D deconvolution microscopy analysis on five different samples (two normozoospermic, two oligo-astheno-teratozoospermic, and one with teratozoospermia) having 40 spermatozoa each (equally split between "top" and vacuolated). Labeling of DNA and acrosome was performed by DAPI and PSA lectin staining, respectively; both methods were then combined and evaluated by simultaneous DIC/epifluorescence observations. As shown by the results, a vacuole can be interpreted as a DAPI negative nuclear concavity surrounded by plasma and acrosomal membranes and intact acrosome (Fig. 10.9) linked to failure of sperm chromatin condensation (85). The above findings were recently confirmed by Cassuto (86) within a study on 5200 spermatozoa from 26 OAT men (count $33.2 \pm 30.0 \times 10^6$/mL; motility $41.3\% \pm 13.2\%$; WHO normal morphology $26.2\% \pm 7.4\%$) with IVF failures, and an equal number of unselected spermatozoa. The chromatin decondensation

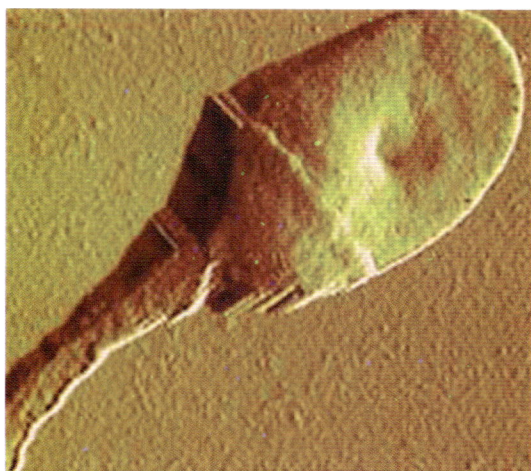

Figure 10.8 A vacuolated spermatozoon observed using Atomic Force Microscopy (AFM) to determine the mean cross-sectional area of both the anterior and posterior portion of the head. *Source*: Adapted from Ref. 85.

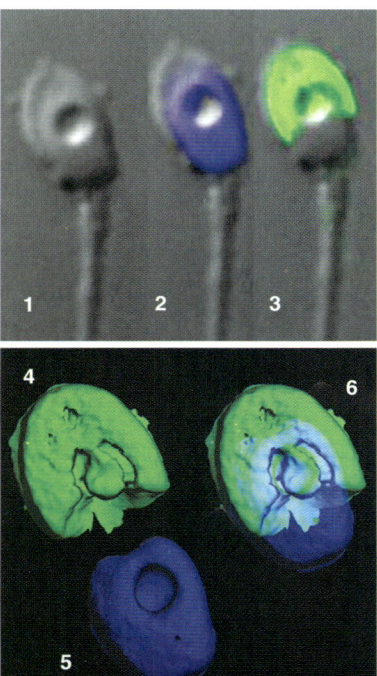

Figure 10.9 Vacuolated spermatozoon, observed under high magnification with Nomarski contrast (DIC): a DIC/DAPI merge (1 and 2) and a DIC/FITC-labeled PSA lectin merge (3). 3D reconstructed images of the same spermatozoa (4–6). DAPI fluoresces blue (4) and PSA lectin fluoresces green (5). Colocalization of fluorescent probes (6). *Abbreviations*: DAPI, 4′,6-diamidino-2-phenylindole; DIC, differential interference contrast; FITC, fluorescein isothiocyanate; PSA, *Pisum sativum* agglutinin. *Source*: Courtesy of Florence Boitrelle.

rate scored 0 according to his classification (highly vacuolated and morphologically abnormal), and turned out to be twice as high as in the control group (19.5% vs. 10.1%; $P < 0.0001$), whereas DNA fragmentation did not significantly differ between the groups (4.2% vs. 3.7%; $P =$ not significant).

A different theory regarding the real meaning of sperm head large vacuoles and their presumed detrimental effect on sperm DNA integrity was made by Watanabe (87). TUNEL assay applied on a heterogeneous population of 12 men (mainly normospermic: 6/12) detected DNA fragmentation in a similar small percentage of both normal nonvacuolated (3.3%) and normal large vacuolated (3.5%) spermatozoa confirming Boitrelle's observations. Moreover when TUNEL fluorescein images are merged with the corresponding DAPI and DIC ones from the same analyzed sperm, it was observed that DAPI negative/fluorescein negative signals (no nuclear content) can correspond to the localization of large nuclear vacuoles and at the same time sperm with normal shaped nuclei without vacuoles can be DAPI positive/Fluorescein positive (fragmented). Thus the author concluded that large vacuoles are craters that do not reflect abnormalities of the sperm head genome but common physiological variations occurring during human spermatogenesis.

On the basis of a positive correlation between DNA fragmentation and sperm nuclear anomalies (7,57,76,83), even other methods capable of selecting mature spermatozoa with no DNA damage as hyaluronic acid (HA) assay (74,88–92) might facilitate the extraction of sperm cells with normal nuclear morphology during MSOME evaluation. Two different methods, namely a medium with HA (SpermSlow™; MediCult) (92) and an HA-binding assay (PICSI®; MidAtlantic Diagnostics) (93), were applied prior to MSOME analysis to prove their effectiveness in the selection of motile spermatozoa with normal morphology. Results were controversial: while Parmegiani (92) found a significantly higher proportion of nuclearly normal spermatozoa in the HA-bounded group than among those collected from PVP (14.5% vs. 11%, respectively), Petersen (93) did not observe any difference in the normal sperm morphology between HA-bound and HA-unbound spermatozoa (2.7% vs. 2.5%, respectively). Given the different characteristics of the samples involved in the studies (normospermic 94; 6/15 oligospermic 93) and different sperm preparation methods (swim-up 94, density gradient 93) used, further investigations are needed in order to determine the actual contribution of that method to MSOME sperm selection.

CONCLUSIONS

Despite the development of various classifications and methods, a rising number of trials have reported IMSI as having significant clinical benefits in terms of fertilization, embryo quality, pregnancy occurrence, and prosecution for delivery (Table 10.1). The underlying reason for such improvements might be linked to high-magnification (>6000×) assessment offering the chance to detect subtle morphological anomalies that would otherwise be unveiled with conventional methods. Among the different malformations identified by MSOME, those affecting nuclear structure, such as large vacuoles, demonstrated to be highly correlated with male, in vivo and in vitro, reproductive impairment (40,43,50,76). There is still

Table 10.2 Sperm DNA Integrity Tests and Positive Correlation with Vacuoles

	N. subjects	Male age	Parameters	Preparation	Comparison	DNA frag.	Aneuploidies	Abnormal chromatin condensation	Structural chromosome aberration
Franco 2008 (76)	30	NP	Infertile	Density gradients	On single sperm: Normal nucleus vs. LV MSOME criteria	Yes	–	–	–
Garolla 2008 (77)	10	28–37	Severe oligozoos. <1 × 10⁶/mL Testicular damage At least 3 ICSI failures	NP	On single immotile sperm: Normal vs. LV Morphology at 13,000×	Yes	Yes (X,Y,18)	–	–
Almeida 2011 (83)	50	31.4 ± 3.7	Teratozoospermia	NP	On same sample	Yes	No (X,Y,13,18,21)	–	–
Perdrix 2011 (84)	20	36.2 ± 1.3	OAT	Washing DNA frag, aneuploidy: Condensation on native samples Density gradients MSOME DNA Frag. Aneuploidy. Condensation on vacuolated sperm	On single sperm: Native sample vs. LV	No	Yes (X,Y,18)	Yes	–
Wilding 2011 (57)	8	NP	NP	Density gradients	On single sperm: Normal vs. Vacuolated MSOME criteria	Yes	–	–	–
Boitrelle 2011 (85)	15	NP	Mixed; 5 OAT 5 Teratozoospermia 5 Normozoospermia	Density gradients	On same single sperm: Top SPZ vs. LV SPZ Morphology at 10,000×	No	No	Yes	–
Watanabe 2011 (44)	3	NP	Mixed 1 OAT 2 Normozoospermia	Density gradient followed by swim-up	On single immotile sperm: Normal head vs. LV Morphology at 1000×	No	–	–	–
	12	NP	1 OAT, 5 Asthenozoospermia 6 Normozoospermia (2 fertile donors)	Density gradient followed by swim-up	On single sperm: Normal head vs. LV Morphology at 1000×	–	–	–	No
Cassuto 2012 (86)	26	37.1 ± 7.7	OAT IVF failures	Density gradients	On single sperm: Native sample vs. Score 0	No	–	Yes	–
Franco 2012 (94)	66	37.8 ± 6.5	Mixed	Density gradients	On single sperm: Normal nucleus vs. LV MSOME criteria	–	–	Yes	–

Abbreviations: Frag., fragmentation; LV, large vacuoles; NP, not present; OAT, oligo-astheno-terato-zoospermia; SPZ, spermatozoa.

disagreement on the meaning of sperm head vacuoles since their both acrosomal and nuclear origins have been advocated (82,85). In the former, consumption of the acrosomal components into the acrosomal reaction might induce a process of "devacuolization" (82). On the other hand, large vacuoles might have even a nuclear content of unclear origin. Current literature agrees on the presence of higher decondensed DNA levels corresponding to vacuolated regions (84–86,94) (Table 10.2); however, when DNA fragmentation and chromosomal aneuploidies are assessed to find out a potential correlation with highly vacuolated spermatozoa, results are controversial (Table 10.2) (57,76,77,83–87). In this respect, the wide heterogeneity of the experiments—using unmatchable male populations, different sperm preparations, and unfixed morphological criteria—still seems to make it hard to come to sound conclusions. Nonetheless, mention should be made of the embryologist's skill playing a crucial prerequisite role in the performance of an accurate selection under high magnification. In this respect, few ART units in Japan have been reported to have experienced a dramatic decrease in their fertilization rates in the first six months of IMSI application (95,96). No doubt that the use of new tools (DIC system, immersion oil objectives, and glass-bottom dish), the prolonged manipulation and work overload are potentially challenging. On the other hand, the existence of different morphological classifications, and hence the lack of standardization still constitute a substantial limitation to learning, research, and clinical practice purposes. All those factors create skeptical attitudes toward the future of IMSI in the field of ART (44). However, based on current results, IMSI can be recognized as a promising technique that has fostered deeper understanding of the mechanisms interfering with male fertility potential in both natural and assisted reproduction. Like any other innovation, only extensive use and availability of larger amounts of data will generate strong assumptions on feasibility, effectiveness, and safety of the IMSI technique.

ACKNOWLEDGMENTS

The author gratefully acknowledges the precious cooperation of Pierre Vanderzwalmen, Yona Barak, Guy Cassuto, and Florence Boitrelle for the images included in this chapter.

REFERENCES

1. Palermo G, Joris H, Devroey P, Van S.A. Pregnancies after intracytoplasmic injection of single spermatozoon into an oocyte. Lancet 1992; 340: 17–18.
2. Oehninger S, Veeck L, Lanzendorf S, et al. Intracytoplasmic sperm injection: achievement of high pregnancy rates in couples with severe male factor infertility is dependent primarily upon female not male factors. Fertil Steril 1995; 64: 977–81.
3. Kupker W, Schulze W, Diedrich K. Ultrastructure of gametes and intracytoplasmic sperm injection: the significance of sperm morphology. Hum Reprod 1998; 13(Suppl 1): 99–106.
4. Host E, Ernst E, Lindenberg S, Smidt-Jensen S. Morphology of spermatozoa used in IVF and ICSI from oligozoospermic men. Reprod BioMed Online 2001; 3: 212–15.
5. Ciler C-O, Attila J, Tamas K, et al. Sperm selection for ICSI: shape properties do not predict the absence or presence of numerical chromosomal aberrations. Human Reprod 2004; 19: 2052–9.
6. Tasdemir I, Tasdemir M, Tavukcuog SKahraman S, Biberog K. Effect of abnormal sperm head morphology on the outcome of intracytoplasmic sperm injection in humans. Human Reprod 1997; 12: 1214–17.
7. Liu J, Nagy Z, Joris H, et al. Successful fertilization and establishment of pregnancies after intracytoplasmic sperm injection in patients with globozoospermia. Hum Reprod 1995; 10: 626–9.
8. Battaglia DE Koehler JK, Klein NA, Tucker MJ. Failure of oocyte activation after intracytoplasmic sperm injection using round-headed sperm. Fertil Steril 1997; 68: 118–22.
9. Kahraman S, Akarsu C, Cengiz G, et al. Fertility of ejaculated and testicular megalohead spermatozoa with intracytoplasmic sperm injection. Hum Reprod 1999; 14: 726–30.
10. De Vos A, Van De Velde H, Joris H, et al. Influence of individual sperm morphology on fertilization, embryo morphology, and pregnancy outcome of intracytoplasmic sperm injection. Fertil Steril 2003; 79: 42–8.
11. Cohen J, Alikani M, Malter H, et al. Partial zona dissection or subzonal sperm insertion: microsurgical fertilization alternatives based on evaluation of sperm and embryo morphology. Fertil Steril 1991; 56: 696–706.
12. Parinaud J, Mieusset R, Vieitez G, Labal B, Richoilley G. Influence of sperm parameters on embryo quality. Fertil Steril 1993; 60: 888–92.
13. Loutradi KE, Tarlatzis BC, Goulis DG, et al. The effects of sperm quality on embryo development after intracytoplasmic sperm injection. J Assist Reprod Genet 2006; 23: 69–74.
14. Miller JE, Smith TT. The effect of intracytoplasmic sperm injection and semen parameters on blastocyst development in vitro. Hum Reprod 2001; 16: 918–24.
15. Nikolettos N, Kupker W, Demirel C, et al. Fertilization potential of spermatozoa with abnormal morphology. Hum Reprod 1999; 14(Suppl 1): 47–70.
16. Glezerman M, Bartoov B. Semen analysis. In: Insler V, Lunenfeld B, eds. Infertility: Male and Female. Edinburgh: Churchill Livingstone, 1993: 285–315.
17. Piomboni P, Strehler E, Capitani S, et al. Submicroscopic mathematical evaluation of spermatozoa in assisted reproduction, in vitro fertilization (notulae seminologicae 7). J Assist Reprod Genet 1996; 13: 635–46.
18. Zamboni L. The ultrastructural pathology of the spermatozoan as a course of infertility: the role of electron microscopy in the evaluation of sperm quality. Fertil Steril 1987; 48: 711–34.
19. Huszar G, Vigue L. Incomplete development of human spermatozoa is associated with increased creatine phosphokinase concentration and abnormal head morphology. Mol Reprod Dev 1993; 34: 292–8.
20. Aitken J, Krausz C, Buckingham D. Relationships between biochemical markers for residual sperm cytoplasm, reactive oxygen species generation, and the presence of leukocytes and precursor germ cells in human sperm suspensions. Mol Reprod Dev 1994; 39: 268–79.

21. Bernardini L, Borini A, Preti S, et al. Study of aneuploidy in normal and abnormal germ cells from semen of fertile and infertile men. Hum Reprod 1998; 13: 3406–13.
22. Rubes J, Lowe X, Moore D 2nd, et al. Smoking cigarettes is associated with increased sperm disomy in teenage men. Fertil Steril 1998; 70: 715–23.
23. Twigg JP, Irvine DS, Aitken RJ. Oxidative damage to DNA in human spermatozoa does not preclude pronucleus formation at intracytoplasmic sperm injection. Hum Reprod 1998; 13: 1864–71.
24. Sakkas D, Mariethoz E, Manicardi G, et al. Origin of DNA damage in ejaculated human spermatozoa. Rev Reprod 1999; 4: 31–7.
25. Griffin DK, Hyland P, Tempest HG, Homa ST. Safety issues in assisted reproduction technology: should men undergoing ICSI be screened for chromosome abnormalities in their sperm? Hum Reprod 2003; 18: 229–35.
26. Carrell DT, Emery BR, Wilcox AL, et al. Sperm chromosome aneuploidy as related to male factor infertility and some ultrastructure defects. Arch Androl 2004; 50: 181–5.
27. Kruger TF, Menkveld R, Stander FSH, et al. Sperm morphologic features as a prognostic factor in vitro fertilization. Fertil Steril 1986; 46: 1118–23.
28. Ménézo Y, Dale B. Paternal contribution to successful embryogenesis. Hum Reprod 1994; 10: 1326–8.
29. Jones GM, Trouson AO, Lolatgis N, Wood C. Factors affecting the success of human blastocyst develoment and pregnancy following in vitro fertilization and embryo transfer. Fertil Steril 1998; 70: 1022–9.
30. Barak Y, Goldman S. Development of in vitro human embryo. In: Allahbadia G, Merchant R, eds. Contemporary Perspectives on Assisted Reproductive Technologies. Reed Elsevier: A division of Elsevier India Private Limited, 2006: 80–8.
31. Rubio C, Simon C, Blanco V, et al. Implications of sperm chromosome abnormalities in recurrent miscarriage. J Assist Reprod Genet 1999; 16: 253–8.
32. Van Steirteghem A, Bonduelle M, Devroey P, Liebaers I. Follow up of children born after ICSI. Hum Reprod Update 2002; 8: 111–16.
33. Hansen M, Kurinczuk JJ, Bower C Webb S. The risk of major birth defects after intracytoplasmic sperm injection and in vitro fertilization. N Engl J Med 2002; 346: 725–30.
34. Van Steirteghem AC, Liu J, Joris H, et al. Higher success rate by intracytoplasmic sperm injection than by subzonal insemination. Report of a second series of 300 consecutive treatment cycles. Human Reprod 1993; 8: 1055–60.
35. Harari O, Bourne H, McDonald M, et al. Intracytoplasmic sperm injection – a major advance in the management of severe male subfertility. Fertil Steril 1995; 64: 360–8.
36. Kuczynski W, Dhont M, Grygoruk C, et al. The outcome of intracytoplasmic injection of fresh and cryopreserved ejaculated spermatozoa—a prospective randomized study. Reprod 2001; 16: 2109–13.
37. Stolwijk AM, Wetzels AM, Braat DD. Cumulative probability of achieving an ongoing pregnancy after in-vitro fertilization and intracytoplasmic sperm injection according to a woman's age, subfertility diagnosis and primary or secondary subfertility. Hum Reprod 2000; 15: 203–9.
38. Olivius K, Friden B, Lundin K, Bergh C. Cumulative probability of live birth after three in vitro fertilization/intracytoplasmic sperm injection cycles. Fertil Steril 2002; 77: 505–10.
39. Bartoov B, Eltes F, Reichart M, et al. Quantitative ultramorphological analysis of human sperm: fifteen years of experience in the diagnosis and management of male factor infertility. Arch Androl 1999; 43: 13–25.
40. Bartoov B, Berkovitz A, Eltes F, et al. Real-time fine morphology of motile human sperm cells is associated with IVF-ICSI outcome. J Androl 2002; 23: 1–8.
41. Kahraman S, Akarsu C, Cengiz G, et al. Fertility of ejaculated and testicular megalohead spermatozoa with intracytoplasmic sperm injection. Hum Reprod 1999; 14: 726–30.
42. Berkovitz A, Eltes F, Yaari S, et al. The morphological normalcy of the sperm nucleus and pregnancy rate of intracytoplasmic injection with morphologically selected sperm. Hum Reprod 2005; 20: 185–90.
43. Berkovitz A, Eltes F, Ellenbogen E, et al. Does the presence of nuclear vacuoles in human sperm selected for ICSI affect pregnancy outcome? Hum Reprod 2006; 21: 1787–90.
44. Palermo GD, Hu JCY, Rienzi L, et al. In: Biennial Review of Infertility. Volume 2 New York: Inc Springer-Verlag, 2011: 277–89.
45. Berkovitz A, Eltes F, Lederman H, et al. How to improve IVF–ICSI outcome by sperm selection. Reprod BioMed Online 2006; 12: 634–8.
46. Cassuto NG, Bouret D, Plouchart JM, et al. A new real-time morphology classification for human spermatozoa: a link for fertilization and improved embryo quality. Fertil Steril 2009; 92: 1616–25.
47. Peer S, Eltes F, Berkovitz A, et al. Is fine morphology of the human sperm nuclei affected by in vitro incubation at 37 degrees C? Fertil Steril 2007; 88: 1589–94.
48. Bartoov B, Eltes F, Pansky M, et al. Improved diagnosis of male fertility potential via a combination of quantitative ultramorphology and routine semen analyses. Hum Reprod 1994; 9: 2069–75.
49. Mundy AJ, Ryder TA, Edmonds DK. A quantitative study of sperm head ultrastructure in subfertile males with excess sperm precursors. Fertil Steril 1994; 61: 751–4.
50. Vanderzwalmen P, Hiemer A, Rubner P, et al. Blastocyst development after sperm selection at high magnification is associated with size and number of nuclear vacuoles. Reprod Biomed Online 2008; 17: 617–27.
51. Bartoov B, Berkovitz A, Eltes F, et al. Pregnancy rates are higher with intracytoplasmic morphologically selected sperm injection than with conventional intracytoplasmic injection. Fertility Steril 2003; 80: 1413–19.
52. Shapiro BS, Richter KS, Harris DC, Daneshmand ST. Dramatic declines in implantation and pregnancy rates in patients who undergo repeated cycles of in vitro fertilization with blastocyst transfer after one or more failed attempts. Fertil Steril 2001; 76: 538–42.
53. Silberstein T, Trimarchi JR, Gonzalez L, Keefe D, Blazar AS. Pregnancy outcome in in vitro fertilization decreases to a plateau with repeated cycles. Fertil Steril 2005; 84: 1043–5.
54. Antinori M, Licata E, Dani G, et al. Intracytoplasmic morphologically selected sperm injection: a prospective randomized trial. Reprod BioMed Online 2008; 16: 835–41.

55. Oliveira JB, Cavagna M, Petersen CG, et al. Pregnancy outcomes in women with repeated implantation failures after intracytoplasmic morphologically selected sperm injection (IMSI). ReprodBiol Endocrinol 2011; 9: 99.
56. Balaban B, Yakin K, Alatas C, et al. Clinical outcome of intracytoplasmic injection of spermatozoa morphologically selected under high magnification: a prospective randomized study. Reprod Biomed Online 2011; 22: 472–6.
57. Wilding M, Coppola G, di Matteo L, et al. Intracytoplasmic injection of morphologically selected spermatozoa (IMSI) improves outcome after assisted reproduction by deselecting physiologically poor quality spermatozoa. J Assist Reprod Genet 2011; 28: 253–62.
58. Knez K, Zorn B, Tomazevic T, Vrtacnik-Bokal E, Virant-Klun I. The IMSI procedure improves poor embryo development in the same infertile couples with poor semen quality: a comparative prospective randomized study. Reprod Biol Endocrinol 2011; 9: 123.
59. Figueira R, de C, Braga DP, et al. Morphological nuclear integrity of sperm cells is associated with preimplantation genetic aneuploidy screening cycle outcomes. Fertil Steril 2011; 95: 990–3.
60. Souza Setti A, Ferreira RC, Paes de Almeida Ferreira Braga D, et al. Intracytoplasmic sperm injection out come versus intracytoplasmic morphologically selected sperm injection outcome: a meta-analysis. Reprod Biomed Online 2010; 21: 450–5.
61. Hazout A, Dumont-Hassan M, Junca AM, Bacrie PC, Tesarik J. High-magnification ICSI overcomes paternal effect resistant to conventional ICSI. Reprod BioMed Online 2006; 12: 19–25.
62. Cassuto NG, Hazout A, Benifla JL, et al. Decreasing birth defect in children by using high magnification selected spermatozoon injection. Fertil Steril 2011; 96(Suppl 3): S85.
63. Kruger TF, Acosta AA, Simmons KF, et al. Predictive value of sperm morphology in in vitro fertilization. Fertil Steril 1988; 49: 112–17.
64. Martin RH, Rademaker A. The relationship between sperm chromosomal abnormalities and sperm morphology in humans. Mutat Res 1988; 207: 159–64.
65. Rosenbusch B, Strehler E, Sterzik K. Cytogenetics of human spermatozoa: correlations with sperm morphology and age of fertile men. Fertil Steril 1992; 58: 1071–2.
66. Lopes S, Jurisicova A, Sun JG, Casper RF. Reactive oxygen species: potential cause for DNA fragmentation in human spermatozoa. Hum Reprod 1998; 13: 896–900.
67. McKenzie LJ, Kovanci E, Amato P, et al. Pregnancy outcome of in vitro fertilization/intracytoplasmic sperm injection with profound teratospermia. Fertil Steril 2004; 82: 847–9.
68. Sailer BL, Jost LK Evenson DP. Bull sperm head morphometry related to abnormal chromatin structure and fertility. Cytometry 1996; 24: 167–73.
69. Virro MR, Larson-Cook KL, Evenson DP. Sperm chromatin structure assay (SCSA) parameters are related to fertilization, blastocyst development, and ongoing pregnancy in in vitro fertilization and intracytoplasmic sperm injection cycles. Fertil Steril 2004; 81: 1289–95.
70. Vicari E, de Palma A, Burrello N, et al. Effect of an abnormal sperm chromatin structural assay (SCSA) on pregnancy outcome following (IVF) with ICSI in previous IVF failures. Arch Androl 2005; 51: 121–4.
71. Nagy ZP, Liu J, Joris H, et al. The result of intracytoplasmic sperm injection is not related to any of the three basic sperm parameters. Hum Reprod 1995; 10: 1123–9.
72. Irvine DS, Twigg JP, Gordon EL, et al. DNA integrity in human spermatozoa: relationships with semen quality. J Androl 2000; 21: 33–44.
73. Seli E, Moffatt O, Kayisli UA, et al. Apoptosis in testis of normal and azoospermic males: a Fas mediated phenomenon. In: Annual Meeting of the Society for Gynecologic Investigation. Los Angeles, CA, 2002.
74. Yagci A, Murk W, Stronk J, Huszar G. Spermatozoa bound to solid state hyaluronic acid show chromatin structure with high DNA chain integrity: an acridine orange fluorescence study. J Androl 2010; 31: 566–72.
75. Lee JD, Kamiguchi Y, Yanagimachi R. Analysis of chromosome constitution of human spermatozoa with normal and aberrant head morphologies after injection into mouse oocytes. Hum Reprod 1996; 11: 1942–6.
76. Franco JG Jr, Baruffi RL, Mauri AL, et al. Significance of large nuclear vacuoles in human spermatozoa: implications for ICSI. Reprod BioMed Online 2008; 17: 42–5.
77. Garolla A, Fortini D, Menegazzo M, et al. High-power microscopy for selecting spermatozoa for ICSI by physiological status. Reprod BioMed Online 2008; 17: 610–16.
78. Nadalini M, Tarozzi N, Distratis V, Scaravelli G, Borini A. Impact of intracytoplasmic morphologically selected sperm injection on assisted reproduction outcome: a review. Reprod Biomed Online 2009; 19(Suppl 3): 45–55.
79. Hoffman R, Gross L. Reflected light differential-interference microscopy: principles, use and image interpretation. J Roy Microscope Soc 1968; 88: 305–49.
80. Hoffman R, Gross L. Demodulation contrast microscope. Nature 1975; 254: 586–8.
81. Padawer J. Denomarski interference-contrast microscope. An experimental basis for image interpretation. J Roy Microscop Soc 1968; 88: 305–49.
82. Kacem O, Sifer C, Barraud-Lange V, et al. Sperm nuclear vacuoles, assessed by motile sperm organellar morphological examination, are mostly of acrosomal origin. Reprod Biomed Online 2010; 20: 132–7.
83. de Almeida Ferreira Braga DP, Setti AS, Figueira RC, et al. Sperm organelle morphologic abnormalities: contributing factors and effects on intracytoplasmic sperm injection cycles outcomes. Urology 2011; 78: 786–91.
84. Perdrix A, Travers A, Chelli MH, et al. Assessment of acrosome and nuclear abnormalities in human spermatozoa with large vacuoles. Hum Reprod 2011; 26: 47–58.
85. Boitrelle F, Ferfouri F, Petit JM, et al. Large human sperm vacuoles observed in motile spermatozoa under high magnification: nuclear thumbprints linked to failure of chromatin condensation. Hum Reprod 2011; 26: 1650–8.
86. Cassuto NG, Hazout A, Hammoud I, et al. Correlation between DNA defect and sperm-head morphology. Reprod Biomed Online 2012; 24: 211–18.
87. Watanabe S, Tanaka A, Fujii S, et al. An investigation of the potential effect of vacuoles in human sperm on DNA damage using a chromosome assay and the TUNEL assay. Hum Reprod 2011; 26: 978–86.
88. Jakab A, Sakkas D, Delpiano E, et al. Intracytoplasmic sperm injection: a novel selection method for sperm with normal frequency of chromosomal aneuploidies. Fertil Steril 2005; 84: 1665–73.

89. Huszar G, Ozenci CC, Cayli S, et al. Hyaluronic acid binding by human sperm indicates cellular maturity, viability, and unreacted acrosomal status. Fertil Steril 2003; 79(Suppl 3): 1616–24.
90. Huszar G, Patrizio P, Vigue L, et al. Cytoplasmic extrusion and the switch from creatine kinase B to M isoform are completed by the commencement of epididymal transport in human and stallion spermatozoa. J Androl 1998; 19: 11–20.
91. Sati L, Ovari L, Demir R, et al. Persistent histones in immature sperm are associated with DNA fragmentation and affect paternal contribution of sperm: A study of aniline blue staining, fluorescence in situ hybridization (FISH) and DNA nick translation. Fertil Steril 2004; 82: S52.
92. Parmegiani L, Cognigni GE, Bernardi S, et al. "Physiologic ICSI": hyaluronic acid (HA) favors selection of spermatozoa without DNA fragmentation and with normal nucleus, resulting in improvement of embryo quality. Fertil Steril 2010; 93: 598–604.
93. Petersen CG, Massaro FC, Mauri AL, et al. Efficacy of hyaluronic acid binding assay in selecting motile spermatozoa with normal morphology at high magnification. Reprod Biol Endocrinol 2010; 8: 149.
94. Franco JG Jr, Mauri AL, Petersen CG, et al. Large nuclear vacuoles are indicative of abnormal chromatin packaging in human spermatozoa. Int J Androl 2012; 35: 46–51.
95. Akimoto S, Kudo T, Abe A, et al. Abstract in the 26th annual meetings of Japanese Society of Reprod Med. Japanese, 2009: 1-A-07.
96. Bonduelle M, Aytoz A, Van Assche et al. Incidence of chromosomal aberrations in children born after assisted reproduction through intracytoplasmic sperm injection. Hum Reprod 1998; 13: 781–2.

11

Use of in vitro maturation in a clinical setting: Patient populations and outcomes

Yoshiharu Morimoto, Aisaku Fukuda, and Manabu Satoh

HISTORY OF IVM

In vitro maturation (IVM) is not a new technology. Its use was first reported by Pincus and Enzmann (1) in mammals in 1935. Preclinical studies were continued in animals by Edwards (2) and Edwards et al. (3) reported clinical application in humans, obtaining immature oocytes from cases with ovarian stimulation. Veeck et al. (4) achieved the first successful birth from immature oocytes produced during an in vitro fertilization (IVF) program. Then Cha et al. (5) initiated the use of immature oocytes from unstimulated ovaries of patients in a donation program. Thereafter, Trounson et al. (6) achieved another breakthrough in the development of IVM. They chose immature oocytes aspirated from patients with polycystic ovary syndrome (PCOS) as a source for the procedure. Gonadotropins, estradiol, and fetal calf serum were supplemented in the medium and a 65% maturation rate was acquired within 43–47 hours of culture. The maturation rate was acceptable, but the pregnancy success rate was only 11.1%. However, IVM has become a main-stream choice for PCOS treatment. Patients with PCOS are hypersensitive to stimulating drugs, and ovarian stimulation for conventional IVF in PCOS patients carries the risk of severe ovarian hyperstimulation syndrome (OHSS), causing some patients to quit treatment. Use of IVM is only the measure that can completely prevent OHSS.

INDICATIONS OF IVM

IVM was originally applied in patients with PCOS without gonadotropin stimulation to avoid OHSS caused by controlled ovarian hyperstimulation (COH) (5,6). IVM is indicated not only for patients with PCOS, but also for women with polycystic ovary (PCO) who are at a higher risk of OHSS by standard COH compared with the regular cycling women. IVM should also be considered in patients who are anxious about the long-term side effects of gonadotropin, since some patients worry about not only the stimulating effect of gonadotropins but also about the prospective events after aging (7,8). Regular cycling women are also successfully treated with IVM with or without gonadotropin administration, but its indication for regular cycling women remains controversial due to the lower number of oocytes available (9–18). The clinical benefits of administering follicle-stimulating hormone (FSH) to regular cycling women are yet to be determined (19,20). Poor embryo quality or repeated failures by conventional IVF is another proposed indication for IVM. Women with the so-called egg factor in which no mature eggs are found in repeated cycles (germinal vesicles only), recurrent fertilization failure, or very poor-quality embryos are also IVM targets (21). Patients who repeatedly failed IVF without distinct causes should also be considered for IVM (22,23). We achieved 88 clinical pregnancies by IVM from 1999 to 2008. Twenty-one pregnancies (24%) resulted from repeated IVF failures. Eight of these 21 pregnancies (38%) were treated by IVM due to poor-quality embryos generated by IVF. Figure 11.1 shows the number of failed IVF cycles and IVM cycles to achieve pregnancy in 18 ongoing cases. They failed 4.9 times with IVF and needed IVM 2.3 times to achieve pregnancy. In conclusion, the primary indication for IVM is PCOS or PCO with high risk of OHSS. Other indications are patients demand not to undergo gonadotropin administration and repeated IVF failures due to impaired oocyte or embryo qualities. IVM is an alternative to the conventional assisted reproductive technique (ART).

FSH PRIMING

The target follicles in IVM being only 5–10 mm, beginners find it quite difficult to puncture these small follicles. Therefore, it is more practical to stimulate and prepare rather easier condition by using bigger follicles. FSH priming prior to IVM has been tried from the initial stage, and FSH is usually administered from day 3 or 5 at a dose of 150–300 IU. Several studies have reported both effectiveness and ineffectiveness of FSH priming. Wynn et al. (19) added recombinant FSH on day 2, 4, and 6 and achieved significant numbers of retrieved oocytes and an increased maturation rate. Mikkelsen et al. (10) found no difference between the two groups of primed and nonprimed patients after a three-day addition of FSH from day 3. On the other hand, the combination of FSH

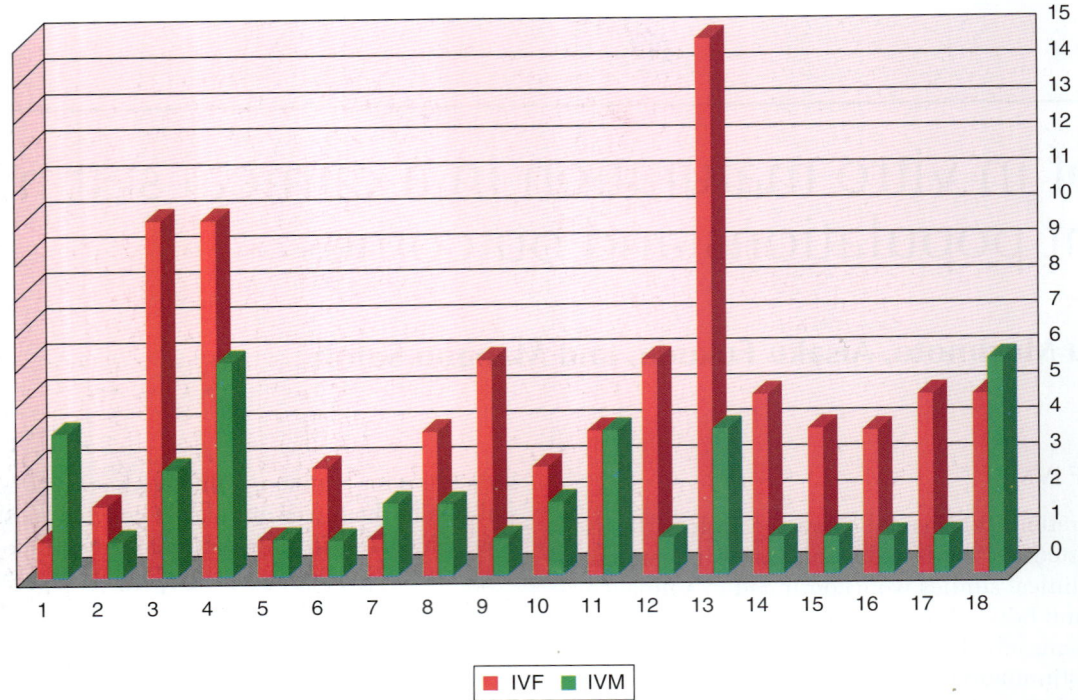

Figure 11.1 The number of failed IVF cycles (red bar) and IVM cycles (green bar) to achieve pregnancy in 18 ongoing cases. *Abbreviations*: IVF, in vitro fertilization; IVM, in vitro maturation.

and human chorionic gonadotropin (hCG) at the same time was reported by Lin et al. (24), and no significant effectiveness was shown in the literature.

The advantage for FSH priming can be described as easier follicular preparation; however, we need to consider its disadvantages. After immature follicles are recruited from the cohort, the dominant follicles start to grow and differentiate. At this moment, apoptosis of follicles and oocytes starts to be atretic in follicles and degenerative in oocytes. This phenomenon may affect both the quality and the developmental competence of oocytes for fertilization and embryogenesis. FSH priming may accelerate the speed of folliculogenesis, that is, the follicles proceed to be atretic in an unusual manner. Therefore, it will be difficult to estimate optimal timing for ovum pickup (OPU) in IVM.

HCG PRIMING

Chian et al. (25) reported the efficacy of hCG administration 36 hours prior to OPU in patients with PCOS. Ten-thousand units of hCG was used for priming. The mean number of oocytes retrieved was equivalent for the hCG-primed and nonprimed groups, but the oocyte maturation rate was significantly improved in the hCG-primed group. The time course changed between the hCG-primed and nonprimed groups. There was no difference in the rates of fertilization and cleavage. The possible presence of luteinizing hormone (LH) or hCG receptors has been described in small follicles. LH induces the rupture of mature follicles; surges in its level offer the optimal conditions for ovulation. Thus, it is obvious that mature follicles possess LH receptors. However, LH receptors are not proven to exist in immature oocytes; rather, they mainly exist in the cumulus–oocyte complexes (COCs). Ge et al. (26) investigated the effect of adding hCG to IVM medium in patients undergoing IVM. Patients with PCO were nonprimed with hCG, and the patients were categorized into three groups according to the medium used; namely the hCG-containing medium, initially non-hCG followed by hCG containing medium, and non-hCG medium groups. No differences were observed between the three groups in the number of retrieved oocytes, maturation rates, fertilization rates, or implantation rates. Surprisingly, high maturation rates of over 60% were obtained without using hCG. Further investigations and clinical data are needed to clarify the effectiveness of hCG priming.

OOCYTE STATUS IN IVM

IVM has been applied not only for PCOS or PCO but also for repeated IVF failures for more than a decade. However, the overall pregnancy rate achieved by IVM is still inferior to that by conventional IVF due to a lower implantation rate (27,28). Therefore, many infertility specialists hesitate to adopt IVM as a routine ART procedure. The major causes of its inferiority to IVF come from the discrepancy of synchronization not only between nuclear and cytoplasmic maturation in the oocytes but also between the developmental speed of the embryos and the endometrial lining. Synchronization of endometrial development with embryonic growth is essential in any ART procedure, but a dominant follicle or corpus luteum does not routinely exist in IVM. Therefore, the contribution of the follicular and luteal sex steroids to

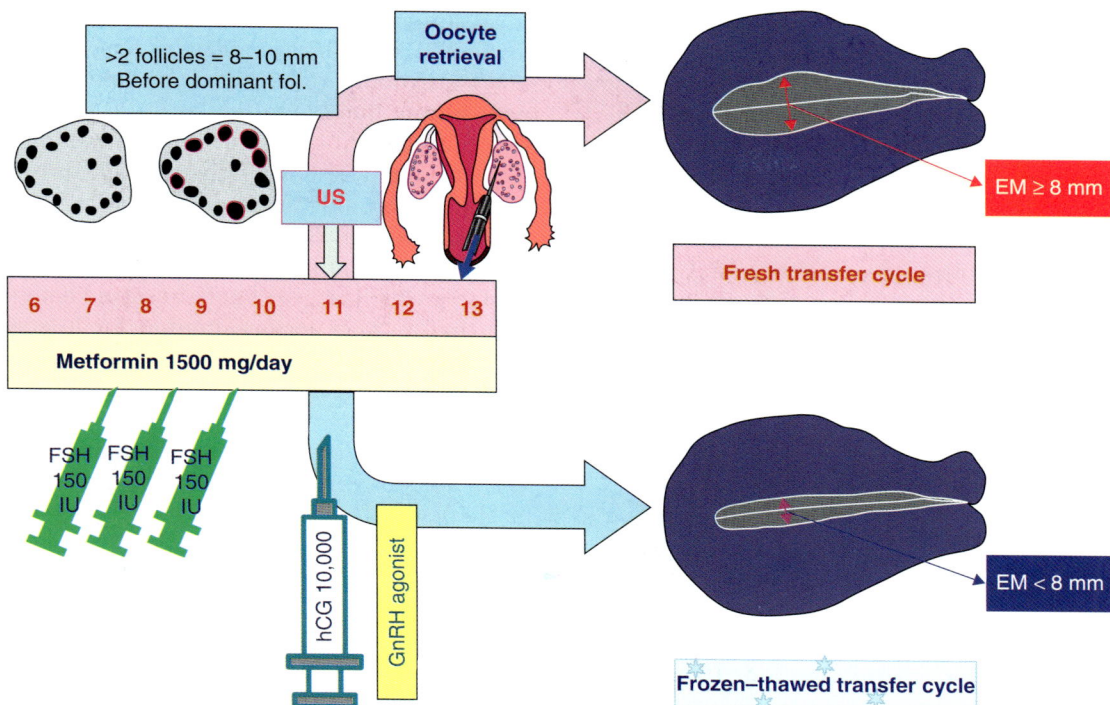

Figure 11.2 This illustration shows how to choose fresh or frozen in vitro maturation cycle by the thickness of endometrial lining on the day of hCG administration. *Abbreviations*: FSH, follicle stimulating hormone; hCG, human chorionic gonadotropin; EM, endometrium; US, ultrasound.

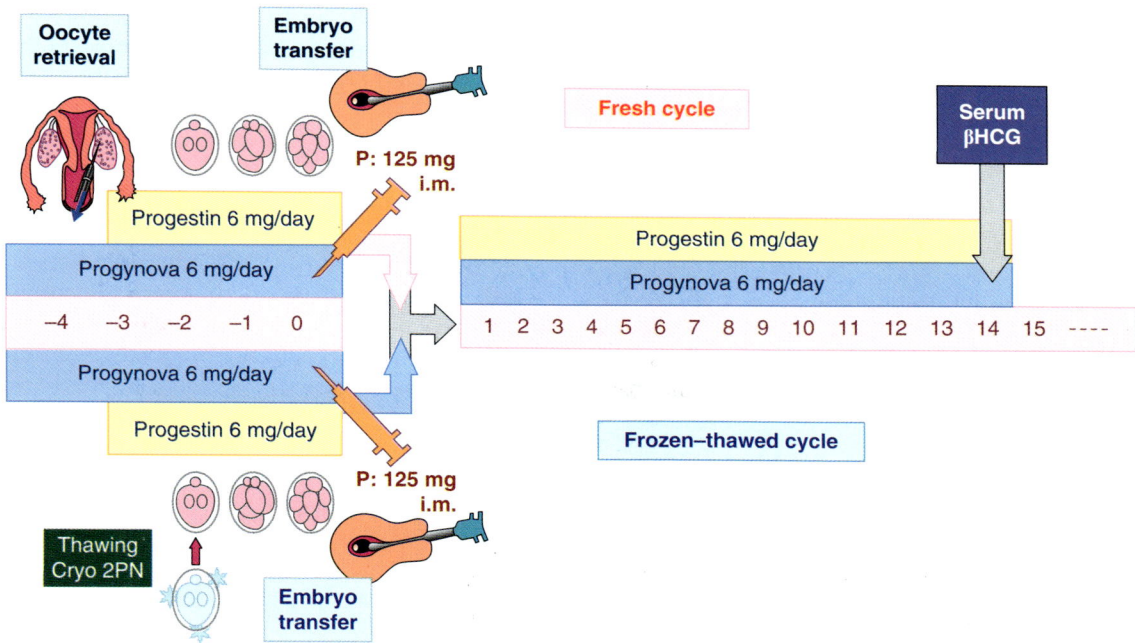

Figure 11.3 This illustration shows the chronological procedures of a fresh and a frozen in vitro maturation cycle after the oocyte retrieval to the embryo transfer. The medication after the transfer until pregnancy test is also shown.

the endometrium is possibly compromised. We achieved the first IVM pregnancy and birth in Japan (29), but the success rate was far less than that of IVF at our institution. To improve IVM pregnancy rates, we included frozen–thawed transfer to the IVM protocol to adjust and facilitate endometrial development (30,31). Our protocol is illustrated in Figures 11.2 and 11.3. Briefly, the scan is started on day 6–8 of the menstrual cycle to measure endometrial thickness and the number and the size of the antral follicles, and to exclude the presence of dominant follicles >14 mm. Pretreatment with metformin for more than a month and low-dose FSH administration are selectively performed. A second evaluation is performed a few days later to determine a suitable day for hCG administration. hCG is given when more than two follicles grow to a size >8 mm. On the day of hCG administration, if the endometrial thickness is ≥8 mm, the transfer of fresh day 3 embryo is usually scheduled. However, if the endometrium thickness is <8 mm, 2 pronuclei (2PN) embryos are cryopreserved for future frozen–thawed embryo transfer as shown in Figures 11.2 and 11.3 (31–34). Frozen–thawed embryo transfer is usually performed under a hormone-supplemented cycle. The medication after transfer was identical in both fresh and frozen cycles (Fig. 11.3). Vitrification of the embryos derived from IVM oocytes is a routine procedure in the clinical application of IVM because of the current prevalence of the techniques (35–40).

OOCYTE CULTURE AND IDENTIFICATION

IVM Medium

Retrieved COCs are transferred to IVM culture medium, cultured for 24–26 hours and assessed for maturity after removal of cumulus cells (CCs) (Fig. 11.4). All IVM cases undergo intracytoplasmic sperm injection (ICSI). IVM culture should be completed without the use of mineral oil to avoid absorption of the steroids secreted by CCs (41).

We compared the MediCult IVM® system (Medicult, Origio, Måløv, Denmark) and tissue culture medium 199 (TCM199, Invitrogen, Carlsbad, California, USA) (Table 11.1). Both the IVM media were supplemented with FSH, hCG, and patient serum. The rates of maturation and pregnancy were significantly increased by changing from TCM199 to MediCult (49.1% vs. 53.3% and 15.9% vs. 30.0%, respectively). Some studies have compared IVM outcomes using different culture media. Söderström-Anttila et al. and Filali et al. reported similar clinical outcomes between MediCult and TCM 199 culturing (42,43). However, de Araujo et al. reported that TCM199 was more suited for human IVM than human tubal fluid (HTF) (44). Therefore, TCM199 or commercialized IVM media are preferred for human IVM.

We also compared different protein sources; patient's own serum, donor's follicular fluid, and Serum Substitute Supplement (SSS™, Irvine Scientific) (Table 11.2). Use of patient serum yielded significantly higher rates of maturation and pregnancy than that of donor's follicular fluid and SSS. Human IVM medium is usually supplemented with patient serum (5,6,45,46). Mikkelsen et al. reported the use of patient serum being more effective than human serum albumin for human IVM (47). Serum may contain factors preferable for oocyte maturation such as epidermal growth factor (EGF), and EGF-like growth factor that improve the maturation of human immature oocytes (48). Further, patient serum is easily available and is not contaminated with foreign viruses or factors.

Oocyte Identification

The follicular aspirate is collected in collection tubes containing HEPES-buffered HTF with 0.4% heparin to prevent blood-clot formation during oocyte retrieval. There are two ways to identify COCs in the follicular aspirates. First, a small volume of follicular aspirates is poured directly into a Petri dish and examined for COCs under a stereomicroscope (25,49). COCs aspirated from IVM cycles have only small amounts of CCs compared with those from COH cycles, and denuded oocytes are sometimes included (Fig. 11.5). Because of the low number of CCs and partially denuded oocytes, it is difficult to identify COCs aspirated from the IVM cycles in a large amount of follicular fluids in a Petri dish. In particular, in the hCG-primed IVM cycles, CC expansion is induced by a high-dose hCG signal, thus making the identification of COCs easier.

Another method of COCs' identification is the use of a cell strainer (70 μm nylon mesh; Becton Dickinson,

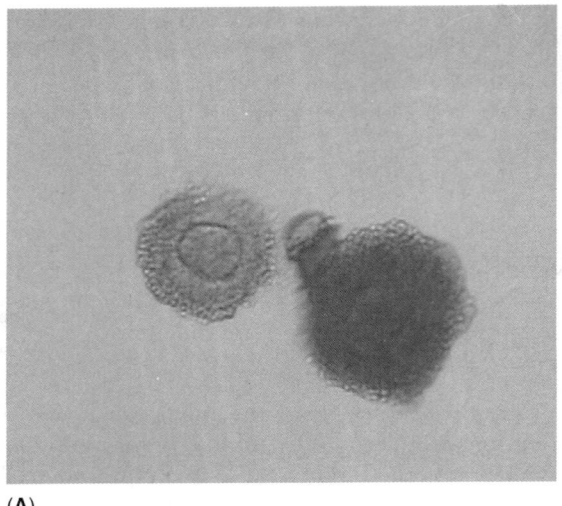
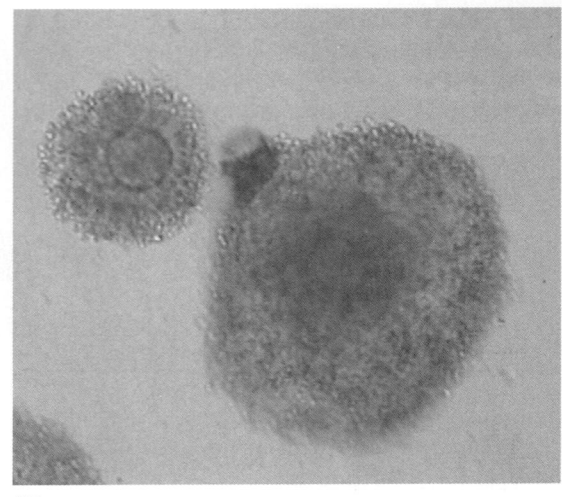

(A)   (B)

Figure 11.4 Morphological changes of cumulus–oocyte complexes (COCs) before and after culture in the in vitro maturation (IVM) medium. (**A**) The immature COCs after oocyte retrieval. (**B**) The same COCs 26 hours after culture in the IVM medium. The cumulus cells have expanded, and COCs volume increased to approximately 2 or 3 times as before culture. Original magnification × 200.

NJ, USA) (50,51). The follicular aspirates in the collection tubes are filtered with the cell strainer (Fig. 11.6), and the collected aspirates are washed with HEPES-buffered HTF containing SSS and 0.4% heparin to remove red blood cells and small cells. The cell strainer is then transferred upside down to a Petri dish, and the collected aspirates are flushed with HTF from the backside of the cell strainer and observed for COCs under a stereomicroscope. The COCs with dispersed CCs are sticky and sometimes block the pores of the cell strainer. It is hard to flush the cell strainer and time consuming to search for the COCs. Therefore, at our center, after identifying the oocytes with dispersed CCs under a stereomicroscope, the remaining aspirates are filtered through a cell strainer to facilitate identification of the oocytes with a less number of CCs.

OPU for IVM

The application of IVM has been limited since its development due to the difficulty in puncturing small follicles. Unstimulated follicles are mobile and therefore, it is not easy to puncture at the correct point of the ovary. The IVM needles for IVM usually range from gauge 21 to gauge 19. Before the procedure, positioning of the large pelvic vessels by color Doppler method is recommended. A careful ultrasonography beforehand makes OPU easier and safer. A complete record of the size and number of follicles is an important resource for further improvement of the procedure.

To facilitate easy puncturing of small follicles, we developed a newly designed needle (IVF OSAKA IVM Needle; Kitazato Medical Co. Ltd., Tokyo, Japan). The needle is composed of two needles, one for puncturing (21G) and one for holding (17G) (Fig. 11.7). The puncture needle is located inside the holding needle. First, the vaginal skin is penetrated without anesthesia and the needle is inserted to reach 1 cm into the ovary to hold it. Second, the puncture needle is smoothly inserted into the holding needle without any resistance from hard skin. Small follicles are sequentially punctured by rotating the needle (Fig. 11.8).

The aspiration pressure used for the puncturing in IVM is an important issue. We compared 180 and 300 mmHg as the puncture pressure for oocyte retrieval (52). The rate of transferable embryos per retrieved oocytes was significantly higher in the lower pressure group (low 23.8%, high 12.8%). The ongoing pregnancy rate was also better in the lower pressure group (low 30.0%, high 4.3%). This finding indicates high-pressure aspiration may affect oocyte quality and developmental competence for embryogenesis.

METFORMIN APPLICATION IN IVM

Metformin, an oral biguanide insulin-sensitizing agent used in Type 2 diabetes mellitus, can reduce the hyperinsulinemia and hyperandrogenemia associated with PCOS and aid in ovulation (53–58). We have tried several approaches, including new needle system, aspiration pressure changes, and frozen–thawed cycles, to improve the clinical outcomes identical to those from conventional IVF (30,31); however, the pregnancy rates did not improve as per expectation. The quality of either the oocyte that matured in vitro or the resulting embryos was an integral factor for achieving this goal. Therefore, we

Table 11.1 Comparison of Clinical Outcomes Between TCH199 and MediCult IVM System

Culture medium	No. of cycles	Mean number of oocytes retrieved	Culture time (hr)	In vitro maturation rate (%)	Pregnancy rate per embryo transfer (%)
TCH199	447	8.4	24	49.1[a]	15.9[A]
MediCult IVM system	591	8.7	26	53.3[b]	30.0[B]

Significant differences between different characters (p < 0.01: a–b, A–B).

Table 11.2 Comparison of Clinical Outcomes Between Three Protein Supplements in MediCult IVM System

Protein supplement	No. of cycles	Mean number of oocytes retrieved	Culture time (hr)	In vitro maturation rate (%)	Pregnancy rate per embryo transfer (%)
Donor's follicular fluid	154	9.2	26	49.6[a]	28.1
Patient's own serum	271	8.9	26	57.7[b]	38.8[A]
Serum Substitute Supplement (Irvine Scientific)	166	7.9	26	52.7[c]	23.1[B]

Significant differences between different characters (p < 0.01: a–b, a–c, A–B; p < 0.05: b–c).

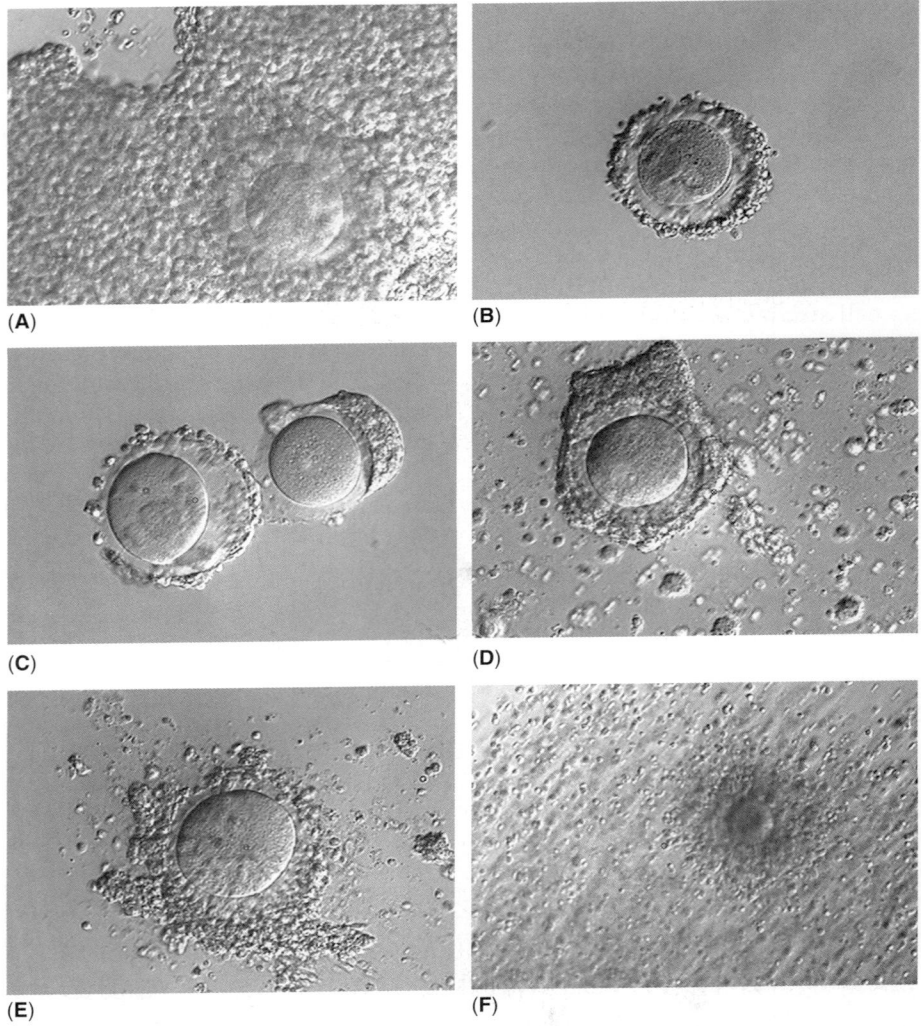

Figure 11.5 Various morphologies of the cumulus–oocyte complexes (COCs) observed at the time of oocyte collection. (**A**) The oocyte with compacted rich CCs. (**B**) germinal vesicle (GV) stage oocyte with <2–3 cumulus cell (CC) layers. (**C**) Metaphase I stage oocyte shows small volume CCs and partially denuded. (**D**) GV stage oocyte with partially dispersed CCs. (**E**) Metaphase-I stage oocyte with dispersed CCs. (**F**) COCs with fully expanded CCs retrieved in controlled ovarian hyperstimulation cycles. Original magnification (**A–E**) × 200, (**F**) × 100.

applied metformin in an IVM protocol as shown in Figure 11.2 (32,33). We then evaluated serum levels of insulin and homeostasis model assessment for insulin resistance (HOMA-R). When HOMA-R was >1, metformin (1500 mg/day) was administrated at least from one month before IVM. If the patient was unable to tolerate the side effects such as diarrhea and nausea, the dose was reduced to 750–1000 mg/day.

Following the initiation of routine metformin use in 2007, the clinical outcomes improved significantly as shown in Figure 11.9. We analyzed the effect of metformin on IVM results (Table 11.1). In the metformin-treated group, the number of oocytes retrieved was significantly higher and the pregnancy rate also had improved significantly in fresh IVM cycles. However, the clinical outcomes of frozen–thawed cycle did not show any significant improvement. Metformin may improve oocyte quality by reducing hyperinsulinemia and by modulating local insulin and IGF levels, but we could not prove this suspicion (59). Although an efficacious implantation in human reproduction is the result of endometrial factors or oocyte and embryonic features (60), our data suggest the beneficial effects of metformin on endometrial development and receptivity as shown by some studies (61–63). In conclusion, metformin pretreatment of patients with PCO before IVM has a positive effect on the clinical outcome of IVM.

CLINICAL OUTCOME AND MALFORMATION RATE

IVM is a relatively new ART technology compared to IVF (64). Although IVM was invented 13 years after IVF and clinically applied two years later (5,6), 20 years have passed since the first IVM baby was born. The clinical outcome of IVM varies not only by institution but also by patient type. The pregnancy rate per IVM transfer for either PCOS or PCO patients is in the range from 21.5% to 52.9% (15,24,25,42,49,65–70). The major reason for this difference might be the different pretreatments such as FSH and hCG used in different patients. Women with normal ovaries or regular cycles experience less success with IVM. Pregnancy rates are as low as 4.0–33.3% per

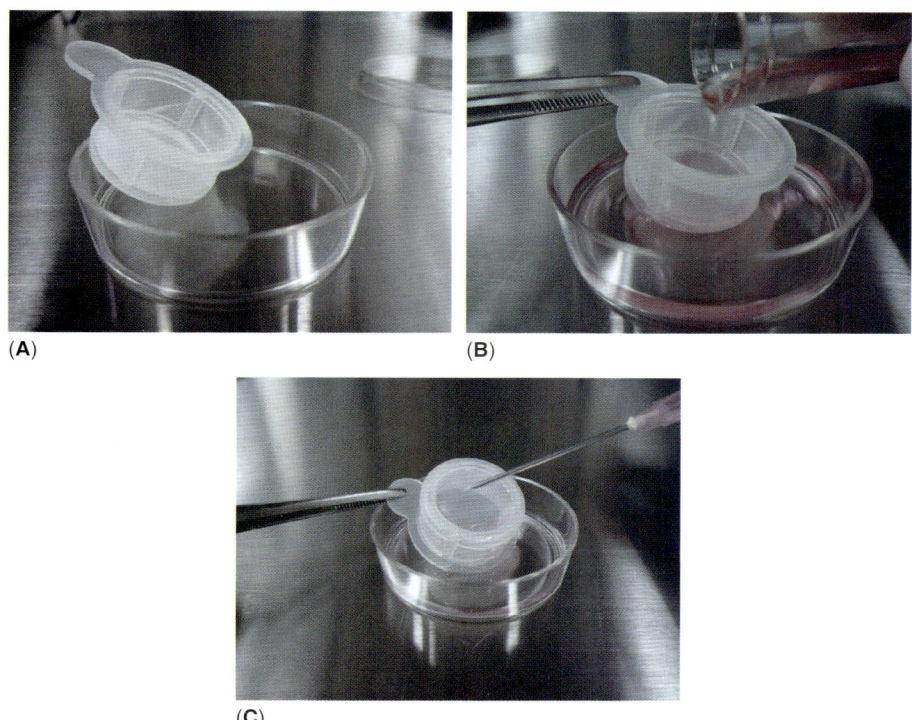

Figure 11.6 The schematic procedure of the oocyte collection using cell strainer. (**A**) The cell strainer is kept in a Petri dish (Falcon, 60 × 15 mm). (**B**) Follicular aspirates containing human tubal fluid with heparin are filtered with a cell strainer. (**C**) After the filtering, the collected aspirates are rinsed and transferred into another Petri dish for identification of cumulus–oocyte complexes under a stereomicroscope.

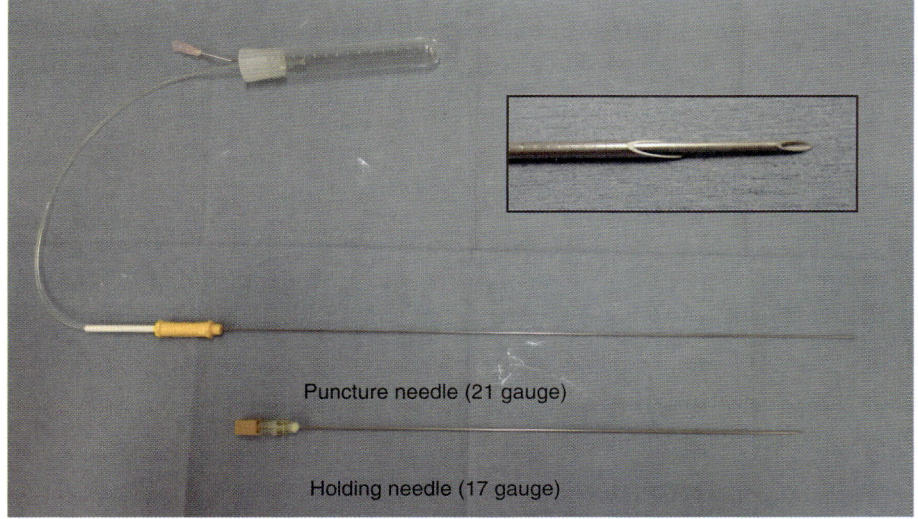

Figure 11.7 The IVF-OSAKA IVM needle comprises a puncture and a holding needle.

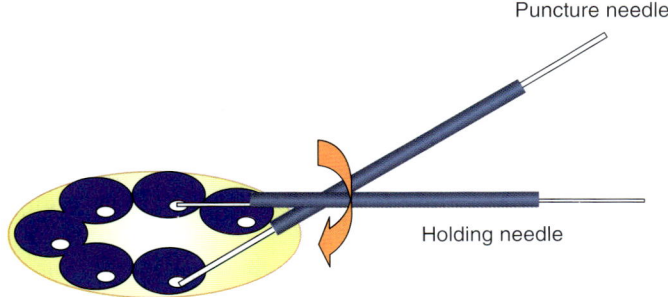

Figure 11.8 After the ovary was fixed by the holding needle, every follicle can be easily punctured by rotation of the puncture needle.

transfer (10,15,17,20,42,50,71,72). To date, FSH priming with hCG administration seems to be common pretreatment for IVM procedure. However, we recommend metformin pretreatment (if possible depending upon the legislation in specific countries) and use of frozen–thawed cycles for patients with poor endometrium development (31–33).

We performed 1071 IVM cycles (638 fresh and 433 frozen cycles); from 1999 to 2011, the pregnancy rate per transfer was 21.3%, while the miscarriage rate was 20.7% (Table 11.2). However, the average pregnancy rate over the last three years was >35%. Various

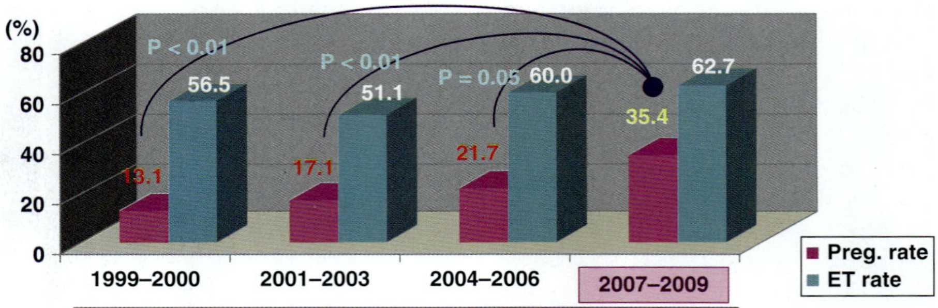

	1999–2000	2001–2003	2004–2006	2007–2009
	Double needle	Double needle	Double needle	Double needle
	Frozen cycle	Frozen cycle	Frozen cycle	Frozen cycle
		hCG	hCG	hCG
			IVM medium	IVM medium
			Aspiration press. 300→150 mmHg	Aspiration press. 300→150 mmHg
			Metformin	Metformin

Figure 11.9 Clinical outcomes of fresh transfer cycle in IVM at IVF Osaka Clinic (*graph*) from 1999 to 2009 and various procedures performed in the meantime (*table*). Abbreviations: ET, embryo transfer; Preg., pregnancy; press., pressure.

attempts have been made to improve the clinical outcome. Several authors' reports have not shown a significant increase in the malformation in IVM babies (42,67,68,73). No differences were observed in the perinatal morbidity, birth weight, gestational age at delivery, APGAR scores, umbilical cord pH, or congenital abnormalities among IVM, IVF, and ICSI treatment outcomes (74). Our data also did not show any increase in the malformation rate by IVM treatment by neither fresh nor frozen cycles.

FOLLOW-UP OF IVM CHILDREN

It is estimated that, globally, >1300 IVM babies have been born in contrast to an estimated 3 million babies conceived by standard IVF/ICSI over the last 33 years (75). However, there may not be much information available about these children in published or unpublished data (67,76,77). In animal models, there have been rising concerns about IVM and its influences on epigenetic disorders (78–81). These theoretical concerns must be recognized in human as well, but such effects have not been confirmed in IVM babies until now. The importance of epigenetics in IVF is still controversial after millions of babies have been born via IVF, so it will take some time to collect the IVM data required for meaningful analysis. We have completed 897 IVM cycles between 1999 and 2010 and achieved 100 pregnancies (70 deliveries and 80 babies born). To date, 51 children born via IVM (36 through fresh cycle and 15 via frozen cycle) were followed until seven years of age so far, through parental questionnaires meant for their parents. The congenital malformation rate, including minor issues, was 3.9% (2/51) that did not differ from that of Japanese natural conception. The physical and mental development of the IVM babies was identical to that of natural conception babies, as determined on the basis of statistical data of cited in the statistics of Japan Ministry of Health, Welfare and Labor (2010 edition). However, one child was normal at birth, but appeared to be Asperger syndrome, and long-term follow-up of IVM babies is warranted.

OOCYTE MATURATION, ULTRASTRUCTURE, AND MITOCHONDRIAL DISTRIBUTION

The IVM procedure has developed and is now used worldwide. Although its simplicity appeals to patients, it is yet an alternative to conventional IVF because of its low or unstable success rates, caused by low maturation rates. To improve the maturation and success rates, it is essential to elucidate the human oocyte maturation process. The oocytes mature in the zona pellucida, cytoplasm, and nucleus; it is also necessary to maintain the harmony of each maturation factor for achieving maturation. The nuclear maturation process has been well investigated, but in contrast, the mechanism and manner of maturation in the cytoplasm remains unclear. Nuclear maturation is identified by germinal vesicle breakdown and the extrusion of polar bodies on light microscopy, unlike cytoplasmic maturation.

Ultrastructural investigation can be used to study the process of cytoplasmic maturation. We observed oocytes during IVM using electron microscopy. In the germinal vesicle stage of unstimulated oocytes, the mitochondria were dense and scattered in the cytoplasm. The volume of smooth endoplasmic reticulum (s-ER) was small. Microvilli had not yet developed at this stage. Within 6–12 hours of culture, the germinal vesicles underwent breakdown and the appearance of cytoplasm changed dramatically. The mitochondria had enlarged and s-ERs ballooned. At this stage of Metaphase I, the communication between the cumulus cells and the oolemma was remarkably activated. The processes from the cumulus cell surface reached the oolemma through the zona pellucida. In the Metaphase II, the mitochondria increased in number and aggregated in the center of the cytoplasm. The microvilli on the surface of the oolemma developed and elongated, extending into the perivitelline space.

At this stage, first and second lysosomes were seen, and the s-ER increased in quantity and ballooned. Mitochondria play an essential role in oocyte maturation. A low oocyte respiration rate indicates that adenosine triphosphate production resulted in maturation failure and atresia in IVF (82). Adenosine triphosphate content is related not only to oocyte maturation, but also to fertilization, embryogenesis, and implantation (83).

Mitochondria migrate and are distributed in each stage of maturation. The mitochondria distribution pattern was found to be homogenous in the germinal vesicles and heterogonous in Metaphase I and II (84,85). Wilding et al. (86) described that the mitochondrial distribution pattern was homogenous in poor-quality embryos. Mitochondrial distribution is controlled by the microtubule network. Inappropriate network formation may cause the mitochondrial distribution abnormal, which indicates the shortage of an energy source to maintain oogenesis and embryogenesis (87). Mitochondria are multifunctioning organelles. They not only create energy, but also transiently store calcium ions and regulate apoptosis for cell death. Further investigation of the mitochondrial function in human oocytes does benefit the better clinical IVM outcome and the improvement in the embryos quality.

FURTHER APPLICATION OF IVM-PREIMPLANTATION GENETIC DIAGNOSIS AND DONOR OOCYTE SOURCES

Although, at present, it may be premature to offer IVM to all types of patients, IVM is definitely a safer option than IVF in patients who are extremely sensitive to gonadotropins, because it avoids the risk of OHSS. From the point of view of safety, IVM should be applied for any male factor-related infertility such as testicular sperm extraction and ICSI cases without female disorders such as PCOS/PCO (15,24,25,42,49,65–69,71) or normal ovaries/regular cycling women (10,17,20,50,71,72). Vitrification of human embryos has become a routine ART method. Not only cleaved embryos but also oocytes have been successfully vitrified (38,39,88,89). Application of frozen cycle on IVM will improve the clinical outcome because of improved uterine receptivity. Moreover, cryopreservation of either immature oocytes or mature oocytes is a safer ART for female cancer patients, especially those with breast cancer (90).

In vitro follicular growth (91) is used with IVM, because it is a necessary step for IVM when ovarian tissue cryopreservation is clinically applied. Other than routine therapeutic ART procedures, IVM benefits oocyte donors by avoiding the risks of both OHSS and unknown longtime side effects (8). Recurrent pregnancy loss patients are also good candidates for IVM, since many of them need several trials to acquire a healthy baby. These patients are usually reluctant to undergo ART treatment because of high cost and the complexities of the ART procedure itself. If patients have sufficient antral follicle counts, IVM is a preferable option for performing a safer preimplantation genetic diagnosis procedure (92). IVM is also a strong tool for repeated IVF failure for many reasons such as premature ovarian failure or insufficiency, poor responders, poor embryo quality, abnormal oocytes, empty follicle syndrome etc. IVM is not only indicated for PCOS/PCO patients to avoid the risk of OHSS but it also plays an integral role in the development of future ART.

REFERENCES

1. Pincus G, Enzmann EV. The comparative behavior of mammalian eggs in vivo and in vitro: I. The activation of ovarian eggs. J Exp Med 1935; 62: 655–75.
2. Edwards R. Maturation in vitro of mouse, sheep, cow, pig, rhesus monkey and human ovarian oocytes. Nature 1965; 20: 349–51.
3. Edwards R, Bavister B, Steptoe P. Early stages of fertilization in vitro of human oocytes matured in vitro. Nature 1969; 221: 632–5.
4. Veeck LL, Wortham JW Jr, Witmyer J, et al. Maturation and fertilization of morphologically immature human oocytes in a program of in vitro fertilization. Fertil Steril 1983; 39: 594–602.
5. Cha KY, Koo JJ, Ko JJ, et al. Pregnancy after in vitro fertilization of human follicular oocytes collected from nonstimulated cycles, their culture in vitro and their transfer in a donor oocyte program. Fertil Steril 1991; 55: 109–13.
6. Trounson A, Wood C, Kaushe A. In vitro maturation and the fertilization and developempental competence of oocytes recovered from untreated polycystic ovarian patients. Fertil Steril 1994; 62: 353–62.
7. Whittemore AS, Harris R, Itnyre J, et al. Characteristics relating to ovarian cancer risk: collaborative analysis of 12 US case-control studies. Am J Epidemiol 1992; 136: 1184–203.
8. Whittemore AS. The risk of ovarian cancer after treatment for infertility. N Engl J Med 1994; 331: 805–6.
9. Barnes FL, Crombie A, Gardner DK, et al. Blastocyst development and birth after in vitro maturation of human primary oocytes, intracytoplasmic sperm injection and assisted hatching. Hum Reprod 1995; 10: 3243–7.
10. Mikkelsen AL, Smith SD, Lindenberg S. In-vitro maturation of human oocytes from regularly menstruating women may be successful without follicle stimulating hormone priming. Hum Reprod 1999; 14: 1847–51.
11. Son WY, Park SJ, Hyun CS, et al. Successful birth after transfer of blastocysts derived from oocytes of unstimulated women with regular menstrual cycle after IVM approach. J Assist Reprod Genet 2002; 19: 541–3.
12. Papanicolaou EG, Platteau P, Albano C, et al. Immature oocyte in-vitro maturation: clinical aspects. Reprod Biomed Online 2005; 10: 587–92.
13. Loutradis D, Kiapekou E, Zapanti E, et al. Oocyte maturation in assisted reproductive technologies. Ann NY Acad Sci 2006; 1092: 235–46.
14. Cobo AC, Requena A, Neuspiller F, et al. Maturation in vitro of human oocytes from unstimulated cycles: selection of the optimal day for ovum retrieval based on follicular size. Hum Reprod 1999; 14: 1864–8.
15. Child TJ, Abdul-Jalil AK, Gulekli B, et al. In vitro maturation of oocytes from unstimulated normal ovaries, polycystic ovaries, and women with polycystic ovary syndrome. Fertil Steril 2001; 76: 936–42.

16. Dal Canto MB, Miginini Renzini M, Brambillasca F, et al. IVM-the first choice for IVF in Italy. Reprod Biomed Online 2006; 13: 159–65.
17. Yoon HG, Yoon SH, Son WY, et al. Pregnancies resulting from in vitro matured oocytes collected from women with regular menstrual cycle. J Assist Reprod Genet 2001; 18: 325–9.
18. Bos-Mikich A, Ferreira M, Höher M, et al. Fertilization outcome, embryo development and birth after unstimulated IVM. J Assist Reprod Geneti 2011; 28: 107–10.
19. Wynn P, Picton HM, Krapez JA, et al. Pretreatment with follicle stimulating hormone promotes the numbers of human oocytes reaching metaphase II by in vitro maturation. Hum Reprod 1998; 13: 3132–8.
20. Fadini R, Dal Canto MB, Miginini Renzini M, et al. Effect of different gonadotrophin priming on IVM of oocytes from women with normal ovaries: a prospective randomized study. Reprod Biomed Online 2009; 19: 343–51.
21. Hourvitz A, Maman E, Brengauz M, et al. In vitro maturation for patients with repeated in vitro fertilization failure due to "oocyte maturation abnormalities." Fertil Steril 2010; 94: 496–501.
22. Gulekli B, Kovali M, Aydiner F, et al. IVM is an alternative for patients with PCO after failed conventional IVF attempt. J Assist Reprod Genet 2011; 28: 495–9.
23. Fukuda A, Kanaya H, Sugihara K, et al. Clinical outcomes of IVM-IVF (In vitro maturation, in vitro fertilization and embryo transfer) as a routine ART treatment and follow up study of IVM-IVF pregnancies in PCO patients. Fertil Steril 2007; 88: S1–261.
24. Lin YH, Hwang JL, Huang LW, et al. Combination of FSH priming and hCG priming for in-vitro maturation of human oocytes. Hum Reprod 2003; 18: 1632–6.
25. Chian RC, Buckett WM, Tulandi T, et al. Prospective randomized study of human chorionic gonadotrophin priming before immature oocyte retrieval from unstimulated women with polycystic ovarian syndrome. Hum Reprod 2000; 15: 165–70.
26. Ge HS, Huang XF, Zhang W, et al. Exposure to human chorionic gonadotropin during in vitro maturation does not improve the maturation rate and developmental potential of immature oocytes from patients with polycystic ovary syndrome. Fertil Steril 2008; 89: 98–103.
27. Edwards RG. IVF, IVM, natural cycle IVF, minimal stimulation IVF – time for a rethink. Reprod Biomed Online 2007; 15: 106–19.
28. Son WY, Chung JT, Herrero B, et al. Selection of the optimal day for oocyte retrieval bassed on the diameter of the dominant follicle in hCG primed in vitro maturation cycles. Hum Reprod 2008; 23: 2680–5.
29. Fukuda A, Kawata A, Tohnaka M, et al. Successful pregnancies by intracytoplasmic sperm injection (ICI) of in vitro matured oocytes from non-stimulated women. J Fertil Implant 2001; 18: 1–4; Japanese.
30. Fukuda A, Tohnaka M, Yamasaki M, et al. Improved pregnancy rate of IVM-IVF by selecting either fresh or frozen-thawed embryo transfer on endometrial thickness in unstimulated cycles. J Fertil Implant 2002; 19: 32–5; Japanese.
31. Fukuda AI, Nakaoka Y, Tohnaka M, et al. Establishment of in vitro maturation system (IVM-IVF) as a routine ART procedure by combination of hCG administration and frozen-thawed embryo transfer. Fertil Steril 2002; 78(Suppl 2): 32.
32. Fukuda AI, Kanaya H, Oku H, et al. Pretreatment of polycystic ovarian syndrome (PCOS) patients with Metformin optimizes results from the clinical application of in vitro maturation, in vitro fertilization and embryo transfer (IVM-IVF. Fertil Steril 2004; 82(Suppl 2): 49–50.
33. Fukuda AI, Kanaya H, Sugihara K, et al. Low dose FSH administration over Metformin pretreatment on polycystic ovarian syndrome (PCOS) patients improves the clinical outcome of in vitro maturation, in vitro fertilization and embryo transfer (IVM-IVF) treatment. Fertil Steril 2004; 84(Suppl 1): 83–4.
34. Fukuda AI, Sato M, Sugihara K, et al. In vitro maturation, in vitro fertilization and embryo transfer (IVM-IVF) combined with low dose FSH administration over Metformin pretreatment and frozen-thawed cycles should be a routine ART option for polycystic ovarian syndrome (PCOS) patients. Fertil Steril 2006; 86(Suppl 2): 128–9.
35. Hashimoto S. Application of in vitro maturation to assisted reproductive technology. J Reprod Dev 2009; 55: 1–5.
36. Hashimoto S, Murata Y, Kikkawa M, et al. Successful delivery after transfer of twice-vitrified embryos derived from in-vitro matured oocytes: a case study. Hum Reprod 2007; 22: 221–3.
37. Godin PA, Gaspard O, Thonon F, et al. Twin pregnancy obtained with frozen thawed embryos after in vitro maturation in a patient with polycystic ovarian syndrome. J Assist Reprod Genet 2003; 20: 347–50.
38. Yang SH, Qin SL, Xu Y, et al. Healthy live birth from vitrified blastocysts produced from natural cycle IVF/IVM. Reprod Biomed Online 2010; 20: 656–9.
39. Vanderzwalmen P, Ectors F, Grobet L, et al. Aseptic vitrification of blastocysts from infertile patients, egg donors and after IVM. Reprod Biomed Online 2009; 19: 700–7.
40. Dowling-Lacey D, Jones E, Bocca S, et al. Two singleton live birth after the transfer of cryopreserved-thawed day-3 embryos following an unstimulated in-vitro oocyte maturation cycle. Reprod Biomed Online 2010; 20: 387–90.
41. Shimada M, Kawano N, Terada T. Delay of nuclear maturation and reduction in developmental competence of pig oocytes after mineral oil overlay of in vitro maturation media. Reproduction 2002; 124: 557–64.
42. Söderström-Anttila V, Mäkinen S, Tuuri T, et al. Favourable pregnancy results with insemination of in vitro matured oocytes from unstimulated patients. Hum Reprod 2005; 20: 1534–40.
43. Filali M, Hesters L, Fanchin R, et al. Retrospective comparison of two media for in-vitro maturation of oocytes. RBM Online 2008; 16: 250–6.
44. de Araujo CH, Nogueira D, de Araujo MC, et al. Supplemented tissue culture medium 199 is a better medium for in vitro maturation of oocytes from women with polycystic ovary syndrome women than human tubal fluid. Fertil Steril 2009; 91: 509–13.
45. Park SE, Son WY, Lee SH, et al. Chromosome and spindle configurations of human oocytes matured in vitro after cryopreservation at the germinal vesicle stage. Fertil Steril 1997; 68: 920–6.
46. Son WY, Tan SL. Laboratory and embryological aspects of hCG-primed in vitro maturation cycles for patients with polycystic ovaries. Hum Reprod Update 2010; 16: 675–89.

47. Mikkelsen AL, Høst E, Blaabjerg J, et al. Maternal serum supplementation in culture medium benefits maturation of immature human oocytes. RBM Online 2001; 3: 112–16.
48. Ben-Ami I, Komsky A, Bern O, et al. In vitro maturation of human germinal vesicle-stage oocytes: role of epidermal growth factor-like growth factors in the culture medium. Hum Reprod 2011; 26: 76–81.
49. Cha KY, Han SY, Chung HM, et al. Pregnancies and deliveries after in vitro maturation culture followed by in vitro fertilization and embryo transfer without stimulation in women with polycystic ovary syndrome. Fertil Steril 2000; 73: 978–83.
50. Mikkelsen AL, Smith S, Lindenberg S. Impact of oestradiol and inhibin A concentrations on pregnancy rate in in-vitro oocyte maturation. Hum Reprod 2000; 15: 1685–90.
51. Son WY, Yoon SH, Park SJ, et al. Ongoing twin pregnancy after vitrification of blastocysts produced by in-vitro matured oocytes retrieved from a woman with polycystic ovary syndrome: case report. Hum Reprod 2002; 17: 2963–6.
52. Hashimoto S, Fukuda A, Murata Y, et al. Effect of aspiration vacuum on the developmental competence of immature human oocytes retrieved using a 20-gauge needle. Reprod Biomed Online 2007; 14: 444–9.
53. Velázquez E, Acosta A, Mendoza SG. Menstrual cyclicity after metformin therapy in polycystic ovary syndrome. Obstet Gynecol 1997; 90: 392–5.
54. Nestler JE, Jakubowicz DJ, Evans WS, et al. Effects of metformin on spontaneous and clomiphene-induced ovulation in the polycycstic ovary syndrome. N Engl J Med 1998; 338: 1876–80.
55. Ehrmann DA, Cavaghan MK, Imperial J, et al. Effects of metformin on insulin secretion, insulin action, and ovarian steroidogenesis in women with polycystic ovary syndrome. J Clin Endocrinol Metab 1997; 82: 524–30.
56. Morin-Papunen LC, Koivunen RM, Ruokonen A, et al. Metformin therapy improves the menstrual pattern with minimal endocrine and metabolic effects in women with polycystic ovary syndrome. Fertil Steril 1998; 69: 691–6.
57. Sattar N, Hopkinson ZE, Greer IA. Insulin-sensitising agents in polycystic-ovary syndrome. Lancet 1998; 351: 305–7.
58. Boomsma CM, Eijkemans MJ, Hughes EG, et al. A meta-analysis of pregnancy outcomes in women with polycystic ovary syndrome. Human Reprod Update 2006; 12: 673–83.
59. Franks S, Gilling-Smith C, Watson H, et al. Insulin action in the normal and polycystic ovary. Endocrinol Metab Clin North Am 1999; 28: 361–78.
60. Schwarz LB, Chiu AS, Courtney M, et al. The embryo versus endometrium controversy revisited as it relates to predicting pregnancy outcome in in-vitro fertilization-embryo transfer cycles. Hum Reprod 1997; 12: 45–50.
61. Jakubowicz DJ, Seppälä M, Jakubowicz S, et al. Insulin reduction with metformin increases luteal phase serum glycodelin and insulin-like growth factor-binding protein 1 concentration and enhances uterine vascularity and blood flow in the polycystic ovary syndrome. J Clin Endocrinol Metab 2001; 86: 1126–33.
62. Kocak M, Caliskan E, Simsir C, et al. Metformin therapy improves ovulatory rates, cervical scores, and pregnancy rates in clomiphene citrate-resistant women with polycystic ovary syndrome. Fertil Steril 2002; 77: 101–6.
63. Palomba S, Russo T, Orio F Jr, et al. Uterine effects of metformin administration in anovulatory cycle women with polycystic ovary syndrome. Hum Reprod 2006; 21: 457–65.
64. Steptoe PC, Edwards RG. Birth after the implantation of a human embryo. Lancet 1978; 2: 366.
65. Son WY, Chung JT, Demirtas E, et al. Comparison of in-vitro maturation cycles with and without in-vivo matured oocytes retrieved. Reprod Biomed Online 2008; 17: 59–67.
66. Lim JH, Yang SH, Xu Y, et al. Selection of patients for natural cycle in vitro fertilization combined with in vitro maturation of immature oocytes. Fertil Steril 2009; 91: 1050–5.
67. Cha KY, Chung HM, Lee DR, et al. Obstetric outcome of patients with polycystic ovary syndrome treated by in vitro maturation and in vitro fertilization-embryo transfer. Fertil Steril 2005; 83: 1461–5.
68. Mikkelsen AL, Lindenberg S. Benefit of FSH priming of women with PCOS to the vitro maturation procedure and outcome: a randomized prospective study. Reproduction 2001; 122: 587–92.
69. Child TJ, Phillips SJ, Abdul-Jalil AK, et al. A comparison of in vitro maturation and in vitro fertilization for women with polycystic ovaries. Obstet Gynecol 2002; 100: 665–70.
70. Le Du A, Kodach IJ, Bourcigaux N, et al. In vitro oocyte maturation for the treatment of infertility associated with polycystic ovarian syndrome. Hum Reprod 2005; 20: 420–4.
71. Mikkelsen AL, Andersson AM, Skakkebaek NE, et al. Basal concentrations of oestradiol may predict the outcome of in-vitro maturation in regularly menstruating women. Hum Reprod 2001; 16: 862–7.
72. Fadini R, Dal Canto MB, Miginini Renzini M, et al. Predictive factors in in-vitro maturation in unstimulated women with normal ovaries. Reprod Biomed Online 2009; 18: 251–61.
73. Suikkari AM, Salokorpi T, Pihlaja M, et al. Healthy children born after in vitro maturation of oocytes. Hum Reprod 2005; 20: i105.
74. Buckett WM, Chian RC, Holzer H, et al. Congenital abnormalities and perinatal outcome in pregnancies following IVM, IVF and ICSI delivered in a single center. Fertil Steril 2005; 84: S80–1.
75. Suikkari AM. In vitro maturation: it's role in fertility treatment. Curr Opin Obstet Gynecol 2008; 20: 242–8.
76. Söderström-Anttila V, Salokorpi T, Pihlaja M, et al. Obstetric and perinatal outcome and preliminary results of development of children born after in-vitro maturation of oocytes. Hum Reprod 2006; 21: 1508–13.
77. Mikkelsen AL. Strategies in human in-vitro maturation and their clinical outcome. Reprod Biomed Online 2005; 10: 593–9.
78. Albertini DF, Sanfins A, Combelles CM. Origins and manifestations of oocyte maturation competencies. Reprod Biomed Online 2003; 6: 410–15.
79. Fauser BC, Bouchard P, Coelingh-Bennink HJ, et al. Alternative approaches in IVF. Human Reprod Update 2002; 8: 1–9.
80. Young LE, Fernandes K, McEvoy TG, et al. Epigenetic change in IGF2R is associated with fetal overgrowth after sheep embryo culture. Nat Genet 2001; 27: 153–4.

81. Kerjean A, Couvert P, Heams T, et al. In vitro follicular growth affects oocyte imprinting establishment in mice. Eur J Hum Genet 2003; 11: 493–6.
82. Scott L, Berntsen J, Davies D, et al. Symposium: innovative techniques in human embryo viability assessment. Human oocyte respiration-rate measurement-potential to improve oocyte and embryo selection? Reprod Biomed Online 2008; 17: 461–9.
83. Van Blerkom J, Davis PW, Lee J. ATP content of human oocytes and developmental potential and outcome after in-vitro fertilization and embryo transfer. Hum Reprod 1995; 10: 415–24.
84. Nishi Y, Takeshita T, Sato K, Araki T. Change of the mitochondrial distribution in mouse ooplasm during in vitro maturation. J Nippon Med Sch 2003; 70: 408–15.
85. Torner H, Brüssow KP, Alm H, et al. Mitochondrial aggregation patterns and activity in porcine oocytes and apoptosis in surrounding cumulus cells depends on the stage of pre-ovulatory maturation. Theriogenology 2004; 61: 1675–89.
86. Wilding M, Dale B, Marino M, et al. Mitochondrial aggregation patterns and activity in human oocytes and preimplantation embryos. Hum Reprod 2001; 16: 909–17.
87. Wang LY, Wang DH, Zou XY, et al. Mitochondrial functions on oocytes and preimplantation embryos. J Zhejiang Univ Sci B 2009; 10: 483–92.
88. Asimakopoulos B, Kotanidis L, Nikolettos N. In vitro maturation and fertilization of vitrified immature human oocytes, subsequent vitrification of produced embryos, and embryo transfer after thawing. Fertil Steril 2011; 95: e1–2.
89. Chian RC, Gilbert L, Huang JYC, et al. Live birth after vitrification of in vitro matured human oocytes. Fertil Steril 2009; 91: 372–6.
90. Oktay K, Buyuk E, Rodrigues-Wallberg KA, et al. In vitro maturation improves oocyte or embryo cryopreservation outcome in breast cancer patients undergoing ovarian stimulation for fertility preservation. Reprod Biomed Online 2010; 20: 634–8.
91. Morimoto Y, Oku Y, Sonoda M, et al. High oxygen atmosphere improves human follicle development in organ cultures of ovarian cortical tissues in vitro. Hum Reprod 2007; 22: 3170–7.
92. Ao A, Jin S, Rao D, et al. First successful pregnancy outcome after preimplantation genetic diagnosis for aneuploidy screening in embryos generated from natural-cycle in vitro fertilization combined with an in vitro maturation procedure. Fertil Steril 2006; 85: e9–11.

12

Micromanipulation

Frank L. Barnes

INTRODUCTION

Over the past 20 years micromanipulation has increased in significance in the livestock and human assisted reproductive technique laboratories. Applications of micromanipulation include embryo bisection for embryo twinning (1), the production of chimeras to investigate cell fate and development (2), nuclear transfer to investigate nuclear equivalence (3), pronuclear DNA injection to establish transgenic animals (4), blastomere biopsy for the diagnosis of genetic disease (5) intracytoplasmic sperm injection (ICSI) for the treatment of infertility (6), and cytoplasmic transfer to investigate and improve embryo development (7,8). While all of these procedures have unique characteristics, they all share some fundamental components. This chapter attempts to provide some insights into the general principles of micromanipulation as recorded from my own experiences.

PRINCIPLES

Micromanipulation of ova refers to the reduction and translation of coarse hand movement to microscopic movement at the level of the egg or embryo. There are five critical pieces of a good micromanipulation system: an inverted microscope of sufficient magnification to visualize clearly the microsurgery to be attempted; a micromanipulator of sufficient refinement to provide smooth translation of movement; microscopic glass tools of appropriate design to effect the surgical procedure; a stereomicroscope to prepare eggs and embryos for manipulation; and appropriate environmental control to maintain the temperature and atmosphere as may be required.

HANDLING CONDITIONS

Air Quality and Temperature

As with any experimental or clinical procedure, day-to-day variation should be minimized, particularly if the product of the procedure is to survive throughout subsequent development. Room conditions should be standardized for temperature, particle count, and humidity if possible. Eggs and embryos prefer a warm and moist environment; therefore, maintenance of the laboratory at 25°C with a clean room status of Class 100–1000 and a humidity of 35–45% is recommended. When conditions are not constant, variation in results can occur, as has been experienced with cloning of cattle embryos. Bovine oocytes are extremely sensitive to temperature fluctuation and can activate when chilled (9). The timing of activation can have a significant effect on the subsequent development of an embryo clone (10). The meiotic spindle of the mammalian egg is temperature sensitive and manipulation of human oocytes should be performed at 37°C to prevent chromosome disassociation and subsequent aneuploidy. The manner in which a manipulation plate is set up may have a similar impact on subsequent embryo development. Thirty-millimeter plates with 2–3 mL of medium without oil overlay will remain 3–5°C cooler than the controlling heat source, owing to evaporation. When there is no heat source a plate will cool precipitously below room temperature within five minutes. Alternatively, microdrops under oil can provide a very stable environment, providing there is a constant heat source, such as a heated microscope stage with very little thermal cycling. The manipulation plate should be designed to handle only a few ova (4–8) to reduce handling times and exposure to room conditions. Recent studies have demonstrated that microtubule depolymerization may occur during the ICSI procedure. Microtubule depolymerization occurs as a result of specimen cooling. The cooling comes from the room temperature objective and the cool air draft from the microscope stage opening (11). New products such as the Tokai Hit Thermo Plate (Zander Medical Supplies, Vero Beach, Florida, USA) are emerging, which eliminate the stage opening and reduce the cooling effect of the objective. Time will tell whether this observation leads to improved ICSI outcomes.

Media

The ionic formulation of handling media can also affect the developmental outcome of an experiment or procedure. Moving eggs and embryos from a complete medium such as Ham's F10 or TCM-199 into Dulbecco's phosphate-buffered saline (PBS), a common manipulation medium, can elicit calcium movement within the cell and ultimately affect development (12). Similarly, medium osmolality is an important parameter to consider when manipulating embryos. Current human embryo culture media range in osmolality from 260 to 285 mOsmol. At first glance this is seemingly of little significance, but changes of this magnitude can lead to visible swelling and shrinking of oocytes or blastomeres. In situations where a cell membrane is breached by the micromanipulation process, such as ICSI, this may lead to increased cell lysis. It is always preferable to manipulate eggs and embryos in a medium that maintains a similar salt balance while keeping temperature constant from incubation to manipulation.

EQUIPMENT AND MATERIALS

Manipulators

The goal of a good micromanipulation system is the efficient, smooth, and confident translation of hand movement to the clearly visualized specimen. Exaggerated hand movement high above the bench top takes time, and the amount of time spent performing micromanipulation potentially exposes your specimens to room conditions that may affect development. There are two basic types of manipulation systems today, motorized and mechanical. I have not used the manipulators by all vendors, and the discussion provided is not intended as an endorsement but rather to point out some of the pros and cons of each system type. Motorized systems have come a long way since their introduction into the market, and I have recently tested a completely motorized system (Eppendorf and the like) and found their action to be smooth and exact. However, we routinely use the Narishige brand of manipulators in most of our ICSI workstations. These set-ups have a blend of motorized coarse movement with a joystick and hydraulic fine movement translated through a separate joystick (Fig. 12.1). This system has the advantage that the joysticks are separate from the microscope and thus do not cause any movement of the specimen during manipulation (Fig. 12.2). Be it a microinjection or blastomere biopsy the hydraulic joystick offers a good range of motion across a 200–400× field and very smooth movement. Moreover, it is nice to be able to raise and lower tools without any dramatic hand movement from the bench top (Fig. 12.2). Hand position on the bench top is very comfortable when using the "drop down" joysticks. A disadvantage of this system is the hydraulic lines (Fig. 12.1). If the lines are pinched in some way, it may be impossible to fix on a location. Additionally, these systems are not very portable, and require a considerable amount of time to assemble and disassemble. Research Instruments (RI) produces completely mechanical systems. The RI system attaches to the microscope, there are no lines or cords or plugs to deal with, and it provides a very clean and neat workstation. The coarse alignment of the manipulator is adjusted with joysticks that protrude upright from the suspended arms of each side of the microscope (Fig. 12.3). The fine-movement joysticks hang down from the suspended arms. They have good three-dimensional movement across a 200–400× field; the joysticks are well oriented to the focus knobs of an inverted microscope. The RI system,

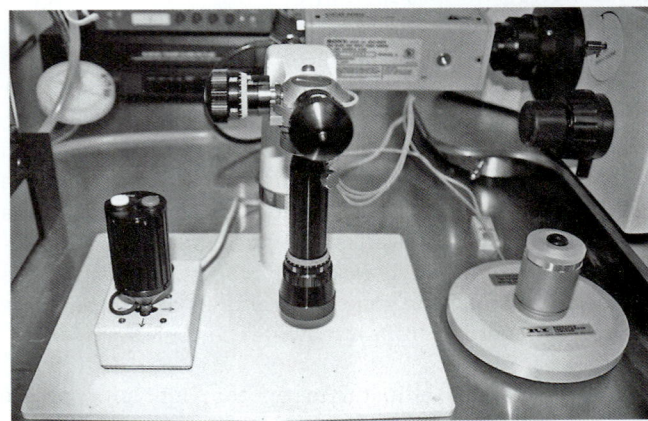

Figure 12.2 Narishige coarse and fine adjustment joysticks are separate from the microscope and prevent operator-induced vibration of the specimen on the microscope stage. Note the position of the screw-actuated syringe (SAS) and the joysticks, which allows even horizontal movement of the left hand to effect the positioning of the specimen and manipulation. The SAS tool chuck is under the control of the right-hand joystick and allows positioning of the glass microtool while the left hand performs the aspiration or injection.

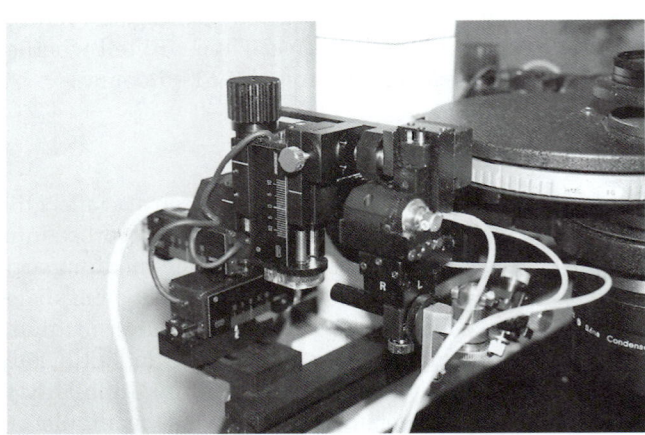

Figure 12.1 Narishige micromanipulator (*left arm*) combines motorized coarse adjustment (*background*) with hydraulic fine adjustment (*foreground*).

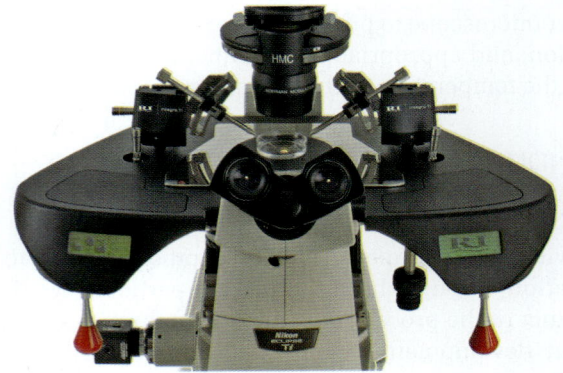

Figure 12.3 Mechanical micromanipulator from Research Instruments, the Integra Ti suspends from the objective pillar of the microscope. Suspension of the joysticks from the mounting arms provides a clean workstation. The small lever on the large upright pillars allows the tool chuck and glass microtools to be raised and lowered easily when changing manipulation plates.

once set, requires almost no coarse adjustment. There are levers on each side of the manipulator above the microscope stage that allow the microtools to be raised and lowered within a fraction of an inch of the bottom of the manipulation plate (Fig. 12.3). This manipulation system can be moved very easily without disassembly. The disadvantage is that you must move your hands from the bench top to a position above the microscope stage to raise and lower glass tools. While this is seldom a problem, the "drop down" joysticks can translate some hand vibration to the manipulation plate and specimen.

Optics

The optics employed should be sufficient to visualize clearly the ova and any components thereof; some type of contrast adjustment is often preferable to bright-field conditions. Micromanipulation is generally conducted using an inverted microscope between 200× and 400×, and therefore 10×, 20×, and 40× objectives are essential for set-up and execution of the procedure. Objective focusing rings make it easier to get a crisp par focal adjustment of the scope. Phase contrast, differential interference contrast, or Hoffman modulation contrast can enhance the specimen image; Hoffman contrast is the popular choice for ICSI where plastic dishes are used. Easy, unobstructed movement between the focus adjustment and the objectives is desirable if a change in the objectives during manipulation is required. Look for inverted microscopes that have a 1.5–2.0× slider just beyond the focus adjustment on the right side of the microscope; you can set the Hoffman condenser to 20 and the objective to 20× at the start of your manipulation session and, with very little hand movement, the magnification increases 1.5× (300×) when the slider is simply pulled out.

Stereomicroscope

Specimens should be quickly moved from the culture plate into the micromanipulation plate, manipulated, and then back again, to reduce the time held at room atmosphere. A stereomicroscope with a magnification range of 10–100× can be valuable for placing specimens into the micromanipulation plate. The "set-up" station should be close to the micromanipulation workstation to avoid unnecessary chair movements (Fig. 12.4).

Heated Stages

Heated stages are required to keep specimens at 37°C. There should be a heated stage on the micromanipulation microscope and on the set-up stereomicroscope. Be aware of hotspots on the stage that may exceed the critical threshold of specimens (greater than 38°C). Thermal cycling can be a problem with some stages; to achieve a 37°C mean temperature the stage may actually cycle between 36°C and 38°C.

Bench-Top Incubators

When performing micromanipulation it is important that the specimen is free of any cellular stress, as much as possible. Therefore, establishing constant conditions for manipulation and culture (temperature, humidity, and gas atmosphere) can improve survival after manipulation. Bench-top incubation systems are important because first, all the specimens may be placed next to the technician at the micromanipulation station so that manipulation plates can be easily and quickly switched, thus reducing the time required to perform a micromanipulation procedure; and secondly, a mixed gas atmosphere with high humidity allows culture in bicarbonate-buffered media and limits exposure to 4-(2-hydroxyethyl)-1- piperazine-ethanesulfonic acid (HEPES) or phosphate-buffered media to the time that specimens are in the micromanipulation plate. It is important to remember to pass the gas mixture through a water bubbler so that the gas atmosphere is stable; anyone who has had the humidity pan in an incubator go dry should be able to acknowledge that one cannot maintain gas atmosphere without humidity. Also, humidity helps to prevent the evaporation of media when working without an oil overlay. Evaporation can decrease the temperature and solution osmolality. There are a variety of bench-top containment systems available that control temperature, humidity, and mixed gas atmosphere (Fig. 12.5).

Containment Systems

Micromanipulation systems are sometimes contained completely within a Perspex or Plexiglas cabinet, complete with temperature and atmosphere regulation. Although these systems appear to be the ultimate in control, they often hinder the microsurgical procedure being attempted owing to space limitation.

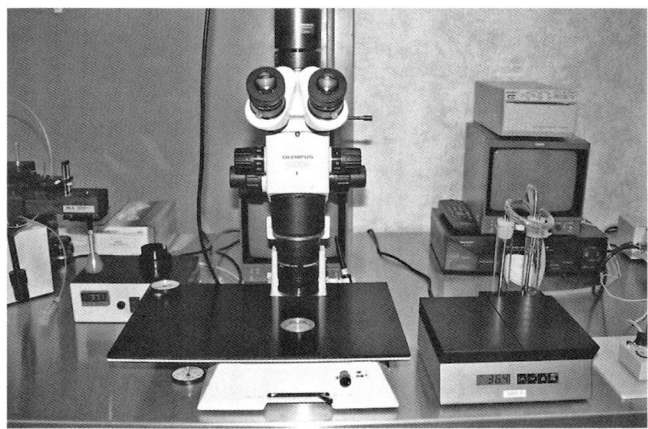

Figure 12.4 A set-up station for micromanipulation should have some type of environmental control for the manipulation and culture plates and be in close proximity to the manipulation microscope. Shown are a stereomicroscope with heated stage and a bench-top incubator with temperature and humidified gas atmosphere control.

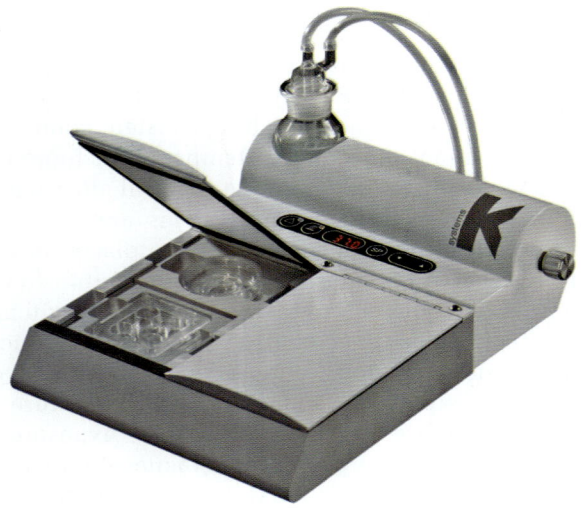

Figure 12.5 The G85 from K-Systems provides temperature regulation and can be set up with humidified mixed gas atmosphere. This system is convenient for short-term incubation at the manipulation bench.

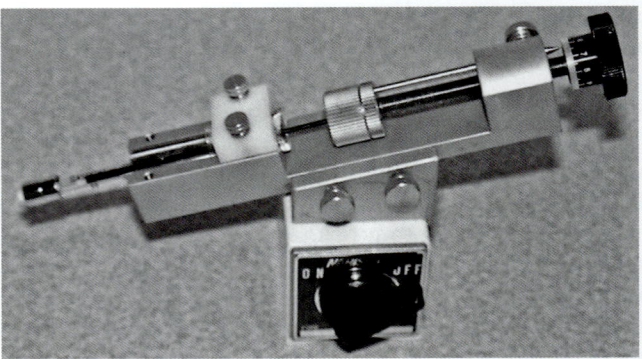

Figure 12.6 Narishige IM 6 syringe commonly used with oil-filled tubing. It is important to use stiff polyethylene tubing to prevent expansion and secondary movement of oil within the line.

Microsyringes, Tubing, and Tool Chucks

Most micromanipulation procedures that have to do with embryos either inject something, such as sperm, or remove something, such as blastomeres. A microsyringe is required to allow for controlled injection or aspiration. Microsyringes have improved significantly over the past 15 years, progressing from poorly controlled systems that can lead to egg and embryo explosion to highly refined instruments of microliter precision. Microsyringes are usually available from micromanipulator manufacturers and are often quite expensive. There are two basic types of microsyringe systems to choose from: those that require hydraulic movement of oil within the tubing that connects the glass microtool to the microsyringe, and those that simply contain air within that tubing (Figs. 12.6 and 12.7). Both types have their advocates, but I prefer the air-filled systems because I feel I have better control and there is essentially no oily mess around the workstation. It is important to point out that one of the control problems with the oil-filled system is the potential for small air bubbles in the tubing, which can compress and cause unexpected fluid movement in the glass microtool, leading to disastrous results. Possibly more important is what to do when you cannot afford an expensive microsyringe or what to do when your microsyringe is not working properly. One workable "homemade" system is a combination of a three-way valve, 10 mL rubber plunger syringe, and 1 mL rubber plunger syringe (Fig. 12.8). Fill the 10 mL syringe with oil and connect it to the three-way valve (Baxter, three-way stop clock, catalog number K75) to which the 1 mL syringe and manipulation tubing are connected. By moving the valve closure between the 1 mL syringe and the tubing, deliberately inject the oil into the system removing all air bubbles. The 1 mL syringe should contain at least 0.5 mL of oil and the tubing should contain oil all the way into the glass microtool; there can be an air space between the oil interface and the medium

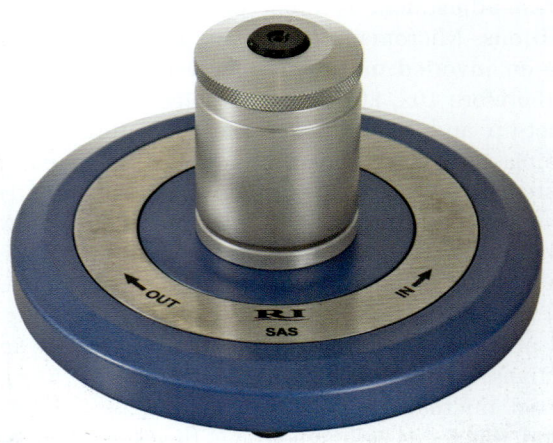

Figure 12.7 Screw-actuated syringe (SAS) from Research Instruments uses air-filled tubing to effect aspiration or injection. It is important to use stiff polyethylene tubing to prevent expansion and secondary movement of medium within the glass microtool during manipulation.

within the glass microtool. Close off the valve at the 10 mL syringe and control the manipulation by gently moving the plunger in and out of the 1 mL syringe. The result is smooth and controlled injection and aspiration. There is another method which requires a great deal more skill by the technician: simply use a 20 mL rubber plunger syringe filled with air, connected to the manipulation line. There may be some benefit to back-loading a small amount of oil into the glass microtool to improve control (Fig. 12.9). The holding pipette also needs some degree of control, and a simple air-filled syringe appears to be appropriate for all types of manipulation. The connection between the micromanipulation line and the syringe can be made with a ureteral catheter connector (French size 3–6, Cook Urological, Inc., Spencer, Indiana, USA; order number 050010). This is the only connector of its type that I have found and it works perfectly. The type of tubing used to connect the microsyringe and the glass microtools is important. Soft tubing allows for too much expansion and ultimately loss of control. Hard polythene tubing will have little expansion capability. Finally, tool chucks or

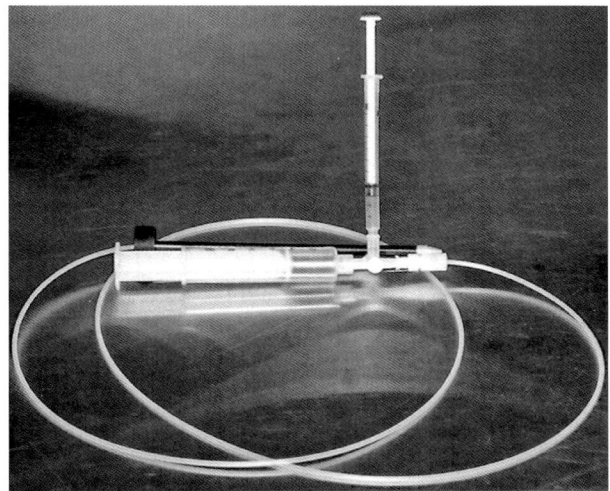

Figure 12.8 Homemade microsyringe to be used with oil-filled tubing. This device can yield extremely sensitive control and is very useful as a back-up system. Shown with polyethylene tubing and tool chuck.

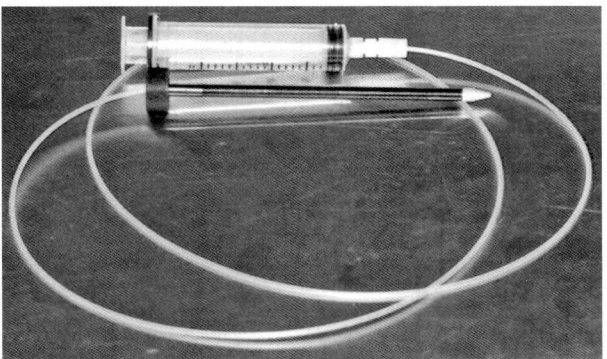

Figure 12.9 Air-filled 20-mL syringe requires additional skills by the operator but it may be useful as a back-up system. This is shown with polyethylene tubing and tool chuck.

holders make the connection between the line and the glass microtool. These are usually acquired through the micromanipulator distributor. Some tool chucks require a small silicon gasket to form a tight seal between the glass microtool and the manipulation tubing, while others simply attach with a type of locknut compression fitting. It is wise to have spare parts of all types to troubleshoot these often delicate, but essential, parts of the micromanipulation system.

Glass Microtools

Five to seven years ago, this section of a laboratory manual would have been the largest because of the extensive equipment and expertise required to make precision glass tools. Fortunately, today, there are as many microtool vendors as media companies. Generally speaking, they all provide a good product, and will make custom tools to meet your specific needs if given the time. The other consideration with regard to glass microtools is whether they should be straight or angled (30°). I prefer using angled pipettes

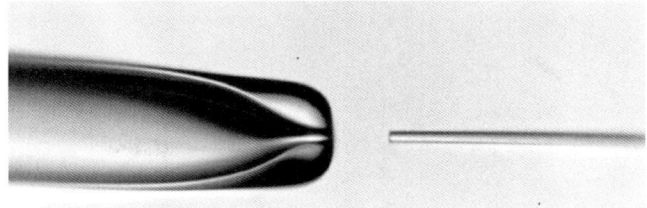

Figure 12.10 Parallel orientation of angled microtools to the bottom of the manipulation plate provides a straight-on approach to the egg or embryo with a clear focus of the tool throughout the observation field (200×). The set-up of the pictured glass microtools is as follows: The tool on the right (acid drilling pipette) is controlled by a joystick on the right and the injection or aspiration control (microsyringe) is on the left side of the microscope; the tool on the left (holder) is controlled by the joystick on the left, and the aspiration microsyringe is on the right side of the microscope. An example of the convenience of this orientation is that the acid-drilling pipette may be moved around inside a secured embryo to allow easy fragment removal without hand crossover at the level of the manipulator.

because one can establish a clear focus on the horizontal section of the tool that provides a straight-on approach to the egg or embryo being manipulated (Fig. 12.10).

Vibration

There is a great deal of concern about how vibration can affect the quality of micromanipulation. Certainly, vibration such as slamming doors or moving cattle through a crush in the next room can cause significant disruption to a micromanipulation procedure. However, with just a little cooperation from the staff outside the manipulation room, expensive vibration tables are not required. To minimize vibration, a couple of things have to be borne in mind: set the manipulator on a separate bench or counter that is not connected to the wall or the bench that might be holding the centrifuge or other vibrating equipment, and prepare your micromanipulation plate with small drops (5 µL) overlaid with oil. Place your microscope on a rubber pad; a typewriter pad works well. These simple adjustments are often all that is needed when performing ICSI. Vibration-free micromanipulation is critical, however, when performing embryo biopsy. There, relatively large manipulation drops (50 µL) are needed to disperse and dilute the acid Tyrode's solution required to breach the zona pellucida. After zona drilling, the embryo is moved to a different area of the manipulation drop and then the blastomere is removed. It is at this point that the larger manipulation drop magnifies any vibration; this can significantly slow the procedure, and potentially lead to a more lethal situation (Fig. 12.11). A great many homemade devices are used to stabilize an inverted microscope and manipulator, and most of these improve the situation. If you are not prone to invention, then you should consider a proper vibration table (Fig. 12.12) or a bench-top variety of the same (Fig. 12.13) if you plan to do an embryo biopsy.

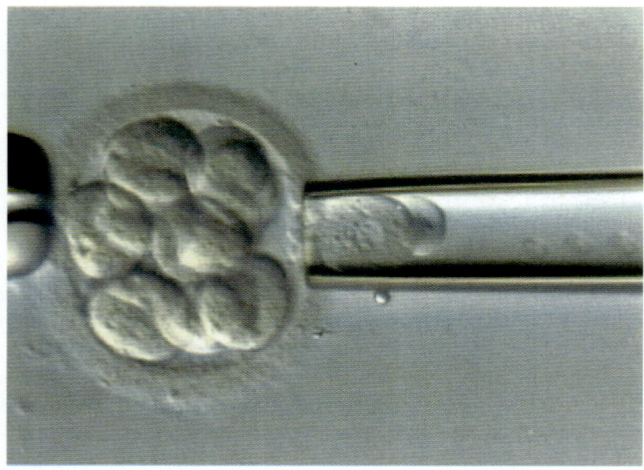

Figure 12.11 An embryo biopsy. *Source*: Photo courtesy of Reproductive Specialties Medical Center, Newport Beach, California, USA.

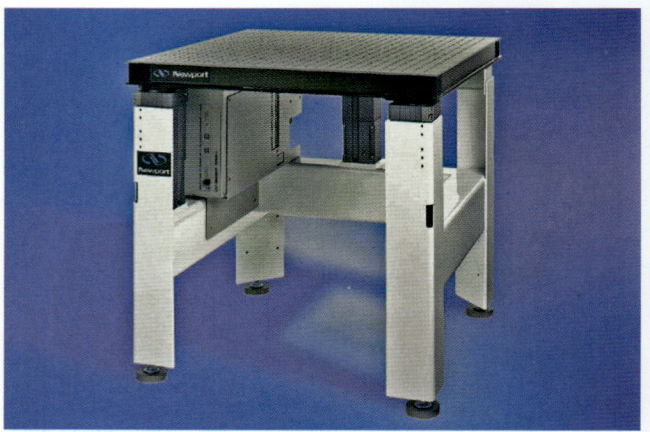

Figure 12.12 Newport Elite 3 series active vibration isolation workstation. *Source*: Photo courtesy of Newport Corporation, Irvine, California, USA, and Newbury, UK (microsyringe distributor).

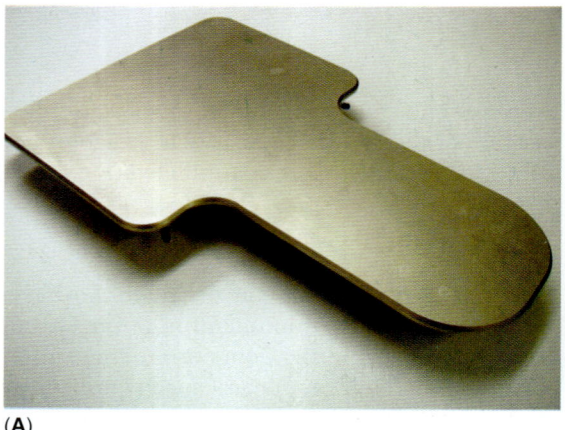

(A)

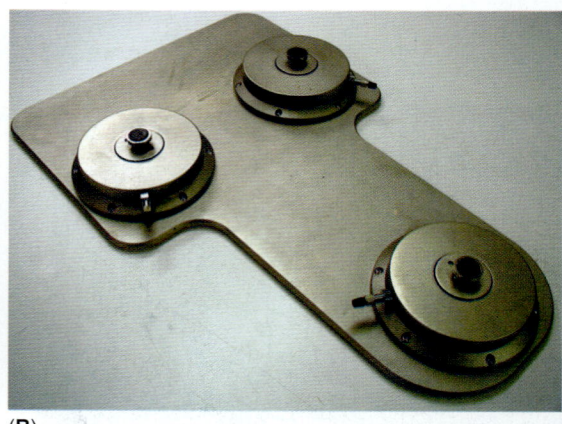

(B)

Figure 12.13 Zander bench-top antivibration table: (**A**) from above; (**B**) from below. *Source*: Photos courtesy of Zander Medical Supplies and Zander IVF, Inc., Vero Beach, Florida, USA.

Laser-Assisted Micromanipulation

Opening the zona pellucida is common to many manipulation procedures and is performed primarily using three methodologies: mechanical zona dissection, zona drilling with acid Tyrode's solution, or laser. All of these methods have their supporters and critics but are effective and do little harm to the developing embryo if performed by an experienced technician. The use of a 1.48 µm diode laser beam (ZILOS-tk® Laser, Hamilton Thorne Research, Beverly, Massachusetts, USA) to open the zona pellucida for assisted hatching or embryo biopsy offers some significant advantages in terms of both efficiency and pregnancy outcomes (13–15). Mechanical zona dissection and zona drilling with acid Tyrode's calls for set-up of specific micromanipulation plates and microtools while assisted hatching with a laser may be performed in an open well or drop without microtools of any kind or additional handling, media steps, and rinses. Also, with the advent of blastocyst vitrification protocols, a single laser pulse can be used to shrink the blastocele which has been demonstrated to improve blastocyst survival following warming (16).

The net outcome is faster manipulation, which can translate into improved outcomes (14). The microtools should be oriented such that they are perpendicular to the microdrop interface at the 9 o'clock and 3 o'clock positions and parallel to the bottom of the manipulation plate (Fig. 12.10).

Common Micromanipulation Applications for the IVF Laboratory

Once considered the most invasive approach to in vitro fertilization (IVF), ICSI is now used in nearly every IVF center in the United States with some centers utilizing it on all their patients (Fig. 12.14). The new area of micromanipulation innovation is embryo biopsy. The standard protocol for nearly two decades has been single-cell biopsy of day 3 embryos using two common methodologies: the blastomere aspiration technique (Fig. 12.11) and the blastomere blow-out technique (Fig. 12.15). The appropriateness of day 3 embryo biopsy has recently been challenged due to concerns of misdiagnosis arising from questions about the robustness

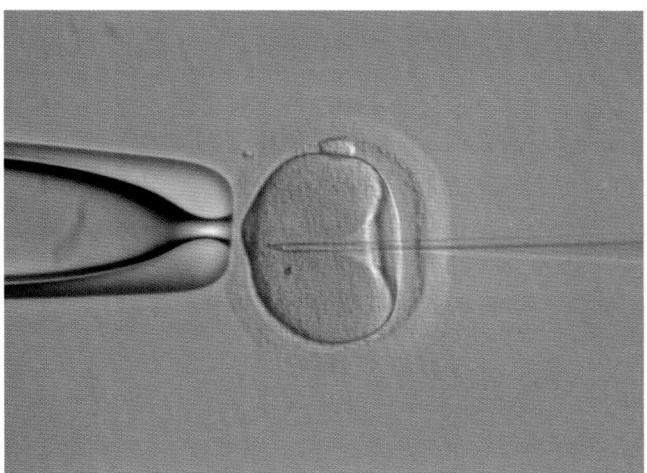

Figure 12.14 Intracytoplasmic sperm injection. Note the focus on the inner lumen of the holding pipette aligned with the focus on the oolemma and the injection pipette. All points of focus keep you in the center of the oocyte.

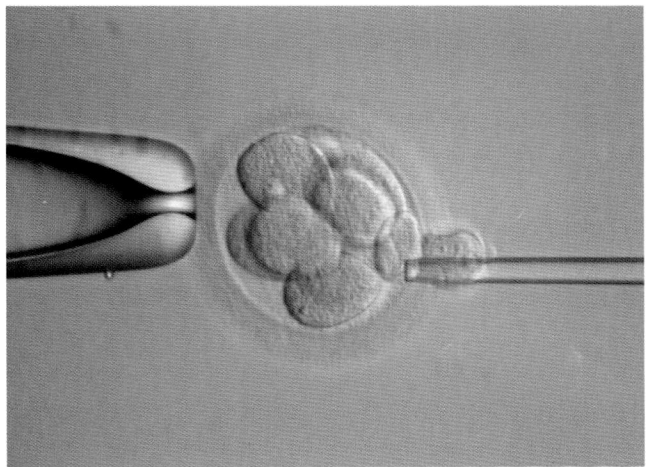

Figure 12.15 Embryo biopsy of a day-3 embryo using the blow-out technique. Note the small pipette just inside the zona pellucida. By injection of small amounts of media the blastomere is forced out of the embryo atraumatically.

of testing methodologies, high rates of blastomere mosaicism on day 3, and the biopsy of poor-quality embryos. These concerns have pushed the laboratory to develop safe and effective methods of blastocyst biopsy. Blastocyst stage embryo biopsy has the advantages of selecting only those embryos that show robust viability and of providing more cells for analysis. Biopsy of the blastocyst is best performed by starting with the day 3 embryo and subjecting it to assisted hatching. By the time of blastocyst formation on day 5/6 the trophoblast is starting to herniate through the assisted hatching site which provides an ample number of cells easily accessible for biopsy (Fig. 12.16). Using a biopsy pipette the cells to be biopsied are stretched to create a thin cellular bundle that can then be dissected with the aid of the laser in two to four pulses (Fig. 12.17).

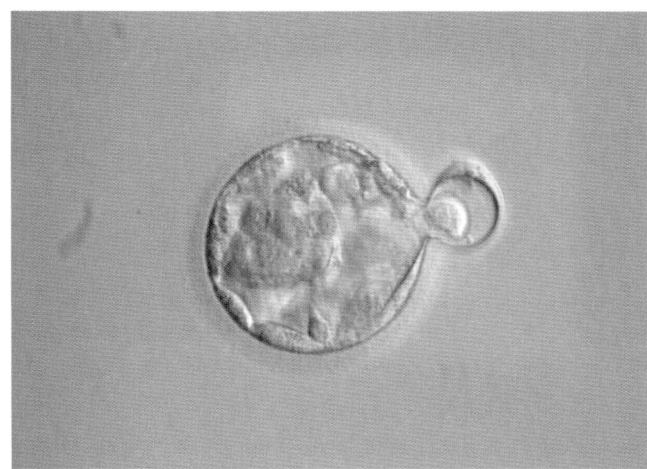

Figure 12.16 Trophoblast cells herniating from the day-5 blastocyst following assisted hatching on day 3; note, make a narrow rent in the zona pellucida on day 3 to produce a tight cellular bundle on day 5 that will facilitate laser cutting of the tissue.

PROCEDURE STEPWISE

Micromanipulator Set-Up

The manipulation workstation is oriented such that the holding pipette is on the left and the manipulation pipette or biopsy pipette is on the right. Their respective controls (syringes) are on the opposing side to avoid hand crossover during the procedure. The holding pipette is attached to a 10 mL syringe via approximately 1 m of polyethylene tubing. The manipulation pipette is attached to a microsyringe via 1 m of polyethylene tubing obtained from the microsyringe distributor. The microtools should be oriented such that they are perpendicular to the microdrop interface at the 9 o'clock and 3 o'clock positions and parallel to the bottom of the manipulation plate (Fig. 12.10).

Manipulation Plate Set-Up

1. Label a Falcon 1006 plate with the identity and/or ownership of the specimen to be manipulated.
2. Place small microdrops in the center of the plate of sufficient size to contain the specimens (5–10 µL). The drops are overlaid with 4–5 mL of mineral oil and placed into a G85 or other suitable incubator to equilibrate the temperature.
3. The micromanipulation plate set-up should be performed at least one hour prior to manipulation so that the temperature is equilibrated at 37°C. It is important that the drops be close together so they fit easily within the objective opening of the microscope stage.
4. Prepare enough manipulation plates such that any given plate is only used once for a given patient or procedure. Care should be taken to keep plates warm. The time that microtools are exposed to air should be minimized when changing plates. Microtools become sticky when exposed to air.

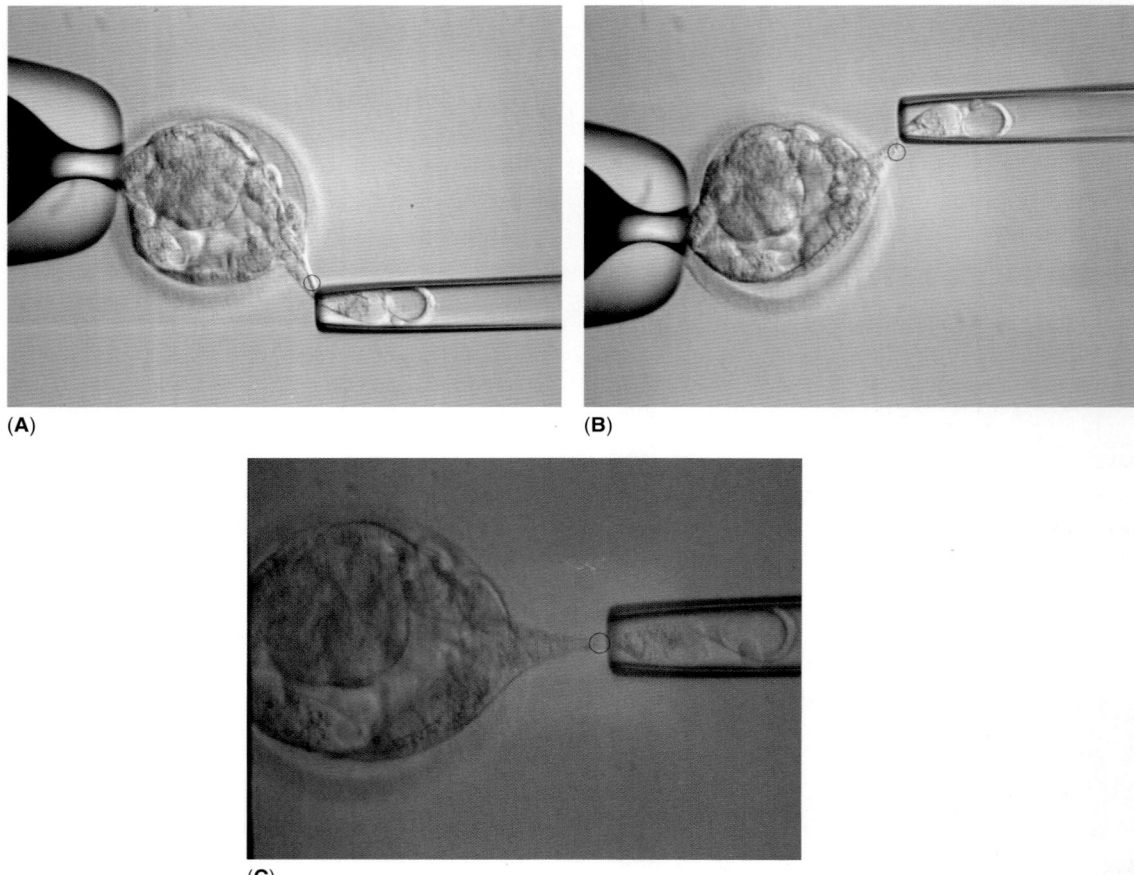

Figure 12.17 Dissection of the cellular bundle; a single laser pulse is performed on each side of the cellular bundle and finally in the center of the bundle; see the area within the circles. Stretching of the cellular bundle easily dissects the tissue after each laser pulse until the tissue pulls free. Care should be taken not to laser the same location twice as this will harden the cellular tissue and make it difficult to separate.

Micromanipulation Technique

1. At 200× magnification, focus on the zona pellucida of the oocyte or embryo.
2. Bring the manipulation pipette into focus.
3. Lower the holding pipette into the drop until it is in focus.
4. With gentle suction, aspirate the oocyte or embryo until it is held firmly without causing distortion of the zona pellucida. When held, the oocyte or embryo should be resting gently on the bottom of the plate with the lumen of the holding pipette and the manipulation pipette and the zona pellucida in sharp focus. If performed exactly in the order described, the microtools will be aligned with the equator of the oocyte or embryo.
5. Change magnification to 400× and focus on the area to be manipulated.
6. Bring the manipulation pipette into focus.
7. Adjust the range of motion of the manipulation pipette. The manipulation pipette should have a range of motion over the area of the oocyte or embryo. Perform the desired manipulation procedure.

REFERENCES

1. Willadsen SM, Lehn-Jensen H, Fehilly CB, Newcomb R. The production of monozygotic twins of preselected parentage by micromanipulation of non-surgically collected cow embryos. Theriogenology 1981; 15: 23–7.
2. Fehilly CB, Willadsen SM, Tucker EM. Interspecific chimaerism between sheep and goat. Nature (London) 1984; 307: 634–6.
3. Willadsen SM. Nuclear transplantation in sheep embryos. Nature (London) 1986; 320: 63.
4. Brinster RL, Chen HY, Trumbauer ME, Yagle MK, Palmiter RD. Factors affecting the efficiency of introducing foreign DNA into mice by microinjecting eggs. Proc Natl Acad Sci USA 1985; 82: 4438–42.
5. Munne S, Magli C, Cohen J, et al. Positive outcome after preimplantation diagnosis of aneuploidy in human embryos. Hum Reprod 1999; 14: 2191–9.
6. Palermo P, Joris H, Devroey P, Van Steirteghem AC. Pregnancies after intracytoplasmic injection of single spermatozoon into an oocyte. Lancet 1992; 340: 17–18.
7. Muggelton-Harris A, Whittingham DG, Wilson L. Cytoplasmic control of preimplantation development in vitro in the mouse. Nature (London) 1982; 299: 460–2.

8. Cohen J, Scott R, Schimmel T, et al. Birth of infant after transfer of anucleate donor oocyte cytoplasm into recipient eggs. Lancet 1997; 350: 186–7.
9. Powell R, Barnes FL. The kinetics of oocyte activation and polar body formation in bovine embryo clones. Mol Reprod Dev 1992; 33: 53–8.
10. Barnes FL, Collas P, Powell R, et al. Influence of recipient oocyte cell cycle stage on DNA synthesis, nuclear envelope breakdown, chromosome constitution and development in nuclear transplant bovine embryos. Mol Reprod Dev 1993; 36: 33–41.
11. Keefe D. New morphologic criteria for imaging viable eggs and embryos. Presented at the 13th Annual in Vitro Fertilization and Embryo Transfer, a Comprehensive Update – 2000, UCLA School of Medicine. Santa Barbara, CA, Mini-symposium on the IVF laboratory; 2000; 83–8.
12. Collas P, Fissore R, Robl JM, Sullivan EJ, Barnes FL. Electrically-induced calcium elevation, activation and parthenogenetic development of bovine oocytes. Mol Reprod Dev 1992; 34: 212–23.
13. Jones AE, Wright G, Kort H, Straub RJ, Nagy ZP. Comparison of laser-assisted hatching and acidified Tyrode's hatching by evaluation of blastocyst development rates in sibling embryos: a prospective randomized trial. Fertil Steril 2006; 85: 487–91.
14. Makrakis E, Angeli I, Agapitou K, et al. Laser versus mechanical assisted hatching: a prospective study of clinical outcomes. Fertil Steril 2006; 86: 1596–600.
15. Lanzendorf SE, Ratts VS, Moley KH, et al. A randomized, prospective study comparing laser-assisted hatching and assisted hatching using acidified medium. Fertil Steril 2007; 87: 1450–7.
16. Mukaida T, Oka C, Goto T, Takahashi K. Artificial shrinkage of blastocoeles using either a micro-needle or a laser pulse prior to the cooling steps of vitrification improves survival rate and pregnancy outcome of vitrified human blastocysts. Hum Reprod 2006; 21: 3246–52.

13

Intracytoplasmic sperm injection: Technical aspects

Queenie V. Neri, Devin Monahan, Zev Rosenwaks, and Gianpiero D. Palermo

BACKGROUND

Spermatozoa sometimes fail to fertilize even when they are artificially placed in close proximity to eggs during conventional in vitro fertilization (IVF). Fertilization failure in IVF is particularly common where there are grossly abnormal semen parameters or when the number of spermatozoa is insufficient. Gamete micromanipulation is the only way to overcome this problem in most cases. The different techniques developed in this regard focused initially on the obstacle to sperm penetration represented by the zona pellucida (ZP), by thinning it through exposure to enzymes or creating an opening through localized chemical digestion, mechanical breach, or even photo ablation (1–3). The placing of the spermatozoon beneath the zona has yielded consistent results, achieving a fertilization rate of ~20% (4). However, these techniques have been abandoned because of limiting factors such as the need for many functional spermatozoa with good progressive motility, and complications like multiple sperm penetration (5).

INTRACYTOPLASMIC SPERM INJECTION

The intracytoplasmic sperm injection (ICSI) procedure entails the deposition of a single spermatozoon directly into the cytoplasm of the oocyte, thus bypassing the ZP and the oolemma. The ability of ICSI to achieve higher fertilization and pregnancy rates regardless of sperm characteristics makes it the most powerful micromanipulation procedure yet with which to treat male factor infertility. In fact, the therapeutic possibilities of ICSI go from cases in which, after sperm selection, the spermatozoa show poor progressive motility, to its application to azoospermic men where spermatozoa are microsurgically retrieved from the epididymis and the testis (6–8). Retrieval of a low number of oocytes represents a further indication for this procedure, because only after cumulus cell removal is it possible to identify the oocytes that have extruded the first polar body and then inseminate them accordingly. In fact, the availability of ICSI has been instrumental in some European countries that include Italy and Germany in circumventing restrictive legislation that limits the number of oocytes inseminated or embryos to be replaced (9,10). ICSI has also made the consistent fertilization of cryopreserved oocytes possible (11) since freezing can lead to a premature exocytosis of cortical granules and so a zona hardening that inhibits natural sperm penetration (12–15). When preimplantation genetic screening is to be performed on oocytes, the removal of the polar body requires the stripping of cumulus corona cells, thus supporting ICSI as the only insemination method to avoid polyspermy. When embryos need to be analyzed for gene defects, the avoidance of contaminating spermatozoa on the ZP reduces the chance of false amplification by polymerase chain reaction. ICSI is the preferred method of insemination by several groups for HIV discordant couples because it virtually avoids the interaction of oocytes with semen, thereby reducing the risk of viral exposure (16–18). Advantages of ICSI over intrauterine insemination for discordant couples also include the considerably higher success rate (16), requiring fewer attempts to achieve a pregnancy with obviously reduced chances to viral exposure (17) for the unaffected partner. Reassuringly, no seroconversions have been reported following assisted reproductive techniques (ARTs) for HIV discordant couples (19).

This chapter is aimed at describing the technical details involved in the appropriate execution of ICSI and depicts the clinical outcome of the different sources of the male gamete.

Semen Collection

When possible, semen samples are collected by masturbation after three days of abstinence and allowed to liquefy for at least 20 minutes at 37°C before analysis. When the semen has high viscosity, this can be reduced within three to five minutes usually by adding it to 2–3 mL of 4–(2-hydroxyethyl)-1-piperazine-ethanesulfonic acid (HEPES)-buffered human tubal fluid (HTF-HEPES) containing 200–300 IU of chymotrypsin (Sigma Chemical Co., St Louis, Missouri, USA). The use of limited proteolytic enzyme with chymotrypsin was shown to effectively disperse hyperviscous samples for semen preparation (20,21). Electroejaculation is applied in cases of spinal cord injury or psychogenic anejaculation (22).

In cases of irreparable obstructive azoospermia, a condition which is often caused by a congenital bilateral absence of the vas deferens and is associated with a cystic fibrosis gene mutation, spermatozoa are retrieved by microsurgical epididymal sperm aspiration or percutaneous epididymal sperm aspiration (23–25). Variable volumes of fluid (1–500 µL) are collected from the epididymal lumen by a glass micropipette or a metal needle. Since spermatozoa are highly concentrated, only microliter quantities are needed. Alternatively, azoospermic patients undergo testicular sperm retrieval when the epididymal approach is not feasible because of scarring or due to impaired sperm production as in nonobstructive situations. An open biopsy or the more recent fine-needle aspiration technique is used for testicular sampling (26). The biopsy specimen of approximately 500 mg is rinsed in medium to remove red blood cells and is divided into small pieces with sterile tweezers under a stereomicroscope (27). Testicular sperm extraction (TESE) and the now-refined micro-TESE (mTESE) procedures retrieve seminiferous tubules with residual spermatogenesis granting a higher probability of sperm retrieval while maintaining a greater anatomical integrity of the testicle (28,29). Motility in place or twitching is then assessed on a microscope at 100–200×, and a second biopsy specimen is obtained if spermatozoa are not found. After the micro-TESE procedure, the testicular samples were maintained overnight in medium at 37°C. Testicular tissue was exposed to collagenase type IV (1000 IU/mL) combined with 25 mg/mL of DNase I (30). The tissue was incubated with collagenase for one hour, and the suspension was mixed every 10–15 minutes to enhance enzymatic digestion. Large portions of undigested tissue such as tubular walls and connective tissues were removed and the digested suspension was centrifuged twice at 500 g for five minutes. When no spermatozoa were identified in the pellet, the supernatant was further centrifuged at 1500–3000 g for five minutes. The pellet from this fraction was also examined. Both pellets were resuspended in a medium ranging from 20 to 200 µL. Sperm presence, viability, and motility characteristics together with the presence of other germ cells were noted. If no spermatozoa were seen, the resuspended sample was placed in individual 8 µL drops under oil and assessed under an inverted microscope at 400×.

Semen Processing: Analysis and Selection

Semen concentration and motility are assessed in a Makler® counting chamber (Sefi Medical Instruments, Haifa, Israel). Morphologic characterization of sperm has a significant correlation with male infertility, and is performed using the Kruger's strict criteria (31). Evaluation is usually made after spreading 5 µL of semen or sperm suspension on pre-stained slides (Testsimplets®; Boehringer, Munster, Germany), which can allow a rapid assessment. The specimen is examined microscopically, and at least 100–200 spermatozoa are categorized. Semen parameters are considered to be impaired when the sperm concentration is $<15 \times 10^6$/mL, the progressive motility is $<40\%$, or a normal morphology is exhibited by $<4\%$ of the spermatozoa (32). For selection of spermatozoa, the sample is washed by centrifugation at 500 g for five minutes in HTF medium supplemented with 6% (v/v) human serum albumin (HSA; Vitrolife, Englewood, Colorado, USA). Semen samples with $<5 \times 10^6$/mL spermatozoa or $<20\%$ motile spermatozoa are washed in HTF medium by a single centrifugation at 500–1800 g for five minutes. The resuspended pellet is layered on a discontinuous ISolate® gradient (Irvine Scientific, Irvine, California, USA) on two layers (90% and 45%) and centrifuged at 300 g for 10 minutes. A one layer ISolate® gradient (90%) is used when samples have a sperm density $<5 \times 10^6$/mL spermatozoa and $<20\%$ motile spermatozoa. The sperm-rich ISolate® fraction is washed by adding 4 mL of HTF medium and centrifuged at 600–800 g for 5–10 minutes to remove the silica gel particles. For spermatozoa with poor kinetic characteristics, the sperm suspension is exposed to a 3 mmol/L solution of pentoxifylline and is centrifuged again. The concentration of the assessed sperm suspension is adjusted to $1–1.5 \times 10^6$/mL, when necessary, by the addition of HTF medium, and subsequently incubated at 37°C in a gas atmosphere of 5% CO_2 in air until utilization for ICSI.

Sperm Cryopreservation

The sperm suspension (adjusted to a concentration of $\sim 30 \times 10^6$/mL) is diluted with at least an equal amount of cryopreservation medium (Freezing Medium-Test Yolk Buffer with Glycerol; Irvine Scientific), and up to 1 mL aliquots of the final solution are placed in 1 mL cryogenic vials (Nalgene Brand Products, Rochester, New York, USA). The vials are exposed to liquid nitrogen (LN_2) vapor at −70°C for 15 minutes, and then plunged into liquid N_2 at −196°C. Vials are thawed at 37°C for 15 minutes when spermatozoa are needed for injection. When in excess, epididymal spermatozoa and testicular tissue were cryopreserved for later use (33). Surgically retrieved samples are cryopreserved similarly to fresh semen with an excess of cryoprotectant and, when appropriate, exposed to a motility enhancer (3 mmol/L pentoxifylline) to facilitate the identification of viable spermatozoa (7).

Collection and Preparation of Oocytes

Baseline blood work and pelvic ultrasound are performed on menstrual cycle day 2 for patients treated with gonadotropin-releasing hormone (GnRH) antagonist protocols and on the menstrual cycle day 3 for patients treated with the long GnRH agonist protocol (34). Normal baseline parameters include FSH less than 12 mIU/mL, estradiol (E_2) less than 75 pg/mL, and progesterone less than 1 ng/mL. Pelvic ultrasound is performed to evaluate endometrial thickness, assess the antral follicle count, and the presence of ovarian cysts.

In the initial IVF cycle, the patient response to controlled hyperstimulation is verified after 2–3 days of gonadotropin stimulation. Tailored doses of human chorionic gonadotropins (hCG) are administered when criteria for oocyte maturity are met, and oocyte retrieval by vaginal ultrasound-guided puncture is performed 35 hours later (34,35). Under the inverted microscope at 100×, the cumulus corona cell complexes are scored as mature, slightly immature, completely immature, or slightly hypermature. Thereafter, the oocytes are incubated for about four hours. Immediately prior to micromanipulation, the cumulus corona cells are removed by exposure to HTF-HEPES-buffered medium containing 40 IU/mL of Cumulase® (Halozyme Therapeutics Inc., San Diego, California, USA). A good cumulus removal is necessary for observation of the oocyte and effective use of the holding and/or injecting pipette during micromanipulation. For final removal of the residual corona cells, the oocytes are repeatedly aspirated in and out of a hand-drawn Pasteur pipette with an inner diameter of ~200 μm. Each oocyte is then examined under the microscope to assess nuclear maturity and morphology; metaphase II (MII) was assessed according to the absence of the germinal vesicle and the presence of an extruded polar body. ICSI is performed only in oocytes that have reached this level of maturity.

Setting for the Microinjection

The holding (HP-120–30; 120 μm OD) and injecting pipettes (IC-C1; 5–7 μm ID) are both made from glass capillary tubes (Vitrolife AB, Göteborg, Sweden). Both pipettes are bent to an angle of approximately 30° at 1 mm from the tip, to be able to perform the injection procedure with the tips of the tools horizontally positioned in a plastic Petri dish (model 351006, Falcon; Becton and Dickinson, Lincoln Park, New Jersey, USA). Immediately before injection, 1 μL of the sperm suspension is diluted with 4 μL of a 7% polyvinylpyrrolidone (PVP) solution with HSA (90121, Irvine Scientific) in HTF-HEPES medium placed in the middle of a plastic Petri dish. It is necessary to use the viscous solution during the procedure in order to slow down the aspiration and prevent the sperm from sticking to the wall of the injection pipette. When there are <100,000 spermatozoa per sample, the sperm suspension is concentrated to approximately 3 μL and transferred directly in drop #8 (Fig. 13.1) where each oocyte is placed in the remaining 8 μL drops G-MOPS (Vitrolife) supplemented with 6% G-MM (Vitrolife). These drops are covered with lightweight oil (Sage Medical, Trumbull, Connecticut, USA). Following immobilization, an individual spermatozoon is aspirated at the 3 o'clock edge of the PVP drop. For low concentration, a spermatozoon is retrieved by the injection tool from drop #8 and moved to the viscous medium central drop in order to remove debris, gain better aspiration control, and to carry out immobilization. The procedure is carried out on a custom-designed heated stage (Eastech Laboratory, Centereach, New York, USA) fitted on a Nikon TE2000U inverted microscope at 400× using Nikon Modulation contrast optics. This microscope is equipped with a customized micromanipulation set-up (NAI-20P, Narishige Co. Ltd., Tokyo, Japan) consisting of two motor-driven coarse control

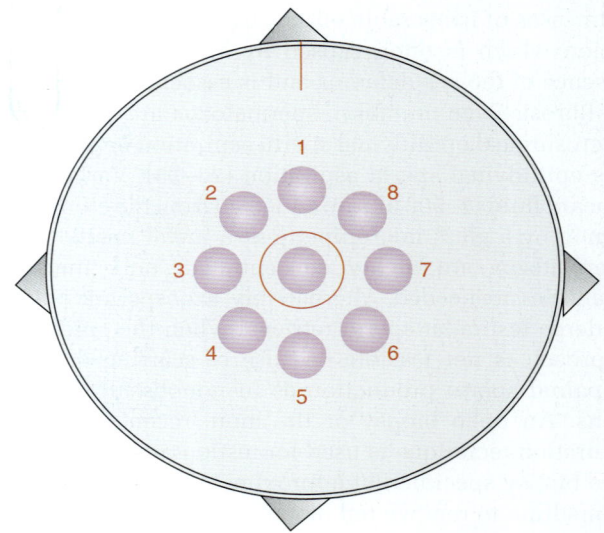

Figure 13.1 Intracytoplasmic sperm injection (ICSI) dish is made of 8 μL drops of ICSI medium plus 1 central drop overlaid with paraffin oil. The drops are labeled with a red pencil that is not embryo toxic: the central drop is marked with a circle while the surrounding drops are numbered 1–8 in a counter clockwise fashion. The central drop is removed and with replaced polyvinylpyrrolidone while drops 1–8 will contain a single oocyte each. Specimens with very few spermatozoa are concentrated to a very small volume and placed on drop #8.

manipulators and two hydraulic micromanipulators. These custom manipulators have a modified low position microscope mounting adaptor, a single power supply for the motor-drive coarse unit, and a tubing-free joystick. The microtools are controlled by two microinjectors, one air control (IM-9B) for the holding pipette and the other IM-6 is oil operated fitted with a metal syringe for the injection tool.

Selection of the Spermatozoon and Immobilization

Normally, at a magnification of 400×, it is not easy to select spermatozoa according to morphologic characteristics while they are in motion in medium. However, selection of a normal spermatozoon can be accomplished by observing its shape, its light refraction, and its motion pattern in viscous medium (6). When 1 μL of sperm suspension was added to the drop containing PVP, motile spermatozoa progress into the viscous medium where debris, other cells, bacteria, and immotile spermatozoa remain at the PVP interface and paraffin oil. The viscous medium, by decelerating the spermatozoon, allows evaluation of its tridimensional motion patterns permitting morphological assessment as well as favoring the aspiration into the pipette.

Although ICSI does not require any specific spermatozoon pretreatment, gentle immobilization achieved through mechanical pressure is needed to permeabilize the membrane that allow the release of a sperm cytosolic factor resulting in oocyte activation and improved fertilization rates (36–38). Human spermatozoa undergo important modifications in the nuclear chromatin where sperm DNA is packed very tightly to protect it during

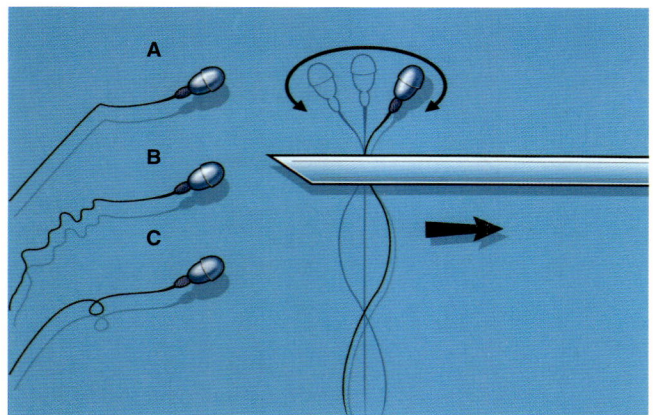

Figure 13.2 Aggressive immobilization of the spermatozoon for intracytoplasmic sperm injection. The correctly immobilized spermatozoon has its tail permanently kinked A, convoluted B, or looped C.

the transition within the male and female genital tracts. Shaping of the male gamete nucleus takes place in late spermiogenesis as its chromatin is undergoing a remarkable condensation that renders the sperm transcriptionally inert and highly resistant to digestion. Following the morphological transformation of the nucleus in the testis, as spermatozoa transit through the epididymis, there occurs a stabilization of the chromatin through establishment of disulfide bonds between the thiol-rich protamines (39). Qualitative and quantitative modifications of the plasma membrane occurring in the lipidic composition and the absorption of specific proteins secreted by the epididymal epithelium result in changes of its electric charge (40,41). The lack of all these changes is associated with a decreased ability of epididymal spermatozoa to bind and penetrate the oocyte (42). Owing to physiologic differences in their membrane characteristics, a more aggressive immobilization technique is necessary when using epididymal and/or testicular spermatozoa.

When the immobilization procedure is performed in a standard fashion, a spermatozoon is positioned at 90° to the tip of the pipette, which is then lowered gently to compress the sperm flagellum. The spermatozoon immobilized in this manner should maintain the shape of its tail. If during the process the latter is damaged or kinked, that spermatozoon is discarded and the procedure repeated with another sperm. An alternative and more effective procedure is aggressive immobilization, where the sperm tail is rolled over the bottom of the Petri dish in a location posterior to the mid-piece. This induces a permanent crimp in the tail section, making it kinked, looped, or convoluted (Fig. 13.2). When these two distinct immobilization methods were applied to immature spermatozoa and the fertilization rates after ICSI were compared, the more extensive sperm tail disruption prior to oocyte injection appeared to improve the outcome. When the fertilization rate was compared within ejaculated spermatozoa, the difference was less remarkable (43,44). The findings were clarified in a later study where spermatozoa were mechanically immobilized and inserted into the perivitelline space of mouse oocytes (44) to allow ultrathin TEM sections that revealed consistent alterations in the acrosomal region including disruption of the plasma membrane, vesiculation, or even loss of the acrosome. All of the sperm assessed had undergone some membrane disorganization of the head, in contrast to the majority of control sperm. Immobilization of sperm immediately prior to the ICSI procedure is fundamental for its consistent success (44–49). A possible explanation of the variation in fertilization rate after aggressive immobilization may lie in the structural membrane differences between mature and immature spermatozoa. Immature gametes probably require additional manipulation to promote membrane permeabilization that enhances the postinjection events involved in sperm nuclear decondensation.

Several studies have shown that suboptimal sperm morphology is often associated with aneuploidy, nuclear DNA damage, and at times, impaired ICSI outcome (50–52). Sperm DNA integrity is currently assessed by invasive methods such as TUNEL, Comet, sperm chromatin dispersion test, or by a sperm chromatin structural assay. All of these require fixation and so destruction of the sperm being assessed (53). It has been postulated that infertile men have compromised DNA integrity as measured by these methods without, however, correlating with sperm concentration and morphology (54,55). However, in a systematic observation performed in our laboratory we identified an inverse relationship, a correlation between DNA fragmentation and motility (56). Perhaps the reason why there is a lack of predictability between DNA integrity and pregnancy outcome with ICSI inseminations may be explained by the fact that only motile spermatozoa are utilized for injection.

Ooplasmic Injection

The oocyte is held in place by the suction applied to the holding pipette. The inferior pole of the oocyte touching the bottom of the dish allows better grip of the egg during the injection procedure. The injection pipette is lowered and focused in accordance with the outer right border of the oolemma on the equatorial plane at 3 o'clock. The spermatozoon is then brought in proximity to the beveled opening of the injection pipette (Fig. 13.3). The latter is pushed against the zona, permitting its penetration and thrusting forward to the inner surface of the oolemma. As the point of the pipette reaches the approximate center of the egg, a break in the membrane should occur. This is reflected by a sudden quivering of the convexities (at the site of invagination) of the oolemma above and below the penetration point, as well as the proximal flow of the cytoplasmic organelles and the spermatozoon moved upward into the pipette (Fig. 13.4). These are then slowly ejected back into the cytoplasm, where the aspiration of the cytoplasm becomes an additional stimulus to activate the egg. To optimize the interaction with the ooplasm, the sperm cell should be ejected past the tip of the pipette to ensure an intimate position among the organelles that will help to maintain the sperm in place while withdrawing the pipette. When the pipette is approximately at the

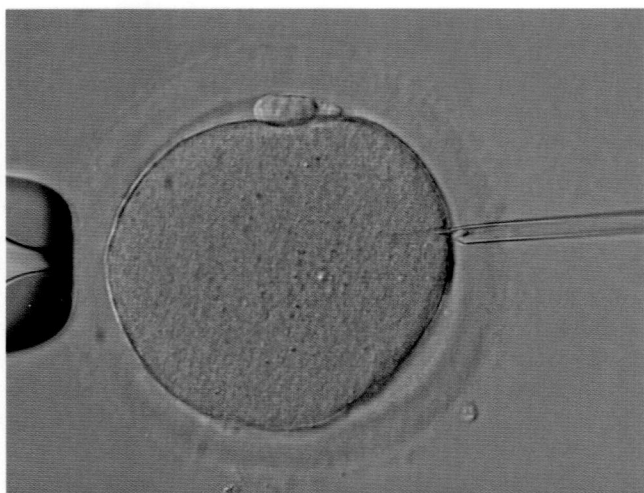

Figure 13.3 Intracytoplasmic sperm injection procedure. Prior to penetrating the oolemma, the spermatozoon is brought in proximity to the beveled opening of the injection pipette.

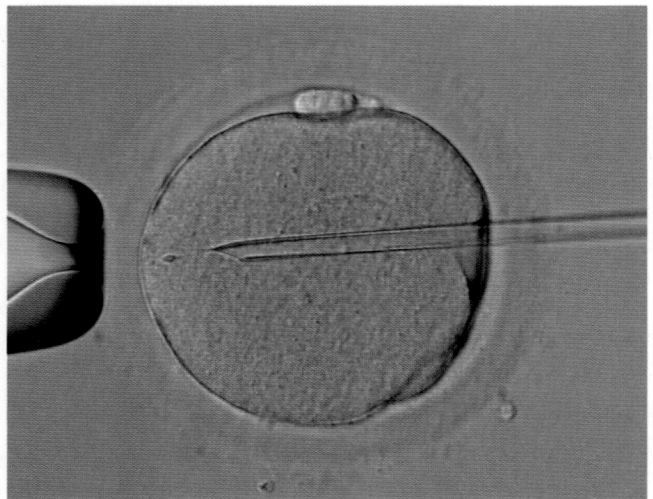

Figure 13.4 Intracytoplasmic sperm injection procedure. After the injection pipette has reached the approximate center of the oocyte, a break in the oolemma is visible as a quivering of the convexities of the membrane above and below the site of penetration.

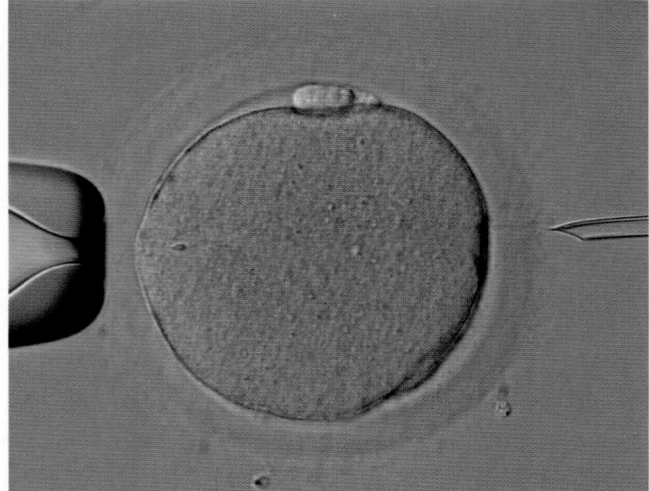

Figure 13.5 Intracytoplasmic sperm injection procedure. After the needle was withdrawn from the oocyte, the breach in the oolemma should be observed as a cone-shaped opening with its vertex toward the center of the oocyte.

center of the egg, eventual surplus medium is reaspirated, with the result that the cytoplasmic organelles tighten around the sperm, thereby reducing the size of the breach produced during penetration. Once the pipette is removed, the breach area is observed, and the order of the opening should maintain a funnel shape with a vertex into the egg (Fig. 13.5). If the border of the oolemma becomes inverted, ooplasmic organelles can leak out (43).

Interestingly, the introduction of sequential media, fashioned with glucose and protein starvation, resulted in complications during the execution of ICSI resulting in increased oocyte damage. This phenomenon was so severe that ICSI operators had to somewhat retrain themselves in performing the procedure paying attention to avoid the eversion of the oolemma due to the adhesion to the injection tool as a consequence of the poor protein content (57). In addition, the low protein content media have also been adopted for sperm incubation with consequential decreased ability of the male gamete to undergo capacitation and related membrane changes. Therefore, when performing ICSI it is necessary to have multiple sequential strikes of the sperm flagellum to obtain effective immobilization and consequent membrane permeabilization (57).

Evaluation of Fertilization, Embryo Development, Culture Conditions, and Embryo Replacement

Around 12–17 hours after injection, oocytes are analyzed with regard to the integrity of the cytoplasm as well as the number and size of pronuclei. First-day cleavage is assessed 24 hours after fertilization, and the number and size of blastomeres recorded for each embryo. After an additional 24 hours, embryos are screened as to their need for assisted hatching. At 72 hours after microinjection (the afternoon of day 3), those with good morphology are transferred into the uterine cavity. The number of embryos transferred depends on embryo quality, availability, and maternal age. When the patient is 30 years old, two or three embryos are usually transferred, whereas in the 31–34, 35–41, and 42-year-old age groups, the number of embryos increases to three, four, and five or more, respectively.

The association between the increased incidence of multiple pregnancies after IVF and the occurrence of maternal and neonatal complications is well documented (58,59). Interest in blastocyst culture and transfer has been recently embraced as a strategy to overcome this problem by the introduction of more sophisticated culture media. The extended culture of embryos to the blastocyst stage allows a "self-embryo selection," indicating the fast-cleaving embryos, and thus permitting the transfer of a lower number of them (60) moving toward a single embryo transfer. The use of sequential culture media, designed not only to allow for changes in nutrient requirements and metabolism as development proceeds, but also to minimize intracellular trauma, can facilitate the development of highly viable blastocysts. Studies have suggested that delaying transfer of embryos to the blastocyst stage (day 4/5) rather than the traditional cleavage stage (day 3) allows for better selection of the best conceptus to maximize pregnancy rates following a single embryo transfer (61).

Patients who are considered candidates for blastocyst culture are young women (<35 years old) with a good ovarian reserve, or older patients with an adequate number of pronuclear embryos. The number of embryos observed on day 3 and the capacity of embryo cleavage are also important criteria to select cases suitable for this procedure. Sequential culture media that meet changing physiologic requirements of the embryos are used, thus supporting viability of the blastocyst. Injected oocytes are rinsed and placed in a culture medium that is a variation of G1 medium, previously described by Barnes et al. and Gardner et al., until assessment of fertilization (62,63). On day 3, after evaluation of embryo cell number and morphology, all embryos are transferred to a modified G2 medium and cultured for 48 hours (60,62). Thereafter, blastocyst formation is assessed and blastocysts are selected according to the established criteria for subsequent transfer (64).

Extended Sperm Search

In cases where no spermatozoa are identified at the initial analysis and followed by high-speed centrifugation and still no sperm cells are found, an extensive search is performed. A dish is made in the same manner as an injection dish, with PVP solution placed in the central drop. The surrounding droplets of medium can be replaced with the actual specimen and pentoxifylline added to each drop to help augment sperm motility. Each drop is browsed and motile spermatozoa that are identified should be picked up and transferred to the PVP drop. The same procedure is performed for surgically retrieved specimens that have been freshly retrieved or recently thawed. Several dishes may have to be made and thoroughly searched for TESE patients until enough spermatozoa are found for injection.

In TESE specimens, sperm may be extremely rare, if not totally absent. In such cases, the extended searches may take greater than three hours to complete, depending on the number of oocytes awaiting injection (65). Unsurprisingly, the level of difficulty in finding and acquiring sperm is negatively related to the clinical outcome. About 60% of testicular biopsies done on nonobstructive azoospermic (NOA) men are successful in retrieving spermatozoa (Fig. 13.6). At our center, when extended search time is used as a parameter and categorized into 30 minutes to one hour, one to two hours, two to three hours, and more than three hours, both fertilization rates (54.2%, 46.3%, 28.0%, and 25.4%, respectively; $R^2 = 0.9315$; $P < 0.001$) of the oocytes and overall pregnancy rates declined ($R^2 = 0.9812$; $P < 0.0001$) as search time increased (Fig. 13.7). Although there is a pronounced decrease in pregnancy outcome as extensive search time increases, the search is still an important and valuable tool overall, as it represents the best opportunity for a male patient with NOA to bear their own biological child. In fact, even in the search of more than three hours, the possibility of achieving pregnancy is still attainable as long as a spermatozoon is identified.

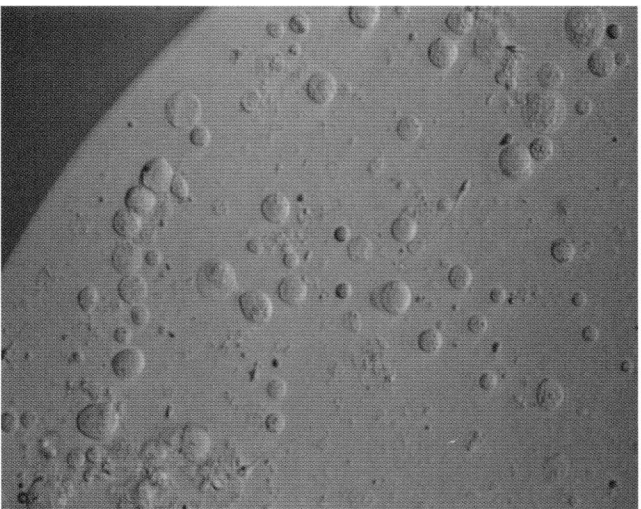

Figure 13.6 An example of a testicular sample for an extensive sperm search that has yielded spermatozoa for pickup and injection.

Optional Sperm Selection Techniques

While ICSI has been the gold standard for most IVF centers for more than 15 years with no proven significant or attributable side effects, some researchers still question the possible deleterious effects of a process that bypasses the natural gamete selecting processes of in vivo human reproduction. Toward that end, several methods have been introduced that expound upon the procedures of ICSI with additional protocols aimed at finding the optimal spermatozoon to inject an oocyte.

IMSI, or intracytoplasmic morphologically selected sperm injection, is a procedure where a high-power magnification is adopted to morphologically screen for optimal spermatozoa (66). This technique referred to as motile sperm organelle morphology examination (MSOME) uses an inverted light microscope with high resolution Nomarski optics followed by computer-assisted magnification up to 6300× or even higher. When using MSOME, the criteria for sperm selection includes a normal nuclear shape with lengths and widths no greater than two standard deviations away from the average measurements of 4.75 µm by 3.28 µm. Spermatozoon with normal nuclear content is identified, meaning that no greater than one vacuole (taking up to <4% of the nuclear area) could be present in the nucleus. Since searching for normal sperm under high magnification and strict criteria takes more time, the sperm sample must be kept at a lower temperature of 21°C to reduce sperm cell metabolism (66). Pregnancy outcomes in trials

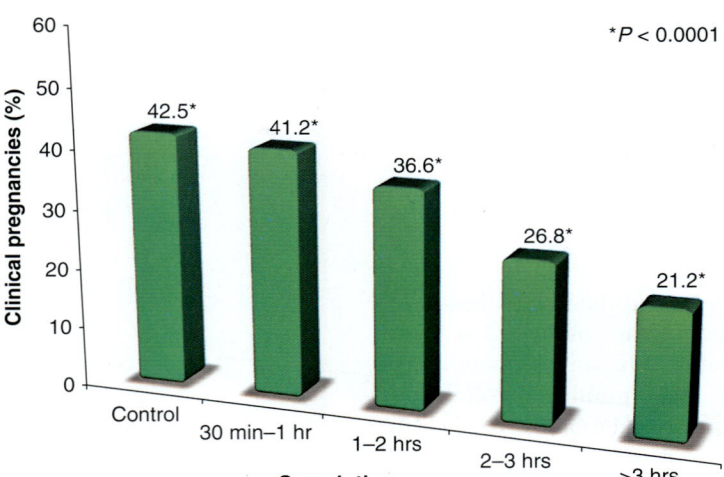

Figure 13.7 Pregnancy outcome according to the amount of time spent searching for spermatozoa.

comparing IMSI and conventional ICSI have garnered controversial results. Some studies have shown an increase in pregnancy outcomes and decrease in pregnancy losses with IMSI, while other centers have seen no difference between the two methods (67). IMSI has shown possible clinical promise, enough so that more research into its efficacy should be performed, however, the fact remains that some inherent characteristics of the procedure may prevent it from being used more routinely in many clinics. With this technique, finding the necessary number of spermatozoa to inject all retrieved oocytes may take hours to complete, as compared to standard ICSI. Complicating matters further is the expensive new equipment necessary for searching, as well as the additional time and costs. Finally, the whole concept of IMSI is best suited for cases where selection of morphologically normal spermatozoa is feasible, but cannot practically be employed in severe oligozoospermic cases such as cryptozoospermia and NOA where only scarce viable cells are present.

PICSI, or "physiologic ICSI," makes use of hyaluronic acid (HA), a substance naturally present in the human body (68). HA can be found in the cumulus oophorus around the oocyte and represents a barrier to the immature gametes by only relenting to "mature" spermatozoa. These so-called "mature" spermatozoa that have undergone the complete process of plasma membrane remodeling, cytoplasmic extrusion, and nuclear maturity will have a significantly higher number of HA receptors and binding sites. Two methods have been proposed on how to perform PICSI. In the first method, a special dish is used in which microdots of hyaluronic acid hydrogel have been attached to the bottom of the dish. When spermatozoa are added, this allows examination of bound spermatozoa. At this point, only HA-bound sperm are recovered using a standard ICSI injection pipette (69). The other method is to use a viscous medium composed partially of HA (68) which would fully replace PVP. Some studies have also shown that spermatozoa capable of HA-binding have lower DNA fragmentation rates than simple post-swim-up spermatozoa. In addition, nucleus normalcy rate (according to MSOME criteria) has been shown to be higher in spermatozoa bound to HA as compared with sperm in PVP (68). Moreover, PICSI correlations to overall results such as pregnancy rate or delivery rate or malformation proportion have been inconsistent. Ultimately, PICSI is still affected by the same major drawbacks as IMSI, where cases with extremely few sperm cells to select from are present.

CLINICAL ICSI OUTCOME

From September 1993 through December 2010 at our Center, ICSI was performed in 18,584 cycles with ejaculated spermatozoa, and in 2045 cycles with surgically retrieved sperm. The mean maternal age was 37.1 ± 4.9 years old for the ejaculated group, and 34.8 ± 5.1 years old in the couples undergoing surgical retrieval of the sperm.

A total of 18,584 ICSI cycles were performed with ejaculated spermatozoa, consisting of 2378 with normal and 16,206 with abnormal semen parameters. A total of 154,279 MII oocytes were obtained from 18,279 oocyte retrievals. After ICSI, 94.5% (145,724/154,166) of these oocytes survived, and 115,701 were fertilized and displayed two pronuclei (2PN). Fertilization and clinical pregnancy rates were not influenced by the condition (fresh or cryopreserved) and collection method (masturbation, electroejaculation, or bladder catheterization) of the spermatozoa used (Table 13.1). When comparing fertilization between ejaculated and surgically retrieved spermatozoa, ejaculated exhibited higher rates ($P=0.0001$); however, surgically retrieved cases had superior clinical pregnancy rates ($P=0.0001$) (Table 13.2) mostly likely due to the younger maternal age ($P=0.001$).

A total of 902 cycles were performed with epididymal spermatozoa and 1143 cycles with testicular samples. When the fertilization and pregnancy characteristics were analyzed according to whether the sample was cryopreserved, we observed that after cryopreservation

Table 13.1 Fertilization Rates According to Semen Origin and Specimen Condition

Semen origin	Cycles	Oocyte fertilized/Oocyte inseminated (%)	Clinical pregnancies (%)
Fresh ejaculate	16,729	103,067/138,161 (74.6)	6650 (39.8)
Frozen ejaculate	1741	10,500/14,327 (73.3)	665 (38.2)
Electroejaculate	58	424/555 (76.4)	30 (51.7)
Frozen electroejaculate	23	141/211 (66.8)	10 (43.5)
Retrograde ejaculate	33	238/313 (76.0)	12 (36.4)

Table 13.2 Fertilization and Pregnancy Rates According to Semen Origin

	Spermatozoa	
No. of items	Ejaculated	Surgically retrieved
Cycles	18,584	2045
Fertilization (%)	114,370/153,567 (74.5)[a]	12,009/18,930 (63.4)[a]
Clinical pregnancies (%)	7367 (39.6)[b]	926 (45.3)[b]

[a] χ^2, 2 × 2, 1 df, effect of spermatozoal source on fertilization rate, $P=0.0001$.
[b] χ^2, 2 × 2, 1 df, effect of spermatozoal source on clinical pregnancy rate, $P=0.0001$.

Table 13.3 Spermatozoal Parameters and Intracytoplasmic Sperm Injection Outcome According to Retrieval Sites and Specimen Condition

	Spermatozoa			
	Epididymal		Testicular	
No. of items	Fresh	Frozen/thawed	Fresh	Frozen/thawed
Cycles	318	584	863	280
Density (10⁶/mL ± SD)	36.9 ± 44	23.5 ± 27	0.4 ± 3.1	0.24 ± 0.7
Motility (% ± SD)	18.8 ± 17[a]	3.6 ± 8[a]	3.6 ± 7.8	1.1 ± 3.6
Morphology (% ± SD)	1.7 ± 2.3	1.3 ± 2	0	0
Fertilization (%)	2302/3185 (72.3)	3743/5258 (71.2)	4565/7939 (57.5)[c]	1399/2548 (54.9)[c]
Clinical pregnancies (%)	195 (61.3)[b]	274 (46.9)[b]	356 (41.3)	101 (36.1)

[a] Student's t-test, two independent samples, effect of epididymal cryopreservation on sperm motility, $P<0.0001$.
[b] χ^2, 2 × 2, 1 df, effect of epididymal cryopreservation on clinical pregnancy rate, $P=0.0001$.
[c] χ^2, 2 × 2, 1 df, effect of testicular cryopreservation on fertilization rate, $P=0.03$.

epididymal samples had lower motility parameters ($P<0.0001$) as well as pregnancy outcome ($P=0.0001$), though without affecting fertilization rate. When testicular samples were used for ICSI, the situation was reversed with zygote formation being higher in the fresh specimens ($P=0.03$) while the ability of the embryo to implant was unaffected (Table 13.3).

Clinical pregnancy was defined as the presence of a gestational sac as well as at least one fetal heartbeat on ultrasonographic examination. The pregnancy outcome of 20,629 ICSI cycles is described in Table 13.4. Of the 10,783 patients presenting with a positive β-hCG (52.3%), 1681 were biochemical (8.1%) and 701 were blighted ova (3.4%). Among 8293 patients in whom a viable fetal heartbeat was observed, 750 had a miscarriage or were therapeutically aborted, and 108 had an ectopic pregnancy. The clinical pregnancy rate was 40.2% per retrieval (8293/20,629) and 43.1% per replacement (8293/19,226). A total of 9717 neonates were born from 7543 deliveries, including 4732 being female and 4985 being male, with an overall frequency of multiple deliveries of 28.8% (2175/7543): 1962 twins (26.0%), 209 triplets (2.8%), and 4 quadruplets (0.05%). Of these deliveries a total of 9150 ICSI live-born infants, 330 (3.6%) of them exhibited congenital abnormalities that was comparable to the IVF babies at 3.6% (187/5183) (Fig. 13.8).

Table 13.4 Evolution of ICSI Pregnancies in 20,629 Cycles

No. of items		Positive outcomes	
ICSI cycles	20,629		
Embryo replacements	19,226		
Positive βhCGs	10,783	Pregnancy	52.3% (10,783/20,629)
Biochemical pregnancies	1681		
Blighted ova	701		
Ectopic pregnancies	108		
Positive fetal heartbeats	8293	Clinical pregnancy	40.2% (8293/20,629)
Miscarriages/therapeutic abortions	750		
Deliveries	7543	Delivery rate	36.6% (7543/20,629)

Abbreviations: hCG, human chorionic gonadotropin; ICSI, intracytoplasmic sperm injection.

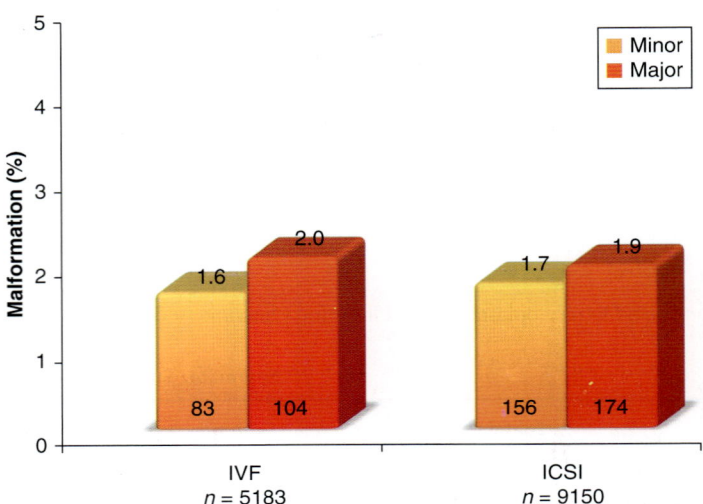

Figure 13.8 Congenital malformation rates of live-born IVF and ICSI neonates. *Abbreviations*: ICSI, intracytoplasmic sperm injection; IVF, in vitro fertilization.

In a cohort of patients from July 1999 through December 2010, blastocyst transfer was performed in 2073 ICSI cycles, 1943 with ejaculated spermatozoa, 75 cycles with epididymal, and 55 with testicular samples. Out of 26,185 injected oocytes at MII stage, 21,362 were successfully fertilized and showed two pronuclei, thus giving a fertilization rate of 81.6%. The cleaving embryos observed at day 3 were 20,582 (96.3%). On day 5, 9356 (45.9%) blastocysts were obtained. Of these, 4275 (53.7%) blastocysts were replaced into the uterine cavity. Additional good-quality blastocysts ($n = 3,695$) were cryopreserved at this stage for later use. Patients presented with a positive β-hCG level (61.8%) were 1281. Of these, 178 (13.9%) pregnancies were biochemical, 67 (5.2%) had a blighted ova, and 6 (0.3%) had an ectopic, while the remaining 1030 cases (49.7%) were clinical pregnancies with a positive fetal heartbeat detected by ultrasound, achieving an implantation rate per embryo of about 35% (Table 13.5). Among these pregnancies, 63.4% were singleton pregnancies, 31.7% twins, and 3.5% were lost to follow-up (Table 13.6).

CHILDREN'S HEALTH

Assisted reproduction treatments, namely IVF and intracytoplasmic sperm injection (ICSI), have become widely used in the treatment of human infertility. At present, 1–3% of children born in developed countries are conceived via assisted reproduction treatments (70,71). It is well established that assisted reproduction is associated with adverse perinatal outcomes, including increased risks of preterm delivery, low birth weight, and neonatal mortality (72–74). In recent years there has been considerable work investigating health outcomes in IVF and ICSI children beyond the neonatal period (75,76). Follow-up of children following ARTs is highly recommended and applied increasingly (77–79), but are extremely time consuming and costly for the family. Therefore, a standardized parent-administered questionnaire namely, Ages and Stages questionnaire (ASQ), has been proposed to screen the children's five key developmental milestones (communication, gross motor, fine motor, problem solving, and personal-social skills) in their own environment (80,81).

Table 13.5 Implantation Rate According to Embryo Culture

No. of items	Embryo replacement	
	Day 3	Day 5
Embryos replaced	52,145	4275
Sacs implanted (%)	12,098 (23.2)[a]	1650 (38.6)[a]
Positive fetal heartbeats (%)	11,003 (21.1)[b]	1485 (34.7)[b]

[a,b]χ^2, 2 × 2, 1 df, effect of extended in vitro culture on implantation, $P = 0.0001$.

Table 13.6 Influence of Embryonic Stage on Pregnancy Outcome and Gestational Order

No. of items	Embryo replacement	
	Day 3	Day 5
Replacements	17,153	2073
Embryos replaced (mean)	3.04	2.06
Clinical pregnancies (+FHB) (%)	7263 (42.3)[a]	1030 (49.7)[a]
Deliveries	6593 (38.4)[b]	950 (45.8)[b]
Singleton births	4548	602
Twin births	1661	301
Triplet births	195	14
Quadruplet births	4	0
Lost to follow-up	185	33

[a]χ^2, 2 × 2, 1 df, effect of embryonic stage on pregnancy rate, $P = 0.0001$.
[b]χ^2, 2 × 2, 1 df, effect of embryonic stage on delivery rate, $P = 0.0001$.
Abbreviations: FHB, fetal heartbeat.

While screening a large number of children using the ASQ, we found that most of the 3-year-old children analyzed in the ICSI and IVF groups had normal cognitive abilities, socio-emotional development, and motor skill scores (82). Of the children that had developmental delays, the large majority originated from high-order gestation ($P<0.01$). This further solidifies the theory that single embryo transfer is essential in ensuring a healthy baby. Interestingly, children whose father's spermatozoa were harvested surgically appeared to score better than those conceived with ejaculated spermatozoa by IVF and ICSI (83). Thus far, studies examining children ranging from 5 to 12 years of age (84–88) have been reassuring in terms of perinatal outcome, IQ, and physical development (75).

The specific concerns in regard to ICSI, whether real or theoretical (89–92), involve the insemination method, the use of spermatozoa with genetic or structural defects, and the possible introduction of foreign genes. Several epidemiological studies of assisted reproduction children report a two-fold increase in infant malformations (93), a recurrent reduction in birth weight (94), certain rare syndromes related to imprinting errors (95–100) and even a higher frequency of some cancers (101). However, current evidence do not prove that there is an increased risk of imprinting disorders and even less so childhood cancers in ICSI children (92).

Epigenetic imbalances have been similarly linked to the exposure of the embryos to long-term culture (75,102). Thus far, Beckwith–Wiedemann Syndrome is the only epigenetic disorder that has been clearly associated with ART procedures (103) and has been found to be equally distributed among the in vitro conception methods. At present, there is no evidence that the ICSI insemination itself is responsible for any increase in epigenetic disorders, findings that have been confirmed in animal studies (104).

CONCLUSIONS

ICSI has established itself as the most reliable technique to overcome fertilization failure. By pinpointing the beginning of fertilization, it has helped to better understand some important aspects of early gamete interaction. The observed high performance of aggressively immobilized spermatozoa suggests a more efficient destabilization and consequent permeabilization of the sperm-membrane, which is responsible for a more prompt release of the oocyte-activating factor (44,45,105). These profound physiologic changes induced on the sperm membrane by the action of the injection needle seem to be critically important for immature, surgically retrieved spermatozoa (8). It has been demonstrated that the positive outcome of ICSI is largely independent of the basic sperm parameters such as concentration, motility, and morphology. This is particularly evident with cryptozoospermia or when no spermatozoa are present in the ejaculate (6). It is in these azoospermic men that the surgical isolation of spermatozoa together with ICSI is able to yield fertilization and support embryo development. The possibility to bypass the steps of testicular and epididymal sperm maturation, acrosome reaction, binding to the ZP, and fusion with the oolemma now permits infertility due to various forms of male factor to be addressed successfully. In fact, in cases of men diagnosed with NOA, as long as a viable spermatozoon is isolated, there is a chance of generating a conceptus. However, we should be cautious about the acquired evidence that subfertile men have a higher frequency of genetic abnormalities that may be passed on through their gametes (8,106). Therefore, the earlier concern focused on ICSI insemination itself has shifted to the screening of the subfertile man who may transmit his genetic defects to the offspring, specifically boys (107). A large worldwide experience suggested that men with extreme male factor conditions caused by a direct genetic component such as Klinefelter's Syndrome or Yq microdeletions can be successfully treated by ICSI and still generate healthy offspring (8).

The current practice of extended embryo culture, made possible by the now established sequential media, is a promising treatment option in conjunction with ICSI, especially for couples with male infertility, where a multifetal pregnancy would represent additional risks. Our experience with blastocyst transfer showed a significant increase in implantation and pregnancy rates. Furthermore, this approach seems to be most effective in curtailing higher-order gestations in addition to provide an option for a successful application of preimplantation genetic diagnosis/preimplantation genetic screening (108,109).

The practice of ICSI has promoted a more careful quest for the ideal spermatozoon to inject. Higher magnification screening of sperm surface irregularities by MSOME is an example of this attempt, even though its claimed benefits remain unproven (67).

The potential effects of ART on child development should always be kept in mind and the monitoring of the child health can be accomplished by a parent administered questionnaire that provides a cost- and time-effective approach to measure their physical and psychological well-being (82). In recent years, a large number of studies have provided information on the health of children born after ART and therefore, current evidence show that the outcome of singletons born at term following ART is generally reassuring (75,110). The increased awareness of the risks related to multiple gestations has supported measures aimed at obtaining singleton births with obvious benefits for the long-term welfare of the offspring.

ACKNOWLEDGMENTS

We thank the clinicians, embryologists, and scientists of The Ronald O Perelman & Claudia Cohen Center for Reproductive Medicine and Urology Department, Weill Cornell Medical College, New York. We are thankful to Justin Kocent, Jennifer Hu, Christopher Chen, Carolyn Daw, Trina Fields, and Bong Kyo Seo for their assistance in ICSI. We are grateful to Kenneth Shen in helping with the preparation of the manuscript and Maryanne Williams-Pitman for kindly recruiting patients for the child study.

REFERENCES

1. Feichtinger W, Strohmer H, Fuhrberg P, et al. Photoablation of oocyte zona pellucida by erbium-YAG laser for in-vitro fertilisation in severe male infertility. Lancet 1992; 339: 811.
2. Gordon JW, Grunfeld L, Garrisi GJ, et al. Fertilization of human oocytes by sperm from infertile males after zona pellucida drilling. Fertil Steril 1988; 50: 68–73.
3. Malter HE, Cohen J. Partial zona dissection of the human oocyte: a nontraumatic method using micromanipulation to assist zona pellucida penetration. Fertil Steril 1989; 51: 139–48.
4. Palermo G, Joris H, Devroey P, Van Steirteghem AC. Induction of acrosome reaction in human spermatozoa used for subzonal insemination. Hum Reprod 1992; 7: 248–54.
5. Cohen J, Alikani M, Malter HE, et al. Partial zona dissection or subzonal sperm insertion: microsurgical fertilization alternatives based on evaluation of sperm and embryo morphology. Fertil Steril 1991; 56: 696–706.
6. Palermo GD, Cohen J, Alikani M, Adler A, Rosenwaks Z. Intracytoplasmic sperm injection: a novel treatment for all forms of male factor infertility. Fertil Steril 1995; 63: 1231–40.
7. Palermo GD, Cohen J, Rosenwaks Z. Intracytoplasmic sperm injection: a powerful tool to overcome fertilization failure. Fertil Steril 1996; 65: 899–908.
8. Palermo GD, Schlegel PN, Hariprashad JJ, et al. Fertilization and pregnancy outcome with intracytoplasmic sperm injection for azoospermic men. Hum Reprod 1999; 14: 741–8.
9. Benagiano G, Gianaroli L. The new Italian IVF legislation. Reprod Biomed Online 2004; 9: 117–25.
10. Ludwig M, Diedrich K. Regulation of assisted reproductive technology: the German experience. In: Brinsden PR, ed. Regulation of Assisted Reproductive Technology: The German Experience. New York: Parthenon Publishing Group Inc 1999; 2: 431–4.
11. Porcu E, Fabbri R, Seracchioli R, et al. Birth of a healthy female after intracytoplasmic sperm injection of cryopreserved human oocytes. Fertil Steril 1997; 68: 724–6.
12. Johnson MH. The effect on fertilization of exposure of mouse oocytes to dimethyl sulfoxide: an optimal protocol. J In Vitro Fert Embryo Transf 1989; 6: 168–75.
13. Schalkoff ME, Oskowitz SP, Powers RD. Ultrastructural observations of human and mouse oocytes treated with cryopreservatives. Biol Reprod 1989; 40: 379–93.
14. Van Blerkom J, Davis PW. Cytogenetic, cellular, and developmental consequences of cryopreservation of immature and mature mouse and human oocytes. Microsc Res Tech 1994; 27: 165–93.

15. Vincent C, Pickering SJ, Johnson MH. The hardening effect of dimethylsulphoxide on the mouse zona pellucida requires the presence of an oocyte and is associated with a reduction in the number of cortical granules present. J Reprod Fertil 1990; 89: 253–9.
16. Mencaglia L, Falcone P, Lentini GM, et al. ICSI for treatment of human immunodeficiency virus and hepatitis C virus-serodiscordant couples with infected male partner. Hum Reprod 2005; 20: 2242–6.
17. Pena JE, Klein J, Thornton M, Chang PL, Sauer MV. Successive pregnancies with delivery of two healthy infants in a couple who was discordant for human immunodeficiency virus infection. Fertil Steril 2002; 78: 421–3.
18. Sauer MV, Chang PL. Establishing a clinical program for human immunodeficiency virus 1-seropositive men to father seronegative children by means of in vitro fertilization with intracytoplasmic sperm injection. Am J Obstet Gynecol 2002; 186: 627–33.
19. van Leeuwen E, Repping S, Prins JM, Reiss P, van der Veen F. Assisted reproductive technologies to establish pregnancies in couples with an HIV-1-infected man. Neth J Med 2009; 67: 322–7.
20. Daw C, Neri QV, Monahan D, et al. Semen hyperviscosity treatment and IUI outcome. Fertil Steril 2011; 96(3 Suppl 1): S266–7.
21. Mortimer D. Sperm recovery techniques to maximize fertilizing capacity. Reprod Fertil Dev 1994; 6: 25–31.
22. Bennett CJ, Seager SW, Vasher EA, McGuire EJ. Sexual dysfunction and electroejaculation in men with spinal cord injury: review. J Urol 1988; 139: 453–7.
23. Schlegel PN, Berkeley AS, Goldstein M, et al. Epididymal micropuncture with in vitro fertilization and oocyte micromanipulation for the treatment of unreconstructable obstructive azoospermia. Fertil Steril 1994; 61: 895–901.
24. Schlegel PN, Cohen J, Goldstein M, et al. Cystic fibrosis gene mutations do not affect sperm function during in vitro fertilization with micromanipulation for men with bilateral congenital absence of vas deferens. Fertil Steril 1995; 64: 421–6.
25. Tsirigotis M, Pelekanos M, Yazdani N, et al. Simplified sperm retrieval and intracytoplasmic sperm injection in patients with azoospermia. Br J Urol 1995; 76: 765–8.
26. Friedler S, Raziel A, Strassburger D, et al. Testicular sperm retrieval by percutaneous fine needle sperm aspiration compared with testicular sperm extraction by open biopsy in men with non-obstructive azoospermia. Hum Reprod 1997; 12: 1488–93.
27. Silber SJ, Van Steirteghem AC, Liu J, et al. High fertilization and pregnancy rate after intracytoplasmic sperm injection with spermatozoa obtained from testicle biopsy. Hum Reprod 1995; 10: 148–52.
28. Ramasamy R, Reifsnyder JE, Bryson C, et al. Role of tissue digestion and extensive sperm search after microdissection testicular sperm extraction. Fertil Steril 2011; 96: 299–302.
29. Schlegel PN. Nonobstructive azoospermia: a revolutionary surgical approach and results. Semin Reprod Med 2009; 27: 165–70.
30. Reis MM, Tsai MC, Schlegel PN, et al. Xenogeneic transplantation of human spermatogonia. Zygote 2000; 8: 97–105.
31. Kruger TF, Menkveld R, Stander FS, et al. Sperm morphologic features as a prognostic factor in in vitro fertilization. Fertil Steril 1986; 46: 1118–23.
32. WHO. WHO laboratory manual for the examination and processing of human semen. World Health Organization, 5th edn. Vol. 5. Cambridge: Cambridge University Press, 2010.
33. Verheyen GI, Pletincx I, Van Steirteghem A. Effect of freezing method, thawing temperature and post-thaw dilution/washing on motility (CASA) and morphology characteristics of high-quality human sperm. Hum Reprod 1993; 8: 1678–84.
34. Huang JY, Kang HJ, Rosenwaks Z. How to monitor for best results. In: Kovacs G, ed. Cup Book: How to Improve IVF Success Rates. 1st edn. Cambridge: Cambridge University Press, 2011.
35. Zarek SM, Muasher SJ. Mild/minimal stimulation for in vitro fertilization: an old idea that needs to be revisited. Fertil Steril 2011; 95: 2449–55.
36. Dozortsev D, Rybouchkin A, De Sutter P, Qian C, Dhont M. Human oocyte activation following intracytoplasmic injection: the role of the sperm cell. Hum Reprod 1995; 10: 403–7.
37. Fishel S, Lisi F, Rinaldi L, et al. Systematic examination of immobilizing spermatozoa before intracytoplasmic sperm injection in the human. Hum Reprod 1995; 10: 497–500.
38. Palermo G, Joris H, Derde MP, et al. Sperm characteristics and outcome of human assisted fertilization by subzonal insemination and intracytoplasmic sperm injection. Fertil Steril 1993; 59: 826–35.
39. Calvin HI, Bedford JM. Formation of disulphide bonds in the nucleus and accessory structures of mammalian spermatozoa during maturation in the epididymis. J Reprod Fertil Suppl 1971; 13(Suppl 13): 65–75.
40. Bedford JM, Calvin H, Cooper GW. The maturation of spermatozoa in the human epididymis. J Reprod Fertil Suppl 1973; 18: 199–213.
41. Kirchhoff C, Osterhoff C, Habben I, Ivell R, Kirchloff C. Cloning and analysis of mRNAs expressed specifically in the human epididymis. Int J Androl 1990; 13: 155–67.
42. Moore HD, Hartman TD, Pryor JP. Development of the oocyte-penetrating capacity of spermatozoa in the human epididymis. Int J Androl 1983; 6: 310–18.
43. Palermo GD, Alikani M, Bertoli M, et al. Oolemma characteristics in relation to survival and fertilization patterns of oocytes treated by intracytoplasmic sperm injection. Hum Reprod 1996; 11: 172–6.
44. Takeuchi T, Colombero LT, Neri QV, Rosenwaks Z, Palermo GD. Does ICSI require acrosomal disruption? An ultrastructural study. Hum Reprod 2004; 19: 114–17.
45. Palermo GD, Schlegel PN, Colombero LT, et al. Aggressive sperm immobilization prior to intracytoplasmic sperm injection with immature spermatozoa improves fertilization and pregnancy rates. Hum Reprod 1996; 11: 1023–9.
46. Fishel S, Lisi F, Rinaldi L, et al. Intracytoplasmic sperm injection (ICSI) versus high insemination concentration (HIC) for human conception in vitro. Reprod Fertil Dev 1995; 7: 169–74; discussion 174–5.
47. Gerris J, Mangelschots K, Van Royen E, et al. ICSI and severe male-factor infertility: breaking the sperm tail prior to injection. Hum Reprod 1995; 10: 484–6.
48. Katayama M, Sutovsky P, Yang BS, et al. Increased disruption of sperm plasma membrane at sperm immobilization promotes dissociation of perinuclear theca

from sperm chromatin after intracytoplasmic sperm injection in pigs. Reproduction 2005; 130: 907–16.
49. Van den Bergh M, Bertrand E, Englert Y. Second polar body extrusion is highly predictive for oocyte fertilization as soon as 3 hr after intracytoplasmic sperm injection (ICSI). J Assist Reprod Genet 1995; 12: 258–62.
50. Tang SS, Gao H, Zhao Y, Ma S. Aneuploidy and DNA fragmentation in morphologically abnormal sperm. Int J Androl 2010; 33: 163–79.
51. Tasdemir I, Tasdemir M, Tavukcuoglu S, Kahraman S, Biberoglu K. Effect of abnormal sperm head morphology on the outcome of intracytoplasmic sperm injection in humans. Hum Reprod 1997; 12: 1214–17.
52. Templado C, Hoang T, Greene C, et al. Aneuploid spermatozoa in infertile men: teratozoospermia. Mol Reprod Dev 2002; 61: 200–4.
53. Zini A, Sigman M. Are tests of sperm DNA damage clinically useful? Pros and cons. J Androl 2009; 30: 219–29.
54. Zini A, Bielecki R, Phang D, Zenzes MT. Correlations between two markers of sperm DNA integrity, DNA denaturation and DNA fragmentation, in fertile and infertile men. Fertil Steril 2001; 75: 674–7.
55. Spano M, Bonde JP, Hjøllund HI, et al. Sperm chromatin damage impairs human fertility. The Danish First Pregnancy Planner Study Team. Fertil Steril 2000; 73: 43–50.
56. Chen C, Li SX, Wang SM, Liang SW. Kinetic characteristics and DNA integrity of human spermatozoa. Hum Reprod 2011; 19(Suppl 1): 30.
57. Palermo GD, Neri QV, Monahan D, Kocent J, Rosenwaks Z. Development and current applications of assisted fertilization. Fertil Steril 2012; 97: 248–59.
58. Society for Assisted Reproductive Technology, American Society for Reproductive Medicine. Assisted reproductive technology in the United States and Canada: 1995 results generated from the American Society for Reproductive Medicine/Society for Assisted Reproductive Technology Registry. Fertil Steril 1998; 69: 389–98.
59. Gardner DK, Schoolcraft WB. Elimination of high order multiple gestations by blastocyst culture and transfer. Female Infertility Therapy: Current Practice. London: Martin Dunitz, 1998.
60. Gardner DK, Lane M. Towards a single embryo transfer. Reprod Biomed Online 2003; 6: 470–81.
61. Zander-Fox DL, Tremellen K, Lane M. Single blastocyst embryo transfer maintains comparable pregnancy rates to double cleavage-stage embryo transfer but results in healthier pregnancy outcomes. Aust NZ J Obstet Gynaecol 2011; 51: 406–10.
62. Barnes FL, Crombie A, Gardner DK, et al. Blastocyst development and birth after in-vitro maturation of human primary oocytes, intracytoplasmic sperm injection and assisted hatching. Hum Reprod 1995; 10: 3243–7.
63. Gardner DK, Vella P, Lane M, et al. Culture and transfer of human blastocysts increases implantation rates and reduces the need for multiple embryo transfers. Fertil Steril 1998; 69: 84–8.
64. Schoolcraft WB, Gardner DK, Lane M, et al. Blastocyst culture and transfer: analysis of results and parameters affecting outcome in two in vitro fertilization programs. Fertil Steril 1999; 72: 604–9.
65. Monahan D, et al. The time spent in searching for testicular spermatozoa influences ICSI outcome. Hum Reprod 2011; 25(Suppl 1): i174–5.
66. Berkovitz A, Eltes F, Yaari S, et al. The morphological normalcy of the sperm nucleus and pregnancy rate of intracytoplasmic injection with morphologically selected sperm. Hum Reprod 2005; 20: 185–90.
67. Palermo GD, Hu JCY, Rienzi L, Maggiulli R, Takeuchi T. Thoughts on IMSI. In: Racowsky C, et al. ed. Biennial Review of Infertility. Vol. 2. New York: Springer, 2011: 296.
68. Parmegiani L, Cognigni GE, Bernardi S, et al. "Physiologic ICSI": hyaluronic acid (HA) favors selection of spermatozoa without DNA fragmentation and with normal nucleus, resulting in improvement of embryo quality. Fertil Steril 2010; 93: 598–604.
69. Yagci A, Murk W, Stronk J, Huszar G. Spermatozoa bound to solid state hyaluronic acid show chromatin structure with high DNA chain integrity: an acridine orange fluorescence study. J Androl 2010; 31: 566–72.
70. Andersen AN, Goossens V, Ferraretti AP, et al. Assisted reproductive technology in Europe, 2004: results generated from European registers by ESHRE. Hum Reprod 2008; 23: 756–71.
71. Wright VC, Chang J, Jeng G, Macaluso M. Assisted reproductive technology surveillance-United States, 2005. MMWR Surveill Summ 2008; 57: 1–23.
72. Helmerhorst FM, Perquin DA, Donker D, Keirse MJ. Perinatal outcome of singletons and twins after assisted conception: a systematic review of controlled studies. BMJ 2004; 328: 261.
73. Jackson RA, Gibson KA, Wu YW, Croughan MS. Perinatal outcomes in singletons following in vitro fertilization: a meta-analysis. Obstet Gynecol 2004; 103: 551–63.
74. McDonald SD, Murphy K, Beyene J, Ohlsson A. Perinatel outcomes of singleton pregnancies achieved by in vitro fertilization: a systematic review and meta-analysis. J Obstet Gynaecol Can 2005; 27: 449–59.
75. Basatemur E, Sutcliffe A. Follow-up of children born after ART. Placenta 2008; 29(Suppl B): 135–40.
76. Sutcliffe AG, Ludwig M. Outcome of assisted reproduction. Lancet 2007; 370: 351–9.
77. Bonduelle M, Bergh C, Niklasson A, Palermo GD, Wennerholm UB. Medical follow-up study of 5-year-old ICSI children. Reprod Biomed Online 2004; 9: 91–101.
78. Leunens L, Celestin-Westreich S, Bonduelle M, Liebaers I, Ponjaert-Kristoffersen I. Cognitive and motor development of 8-year-old children born after ICSI compared to spontaneously conceived children. Hum Reprod 2006; 21: 2922–9.
79. Ombelet W, Peeraer K, De Sutter P, et al. Perinatal outcome of ICSI pregnancies compared with a matched group of natural conception pregnancies in Flanders (Belgium): a cohort study. Reprod Biomed Online 2005; 11: 244–53.
80. Neri QV, Tanaka N, Wang A, et al. Intracytoplasmic sperm injection. Accomplishments and qualms. Minerva Ginecol 2004; 56: 189–96.
81. Squires J, Carter A, Kaplan P. Developmental monitoring of children conceived by intracytoplasmic sperm injection and in vitro fertilization. Fertil Steril 2003; 79: 453–4.
82. Palermo GD, Neri QV, Takeuchi T, et al. Genetic and epigenetic characteristics of ICSI children. Reprod Biomed Online 2008; 17: 820–33.
83. Neri QV, Williams-Pitman M, Rosenwaks Z, Squires J, Palermo GD. Cognitive and behavioral developmental profiles of ICSI children conceived

from surgically retrieved spermatozoa. Fertil Steril 2007; 88(Suppl 1): S39.
84. Basatemur E, Shevlin M, Sutcliffe A. Growth of children conceived by IVF and ICSI up to 12years of age. Reprod Biomed Online 2010; 20: 144–9.
85. Belva F, Henriet S, Liebaers I, et al. Medical outcome of 8-year-old singleton ICSI children (born >or=32 weeks' gestation) and a spontaneously conceived comparison group. Hum Reprod 2007; 22: 506–15.
86. Goldbeck L, Gagsteiger F, Mindermann I, Strobele S, Izat Y. Cognitive development of singletons conceived by intracytoplasmic sperm injection or in vitro fertilization at age 5 and 10 years. J Pediatr Psychol 2009; 34: 774–81.
87. Knoester M, Helmerhorst FM, Vandenbroucke JP, et al. Perinatal outcome, health, growth, and medical care utilization of 5- to 8-year-old intracytoplasmic sperm injection singletons. Fertil Steril 2008; 89: 1133–46.
88. Leunens L, Celestin-Westreich S, Bonduelle M, Liebaers I, Ponjaert-Kristoffersen I. Follow-up of cognitive and motor development of 10-year-old singleton children born after ICSI compared with spontaneously conceived children. Hum Reprod 2008; 23: 105–11.
89. Cummins JM, Jequier AM. Treating male infertility needs more clinical andrology, not less. Hum Reprod 1994; 9: 1214–19.
90. de Kretser DM. The potential of intracytoplasmic sperm injection (ICSI) to transmit genetic defects causing male infertility. Reprod Fertil Dev 1995; 7: 137–41; discussion 141–2.
91. De Rycke M, Liebaers I, Van Steirteghem A. Epigenetic risks related to assisted reproductive technologies: risk analysis and epigenetic inheritance. Hum Reprod 2002; 17: 2487–94.
92. Edwards RG, Ludwig M. Are major defects in children conceived in vitro due to innate problems in patients or to induced genetic damage? Reprod Biomed Online 2003; 7: 131–8.
93. Hansen M, Kurinczuk J, Bower C, Webb S. The risk of major birth defects after intracytoplasmic sperm injection and in vitro fertilization. N Engl J Med 2002; 346: 725–30.
94. Schieve LA, Meikle SF, Ferre C, et al. Low and very low birth weight in infants conceived with use of assisted reproductive technology. N Engl J Med 2002; 346: 731–7.
95. Cox GF, Burger J, Lip V, et al. Intracytoplasmic sperm injection may increase the risk of imprinting defects. Am J Hum Genet 2002; 71: 162–4.
96. DeBaun MR, Niemitz EL, Feinberg AP. Association of in vitro fertilization with Beckwith-Wiedemann syndrome and epigenetic alterations of LIT1 and H19. Am J Hum Genet 2003; 72: 156–60.
97. Gicquel C, Gaston V, Mandelbaum J, et al. In vitro fertilization may increase the risk of Beckwith-Wiedemann syndrome related to the abnormal imprinting of the KCN1OT gene. Am J Hum Genet 2003; 72: 1338–41.
98. Halliday J, Oke K, Breheny S, Algar E, J Amor D. Beckwith-Wiedemann syndrome and IVF: a case-control study. Am J Hum Genet 2004; 75: 526–8.
99. Maher ER, Brueton LA, Bowdin SC, et al. Beckwith-Wiedemann syndrome and assisted reproduction technology (ART). J Med Genet 2003; 40: 62–4.
100. Orstavik KH. Intracytoplasmic sperm injection and congenital syndromes because of imprinting defects. Tidsskr Nor Laegeforen 2003; 123: 177.
101. Moll AC, Imhof SM, Schouten-van Meeteren AY, van Leeuwen FE. In-vitro fertilisation and retinoblastoma. Lancet 2003; 361: 1392.
102. Rivera RM, Stein P, Weaver JR, et al. Manipulations of mouse embryos prior to implantation result in aberrant expression of imprinted genes on day 9.5 of development. Hum Mol Genet 2008; 17: 1–14.
103. Sutcliffe AG, Peters CJ, Bowdin S, et al. Assisted reproductive therapies and imprinting disorders — a preliminary Britsh survey. Hum Reprod 2006; 21: 1009–1011.
104. Wilson TJ, Lacham-Kaplan O, Gould J, et al. Comparison of mice born after intracytoplasmic sperm injection with in vitro fertilization and natural mating. Mol Reprod Dev 2007; 74: 512–19.
105. Wolny YM, Fissore RA, Wu H, et al. Human glucosamine-6-phosphate isomerase, a homologue of hamster oscillin, does not appear to be involved in Ca2+ release in mammalian oocytes. Mol Reprod Dev 1999; 52: 277–87.
106. De Kretser DM, Burger HG, Fortune D, et al. Hormonal, histological and chromosomal studies in adult males with testicular disorders. J Clin Endocrinol Metab 1972; 35: 392–401.
107. Katagiri Y, Neri QV, Takeuchi T, et al. Y chromosome assessment and its implications for the development of ICSI children. Reprod Biomed Online 2004; 8: 307–18.
108. Alfarawati S, Fragouli E, Colls P, et al. The relationship between blastocyst morphology, chromosomal abnormality, and embryo gender. Fertil Steril 2011; 95: 520–4.
109. Munne S, Fragouli E, Colls P, et al. Improved detection of aneuploid blastocysts using a new 12-chromosome FISH test. Reprod Biomed Online 2010; 20: 92–7.
110. Steel AJ, Sutcliffe A. Long-term health implications for children conceived by IVF/ICSI. Hum Fertil (Camb) 2009; 12: 21–7.

14

Assisted hatching

Anna Veiga and Itziar Belil

INTRODUCTION

The Zona Pellucida

The zona pellucida (ZP) of mammalian eggs and embryos is an acellular matrix composed of sulfated glycoproteins with different roles during fertilization and embryo development (1).

Three distinct glycoproteins have been described both in mice and in humans (ZP1, ZP2, and ZP3) (2). Acrosome-reacted spermatozoa bind to ZP receptors, and biochemical changes have been observed after fertilization (3) that are responsible for the prevention of polyspermic fertilization.

The main function of the ZP after fertilization is the protection of the embryo and the maintenance of its integrity (4). It has been postulated that blastomeres may be weakly connected, and that the ZP is needed during the migration of embryos through the reproductive tract to maintain the embryo structure. Implantation has been observed after replacement of zona-free mouse morulae or blastocysts, while the transfer of zona-free precompacted embryos results in the adherence of transferred embryos to the oviductal walls or to one another. A possible protective role against hostile uterine factors has also been described (4). Degeneration of sheep eggs after a complete or partial ZP removal that could be ascribed to an immune response was described by Trounson and Moore (5).

Hatching

Once in the uterus, the blastocysts must get out of the ZP (hatching) so that the trophectoderm cells can interact with endometrial cells and implantation can occur. The loss of the ZP in utero is the result of embryonic and uterine functions.

Zona hardening after zona reaction subsequent to fertilization occurs, and is evidenced by an increased resistance to dissolution by different chemical agents. A loss of elasticity is also observed. This physiological phenomenon is essential for polyspermy block and for embryo protection during transport through the reproductive tract.

It has been postulated that additional ZP hardening may occur in both mice and humans as a consequence of in vitro culture (4,6,7). Hatching could be inhibited in some in vitro cultured human embryos owing to the inability of the blastocysts to escape from a thick or hardened ZP (8).

Schiewe et al. performed a study to characterize ZP hardening in unfertilized and abnormal embryos and to correlate it with culture duration, patient age, and ZP thickness (9). Dispersion of ZP glycoproteins and the time needed for complete digestion after α-chymotrypsin treatment were assessed. The results obtained proved that zona hardening of fertilized eggs was increased, compared with inseminated unfertilized eggs. Wide patient-to-patient variation in zona hardness was observed, but no correlation was established between zona hardness or thickness and patient age. Furthermore, the data obtained did not support the concept that additional ZP hardening occurred during extended culture.

Expansion and ZP thinning occur in mammalian blastocysts prior to hatching.

Cycles of contraction and expansion have been described in mice, sheep, cattle, and human blastocysts in vitro prior to ZP hatching. As a result of several cycles of contraction and expansion and because of its elasticity, the ZP thins. Contraction–expansion cycles as well as cytoplasmic extensions of trophectoderm (trophectoderm projections, TEPs) have been documented by time-lapse video recording (10) in human blastocysts. TEPs could be a component of zona escape in cultured embryos. It is not clear whether TEPs are needed in vivo for ZP hatching, but they seem to have a role in attachment, implantation, and possibly embryo locomotion (11).

Lysins of embryonic and/or uterine origin are involved in ZP thinning and hatching. Gordon and Dapunt showed that, in mice, hatching is predominantly the result of zona lysis, and that the pressure exerted against the zona by the expanding blastocyst plays little or no part in the escape of the embryo from the ZP (12).

Schiewe et al. demonstrated, with the use of a mouse antihatching model, the involvement of zona lysins in the mechanism of hatching; (13) physical expansion of the blastocyst, even though involved in hatching, does not seem to be the primary mechanism. Their results also show that trophectoderm cells are responsible for secreting the zona lysins required for hatching. On the other hand, two observational studies demonstrate that a natural hatching site usually develops in close proximity of the inner cell mass (ICM) of blastocysts in humans, whereas that of the mouse is at the opposite side to the ICM (14,15).

A study on mouse blastocysts indicates that hatching in vitro is dependent on a sufficient number of cells constituting the embryo. Hatching in vivo must be different from that in vitro, the difference involving uterine and/or uterine-induced trophectoderm lytic factors (16).

ASSISTED HATCHING

The first report of the use of assisted hatching (AH) in human embryos was published by Cohen et al. in 1990 (7). These authors documented an important increase of implantation rates with mechanical AH in embryos from unselected in vitro fertilization (IVF) patients.

Why Perform Assisted Hatching?

The ratio of lysin production to ZP thickness could determine whether the embryo will lyse the zona and undergo hatching. Embryos with thick zonae or those that present extensive fragmentation or cell death after freezing and thawing may benefit from AH (17).

Both quantitative and qualitative deficiencies in lysin secretion could result in hatching impairment. Suboptimal culture conditions may cause such deficiencies. The trophectoderm of some embryos may not be able to secrete the "hatching factor," and lysin production could be influenced by a patient's age (8,13). Uterine lysin action could also be impaired in some patients or cycles (18).

It is believed that ZP hardening may be exacerbated at any stage of embryo development after long-term in vitro culture and cryopreservation of embryos (19). Furthermore, experiments on mouse embryos have demonstrated that damaged blastomeres have a toxic effect, reducing dramatically the rate of hatching (20). However, embryo viability was restored after microsurgical removal of the degenerating material (21). Removal of necrotic blastomeres from frozen–thawed, partially damaged human embryos significantly increased the implantation rate (22).

It has been stated that overall zona thickness varies between age groups and types of infertility (23). The variability of zona thickness in the same embryo is one of the most significant morphologic predictive factors of implantation (24). Palmstierna et al. demonstrated that human embryos with zona thickness variation of >20% resulted in a 76% pregnancy rate with two embryos transferred (25). Zona-assisted thinning of a substantial area may favor complete hatching in embryos with invariable zona thickness (26). Khalifa et al. have shown that ZP thinning significantly increases the complete hatching of mouse embryos (27). Gordon and Dapunt demonstrated the usefulness of ZP thinning with acid Tyrode's to improve hatching in hatching-defective mouse embryos created by the destruction of one-quarter of the blastomeres (17). They reported normal implantation rates in pseudopregnant female mice after the transfer of assisted-hatched embryos that had cell numbers reduced.

The mechanism by which AH promotes embryo implantation remains unclear. The implantation window is the critical period when the endometrium reaches its ideal receptive state for implantation. Precise synchronization between the embryo and the endometrium is essential. In a randomized study, Liu et al. demonstrated that implantation occurred significantly earlier in patients whose embryos were submitted to AH when compared with the control group, possibly by allowing an earlier embryo–endometrium contact (28). Furthermore, although most molecules are able to cross the ZP, the rate of transport may be related to zona thickness. The presence of an artificial gap may alter the two-way transport of metabolites and growth factors across the ZP, permitting earlier exposure of the embryo to vital growth factors (8).

It has been also reported that the location of herniation of fresh, human hatched blastocysts can predict their implantation behavior (29). Significantly higher clinical pregnancy rates were observed if blastocysts that hatched close to the ICM were transferred (72%) as compared with those that herniated from the mural trophectoderm (51%). A recent study suggested the existence of polarity in the hatching process of vitrified–thawed human blastocysts. Laser AH performed close to the ICM improved complete hatching rates, whereas AH at the anembryonic site caused embryo trapping within the ZP (30). It is likely that in vitrified and warmed blastocysts the complete opening of the ZP by means of laser pulses changes the pressure conditions that would be one of the prerequisites for optimal hatching (31). Applying AH at a specific site of ZP may enhance vitrified blastocyst implantation.

Methods

When breaches are made in the ZP of early-cleavage IVF embryos, embryonic cell loss may occur through the zona as a result of uterine contractions after replacement of the embryos. It is advisable to manipulate embryos for AH after the adherence between blastomeres has increased, just before compaction (32). Artificial opening of the ZP of blastocysts can also be performed to promote complete blastocyst hatching (33,34). Embryos at the six to eight-cell stage at day 3 after insemination, or at the blastocyst stage, at day 5 or 6 after insemination, can be manipulated with different methods for the performance of AH.

Microtools for AH can be made by means of a pipette puller and microforge, but are also commercially available. Micropipettes are mounted on micromanipulators. It is very important to minimize the time that the embryo is out of the incubator, and to optimize methodologies to reduce pH and temperature variations that can be detrimental for embryo development.

To reduce environmental variations, AH has to be performed in microdrops of 4-(2-hydroxyethyl)-1-piperazine-ethanesulfonic acid (HEPES) or equivalent buffered medium covered with oil, under an inverted microscope with Nomarski or Hoffman optics, on a heated microscope stage, at 37°C.

It is important that the size of the hole created in the zona is large enough to avoid trapping of the embryo during hatching, but not so large that it permits blastomere loss (35–38). Monozygotic twinning has been described as a consequence of AH (39). The adequate size of the hole seems to be 30–40 μm when AH is performed on day 3 embryos. Nevertheless, AH applied to cryopreserved blastocysts seems to give better results when Þ50% of the ZP is opened or ZP is totally removed (40,41). Half of ZP thinning in early-stage vitrified embryos seems to be associated with higher pregnancy rates than quarter thinning (42).

Different protocols have been described, but a minimum 30-minute culture period seems to be sufficient before the transfer of the manipulated embryos.

Embryo transfer to the uterus has to be performed as atraumatically as possible to avoid damage of ZP-manipulated embryos.

Treatment during four days, starting on the day of oocyte retrieval, with broad-spectrum antibiotics and corticosteroids (methyl prednisolone, 16 mg daily) has been postulated. Cohen et al. suggested that such treatment may be useful for patients whose embryos have been assisted-hatched, to avoid infection and immune cell invasion of the embryos (7).

Partial Zona Dissection

The method of partial zona dissection (PZD) is similar to that described for oocytes, to assist oocyte ZP penetration by spermatozoa with no preincubation of the embryos in sucrose (43).

Embryos denuded of corona cells are micromanipulated in microdrops of HEPES-buffered medium under paraffin oil. As mentioned above, the procedure is performed at 37°C, under an inverted microscope. The embryo is held with a holding pipette, and the ZP is tangentially pierced with a microneedle from the 1 o'clock to the 11 o'clock position. The embryo is released from the holding pipette, and the part of the ZP between the two points is rubbed against the holding pipette until a slit is made in the zona. The embryo is washed twice in a fresh culture medium and placed in the transfer dish.

A 3D-PZD in the shape of a cross has been described (38). The procedure starts as conventional PZD and a second cut is made in the ZP under the first slit. A cross-shaped cut can be seen on the surface of the ZP. This method allows the creation of larger openings while permitting protection of the embryo by the ZP flaps during embryo transfer.

A new technique called "controlled zona dissection" has been recently described as a variation of PZD (34). The embryo is held at the 8 o'clock position by a bevel opened holding pipette, and a thin angled hatching needle with a blunted tip pierces the ZP at the 5 o'clock position. The hatching needle is inserted deeply into the holding pipette until the embryo is pushed to the angle of the hatching needle. The curve of the needle is then pressed against the bottom of the dish to cut the pierced ZP. A large slit (two-thirds of embryo's diameter) created by controlled zona dissection enhances significantly the rate of complete in vitro hatching of blastocysts compared with the 3D-PZD.

Acid Tyrode's Assisted Hatching

It has been described that zona hardening and the increase in volume of the perivitelline space in zygotes and embryos allow an efficient and safe use of acid Tyrode's (AT) solution in human embryos for ZP drilling, compared with oocytes. Nevertheless, it has to be taken into account that the use of acidic solutions for AH may be detrimental for the blastomere(s) adjacent to the drilled portion of the ZP. Limiting embryo exposure to AT by adequate and quick manipulation is necessary to avoid harmful effects on embryo development.

AT solution can be prepared in the laboratory based on the protocol of Hogan et al. (44) and adjusted to a pH of 2.5, or can be purchased commercially.

One advantage of AT drilling compared with PZD is the possibility of increasing the size of the hole in the ZP. Large holes have proved to be more efficient for enhancing hatching and avoiding embryo entrapment (7,37,45).

The embryo is held with a holding pipette in such a way that the micropipette containing AT solution (internal diameter 3–5 μm) at the 3 o'clock position faces a large perivitelline space or an area with cytoplasmic fragments of the embryo. The acidic solution is gently delivered with the help of a microinjector over a small area of the ZP, with the tip of the pipette positioned very close to the zona. Accumulation of AT solution in a single area must be avoided. Extracellular fragments can also be removed during the procedure (8). As soon as a hole is created in the ZP, suction is applied to avoid excess AT solution entering the perivitelline space. If the inner region of the ZP is difficult to breach, creation of the hole can be facilitated by pushing the AT micropipette against the ZP (46).

It is necessary to rinse the embryo several times in fresh culture medium.

Laser-Assisted Hatching

The use of laser techniques in the field of assisted reproduction for application in gametes or embryos was first described by Tadir et al. (47,48). For a fast and an efficient clinical use of laser systems in AH, it is important that the laser is accurately controlled and produces precise ZP openings without thermal or mutagenic effects. The application of a laser on the ZP for AH results in the photoablation of the ZP.

Contact Lasers

The procedure is performed on a microscope slide, and the embryo is placed on a drop of the medium covered with paraffin oil. The embryo is held with a holding pipette, and the laser is delivered through a microscopic laser glass fiber, fitted to the manipulator by a pipette holder, in direct contact with the ZP. Several pulses are necessary to penetrate the ZP. Because each laser pulse removes only small portions of the ZP, the fiber tip has to be continuously readjusted to guarantee that the laser is in close contact with the remaining zona.

The first use of a laser for ZP drilling was reported by Palanker et al. with an ArF excimer laser (UV region, 193 nm wavelength) (49). This laser system makes it necessary to touch the ZP with the laser-delivering pipette (contact mode laser). The erbium:yttrium–aluminum–garnet (Er:YAG) laser (2940 nm radiation), also working in contact mode, has been used for ZP AH and thinning, and its safety and efficacy have been demonstrated in clinical practice (50,51). Obruca et al. performed a study to evaluate the ultrastructural effects of the Er:YAG laser on the ZP and membrane of oocytes and embryos (52). No degenerative alterations were observed using light and scanning electron microscopy after ZP drilling with such a system. Antinori et al. (53) described the method for ZP thinning with the use of an Er:YAG laser. Five to eight pulses were needed to ablate 50% of the ZP thickness in a length of 20 μm. The necessity of sterile micropipettes and optical fibers to deliver the laser beam to the target is the main disadvantage of contact mode lasers (54).

Noncontact Lasers

Noncontact laser systems allow microscope objective–delivered accessibility of laser light to the target. Laser propagation is made through water, and as it avoids the UV absorption peak of DNA, no mutagenic effect on the oocyte or embryo is expected. Blanchet et al. first reported the use of a noncontact laser system (248 nm KrF excimer) for mouse ZP drilling (55). Neev et al. described the use of a noncontact laser holmium:yttrium scandium–gallium–garnet (Ho:YSGG) laser (2.1 μm wavelength) for AH in mice (56). The study showed a lack of embryotoxic effects as well as improved blastocyst hatching. Similar results were reported by Schiewe et al. (57).

Rink et al. designed and introduced a noncontact infrared diode laser (1.48 μm) that delivers laser light through the microscope objective (58). The drilling mechanism is explained by a thermal effect induced at the focal point by absorption of the laser energy by water and/or ZP macromolecules, leading to the thermolysis of the ZP matrix. Laser absorption by the culture dish and medium is minimal. The effect on the ZP is greatly localized, and the holes are cylindrical and precise. Exposure time (1–40 msec) can be minimized. The safety and usefulness of the system was demonstrated in mice and humans (59–61). Its use for polar body as well as blastomere and blastocyst biopsy has also been reported (62–64). The system is compact and easily adapted to all kinds of microscopes. The size of the hole is related to the laser exposure time, and thus the system is simple, quick, and easy to use. Figure 14.1 shows an eight-cell embryo in which laser AH has been performed.

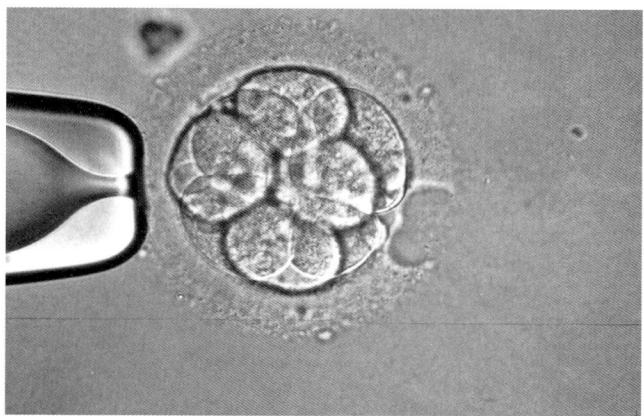

Figure 14.1 Day 3 embryo in which the zona pellucida has been drilled with two laser shots (Fertilase®, MTM, Montreaux, Switzerland).

Antinori et al. have reported the use of a compact, noncontact UV (337 nm wavelength) laser microbeam system to create holes in the ZP of human embryos (65,66). This equipment requires the manipulation of the oocytes and embryos in Petri dishes with a membrane bottom.

Depending on the laser equipment, different methods are used, varying in energy, time, and number of pulses needed to open the ZP. Two studies have reported the immediate effects of localized heating after the use of noncontact infrared lasers in animal models (67,68). The diode laser beam produces superheated water approaching 200°C on the beam axis. The action of the laser must be strictly limited to the targeted region of the ZP, since focused laser irradiation on a specific cell will cause damage and probably be lethal to that cell. Following irradiation, the heat is conducted away from the target and is dissipated into the surrounding medium. The potential to damage blastomeres adjacent to the hole created by the laser is minimized by using pulse durations of ≤5 msec and laser power ~100 mW at a safe distance from the blastomeres.

In a recent study made on the murine model to determine the optimal technical settings for laser AH—changing laser intensity, pulse duration, number of pulses, as well as the depth of disruptions—the highest hatching rate seemed to be achieved when laser intensity was reduced (69).

There are studies that compare laser AH with other AH methods (70,71). Sister embryos of patients undergoing preimplantation genetic diagnosis, randomly assigned on day 3 to AT solution zona drilling or to laser zona drilling, showed similar blastocyst development rates (70). However, implantation rates of laser ZP-drilled embryos were significantly higher than those of mechanically treated embryos, when the embryos of women of advanced age (39 years) underwent AH (71).

Zona Pellucida Thinning

The aim of ZP thinning is to thin the ZP without complete lysis and perforation. By not breaching the zona, the potential risk of blastomere loss and embryonic infection is minimized.

ZP thinning with AT has been described in mice and humans (27,72). It involves bidirectional thinning of a cross-shaped area of the ZP over about one-quarter of the embryo circumference. Care has to be taken not to rupture the ZP completely. Embryos are washed in fresh droplets of the medium and cultured before transfer. This methodology has proved useful for hatching enhancement in mice but not in humans, probably because of differences observed in both the morphologic and the biophysical characteristics of the ZP between the two species. The mouse ZP has a monolayer structure whereas the human ZP, as shown by electron microscopy, is composed of a less dense, easily digestible, thick outer layer and a more compact but resilient inner layer (72).

The use of laser technology for ZP thinning at the cleavage stage seems to be beneficial for embryo implantation for certain authors (26,53,73–75). Antinori et al. demonstrated a significant increase in implantation and pregnancy rate when 50% of the zona thickness from 2-day-old embryos was thinned to a length of 20 μm using a YAG contact laser (53). Diode laser ZP thinning enhances the variation of zona thickness in human embryos, allows natural zona thinning, and increases significantly the rate of blastocyst hatching (26).

Acceptable clinical pregnancy rates were obtained after transfer of frozen–thawed blastocysts that underwent laser-assisted thinning at the day 3 cleaving stage before freezing (73).

Laser partial zona thinning has been associated with higher implantation and pregnancy rates than total laser AH, especially in women who suffer from recurrent implantation failure (76).

The enzymatic action of pronase to thin the ZP of human early-cleaving embryos yields similar benefit to other AH methods (77).

Nevertheless, zona thinning for cryopreserved–thawed embryos, using pronase action or laser methodology, has failed to show improvement in the implantation rate (78–81).

A new method for mechanical AH, inspired by the natural expanding effects of blastocysts on the ZP, has been described (82). This mechanical AH method expands/stretches the ZP by injecting hydrostatic pressure into the perivitelline space using an ICSI injection needle and culture medium, inducing a short time (≤30 seconds) ZP thinning. Mechanically expanding the ZP of frozen–thawed day 3 human embryos with injected hydrostatic pressure has shown to increase implantation and clinical pregnancy rate when compared with control embryos.

Blastocyst Assisted Hatching

Even though AH is usually performed on early-cleavage embryos (day 3, six to eight-cell stage), it can also be applied to blastocysts to increase implantation rates. A monozygotic twin pregnancy was achieved after transfer of a frozen–thawed human blastocyst, on which ZP rubbing was applied with a microneedle (83). The size of the hole made on the human blastocyst's ZP during AH

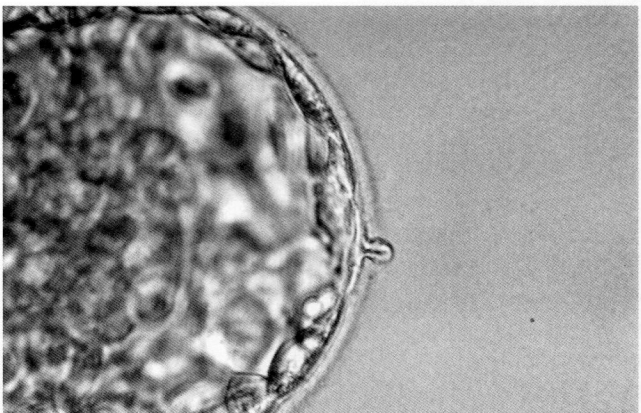

Figure 14.2 Laser-assisted hatching (Fertilase®) in an expanded blastocyst. A trophectoderm cell is protruding through the thin zona pellucida.

seems to be important for the final hatching development. A large slit created on the ZP of human blastocysts after mechanical AH with CZD enhanced significantly total blastocyst hatching in vitro compared to a moderate size slit (two-fifths of ZP diameter) (34). Zona opening of small or moderate size induced the hatching blastocyst into an "8" shape and often trapped the ICM.

AH can be also applied on frozen–thawed blastocysts. Artificial opening of the ZP by 3D-PZD or by laser and a total ZP removal after the warming of vitrified blastocysts significantly improved the implantation and pregnancy rates (33,40,41). Fong et al. described a method for enzymatic treatment of the ZP of blastocysts (84). Culture to the blastocyst stage was achieved with the use of sequential media; early and expanding blastocysts were treated with 10 IU/ml pronase for 1 minute at 37°C. Just before complete disappearance of the ZP in the pronase solution, the blastocysts were placed in a fresh medium and washed twice. They were cultured for a few hours before transfer. The results obtained have shown that ZP-manipulated blastocysts have a high implantation rate (33%), and there is a need to limit the number of AH blastocysts to be transferred to one or two to reduce multiple pregnancies.

Park et al. reported the use of a 1.48 μm noncontact diode laser for AH of in vitro matured/in vitro fertilized/in vitro cultured (IVM/IVF/IVC) blastocysts (85). Short irradiation exposure times (3–5 msec) were applied, and a significant increase in the hatching rate was observed.

We have described the use of a 1.48 μm diode laser for AH in human blastocysts (86). Even though no statistically significant differences were observed, a trend toward higher pregnancy and implantation rates was obtained when laser-drilled AH blastocysts were replaced, compared with nondrilled blastocysts (44.4% vs. 23.8% and 30.6% vs. 11.6%) (Fig. 14.2).

RESULTS AND CONCLUSIONS

Several studies have been performed to demonstrate the usefulness and efficacy of AH in different groups of patients using the various methods described. Most of the studies have been done in patients with poor prognosis, including advanced-age patients, patients with elevated concentrations of follicle-stimulating hormone (FSH), patients with previous implantation failures, or with embryos with thick ZP, some of them with contradictory results. One study included women with endometriosis, not showing improvement after AH (87). AH has been applied to fresh early-cleavage stage embryos and blastocysts and also to frozen–thawed embryos and vitrified–warmed blastocysts. Removal of necrotic blastomeres from partially damaged cryopreserved–thawed embryos may help to maintain their development potential (22,88).

Tables 14.1 and 14.2 show the results reported by different authors.

The variability of methodologies, study design, and groups of patients, described on the published AH studies, makes it very difficult to come to a definitive conclusion on the possible effect of AH on embryo implantation. The last Cochrane review "AH on Assisted Conception" concludes that even though live birth should be considered the primary outcome, available data do not show any positive effect of AH on live birth rates (89). On the other hand, a recent systematic review and meta-analysis of medical literature used to evaluate the effect of AH on assisted reproduction outcomes concluded that AH was related with increased clinical pregnancy and multiple pregnancy rates in women with previous repeated failure or in frozen–thawed embryo transfer (90). From the published results and taking into account the variability in

Table 14.1 Assisted Hatching Results Reported by Different Authors (1992–1999)

Author	Study method	Population	Randomized	Pregnancy rate increase
Cohen 1992 (8)	AT	Normal FSH	Yes	Yes, NS
		≥15 μm ZP	Yes	Yes, sig.
Tucker 1993 (72)	AT	All IVF	Yes	No
	ZP thinning			
Olivennes 1994 (91)	PZD	Impl. failures	No (no control)	—
		Day 3, FSH >15	Yes	Yes, sig.
Obruca 1994 (51)	Er:YAG laser	Impl. failures	No	Yes, sig.
Tucker 1994 (92)	AT, CC	Age ≥38 yrs, impl. Failures	Yes (control: AT)	Yes, sig.
Schoolcraft 1994 (46)	AT	Elevated FSH, ≥39 yrs	No	Yes, sig.
		Impl. failures		
Schoolcraft 1995 (93)	AT	≥40 yrs	No, retrosp.	Yes, sig.
Stein 1995 (94)	PZD	≥3 impl. failures	Yes	Yes, sig. >38 yrs
Hellebaut 1996 (74)	PZD	1st cycle	Yes	No
Antinori 1996 (53)	UV laser	Impl. failures	No	Yes, sig.
Check 1996 (95)	AT	Frozen ET	No	Yes, NS
Antinori 1996 (65)	Er:YAG laser	1st cycle	Yes	Yes, sig.
		Impl. failures	Yes	Yes, sig.
Tucker 1996 (96)	AT	ICSI, ≥35 yrs	No	Yes, sig.
Bider 1997 (97)	AT	≥38 yrs	No	No
Chao 1997 (98)	PZD	Impl. Failures	Yes	Yes, IVF
				No, TET
Hurst 1998 (99)	AT	1st cycle	Yes	No
Magli 1998 (100)	AT	≥38 yrs	No	Yes, sig.
		≥3 Impl. failures		Yes, sig.
		Both		No
Lanzendorf 1998 (101)	AT	≥36 yrs	Yes	No
Meldrum 1998 (102)	AT	≥35 yrs	No	Yes, NS
Antinori 1999 (66)	Er:YAG laser	1st cycle	Yes	Yes (?)
		≥6 Impl. failures	Yes	Yes (?)
Edirisinghe 1999 (103)	PZD	≥38 yrs, ZP ≥15, ≥1 impl. failure	No	No
Baruffi 1999 (61)	Diode laser, ZP thinning	<37 yrs, 1st cycle	Yes	No
Veiga 1999 (86)	Diode laser	Impl. failure, CC	Yes	Yes, NS
		1st cycle	Yes	No (unpubl.)
Cieslak 1999 (38)	3D PZD	All IVF	Yes (control: conv. PZD)	Yes, NS
Alikani 1999 (104)	PZD + frag. removal	≥6% frag.	No, retrosp.	Yes, sig.
Nakayama 1999 (105)	Piezomicromanipulator	≥2 Impl. failures	Yes	Yes, sig.

Abbreviations: AT, acid Tyrode's; blast., blastomere; CC, co-culture; conv., conventional; D, day; Er:YAG, erbium:yttrium–aluminum–garnet; ET, embryo transfer; frag., fragment/ed; FSH, follicle-stimulating hormone; ICSI, intracytoplasmic sperm injection; impl. implantation; IVF, in vitro fertilization; NS, not significant; PZD, partial zona dissection; retrosp., retrospective; sig., significant; TET, thawed embryo transfer; unpubl., unpublished; UV, ultraviolet; ZP, zona pellucida.

Table 14.2 Assisted Hatching Results Reported by Different Authors (2000–2007)

Author	Study method	Population	Randomized	Pregnancy rate increase
Mansour 2000 (106)	ZP removal, AT	1st cycle	Yes	No
		≥40 yrs ≥2 impl. failures	Yes	Yes, sig.
Mantoudis 2001 (107)	Diode laser	Poor responders ≥38 yrs, ≥2 impl. failures, Frozen ET	No	Yes, sig. (for ZP thinning)
	Total AH, Partial AH, ZP thinning			
Malter 2001 (108)	Diode laser versus AT	All IVF/ICSI	Yes (control: AT)	No
Balaban 2002 (77)	PZD	All IVF/ICSI	No, retrosp.	No
	AT			No
	Diode laser			No
	Pronase thinning			No
Rienzi 2002 (22)	Diode laser	Frozen ET	Yes	Yes, sig.
	Necrotic blast. removal			
Hsieh 2002 (109)	Diode laser versus AT	≥38 yrs	Yes	Yes, sig. (for laser)
Milki 2002 (110)	AH D + 3 versus CC	40–43 yrs	No, retrosp.	No
Vanderzwalmen 2003 (33)	PZD blastocysts	Frozen (vitrif.) ET	No, retrosp	Yes, sig.
Gabrielsen 2004 (111)	AT	Frozen ET	Yes	No
Petersen 2005 (75)	Diode laser, ZP thinning	≥2 Impl. failures	Yes	Yes, NS
Ng 2005 (79)	Diode laser, ZP thinning	Frozen ET	Yes	No
Nadir 2005 (87)	Diode laser, ZP thinning	Endometriosis	Yes	No
Frydman 2006 (112)	Diode laser, ZP thinning	≥37 yrs	Yes	No
Balaban 2006 (113)	Diode laser	Frozen ET	Yes	Yes, sig.
Sifer 2006 (78)	Pronase, ZP thinning	Frozen ET	Yes	No
Petersen 2006 (80)	Diode laser, ZP thinning	Frozen ET from OHSS IVF cycles	Yes	Yes, NS
Sagoskin 2007 (114)	Diode laser	Good prognosis	Yes	No
Hiraoka 2007 (41)	Diode laser versus AT	≥2 Impl. failures	No, retrosp.	Yes, sig. (for total removal)
	Total ZP removal versus partial drilling	Frozen ET		
	Blastocyst AH			
Hiraoka 2008 (40)	Diode laser	≥2 Impl. failures	No, retrosp.	Yes, sig. (for 50%)
	ZP drilling	Frozen ET		
	50% versus 40 μm			
Hiraoka 2009 (42)	Diode laser, ZP thinning	Frozen ET	Yes	Yes, sig. (for 50%)
	D + 3 50% versus 25%			
Valojerdi 2010 (81)	Diode laser, ZP thinning	Frozen ET	Yes	No, (sig. decrease)
	D + 3 vitrified			
Fang 2010 (82)	Mechanical expansion	Frozen ET	Yes	Yes, sig.
	D + 3			

Abbreviations: AT, acid Tyrode's; AH, assisted hatching; blast., blastomere; CC, co-culture; D, day; ET, embryo transfer; FSH, follicle-stimulating hormone; ICSI, intracytoplasmic sperm injection; impl. implantation; IVF, in vitro fertilization; PZD, partial zona dissection; retrosp., retrospective; NS, not significant; sig., significant; OHSS, ovarian hyperstimulation syndrome; vitrif., vitrification; ZP, zona pellucida.

methods and study designs, the conclusions concerning AH benefits are as follows:

1. AH does not increase the pregnancy and implantation rate in patients in their first IVF attempt.
2. AH increases the pregnancy and implantation rate in patients with previous implantation failures.
3. There is some evidence that AH may enhance embryo implantation and pregnancy rate in patients undergoing frozen–thawed embryo transfer.
4. It is not clear whether AH is beneficial for patients of an advanced age, for patients with a thick ZP.
5. Currently, there is insufficient evidence to recommend AH as a routine technique in patients undergoing assisted reproductive techniques.

The potential of AH in assisted conception makes it imperative that studies of adequate methodological quality (preferably multicenter trials with appropriate design, adequate power, and appropriate duration of follow-up) are undertaken to investigate the role of the various methods of AH, when applying at different development stages of the embryo, and in different subgroups of population to provide the urgently needed answers: women undergoing frozen embryo transfers, women in older age groups, following repeated implantation failure, those with high early proliferative phase serum FSH levels and embryos with thick or hardened ZP.

It is questionable whether different methods of AH yield similar outcomes. Large randomized studies comparing AH methods with regard to embryo implantation rate and live birth rate are needed and follow-up of obstetrical and post-natal outcome is far recommended. Mechanical hatching by PZD is limited by the difficulty of creating a hole of consistent size. The variability and possible embryotoxicity are potential problems with the use of AT for zona drilling. Enzymatic methods to dissolve or thin the zona seem to be effective and safe. Although the equipment may be expensive, the use of a 1.48 μm diode infrared laser system for zona drilling offers a low potential risk, it is quick and relatively simple to perform with high consistency between operators, and appears to be the most suitable method for AH in the IVF laboratory.

REFERENCES

1. Dean J. Biology of mammalian fertilization: the role of the zona pellucida. J Clin Invest 1992; 89: 1055–9.
2. Shabanowitz RB, O'Rand MG. Characterization of the human zona pellucida from fertilized and unfertilized eggs. J Reprod Fert 1988; 82: 151–61.
3. Ducibella T, Kurasawa S, Ramgarajan S, Kopf GS, Schultz RM. Precocious loss of cortical granules during oocyte meiotic maturation and correlation with an egg-induced modification of the zona pellucida. Dev Biol 1990; 137: 46–55.
4. Cohen J. Assisted hatching of human embryos. J In Vitro Fert Embryo Transfer 1991; 8: 179–90.
5. Trounson AO, Moore NW. The survival and development of sheep eggs following complete or partial removal of the zona pellucida. J Reprod Fert 1974; 41: 97–105.
6. De Felici M, Siracusa G. Spontaneous hardening of the zona pellucida of mouse oocytes during in vitro culture. Gamete Res 1982; 6: 107–13.
7. Cohen J, Elsner C, Kort H, et al. Impairment of the hatching process following IVF in the human and improvement of implantation by assisted hatching using micromanipulation. Hum Reprod 1990; 5: 7–13.
8. Cohen J, Alikani M, Trowbridge J, Rosenwaks Z. Implantation enhancement by selective assisted hatching using zona drilling of human embryos with poor prognosis. Hum Reprod 1992; 7: 685–91.
9. Schiewe MC, Araujo JR, Asch RH, Balmaceda JP. Enzymatic characterization of zona pellucida hardening in human eggs and embryos. J Assist Reprod Genet 1995; 12: 2–7.
10. Gonzales D, Bavister B. Zona pellucida escape by hamster blastocysts in vitro is delayed and morphologically different compared with zona escape in vivo. Biol Reprod 1995; 52: 470–80.
11. Gonzales DS, Jones JM, Pinyopumintr P, et al. Trophectoderm projections: a potential means for locomotion, attachment and implantation of bovine, equine and human blastocysts. Hum Reprod 1996; 11: 2739–45.
12. Gordon J, Dapunt U. A new mouse model for embryos with a hatching deficiency and its use to elucidate the mechanism of blastocyst hatching. Fertil Steril 1993; 59: 1296–301.
13. Schiewe MC, Hazeleger NL, Sclimenti C, Balmaceda JP. Physiological characterization of blastocyst hatching mechanisms by use of a mouse antihatching model. Fertil Steril 1995; 63: 288–94.
14. Veeck LL, Zaninovic N. Blastocyst hatching. In: Veeck LL, Zaninovic N, eds. An Atlas of Human Blastocysts. London: Informa Healthcare, 2003: 159–71.
15. Gonzales DS, Jones JM, Pinyopumintr T, et al. Trophectoderm projections: a potential means for locomotion, attachment and implantation of bovine, equine and human blastocysts. Hum Reprod 1996; 11: 2739–45.
16. Montag M, Koll B, Holmes P, Van der Ven H. Significance of the number of embryonic cells and the state of the zona pellucida for hatching of mouse blastocysts in vitro versus in vivo. Biol Reprod 2000; 62: 1738–44.
17. Gordon J, Dapunt U. Restoration of normal implantation rates in mouse embryos with a hatching impairment by use of a new method of assisted hatching. Fertil Steril 1993; 59: 1302–7.
18. Mandelbaum J. The effects of assisted hatching on the hatching process and implantation. Hum Reprod 1996; 11: 43–50.
19. Ludwig M, Al-Hasani S, Felderbaum DK. New aspects of crypreservation of oocytes and embryos in assisted reproduction and future perspectives. Hum Reprod 1999; 14(Suppl 1): 162–85.
20. Alikani M, Oliviennes F, Cohen J. Microsurgical correction of partially degenerate mouse embryos promotes hatching and restores their viability. Hum Reprod 1993; 8: 1723–8.
21. Elliot TA, Colturato LFA, Taylor TA, et al. Lysed cell removal promotes frozen-thawed embryo development. Fertil Steril 2007; 87: 1444–9.
22. Rienzi L, Nagy ZP, Ubaldi F, et al. Laser-assisted removal of necrotic blastomeres from cryopreserved embryos that were partially damaged. Fertil Steril 2002; 77: 1196–201.
23. Loret de Mola JR, Garside WT, Bucci J, et al. Analysis of the human zona pellucida during culture; correlation with diagnosis and the preovulatory hormonal environment. Assist Reprod Genet 1997; 14: 332–6.
24. Cohen J, Wiker SR, Inge KL, et al. Videocinematography of fresh and cryopreserved embryos: a retrospective analysis of embryonic morphology and implantation. Fertil Steril 1989; 51: 821–7.
25. Palmstierna M, Murkes D, Csemiczdy G, et al. Zona pellucida thickness variation and occurrence of visible mononucleated blastomeres in preembryos are associated with a high pregnancy rate in IVF treatments. J Assist Reprod Genet 1998; 15: 70–5.
26. Blake DA, Forsberg AS, Johansson BR, Wikland M. Laser zona pellucida thinning—an alternative approach to assisted hatching. Hum Reprod 2001; 16: 1959–64.
27. Khalifa EAM, Tucker MJ, Hunt P. Cruciate thinning of the zona pellucida for more successful enhancement of blastocyst hatching in the mouse. Hum Reprod 1992; 7: 532–6.
28. Liu HC, Cohen J, Alikani M, Noyes N, Rosenwaks Z. Assisted hatching facilitates earlier implantation. Fertil Steril 1993; 60: 871–5.
29. Ebner T, Gruber I, Moser M. Location of herniation predicts implantation behaviour of hatching blastocysts. J.Turkish-German Gynecol Assoc 2007; 8: 184–8.
30. Miyata H, Matsubayashi H, Fukutomi N, et al. Relevance of the site of assisted hatching in thawed human

blastocysts: a preliminary report. Fertil Steril 2010; 94: 2444–7.
31. Ebner T, Shebl O, Mayer RB, et al. Relevance of the site of assisted hatching in thawed human blastocysts (Letter to the editor). Fertil Steril 2010; 94: e65.
32. Dale B, Talevi R, Gualtieri R, et al. Intercellular communication in the early human embryo. Mol Reprod Dev 1991; 29: 22–8.
33. Vanderzwalmen P, Bertin G, Debauche Ch, et al. Vitrification of human blastocysts with the Hemi-Straw carrier: application of assisted hatching after thawing. Hum Reprod 2003; 18: 1504–11.
34. Lyu QF, Wu LQ, Li YP, et al. An improved mechanical technique for assisted hatching. Hum Reprod 2005; 20: 1619–23.
35. Talansky BE, Gordon JW. Cleavage characteristics of mouse embryos inseminated and cultures after zona pellucida drilling. Gamete Res 1998; 21: 277–8.
36. Nichols J, Garner RL. Effect of damage of the zona pellucida on development of preimplantation embryos in the mouse. Hum Reprod 1989; 4: 180–7.
37. Cohen J, Feldberg D. Effects of the size and number of zona pellucida openings on hatching and trophoblast outgrowth in the mouse embryo. Mol Reprod Dev 1991; 30: 70–8.
38. Cieslak J, Ivakhnenko V, Wolf G, Sheleg S, Verlinsky Y. Three dimensional partial zona dissection for preimplantation genetic diagnosis and assisted hatching. Fertil Steril 1999; 71: 308–13.
39. Alikani M, Noyes N, Cohen J, Rosenwaks Z. Monozygotic twinning in the human is associated with the zona pellucida architecture. Hum Reprod 1994; 9: 1318–21.
40. Hiraoka K, Fuchiwaki M, Horaoka K, et al. Effect of the size of zona pellucida outcome of frozen cleaved embryos that were cultured to blastocyst after thawing in women with multiple implantation failures of emryo transfer: a retrospective study. J Assist Reprod Genet 2008; 25: 129–35.
41. Hiraoka K, Fuchiwaki M, Horaoka K, et al. Zona pellucida removal and vitrified blastocyst transfer outcome: a preliminary study. RBM Online 2007; 15: 68–75.
42. Hiraoka K, Hiraoka K, Horiuchi T, et al. Impact of the size of zona pellucida on vitrified-warmed cleavage-stage embryo transfers: a prospective, randomized study. J Assist Reprod Genet 2009; 26: 515–21.
43. Malter HE, Cohen J. Partial zona dissection of the human oocyte: a no traumatic method using micromanipulation to assist zona pellucida penetration. Fertil Steril 1989; 51: 139–48.
44. Hogan B, Constantini F, Lacy E. Manipulating the Mouse Embryo: a Laboratory Manual. New York: Cold Spring Harbor Laboratory Press, 1986.
45. Malter H, Cohen J. Blastocyst formation and hatching in vitro following zona drilling of mouse and human embryos. Gamete Res 1989; 24: 67–80.
46. Schoolcraft W, Schenker T, Gee M, Jones GS, Jones HW. Assisted hatching in the treatment of poor prognosis in vitro fertilization candidates. Fertil Steril 1994; 62: 551–4.
47. Tadir Y, Wright WH, Vafa O, et al. Micromanipulation of sperm by a laser generated optical trap. Fertil Steril 1989; 52: 870–3.
48. Tadir Y, Wright WH, Vafa O, et al. Micromanipulation of gametes using laser microbeams. Hum Reprod 1991; 6: 1011–16.
49. Palanker D, Ohad S, Lewis A, et al. Technique for cellular microsurgery using the 193 nm excimer laser. Laser Surg Med 1991; 11: 589–6.
50. Strohmer H, Feichtinger W. Successful clinical application of laser for micromanipulation in an in vitro fertilization program. Fertil Steril 1992; 58: 212–14.
51. Obruca A, Strohmer H, Sakkas D, et al. Use of lasers in assisted fertilization and hatching. Hum Reprod 1994; 9: 1723–6.
52. Obruca A, Strohmer H, Blaschitz A, et al. Ultrastuctural observations in human oocytes and preimplantation embryos after zona opening using an Er:YAG laser. Hum Reprod 1997; 12: 2242–5.
53. Antinori S, Panci C, Selman HA, et al. Zona thinning with the use of laser: a new approach to assisted hatching in humans. Hum Reprod 1996; 11: 590–4.
54. Neev J, Tadir Y, Ho P, et al. Microscope-delivered ultraviolet laser zona dissection: principles and practices. J Assist Reprod Genet 1992; 9: 513–23.
55. Blanchet GB, Russell JB, Fincher CR, Portman M. Laser micromanipulation in the mouse embryo: a novel approach to zona drilling. Fertil Steril 1992; 57: 1337–41.
56. Neev J, Schiewe M, Sung VW, et al. Assisted hatching in mouse embryos using a noncontact Ho:YSGG laser system. J Assist Reprod Genet 1995; 12: 288–93.
57. Schiewe M, Neev J, Hazeleger NL, et al. Developmental competence of mouse embryos following zona drilling using a non-contact Ho:YSGG laser system. Hum Reprod 1995; 10: 1821–4.
58. Rink K, Delacretaz G, Salathe RP, et al. Non-contact microdrilling of mouse zona pellucida with an objective-delivered 1.48-microns diode laser. Laser Surg Med 1996; 18: 52–62.
59. Germond M, Nocera D, Senn A, et al. Microdissection of mouse and human zona pellucida using a 1.48 μm diode laser beam: efficacy and safety of the procedure. Fertil Steril 1995; 64: 604–11.
60. Germond M, Nocera D, Senn A, et al. Improved fertilization and implantation rates after non touch zona pellucida microdrilling of mouse oocytes with a 1.48 μm diode laser beam. Hum Reprod 1996; 11: 1043–8.
61. Baruffi R, Mauri AL, Petersen C, et al. Assisted hatching with a laser diode in patients <37 years old with no previous failure of implantation: a prospective randomized study [Abstracts of the 15th Annual meeting of the ESHRE, Tours, France]. Hum Reprod 1999; 14: abstr book 1.
62. Montag M, Van der Ven K, Delacretaz G, et al. Laser assisted microdissection of the zona pellucida facilitates polar body biopsy. Fertil Steril 1998; 69: 539–42.
63. Boada M, Carrera M, de la Iglesia C, et al. Successful use of a laser for human embryo biopsy in preimplantation genetic diagnosis: report of two cases. J Assist Reprod Genet 1998; 15: 302–7.
64. Veiga A, Sandalinas M, Benkhalifa M, et al. Laser blastocyst biopsy for preimplantation diagnosis in the human. Zygote 1997; 5: 351–4.
65. Antinori S, Selman HA, Caffa B, et al. Zona opening of human embryos using a non contact UV laser for assisted hatching in patients with poor prognosis of pregnancy. Hum Reprod 1996; 11: 2488–92.
66. Antinori S, Versaci C, Dani L, et al. Laser assisted hatching at the extremes of the IVF spectrum: first cycle and after 6 cycles: a randomized prospective

trial [Abstracts of the 15th Annual Meeting of the ESHRE, Tours, France]. Hum Reprod 1999; 14: abstr book 1.
67. Douglas-Hamilton DH, Conia J. Thermal effects in laser-assisted pre-embryo zona drilling. J Biomed Optics 2001; 6: 205–13.
68. Chatzimeletiou K, Picton HM, Handyside AH. Use of a non-contact, infrared laser for zona drilling of mouse embryos: assessment of immediate effects on blastomere viability. Reprod Biomed Online 2001; 2: 178–87.
69. Tinney GM, Windt ML, Kruger TF, Lombard CJ. Use of a zona laser treatment system in assisted hatching: optimal laser utilization parameters. Fertil Steril 2005; 84: 1737–41.
70. Jones AE, Wright G, Kort HI, et al. Comparison of laser-assisted hatching and acidified Tyrode's hatching by evaluation of blastocyst development rates in sibling embryos: a prospective randomized trial. Fertil Steril 2006; 85: 487–91.
71. Makrakis E, Angeli I, Agapitou K, et al. Laser versus mechanical assisted hatching: a prospective study of clinical outcomes. Fertil Steril 2006; 86: 1596–600.
72. Tucker MJ, Luecke NM, Wiker SR, Wright G. Chemical removal of the outside of the zona pellucida of day 3 human embryos has no impact on implantation rate. J Assist Reprod Genet 1993; 10: 187–91.
73. Kung FT, Lin YC, Tseng YJ, et al. Transfer of frozen–thawed blastocysts that underwent quarter laser-assisted hatching at the day 3 cleaving stage before freezing. Fertil Steril 2003; 79: 893–9.
74. Hellebaut S, De Sutter P, Dozortsev D, et al. Does assisted hatching improve implantation rates after in vitro fertilization or intracytoplasmic sperm injection in all patients? A prospective randomized study. J Assist Reprod Genet 1996; 13: 19–22.
75. Petersen CG, Mauri AL, Baruffi RL, et al. Implantation failures: success of assisted hatching with quarter-laser zona thinning. RBM Online 2005; 10: 224–9.
76. Ghobara TS, Cahill DJ, Ford WCL, et al. Effects of assisted hatching method and age on implantation rates of IVF and ICSI. RBM Online 2006; 13: 261–7.
77. Balaban B, Urman B, Alatas C, et al. A comparison of four different techniques of assisted hatching. Hum Reprod 2002; 17: 1239–43.
78. Sifer C, Sellami A, Poncelet C, et al. A prospective randomized study to assess the benefit of partial zona pellucida digestion before frozen-thawed embryo. Hum Reprod 2006; 21: 2384–9.
79. Ng EHY, Naveed F, Lau EYL, et al. A randomized double-blind controlled study of the efficacy of laser-assisted hatching on implantation and pregnancy rates of frozen-thawed embryo transfer at the cleavage stage. Hum Reprod 2005; 20: 979–85.
80. Petersen CG, Mauri AL, Baruffi RL, et al. Laser-assisted hatching of cryopreserved-thawed embryos by thinning one quarter of the zona. RBM Online 2006; 13: 668–75.
81. Valojerdi MR, Eftekhari-Yazdi P, Karimian L, et al. Effect of laser zona thinning on vitrified-warmed embryo transfer at the cleavage stage: a prospective, randomized study. RBM Online 2010; 20: 234–42.
82. Fang C, Li T, Miao BY, et al. Mechanically expanding the zona pellucida of human frozen thawed embryos: a new method of assisted hatching. Fertil Steril 2010; 94: 1302–7.
83. Nijs M, Vanderzwalmen P, Segal-Berti G, et al. A monozygotic twin pregnancy after application of zona rubbing on a frozen–thawed blastocyst. Hum Reprod 1993; 8: 127–9.
84. Fong CY, Bongso A, Ng SC, et al. Blastocyst transfer after enzymatic treatment of the zona pellucida: improving in vitro fertilization and understanding implantation. Hum Reprod 1998; 13: 2926–32.
85. Park S, Kim EY, Yoon SH, Chung KS, Lim JH. Enhanced hatching rate of bovine IVM/IVF/IVC blastocysts using a 1.48 μm diode laser beam. J Assist Reprod Genet 1999; 16: 97–101.
86. Veiga A, Torelló MJ, Ménézo Y, et al. Use of co-culture of human embryos on Vero cells to improve clinical implantation rate. Hum Reprod 1999; 14: 112–20.
87. Nadir H, Bener F, Karagenc L, et al. Impact of assisted hatching on ART outcome in women with endometriosis. Hum Reprod 2005; 20: 2546–9.
88. Rienzi L, Ubaldi F, Iacobelli M, et al. Developmental potential of fully intact and partially damaged cryopreserved embryos after laser-assisted removal of necrotic blastomeres and post-thaw culture selection. Fertil Steril 2005; 84: 888–94.
89. Das S, Blake D, Farquhar C, et al. Assisted hatching on assisted conception (IVF and ICSI). Cochrane Database Syst Rev 2009: CD001894.
90. Martins WP, Rocha IA, Ferriani RA, et al. Assisted hatching of human embryos: a systematic review and meta-analysis of randomized controlled trials. Hum Reprod Update 2011; 17: 438–53.
91. Oliviennes F, Bergere M, Fanchin R, et al. L'éclosion embryonnaire assistée. Contracept Fertil Sex 1994; 22: 493–7.
92. Tucker M, Ingargiola P, Massey JB, et al. Assisted hatching with or without bovine oviductal epithelial cell co-culture for poor prognosis in vitro fertilization patients. Hum Reprod 1994; 9: 1528–31.
93. Schoolcraft WB, Schlenker T, Jones GS, Jones HW. In vitro fertilization in women age 40 and older: the impact of assisted hatching. J Assist Reprod Genet 1995; 12: 581–4.
94. Stein A, Rufas O, Amit S, et al. Assisted hatching by partial zona dissection of human pre-embryos in patients with recurrent implantation failure after in vitro fertilization. Fertil Steril 1995; 63: 838–41.
95. Check JH, Hoover L, Nazari A, O'Shaughnessy A, Summers D. The effect of assisted hatching on pregnancy rates after frozen embryo transfer. Fertil Steril 1996; 65: 254–7.
96. Tucker MJ, Morton PC, Wright G, et al. Enhancement of outcome from intracytoplasmic sperm injection: does co-culture or assisted hatching improve implantation rates? Hum Reprod 1996; 11: 2434–7.
97. Bider D, Livshits A, Yonish M, et al. Assisted hatching by zona drilling of human embryos in women of advanced age. Hum Reprod 1997; 12: 317–20.
98. Chao KH, Chen SU, Chen HF, et al. Assisted hatching increases the implantation and pregnancy rate of in vitro fertilization (IVF)– embryo transfer (ET), but not that of IVF–tubal ET in patients with repeated IVF failures. Fertil Steril 1997; 67: 904–8.
99. Hurst BS, Tucker KE, Awoniyi CA, Schlaff WD. Assisted hatching does not enhance IVF success in good-prognosis patients. J Assist Reprod Genet 1998; 15: 62–4.

100. Magli MC, Gianaroli L, Ferraretti AP, et al. Rescue of implantation potential in embryos with poor prognosis by assisted zona hatching. Hum Reprod 1998; 13: 1331–5.
101. Lanzendorf SE, Nehchiri F, Mayer JF, Oehninger S, Muasher SJ. A prospective, randomized, double-blind study for the evaluation of assisted hatching in patients with advanced maternal age. Hum Reprod 1998; 13: 409–13.
102. Meldrum DR, Wisot A, Yee B, et al. Assisted hatching reduces the age-related decline in IVF outcome in women younger than age 43 without increasing miscarriage or monozygotic twinning. J Assist Reprod Genet 1998; 15: 418–21.
103. Edirisinghe WR, Ahnonkitpanit V, Promviengchai S, et al. A study failing to determine significant benefits from assisted hatching: patients selected for advanced age, zonal thickness of embryos, and previous failed attempts. J Assist Reprod Genet 1999; 16: 294–301.
104. Alikani M, Cohen J, Tomkin G, et al. Human embryo fragmentation in vitro and its implications for pregnancy and implantation. Fertil Steril 1999; 71: 836–42.
105. Nakayama T, Fujiwara H, Yamada S, et al. Clinical application of a new assisted hatching method using a piezo-micromanipulator for morphologically low-quality embryos in poor-prognosis infertile patients. Fertil Steril 1999; 71: 1014–18.
106. Mansour RT, Rhodes CA, Aboulghar MA, Serour GI, Kamal A. Transfer of zona-free embryos improves outcome in poor prognosis patients: a prospective randomized controlled study. Hum Reprod 2000; 15: 1061–4.
107. Mantoudis E, Podsiadly BT, Gorgy A, Venkat G, Craft IL. A comparison between quarter, partial and total laser assisted hatching in selected infertility patients. Hum Reprod 2001; 16: 2182–6.
108. Malter H, Schimmel T, Cohen J. Zona dissection by infrared laser: developmental consequences in the mouse, technical considerations, and controlled clinical trial. Reprod BioMed Online 2001; 3: 117–23.
109. Hsieh YY, Huang CC, Cheng TC, et al. Laser-assisted hatching of embryos is better than the chemical method for enhancing the pregnancy rate in women with advanced age. Fertil Steril 2002; 78: 179–82.
110. Milki AA, Hinckley MD, Behr B. Comparison of blastocyst transfer to day 3 transfer with assisted hatching in the older patient. Fertil Steril 2002; 78: 1244–7.
111. Gabrielsen A, Agerholm I, Toft B, et al. Assisted hatching improves implantation rates on cryopreserved-thawed embryos. A randomized prospective study. Hum Reprod 2004; 19: 2258–62.
112. Frydman N, Madoux S, Hesters L, et al. A randomized double-blind controlled study on the efficacy of laser zona pellucida thinning on live birth rates in cases of advanced female age. Hum Reprod 2006; 21: 2131–5.
113. Balaban B, Urman B, Yakin K, Isiklar F. Laser-assisted hatching increases pregnancy and implantation rates in cryopreserved embryos that were allowed to cleave in vitro after thawing: a prospective randomized study. Hum Reprod 2006; 21: 2136–40.
114. Sagoskin AW, Levy MJ, Tucker MJ, et al. Laser assisted hatching in good prognosis patients undergoing in vitro fertilization-embryo transfer: a randomized controlled trial. Fertil Steril 2007; 87: 283–7.

15

Human embryo biopsy procedures

Alan R. Thornhill, Christian Ottolini, and Alan H. Handyside

INTRODUCTION

In the mid-1980s, the development of polymerase chain reaction (PCR) strategies for amplification of specific fragments of DNA from single cells (1–3) facilitated preimplantation genetic diagnosis (PGD) of inherited disease using one or more cells biopsied from embryos at preimplantation stages after in vitro fertilization (IVF) (4). Currently, PGD requires the removal of one or more cells from each embryo, making embryo biopsy comparable to amniocentesis or chorionic villus sampling at fetal stages, since the primary aim is the removal of sufficient embryonic tissue to allow diagnosis.

Embryo biopsy is a two-step micromanipulation process involving the penetration or removal of part of the zona pellucida surrounding the oocyte or embryo followed by removal of one or more cells. Theoretically, this can be accomplished at any developmental stage between the mature oocyte and blastocyst, but to date only three discrete stages have been proposed: polar body, cleavage stage, and blastocyst. Clearly, each of these stages is biologically different, and thus the strategic considerations have both advantages and disadvantages (Table 15.1). Furthermore, the different biopsy strategies, both between and within developmental stages, require different technical approaches (Table 15.2), each providing varying prospects of success.

Many of the biopsy techniques currently in use for human embryos were pioneered in animal models, notably the mouse (5,6), rabbit, (7,8) cow, (9) and marmoset (10). While the total number of human embryos biopsied in clinical cases is vast, relatively little work has been published to define the relative merits of different biopsy methods and their safety and efficacy in clinical application. This chapter describes the three stages of biopsy – polar body, cleavage stage (blastomere) and blastocyst (trophectoderm) – routinely used in clinical practice (11).

PENETRATION OF THE ZONA PELLUCIDA

Until the advent of noncontact lasers for use in micromanipulation (see below), two basic methods were employed for penetrating the zona. Both of these were pursued initially as a means to enhance fertilization rates with oligozoospermic men, and have now been overtaken for this purpose by the use of intracytoplasmic sperm injection (ICSI).

The first approach, partial zona dissection, involves using a fine needle to penetrate through the zona and, avoiding damage to the oocyte or embryo, penetrating out through the zona again at a distance around the circumference (12). The embryo can then be detached from the holding pipette as it is effectively held on the needle, and a gentle rubbing action against the side of the holding pipette used to make a slit between the two apertures generated by the needle. Although a narrow-diameter micropipette can be pushed through such a slit, it is difficult to use one large enough to aspirate cleavage-stage blastomeres, and with the human embryo, pressure on the zona can lead to lysis of blastomeres and/or, where a slit has been made, force blastomeres out through the slit.

The second approach is used for embryo biopsy in some centers, but requires highly skilled micromanipulation, can be difficult to control, does not allow precise selection of blastomeres, and the risk of lysis can be high. A modification is to make two slits to create a "flap" or "cross" in the zona that can be flipped open, allowing more flexibility in the size of the opening created. This method is effective for both polar body and blastomere biopsy (13).

In general, mechanical methods for zona penetration are time consuming and require skillful micromanipulation, possibly making them inaccessible to some IVF laboratories. As an alternative, zona drilling using acid Tyrode's solution (pH 2.2–2.4) to dissolve the zona glycoproteins has been extensively used and is commercially available from most culture media manufacturers. Again, this method was developed in the mouse embryo model, as a possible means to improve fertilization rates with low sperm densities (14). However, its use with human oocytes, while increasing the incidence of fertilization, arrested the further development of the zygote, presumably consequent to changes in intracellular pH (15). With zona drilling, the effect of the acid Tyrode's solution is localized to a small area of the zona using a fine micropipette with an inner diameter of 5–10 μm.

The micropipette filled with acid Tyrode's solution is brought into direct contact with the zona at the appropriate position, and a combination of slight pulling away and "stroking" movements is used to control the flow of acid

Table 15.1 Strategic Considerations of Biopsy at Different Developmental Stages for Preimplantation Genetic Diagnosis

Developmental stage	Advantages	Disadvantages
Oocyte (1st polar body)	Cell removal has no effect on embryo development	Only 1 cell available for analysis
	Increased time to perform diagnosis prior to transfer	Increased risk of diagnostic error
	Can transfer between PN stage and day 2 or beyond	Gender determination not possible
	~85% aneuploidy originates in maternal meiosis	Diagnose maternal aneuploidy (MI) and inherited disease only
	Homogeneous oocyte quality at biopsy	Misses meiosis II errors (30%) and post-zygotic aneuploidy
	High proportion of oocyte cohort available for biopsy	Single cell sensitive analysis required
	Favored for some ethical, legal and societal frameworks	Relatively labor-intensive/high cost to test all samples
	Facilitates fresh cleavage/blastocyst stage embryo transfer	Additional follow-up confirmatory testing often needed
(1st + 2nd polar bodies)	2 cells for analysis (greater accuracy/reliability)	Diagnose maternal aneuploidy (MI/MII) & inherited disease only
	Cell removal has no effect on embryo development	Gender determination not possible
	Increased time to perform diagnosis prior to transfer	Simultaneous biopsy (1st polar body may degenerate)
	Allows embryo transfer from day 2 onwards	Sequential biopsy (extra manipulations required)
	Homogeneous oocyte quality at biopsy	Single cell sensitive analysis required
	High proportion of oocyte cohort available for biopsy	Labor-intensive/high cost to test all samples
	Favored for some ethical, legal and societal frameworks	Additional follow-up confirmatory testing often needed
	Facilitates fresh cleavage/blastocyst stage embryo transfer	Misses post-zygotic aneuploidy
Cleavage stage (blastomeres)	Diagnose maternal/paternal aneuploidy & inherited disease	Chromosomal mosaicism compromises accuracy
	Gender determination possible	Choice of blastomere is critical
	Large body of clinical data available	Time for analysis limited to 48–72 hrs (fresh transfer)
	1–3 cells available for analysis	Most cells in interphase (no karyotypic data)
	Biopsied embryos develop into normal blastocysts	Reduced embryo implantation potential post-biopsy
		Single cell sensitive analysis required
		Heterogeneous embryo quality/stage at biopsy
		Requires extended culture for fresh embryo transfer
		Additional follow-up confirmatory testing often needed
		Requires biopsy of large proportion of cell mass
		Relatively labor-intensive/high cost to test all cells
Blastocyst (Trophectoderm)	Sample multiple (up to 10) cells on day 5/6	Time for analysis may be limited
	Increased amplification efficiency and accuracy (reduce ADO)	Blastocysts may need cryopreservation
	Increased scope for diagnostic testing (genes + chromosomes)	Requires extended culture for fresh embryo transfer
	Homogeneous embryo quality preselected (high implantation rate)	High rate of cancellation prior to embryo transfer
	Trophectoderm sampled rather than inner cell mass	TE cells may not represent embryo proper
	Fewer embryos (reduces diagnostic burden and cost)	Few embryos (compromises aneuploidy risk assessment)
	Post-zygotic aneuploidy detection	Operator dependent biopsy success and safety
	Gender determination possible	Avoidance of inner cell mass critical
	Embryo more robust to withstand biopsy	
	Embryo has 'genetic stability'	
	Lowest diagnostic failure rate	
	Highest positive predictive value (PPV)	

and the area to be drilled, respectively. Medium pH was originally maintained by employing phosphate-buffered saline but is now routinely maintained using a modified culture medium buffered with either 4-morpholinopropanesulfonic acid (MOPS) or 4-(2-hydroxyethyl)-1-piperazineethane sulfonic acid (HEPES). When the drilling is complete, the micropipette is immediately withdrawn.

The shift across centers worldwide from zona drilling using acid Tyrode's solution (16) to laser ablation of the zona pellucida has been dramatic. Indeed, according to a survey of PGD centers, the laser has overtaken acid Tyrode's solution as the most popular form of zona ablation, accounting for 60% cleavage-stage embryo biopsies (11). This shift is likely associated with ease of use and the elimination of the need for a double tool holder rather than any measurable improvement in safety or efficacy.

The preferred model of laser is the near-infrared solid-state compact diode 1.48 µm laser. The advantage of using light as a cutting tool is that it obviates the need for disposable or reusable cutting tools, it is extremely precise; if used appropriately it provides consistent, repeatable, and rapid results. Moreover, since neither microtools nor reagents are required to dissect the zona, the opportunity

Table 15.2 Embryo Biopsy Methods – Benefits, Limitations and Factors Critical to Success

Zona penetration method	Benefits	Limitations	Factors critical to success
Mechanical	Least invasive to embryo (safer)	Steep learning curve	Operator skill and speed
	Inexpensive, portable technique	Operator dependent	Appropriate microtools needed
	Improved survival after freeze-thaw?	Time consuming	Double tool holder optimal
Chemical (acidified tyrodes)	Relatively inexpensive	Operator dependent	Acidified tyrodes pH 2.2–2.4
	Widespread clinical use	Effect on cryopreservation	Sensitive control of acid flow
	Portable technique	Difficult to limit aperture size	Rinsing acid from embryos
			Double tool holder optimal
Laser (1.48 µm non-contact)	Rapid and reproducible	Cost (30–60,000 US dollars)	Laser alignment and calibration
	Simple to use	Not all systems portable	Pulse number, location & duration
	Integrated archiving/analysis software	Invisible thermal damage/stress	Distance between laser and zona
			Appropriate training and validation

Cell removal method

Cleavage stage blastomere biopsy

Aspiration	Ability to select a specific cell for analysis	Cell lysis during aspiration	Appropriate microtools needed
			Sensitive suction device needed
Fluid displacement	No contact between pipette and cells	Limited ability to select cell	Operator skill essential
	Rapid		
Mechanical displacement	No contact between pipette and cells	Limited ability to select cell	Operator skill essential
	Rapid	Damage to non-biopsied cells	

Trophectoderm sampling

Spontaneous hatching/herniation	Non-invasive (cells undisturbed within zona)	No control over timing/cell numbers	High blastocyst development rate
		Time for analysis very limited Asynchronous development/hatching	Hatching blastocyst in vitro
Zona penetration + herniation **or**	Pre-empts spontaneous hatching	As above	
Stitch and pull **or**	Rapid/some control over cells sampled	Biopsied/non-biopsied cell damage	Operator skill essential
aspiration/laser ablation	Rapid/some control over cells sampled	Biopsied/non-biopsied cell damage	Operator skill essential
Zona ablation and immediate aspiration with laser dissociation of sampled cells	Blastocysts biopsied at optimal stages	Laser damage may reduce diagnostic reliability of sampled cells	Operator skill essential
	Control over hatching site (away from ICM)		

for introducing contamination or pH changes in the medium surrounding the embryo is greatly reduced. The 1.48 µm diode laser is small but at the appropriate pulse duration can emit light at power levels sufficient to cause selective thermal disruption of the zona pellucida glycoproteins and is not absorbed by water.

This noncontact laser can be inserted into the body of the microscope on which the manipulations take place or it can be integrated in a special objective and the beam delivered to the target through the dish. Since the laser beam travels up through an objective which lies below the sample, localized heating causes denaturation of the zona proteins in a cylindrical spot where the laser beam is focused, and the size of the aperture created is controlled by adjusting the duration of the laser pulse. The thermal energy created produces a groove in the zona perpendicular to the microscope stage, rather than a circular aperture. However, an "aperture" is produced in the zona at the point at which the zona is perpendicular to the microscope stage. The size of the aperture (or more accurately the width of the groove at its widest point) created in the zona ranges from 5 to 20 µm and is governed by the pulse irradiation time (ranging from 3 to 100 msec) or the accumulation of pulses along the length of the zona margin. The precision of the laser is illustrated by the fact that drilled mouse and human embryos show no sign of extraneous thermal damage under light or scanning microscopy (17).

Many centers use this equipment for assisted hatching as well as PGD (18) and there appears to be no detrimental effect of the laser itself on the development to the blastocyst stage or pregnancy rates in animal and human studies (19–23). However, studies of the immediate effects at the blastomere level in a mouse model have shown that the laser can cause damage if used inappropriately (24). Certainly, if the laser beam is fired in an area in direct contact with a blastomere, its viability is always compromised. However, as the pulse length and therefore localized heating is increased, the distance between the laser beam and blastomere required to avoid damage increases. Hence, care is required to drill the zona away from underlying blastomeres and from as far away as possible, and also to use minimum pulse lengths to restrict any damaging effects.

Several practical guidelines have emerged to ensure safe and effective use of the laser for human embryo biopsy as follows. A single aperture is used for cellular aspiration as double or multiple apertures may cause problems during embryo hatching as the embryo will attempt to hatch out of multiple openings, which could compromise further inner cell mass (ICM) development or lead to an increased monozygotic twinning rate. To generate the desired aperture, it is preferable to use several pulses of short duration rather than a single pulse of long duration and high energy, which could cause thermal damage. During laser use, it is imperative to maintain the oocyte or embryo as close to the bottom of the biopsy dish as possible to allow a focused beam to ablate the zona pellucida. As the embryo is raised above the dish surface, the beam energy is diffused and can create localized heating or simply prevent effective ablation of the zona.

POLAR BODY BIOPSY

Neither the first nor second polar body is required for successful fertilization or normal embryonic development. Thus, removal of either the first or second polar body or both for the purposes of genetic diagnosis should have no deleterious effect per se on the developing embryo. Originally, it was suggested that biopsy and genetic analysis of the first polar body would allow PGD of maternal defects prior to conception (25). Apart from some arguable practical advantages (see below), this concept was also attractive as it involves manipulation of only the human egg and not the fertilized embryo, and would therefore be more acceptable to those with moral or ethical objections to screening embryos, as is the legal situation in some European countries including Switzerland (26). For preconception diagnosis, either the first polar body alone or both the first and second polar bodies may be biopsied to provide genetic information relating to a particular embryo.

Initially, preconception diagnosis focused on the former approach. However, biopsy of the first polar body has limited applicability for PGD for a number of reasons. The process of polar body biopsy is relatively labor-intensive and may involve the micromanipulation of oocytes that ultimately do not develop into therapeutic quality embryos. The procedure only allows the detection of maternal genetic defects, and crossing-over of homologous chromosomes during meiosis I can prevent identification of the maternal allele remaining in the oocyte, leading to a reduction in the number of embryos available for transfer (27). Also there is only the possibility of a single cell for analysis, leading to a lower overall reliability (in contrast to cleavage-stage biopsy in which two cells may be taken for independent analysis). As a consequence, it was suggested that more misdiagnoses would result from polar body analyses when compared with blastomere analysis (28) and, to overcome these disadvantages, both the first and second polar bodies were removed for analysis (29) after first assessing the safety of removing the second polar body in a mouse model (30). This approach has been successfully applied to PGD for the detection of a large number and variety of different single gene disorders, chromosomal aneuploidies, and maternal chromosome translocations (29,31).

The first polar body can be removed from the oocyte on the day of the oocyte collection between 36 and 42 hours after injection of human chorionic gonadotropin (hCG), as long as the oocyte has entered metaphase II and fully extruded the first polar body (25). To perform polar body biopsy by mechanical means, a holding pipette and a beveled micropipette (12–15 µm in diameter) are needed. The oocyte is held in place with the polar body at the 12 o'clock position. The beveled micropipette is passed through the zona and into the perivitelline space tangentially toward the polar body. The polar body may then be aspirated into the pipette. Alternatively, after mechanical zona dissection to form a flap or cross or laser ablation, an aspiration micropipette is introduced into the perivitelline space, and the polar body removed. If the polar body is still attached to the ooplasm, further incubation may be required to permit complete extrusion (25).

Most approaches to polar body biopsy have adopted mechanical or laser techniques rather than chemical methods. While live offspring resulted after treating the zona pellucida of mouse oocytes with acid Tyrode's solution, studies using human oocytes showed that, despite fertilization, there was an inhibitory effect on embryonic development (15) due to a direct effect of acid on the oocyte spindle, possibly as a result of the difference in thickness of the human and mouse zona pellucida.

The first and second polar body can be removed simultaneously (29) from the zygote between 18 and 22 hours post-insemination, but the first polar body may have degenerated by this time, causing possible diagnostic failure and leading practitioners to aim for much earlier simultaneous biopsy at 8–9 hours post-ICSI (32). Simultaneous biopsy of the two polar bodies is acceptable for fluorescent in situ hybridization (FISH) analysis, since they can provide distinguishable results (32). Moreover, the polar bodies are morphologically distinguishable: the first polar body tends to have a crinkled surface and may fragment; the second polar body is generally smooth and may have a visible interphase nucleus under interference contrast. However, a sequential biopsy of polar bodies, where the first polar body is removed on day 0 and the second polar body on day 1 is recommended for PCR analysis to determine recombination events between the first and second polar body. In addition to the obvious advantages of not damaging the embryo and allowing a maximum time for genetic analysis, at a technical level, analysis of both polar bodies allows detection of allele drop-out (ADO). ADO is the random amplification failure of one parental allele after PCR from single cells (33), and is therefore a significant source of potential error in PGD. Despite the removal of both polar bodies, in many cases, cleavage-stage biopsy may also be required to confirm the polar body diagnosis.

Despite the large number of cycles reported using polar body biopsy and analysis, relatively few centers have used the approach. This may be the result of a number of factors. First, the approach can only be applied to maternally inherited diseases. Secondly, diseases that are detected by assessing changes in gene product (34) are not candidates for this approach. Thirdly, polar body biopsy cannot be used for gender determination. Finally, biopsy of both the first and second polar bodies is required for optimal diagnostic efficiency and, although this can be achieved by either sequential or simultaneous biopsy with successful results, it is labor-intensive and may involve oocytes and zygotes, which, ultimately, do not develop into therapeutic-quality embryos. If polar bodies are sampled sequentially and cleavage-stage blastomere confirmation is required, three independent manipulations are needed, with the possibility of ICSI inbetween (for PCR-based cases), making a total of four manipulations on the same oocyte and embryo. However, in experienced hands, the three independent biopsy manipulations appear to have no deleterious effect on development (35,36).

CLEAVAGE-STAGE EMBRYO BIOPSY

The first PGD cycles were carried out in late 1989 in a series of couples at risk of X-linked disease and involved cleavage-stage embryo biopsy (37). Cleavage-stage biopsy has remained the most widely practiced form of embryo biopsy worldwide (according to ESHRE PGD Consortium, it accounts for around 90% of all reported PGD cycles (11)). However, there have been a number of modifications and improvements since 1989. In the first cases, a tapered micropipette with a narrow lumen (internal diameter 5–7 µm) containing acidified Tyrode's solution (pH 2.2–2.4) was used to drill relatively large apertures (20–30 µm) in the zona.

The pipette is placed close to the zona pellucida and the acidified solution gently expelled from the pipette until the zona thins and an aperture is drilled (in some cases, the zona can be seen to "pop" as an aperture is made). The flow can be controlled via an oil-filled syringe (hydraulic), air-filled syringe (pneumatic), or by using a mouth pipette. The human zona is bilayered and the zona drilling process must be carefully monitored as the outer layer dissolves more rapidly than the inner layer. Moreover, there is great variation in zonae pellucidae, between and within cohorts of human oocytes and embryos. The final diameter of the aperture made will be determined by a combination of the above factors. An excessively large aperture may result in the unwanted loss of blastomeres but, more significantly, may indicate that the blastomeres were exposed to potentially damaging quantities of acid, which could compromise further development. A second micropipette, filled with the biopsy medium and held in a double holder alongside the acid Tyrode's pipette, can be used to aspirate single cells (38–40).

It is possible to use a single micropipette for both drilling and aspiration, but care is needed to prevent overexposure to acid (41,42). Any advantage accrued in terms of speed of the procedure may be offset by potential damage as a result of overexposure to acid.

Cleavage stage biopsy using laser and blastomere aspiration is typically performed as follows: following laser ablation of the zona pellucida adjacent to the blastomere selected for analysis, the blastomere is aspirated by gentle suction using a polished pipette. The aperture may be sited adjacent to either a selected blastomere or a subzonal space between blastomeres. A finely polished "sampling" pipette (internal diameter of 30–40 µm, depending on the cell size) is used to aspirate the blastomere. The pipette is placed through the aperture, close to the blastomere to be aspirated. By gentle suction, the blastomere is drawn into the pipette while the pipette is withdrawn from the aperture. The aperture of the sampling pipette is critical for successful biopsy. If the internal diameter is too large for the cell being removed, the pipette will have little purchase on that cell, which may result in unwanted suction of nonbiopsied cells. Conversely, an undersized pipette will cause the biopsied cell to be squeezed unnecessarily, resulting in blebbing on the cell membrane and ultimately lysis, which will probably reduce the chances of a successful diagnosis in that embryo. Similarly, use of a holding pipette with an internal diameter of 30 µm (i.e., larger than a regular ICSI holding pipette) ensures safe and reliable suction on the zona, particularly during difficult biopsies.

Once the blastomere is free of the embryo, it is gently expelled from the sampling pipette. Following biopsy, the embryo should be rinsed in the culture medium at least twice to remove residual embryo biopsy medium and acid Tyrode's solution (if applicable) before returning to culture. The blastomere should be washed extensively in the handling medium before proceeding with the analysis. The most frequently used method of blastomere removal is aspiration, but other methods have been described and used clinically, although no studies have been conducted to compare their relative safety and efficacy. In the extrusion method, after zona pellucida drilling, the blastomere is extruded through the aperture by pushing against the zona at another site (usually at 90° to the aperture) using a blunt pipette (43). The slit in the zona pellucida can be introduced using mechanical means, chemical (acid Tyrode's solution) exposure or laser ablation. Another variation in the method of cell removal involves fluid displacement, whereby the culture medium surrounding the embryo is used to displace individual cells following a zona breach. This method was pioneered in mouse embryos by introducing a slit in the zona with a sharpened needle and, through a second puncture site, injecting medium to dislodge the blastomere through the first puncture site (44). This method requires the production of two separate apertures and considerable skill to displace the blastomere of choice, but was modified for clinical application (45). Challenges common to both of these methods are to ensure the selected cell is removed and the difficulties encountered when two different cells are required for analysis.

Practical Considerations for Embryo Biopsy

Preparation Before Biopsy

ICSI is recommended for all PCR cases to reduce the chance of paternal contamination from extraneous sperm attached to the zona pellucida or nondecondensed sperm within blastomeres. Similarly, all cumulus cells should be removed before biopsy, as these cells can contaminate both FISH and PCR diagnosis. Embryo and blastomere identity (individual drops or dishes) should be checked throughout the procedure so that diagnostic results can be reliably linked to specific embryos (46,47). The use of a standard IVF culture medium during biopsy is acceptable, but its effectiveness may be highly dependent upon the developmental stage of the embryo biopsied. Commercially produced calcium- and magnesium-free (Ca^{2+}/Mg^{2+} free) medium is widely available and is used by many centers for routine clinical cleavage-stage biopsy, with the benefit of reducing the frequency of cell lysis combined with a shorter time needed to perform the biopsy procedure (46,48).

Timing of Biopsy

Since the first clinical application of PGD, culture media have been improved and optimized, and the new generation of media are designed, tested, and manufactured to high-quality control standards specifically for clinical use. Although embryos developed to the blastocyst stage, pregnancy rates after transfer were very low and, importantly for embryo biopsy, most embryos did not appear to compact. With the newer media, compaction on day 3 is much more pronounced, which has necessitated the use of calcium and magnesium-free (Ca^{2+}/Mg^{2+} free) medium to reverse the initial calcium-dependent adhesion (48). The use of Ca^{2+}/Mg^{2+} free medium also facilitates later biopsy (i.e., beyond the eight-cell stage), making the timings more flexible. Most cleavage-stage biopsy takes place on the third morning following insemination, although the exact timing varies according to timings of procedures in different laboratories.

One variation is to alter the timing of ICSI to allow cleavage-stage biopsy at the same embryonic stage, but late on day 2 (biopsy at earlier cleavage stages on day 2 may adversely affect embryo development (49)), allowing more time for genetic analysis. In cases where retarded development is observed, the possibility of delaying the biopsy procedure to allow diagnosis of a larger proportion of the embryo cohort should be considered. Furthermore, as a result of increased use of sequential media and experience with blastocyst culture and transfer, most groups routinely delay transfer until day 4 or 5, allowing more time for analysis and with the additional aim of improving pregnancy and implantation rates, because developing embryos that have undergone further cleavage divisions following biopsy can be preferentially selected for transfer.

Most laboratories exclude very poor-quality embryos or those not reaching a predefined cell stage from the embryo biopsy procedure. Of centers surveyed, most will consider only embryos at the five-cell stage and beyond for biopsy (16). Biopsy at the four-cell stage in mice results in a distorted allocation of cells to the ICM, and trophectoderm (TE) and abnormal post-implantation development (50), whereas human embryos biopsied on day 2 show cleavage rate retardation and smaller blastocysts (49). Conversely, four-cell stage human embryos surviving freeze–thaw procedures with the loss of one or more blastomeres can develop, implant, and result in live birth, albeit at a reduced rate compared with nonfrozen embryos. Stringent biopsy policies have the benefits that fewer embryos need to be biopsied and fewer cells prepared and tested, with only developmentally competent embryos considered. On the down side, an opportunity to identify genotypes on a full cohort of embryos may be lost.

Number of Cells to be Removed During Cleavage-Stage Biopsy

To decide how many cells to biopsy from cleavage-stage embryos, it is necessary to balance diagnostic accuracy with potential to implant and develop, which is progressively compromised as a greater proportion of the embryo is removed (51). There is no consensus on the number of blastomeres that can be safely removed during cleavage-stage embryo biopsy. In many centers, a second blastomere is removed from embryos having seven or more cells, regardless of the type of analysis involved, but this approach has been criticized as compromising the implantation potential of the biopsied embryo based on extrapolation from frozen–thaw embryo implantation rates (52).

The decision to remove one or two cells is based on many factors, including the embryo cell number and the accuracy and reliability of the diagnostic test used. If removal of two cells is considered, it is recommended that it is undertaken only on embryos with six or more cells (53). While removal of two blastomeres decreases the likelihood of blastocyst formation, compared with removal of one blastomere, day 3 in vitro developmental stage is a stronger predictor for day 5 developmental potential than the removal of one or two cells. The biopsy of only one cell significantly lowers the efficiency of a

PCR-based diagnosis, whereas the efficiency of the FISH PGD procedure remains similar whether one or two cells are removed. However, a randomized trial demonstrated that live-birth rate was compromised at a level of one birth for every 33 cycles of two-cell embryo biopsy, suggesting that, ideally, one-cell biopsy should always be performed unless the diagnostic test is suboptimal (54). In the case of lost or anucleate blastomeres and failed diagnosis, rebiopsy of embryos is possible but embryo cell number and timing of rebiopsy should be considered to avoid excessive harm to the embryo. Although technically challenging, the original zona breach site should be accessed to prevent later problems with embryos hatching via multiple hatching sites. No specific recommendations for time limits for embryos out of the incubator are available but, ideally, biopsy should be performed as quickly as possible to ensure pH, temperature, and osmolality are maintained. A documented record for biopsy timings is recommended for quality control/quality assurance purposes (46,55).

Safety and Success Rates after Biopsy

The reliability of cleavage-stage biopsy has been established in many centers, and the ESHRE PGD Consortium reported the efficiency of successful embryo biopsy as 99% in over 150,000 cleavage-stage embryos in clinical PGD cycles (55). Pregnancy rates after PGD are notoriously difficult to assess between different indications and centers. Nevertheless, in the largest series analyzed in detail to date, mostly following cleavage-stage biopsy, pregnancy rates are only 17–22% per oocyte retrieval and 26–29% per embryo transfer depending on the indication (11). The reasons for the apparently low success rates are manyfold, but unsurprising, considering that a proportion of embryos cannot be transferred because they are diagnosed as affected, and in many countries the number of embryos transferred is limited to a maximum of two. It is anticipated that pregnancy rates per embryo transfer will be significantly higher regardless of indication following blastocyst biopsy, primarily because of the higher implantation potential per biopsied embryo, but a rigorous assessment of pregnancies per started cycle will provide a true assessment of the value of blastocyst biopsy. The potentially detrimental effects of embryo biopsy, particularly if performed poorly also contribute to reduced success rates. Data from a randomized trial provides some insight into the possible detrimental effects of biopsy with a reduction in implantation potential evident in undiagnosed biopsied embryos compared with non-biopsied control embryos (52,56). A separate trial with dramatically reduced implantation rates from biopsied versus non-biopsied cleavage stage embryos (without any genetic selection) further supports the notion that cleavage stage embryo biopsy is costly to the embryo particularly if poorly performed (57).

It is well established in mammalian embryos that as an increasing proportion of the embryo is removed or destroyed before transfer, implantation and fetal development rates decline, suggesting a lower limit of embryo mass compatible with implantation and development (58). Reduction of 50% or more of the cell mass frequently results in cell proliferation in the absence of normal differentiation; thus, it is important to minimize the cellular mass removed at biopsy. However, cell reduction within this limit is compatible with normal embryo metabolism, blastocyst development, and fetal growth, while cell numbers in the TE and ICM of blastocysts were in proportion to the cellular mass removed at biopsy, making cleavage-stage biopsy for PGD a viable option (38). Hence, human cleavage-stage biopsy is delayed until just before the beginning of compaction, the process of intercellular adhesion and junction formation, which progressively makes the removal of blastomeres more difficult and eventually impossible without causing damage to the embryo.

Generally, cells identified as having completed the third cleavage division (on the basis of their size) are selected for biopsy. Theoretically, therefore, each blastomere removes only one-eighth of the cellular mass of the embryo. As zona drilling for assisted hatching may be beneficial, it is also possible that this offsets to some extent the adverse effects of reducing the cell mass of the embryo. In frozen embryo transfer (FET) cases, viable pregnancies can be achieved and no increase in fetal abnormalities has been reported following transfer of cryopreserved embryos in which some cells have been destroyed by freezing and subsequent thawing (59). Indeed, estimates of the loss of implantation potential have been made based on outcomes following FET involving embryos with one or more nonviable cells after thawing (52). It is now apparent that cleavage-stage biopsy should be considered a "cost" to the embryo, and this must always be weighed against the potential benefit to the embryo of any diagnostic testing.

Selection of Cells in the Cleavage-Stage Embryo

Biopsy at cleavage stages is based on the principle that at these stages the blastomeres remain totipotent and equivalent, such that the removal of a single blastomere will (*i*) provide a representative sample of the entire embryo and (*ii*) compromise the embryo only to the extent of one-eighth of the embryo mass rather than removal of a developmentally important blastomere.

The importance of selecting a blastomere with a single visible interphase nucleus cannot be stressed enough. It is probably the most challenging aspect of cleavage-stage biopsy, and time spent in careful examination of the embryo and orienting it to selectively remove specific blastomeres is essential to attain the high diagnostic efficiencies required for clinical effectiveness.

The reasons for this are that, first, an interphase nucleus is essential for FISH analysis, since the nucleus is prepared on a slide by a process of cell lysis in which individual chromosomes will not be visible and are likely to be lost (60). Secondly, post-zygotic chromosomal mosaicism arising during cleavage is known to be associated with nuclear abnormalities (61). The exception is binucleate blastomeres, in which there are two normal sized nuclei. In most cases, these are generated through failure of cytokinesis, and both nuclei contain the normal diploid chromosomal complement for that embryo. In general, multinucleate cells should not be selected for biopsy if FISH analysis for aneuploidy detection follows, and the removal of only mononucleate cells is recommended (62).

For accuracy during FISH-based diagnosis, it is advisable to use only bi- or multinucleated cells as a backup to biopsied mononucleated cells. This may be less critical for PCR-based testing in which presence or absence of a specific parental chromosome is important rather than copy number per se. However, even with careful blastomere selection, diagnostic efficiency is not 100%, and aneuploid results are common even in mononucleate blastomeres primarily as a result of chromosomal mosaicism (62). Biopsy of two nucleated blastomeres is only possible in good-quality embryos at a sufficiently advanced stage, such that even with a two-cell biopsy policy, a mixture of embryos with one or two blastomeres for analysis is common (53). Where possible, one of the smaller blastomeres should be selected to minimize the reduction in mass and the relative sizes of cells may provide an indication of recent mitosis. This may also reduce the risk that a cell in metaphase will be taken, the chromosomes of which could be lost during the fixation process.

Concerns Surrounding Cleavage-Stage Embryo Biopsy

As with any micromanipulation procedure involving human gametes or embryos, every reasonable precaution should be taken to minimize damage and stress during the procedure. General precautions include the correct installation, calibration, and maintenance of all micromanipulation equipment (particularly the laser). In advance of all clinical procedures, one should ensure that all appropriate reagents and micromanipulation tools are available, sterile, and within their expiration date.

Biopsy should be performed by a suitably qualified and trained person. Regular reviews of biopsy efficiency, post-biopsy morphology, and cell numbers of untransferred embryos provide an indication of the possible harm as a result of biopsy, as do pregnancy rates after biopsy (particularly those not developing beyond the biochemical stage). Clearly, effects on post-implantation development should also be closely monitored, as any increase in fetal malformations or congenital abnormalities would be unacceptable. To date, studies of pregnancies and children born after PGD have identified no significant increase in abnormalities above the rate seen in routine IVF (11,55,63–65).

The main problem in terms of diagnostic efficiency with cleavage-stage biopsy is the presence of chromosomal mosaicism, which has been reported to occur in up to 80% embryos using FISH for limited chromosomes (66–68). A full discussion of the impact of chromosomal mosaicism on the accuracy of PGD is beyond the scope of this review, but its impact can be significant. Mosaicism is thought to be the primary reason for the high rate of false positives depleting the pool of chromosomally "normal" embryos for transfer and hence significantly lowering the chance of live births following preimplantation genetic screening for chromosomal aneuploidy compared with controls in a randomized controlled trial (56). Preliminary work using more accurate array comparative genomic hybridization techniques to compare individual blastomere comprehensive chromosomal constitutions from 'normal' cleavage stage embryos from young patients suggests that the false positive rate in diploid/aneuploid mosaic embryos may be as low as 7% but this requires larger scale corroboration (69).

BLASTOCYST-STAGE BIOPSY (TE BIOPSY)

The number of cells present at the blastocyst stage make blastocyst biopsy more akin to early prenatal diagnosis and therefore, to some, more ethically acceptable (Figure 15.1). In theory, TE cells, which form the spherical outer epithelial monolayer of the blastocyst, can be removed without harming or depleting the ICM from which the fetus is derived. For blastocyst biopsy, it is therefore possible to remove up to 10 TE cells for analysis, which would overcome many of the problems encountered in single-cell DNA amplification and FISH. FISH analysis would be more successful with a virtual guarantee of a result for each sample and the problems of split signal, signal overlap, or probe failure would be significantly less misleading. In the case of PCR, the problems of amplification failure and ADO or preferential amplification would be much reduced. Indeed, when more than two cells are present in the same sample tube, these problems have been shown to virtually disappear, particularly if using whole genome amplification (WGA) techniques (69,70). With or without WGA, the availability of more cells automatically increases the diagnostic possibilities (more chromosomes analyzed with FISH or more specific sequences with PCR, or both).

In the mouse, TE biopsy is easily achieved by partial zona dissection using mechanical means, followed by a period in culture during which the expansion of the blastocele cavity forces the TE to herniate out of the slit (71). The herniating TE vesicle can then be excised on a bed of agarose by using a needle (which can be handheld or attached to a micromanipulator) and a cutting action close to the zona, which causes the embryo to roll. Both the biopsied embryo and TE vesicles often remain expanded, since they appear to be resealed, possibly as a consequence of twisting at the constriction. Furthermore, to some extent, the size of the TE biopsy can be controlled by the size of the slit and the length of incubation.

A similar approach was used to biopsy human blastocysts on day 5 or 6 post-insemination and was later used to examine effects on viability following biopsy, with the finding that hCG production was equivalent for biopsied and nonbiopsied controls (72). Another more aggressive technique to remove TE cells during blastocyst biopsy is the mechanical stitch and pull method (73). The best technique seems to be to stabilize the blastocyst by gentle suction and make an incision at the pole opposite to the ICM mass using a 2 μm beveled pipette. The pipette is pushed in and out through the

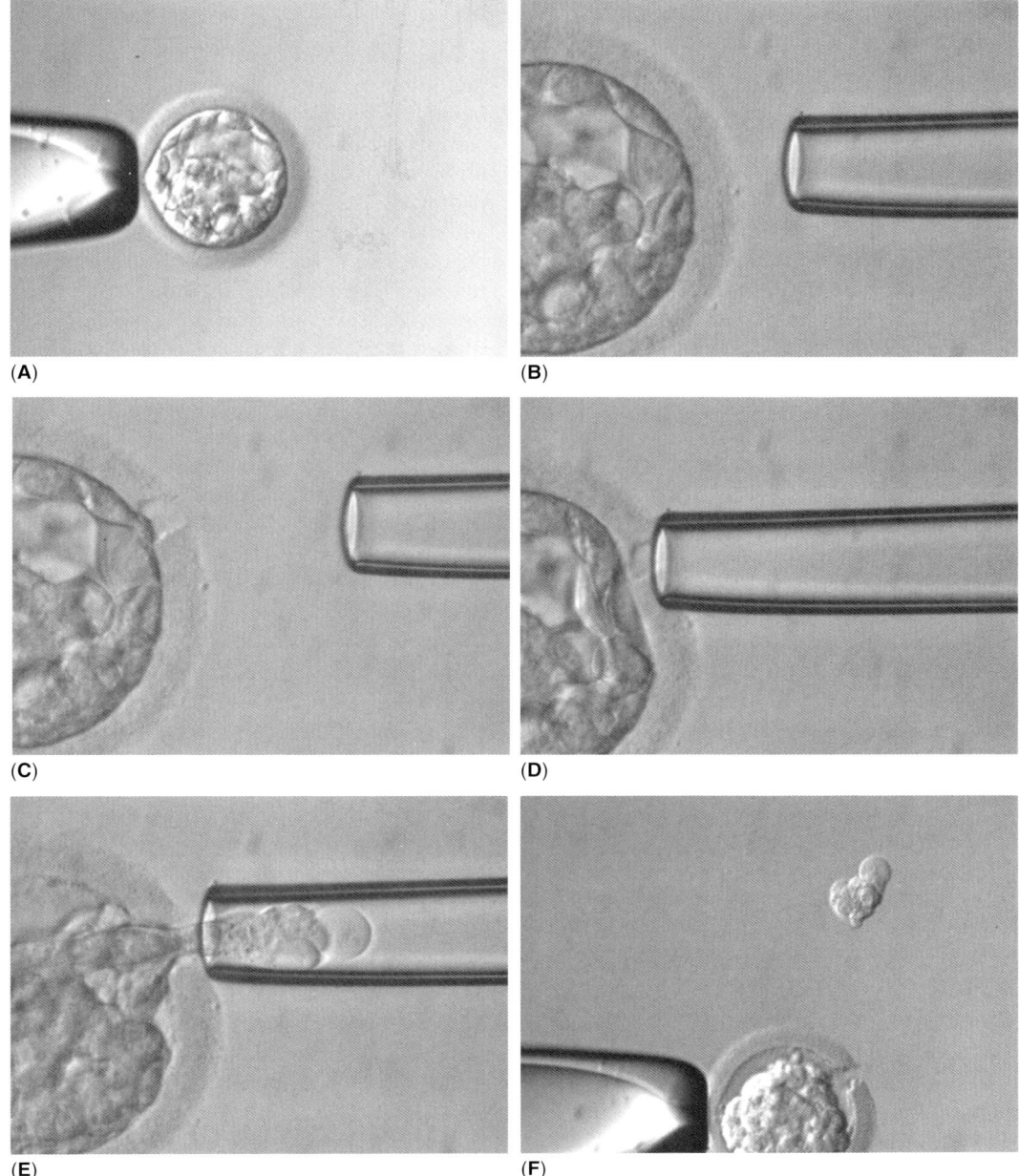

Figure 15.1 Blastocyst biopsy following laser ablation of the zona pellucida on a day 5 human embryo. Aspiration of trophectodermal cells follows immediately after ablation without additional embryo culture prior to biopsy. For a more detailed account see Appendix.

zona and pulled upward to make the incision. The blastocysts are then left for 6–24 hours until some TE herniates through the slit. When herniation involves about 10–25% of the blastocyst (10–30 cells), the TE is excised using a glass needle.

As with the other stages of embryo biopsy, noncontact infrared lasers are now routinely used to not only create an opening in the zona pellucida but also to excise the herniating trophectoderm (74) (see Appendix for a clinical protocol describing this method in more detail).

Originally, blastocyst development rates were not consistently high in laboratories and pregnancy rates following blastocyst-stage transfers were too low to consider biopsy at this stage. With improvements in culture systems, the proportion of embryos developing to the blastocyst stage has increased, and implantation rates per blastocyst transferred are significantly better than those at cleavage stages (75). Another concern was the effect that the removal of a proportion of the TE cells and damage of additional cells in the process would have on implantation. However, skilled practitioners are able to reliably biopsy up to 10 TE cells from blastocysts on day 5 using a noncontact infrared laser for zona drilling and excision of herniating TE cells, and achieve pregnancy and implantation rates that are comparable to those for nonbiopsied controls (76). The high incidence of multiple pregnancies in PGD demands efforts to reduce the number of unaffected embryos transferred, and transfer of blastocysts with high implantation potential is an effective strategy (77).

Challenges Associated with Blastocyst Biopsy

The main limitation of blastocyst biopsy is the low or unpredictable number of embryos that reach the blastocyst stage in vitro for unselected patients, even with improved culture conditions. Since a high number of embryos are needed for successful PGD to allow for sufficient embryo selection from the desired genotype, blastocyst culture may not produce enough embryos for diagnosis, and transfer to make PGD at this stage effective for all patients and may be more appropriate for younger, good prognosis patients. An additional obstacle to the widespread adoption of blastocyst biopsy is the concern that TE cells may have diverged genetically from the ICM because, in approximately 2% of human conceptions, confined placental mosaicism is observed (78) in which the chromosome status of the embryo is different from that of the placenta. In a mouse model, abnormal cells were shown to be preferentially allocated to the TE (79) but the situation is less clear in the human.

The level of mosaicism in the human blastocyst is lower than that in cleavage-stage embryos (80) and, where present, often takes the form of polyploidy in the trophectodermal lineage (81) with no obvious preferential allocation of aneuploid cells to the TE lineage (82). Considering polyploidy cells for PGD analyses using FISH, if enough chromosomes are analyzed then any underlying abnormality (such as trisomy 21) may be recognized within the polyploidy (HC Kuo and AH Handyside, unpublished observation). Similarly, for PCR-based diagnoses, the presence of multiple copies of each chromosome in polyploid cells should pose few problems, so long as both parental copies of the chromosome are represented. Clearly, chromosomal differences between the ICM and TE as a consequence of high levels of mosaicism at the cleavage stage would reduce the accuracy of diagnosis even when multiple biopsied TE cells are available. However, comparisons between biopsied trophectoderm and inner cell mass cells using more accurate molecular techniques demonstrate high concordance in chromosomal status (83,84).

In summary, blastocyst biopsy is rapidly becoming a popular choice for embryo biopsy (18,85–88) and, in contrast to previous practice focusing on poor prognosis patients, is particularly promising for younger patients aiming for single embryo transfer, with a randomized controlled trial demonstrating a 66% relative increase in ongoing pregnancy rate following 24 chromosome aneuploidy screening (77). Its widespread adoption in laboratories previously performing biopsy at other developmental stages is predicted allowing large-scale clinical assessment. At present, the logistics of blastocyst biopsy dictate a limited time-frame in which to perform diagnosis that might necessitate cryopreservation of biopsied blastocysts for transfer in a later unstimulated thaw cycle which, despite growing evidence of safety and efficacy (88–91), will require a cultural shift for both patients and providers.

FUTURE DEVELOPMENTS

A major challenge in PGD, where high value test normal embryos are available and single embryo transfer is becoming common, has been to develop an effective standardized method for cryopreservation of biopsied embryos. Attempts to use conventional slow-freezing protocols either in the mouse model or in humans have shown extensive damage after thawing, presumably because of the loss of protection from ice crystals in the medium provided by an intact zona pellucida (92,93). Several improved slow-freezing protocols have been reported in which damage is much reduced (94,95). However, following a successful application in animal models, (96–98) vitrification looks set to replace slow freezing for both cleavage- and blastocyst-stage embryos after polar body or embryo biopsy (88). With the high rate of multiple pregnancies reported after PGD, it is imperative to develop effective methods of cryopreservation that will (*i*) allow storage of unaffected embryos for later transfer so that the numbers transferred can be limited to two- or even single-embryo transfers and (*ii*) provide additional time to perform more extensive diagnostic tests. Indeed, the growing body of evidence suggesting comparable success rates (88) and normalized birthweights (89) from frozen-thaw transfer cycles (compared with fresh stimulated transfer cycles) may lead to a new era in which PGD cycles separate the stimulation and embryo production phase of treatment from diagnostic testing and embryo transfer phase. As a consequence, outcomes may improve overall with the added benefit to patients of having sufficient time for informed decision making.

With the introduction of quality management systems and accreditation in IVF laboratories (46,47) safer methods of biopsy can be anticipated through agreed definitions of successful and safe biopsy, standardized training and procedures, validation of new techniques, as well as calibration of new and existing instruments such as the laser. It has become clear that embryo biopsy, like any form of invasive testing or manipulation, exacts a cost to the embryo in the form of either cellular depletion, or metabolic stress, or both. Thus, it is imperative to assess the potential benefit to the embryo itself in terms of improved selection or disease-free status before performing an embryo biopsy. However, in the future it may be possible to diagnose inherited diseases or chromosomal imbalance in early human embryos by a noninvasive analysis of the secretome or metabolome in a spent culture medium (99), or possibly by changes in developmental growth rates as measured by time-lapse photographic methods (100,101). Both approaches would shift the cost-benefit ratio away from the cost of invasive biopsy heavily towards potential benefit.

ACKNOWLEDGMENTS

The authors are grateful to Drs Antonio Capalbo and Laura Rienzi (Genera, Rome, Italy) for the images in Figure 15.1.

APPENDIX 1

Clinical Protocol for Blastocyst Stage Embryo Biopsy

This clinical protocol describes the biopsy of human blastocysts on day 5 or day 6 of development to obtain multicellular samples for DNA amplification and genetic testing. The protocol is suitable for both hatching and non-hatching blastocysts and requires no zona breach during cleavage stages or period of culture prior to biopsy. For brevity all culture media reagents described below are from the Quinn's Advantage Culture Media Suite (Sage, Cooper Surgical, Inc. Trumbull, CT, USA).

A. Preparation Prior to Biopsy

1. Prepare sufficient Embryo GPS culture dishes (EGPS-100, LifeGlobal) with blastocyst medium for all embryos eligible for biopsy on the day prior to biopsy to allow for equilibration in the patient-allocated incubator section. Dish(es) should have sufficient 30 μL outer wells to allow individual culture of every embryo that has undergone biopsy. Spare medium in the 60 μL inner wells should also be available for washing embryos after biopsy to remove buffered medium.
2. Turn on workstation, micromanipulators and heated stage (perform routine QC checks for temperature, etc.)
3. Ensure anti-vibration table is inflated and functioning.
4. Set up one biopsy dish per embryo with QA HEPES buffered medium + 10% Synthetic Serum Replacement (buffered biopsy medium - BBM) and oil for tissue culture. In Falcon 50 × 9 mm Petri dish (code 351006, BD Biosciences), 3 × 10 μL drops of BBM are aliquoted and covered with 4 mL oil. These should be kept on a heated stage to equilibrate to 37°C for at least 15 minutes prior to use and used within 120 minutes.
5. Turn on SATURN laser (Research Instruments Ltd, Falmouth, UK) and workstation computer. Open CRONUS software and follow instruction booklet for alignment of laser using 'pilot' to check target is correct (refer to SATURN laser manual for additional guidance).
6. Pipette set up is essentially the same as that done for ICSI, however in the place of the injection pipette, a blastomere aspiration pipette (code K-EBPH-3035, Cook Medical Europe Ltd, Limerick, Ireland) is inserted into the holder. Biopsy pipettes are available in a range of diameters and can be bevelled if required. Current diameters used are between 25 and 35 μm and are available commercially from a number of different providers.
7. If required the angle of the biopsy pipette can be adjusted between 30° to 40° to allow optimal movement during biopsy.

B. Biopsy

1. Label the biopsy dish with the patient details, embryo number and attach a Radio Frequency Identification (RFID) tag for use with the RI Witness™ system (Research Instruments, UK)
2. Allocate the biopsy dish appropriately on the witness system and transfer one embryo to the central drop in the dish. The embryos should be 'rinsed' in the extra 'wash' drops so that excess culture media does not dilute the BBM. This also reduces the chance of debris carry over and allows removal of loose cumulus cells that may otherwise present a risk of false diagnosis.
3. Place the dish on the heated stage of the micromanipulator workstation.
4. Carefully lower the holding and aspiration pipettes into the central drop (with the embryo) taking care to avoid damaging the embryo using a low powered objective (Fig. 15.1a).
5. Ensure both pipettes have equilibrated and are offering sensitive control then, with gentle aspiration, secure the embryo to the holding pipette avoiding any herniating cells.

For hatching blastocysts go directly to step 9.
For non-hatching blastocysts continue with step 6.

6. Position the embryo on the holding pipette to give a clear view of the inner cell mass at 9 o'clock (i.e. away from the biopsy pipette) under high power magnification (Fig. 15.1b).
7. Select appropriate laser pulse duration for the desired aperture size (Fig. 15.1c) and, after selecting the laser objective, begin to make an opening in the embryo zona with a series of laser pulses working inwards from the outer surface of the zona taking care to avoid damaging the embryo. Zona thickness variation between embryos will mean that pulse time are number of pulses will vary. Pulse duration can be altered manually if required. The exact duration and number of pulses varies with different commercially available lasers and should be validated within each centre.
8. As soon as the aperture is wide enough to accommodate the passage of several trophectoderm cells (~10 μm), carefully press the biopsy pipette against the zona, gently expelling medium through the breach to release the cells from the internal surface of the zona (Fig. 15.1d).
9. Once the trophectoderm is free from the zona, aspirate 3–10 cells into the biopsy pipette with gentle suction (Fig. 15.1e). In the case of hatching blastocysts, aspirate herniating cells into the biopsy pipette.
10. Direct the laser to the thinnest part of the aspirated cells and use several laser pulses at the junctions between cells to disconnect the aspirated cells from the body of the embryo. It may be necessary to apply more suction with the biopsy pipette taking care not to inadvertently aspirate additional cells into the biopsy pipette.
11. When the biopsied cells are free from the embryo (i.e. within the biopsy pipette), move the biopsy

pipette away from the embryo and gently release the aspirated cells (Fig. 15.1f). Record the approximate number of cells, their appearance and location in the drop to aid relocation at time of cell preparation.
12. Label a pre-equilibrated post-biopsy (GPS) culture dish clearly with the patient's details and attach an RFID tag. Mark the embryo number adjacent to each culture well, on the dish base with indelible marker.
13. Allocate the culture dish appropriately on the witness system and return the biopsied embryo to this culture dish - each numbered embryo in the biopsy dish should be moved to the culture well with the corresponding number. Ensure that wash drops are used to minimise any carry-over of HEPES medium into the culture drop. Use a 275 μm pipette tip to minimise any additional stress to the embryo during this movement. Manual human double witnessing must be performed and recorded for every embryo that is moved following biopsy to ensure appropriate identification.
14. Return the dish to the patient incubator section and culture until embryo transfer, vitrification or disposal.
15. The dish containing the aspirated cells for analysis should be given to the scientist performing the cell preparation (tubing or cell fixation) immediately or can be placed in the workstation for later preparation (if validated) once the biopsy is completed.
16. Perform biopsy procedure on the next eligible embryo.
17. Biopsy all embryos that are of suitable quality and have reached the appropriate stage of development. This is normally a full blastocyst of average quality or above (grade 3BB or better using Gardner's blastocyst scoring system).

C. Special Considerations

1. In many cases results of the genetic analysis can be ready within 24 hours. Embryos biopsied early on Day 5 may be transferred fresh on day 6. Any embryos biopsied later on day 5 or day 6 should be vitrified and transferred in a frozen embryo transfer cycle pending genetics results.
2. If the majority of embryos have not reached the full blastocyst stage by day 6 or no embryos are suitable for biopsy the case should be reviewed by the appropriate team members. Considerations can be made to perform embryo transfer without biopsy and subsequent genetic testing. For example, patients for aneuploidy screening may elect to not proceed with biopsy depending on the specific indication.

REFERENCES

1. Li A, Gyllenstein UB, Cui X, et al. Amplification and analysis of DNA sequences in single human sperm and diploid cells. Nature (London) 1988; 335: 414–19.
2. Coutelle C, Williams C, Handyside A, et al. Genetic analysis of DNA from single human oocytes: a model for preimplantation diagnosis of cystic fibrosis. Br Med J 1989; 299: 22–4.
3. Holding C, Monk M. Diagnosis of thalassaemia by DNA amplification in single blastomeres from mouse preimplantation embryos. Lancet 1989; 2: 532–5.
4. Tarin JJ, Handyside AH. Embryo biopsy strategies for preimplantation diagnosis. Fertil Steril 1993; 59: 943–52.
5. Monk M, Muggleton-Harris AL, Rawlings E, Whittingham DG. Pre-implantation diagnosis of HPRT-deficient male and carrier female mouse embryos by trophectoderm biopsy. Hum Reprod 1988; 3: 377–81.
6. Wilton LJ, Shaw JM, Trounson AO. Successful single-cell biopsy and cryopreservation of preimplantation mouse embryos. Fertil Steril 1989; 51: 513–17.
7. Edwards RG, Gardner RL. Sexing of live rabbit blastocysts. Nature 1967; 214: 576–7.
8. Yang X, Foot RH. Production of identical twin rabbits by micromanipulation of embryos. Biol Reprod 1987; 37: 1007–14.
9. Ozil JP. Production of identical twins by bisection of blastocysts in the cow. J Reprod Fertil 1983; 69: 463–8.
10. Summers PM, Campbell JM, Miller MW. Normal in vivo development of marmoset monkey embryos after trophectoderm biopsy. Human Reprod 1988; 3: 389–93.
11. Harper JC, Wilton L, Traeger-Synodinos J, et al. The ESHRE PGD Consortium: 10 years of data collection. Hum Reprod Update 2012; 18: 234–47.
12. Cohen J, Malter H, Wright G, et al. Partial zona dissection of human oocytes when failure of zona pellucida penetration is anticipated. Hum Reprod 1989; 4: 435–42.
13. Cieslak J, Ivakhnenko V, Wolf G, Sheleg S, Verlinsky Y. Three-dimensional partial zona dissection for preimplantation genetic diagnosis and assisted hatching. Fertil Steril 1999; 71: 308–13.
14. Gordon JW, Talansky BE. Assisted fertilization by zona drilling: a mouse model for correction of oligospermia. J Exp Zool 1986; 239: 347–54.
15. Malter HE, Cohen J. Partial zona dissection of the human oocyte: a nontraumatic method using micromanipulation to assist zona pellucida penetration. Fertil Steril 1989; 51: 139–48.
16. Geraedts J, Handyside A, Harper J, et al. ESHRE Preimplantation Genetic Diagnosis (PGD) Consortium: preliminary assessment of data from January 1997 to September 1998. ESHRE PGD Consortium Steering Committee. Hum Reprod 1999; 14: 3138–48.
17. Germond M, Nocera D, Senn A, et al. Microdissection of mouse and human zona pellucida using a 1.48-microns diode laser beam: efficacy and safety of the procedure. Fertil Steril 1995; 64: 604–11.
18. Boada M, Carrera M, De La Iglesia C, et al. Successful use of a laser for human embryo biopsy in preimplantation genetic diagnosis: report of two cases. J Assist Reprod Genet 1998; 15: 302–7.
19. Montag M, Van der Ven H. Laser-assisted hatching in assisted reproduction. Croat Med J 1999; 40: 398–403.
20. Montag M, Van der Ven K, Delacretaz G, Rink K, Van der Ven H. Laser-assisted microdissection of the zona pellucida facilitates polar body biopsy. Fertil Steril 1998; 69: 539–42.
21. Park S, Kim EY, Yoon SH, Chung KS, Lim JH. Enhanced hatching rate of bovine IVM/IVF/IVC

blastocysts using a 1.48-micron diode laser beam. J Assist Reprod Genet 1999; 16: 97–101.
22. Han TS, Sagoskin AW, Graham JR, Tucker MJ, Liebermann J. Laser-assisted human embryo biopsy on the third day of development for preimplantation genetic diagnosis: two successful case reports. Fertil Steril 2003; 80: 453–5.
23. Joris H, De Vos A, Janssens R, et al. Comparison of the results of human embryo biopsy and outcome of PGD after zona drilling using acid Tyrode medium or a laser. Hum Reprod 2003; 18: 1896–902.
24. Chatzimeletiou K, Picton HM, Handyside AH. Use of a non-contact, infrared laser for zona drilling of mouse embryos: assessment of immediate effects on blastomere viability. Reprod BioMed Online 2001; 2: 178–87.
25. Verlinsky Y, Ginsberg N, Lifchez A, et al. Analysis of the first polar body: preconception genetic diagnosis. Hum Reprod 1990; 5: 826–9.
26. Corveleyn A, Morris MA, Dequeker E, et al. Provision and quality assurance of preimplantation genetic diagnosis in Europe. Eur J Hum Genet 2008; 16: 290–9.
27. Dreesen JC, Geraedts JP, Dumoulin JC, Evers JL, Pieters MH. RS46(DXS548) genotyping of reproductive cells: approaching preimplantation testing of the fragile-X syndrome. Hum Genet 1995; 96: 323–9.
28. Navidi W, Arnheim N. Using PCR in preimplantation genetic disease diagnosis. Hum Reprod 1991; 6: 836–49.
29. Verlinsky Y, Rechitsky S, Cieslak J, et al. Preimplantation diagnosis of single gene disorders by two-step oocyte genetic analysis using first and second polar body. Biochem Mol Med 1997; 62: 182–7.
30. Kaplan B, Wolf G, Kovalinskaya L, Verlinsky Y. Viability of embryos following second polar body removal in a mouse model. J Assist Reprod Genet 1995; 12: 747–9.
31. Verlinsky Y, Cieslak J, Ivakhnenko V, et al. Preimplantation diagnosis of common aneuploidies by the first- and second-polar body FISH analysis. J Assist Reprod Genet 1998; 15: 285–9.
32. Magli MC, Montag M, Koster M, et al. Polar body array CGH for prediction of the status of the corresponding oocyte. Part II: technical aspects. Hum Reprod 2011; 26: 3181–5.
33. Ray P, Winston R, Handyside A. Reduced allele dropout in single-cell analysis for preimplantation genetic diagnosis of cystic fibrosis. J Assist Reprod Genet 1996; 13: 104–6.
34. Eldadah ZA, Grifo JA, Dietz HC. Marfan syndrome as a paradigm for transcript-targeted preimplantation diagnosis of heterozygous mutations. Nat Med 1995; 1: 798–803.
35. Magli MC, Gianaroli L, Ferraretti AP, et al. The combination of polar body and embryo biopsy does not affect embryo viability. Hum Reprod 2004; 19: 1163–9.
36. Cieslak-Janzen J, Tur-Kaspa I, Ilkevitch Y, et al. Multiple micromanipulations for preimplantation genetic diagnosis do not affect embryo development to the blastocyst stage. Fertil Steril 2006; 85: 1826–9.
37. Handyside AH, Kontogianni EH, Hardy K, Winston RM. Pregnancies from biopsied human preimplantation embryos sexed by Y-specific DNA amplification. Nature 1990; 344: 768–70.
38. Hardy K, Martin KL, Leese HJ, Winston RML, Handyside AH. Human preimplantation development in vitro is not adversely affected by biopsy at the 8-cell stage. Hum Reprod 1990; 5: 708–14.
39. Ao A, Handyside AH. Cleavage stage human embryo biopsy. Hum Reprod Update 1995; 1: 3.
40. Handyside AH, Thornhill AR. Cleavage stage embryo biopsy for preimplantation genetic diagnosis. In: Kempers RD, Cohen J, Haney AF, Younger JB, eds. Fertility and Reproductive Medicine. Amsterdam: Elsevier, 1998: 223–9.
41. Chen SU, Chao KH, Wu MY, et al. A simplified twopipette technique is more efficient than the conventional three-pipette method for blastomere biopsy in human embryos. Fertil Steril 1998; 69: 569–75.
42. Inzunza J, Iwarsson E, Fridstrom M, et al. Application of single-needle blastomere biopsy in human preimplantation genetic diagnosis. Prenat Diagn 1998; 8: 1381–8.
43. Levinson G, Fields RA, Harton GL, et al. Reliable gender screening for human preimplantation embryos, using multiple DNA target-sequences. Hum Reprod 1992; 7: 1304–13.
44. Roudebush WE, Kim JG, Minhas BS, Dodson MG. Survival and cell acquisition rates after preimplantation embryo biopsy: use of two mechanical techniques and two mouse strains. Am J Obstet Gynecol 1990; 162: 1084–90.
45. Pierce KE, Michalopoulos J, Kiessling AA, Seibel MM, Zilberstein M. Preimplantation development of mouse and human embryos biopsied at cleavage stages using a modified displacement technique. Hum Reprod 1997; 12: 351–6.
46. Thornhill AR, deDie-Smulders CE, Geraedts JP, et al. ESHRE PGD Consortium 'Best practice guidelines for clinical preimplantation genetic diagnosis (PGD) and preimplantation genetic screening (PGS)'. Hum Reprod 2005; 20: 35–48.
47. Preimplantation Genetic Diagnosis International Society (PGDIS). Guidelines for good practice in PGD: programme requirements and laboratory quality assurance. Reprod Biomed Online 2008; 16: 134–47.
48. Dumoulin JC, Bras M, Coonen E, et al. Effect of Ca^{2+}/Mg^{2+}-free medium on the biopsy procedure for preimplantation genetic diagnosis and further development of human embryos. Hum Reprod 1998; 13: 2880–3.
49. Tarin JJ, Conaghan J, Winston RM, Handyside AH. Human embryo biopsy on the 2nd day after insemination for preimplantation diagnosis: removal of a quarter of embryo retards cleavage. Fertil Steril 1992; 58: 970–6.
50. Tsunoda Y, McLaren A. Effect of various procedures on the viability of mouse embryos containing half the normal number of blastomeres. J Reprod Fertil 1983; 69: 315–22.
51. Liu J, Van den Abbeel E, Van Steirteghem A. The in-vitro and in-vivo developmental potential of frozen and non-frozen biopsied 8-cell mouse embryos. Hum Reprod 1993; 8: 1481–6.
52. Cohen J, Wells D, Munne S. Removal of 2 cells from cleavage stage embryos is likely to reduce the efficacy of chromosomal tests that are used to enhance implantation rates. Fertil Steril 2007; 87: 496–503.

53. Van de Velde H, De Vos A, Sermon K, et al. Embryo implantation after biopsy of one or two cells from cleavage-stage embryos with a view to preimplantation genetic diagnosis. Prenat Diagn 2000; 20: 1030–7.
54. Goossens V, De Rycke M, De Vos A, et al. Diagnostic efficiency, embryonic development and clinical outcome after the biopsy of one or two blastomeres for preimplantation genetic diagnosis. Hum Reprod 2008; 23: 481–92.
55. Goossens V, Traeger-Synodinos J, Coonen E, et al. ESHRE PGD Consortium data collection XI: cycles from January to December 2008 with pregnancy follow-up to October 2009. Hum Reprod 2012; [Epub ahead of print].
56. Mastenbroek S, Twisk M, van Echten-Arends J, et al. In vitro fertilization with preimplantation genetic screening. N Engl J Med 2007; 357: 9–17.
57. Treff N, Ferry KM, Zhao T, et al. Cleavage stage embryo biopsy significantly impairs embryonic reproductive potential while blastocyst biopsy does not: a novel paired analysis of cotransferred biopsied and non-biopsied sibling embryos. Fertil Steril 2011; 96: S2.
58. Rossant J. Postimplantation development of blastomeres isolated from 4 and 8cell mouse eggs. J Embryol Exp Morphol 1976; 36: 283–90.
59. Sutcliffe AG, D'Souza SW, Cadman J, et al. Outcome in children from cryopreserved embryos. Arch Dis Child 1995; 72: 290–3.
60. Harper JC, Coonen E, Ramaekers FC, et al. Identification of the sex of human preimplantation embryos in two hours using an improved spreading method and fluorescent in situ hybridization (FISH) using directly labelled probes. Hum Reprod 1994; 9: 721–4.
61. Munné S, Cohen J. Unsuitability of multinucleated human blastomeres for preimplantation genetic diagnosis. Hum Reprod 1993; 8: 1120–5.
62. Kuo HC, Ogilvie CM, Handyside AH. Chromosomal mosaicism in cleavage-stage human embryos and the accuracy of single-cell genetic analysis. J Assist Reprod Genet 1998; 15: 276–80.
63. Strom CM, Levin R, Strom S, et al. Neonatal outcome of preimplantation genetic diagnosis by polar body removal: the first 109 infants. Pediatrics 2000; 106: 650–3.
64. Banerjee I, Shevlin M, Taranissi M, et al. Health of children conceived after preimplantation genetic diagnosis: a preliminary outcome study. Reprod Biomed Online 2008; 16: 376–81.
65. Nekkebroeck J, Bonduelle M, Desmyttere S, Van den Broeck W, Ponjaert-Kristoffersen I. Mental and psychomotor development of 2-year-old children born after preimplantation genetic diagnosis/screening. Hum Reprod 2008; 23: 1560–6.
66. Harper JC, Coonen E, Handyside AH, et al. Mosaicism of autosomes and sex chromosomes in morphologically normal,monospermic preimplantation human embryos. Prenat Diagn 1995; 15: 41–9.
67. Magli MC, Jones GM, Gras L, et al. Chromosome mosaicism in day 3 aneuploid embryos that develop to morphologically normal blastocysts in vitro. Hum Reprod 2000; 15: 1781–6.
68. Bielanska M, Tan SL, Ao A. Chromosomalmosaicism throughout human preimplantation development in vitro: incidence, type, and relevance to embryo outcome. Hum Reprod 2002; 17: 413–19.
69. Wilton L. Chromosomal mosaicism in the cleavage stage embryo revisited. Reproductive Biomedicine Online 2012; 24(Suppl 2): PS35, S-11.
70. Handyside AH, Robinson MD, Simpson RJ, et al. Isothermal whole genome amplification from single and small numbers of cells: a new era for preimplantation genetic diagnosis of inherited disease. Mol Hum Reprod 2004; 10: 767–72.
71. Nijs M, Van Steirteghem A. Developmental potential of biopsied mouse blastocysts. J Exp Zool 1990; 256: 232–6.
72. Dokras A, Sargent IL, Ross C, Gardner RL, Barlow DH. The human blastocyst: morphology and human chorionic gonadotrophin secretion in vitro. Hum Reprod 1991; 6: 1143–51.
73. Muggleton-Harris AL, Glazier AM, Pickering SJ. Biopsy of the human blastocyst and polymerase chain reaction (PCR) amplification of the beta-globin gene and a dinucleotide repeat motif from 2–6 trophectoderm cells. Hum Reprod 1993; 8: 2197–205.
74. Veiga A, Sandalinas M, Benkhalifa M, et al. Laser blastocyst biopsy for preimplantation diagnosis in the human. Zygote 1997; 5: 351–4.
75. Papanikolaou EG, Kolibianakis EM, Tournaye H, et al. Live birth rates after transfer of equal number of blastocysts or cleavage-stage embryos in IVF. A systematic review and meta-analysis. Hum Reprod 2008; 23: 91–9.
76. Kokkali G, Traeger-Synodinos J, Vrettou C, et al. Blastocyst biopsy versus cleavage stage biopsy and blastocyst transfer for preimplantation genetic diagnosis of beta-thalassaemia: a pilot study. Hum Reprod 2007; 22: 1443–9.
77. Yang Z, Liu J, Collins GS, et al. Selection of single blastocysts for fresh transfer via standard morphology assessment alone and with array CGH for good prognosis IVF patients: results from a randomized pilot study. Mol Cytogenet 2012; 5: 24.
78. Kalousek D, Vekemans M. Confined placental mosaicism. J Med Genet 1996; 33: 529–33.
79. James R, West J. A chimaeric animal model for confined placental mosaicism. Hum Genet 1994; 93: 603–4.
80. Ruangvutilert P, Delhanty JD, Serhal P, et al. FISH analysis on day 5 post-insemination of human arrested and blastocyst stage embryos. Prenat Diagn 2000; 20: 552–60.
81. Evsikov S, Verlinsky Y. Mosaicism in the inner cell mass of human blastocysts. Hum Reprod 1998; 13: 3151–5.
82. Derhaag JG, Coonen E, Bras M, et al. Chromosomally abnormal cells are not selected for the extra-embryonic compartment of the human preimplantation embryo at the blastocyst stage. Hum Reprod 2003; 18: 2565–74.
83. Johnson DS, Cinnioglu C, Ross R, et al. Comprehensive analysis of karyotypic mosaicism between trophectoderm and inner cell mass. Mol Hum Reprod 2010; 16: 944–9.
84. Capalbo A, Wright G, Themaat L, et al. FISH reanalysis of inner cell mass and trophectoderm samples of previously array CGH screened blastocysts reveals high accuracy of diagnosis and no sign of mosaicism or preferential allocation. Fertil Steril 2011; 96: S22.
85. McArthur SJ, Leigh D, Marshall JT, de Boer KA, Jansen RP. Pregnancies and live births after trophectoderm

biopsy and preimplantation genetic testing of human blastocysts. Fertil Steril 2005; 84: 1628–36.
86. Kokkali G, Vrettou C, Traeger-Synodinos J, et al. Birth of a healthy infant following trophectoderm biopsy from blastocysts for PGD of beta-thalassaemia major. Hum Reprod 2005; 20: 1855–9.
87. de Boer KA, Catt JW, Jansen RP, Leigh D, McArthur S. Moving to blastocyst biopsy for preimplantation genetic diagnosis and single embryo transfer at Sydney IVF. Fertil Steril 2004; 82: 295–8.
88. Schoolcraft WB, Treff NR, Stevens JM, et al. Live birth outcome with trophectoderm biopsy, blastocyst vitrification, and single-nucleotide polymorphism microarray-based comprehensive chromosome screening in infertile patients. Fertil Steril 2011; 96: 638–40.
89. Henningsen AK, Pinborg A, Lidegaard O, et al. Perinatal outcome of singleton siblings born after assisted reproductive technology and spontaneous conception: Danish national sibling-cohort study. Fertil Steril 2011; 95: 959–63.
90. Magli MC, Gianaroli L, Grieco N, et al. Cryopreservation of biopsied embryos at the blastocyst stage. Hum Reprod 2006; 21: 2656–60.
91. Parriego M Sole M, Aurell R, Barri PN, Veiga A. Birth after transfer of frozen-thawed vitrified biopsied blastocysts. J Assist Reprod Genet 2007; 24: 147–9.
92. Joris H, Van den Abbeel E, Vos AD, Van Steirteghem A. Reduced survival after human embryo biopsy and subsequent cryopreservation. Hum Reprod 1999; 14: 2833–7.
93. Magli MC, Gianaroli L, Fortini D, Ferraretti AP, Munné S. Impact of blastomere biopsy and cryopreservation techniques on human embryo viability. Hum Reprod 1999; 14: 770–3.
94. Jericho H, Wilton L, Gook DA, Edgar DH. A modified cryopreservation method increases the survival of human biopsied cleavage stage embryos. Hum Reprod 2003; 18: 568–71.
95. Stachecki JJ, Cohen J, Munné S. Cryopreservation of biopsied cleavage stage human embryos. Reprod Biomed Online 2005; 11: 711–15.
96. Agca Y, Monson RL, Northey DL, et al. Normal calves from transfer of biopsied, sexed and vitrified IVP bovine embryos. Theriogenology 1998; 50: 129–45.
97. Baranyai B, Bodo S, Dinnyes A, Gocza E. Vitrification of biopsied mouse embryos. Acta Vet Hung 2005; 53: 103–12.
98. Isachenko V, Montag M, Isachenko E, van der Ven H. Vitrification of mouse pronuclear embryos after polar body biopsy without direct contact with liquid nitrogen. Fertil Steril 2005; 84: 1011–16.
99. Edwards R, Hollands P. New advances in human embryology: implications of the preimplantation diagnosis of genetic disease. Hum Reprod 1988; 3: 549–56.
100. Wong CC, Loewke KE, Bossert NL, et al. Non-invasive imaging of human embryos before embryonic genome activation predicts development to the blastocyst stage. Nat Biotechnol 2010; 28: 1115–21.
101. Meseguer M, Herrero J, Tejera A, et al. The use of morphokinetics as a predictor of embryo implantation. Hum Reprod 2011; 26: 2658–71.

16

Analysis of fertilization

Thomas Ebner

INTRODUCTION

In vitro fertilization (IVF) and intracytoplasmic sperm injection (ICSI) cycles have shown that women have only a finite number of gametes out of a pool of collected oocytes which are capable of generating a term pregnancy. This demonstrates the need for simple methods of preimplantation embryo assessment in the prediction of pregnancy rates. In this respect intensive research has been done at zygote stage on day 1 of preimplantation development.

While conventional IVF more or less mimics natural fertilization, ICSI is a rather invasive procedure circumventing some of the major steps in the process of oocyte activation and fertilization. Consequently, the ICSI schedule differs slightly from the IVF one (1). This delay is attributed to the time needed for the sperm to pass through the oocyte outer complex, in particular the cumulus and corona cells as well as the zona pellucida. Fusion of the spermatozoon with the oolemma and incorporation into the oocyte plasma, on the other hand, seem to occur very rapidly (2).

In ICSI, fertilization usually has to be assessed approximately two hours earlier (e.g., 16–18 hours post insemination) than in IVF (18–20 hours) in order to face identical developmental stages (3).

TIMING OF FERTILIZATION EVENTS

Either active propulsion (conventional IVF) or direct deposition (ICSI) ensures presence of a spermatozoon in the cytoplasm. Elegant time-lapse video cinematography of ICSI gametes has proven that regular fertilization follows a definite course of events, though timing of these events may vary between eggs (4). In the study of Payne and colleagues (4), approximately 90% of the oocytes showed circular waves of granulation within the cytoplasm after ICSI (periodicity of 20–53 minutes). During this granulation phase the head of the spermatozoon decondensed. Subsequently, the second polar body was extruded, which was followed by the central formation of the male pronucleus. At about the same time, the female counterpart formed and was drawn toward the male pronucleus until the two abutted. Data from literature suggest (5) that during this process, the male pronucleus rotates onto the female one, in which the chromatin condenses on the side facing the center of the egg, in order to also align its chromatin toward the spindle that forms between both pronuclei. Then both pronuclei increase in size and their nucleoli move around and arrange themselves near the common junction (4).

Within both nuclei, nucleoli form at sites on the DNA known as the "nucleolar organizing regions" located on the chromosomes where the ribosomal genes are situated (6). This means that the nucleoli are the active sites of rRNA synthesis. During the course of development, nucleoli tend to fuse due to an increase in protein synthesis (4,7). It should be emphasized once again that IVF zygotes reach the final stage of nucleolar organization at a later time than ICSI zygotes.

The size and distribution patterns of the nucleoli may serve as prognostic parameters of the events of fertilization, the completion of meiosis and the cell cycle leading to the first mitotic division, the normality of the chromatin complement in the two nuclei, and the formation with chromosome attachment of the mitotic spindle (6).

In particular, asynchrony in the formation and polarization of nucleoli (Fig. 16.1A) may severely impair further development of the preimplantation embryo (8–12). Consequently, good quality embryos can arise from oocytes that have more uniform timing from injection to pronuclear abuttal (4).

PRONUCLEAR GRADING

Since nucleolar arrangement and morphology is strictly time-dependent, embryologists have to face several pronuclear patterns at the time of fertilization assessment. Based on original data from Wright et al. (13), Scott and Smith (9) were amongst the first to attribute zygote morphology a certain prognostic value for subsequent implantation. In particular, the alignment of nucleoli at the junction of the two pronuclei was found to be a selection criterion for embryo transfer. Since this zygote score did not exclusively rely on pronuclear pattern but also comprised multiple other parameters, including appearance of cytoplasm and timing of nuclear membrane breakdown, the actual impact of pronuclear morphology on further outcome remained unclear.

Thus, Tesarik and Greco (10) were the pioneers in predicting preimplantation development by focusing exclusively on the number and the distribution of nucleoli (nucleolar precursor bodies, NPBs) in each pronucleus. They considered interpronuclear synchrony, evaluated 12–20 hours post IVF/ICSI, as being more important than the actual NPB polarity at the site of pronuclear apposition since they presumed that the polarization of nucleoli is not evident from the beginning of pronuclei formation, but much rather appears progressively with time (7). According to Tesarik and Greco (10) the optimal synchronized pattern 0 yields 37.3% of good-quality embryos compared with all other patterns (27.8%). In addition, the frequency of developmental arrest of pattern 0 zygotes was only 8.5% as compared with 25.6%.

Since all these previous reports had been of retrospective character, particular importance must be assigned to a prospective multicenter study of Montag and Van der Ven (3). These authors highlighted that cycles with transfer of at least one embryo derived from pattern 0B (Fig. 16.1B), but not pattern 0A, resulted in significantly higher rates of pregnancy (37.9%) and implantation (20.5%) than non-pattern 0B cycles (26.4% and 15.7%). Similar results have been published by others (11) who found significantly increased pregnancy rates (44.8% vs. 30.2%) if embryos derived from zygotes with pattern 0 were transferred. Of significance, NPB polarization at the area of pronuclear contact outdoes pronuclear symmetry.

Recently, Scott et al. (12,14) further refined their score, also creating a single observation zygote score. This so-called Z-score was comparable with the score introduced by Tesarik and Greco (10), since patterns Z1 and Z2 resemble patterns 0B and 0A. Several other authors successfully used the zygote scores of Scott et al. (9,12) and Tesarik and Greco (10) for prognostic purposes (3,11, 15–18). Though the grading systems differ slightly in some of these papers, the conclusion is a common one. Zygotes showing pronuclei with approximately the same number and alignment of NPBs in the furrow between the nuclei had the best prognosis in terms of subsequent implantation.

It is noteworthy that Salumets et al. (19) failed to show any correlation between zygote score and pregnancy rate. This is of particular interest because this group analyzed only single embryo transfers and, consequently, the actual implantation potential could be accurately estimated. Though two different scores were applied (9,10) no correlation to treatment outcome could be demonstrated.

This discrepancy in literature results may be explained by different culture media, stimulation protocols, and differences in the timing of fertilization assessments, for example, the inclusion of early cleavage in the Scott and Smith (9) scoring system.

An increased incidence of subsequent blastocyst formation in zygotes with optimal pattern of the pronuclei (12,17,20) seems to be consistent with the reported increase in terms of pregnancy rate. Theoretically, a lower blastocyst formation rate in abnormal zygotes could be related to their chromosomal status since there is information from literature that several pronuclear patterns seem to be associated with aneuploidy (21–24).

In detail, Kahraman and colleagues (23) found a 52.2% rate of chromosomal abnormality in biopsied embryos derived from suspicious zygotes (showing an asymmetric distribution of NPB) which was significantly lower than the observed 37.6% in the normal control zygotes. Others (24) also confirmed that the position of pronuclei within the cytoplasm, the size and distribution of nucleoli, and the orientation of polar bodies with respect to pronuclei were highly predictive for the presence of chromosomal abnormalities in the corresponding embryos. In this study (24), zygotes with abutted pronuclei, large-size nucleoli, and polar bodies with small angles subtended by pronuclei and polar bodies were the configurations associated with the highest rates of euploidy. Using the Z-score it could be shown (22) that Z1 patterns had a significantly higher rate of euploidy (71%) than Z3 (35%) and Z4 (36%) patterns. The same also holds true for the score of Tesarik and Greco (10) since pattern 0 was associated with a minimal rate of aneuploidy (26%), whereas patterns with poor prognosis showed higher rates of up to 83% (21).

Although not all studies published to date suggest complete reliance on zygote morphology (19,25) the vast majority of papers do so, and it may be concluded that PN morphology predicts the risk of both embryo developmental arrest and chromosomal abnormalities.

A definite difference between IVF and ICSI cycles with regard to the frequency of good patterns (pattern 0 according to Tesarik and Greco (10)) was reported (3). In particular,

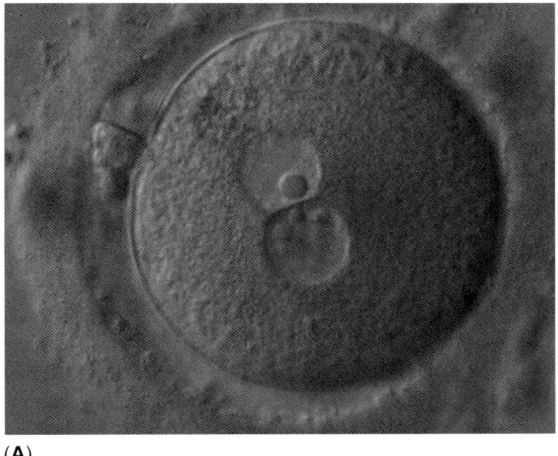
(A)

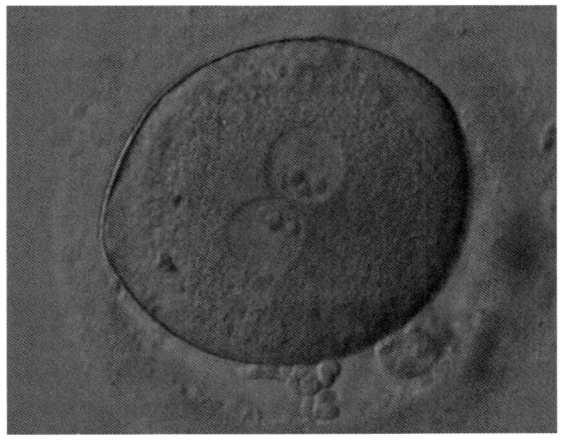
(B)

Figure 16.1 Different pronuclear formation and patterns. (**A**) A bad prognosis zygote with asymmetric pronuclear pattern corresponding to pattern 4 (10) or Z3 (12), respectively. (**B**) A zygote showing an optimal pronuclear pattern 0B (10) or Z1 (12), respectively, and a clear halo.

superior pronuclear patterns were observed in ICSI cycles. This phenomenon may be due to the above-mentioned accelerated course of development in ICSI (1,26). Zygotes showing this most advanced stage of nuclear polarization seem to reach that stage earlier after ICSI than after conventional IVF (3). However, the study did not evaluate the position of the pronuclei relative to the presumed polar axis. This arrangement has been reported to relate to embryo quality (27,28). Edwards and Beard (29) suggested that the oocyte might establish this polarity by either ooplasmic or pronuclear rotation toward the second polar body. Such a resetting of a new axis after fertilization is governed by cytoplasmic contraction waves organized by the sperm centrosome (29). Embryos unable to achieve optimal pronuclear orientation, possibly due to shorter cytoplasmic waves (4), may exhibit poor morphology, for example, uneven cleavage or fragmentation (27).

ABNORMAL PRONUCLEAR FORMATION AND PATTERNS

Single pronucleate zygotes (1PN) can be obtained following IVF and ICSI at frequencies ranging from 2% to 5% (30). They were reported to show a trend toward a higher frequency in ICSI. Karyotyping has indicated that following IVF more than half of 1PN embryos are in fact diploid, but in these studies (31,32) it was not differentiated between diploidy produced by fusion of both pronuclei and through fertilization by parthenogenetic activation. However, in further studies it could be demonstrated that when embryos were proven to be diploid approximately half of them were fertilized (33,34). Two mechanisms could be responsible for this observation, asynchronous appearance or fusion of both pronuclei (35). If there is no other choice such IVF-embryos could be considered for transfer, in particular, if the single pronucleus is larger than the regular size. Both studies dealing with one-pronucleate zygotes generated by ICSI indicated that the vast majority of these were activated but not fertilized (34,35). Consequently, such embryos should not be re-placed into the patient.

The presence of 3PN after IVF is the most common fertilization anomaly in humans. This is mostly caused by dispermy (3PN, 2 polar bodies) and the majority of the corresponding embryos will cleave but stop development at later stages (30). In ICSI some 4% (30) of zygotes show digynic triploidy, meaning that a single sperm is present in the egg but the second polar body was not extruded (non-disjunction). In this case the chromosomes of the three pronuclei are organized in a single bipolar spindle at syngamy indicating that only one centrosome deriving from one sperm is active.

Within 3PN zygotes a special case is the presence of 2PN with a third additional small nucleus (Fig. 16.2). Since it was shown that this smaller nucleus may contain chromosomal material (unpublished data) it is particularly important not to transfer embryos or blastocysts stemming from such abnormal zygotes. Due to the sometimes small size of these additional nuclei there is of course a high risk of missing them during routine fertilization checks, especially when using objectives of lower magnification.

Regardless of the pronuclear pattern the oocyte reflects, it is generally accepted that both pronuclei should be located in the center of the female gamete. Cytoplasmic inclusions, such as dense granularity, large refractile bodies, and/or vacuoles may displace both pronuclei. However, this scenario can also happen in zygotes with normal homogeneous ooplasm. Any deviation from the presumed optimal central arrangement, for example, peripheral apposition of both pronuclei (Fig. 16.3), is most likely associated with reduced developmental capacity (27). Considering the fact that the first cleavage plane runs through the contact zone of both pronuclei it is a frequent phenomenon that the corresponding embryo will show uneven cleavage. This scenario is more frequent in conventional IVF than in ICSI (3.3% vs. 11.8%), probably due to varying sites of sperm entrance in IVF (27); for example, spindle-near penetration of the zona which in turn could force an eccentric formation of pronuclei (5).

Another problem occasionally arising during fertilization is a failure in alignment of both pronuclei (Fig. 16.4),

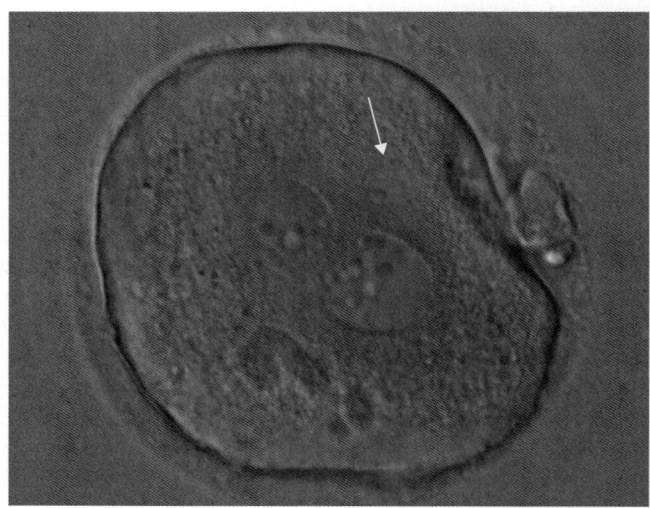

Figure 16.2 A zygote showing 2PN with additional smaller nucleus (*arrow*) possibly containing chromosomal material.

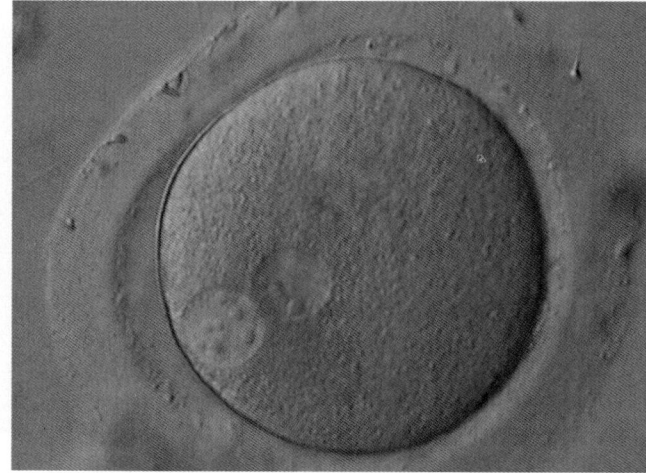

Figure 16.3 An IVF zygote showing peripheral apposition of both pronuclei.

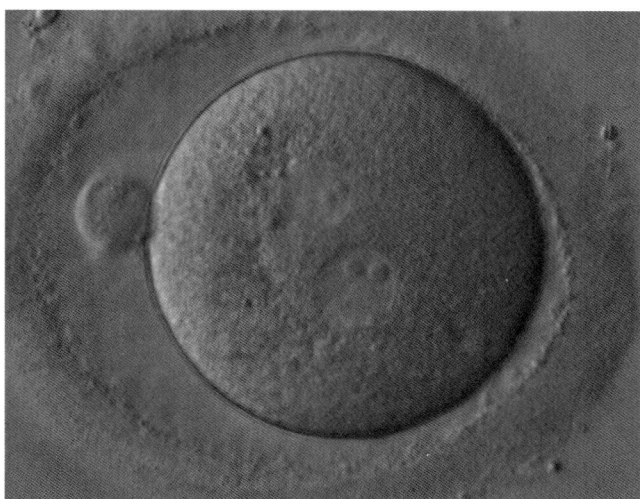

Figure 16.4 A zygote with failure in the alignment of both pronuclei.

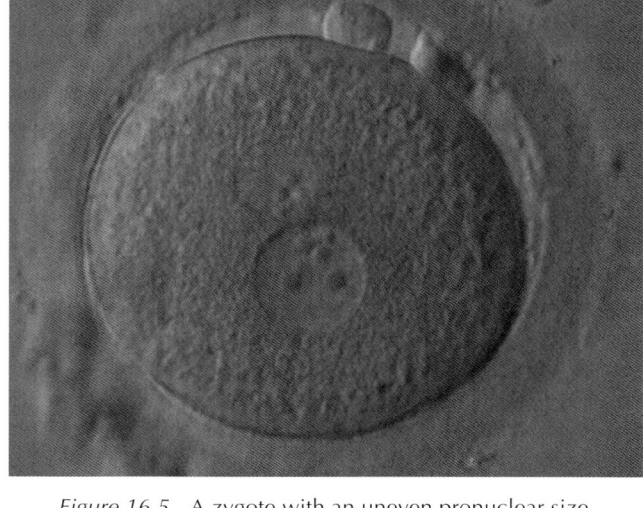

Figure 16.5 A zygote with an uneven pronuclear size.

which is caused by an intrinsic defect of the cytoskeleton, or the parental centrosome may cause a complete failure in alignment (9). While it is rather uncommon in assisted reproductive techniques (approximately 1%) it is rather detrimental since the vast majority of zygotes with unaligned pronuclei fail to cleave or show developmental arrest at early stages (10) if not resulting in chromosomal aberrations at all (24).

Though the female pronucleus usually is smaller than its male counterpart (4), more extensive differences in size (>4 µm) may be observed in vitro (Fig. 16.5). This divergence most likely is the result of problems arising during male pronucleus formation since in vitro matured oocytes ICSI with labeled spermatozoa showed proximity of the fluorescent sperm mid-piece remnant to the smaller pronucleus (36). Uneven pronuclear size severely affects viability of the corresponding embryos since more than 87% were found to be aneuploid, mostly mosaics (37,38). This fact probably led them to arrest at a significantly higher rate than zygotes with pronuclear diameters showing no excessive differences. In addition, a higher incidence of day 2 multinucleation was observed (37).

Interestingly, 1% of all zygotes do not show pronuclei at all (30). Manor et al. (38) demonstrated that 57% of such undocumented zygotes are normally diploid. If two polar bodies are present on day 1, corresponding embryos may be considered for transfer in case insufficient bipronucleated embryos are available. The most probable reason for this failure in detection is an abnormal developmental speed and/or inaccurate timing of fertilization control. It has also been reported that pronuclei may be hidden to extensive cytoplasmic granularity (30).

CYTOPLASMIC HALO

Immediately prior to pronuclear growth, a microtubule-mediated withdrawal of mitochondria and other cytoplasmic components contracts from the cortex toward the center of the oocyte leaving a clear halo around the cortex (4). Since the presence of a halo effect (Fig. 16.1B) within the ooplasm may be recognized in 65–85% of all zygotes (17,19,39) it is less applicable for scoring purposes than pronuclear pattern. Nevertheless, this particular morphism was found to be correlated with better embryo quality (14,19), increased blastocyst formation on day 5 (40), and a higher pregnancy rate (39). The physiological role of mitochondrial redistribution in zygotes is still unknown but it has been speculated that clustering of mitochondria to perinuclear regions may be involved in cell cycle regulation (41–43), for example, by means of calcium mobilization and ATP liberation (44–46). In addition, location of mitochondria next to the pronuclei will allow immature mitochondria, as seen in zygotes (47), to complete maturation presuming that some input from the nucleus is needed (43).

There is a certain disagreement among most of the studies dealing with cytoplasmic appearance at zygote stage. Some did not distinguish between several types of haloes, thus pooling symmetrical and polar haloes (9,19), whereas others presuppose that symmetrical (39) or extreme haloes (40) are abnormal. In view of this lack of uniformity our working group (17) set up a prospective trial to investigate the actual influence of certain subtypes of haloes on preimplantation development of IVF and ICSI embryos. In this paper, haloes were measured accurately in order to see whether a light or extreme halo effect would have any impact on subsequent developmental stages. Based on our findings it was concluded that any halo effect, irrespective of its grade and dimension, is of positive predictive power in terms of blastocyst quality and, consequently, clinical pregnancy rate (17). Neither the method used for insemination (IVF or ICSI) nor the presence of areas of dense cytoplasmic granulation or larger vacuoles affected the zygote in terms of halo performance. Furthermore, it was demonstrated that pronuclear pattern and halo formation are two distinct parameters (17).

CONCLUSION

During the evaluation of zygote morphology it has to be considered that halo and pronuclear formation follow a fixed schedule. Since direct ooplasmic placement of a viable spermatozoon is performed in ICSI, thus bypassing most steps of fertilization (including acrosome reaction and zona binding), the further course of development will be somewhat accelerated as compared with conventional IVF.

Pronuclear morphology and halo characteristics have turned out to be unstable independent factors within the dynamic process of fertilization. The degree and morphology of the halo per se has no influence on further outcome. However, presence of such a halo was of positive predictive power. Consequently, halo formation in combination with optimal pronuclear patterns, for example, those with alignment of fused nucleoli, will characterize a subgroup of oocytes showing a developmental advantage over zygotes which do not show these positive predictors. This is in line with recent findings indicating that during syngamy those zygotes with an accelerated breakdown of the pronuclear membranes 22–25 hours post insemination or injection implanted significantly more frequently than those with delayed dissolution (48). Furthermore, one should not forget the reported positive correlation between the occurrence of the first mitotic division and the rates of implantation and clinical pregnancy (49–51).

Recently, promising strategies have been published combining morphological information of zygote stage with other developmental stages (52–56). In detail, a sequential assessment of cultured human embryos allowed for accurate prognosis in terms of good quality blastocyst development (54,55). Others (52) found relatively high outcome predictability after IVF using a combined score for zygote and embryo morphology, and growth rate. Finally, day 3 embryo transfer with combined evaluation at the pronuclear and cleavage stage compared favorably with day 5 blastocyst transfer (53) (see chap. 18 by Sakkas and Gardner for further details). It is proposed that zygote stage, although being an important developmental phase, should not be used solitarily as a prognostic parameter but much rather morphological information from day 1 should be pooled with that of earlier and/or later stages in order to maximize benefit and minimize the numbers of embryos transferred.

REFERENCES

1. Nagy ZP, Janssenswillen C, Janssens R, et al. Timing of oocyte activation, pronucleus formation, and cleavage in humans after intracytoplasmic sperm injection (ICSI) with testicular spermatozoa and after ICSI or in-vitro fertilization on sibling oocytes with ejaculated spermatozoa. Hum Reprod 1998; 13: 1606–12.
2. van Wissen B, Wolf JP, Bomsel-Helmreich O, et al. Timing of pronuclear development and first cleavages in human embryos after subzonal insemination: influence of sperm phenotype. Hum Reprod 1995; 10: 642–8.
3. Montag M, Van der Ven H. Evaluation of pronuclear morphology as the only selection criterion for further embryo culture and transfer: results of a prospective multicentre study. Hum Reprod 2001; 16: 2384–9.
4. Payne D, Flaherty SP, Barry MF, et al. Preliminary observations on polar body extrusion and pronuclear formation in human oocytes using time-lapse video cinematography. Hum Reprod 1997; 12: 532–41.
5. Van Blerkom J, Davis P, Merriman J, et al. Nuclear and cytoplasmic dynamics of sperm penetration, pronuclear formation and microtubule organization during fertilization and early preimplantation development in the human. Hum Reprod Update 1995; 1: 429–61.
6. Scott L. The biological basis of non-invasive strategies for selection of human oocytes and embryos. Hum Reprod Update 2003; 9: 137–249.
7. Tesarik J, Kopecny V. Development of human male pronucleus: ultrastructure and timing. Gamete Res 1989; 24: 135–49.
8. Van Blerkom J. Occurrence and developmental consequences of aberrant cellular organization in meiotically mature oocytes after exogeneous ovarian hyperstimulation. J Electron Microsc Technique 1990; 16: 324–46.
9. Scott LA, Smith S. The successful use of pronuclear embryo transfers the day following oocyte retrieval. Hum Reprod 1998; 13: 1003–13.
10. Tesarik J, Greco E. The probability of abnormal preimplantation development can be predicted by a single static observation on pronuclear stage morphology. Hum Reprod 1999; 14: 1318–23.
11. Tesarik J, Junca AM, Hazout A, et al. Embryos with high implantation potential after intracytoplasmic sperm injection can be recognized by a simple, non-invasive examination of pronuclear morphology. Hum Reprod 2000; 15: 1396–9.
12. Scott LA, Alvero R, Leondires M. The morphology of human pronuclear embryos is positively related to blastocyst development and implantation. Hum Reprod 2000; 15: 2394–403.
13. Wright G, Wiker S, Elsner C, et al. Observations on the morphology of pronuclei and nucleoli in human zygotes and implications for cryopreservation. Hum Reprod 1990; 5: 109–15.
14. Scott L. Pronuclear scoring as a predictor of embryo development. Reprod Biomed Online 2003; 6: 201–14.
15. Ludwig M, Schöpper B. Al-Hasani. Clinical use of a PN stage score following intracytoplasmic sperm injection: impact on pregnancy rates under the conditions of the German embryo protection law. Hum Reprod 2000; 15: 325–9.
16. Wittemer C, Bettahar-Lebugle K, Ohl J. Zygote evaluation: an efficient tool for embryo selection. Hum Reprod 2000; 15: 2591–7.
17. Ebner T, Moser M, Sommergruber M, et al. Presence, but not type or degree of extension, of a cytoplasmic halo has a significant influence on preimplantation development and implantation behaviour. Hum Reprod 2003; 18: 2406–12.
18. Arroyo G, Veiga A, Santaló J, et al. Developmental prognosis for zygotes based on pronuclear pattern: usefulness of pronuclear scoring. J Assist Reprod Genetics 2007; 14: 173–81.
19. Salumets A, Hydén-Granskog C, Suikkari AM, et al. The predictive value of pronuclear morphology of zygotes in the assessment of human embryo quality. Hum Reprod 2001; 16: 2177–81.
20. Balaban B, Urman B, Isiklar A, et al. The effect of pronuclear morphology on embryo quality parameters and blastocyst transfer outcome. Hum Reprod 2001; 16: 2357–61.

21. Balaban B, Yakin K, Urman B, et al. Pronuclear morphology predicts embryo development and chromosome constitution. Reprod Biomed Online 2004; 8: 695–700.
22. Chen CK, Shen GY, Horng SG, et al. The relationship of pronuclear stage morphology and chromosome status at cleavage stage. J Assist Reprod genetics 2003; 20: 413–20.
23. Kahraman S, Kumtepe Y, Sertyel S, et al. Pronuclear morphology scoring and chromosomal status of embryos in severe male infertility. Hum Reprod 2002; 17: 3193–200.
24. Gianaroli L, Magli MC, Ferraretti AP, et al. Pronuclear morphology and chromosomal abnormalities as scoring criteria for embryo selection. Fertil Steril 2003; 80: 341–9.
25. Arroyo G, Santaló J, Parriego M, et al. Pronuclear morphology, embryo development and chromosome constitution. Reprod Biomed Online 2010; 20: 649–55.
26. Sakkas D, Shoukir Y, Chardonnens D, et al. Early cleavage of human embryos to the two-cell stage after intracytoplasmic sperm injection as an indicator of embryo viability. Hum Reprod 1998; 13: 182–7.
27. Garello C, Baker H, Rai J, et al. Pronuclear orientation, polar body placement, and embryo quality after intracytoplasmic sperm injection and in-vitro fertilization: further evidence for polarity in human oocytes? Hum Reprod 1999; 14: 2588–94.
28. Kattera S, Chen C. Developmental potential of human pronuclear zygotes in relation to their pronuclear orientation. Hum Reprod 2004; 19: 294–9.
29. Edwards RG, Beard HK. Oocyte polarity and cell determination in early mammalian embryos. Mol Hum Reprod 1997; 3: 863–905.
30. Munné S, Cohen J. Chromosome abnormalities in human embryos. Hum Reprod Update 1997; 6: 842–55.
31. Plachot M. Chromosome analysis of oocytes and embryos. In: Verlinsky Y, Kuliev AM, eds. Preimplantation Genetics. New York: Plenum Press, 1991: 103–12.
32. Staessen C, janssenwillen C, Devroey P, et al. Cytogenetic and morphological observations of single pronucleated human oocytes after in-vitro fertilization. Hum Reproduction 1993; 8: 221–3.
33. Sultan KM, Munné S, Palermo GD, et al. Chromosomal status of uni-pronuclear human zygotes following in-vitro fertilization and intracytoplasmic sperm injection. Hum Reprod 1995; 10: 132–6.
34. Staessen C, Van Steirteghem AC. The chromosomal constitution of embryos developing from abnormally fertilized oocytes after intracytoplasmic sperm injection and conventional in-vitro fertilization. Hum Reprod 1997; 12: 321–7.
35. Levron J, Munné S, Willadsen S, et al. Male and female genomes associated in a single pronucleus in human zygotes. Biol Reprod 1995; 52: 653–7.
36. Goud P, Goud A, Van Oostveldt P, et al. Fertilization abnormalities und pronucleus size asynchrony after intracytoplasmic sperm injection are related to oocyte post maturity. Fertil Steril 1999; 72: 245.
37. Sadowy S, Tomkin G, Munné S, et al. Impaired development of zygotes with uneven pronuclear size. Zygote 1998; 6: 137–41.
38. Manor D, Drugan A, Stein D, et al. Unequal pronuclear size – a powerful predictor of embryonic chromosome anomalies. J Assist Reprod Genetics 1999; 16: 385–9.
39. Stalf T, Herrero J, Mehnert C, et al. Influence of polarization effects and pronuclei on embryo quality and implantation in an IVF program. J Assist Reprod Genetics 2002; 19: 355–62.
40. Zollner U, Zollner KP, Hartl G, et al. The use of a detailed zygote score after IVF/ICSI to obtain good quality blastocysts: the German experience. Hum Reprod 2002; 17: 1327–33.
41. Barnett DK, Kimura J, Bavister BD. Translocation of active mitochondria during hamster preimplantation embryo development studied by confocal laser scanning microscopy. Dev Dyn 1996; 205: 64–72.
42. Wu GJ, Simerly C, Zoran SS, et al. Microtubule and chromatin dynamics during fertilization and early development in rhesus monkeys, and regulation by intracellular calcium ions. Biol Reprod 1996; 55: 260–70.
43. Bavister BD, Squirrell JM. Mitochondrial distribution and function in oocytes and early embryos. Hum Reprod 2000; 15(Suppl 2): 189–98.
44. Sousa M, Barros A, Silva J, et al. Developmental changes in calcium content of ultrastructurally distinct subcellular compartments of pre-implantation human embryos. Mol Hum Reprod 1997; 3: 83–90.
45. Diaz G, Setzu M, Zucca A, et al. Subcellular heterogeneity of mitochondrial membrane potential: relationship with organelle distribution and intercellular contacts in normal, hypoxic and apoptotic cells. J Cell Sci 1999; 112: 1077–84.
46. Van Blerkom J, Davis P, Alexander S. Differential mitochondrial distribution in human pronuclear embryos leads to disproportionate inheritance between blastomeres: relationship to microtubular organization, ATP content and competence. Hum Reprod 2000; 15: 2621–33.
47. Motta PM, Nottola SA, Makabe S, et al. Mitochondrial morphology in human fetal and adult gene cells. Hum Reprod 2000; 15(Suppl 2): 129–47.
48. Fancsovits P, Toth L, Takacz ZF, et al. Early pronuclear breakdown is a good indicator of embryo quality and viability. Fertil Steril 2005; 84: 881–7.
49. Shoukir Y, Campana A, Farley T, et al. Early cleavage of in-vitro fertilized human embryos to the 2-cell stage: a novel indicator of embryo quality und viability. Hum Reprod 1997; 12: 1531–6.
50. Sakkas D, Percival G, D´Arcy Y, et al. Assessment of early cleaving in in vitro fertilized human embryos at the 2-cell stage before transfer improves embryo selection. Fertil Steril 2001; 76: 1150–6.
51. Lundin K, Bergh C, Hardarson T. Early embryo cleavage is a strong indicator of embryo quality in human IVF. Hum Reprod 2001; 16: 2652–7.
52. De Placido G, Wilding M, Strina I, et al. High outcome predictability after IVF using a combined score for zygote und embryo morphology und growth rate. Hum Reprod 2002; 17: 2402–9.
53. Rienzi L, Ubaldi F, Iacobelli M, et al. Day 3 embryo transfer with combined evaluation at the pronuclear and cleavage stage compares favourably with day 5 blastocyst transfer. Hum Reprod 2002; 17: 1852–5.
54. Lan KC, Huang FJ, Lin YC, et al. The predictive value of using a combined Z-score und day 3 embryo morphology score in the assessment of embryo survival on day 5. Hum Reprod 2003; 18: 1299–306.
55. Neuber E, Rinaudo P, Trimarchi JR, et al. Sequential assessment of individually cultured human embryos as an indicator of subsequent good quality blastocyst development. Hum Reprod 2003; 18: 1307–12.
56. Alvarez C, Taronger R, Garcia-Garrido C, et al. Zygote score and status 1 or 2 days after cleavage and assisted reproduction outcome. Int J Gynaecol Obstet 2008; 101: 16–20.

17
Culture systems for the human embryo

David K. Gardner and Michelle Lane

INTRODUCTION

Embryo culture is often mistaken for a relatively simple procedure. In reality, it is a complex task, requiring proactive quality control and quality assurance programs, together with a high level of training for embryologists. Furthermore, a sufficient number of incubation chambers are required to maintain a stable environment for development in vitro. Consequently, embryo culture is far more involved than simply using the appropriate culture media formulations. In order to optimize embryo development in vitro and maintain the viability of the conceptus, it is essential to consider the embryo culture system in its entirety. The embryo culture system consists of the media, gas phase, type of medium overlay, the culture vessel, the incubation chamber, ambient air quality, and the embryologists themselves. The concept of an embryo culture system highlights the interactions that exist not only between the embryo and its physical surroundings, but between all parameters within the laboratory (Fig. 17.1). Only by taking such a holistic approach can one optimize embryo development in vitro.

It is also important to appreciate that it is not possible to make a good embryo from poor-quality gametes. Rather, the role of the laboratory is to maintain the inherent viability of the oocyte and sperm from which the embryo is derived. Ultimately, the in vitro fertilization (IVF) laboratory is dependent on the quality of the ovarian stimulation decided by the physician, the development of a receptive endometrium, as well as on patient factors including the impact of their lifestyle choices, and hence emphasizes the need for a broader perspective of patient management as well as laboratory management. In order to ensure consistent successful outcomes adequate communication pathways need to exist between physicians and scientists to ensure all variables are monitored, and action plans put in place, should changes need to be implemented.

THE HUMAN EMBRYO IN CULTURE

Serendipitously for the field of human IVF, the human embryo exhibits a considerable degree of plasticity, enabling it to develop under a wide variety of culture conditions. Indeed it appears that the human preimplantation embryo is the most resilient of all mammalian species studied to date. However, this should be perceived as a testament of the ability of the human embryo to adapt to its surroundings and not our ability to culture it. Undoubtedly, having to adapt to suboptimal collection and/or culture conditions comes at the cost of impaired viability and potentially compromised pregnancy outcomes (1,2). Therefore, it is important to focus on the generation of healthy embryos, as it is evident that embryo development in culture, even to the blastocyst stage per se, does not necessarily equate to the development of a viable embryo (3). The definition of viability is best defined as the ability of the embryo to implant successfully and give rise to a normal healthy term baby. Subsequently, implantation rate (fetal heart rate, as opposed to fetal sac), and ideally live birth rates, should always be reported and considered, as they reflect the true efficacy of a given IVF system.

Today, clinics are not only faced with a multitude of embryo culture media to choose from, whether to employ a reduced oxygen concentration etc. but also have to make a decision of whether to transfer at the cleavage or the blastocyst stage. However, with the publication of an evidence-based Cochrane review (4) and subsequent meta-analysis (5), demonstrating a clear increase in pregnancy and implantation rates and reduced pregnancy loss following blastocyst culture in sequential media, and with morphological selection being more predictive at the blastocyst stage, there is an increasing awareness and need for laboratories to be able to support extended culture (3). It is the aim of this chapter to discuss the types of media and culture systems currently available, and to describe how they can be implemented in a clinical setting irrespective of the day of transfer.

IMPACT OF SINGLE EMBRYO TRANSFER ON THE LABORATORY

It is evident that with the development of enhanced culture systems and better methods for embryo selection (chap. 18 by Sakkas and Gardner) and cryopreservation (chaps. 23 by Zaninovic and 24 by Nagy), the move to single embryo transfer (SET) for a significant number of patients is now a practical reality. Indeed, in several countries this is mandated. Far from being exceptional, SET (or single blastocyst transfer) is becoming the primary

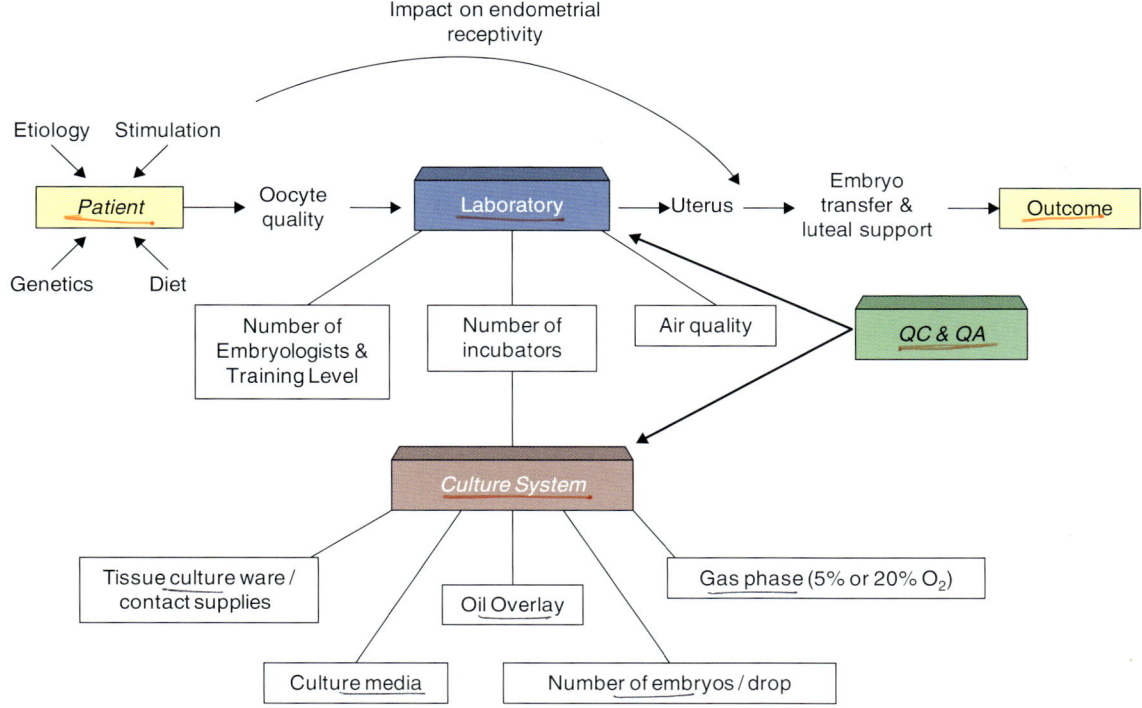

Figure 17.1 The relationship between patient stimulation, the laboratory, and transfer outcome in human in vitro fertilization (IVF). This figure serves to illustrate the complex and interdependent nature of human IVF treatment. For example, the stimulation regimen used not only impacts on oocyte quality (and hence embryo physiology and viability (186)), but can also affect subsequent endometrial receptivity ((131, 187–189). Furthermore, the health and dietary status of the patient can have a profound effect on the subsequent developmental capacity of the oocyte and embryo (66,190). The dietary status of patients attending IVF is typically not considered as a compounding variable, but growing evidence would indicate otherwise. In the schematic, the laboratory has been broken down into its core components, only one of which is the culture system. The culture system has in turn been broken down to its components, only one of which is the culture media. Therefore, it will appear rather simplistic to assume that by changing only one part of the culture system (i.e., culture media), that one is going to mimic the results of a given laboratory or clinic. One of the biggest impacts on the success of a laboratory and culture system is the level of quality control (QC) and quality assurance (QA) in place. For example, one should never assume that anything coming into the laboratory that has not been pre-tested with a relevant bioassay (e.g., mouse embryo assay), is safe merely because a previous lot has performed satisfactorily. Only a small percentage of the contact supplies and tissue culture ware used in IVF comes suitably tested. Therefore it is essential to assume that everything entering the IVF laboratory without a suitable pre-test is embryotoxic until proven otherwise. In our program the 1-cell mouse embryo assay (MEA) is employed to prescreen every lot of tissue culture ware that enters the program. Around 25% of all such material fail the 1-cell MEA (in a simple medium lacking protein after the first 24 hrs) (118). Therefore, if one does not perform QC to this level, 1 in 4 of all contact supplies used clinically will compromise embryo development. In reality many programs cannot allocate the resources required for this level of QC and when embryo quality is compromised in the laboratory it is the media that are held responsible, when in fact the labware are more often the culprit. *Source*: Adapted from Ref. 92.

standard of care for the majority of patients that seek IVF treatment (6) (chap. 54 by Hovatta). One of the impacts of SET is the increased reliance on a successful frozen embryo program. Therefore, an important consideration in assessing the efficacy of any culture system is of its ability to produce high-quality embryos that can survive cryopreservation by freezing and thawing, or by vitrification followed by warming. This has significant implications for cumulative pregnancy rates per retrieval.

DYNAMICS OF EMBRYO AND MATERNAL PHYSIOLOGY

Before attempting to culture any cell type, be it embryonic or somatic, it is important to consider the physiology of the cell in order to establish its nutrient requirements. The mammalian embryo represents an intriguing situation in that it undergoes significant changes in its physiology, molecular regulation, and metabolism during the preimplantation period. The preimplantation human embryo is, therefore, a highly dynamic entity with its needs changing as development proceeds. Indeed, it goes from being one of the most quiescent tissues in the body (the oocyte), to being among the most metabolically active (the blastocyst) within just four days (1). Interestingly, the pronucleate oocyte, like the MII oocyte from which it was derived, exhibits relatively low levels of oxygen consumption and has a preference for carboxylic acids, such as pyruvate, as its primary energy source (7,8). Glucose is only consumed and utilized in relatively small amounts by the early embryo (9). In particular, the balance of mitochondrial and cytoplasmic metabolism is critical at these early stages of development to maintain adequate levels of ATP production (10). However, despite the low levels of biosynthetic activity at these early stages of development there is an increasing awareness of a significant amount

Table 17.1 Differences in Embryo Physiology Pre- and Postcompaction

Pre-compaction	Postcompaction
Low biosynthetic activity	High biosynthetic activity
Low oxygen utilisation	High oxygen utilisation
Preferred nutrient, pyruvate	Preferred nutrient, glucose
Nonessential amino acids	Nonessential + essential amino acids
Maternal genome	Embryonic genome
Individual cells	Transporting epithelium
1 cell type	2 distinct cell types: inner cell mass and trophectoderm

- Highly susceptible to stress
- limited capacity to maintain cellular functions as intracellular pH, ionic haemostasis
- less susceptible

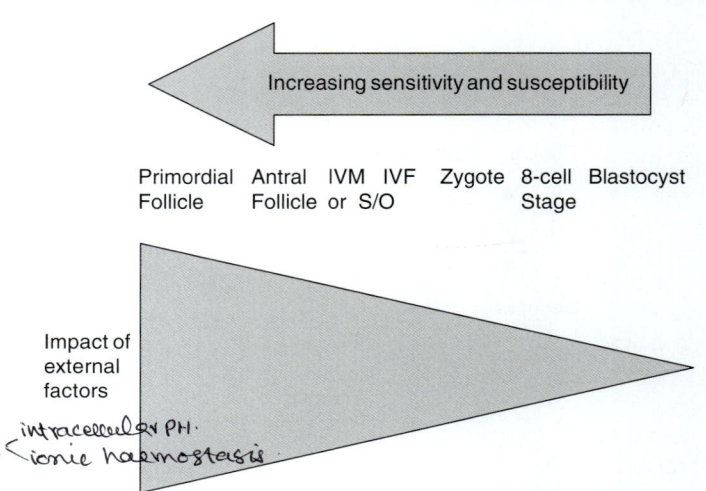

Figure 17.2 Sensitivity and susceptibility of germ cells and embryos to external factors. *Abbreviations*: IVF, in vitro fertilization; IVM, in vitro maturation; S/O, superovulation.

of remodeling of the nucleus. For example, there are major changes in methylation and acetylation levels, with many of the processes involved still to be elucidated (11–13). Nevertheless, what is critical is that many key developmental events, such as activation of the egg and regulation of methylation and acetylation, are regulated by proteins whose activity is dependent on metabolic regulation (14–16). Therefore, maintenance of metabolic homeostasis at these early stages is paramount for the maintenance of viability. Consequently, the environment of the early embryo continues to be a major focus of the culture system in the laboratory (1).

As development proceeds and energy demands increase with cell multiplication, transcription following activation of the embryonic genome, and subsequent increase in protein synthesis, there is a concomitant increase in energy requirement and glucose utilization. By the blastocyst stage, the embryo exhibits high oxygen utilization and an ability to readily utilize glucose, along with other energy sources. Table 17.1 highlights some of the differences between the pre- and postcompacted embryo. In many ways the physiology of the cells of the embryo prior to compaction, hence before the formation of a transporting epithelium, can be likened to unicellular organisms (17). This in part explains why those amino acids classified as nonessential for tissue culture purposes are beneficial to the cleavage-stage embryo, as they confer stability to several key cell functions.

Significantly, the nutrients available within the human female reproductive tract mirror the changing nutrient preference of the embryo. At the time when the embryo resides in the oviduct the fluid within is characterized by relatively high concentrations of pyruvate (0.32 mM) and lactate (10.5 mM), and a relatively low concentration of glucose (0.5 mM) (18). In contrast, uterine fluid is characterized by relatively low levels of pyruvate (0.1 mM) and lactate (5.87 mM), and a high concentration of glucose (3.15 mM), consistent with the changes in embryo energy production.

SUSCEPTIBILITY OF THE PREIMPLANTATION EMBRYO TO STRESS

There is an increasing understanding in mammalian embryology that the early embryo is highly adaptive to its environment. The embryo appears to have the ability to continue development, even to the blastocyst stage, at the cost of normal cellular processes and checkpoints that may be essential for viability. Therefore, as a result many embryos can appear to be morphologically normal while at a cellular level are actually highly perturbed and unlikely to be viable (2,17). Consequently, one of the key focuses of the embryology laboratory should be to ensure its gamete collection and culture system are able to maintain normal development at a cellular level. Although the human embryo has a plasticity to adapt to its environment, as already highlighted, this is at a cost of cellular regulation either through metabolic adaptations or adaptations at a molecular level. Therefore, the laboratory should seek to employ systems that reduce these adaptations, thereby maintaining viability.

Cleavage Stages Versus Postcompaction Embryo and Stress

As a result of its more "primitive" physiology, the precompaction stage embryo is highly susceptible to stress compared to the postcompaction stage embryo. A stress applied in vitro at the 2PN to the eight-cell stage can have devastating effects on normal cellular physiology and viability of the subsequent blastocyst and fetus (Fig. 17.2) (17,19–21). At these early stages of development prior to activation of the embryonic genome, the embryo possesses only limited capacity at a molecular level to respond to a stress. In somatic cells, when a cell finds itself in a hostile environment it can activate a cascade of molecular signaling pathways to engage systems to maintain normal development. However, the precompaction stage embryo has a limited capacity for gene transcription (22) and therefore, the human embryo prior to the eight-cell stage is highly vulnerable to any perturbed environment. At these early stages of embryo development prior to compaction, there is limited capacity to maintain normal cellular functions such as regulation of intracellular pH (pHi) and alleviation of oxidative stress and ionic homeostasis (2,17). Therefore, a stress applied at these early stages of development can result in major disruptions to subsequent viability. In contrast, the application of the same stress postcompaction and postembryonic genome activation typically has a limited negative impact on subsequent developmental competence (17,20,21).

It is evident that stress can be masked at the level of morphological assessment and may only become evident downstream of the stress itself. It has been shown that the detrimental effects of a stress applied at the early stage of development during handling and culture of the oocyte and 2PN may not be evident until the blastocyst stage. Even then, the effects may only be at a subcellular level with the embryo having reduced metabolic capacity, high levels of apoptosis, and altered molecular profile, which ultimately result in a reduction in pregnancy rates (19–21). Therefore, the conditions employed for the collection and culture of the human cleavage-stage embryo directly affect the ability of the embryo to implant and form a viable pregnancy, independent of morphological assessments within the laboratory. The inability of morphology alone to distinguish viable and nonviable embryos highlights a major limitation in the field and reaffirms the need for the development of more diagnostic procedures to quantitate normal development (chap. 18 by Sakkas and Gardner).

COMPOSITION OF CULTURE MEDIA

There are several extensive treatise on the composition of embryo culture media (8,23–27), and it is beyond the scope of this chapter to discuss in detail the role of individual medium components. However, two key components, amino acids and macromolecules, will be discussed due to their significant impact on cycle outcome. Understanding their effects on embryo physiology will greatly assist clinics to make a more informed decision regarding their choice of culture media.

Amino Acids

It is certainly the case that the human embryo can grow in the absence of amino acids. The real question is: how well do they develop in their absence and how viable are the resultant embryos? There are several reasons for the inclusion of amino acids in embryo culture media. Oviduct and uterine fluids contain significant levels of free amino acids (28–33), while oocytes and embryos possess specific transport systems for amino acids (34) to maintain an endogenous pool (35). Amino acids are readily taken up and metabolized by the embryo (36,37). Table 17.2 lists the roles amino acids can fulfill during the pre- and peri-implantation period of mammalian embryo development.

Oviduct and uterine fluids are characterized by high concentrations of the amino acids such as alanine, aspartate, glutamate, glycine, serine, and taurine (28–33). With the exception of taurine, the amino acids at high concentrations in oviduct fluid bear a striking homology to those amino acids present in Eagle's nonessential amino acids (38). Studies on the embryos of several mammalian species, such as mouse (39–42), hamster (43,44), sheep (45,46), cow (47,48), and human (49,50), have all demonstrated that the inclusion of amino acids in the culture medium enhances embryo development to the blastocyst stage.

Table 17.2 Functions of Amino Acids During Preimplantation Mammalian Embryo Development

Role	Reference
Biosynthetic precursors	(177)
Energy source	(178)
Regulators of energy metabolism	(1,10)
Osmolytes	(179)
Buffers of pHi	(54)
Antioxidants	(180)
Chelators	(181)
Signaling	(182,183)
Regulation of differentiation	(51,184)

More significantly, it has been demonstrated that the preimplantation embryo exhibits a switch in amino acid requirements as development proceeds. Up to the eight-cell stage nonessential amino acids and glutamine increase cleavage rates (48,51,52); that is, those amino acids present at the highest levels in oviduct fluid stimulate the cleavage-stage embryo. However, after compaction, nonessential amino acids and glutamine increase blastocele formation and hatching, while the essential amino acids stimulate cleavage rates and increase development of the inner cell mass (ICM) in the blastocyst (19,51). Recently, the essential amino acid threonine has been shown to be important in the maintenance of pluripotency in mouse embryonic stem cells (53). Importantly, amino acids have been reported to increase viability of cultured embryos from several species after transfer to recipients (23,46,51) as well as increasing embryo development in culture. In the mouse, equivalent implantation rates to in vivo developed blastocysts have been achieved when pronucleate embryos were cultured with nonessential amino acids to the 8-cell stage followed by culture with all 20 amino acids from the 8-cell stage to the blastocyst (51).

The terms nonessential and essential have little meaning in terms of embryo development and differentiation; rather they reflect the requirements of certain somatic cells in vitro (38). More appropriate terminology will reflect the ability of the nonessential group to stimulate early cleavage (cleavage amino acids or CAA), while the essential group stimulate the development of the ICM (ICM amino acids). The reasons for this switch undoubtedly stem from the nature of the nonessential amino acids; they act as good intracellular buffers of pH due to their zwitterionic nature (43), and they are able to chelate toxins. As discussed, prior to compaction the blastomeres of the mammalian embryo appear to behave like unicellular organisms and use exogenous amino acids to help regulate their homeostasis. In contrast, postcompaction and the generation of a transporting epithelium, the embryo is able to regulate its internal environment and is not as dependent on the nonessential amino acids to regulate intracellular function as it did before (54).

It has been shown that even a transient exposure (~5 minutes) of mouse zygotes to medium lacking amino acids impairs subsequent developmental potential, providing further evidence of the significance of amino acids (55). During this five-minute period, in a simple medium the zygote loses its entire endogenous pool of amino acids, which takes several hours of transport to replenish after returning the embryo to medium with amino acids. This has direct implications for the collection of oocytes, and more importantly the manipulation of denuded oocytes during intracytoplasmic sperm injection (ICSI), where the inclusion of amino acids in the holding medium will decrease or prevent intracellular stress.

Similarly, the work of Ho et al. (56) on gene expression in mouse embryos goes some way to confirm this hypothesis, in that gene expression in mouse embryos cultured in the presence of amino acids was comparable to that of embryos developed in vivo. In contrast, mouse embryos cultured in the absence of amino acids, that is, in a medium based on a simple salt solution, exhibited aberrant gene expression and altered the imprinting of the H19 gene (57).

Cautionary Tale

Even though the formulations of embryo culture media have improved significantly over the years, and for the most part have become more physiological in their basis, there is nothing physiological about a polystyrene culture dish. Therefore, one has to be careful about in vitro artifacts induced by a static environment. A good example of this is the production of ammonium by both embryo metabolism of amino acids (58) and by the spontaneous breakdown of amino acids in the culture medium once incubated at 37°C (Fig. 17.3) (39). Although amino acids are used by human embryos, which in turn produce ammonium, it is the spontaneous breakdown of amino acids at 37°C that results in the majority of ammonium produced in the medium. Ammonium buildup in culture medium can not only have negative effects on embryo development and differentiation in culture (39,45,59), but can affect subsequent fetal growth rates and normality at a concentration of around 300 μM (19,60). Furthermore, it has been shown that ammonium affects embryo metabolism, pHi regulation, and gene expression (61). As amino acids are such important regulators of embryo development it is essential to alleviate this in vitro problem. The immediate answer is to renew the culture medium, thereby bringing the ammonium concentration under control. A second, and complementary, solution is to replace the most labile amino acid, glutamine, with a dipeptide form such as alanyl-glutamine or glycyl-glutamine. These dipeptides are just as effective as glutamine and have the

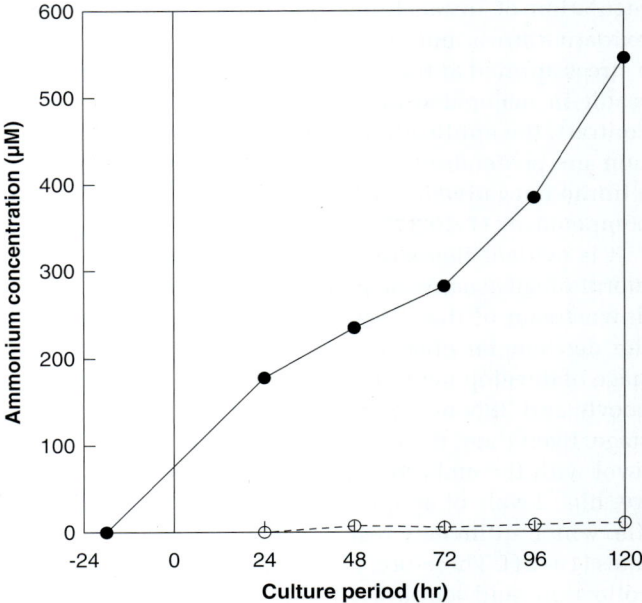

Figure 17.3 Production of ammonium into the culture medium (lacking embryos) by the spontaneous breakdown of amino acids in culture media. Solid circles, KSOM^{AA}; Open circles, G1/G2. The media were placed in the incubator at 4 pm the day before culture for equilibration purposes. The line at time zero represents when embryos would be placed into culture (although these measurements were taken in the absence of embryos). Medium KSOM^{AA} contains 1 mM glutamine and therefore releases significant levels of ammonium into the culture medium. Media G1 and G2 do not contain glutamine, but rather the stable dipeptide form, alanyl-glutamine; therefore, these media do not release significant levels of ammonium. At a concentration of just 75 μmol/L ammonium can induce a 24-hour developmental delay in mouse fetal development by day 15 and induces the neural tube defect exencephaly in 20% of all fetuses (53,61). It is therefore evident that dangerously high levels of ammonium are produced by media containing glutamine. *Source*: Adapted from Ref. 137.

advantage of not breaking down at 37°C. Therefore, media containing such stable forms of glutamine produce significantly lower levels of ammonium.

Although there is some debate as to the level of concern one should place on ammonium toxicity in culture medium (62,63), there is growing data to support the appearance of ammonium in the culture medium over time (39,59,64,65) and its toxicity to embryos, including the human (59). Furthermore, exposure of gametes and embryos to increasing concentrations of ammonium in vivo is not consistent with maintained embryo viability (66–68). It is, therefore, the authors' humble opinion that one should err on the side of caution, consider the data from animal and human in vitro and in vivo studies, and take the appropriate action, that is, renew the culture medium at least every 48 hours. Medium renewal should take place for any culture system that employs amino acids.

Macromolecules

Most culture media for the human embryo contain serum albumin as the protein source. The use of whole serum can no longer be condoned due its documented detrimental effects on embryos (46,69–72).

Although serum albumin is a relatively pure fraction, it is still contaminated with fatty acids and other small molecules. The latter has been shown to include an embryotrophic factor, namely citrate, which stimulates cleavage and growth in rabbit morulae and blastocysts (73). Not only are there significant differences between sources of serum albumin (74,75), but also between batches from the same source (74,76). Therefore, when using serum albumin or any albumin preparation, it is essential that each batch is screened for its ability to adequately support mouse embryo development and human sperm survival prior to clinical use.

Recombinant human albumin is available, which should eliminate the problems inherent with using blood-derived products, and lead to the standardization of media formulations. Recombinant human albumin has now been shown to be as effective as blood-derived albumin in supporting fertilization (77) and embryo development, and its efficacy has been proven in a prospective randomized trial (78). Significantly, embryos cultured in the presence of recombinant albumin exhibit an increased tolerance to cryopreservation (79).

A further macromolecule present in the female reproductive tract is hyaluronan, which in the mouse uterus increases at the time of implantation (80). Hyaluronan is a high molecular mass polysaccharide that can be obtained free of endotoxins and prions from a yeast fermentation procedure. It has been demonstrated that not only can hyaluronan improve mouse and bovine embryo culture systems (81,82), but that its use for embryo transfer results in a significant increase in embryo implantation (81,83,84). In the largest prospective trial to date, which enrolled 1282 cycles of IVF, it was determined that the use of hyaluronan-enriched medium was associated with significant increases in clinical pregnancy rates and implantation rates, both for day 3 and day 5 embryo transfers. The beneficial effect was most evident in women who were >35 years of age, in women who had only poor-quality embryos available for transfer, and in women who had previous implantation failures (84,85).

However, another highly significant effect of the inclusion of hyaluronan in the culture medium is its beneficial effects on cryosurvivability of cultured embryos from a number of species including the human, mouse, sheep, and cow (79,83,86–88). As IVF programs are moving to transfer fewer embryos, there is an increasing need to be able to cryopreserve supernumerary embryos. The ability of culture systems that support increased cryosurvival, therefore increased cumulative pregnancy outcomes, is an important factor in deciding which culture system to use in the laboratory. In Fig. 17.4 the effects of culture medium composition on the cryosurvival and subsequent implantation of human embryos is shown. Embryos were cultured in media with or without hyaluronan prior to slow freezing at the cleavage stage. Both survival and viability were higher if the embryos had been cultured in the presence of hyaluronan.

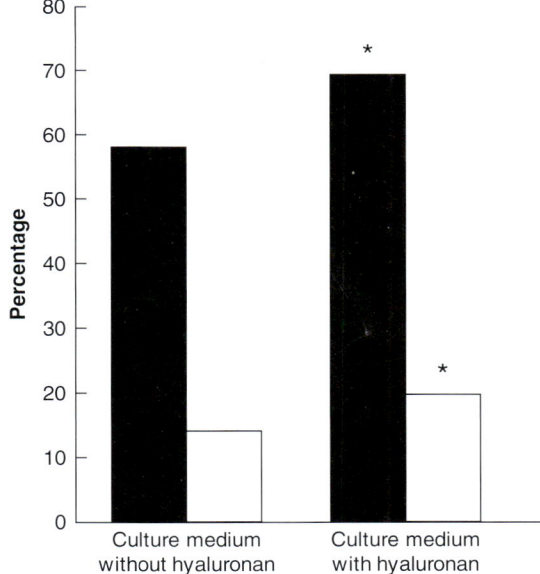

Figure 17.4 Effect of culture medium on the subsequent cryosurvival of cleavage-stage human embryos. Embryos were cultured in a medium either without hyaluronan (n = 1235) or with elevated hyaluronan (n = 1351). Solid bars represent survival rate assessed as greater or equal to 50% of blastomeres being intact post-thaw. Open bars represent implantation rates as assessed by fetal heart beat at an 8-week scan. *Significantly different $P < 0.05$.

MONOCULTURE OR SEQUENTIAL MEDIA?

It was established in the 1960s that it was feasible to culture the one-cell mouse embryo to the blastocyst stage in medium lacking amino acids. In the intervening decades, it has become apparent that amino acids have a significant role to play during embryo development (discussed earlier), and that medium needs to be renewed at least every 48 hours to ensure minimal accumulation of embryotoxic ammonium. Subsequently, all culture systems have become, by default, dynamic (89). From a practical point of view, therefore, the amount of work and embryo manipulations required are the same whether one is working with sequential media or a monophasic system (i.e., one medium formulation for the entire preimplantation period).

However, the two approaches to embryo culture do have some fundamental differences. Specifically, monoculture is based on the principle of letting the embryo choose what it wants during development. In contrast, sequential media were developed to accommodate the dynamics of embryo nutrition and to mirror the environment of the female reproductive tract (in which the embryo is exposed to a gradient of nutrients as it passes along the oviduct into the uterus) (18,32,33). The significance of these nutrient gradients to the embryo in culture warrants further research as existing data on the mouse indicate that such gradients in vitro do impact embryo viability following transfer. For example, when the mouse zygote is cultured to the eight-cell stage and then transferred, embryo viability is highest after exposure of the embryo to a high lactate concentration (>20 mM D/L-lactate). However, when the embryo is cultured postcompaction to the blastocyst stage, viability is highest after exposure to lower levels of lactate (<5 mM D/L-lactate) (90). These data support the hypothesis that the physiology of the developing conceptus is regulated by the concentration of nutrients available at specific stages of development (91). Therefore, sequential media are better able to meet the changing needs of the embryo compared with a single culture medium, which must make a compromise between supporting the pre- or postcompaction stage embryo.

Sequential media have now proven themselves to be highly effective in clinical settings. Assessments of the literature using an evidence-based Cochrane review (4) has determined that the benefit of blastocyst culture over cleavage-stage culture is only evident in a sequential culture system, thereby indicting that there is a compromise in developmental competence when embryos are grown beyond the cleavage stage in a single medium. This finding for human IVF cycles mirrors the literature on animal embryos that have established developmental outcomes more similar to in vivo results after culture in sequential culture media compared with a monoculture system (92).

HOW FAR BEHIND EMBRYO DEVELOPMENT IN VIVO IS TO DEVELOPMENT IN VITRO?

Historically, embryos cultured in vitro lag behind their in vivo developed counterparts (93,94). However, with the development of sequential media based on the premise of meeting the changing requirements of the embryo and minimizing trauma coupled with use of reduced oxygen concentrations in the gas phase, in vivo rates of embryo development can now be attained in vitro in the mouse (1,95). The one proviso is that each laboratory must have sufficient quality systems in place to ensure the optimum operation of a given culture system. Such advances in culture systems represent a significant development for the laboratory, for now there exists a means of producing blastocysts at the same time and with the same cell number and allocation to the ICM as embryos developed in the female tract (89,92). Using sequential media in a highly controlled environment, as detailed throughout this book, it is possible to attain high rates of human embryo development to the blastocyst stage. Using an oocyte donor model to evaluate the efficacy of culture approaches, where the age of the oocytes is typically under 30 years, it is possible not only to obtain a blastocyst formation rate of 65%, but the resultant viability (as determined by fetal heart beat following transfer) is >65% (Table 17.3). As such, oocyte donors represent as close to a human "gold standard" as one can have in an infertility clinic. With this in mind, ensuring one can attain blastocyst development of >50% and implantation rates of over 50% when using donated oocytes is a good potential starting point for introducing blastocyst culture clinically, or patients under 35 years of age.

Table 17.3 Viability of Human Embryos Conceived in Vitro Using an Oocyte Donor Model

Mean blastocyst development (%)	65.1
Mean number of blastocysts transferred	2.05
Mean age of recipient	40.3
Fetal heart beat (per blastocyst transferred) (%)	68.0
Clinical pregnancy rate (per retrieval) (%)	85.2
Twins (%)	59.9

All pronucleate oocytes were cultured for 48 hours in medium G1 at 5% O_2, 6% CO_2, and 89% N_2. On day 3 of development embryos were washed and transferred into medium G2 under the same gaseous environment. Embryos were cultured in groups of 4 in 50 μL drops of medium under Ovoil™ (Vitrolife AB, Gothenburg, Sweden) in 60 mm Falcon Primaria (Becton Dickinson) dishes. All embryos were transferred on day 5 of development. n = 950 patients (185).

CULTURE SYSTEMS

Several key components of the culture system are reviewed here, none of which should be considered in isolation as all directly impact upon media performance.

Incubation Chamber

Whatever incubation chamber is chosen, a key to successful embryo culture is to minimize perturbations in the atmosphere around the embryo. The two key perturbations to avoid are pH and temperature changes. This means that ideally the environment in which the embryo is placed is not disturbed during the culture period. Practically this is difficult to achieve in a busy clinical laboratory. The use of an individual incubation chamber, such as a modular incubator chamber or a glass desiccator which can be purged with the appropriate gas mix, can alleviate such concerns. Using such incubator chambers, each patient's embryos can be completely isolated within an incubator, the gas phase and for the most part temperature, being unaffected when the incubator door is opened. We like to consider such chambers as "a womb with a view." However, a downside of this approach is that only three modular chambers can be placed in one incubator, thereby necessitating the acquisition of sufficient incubators. An alternative to the use of modular chambers is the use of inner doors within an incubator to significantly reduce fluctuations in the gaseous environment upon opening the incubator door. Several incubator manufacturers make incubators with inner doors. A more recent move has been the production of incubators with a greatly reduced working volume, such that rather than two double stacks of conventional incubators (giving four working chambers), one can now have three rows of smaller incubators, stacked three high, giving a total of nine chambers. This approach allows the successful allocation of one chamber to just one or two patients, thereby stabilizing the culture environment.

Incubators with infrared as opposed to thermo couple CO_2 sensors are quicker at regulating the internal environment of the chamber, and are less sensitive to environmental factors such as humidity and subsequently are better able to maintain a constant CO_2 level in the incubator. Therefore, incubators equipped with infrared sensors will provide a more stable environment for embryo development.

With regards to temperature changes, incubators with an air jacket are less susceptible to large temperature fluctuations as those with a water jacket. Again the use of inner doors will aid in minimizing environmental fluctuations within the chamber.

Alternatives to classic tissue culture incubators are the mini incubators with constant flow chambers, which allow for direct heat transfer between the chamber and culture vessel. Such chambers also allow for a direct flow of premixed gas and therefore minimize changes in pH. However, such systems come at relatively high running costs (using premixed gas cylinders) and have limited ability to maintain temperature or pH in the event of an emergency.

What is evident is that it is imperative to have sufficient numbers of incubator chambers to match the caseload. This is especially true when performing extended culture. It is important to consider the number of times an incubator will be opened in a day and to keep this to a minimum. It is advisable to have separate incubators for media equilibration and for embryo culture, thereby minimizing the amount of access to incubators containing embryos. It can also be useful to have a mixture of incubator chambers for overnight or longer-term cultures, and desktop models which recover quickly for manipulations such as denuding and ICSI. Consistent high rates of implantation are achieved if an incubation chamber is used for just two to three patients per week. Space can be optimized through the use of smaller incubation chambers.

pH and Carbon Dioxide

When discussing pH it is worth considering that the pHi of the embryo is around 7.2 (96–98) while the pH of the media routinely ranges from 7.25 to 7.40. Specific media components, such as lactic and amino acids directly affect and buffer pHi respectively. Of the two isomers of lactate, D- and L-, only the L-form is biologically active. However, both the D- and L-forms decrease pHi of the embryo (98). Therefore, it is advisable to use only the L-isomer of lactate and not a medium containing both the D- and L-forms. While high concentrations of lactate in the culture medium can drive pHi down (98), amino acids increase the intracellular buffering capacity and help maintain the pHi at around 7.2 (54). As the embryo has to maintain pHi against a gradient when incubated at pH 7.4, it would seem prudent to culture embryos at a lower pH. The pH of a CO_2/bicarbonate buffered medium is not easy to quantitate. A pH electrode can be used, but one must be quick and the same technician must take all readings to ensure consistency. An alternative approach is to take samples of the medium and measure the pH with a blood–gas analyzer. A final method necessitates the presence of phenol red in the culture medium and the use of Sorensons's phosphate buffer standards. This method allows visual inspection of a medium's pH with a tube in the incubator and is accurate to 0.2 pH units (8,26).

When using bicarbonate buffered media, the concentration of CO_2 has a direct impact on medium pH (26). Although most media work over a wide range of pH (7.2–7.4), it is preferable to ensure that pH does not go over 7.4. Therefore, it is advisable to use a CO_2 concentration of between 6% and 7% to yield a medium pH of around 7.3. The amount of CO_2 in the incubation chamber can be calibrated with a Fyrite® (Bacharach, New Kensington, Pennsylvania, USA), although such an approach is only accurate to ±1%. A more suitable method is to use a hand-held infrared metering system, such as that made by Vaisala, which can calibrate and is accurate to around 0.2%.

When using a CO_2/bicarbonate-buffered medium it is essential to minimize the amount of time the culture dish is out of a CO_2 environment to prevent increases in pH. To facilitate this modified pediatric isolettes designed to maintain temperature, humidity and CO_2 concentration can be used. However, should it not be feasible to use an isolette, then the media used can be buffered with either 20–23 mM 4-(2-hydroxyethyl)-1-piperazine-ethanesulfonic acid (HEPES) (99) or 4-morpholinopropanesulfonic acid (MOPS) (100) together with 5–2 mM bicarbonate. Such buffering systems do not require a CO_2 environment. An oil overlay also reduces the speed of CO_2 loss and the associated increase in pH.

Oxygen

The concentration of oxygen in the lumen of the rabbit oviduct is reported to be 2–6% (101,102), whereas the oxygen concentration in the oviduct of hamster and rhesus monkey is ~8% (103). Interestingly, the oxygen concentration in the uterus is significantly lower than in the oviduct, ranging from 5% in the hamster and rabbit to 1.5% in the rhesus monkey (103).

Significantly, it has been demonstrated that optimum embryo development of all non-human mammalian species occurs at an oxygen concentration below 10% (74,104,105). The fact that human embryos can grow at an atmospheric oxygen concentration (~20%) and give rise to viable pregnancies, has led to some confusion regarding the optimal concentration for embryo culture. Consequently, the validity of having to use a reduced oxygen concentration for human embryo culture is continually challenged. The continued use of 20% oxygen in a human IVF culture system is a good example of something that has been used for over three decades and does give results; however, the question remains, does 20% oxygen adversely affect the physiology of the developing embryo before implantation?

In the mouse model it has been established that 20% oxygen impacts embryo development as early as the first cleavage (Fig. 17.5) (106). Of great interest is that 20% oxygen is found to be detrimental to embryo development at all stages, but with the greatest detrimental effects being imparted at the cleavage stages (106).

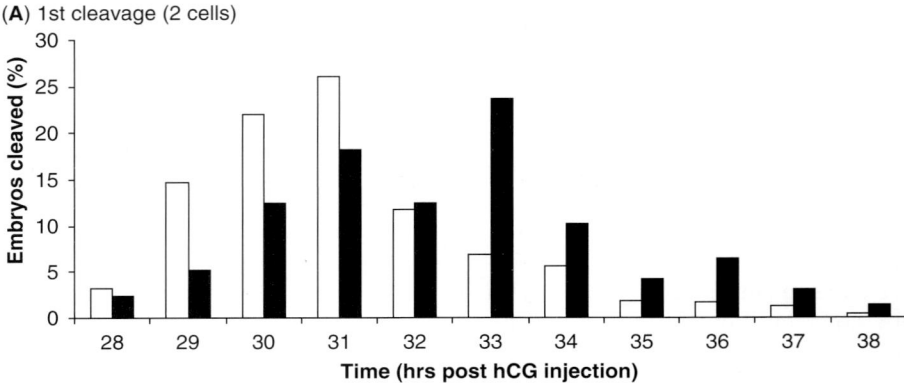
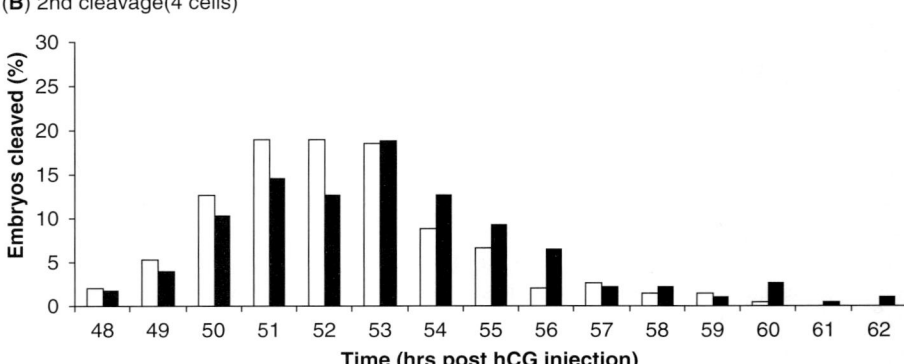
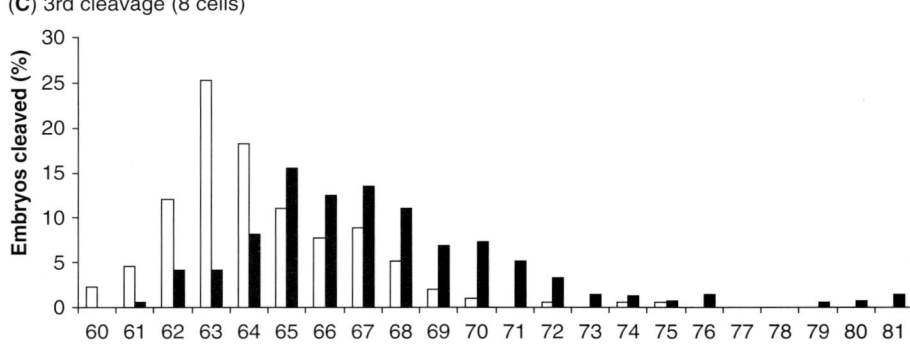

Figure 17.5 Distribution of cleavage timing for 1st, 2nd, and 3rd cleavage divisions of mouse pronucleate oocytes cultured in either 5% or 20% oxygen. White bars represent 5% oxygen concentration and black bars represent 20% oxygen concentration. As development progresses, there is a significant cumulative delay in embryo development induced by 20% oxygen. *Source*: Adapted from Ref. 106.

Furthermore, embryos cultured to the blastocyst stage in the presence of 20% oxygen have altered gene expression and perturbed proteome compared with embryos developed in vivo (17,107,108). In contrast, culture in 5% oxygen had significantly less effect on both embryonic gene expression and proteome. Similarly, 20% oxygen has been shown to adversely affect embryonic metabolism (2).

These data from animal models clearly indicate that 20% oxygen induces significant trauma at the genomic, proteomic, and metabolomic level. Consequently, it is strongly recommended to culture embryos at low oxygen concentrations (~5%). This can easily be achieved with modern tri-gas incubators or by using a premixed cylinder to purge a modular chamber/direct contact incubator.

Recent clinical data, including a randomized controlled trial, support this move to more physiological conditions where lower oxygen concentrations increased both implantation and live birth rates (109–111).

Incubation Vessel and the Embryo:Volume Ratio

Culture of embryos in drops of culture medium under an oil overlay is the preferred and effective method of culturing embryos. Within the lumen of the female reproductive tract the developing embryo is exposed to microliter volumes of fluid (112). In contrast, the embryo grown in vitro is subject to relatively large volumes of medium of up to 1 mL. Consequently, any autocrine factor(s) produced by the developing embryo will be diluted and may therefore become ineffectual. It has been demonstrated in the mouse that cleavage rate and blastocyst formation increase when embryos are grown in groups (up to 10) or reduced volumes (around 20 µL) (113–115). Of greatest significance is the observation that decreasing the incubation volume significantly increases embryo viability (115) due to an increase in ICM development. Similar results have been obtained with sheep (45) and cow embryos (116). It is therefore apparent that the preimplantation mammalian embryo produces a factor(s) capable of stimulating development of both itself and surrounding embryos. Furthermore, embryos of one species can be used to promote development and differentiation of another (117).

In order to culture in such reduced volumes (of 20–50 µL) an oil overlay is required. Although the use of an oil overlay is time consuming, it prevents the evaporation of media, thereby reducing the harmful effects of increases in osmolality, and reduces changes in pH caused by a loss of CO_2 from the medium when culture dishes are taken out of the incubator for embryo examination. Embryo-tested paraffin oil is highly recommended. Such an overlay also serves another purpose in being able to trap a number of volatile organic compounds.

The benefits of using drops of medium under oil would obviously be negated should the oil be embryo toxic. Therefore, care must be taken in selecting and storing oil, which if done incorrectly will lead to it becoming toxic. Oil should be stored in the dark and in glass. It should not be stored for extended periods in the incubator. Oil should never be aliquoted into tissue culture flasks as these are styrene based and oils are able to leach styrene from such containers at high rates over time. Always use a batch of oil prescreened with an appropriate mouse embryo bioassay before clinical use. Oil toxicity may not necessarily show up by simply culturing mouse embryos to the blastocyst stage. Rather, one should also look for signs of necrosis, which is most evident at the blastocyst stage, and perform cell counts on the blastocysts developed.

Medium Storage

Commercially available culture media have several labile components and it is therefore important to know how to handle and store such solutions. Two of the most labile components are amino acids and vitamins. Glutamine is the most labile amino acid and produces the highest levels of ammonium of any amino acid. Therefore, it is paramount that when using culture media containing amino acids they are placed in the incubator for the minimum time required for equilibration, and they should certainly never be stored in the incubator. Fortunately, glutamine can be replaced with alanyl-glutamine or glycyl-glutamine, dipeptides that are stable at 37°C. Vitamins are light sensitive and therefore care should be taken to minimize exposure to light by storing culture media in the dark.

Quality Control

Setting up an appropriate quality control system for the IVF laboratory is a pre-requisite in the establishment of a successful laboratory (chap. 2). The types of bioassays conducted for this have been the focus of much discussion (118). In reality there is no perfect model for the human, save for the very patients we treat. Consequently, it is important to understand the limitations of the assays performed and to use data obtained from bioassays in an appropriate fashion. Quality control should not be limited to the culture media used, but should include all contact supplies and gases used in an IVF procedure. The bioassay we favor is the culture of pronucleate mouse oocytes in protein-free media. There has been a lot of conflicting data regarding the use of the mouse embryo bioassay, but by adjusting conditions, one can not only increase the sensitivity of the assay, but can also quantitate quality with it.

First of all the stage at which the embryo is cultured from has an impact on development. Mouse embryos collected at the pronucleate stage do not tend to fair as well in culture as those collected at the two-cell stage. Second, the strain of mice is important. Embryos from hybrid parents have a decided advantage in culture, and do not represent the diverse genetic background one is dealing with in an infertility clinic. Therefore, a random bred strain of mice provides greater genetic diversity. Third, the embryo cultures should be performed in the absence of protein, as protein has the ability to mask the effects of any potential toxins present. Reports that mouse embryos can develop in culture in a medium prepared using tap water (119,120) should be interpreted carefully after taking into account the strain of mouse, types of media used, and the supplementation of medium with protein. Silverman et al. (119) used Ham's F-10. This medium contains amino acids, which can chelate any possible toxins present in the tap water, for example heavy metals. George et al. (120) included high levels of BSA in their zygote cultures to the blastocyst. Albumin can chelate potential embryo toxins and thereby mask the effect of any present in the culture medium (121,122). Furthermore, all such studies used blastocyst development as the sole criterion for assessing embryo development. Blastocyst development is a poor indicator of embryo quality and does not accurately reflect developmental potential (51). Therefore, rates of development should be determined by scoring the embryos at specific times during culture. Key times to examine the embryos include the morning of day 3, to determine the extent of compaction, the afternoon of day 4, to determine the degree of blastocyst formation, and the morning of day 5, to assess the initiation of hatching.

Finally, the embryos that form blastocysts in a given time, typically on the morning of day 5, should have their cell numbers determined, as blastocyst cell number is a good indicator of subsequent development potential. When new components of certain culture media can affect the development of the ICM directly, such as essential amino acids, a differential nuclear stain should be performed in order to determine the extent of ICM development. Using such an approach it is possible to identify potential problems in culture media before they are used clinically. In our experience around 25% of all contact supplies fail such pre-screening (118). Although some of the contact supplies that fail the bioassay are not outright lethal, they do compromise embryo development. If undetected this would result in reduced clinical pregnancy rates. Consequently, this helps to explain periodic changes in clinical pregnancy rates and emphasizes the significance of an ongoing quality control program. There are an increasing number of products on the market that are pre-screened for embryo toxicity. However, it is worthy to note that not all testing methods are the same and that it is worth understanding the sensitivity of the assay used before introduction of an item into the laboratory. However, irrespective of the testing, all supplies should be tracked by lot number as they enter the laboratory to confirm the efficacy for human embryos.

ON WHAT DAY SHOULD EMBRYO TRANSFER BE PERFORMED?

For the past three decades the majority of embryos conceived through IVF have been transferred between days 1 and 3 at either the pronucleate or the cleavage stage. The reason for this stems primarily from the inability of past culture systems to support the development of viable blastocysts at acceptable rates. However, with the advent of sequential culture media (3) it is feasible to perform day 5 blastocyst transfers as a matter of routine in an IVF clinic (123,124). This now facilitates an answer to the question; on which day of embryo development should embryos be transferred? Before answering this question, the potential advantages and disadvantages of blastocyst culture and transfer are considered.

Blastocyst Transfer: Advantages and Disadvantages

The potential advantages of blastocyst culture and transfer have been well documented (125–128). Advantages include the following:

1. Synchronizing embryonic stage with the female tract. This is important as the levels of nutrients within the fallopian tube and uterus do differ, and therefore the premature transfer of the cleavage-stage embryo to the uterus could result in metabolic stress (1). Furthermore, the uterine environment during a stimulated cycle cannot be considered normal. Certainly it is known from animal studies that the hyperstimulated female tract is a less than an optimal environment for the developing embryo, resulting in impaired embryo and fetal development (129–131). Therefore, it would seem prudent to shorten the length of time an embryo is exposed to such an environment before implantation.
2. When embryos are selected for transfer at the two- to eight-cell stage the embryonic genome has only just begun to be transcribed (22,132), and therefore it is not possible to identify from within a given cohort those embryos with the highest developmental potential. Only by culturing embryos past the maternal/embryonic genome transition and up to the blastocyst does it become realistic to identify those embryos with limited or no developmental potential. Assessment of pronucleate stage oocytes in order to select embryos for transfer (133) has reported increased implantation rates while others (134) have used a scoring system for use on day 3 to increase implantation rates. However, assessment of the embryos at either the pronucleate oocyte or cleavage stages can at best be considered as an assessment of the oocyte. The quality of the oocyte is important, as the quality of the developing embryo is ultimately dependent on the quality of gametes from which it is derived, but it provides limited information regarding true embryo developmental potential and eliminates the impact of the male gamete on development.
3. Not all fertilized oocytes are normal, and therefore a percentage always exists that is not destined to establish a pregnancy or go to term. Factors contributing to embryonic attrition include an insufficiency of stored oocyte-coded gene products, and a failure to activate the embryonic genome (135). The culmination of this is that many abnormal embryos arrest during development in vitro. So by culturing embryos to the blastocyst stage, one has already selected against those embryos with little, if any, developmental potential. Sandalinas and colleagues (136) have confirmed that some chromosomally abnormal human embryos can reach the blastocyst stage in vitro. However, even though aneuploid embryos form blastocysts at lower rates than their euploid counterparts, this means blastocyst culture cannot be used as the sole means in identifying chromosomally abnormal embryos.
4. Uterine contractions have been negatively correlated with embryo transfer outcome, possibly by the expulsion of embryos from the uterine cavity (137). Uterine junctional zone contractions have been quantitated and found to be strongest on the day of oocyte retrieval (138). All patients exhibited such contractions on day 2 and 3 after retrieval, but contractility decreased and was barely evident on day 4. It is therefore feasible that the transfer of blastocysts on day 5 is, by default, associated with reduced uterine contractions and therefore there is less chance for embryonic expulsion and loss (139).
5. Cryopreservation of embryos at the blastocyst stage appears more successful than at earlier stages (140).
6. Trophectoderm biopsy and analysis may prove to be more reliable than current procedures performed on cleavage-stage embryos (141,142).

The potential disadvantage of extended embryo culture in a program where only blastocyst culture and transfer is offered is the possibility that a patient will not have a morula or blastocyst for transfer. Certainly there has been an increase in the percentage of patients who do not have an embryo transfer from 2.9% on day 3 to 6.7% on day 5 in one clinic (124), and from 1.3% on day 3 to 2.8% on day 5 in another (123). Interestingly, in spite of the increase in patients not having an embryo transfer, there was a significant increase in pregnancy rate per retrieval with blastocyst culture, due to a significant increase in implantation rates.

In support of the move to blastocyst transfer, as opposed to the transfer of embryos at the cleavage stage, 17 prospective randomized trials on blastocyst transfer following the use of sequential media have been published (Table 17.4) (143–159). Eight have reported a significant increase in implantation/pregnancy rates when embryos were transferred at the blastocyst stage on day 5 rather than at the cleavage stage. Eight of the trials reported no difference in implantation rate with respect to day of transfer, while only one clinic reported a lower implantation rate with day 5 transfer.

Table 17.4 Outcome of Prospective Randomized Trials on Embryo Transfer at the Cleavage and Blastocyst Stages When Sequential Media Have Been Used for Embryo Culture

Author	Patient population	Cleavage stage			Blastocyst		
		No. of embryos transferred	Implantation rate (%)	Pregnancy (%)	No. of embryos transferred	Implantation rate (%)	Pregnancy (%)
Gardner et al. (143)	>10 follicles of >12 mm on the day of hCG	3.7	37.0	66	2.2	55.4[b]	71
Coskun et al. (144)	≥4 2PN	2.3	21	39	2.2	24	39
Karaki et al. (145)	≥5 2PN	3.5	13	26	2.0	26[b]	29
Levron et al. (146)	<38 years old and >5 2PN	3.1	38.7[b]	45.5	2.3	20.2	18.6
Utsunomiya et al. (147)	All	2.9	11.7	26.3	3.0	9.2	24.9
Rienzi et al. (148)	<38 years old and ≥8 2PN by ICSI	2	35	58	2	38	62
Van der Auwera et al. (149)	All (day 2 transfers)	1.86	29	32	1.87	46[a]	44
Frattarelli et al. (150)	<35 years old, no previous IVF and ≥10 follicles of ≥14 mm on the day of hCG	2.96	26.1	43.5	2.04	43.4[a]	69.2
Emiliani et al. (151)	<39 (day 2 transfers)	2.1	29	49	1.9	30	44
Margreiter et al. (152)	Mean age of 32.1 with a mean of 7 pronucleate oocytes (days 1–5 transfers)			20 on day 1 and 30.4 on days 2 & 3			50[a] on days 4 & 5
Bungum et al. (153)	<40 years old, FSH <12 IU/L, >2 eight-cell embryo with <20% fragmentation	2.0	43.9	61	1.96	36.7	51
Pantos et al. (154)	<40 years old, <4 previous failures, day 2 and 3	4.0	15.7 and 16	46.9 and 48.1	3.39	15.6	37
Levitas et al. (155)	<37-years old and 3 failed IVF attempts	3.4	6.0	12.9	1.9	21.2[b]	21.7
Hreinsson et al. (156)	>5 follicles, day 2 and 3	1.8	20.9	36.7	1.9	21.1	32.5
Kolibianakis et al. (157)	<43-years old	1.9	24.5	33.1	1.8	24.5	33.2
Papanikolaou et al. (158)	<37-years old, >3 embryos with >5 cells and <20% fragmentation	2.0	20.6	27.4	1.97	37.0[b]	51.3[b]
Papanikolaou et al. (159)	<36-years old, 1st or 2nd cycle, FSH <13	1	23.3	21.6	1	33.1[a]	33.1[a]

Significantly different from the cleavage stage; [a]$P < 0.05$; [b]$P < 0.01$. *Abbreviations*: ICSI, intracytoplasmic sperm injection; IVF, in vitro fertilization; FSH, follicle-stimulating hormone; hCG, human chorionic gonadotrophin.

Interestingly, of the trials listed in Table 17.4, there is incomplete information published on the culture system used. Although the media types are listed, there is limited other information available on the other components of the culture system used. Furthermore, the number and type of incubators in each laboratory, nor the types of air handling systems are documented. It is important to encourage clinics to report such parameters in order to be able to assess the merits and impacts of such variables on IVF outcome.

In a meta-analysis of prospective trials, in which equal numbers of embryos were transferred, it was concluded that "the best available evidence suggests that the probability of live birth after fresh IVF is significantly higher after blastocyst-stage embryo transfer as compared to cleavage-stage embryo transfer when equal numbers of embryos are transferred ...." (5). Additionally, in the most recent Cochrane report on blastocyst transfer it was concluded: ".....there is a significant difference in pregnancy and live birth rates in favour of blastocyst transfer with good prognosis patients. There is emerging data to suggest that in selected patients, blastocyst culture maybe applicable for single embryo transfer" (4).

In support of such analyses, from a model previously developed to determine which patients should have a SET, it was determined that pregnancy outcome was more favorable with day 5 than day 3 transfer (160).

Along with the published prospective randomized trials, there are retrospective studies that have concluded that day 5 transfer exhibits significant benefits for human assisted reproductive technique in both nonselected and specific patient populations (123,124,161).

For patients having oocyte donation, blastocyst culture and transfer is the most effective course of treatment (162). Oocytes from donors generally represent a more viable cohort of gametes, as they tend to come from young fertile women. Embryos derived from oocyte donors tend to reach the blastocyst stage at a higher frequency than those from IVF patients, and be of higher quality. It is possible to attain an implantation rate of >65% when transferring blastocysts to recipients whose mean age is over 40 (Table 17.3) (163). Such data not only reflect the competency of modern embryo culture systems, but emphasize the need to move to SETs, especially when performing day 5 transfers (164).

TOWARD SINGLE EMBRYO TRANSFER

Several reviews have discussed the development of scoring systems used in clinical IVF and their significance in identifying the most viable embryo(s) for transfer (165–167) (chap. 18). Certainly with newer types of embryo culture media, implantation rates are increasing whether embryos are transferred at the cleavage stage or blastocyst. It is envisaged that for a significant number of patients, blastocyst culture and transfer will be the most effective means of being able to transfer a single embryo while maintaining high pregnancy rates, as it is evident that blastocyst score is highly predictive of implantation potential. A prospective randomized trial of one versus two blastocysts transferred in patients with 10 or more

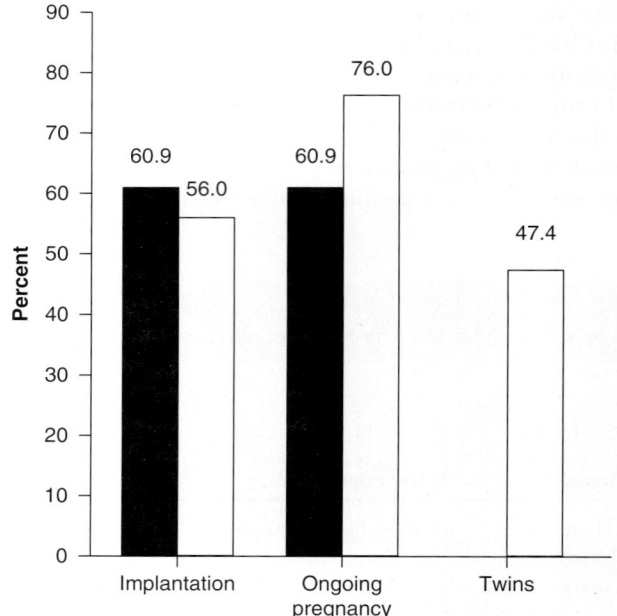

Figure 17.6 In vitro fertilization outcomes following the transfer of either 1 or 2 blastocysts. Dark bars represent the transfer of a single blastocyst (Group I); open bars represent the transfer of 2 blastocysts (Group II). Implantation and pregnancy rates were not statistically different between the two groups of patients. There were no twins in Group I in contrast to 47.4% twins in Group II. The biochemical pregnancy rate was equivalent between the two groups (Group I, 12.5%; Group II, 5%). *Source*: Adapted from Ref. 164.

follicles has been performed. The data in Fig. 17.6 indicate that it is possible to transfer a single blastocyst and obtain an ongoing pregnancy rate of 60% (164). Subsequent trials of single blastocyst transfer versus cleavage-stage embryo transfer have confirmed the higher implantation rate of the later-stage embryo. It has also been established that fetal loss is significantly less following blastocyst transfer (168).

CUMULATIVE PREGNANCY RATES PER RETRIEVAL: THE SIGNIFICANCE OF CRYOPRESERVATION

The introduction of blastocyst culture was met with much speculation as not all laboratories were able to cryopreserve blastocysts that were not transferred. However, with the development of more suitable cryopreservation procedures, it is now possible to obtain implantation and ongoing pregnancy rates of greater than 30% and 60%, respectively, using frozen–thawed blastocysts (140). Clinical data following blastocyst vitrification are also most encouraging (169). Consequently, the ability of a given culture system to support embryo cryosurvival is of great significance. Media containing hyaluronan appear to confer great advantage in this regard (86).

FUTURE DEVELOPMENTS IN EMBRYO CULTURE SYSTEMS

An area not discussed in this text has been the role of growth factors in regulating embryo development

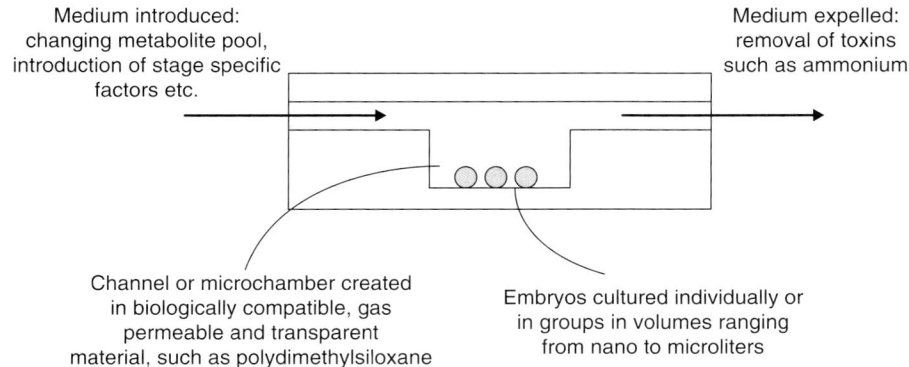

Figure 17.7 A schematic representation of an embryo perfusion culture system. Culture media are continuously passed over the embryo(s). The composition of the culture media can be changed according to the specific requirements of each stage of embryonic development. Toxins such as ammonium are not able to build up and impair embryo development, while more labile components of the culture system are not denatured. *Source*: Adapted from Ref. 23.

in culture and subsequent fetal development. Although numerous growth factors in isolation have been shown to modulate embryo development in culture (170,171), we currently do not know their optimal concentration for clinical use, nor are we aware which groups of growth factors should be present together in the medium. However, growing research on the effects of such factors at the physiological, genomic, and proteomic levels could lead to their introduction into clinical IVF over the next few years.

As discussed previously, there is nothing physiological about the physical conditions in which embryos are cultured. Rather than a static drop of medium, the future may engage perfusion culture systems, enabling the embryo to be exposed to a flux of nutrients and factors (Fig. 17.7) (23,162,172) (chap. 31). This latter approach has the advantage of being able to expose embryos to numerous gradients and fresh media throughout development. Furthermore, samples of medium can be taken and analyzed for carbohydrates (173), amino acids (174), and other factors related to implantation potential post-transfer (175) (chap. 18). Research in this area is growing, and the application of novel elastomers together with soft lithography, is starting to produce new generations of chips capable of moving sub-microliter volumes accurately for both culture and analysis (172,176).

CONCLUSIONS

The culture system in the clinical laboratory is one part of the overall treatment cycle. Good oocytes, derived from appropriate stimulation regimes, are able to give rise to good embryos. However, it is not feasible to obtain good embryos from poor oocytes. Consequently, the embryo transfer technique and subsequent luteal support administered have an impact on the cycle outcome.

Significant improvements in culture media formulations and embryo culture systems have conclusively provided better conditions for the human embryo to develop in the laboratory, and have facilitated the routine culture of blastocyst stage embryos and a reduction in the numbers of embryos transferred. Increasing evidence supports the move to day 5 transfers for a significant number of patients attending an infertility program, especially those undergoing oocyte donation, or who are <38 and in their first cycle. However, there are certain exceptions to this, such as clinics in countries like Germany, who are only able to culture as many pronucleate embryos as they will transfer and this can be no more than three. In such cases, people may be deterred from trying blastocyst culture, as certainly there will be an increase in the number of patients not having an embryo transfer.

It is evident that culture conditions affect the ability of embryos to survive cryopreservation. As we move closer to the day when single embryo/blastocyst transfer is considered the standard of care, it becomes more important than ever to ensure embryos are given the best chance of being cryopreserved for transfer at a later date, thereby increasing the efficiency of each oocyte retrieval procedure.

In this chapter we have outlined how human embryos can be successfully cultured. The systems outlined work extremely effectively, as reflected in the high implantation and pregnancy rates that can be attained, especially in an oocyte donation model. Ongoing investment in Quality Management and Quality Control ensure that an IVF laboratory will run at its highest level of performance and that results will remain consistent over time.

EMBRYO CULTURE PROTOCOL

In order to perform oocyte isolation, preparation for ICSI, or embryo manipulation outside a CO_2 incubator there are two distinct approaches; one can use media that have a second buffer system in them, such as MOPS or HEPES (both of which will keep the pH of the medium relatively constant in air), or one can employ a pediatric isolette-type system. The latter maintains both temperature and CO_2, and negates the use of buffer systems other than bicarbonate. Both approaches can be made to work effectively; the choice is one of preference and cost.

Embryo culture should be performed in a reduced O_2 environment (typically 5%, but the optimum value below 10% is yet to be determined) and 5–7% CO_2 depending on the media system chosen and altitude. This multigas environment can be created using either a tri-gas incubator or a modular incubator chamber/dissector, and a cylinder of special gas mix. It is advisable to minimize the number of observations made during embryo development, and to minimize the number of cases per incubator. It is also essential that all contact supplies, media, oil etc. are prescreened with a suitable assay (118).

PRONUCLEATE OOCYTES TO DAY 3 CULTURE

Embryo Manipulation (Following Fertilization Assessment)

Once the cumulus is removed (chap. 7 by Rienzi) then all manipulations should be performed using a glass capillary-style pipette or a displacement pipette. Fine control can be attained with both approaches. It is important to use a pipette with the appropriate size tip (day 1–3; around 200 µM). Using the appropriate size tip minimizes the volumes of culture medium moved with each embryo, which typically should be less than one microliter. Such volume manipulation is a prerequisite for successful culture.

Setting Up Culture Dishes (Day 1–Day 3)

At around 4 pm on the day of oocyte retrieval, label pretested 60 mm dishes with the patient's name. Using a single-wrapped tip, rinse the tip once first, then place 6 × 25 µL drops of phase 1 medium into the plate. Four drops should be placed at the 3, 6, 9, and 12 o'clock positions (for embryo culture), the fifth and sixth drops should be in the middle of the dish (wash drops). Immediately cover drops with 9 mL of prescreened paraffin oil. Prepare no more than two plates at one time. Using a new tip for each drop, first rinse the tip and then add a further 25 µL of medium to each original drop. Immediately place the dish in the incubator. Gently remove the lid of the dish and set at an angle on the side of the plate. Dishes must gas in the incubator for a minimum of four hours (this is the minimal measured time for the media to reach the correct pH under oil).

For each patient, set up a wash dish at the same time as the culture dishes. Place 1 mL of phase 1 medium into the center of an organ well dish. Place 2 mL of medium into the outer well. Place the dish immediately into the incubator. If working outside an isolette, use HEPES/MOPS-buffered medium with amino acids. This should not be placed in a CO_2 incubator, but rather warmed on a heated stage.

MORNING OF DAY 1

Culture in Phase 1 Medium

Following removal of the cumulus cells, embryos are transferred to the organ well dish and washed in the center well drop of medium in the culture dish. Washing entails picking up the embryo two to three and moving it around within the well. Embryos should then be washed in the two center drops in the culture dish and up to four embryos placed in each drop of the culture medium. Four is the maximum number of embryos that can be cultured in each drop due to their nutrient requirements. More than four embryos may result in a significant depletion of the nutrient pool by the embryos. This will result in no more than 16 embryos per dish. Return the dish to the incubator immediately. It is advisable to culture embryos in at least groups of 2. Therefore for example, for a patient with 6 embryos it is best to culture in 2 groups of 3 and not 4 and 2 or 5 and 1. On day 3, embryos can be transferred to the uterus in an appropriate hyaluronan-enriched transfer medium.

DAY 3 EMBRYOS TO THE BLASTOCYST

Setting Up Culture Dishes (Day 3–Day 5)

On day 3 before 8:30 am, label a 60 mm dish with the patient's name. Using a single-wrapped tip, rinse the tip once first, then place 6 × 25 µL drops of the second-phase medium into the plate. Immediately cover them with 9 mL of oil. Never prepare more than two plates at one time. Using a new tip for each drop, rinse the tip and then add a further 25 µL of medium to each original drop. Immediately place the dish in the incubator. Gently remove the lid and set on the side of the plate.

For each patient, set up one wash dish for 10 embryos. Place 1 mL of the second phase medium into the center of an organ well dish. Place 2 mL of medium into the outer well. Place the dishes immediately into the incubator. Dishes must gas in the incubator for a minimum of four hours. If working outside an isolette, use HEPES/MOPS-buffered medium with amino acids. This should not be placed in a CO_2 incubator, but rather warmed on a heated stage.

For each patient, set up one sorting dish before 8:30 am. Place 1 mL of the second phase medium into the center of an organ well dish. Place 2 mL of the medium into the outer well. Place immediately into the incubator. If working outside an isolette, use HEPES/MOPS-buffered medium with amino acids. This should not be placed in a CO_2 incubator, but rather warmed on a heated stage.

Culture in the Second Phase Medium

Moving embryos from the first phase to second phase medium should occur between 9 am and mid-day. Wash embryos in the organ well very well. Washing entails picking up the embryo two to three times and moving it around within the well.

Transfer embryos to the sorting dish and group likeembryos together. Rinse through the wash drops of medium and again place up to four embryos in each drop of the second phase medium. This will result in no more than 16 embryos per dish. Return the dish to the low O_2 incubator immediately. If working outside an isolette, use HEPES/MOPS-buffered medium with amino acids in the sorting dish. This should not be placed in a CO_2 incubator, but rather warmed on a heated stage.

On the morning of day 5 embryos should be scored (Fig. 17.8; (191); chap. 18) and the top scoring embryo is selected for transfer. Transfers should be performed in a medium enriched with hyaluronan. Any blastocysts not transferred can be cryopreserved. Should an embryo not have formed a blastocyst by day 5 then it should be cultured in a fresh drop of the second phase medium for 24 hours and assessed on day 6. Embryos at different stages of development are shown in Fig. 17.8. For more details on blastocyst grading, see chap. 18 and Ref. (192).

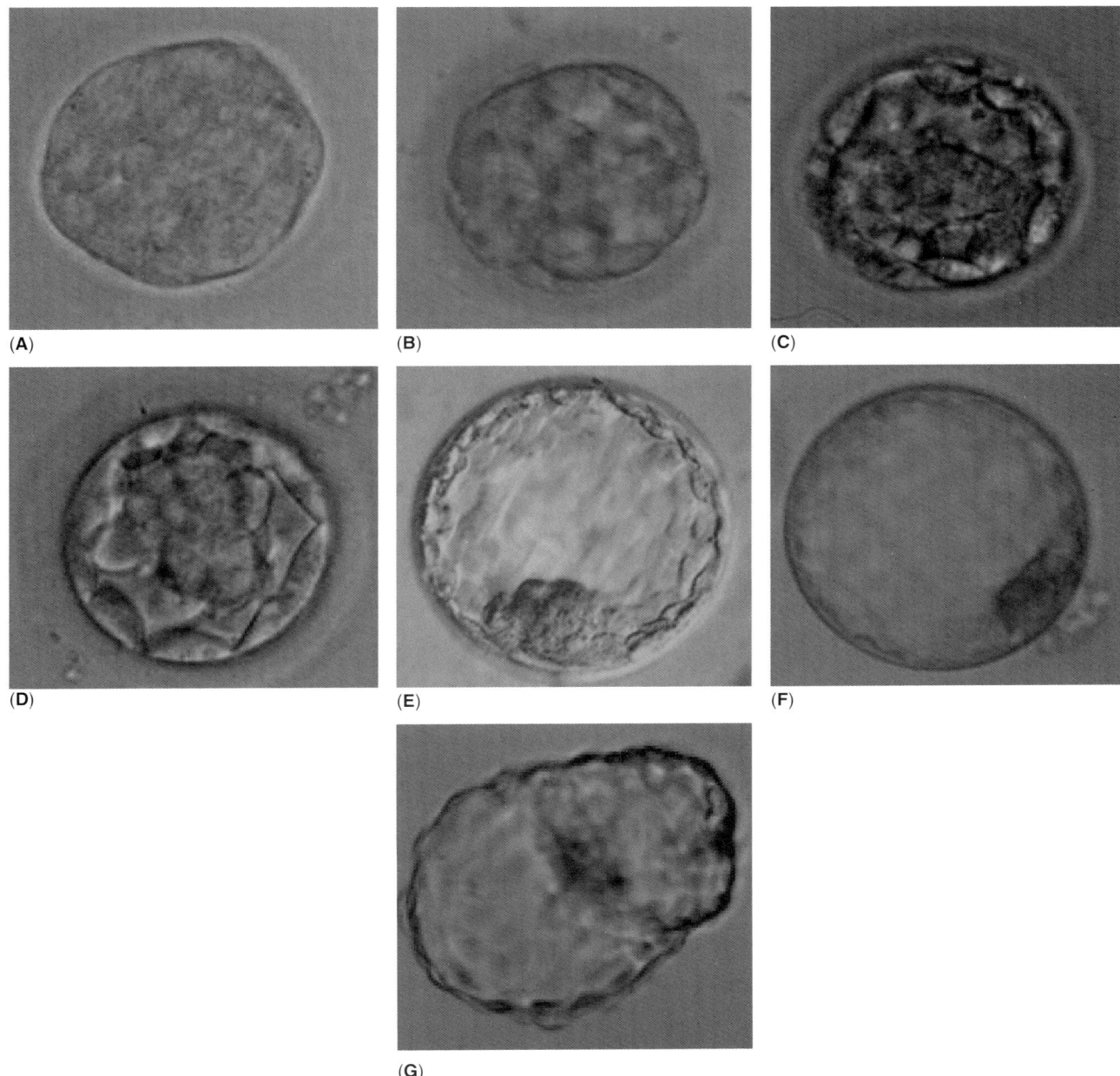

Figure 17.8 Human embryos the morning of day 5 (4 days of culture from the pronucleate stage). Embryos were cultured from the pronucleate oocyte until midday on day 3 in medium G1. Cleavage-stage embryos were then washed in medium G2 and cultured in G2 for a further 48-hours.

A	0 – Morula or a lesser stage		No blastocoel cavity seen
B	1 – Early blastocyst		Blastocoel less than half the volume of the embryo
C	2 – Blastocyst		Blastocoel ≥ half of the volume of the embryo
D	3 – Full blastocyst		Blastocoel completely fills the embryo
E	4 – Expanded		Blastocyst zona thinning and overall increase in size
F	5 – Hatching		Blastocyst trophectoderm has started to herniate through the zona
G	6 – Hatched blastocyst		Blastocyst has completely escaped from the zona

REFERENCES

1. Gardner DK. Changes in requirements and utilization of nutrients during mammalian preimplantation embryo development and their significance in embryo culture. Theriogenology 1998; 49: 83–102.
2. Lane M, Gardner DK. Understanding cellular disruptions during early embryo development that perturb viability and fetal development. Reprod Fertil Dev 2005; 17: 371–8.
3. Gardner DK, Lane M. Culture and selection of viable blastocysts: a feasible proposition for human IVF? Hum Reprod Update 1997; 3: 367–82.
4. Blake DA, Farquhar CM, Johnson N, Proctor M. Cleavage stage versus blastocyst stage embryo transfer in assisted conception. Cochrane Database Syst Rev 2007; 4: CD002118.
5. Papanikolaou EG, Kolibianakis EM, Tournaye H, et al. Live birth rates after transfer of equal number of blastocysts or cleavage-stage embryos in IVF. A systematic review and meta-analysis. Hum Reprod 2008; 23: 91–9.
6. Adashi EY, Barri PN, Berkowitz R, et al. Infertility therapy-associated multiple pregnancies (births): an ongoing epidemic. Reprod Biomed Online 2003; 7:515–42.
7. Leese HJ. Metabolism of the preimplantation mammalian embryo. Oxf Rev Reprod Biol 1991; 13: 35–72.
8. Gardner DK, Lane M. Embryo culture systems. In: Gardner DK, ed. In Vitro Fertilization a Practical Approach. New York: Informa Healthcare, 2007: 221–82.
9. Hardy K, Hooper MA, Handyside AH, et al. Noninvasive measurement of glucose and pyruvate uptake by individual human oocytes and preimplantation embryos. Hum Reprod 1989; 4: 188–91.
10. Lane M, Gardner DK. Mitochondrial malate-aspartate shuttle regulates mouse embryo nutrient consumption. J Biol Chem 2005; 280: 18361–7.
11. Ratnam S, Mertineit C, Ding F, et al. Dynamics of Dnmt1 methyltransferase expression and intracellular localization during oogenesis and preimplantation development. Dev Biol 2002; 245: 304–14.
12. Huang JC, Lei ZL, Shi LH, et al. Comparison of histone modifications in in vivo and in vitro fertilization mouse embryos. Biochem Biophys Res Commun 2007; 354: 77–83.
13. Lucifero D, La Salle S, Bourc'his D, et al. Coordinate regulation of DNA methyltransferase expression during oogenesis. BMC Dev Biol 2007; 7: 36.
14. Dumollard R, Marangos P, Fitzharris G, et al. Sperm-triggered [Ca2+] oscillations and Ca2+ homeostasis in the mouse egg have an absolute requirement for mitochondrial ATP production. Development 2004; 131: 3057–67.
15. Gangaraju VK, Bartholomew B. Mechanisms of ATP dependent chromatin remodeling. Mutat Res 2007; 618: 3–17.
16. Pepin D, Vanderhyden BC, Picketts DJ, Murphy BD. ISWI chromatin remodeling in ovarian somatic and germ cells: revenge of the NURFs. Trends Endocrinol Metab 2007; 18: 215–24.
17. Gardner DK, Lane M. Ex vivo early embryo development and effects on gene expression and imprinting. Reprod Fertil Dev 2005; 17: 361.
18. Gardner DK, Lane M, Calderon I, Leeton J. Environment of the preimplantation human embryo in vivo: metabolite analysis of oviduct and uterine fluids and metabolism of cumulus cells. Fertil Steril 1996; 65: 349–53.
19. Lane M, Gardner DK. Increase in postimplantation development of cultured mouse embryos by amino acids and induction of fetal retardation and exencephaly by ammonium ions. J Reprod Fertil 1994; 102: 305–12.
20. Zander DL, Thompson JG, Lane M. Perturbations in mouse embryo development and viability caused by ammonium are more severe after exposure at the cleavage stages. Biol Reprod 2006; 74: 288–94.
21. Rooke JA, McEvoy TG, Ashworth CJ, et al. Ovine fetal development is more sensitive to perturbation by the presence of serum in embryo culture before rather than after compaction. Theriogenology 2007; 67: 639–47.
22. Braude P, Bolton V, Moore S. Human gene expression first occurs between the four- and eight-cell stages of preimplantation development. Nature 1988; 332: 459–61.
23. Gardner DK. Mammalian embryo culture in the absence of serum or somatic cell support. Cell Biol Int 1994; 18: 1163–79.
24. Bavister BD. Culture of preimplantation embryos: facts and artifacts. Hum Reprod Update 1995; 1: 91–148.
25. Leese HJ. Metabolic control during preimplantation mammalian development. Hum Reprod Update 1995; 1: 63–72.
26. Gardner DK, Lane M. Embryo culture systems, 2nd edn. In: Trounson A, Gardner DK, eds. Handbook of In Vitro Fertilization. Boca Raton, FL: CRC Press, 1999: 205–64.
27. Pool TB. Recent advances in the production of viable human embryos in vitro. Reprod Biomed Online 2002; 4: 294–302.
28. Perkins JL, Goode L. Free amino acids in the oviduct fluid of the ewe. J Reprod Fertil 1967; 14: 309–11.
29. Casslen BG. Free amino acids in human uterine fluid. Possible role of high taurine concentration. J Reprod Med 1987; 32: 181–4.
30. Miller JG, Schultz GA. Amino acid content of preimplantation rabbit embryos and fluids of the reproductive tract. Biol Reprod 1987; 36: 125–9.
31. Gardner DK, Leese HJ. Concentrations of nutrients in mouse oviduct fluid and their effects on embryo development and metabolism in vitro. J Reprod Fertil 1990; 88: 361–8.
32. Harris SE, Gopichandran N, Picton HM, et al. Nutrient concentrations in murine follicular fluid and the female reproductive tract. Theriogenology 2005; 64: 992–1006.
33. Hugentobler SA, Diskin MG, Leese HJ, et al. Amino acids in oviduct and uterine fluid and blood plasma during the estrous cycle in the bovine. Mol Reprod Dev 2007; 74: 445–54.
34. Van Winkle LJ. Amino acid transport regulation and early embryo development. Biol Reprod 2001; 64: 1–12.
35. Schultz GA, Kaye PL, McKay DJ, Johnson MH. Endogenous amino acid pool sizes in mouse eggs and preimplantation embryos. J Reprod Fertil 1981; 61: 387–93.

36. Gardner DK, Clarke RN, Lechene CP, Biggers JD. Development of a noninvasive ultramicrofluorometric method for measuring net uptake of glutamine by single preimplantation mouse embryos. Gamete Res 1989; 24: 427–38.
37. Rieger D, Loskutoff NM, Betteridge KJ. Developmentally related changes in the metabolism of glucose and glutamine by cattle embryos produced and co-cultured in vitro. J Reprod Fertil 1992; 95: 585–95.
38. Eagle H. Amino acid metabolism in mammalian cell cultures. Science 1959; 130: 432–7.
39. Gardner DK, Lane M. Amino acids and ammonium regulate mouse embryo development in culture. Biol Reprod 1993; 48: 377–85.
40. Dumoulin JC, Evers JL, Bakker JA, et al. Temporal effects of taurine on mouse preimplantation development in vitro. Hum Reprod 1992; 7: 403–7.
41. Dumoulin JC, Evers JL, Bras M, et al. Positive effect of taurine on preimplantation development of mouse embryos in vitro. J Reprod Fertil 1992; 94: 373–80.
42. Gardner DK, Lane M. The 2-cell block in CF1 mouse embryos is associated with an increase in glycolysis and a decrease in tricarboxylic acid (TCA) cycle activity: alleviation of the 2-cell block is associated with the restoration of in vivo metabolic pathway activities. Biol Reprod 1993; 49(Suppl 1): 152.
43. Bavister BD, McKiernan SH. Regulation of hamster embryo development in vitro by amino acids. In: Bavister BD. ed Preimplantation Embryo Development. New York: Springer-Verlag, 1992: 57–72.
44. McKiernan SH, Clayton MK, Bavister BD. Analysis of stimulatory and inhibitory amino acids for development of hamster one-cell embryos in vitro. Mol Reprod Dev 1995; 42: 188–99.
45. Gardner DK, Lane M, Spitzer A, Batt PA. Enhanced rates of cleavage and development for sheep zygotes cultured to the blastocyst stage in vitro in the absence of serum and somatic cells: amino acids, vitamins, and culturing embryos in groups stimulate development. Biol Reprod 1994; 50: 390–400.
46. Thompson JG, Gardner DK, Pugh PA, et al. Lamb birth weight is affected by culture system utilized during in vitro pre-elongation development of ovine embryos. Biol Reprod 1995; 53: 1385–91.
47. Takahashi Y, First NL. In vitro development of bovine one-cell embryos influence of glucose, lactate, amino acids and vitamins. Theriogenology 1992; 37: 963–78.
48. Steeves TE, Gardner DK. Temporal and differential effects of amino acids on bovine embryo development in culture. Biol Reprod 1999; 61: 731–40.
49. Devreker F, Winston RM, Hardy K. Glutamine improves human preimplantation development in vitro. Fertil Steril 1998; 69: 293–9.
50. Devreker F, Van den Bergh M, Biramane J, et al. Effects of taurine on human embryo development in vitro. Hum Reprod 1999; 14: 2350–6.
51. Lane M, Gardner DK. Differential regulation of mouse embryo development and viability by amino acids. J Reprod Fertil 1997; 109: 153–64.
52. Lane M, Gardner DK. Nonessential amino acids and glutamine decrease the time of the first three cleavage divisions and increase compaction of mouse zygotes in vitro. J Assist Reprod Genet 1997; 14: 398–403.
53. Wang J, Alexander P, Wu L, et al. Dependence of mouse embryonic stem cells on threonine catabolism. Science 2009; 325: 435–9.
54. Edwards LJ, Williams DA, Gardner DK. Intracellular pH of the mouse preimplantation embryo: amino acids act as buffers of intracellular pH. Hum Reprod 1998; 13: 3441–8.
55. Gardner DK, Lane M. Alleviation of the '2-cell block' and development to the blastocyst of CF1 mouse embryos: role of amino acids, EDTA and physical parameters. Hum Reprod 1996; 11: 2703–12.
56. Ho Y, Wigglesworth K, Eppig JJ, Schultz RM. Preimplantation development of mouse embryos in KSOM: augmentation by amino acids and analysis of gene expression. Mol Reprod Dev 1995; 41: 232–8.
57. Doherty AS, Mann MR, Tremblay KD, et al. Differential effects of culture on imprinted H19 expression in the preimplantation mouse embryo. Biol Reprod 2000; 62: 1526–35.
58. Gardner DK, Lane M, Stevens J, Schoolcraft WB. Noninvasive assessment of human embryo nutrient consumption as a measure of developmental potential. Fertil Steril 2001; 76: 1175–80.
59. Virant-Klun I, Tomazevic T, Vrtacnik-Bokal E, et al. Increased ammonium in culture medium reduces the development of human embryos to the blastocyst stage. Fertil Steril 2006; 85: 526–8.
60. Sinawat S, Hsaio WC, Flockhart JH, et al. Fetal abnormalities produced after preimplantation exposure of mouse embryos to ammonium chloride. Hum Reprod 2003; 18: 2157–65.
61. Lane M, Gardner DK. Ammonium induces aberrant blastocyst differentiation, metabolism, pH regulation, gene expression and subsequently alters fetal development in the mouse. Biol Reprod 2003; 69: 1109–17.
62. Biggers JD, McGinnis LK, Summers MC. Discrepancies between the effects of glutamine in cultures of preimplantation mouse embryos. Reprod Biomed Online 2004; 9: 70–3.
63. Menezo YR, Guerin P. Preimplantation embryo metabolism and embryo interaction with the in vitro environment. In: Elder K, Cohen J, eds. Human Preimplantation Embryo Selection. London: Informa healthcare, 2007: 191–200.
64. Nakazawa T, Ohashi K, Yamada M, et al. Effect of different concentrations of amino acids in human serum and follicular fluid on the development of one-cell mouse embryos in vitro. J Reprod Fertil 1997; 111: 327–32.
65. Lane M, Gardner DK. Removal of embryo-toxic ammonium from the culture medium by in situ enzymatic conversion to glutamate. J Exp Zool 1995; 271: 356–63.
66. Gardner DK, Stilley KS, Lane M. High protein diet inhibits inner cell mass formation and increases apoptosis in mouse blastocysts developed in vivo by increasing the levels of ammonium in the reproductive tract. Reprod Fertil Dev 2004; 16: 190.
67. He Y, Hakvoort TB, Vermeulen JL, et al. Glutamine synthetase is essential in early mouse embryogenesis. Dev Dyn 2007; 236: 1865–75.
68. McEvoy TG, Robinson JJ, Aitken RP, et al. Dietary excesses of urea influence the viability and metabolism of preimplantation sheep embryos and may

affect fetal growth among survivors. Anim Reprod Sci 1997; 47: 71–90.
69. Dorland M, Gardner DK, Trounson A. Serum in synthetic oviduct fluid causes mitochondrial degeneration in ovine embryos. Reprod Fertil (Abstr Ser) 1994; 13: 70.
70. Khosla S, Dean W, Brown D, et al. Culture of preimplantation mouse embryos affects fetal development and the expression of imprinted genes. Biol Reprod 2001; 64: 918–26.
71. Wrenzycki C, Herrmann D, Keskintepe L, et al. Effects of culture system and protein supplementation on mRNA expression in pre-implantation bovine embryos. Hum Reprod 2001; 16: 893–901.
72. Young LE, Fernandes K, McEvoy TG, et al. Epigenetic change in IGF2R is associated with fetal overgrowth after sheep embryo culture. Nat Genet 2001; 27: 153–4.
73. Gray CW, Morgan PM, Kane MT. Purification of an embryotrophic factor from commercial bovine serum albumin and its identification as citrate. J Reprod Fertil 1992; 94: 471–80.
74. Batt PA, Gardner DK, Cameron AW. Oxygen concentration and protein source affect the development of preimplantation goat embryos in vitro. Reprod Fertil Dev 1991; 3: 601–7.
75. McKiernan SH, Bavister BD. Different lots of bovine serum albumin inhibit or stimulate in vitro development of hamster embryos. In Vitro Cell Dev Biol 1992; 28A: 154–6.
76. Kane MT. Variability in different lots of commercial bovine serum albumin affects cell multiplication and hatching of rabbit blastocysts in culture. J Reprod Fertil 1983; 69: 555–8.
77. Bavister BD, Kinsey DL, Lane M, Gardner DK. Recombinant human albumin supports hamster in-vitro fertilization. Hum Reprod 2003; 18: 113–16.
78. Bungum M, Humaidan P, Bungum L. Recombinant human albumin as protein source in culture media used for IVF: a prospective randomized study. Reprod Biomed Online 2002; 4: 233–6.
79. Lane M, Maybach JM, Hooper K, et al. Cryo-survival and development of bovine blastocysts are enhanced by culture with recombinant albumin and hyaluronan. Mol Reprod Dev 2003; 64: 70–8.
80. Zorn TM, Pinhal MA, Nader HB, et al. Biosynthesis of glycosaminoglycans in the endometrium during the initial stages of pregnancy of the mouse. Cell Mol Biol 1995; 41: 97–106.
81. Gardner DK, Rodriegez-Martinez H, Lane M. Fetal development after transfer is increased by replacing protein with the glycosaminoglycan hyaluronan for mouse embryo culture and transfer. Hum Reprod 1999; 14: 2575–80.
82. Palasz AT, Rodriguez-Martinez H, Beltran-Brena P, et al. Effects of hyaluronan, BSA, and serum on bovine embryo in vitro development, ultrastructure, and gene expression patterns. Mol Reprod Dev 2006; 73: 1503–11.
83. Dattena M, Mara L, Bin TA, Cappai P. Lambing rate using vitrified blastocysts is improved by culture with BSA and hyaluronan. Mol Reprod Dev 2007; 74: 42–7.
84. Urman B, Yakin K, Ata B, et al. Effect of hyaluronan-enriched transfer medium on implantation and pregnancy rates after day 3 and day 5 embryo transfers: a prospective randomized study. Fertil Steril 2008; 90: 604–12.
85. Bontekoe S, Blake D, Heineman MJ, et al. Adherence compounds in embryo transfer media for assisted reproductive technologies. Cochrane Database Syst Rev 2010; 7: CD007421.
86. Balaban B, Urman B. Comparison of two sequential media for culturing cleavage-stage embryos and blastocysts: embryo characteristics and clinical outcome. Reprod Biomed Online 2005; 10: 485–91.
87. Stojkovic M, Kolle S, Peinl S, et al. Effects of high concentrations of hyaluronan in culture medium on development and survival rates of fresh and frozen-thawed bovine embryos produced in vitro. Reproduction 2002; 124: 141–53.
88. Palasz AT, Brena PB, Martinez MF, et al. Development, molecular composition and freeze tolerance of bovine embryos cultured in TCM-199 supplemented with hyaluronan. Zygote 2008; 16: 39–47.
89. Gardner DK. Dissection of culture media for embryo: the most important and less important components and characteristics. Reprod Fertil Dev 2008; 20: 1–10.
90. Gardner DK, Sakkas D. Mouse embryo cleavage, metabolism and viability: role of medium composition. Hum Reprod 1993; 8: 288–95.
91. Lane M, Gardner DK. Lactate regulates pyruvate uptake and metabolism in the preimplantation mouse embryo. Biol Reprod 2000; 62: 16–22.
92. Gardner D, Lane M. Towards a single embryo transfer. Reprod Biomed Online 2003; 6: 470–81.
93. Bowman P, McLaren A. Cleavage rate of mouse embryos in vivo and in vitro. J Embryol Exp Morphol 1970; 24: 203–7.
94. Harlow GM, Quinn P. Development of preimplantation mouse embryos in vivo and in vitro. Aust J Biol Sci 1982; 35: 187–93.
95. Gardner DK, Lane M. Development of viable mammalian embryos in vitro: evolution of sequential media. In: Cibelli R, Lanza K, Campbell AK, West MD, eds. Principles of Cloning. New York: Elsevier Science. 2002: 187–213.
96. Phillips KP, Leveille MC, Claman P, Baltz JM. Intracellular pH regulation in human preimplantation embryos. Hum Reprod 2000; 15: 896–904.
97. Lane M, Baltz JM, Bavister BD. Regulation of intracellular pH in hamster preimplantation embryos by the sodium hydrogen (Na+/H+) antiporter. Biol Reprod 1998; 59: 1483–90.
98. Edwards LJ, Williams DA, Gardner DK. Intracellular pH of the preimplantation mouse embryo: effects of extracellular pH and weak acids. Mol Reprod Dev 1998; 50: 434–42.
99. Quinn P, Barros C, Whittingham DG. Preservation of hamster oocytes to assay the fertilizing capacity of human spermatozoa. J Reprod Fertil 1982; 66: 161–8.
100. Lane M, Gardner DK. Preparation of gametes, in vitro maturation, in vitro fertilization, embryo recovery and transfer. In: Gardner DK, Lane M, Watson AJ, eds. A Laboratory Guide to the Mammalian Embryo. New York: Oxford Press, 2004: 24–40.
101. Mastroianni L Jr, Jones R. Oxygen tension within the rabbit fallopian tube. J Reprod Fertil 1965; 147: 99–102.
102. Ross RN, Graves CN. O_2 levels in female rabbit reproductive tract. J Anim Sci 1974; 39: 994.

103. Fischer B, Bavister BD. Oxygen tension in the oviduct and uterus of rhesus monkeys, hamsters and rabbits. J Reprod Fertil 1993; 99: 673–9.
104. Quinn P, Harlow GM. The effect of oxygen on the development of preimplantation mouse embryos in vitro. J Exp Zool 1978; 206: 73–80.
105. Thompson JG, Simpson AC, Pugh PA, et al. Effect of oxygen concentration on in-vitro development of preimplantation sheep and cattle embryos. J Reprod Fertil 1990; 89: 573–8.
106. Wale PL, Gardner DK. Time-lapse analysis of mouse embryo development in oxygen gradients. Reprod Biomed Online 2010; 21: 402–10.
107. Katz-Jaffe MG, Linck DW, Schoolcraft WB, Gardner DK. A proteomic analysis of mammalian preimplantation embryonic development. Reproduction 2005; 130: 899–905.
108. Rinaudo PF, Giritharan G, Talbi S, et al. Effects of oxygen tension on gene expression in preimplantation mouse embryos. Fertil Steril 2006; 86(4 Suppl): 1252–65.
109. Meintjes M, Chantilis SJ, Douglas JD, et al. A controlled randomized trial evaluating the effect of lowered incubator oxygen tension on live births in a predominantly blastocyst transfer program. Hum Reprod 2009; 24: 300–7.
110. Nanassy L, Peterson CA, Wilcox AL, et al. Comparison of 5% and ambient oxygen during days 3–5 of in vitro culture of human embryos. Fertil Steril 2010; 93: 579–85.
111. Waldenstrom U, Engstrom AB, Hellberg D, Nilsson S. Low-oxygen compared with high-oxygen atmosphere in blastocyst culture, a prospective randomized study. Fertil Steril 2009; 91: 2461–5.
112. Leese HJ. The formation and function of oviduct fluid. J Reprod Fertil 1988; 82: 843–56.
113. Wiley LM, Yamami S, Van Muyden D. Effect of potassium concentration, type of protein supplement, and embryo density on mouse preimplantation development in vitro. Fertil Steril 1986; 45: 111–19.
114. Paria BC, Dey SK. Preimplantation embryo development in vitro: cooperative interactions among embryos and role of growth factors. Proc Natl Acad Sci 1990; 87: 4756–60.
115. Lane M, Gardner DK. Effect of incubation volume and embryo density on the development and viability of mouse embryos in vitro. Hum Reprod 1992; 7: 558–62.
116. Ahern TJ, Gardner DK. Culturing bovine embryos in groups stimulates blastocyst development and cell allocation to the inner cell mass. Theriogenology 1998; 49: 194.
117. Spindler RE, Crichton EG, Agca Y, et al. Improved felid embryo development by group culture is maintained with heterospecific companions. Theriogenology 2006; 66: 82–92.
118. Gardner DK, Reed L, Linck D, et al. Quality control in human in vitro fertilization. Semin Reprod Med 2005; 23: 319–24.
119. Silverman IH, Cook CL, Sanfilippo JS, et al. Ham's F-10 constituted with tap water supports mouse conceptus development in vitro. J In Vitro Fert Embryo Transf 1987; 4: 185–7.
120. George MA, Braude PR, Johnson MH, Sweetnam DG. Quality control in the IVF laboratory: in-vitro and in-vivo development of mouse embryos is unaffected by the quality of water used in culture media. Hum Reprod 1989; 4: 826–31.
121. Fissore RA, Jackson KV, Kiessling AA. Mouse zygote development in culture medium without protein in the presence of ethylenediaminetetraacetic acid. Biol Reprod 1989; 41: 835–41.
122. Flood LP, Shirley B. Reduction of embryotoxicity by protein in embryo culture media. Mol Reprod Dev 1991; 30: 226–31.
123. Wilson M, Hartke K, Kiehl M, et al. Integration of blastocyst transfer for all patients. Fertil Steril 2002; 77: 693–6.
124. Marek D, Langley M, Gardner DK, et al. Introduction of blastocyst culture and transfer for all patients in an in vitro fertilization program. Fertil Steril 1999; 72: 1035–40.
125. Menezo YJ, Guerin JF, Czyba JC. Improvement of human early embryo development in vitro by coculture on monolayers of Vero cells. Biol Reprod 1990; 42: 301–6.
126. Lopata A. The neglected human blastocyst. J Assist Reprod Genet 1992; 9: 508–12.
127. Olivennes F, Hazout A, Lelaidier C, et al. Four indications for embryo transfer at the blastocyst stage. Hum Reprod 1994; 9: 2367–73.
128. Scholtes MC, Zeilmaker GH. A prospective, randomized study of embryo transfer results after 3 or 5 days of embryo culture in in vitro fertilization. Fertil Steril 1996; 65: 1245–8.
129. Ertzeid G, Storeng R. Adverse effects of gonadotrophin treatment on pre- and postimplantation development in mice. J Reprod Fertil 1992; 96: 649–55.
130. Ertzeid G, Storeng R, Lyberg T. Treatment with gonadotropins impaired implantation and fetal development in mice. J Assist Reprod Genet 1993; 10: 286–91.
131. Van der Auwera I, Pijnenborg R, Koninckx PR. The influence of in-vitro culture versus stimulated and untreated oviductal environment on mouse embryo development and implantation. Hum Reprod 1999; 14: 2570–4.
132. Taylor DM, Ray PF, Ao A, et al. Paternal transcripts for glucose-6-phosphate dehydrogenase and adenosine deaminase are first detectable in the human preimplantation embryo at the three- to four-cell stage. Mol Reprod Dev 1997; 48: 442–8.
133. Scott LA, Smith S. The successful use of pronuclear embryo transfers the day following oocyte retrieval. Hum Reprod 1998; 13: 1003–13.
134. Gerris J, De Neubourg D, Mangelschots K, et al. Prevention of twin pregnancy after in-vitro fertilization or intracytoplasmic sperm injection based on strict embryo criteria: a prospective randomized clinical trial. Hum Reprod 1999; 14: 2581–7.
135. Tesarik J. Developmental failure during the preimplanation period of human embryogenesis. In: Van Blerkom J, ed. The Biological Basis of Early Human Reproductive Failure. New York: Oxford University Press, 1994: 327–44.
136. Sandalinas M, Sadowy S, Alikani M, et al. Developmental ability of chromosomally abnormal human embryos to develop to the blastocyst stage. Hum Reprod 2001; 16: 1954–8.
137. Fanchin R, Righini C, Olivennes F, et al. Uterine contractions at the time of embryo transfer alter pregnancy

rates after in-vitro fertilization. Hum Reprod 1998; 13: 1968–74.
138. Lesny P, Killick SR, Tetlow RL, et al. Uterine junctional zone contractions during assisted reproduction cycles. Hum Reprod Update 1998; 4: 440–5.
139. Fanchin R, Ayoubi JM, Righini C, et al. Uterine contractility decreases at the time of blastocyst transfers. Hum Reprod 2001; 16: 1115–19.
140. Veeck LL. Does the developmental stage at freeze impact on clinical results post-thaw? Reprod Biomed Online 2003; 6: 367–74.
141. Fragouli E, Lenzi M, Ross R, et al. Comprehensive molecular cytogenetic analysis of the human blastocyst stage. Hum Reprod 2008; 23: 2596–608.
142. Schoolcraft WB, Fragouli E, Stevens J, et al. Clinical application of comprehensive chromosomal screening at the blastocyst stage. Fertil Steril 2010; 94: 1700–6.
143. Gardner DK, Schoolcraft WB, Wagley L, et al. A prospective randomized trial of blastocyst culture and transfer in in-vitro fertilization. Hum Reprod 1998; 13: 3434–40.
144. Coskun S, Hollanders J, Al-Hassan S, et al. Day 5 versus day 3 embryo transfer: a controlled randomized trial. Hum Reprod 2000; 15: 1947–52.
145. Karaki RZ, Samarraie SS, Younis NA, et al. Blastocyst culture and transfer: a step toward improved in vitro fertilization outcome. Fertil Steril 2002; 77: 114–18.
146. Levron J, Shulman A, Bider D, et al. A prospective randomized study comparing day 3 with blastocyst-stage embryo transfer. Fertil Steril 2002; 77: 1300–1.
147. Utsunomiya T, Naitou T, Nagaki M. A prospective trial of blastocyst culture and transfer. Hum Reprod 2002; 17: 1846–51.
148. Rienzi L, Ubaldi F, Iacobelli M, et al. Day 3 embryo transfer with combined evaluation at the pronuclear and cleavage stages compares favourably with day 5 blastocyst transfer. Hum Reprod 2002; 17: 1852–5.
149. Van der Auwera I, Debrock S, et al. A prospective randomized study: day 2 versus day 5 embryo transfer. Hum Reprod 2002; 17: 1507–12.
150. Frattarelli JL, Leondires MP, McKeeby JL, et al. Blastocyst transfer decreases multiple pregnancy rates in in vitro fertilization cycles: a randomized controlled trial. Fertil Steril 2003; 79: 228–30.
151. Emiliani S, Delbaere A, Vannin AS, et al. Similar delivery rates in a selected group of patients, for day 2 and day 5 embryos both cultured in sequential medium: a randomized study. Hum Reprod 2003; 18: 2145–50.
152. Margreiter M, Weghofer A, Kogosowski A, et al. A prospective randomized multicenter study to evaluate the best day for embryo transfer: does the outcome justify prolonged embryo culture? J Assist Reprod Genet 2003; 20: 91–4.
153. Bungum M, Bungum L, Humaidan P, Yding Andersen C. Day 3 versus day 5 embryo transfer: a prospective randomized study. Reprod Biomed Online 2003; 7: 98–104.
154. Pantos K, Makrakis E, Stavrou D, et al. Comparison of embryo transfer on day 2, day 3, and day 6: a prospective randomized study. Fertil Steril 2004; 81: 454–5.
155. Levitas E, Lunenfeld E, Har-Vardi I, et al. Blastocyst-stage embryo transfer in patients who failed to conceive in three or more day 2–3 embryo transfer cycles: a prospective, randomized study. Fertil Steril 2004; 81: 567–71.
156. Hreinsson J, Rosenlund B, Fridstrom M, et al. Embryo transfer is equally effective at cleavage stage and blastocyst stage: a randomized prospective study. Eur J Obstet Gynecol Reprod Biol 2004; 117: 194–200.
157. Kolibianakis EM, Zikopoulos K, Verpoest W, et al. Should we advise patients undergoing IVF to start a cycle leading to a day 3 or a day 5 transfer? Hum Reprod 2004; 19: 2550–4.
158. Papanikolaou EG, D'Haeseleer E, Verheyen G, et al. Live birth rate is significantly higher after blastocyst transfer than after cleavage-stage embryo transfer when at least four embryos are available on day 3 of embryo culture: a randomized prospective study. Hum Reprod 2005; 20: 3198–203.
159. Papanikolaou EG, Camus M, Kolibianakis EM, et al. In vitro fertilization with single blastocyst-stage versus single cleavage-stage embryos. N Engl J Med 2006; 354: 1139–46.
160. Hunault CC, Eijkemans MJ, Pieters MH, et al. A prediction model for selecting patients undergoing in vitro fertilization for elective single embryo transfer. Fertil Steril 2002; 77: 725–32.
161. Balaban B, Urman B, Alatas C, et al. Blastocyst-stage transfer of poor-quality cleavage-stage embryos results in higher implantation rates. Fertil Steril 2001; 75: 514–18.
162. Kresowik JD, Stegmann BJ, Sparks AE, et al. Five-years of a mandatory single-embryo transfer (mSET) policy dramatically reduces twinning rate without lowering pregnancy rates. Fertil Steril 2011; 96: 1367–9.
163. Schoolcraft WB, Gardner DK. Blastocyst culture and transfer increases the efficiency of oocyte donation. Fertil Steril 2000; 74: 482–6.
164. Gardner DK, Surrey E, Minjarez D, et al. Single blastocyst transfer: a prospective randomized trial. Fertil Steril 2004; 81: 551–5.
165. Cummins JM, Breen TM, Harrison KL, et al. A formula for scoring human embryo growth rates in in vitro fertilization: its value in predicting pregnancy and in comparison with visual estimates of embryo quality. J In Vitro Fert Embryo Transf 1986; 3: 284–95.
166. Steer CV, Mills CL, Tan SL, et al. The cumulative embryo score: a predictive embryo scoring technique to select the optimal number of embryos to transfer in an in-vitro fertilization and embryo transfer programme. Hum Reprod 1992; 7: 117–19.
167. Scott L. The biological basis of non-invasive strategies for selection of human oocytes and embryos. Hum Reprod Update 2003; 9: 237–49.
168. Papanikolaou V. Early pregnancy loss is significantly higher after day 3 single embryo transfer that after day 5 single blastocyst transfer in GnRH antagonist stimulated IVF cycles. RBM Online 2006; 12: 60–5.
169. Takahashi K, Mukaida T, Goto T, Oka C. Perinatal outcome of blastocyst transfer with vitrification using cryoloop: a 4-year follow-up study. Fertil Steril 2005; 84: 88–92.
170. Kane MT, Morgan PM, Coonan C. Peptide growth factors and preimplantation development. Hum Reprod Update 1997; 3: 137–57.
171. Hardy K, Spanos S. Growth factor expression and function in the human and mouse preimplantation embryo. J Endocrinol 2002; 172: 221–36.

172. Wheeler MB, Walters EM, Beebe DJ. Toward culture of single gametes: the development of microfluidic platforms for assisted reproduction. Theriogenology 2007; 68(Suppl 1): S178–89.
173. Lane M, Gardner DK. Selection of viable mouse blastocysts prior to transfer using a metabolic criterion. Hum Reprod 1996; 11: 1975–8.
174. Brison DR, Houghton FD, Falconer D, et al. Identification of viable embryos in IVF by non-invasive measurement of amino acid turnover. Hum Reprod 2004; 19: 2319–24.
175. Gardner DK, Sakkas D. Assessment of embryo viability: the ability to select a single embryo for transfer—a review. Placenta 2003; 24(Suppl B): S5–12.
176. Urbanski JP, Thies W, Rhodes C, et al. Digital microfluidics using soft lithography. Lab Chip 2006; 6: 96–104.
177. Crosby IM, Gandolfi F, Moor RM. Control of protein synthesis during early cleavage of sheep embryos. J Reprod Fertil 1988; 82: 769–75.
178. Rieger D, Loskutoff NM, Betteridge KJ. Developmentally related changes in the uptake and metabolism of glucose, glutamine and pyruvate by cattle embryos produced in vitro. Reprod Fertil Dev 1992; 4: 547–57.
179. Van Winkle LJ, Haghighat N, Campione AL. Glycine protects preimplantation mouse conceptuses from a detrimental effect on development of the inorganic ions in oviductal fluid. J Exp Zool 1990; 253: 215–19.
180. Liu Z, Foote RH. Development of bovine embryos in KSOM with added superoxide dismutase and taurine and with five and twenty percent O_2. Biol Reprod 1995; 53: 786–90.
181. Lindenbaum A. A survey of naturally occurring chelating ligands. Adv Exp Med Biol 1973; 40: 67–77.
182. Wu G, Morris SM Jr. Arginine metabolism: nitric oxide and beyond. Biochem J 1998; 336: 1–17.
183. Martin PM, Sutherland AE, Van Winkle LJ. Amino acid transport regulates blastocyst implantation. Biol Reprod 2003; 69: 1101–8.
184. Martin PM, Sutherland AE. Exogenous amino acids regulate trophectoderm differentiation in the mouse blastocyst through an mTOR-dependent pathway. Dev Biol 2001; 240: 182–93.
185. Gardner DK. Dissection of culture media for embryos: the most important and less important components and characteristics. Reprod Fertil Dev 2008; 20: 9–18.
186. Hardy K, Robinson FM, Paraschos T, et al. Normal development and metabolic activity of preimplantation embryos in vitro from patients with polycystic ovaries. Hum Reprod 1995; 10: 2125–35.
187. Simon C, Garcia Velasco JJ, Valbuena D, et al. Increasing uterine receptivity by decreasing estradiol levels during the preimplantation period in high responders with the use of a follicle-stimulating hormone step-down regimen. Fertil Steril 1998; 70: 234–9.
188. Ertzeid G, Storeng R. The impact of ovarian stimulation on implantation and fetal development in mice. Hum Reprod 2001; 16: 221–5.
189. Kelley RL, Kind KL, Lane M, et al. Recombinant human follicle-stimulating hormone alters maternal ovarian hormone concentrations and the uterus and perturbs fetal development in mice. Am J Physiol Endocrinol Metab 2006; 291: E761–70.
190. Kwong WY, Wild AE, Roberts P, et al. Maternal undernutrition during the preimplantation period of rat development causes blastocyst abnormalities and programming of postnatal hypertension. Development 2000; 127: 4195–202.
191. Gardner DK, Schoolcraft WB. In vitro culture of human blastocyst. In: Jansen R, Mortimer D, eds. Towards Reproductive Certainty: Fertility and Genetics Beyond 1999. Carnforth, UK: Parthenon Publishing, 1999: 378–88.
192. Gardner DK, Stevens J, Sheehan CB, Schoolcraft WB. Analysis of blastocyst morphology. In: Elder K, Jacques C, eds. Human Preimplantation Embryo Selection. London: Informa Healthcare, 2007: 79–87.

18

Evaluation of embryo quality: Analysis of morphology and quantification of nutrient utilization and the metabolome

Denny Sakkas and David K. Gardner

INTRODUCTION

Utilization of assisted reproductive techniques (ARTs) continues to increase annually, with well over half a million treatment cycles being initiated in the United States, Europe, Australia, and New Zealand alone in 2006 (1–3). This trend is driven by the steady improvement in ART delivery rates, improving access to care in many areas, and the relative ineffectiveness of other treatment options. The proportion of infants born after ART in Europe now ranges from 0.1% to 3.9% of all live born children (4,5).

The high success rates established through in vitro fertilization (IVF) are attained, in many cases, only through the simultaneous transfer of multiple embryos. In 2009 (5) in the United States, a mean number of more than two embryos per patient were transferred leading to an overall multiple birth rate of approximately 30% in women under 38 years of age.

The risks to both mother and baby related to multiple gestations are well documented and include maternal hypertension, preterm delivery, low birth weight, and a dramatic increase in the relative risk for cerebral palsy (reviewed by Ref. (6)). These complications lead to a higher incidence of medical, perinatal, and neonatal complications and a 10-fold increase in health care costs compared with a singleton delivery (7). Decreasing the prevalence of multiple gestations while maintaining or improving overall pregnancy rates remains the most significant contemporary goal of infertility research.

In many countries including Norway, Sweden, Denmark, Belgium, England, Italy, and Germany, the dangers associated with multiple pregnancies have been allayed by legal restrictions on the number of embryos that can be transferred in a given IVF cycle. For example, in most Scandinavian countries and Belgium the government has set a legal limit of single embryo transfer (i.e., only one embryo to be transferred per cycle) for specific patient groups, while many other European countries have restricted the number of transferred embryos to a maximum of two. In other parts of the world, where no legal restrictions exist, the onus is on the individual clinic (as well as the couple) to decrease the number of embryos transferred so that an acceptable balance can be achieved between the risks associated with multiple gestations and "acceptable" pregnancy rates. The current indications are that in the future, clinics in the United States, and other countries currently lacking legislation, will be compelled via legal, financial and/or, moral obligation to restrict the number of embryos transferred in order to minimize the risk of multiple gestations.

A major issue in limiting the number of embryos transferred is the apparent inability to accurately estimate the reproductive potential of individual embryos within a cohort of embryos using the existing selection techniques, which largely encompasses morphological evaluation. Faced with the scenario that we, the worldwide IVF community, will in the future have to select only one or two embryos for transfer, we will be forced to make certain choices. The first may be to rely on less aggressive stimulation protocols thus generating a lower number of eggs at collection. Paradoxically, the generation of a smaller number of oocytes could lead to a greater percentage of viable embryos within a given cohort (8,9) and a more receptive endometrium. The second choice (which is not exclusive from the first) is to improve the selection process for defining the quality of individual embryos so that the ones we choose for transfer are more likely to implant. This chapter will discuss several strategies in selection criteria that will help us achieve this second choice.

MORPHOLOGY AS AN ASSESSMENT TOOL

For over 30 years, morphological assessment has been the primary means of the embryologist for selecting which embryo(s) to replace. Since the early years of IVF it was noted that embryos cleaving faster and those of better morphological appearance were more likely to lead to a pregnancy (10,11). Morphological assessment systems have evolved over the past decade and in addition to the classical parameters of cell number and fragmentation, numerous other characteristics have been examined including: pronuclear morphology, early cleavage to the two-cell stage, top quality embryos on successive days, and various forms of sequential assessment of embryos (see reviews by Refs. (12–14)). In addition, the ability to culture and assess blastocyst stage embryos has also significantly improved the ability to select embryos on the basis of morphology (15). Here, we describe key morphogenic events and the key times at which they should take place in the laboratory.

THE PRONUCLEATE OOCYTE

The many transformations that take place during the fertilization process make this a highly dynamic stage to assess. The oocyte contains the majority of the developmental material, maternal mRNA, for ensuring that the embryo reaches the four- to eight-cell stage. In human embryos, embryonic genome activation has been shown to occur between the four- and eight-cell stages (16). The quality of the oocyte therefore, plays the lead role for determining embryo development and subsequent viability.

A number of studies have postulated that embryo quality can be predicted at the pronucleate oocyte stage. Separate studies by Tesarik and Scott (17,18) concentrated on the predictive value of the nucleoli. Tesarik and Greco (17) postulated that the normal and abnormal morphology of the pronuclei were related to the developmental fate of human embryos. They retrospectively assessed the number and distribution of nucleolar precursor bodies (NPBs) in each pronucleus of fertilized oocytes that led to embryos that implanted. The characteristics of these concepti were then compared with those that led to failures in implantation. The features that were shared by zygotes that had the 100% implantation success were (*i*) the number of NPBs in both pronuclei never differed by more than 3 and (*ii*) the NPBs were always polarized or not polarized in both pronuclei but never polarized in one pronucleus and not in the other. Pronucleate oocytes not showing the above criteria were more likely to develop into preimplantation embryos that had poor morphology and/or experienced cleavage arrest. The presence of at least one embryo, which had shown the above criteria at the pronuclear stage in those transferred, led to a pregnancy rate of 22/44 (50%) compared to only 2/23 (9%) when none were present.

A further criterion of pronucleate oocytes that may affect embryo morphology is the orientation of pronuclei relative to the polar bodies. Oocyte polarity is clearly evident in non-mammalian species. In mammals, the animal pole of the oocyte may be estimated by the location of the first polar body, whereas after fertilization, the second polar body marks the embryonic pole (19). In human oocytes a differential distribution of various factors within the oocyte has been described and anomalies in the distribution of these factors, in particular the side of the oocyte believed to contain the animal pole, are thought to affect embryo development and possibly fetal growth (20,21). Following from this hypothesis Garello et al. (22) examined pronuclear orientation, polar body placement, and embryo quality to ascertain if a link existed between a plausible polarity of oocytes at the pronuclear stage and further development. The most interesting observation involved the calculation of angle β (Fig. 18.1), which represented the angle between a line drawn through the axis of the pronuclei and the position of the furthest polar body. They found that as the angle β increased there was a concurrent decrease in the morphological quality of preimplantation stage human embryos. They postulated that the misalignment of the polar body might be linked to cytoplasmic turbulence thus disturbing the delicate polarity of the zygote.

A further study by Scott and Smith (23) devised an embryo score on day 1 on the basis of alignment of pronuclei and nucleoli, the appearance of the cytoplasm, nuclear membrane breakdown, and cleavage to the two-cell stage. Patients who had an overall high embryo score ($\geq$15) had a pregnancy and implantation rate of 34/48 (71%) and 49/175 (28%), respectively, compared with only 4/49 (8%) and 4/178 (2%) in the low embryo score group. The use of pronuclear scoring has been reviewed by Scott (24). A recent report by Wong et al. (25) has also shown that success in progression to the blastocyst stage

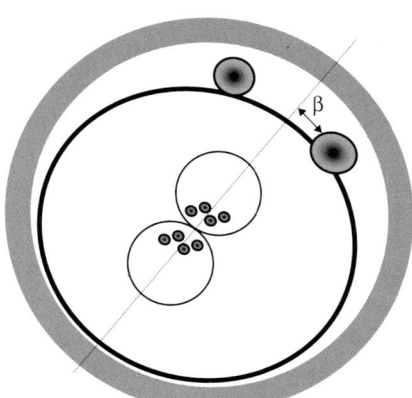

Ideal features shared by pronucleate oocytes that have high viability:

(i) the number of nucleolar precursor bodies (NPBs) in both pronuclei never differed by more than three

(ii) the NPBs are always polarized or nonpolarized in both pronuclei but never polarized in one pronucleus and not in the other

(iii) the angle β from the axis of the pronuclei and the furthest polar body is less than 50°

18–19 hrs post insemination/injection

Figure 18.1 Ideal features shared by pronucleate oocytes that have high viability as described by Tesarik and Greco (17), Garello et al. (22), and Scott and Smith (23).

can be predicted with >93% sensitivity and specificity by measuring three dynamic, noninvasive imaging parameters to the four-cell stage.

CLEAVAGE-STAGE EMBRYOS

The most widely used criteria for selecting the best embryos for transfer have been based on cell number and morphology (10). A vast number of variations on the theme have been published. Some of the key studies have been presented by Gerris et al. (26) and Van Royen et al. (27) who employed strict embryo criteria to select single embryos for transfer. The necessary characteristics of their "top" quality embryos were established by retrospectively examining embryos that had a very high implantation potential (27). These "top" quality embryos had the following characteristics: 4 or 5 blastomeres on day 2 and at least 7 blastomeres on day 3 after fertilization; absence of multinucleated blastomeres and <20% of fragments on day 2 and day 3 after fertilization. When these criteria were utilized in a prospective, randomized clinical trial comparing single and double embryo transfers it was found that in (26) single embryo transfers where a top quality embryo was available an implantation rate of 42.3% and an ongoing pregnancy rate of 38.5% were obtained. In (27) double embryo transfers an implantation rate of 48.1% and an ongoing pregnancy rate of 74% were obtained. A larger study analyzing the outcome of 370 consecutive single top quality embryo transfers in patients younger than 38 years for pregnancy showed that the pregnancy rate after single top quality embryo transfer was 51.9% (28). Recently, the same group of authors has provided further evidence of the importance of multinucleation as part of the equation in selecting top quality embryos (29).

The majority of studies that have used and report embryo selection criteria on the basis of cell number and morphology do so by stating that embryos were selected on day 2 or day 3. As discussed by Bavister (30) one of the most critical factors in determining selection criteria is to ascertain strict time points to compare the embryos. A four-cell embryo scored in the morning of day 2 is definitely not the same as one that was scored as a four-cell embryo in the afternoon. Sakkas and colleagues have therefore used cleavage to the two-cell stage at 25-hour post insemination or microinjection as the critical time point for selecting embryos (31–33). In a larger series of patients it was found that 45% of patients undergoing IVF or intracytoplasmic sperm injection (ICSI) have early cleaving two-cell embryos. Patients who have early cleaving two-cell stage embryos allocated for transfer on day 2 or 3 have significantly higher implantation and pregnancy rates (33). Furthermore, nearly 50% of the patients who have two early cleaving two-cell embryos transferred achieve a clinical pregnancy (Fig. 18.2). The most convincing data supporting the usefulness of early cleaving two-cell embryos is that provided by single embryo transfer (34,35). In one such study Salumets et al. (34) showed that when transferring single embryos, a significantly higher clinical pregnancy rate was observed after transfer

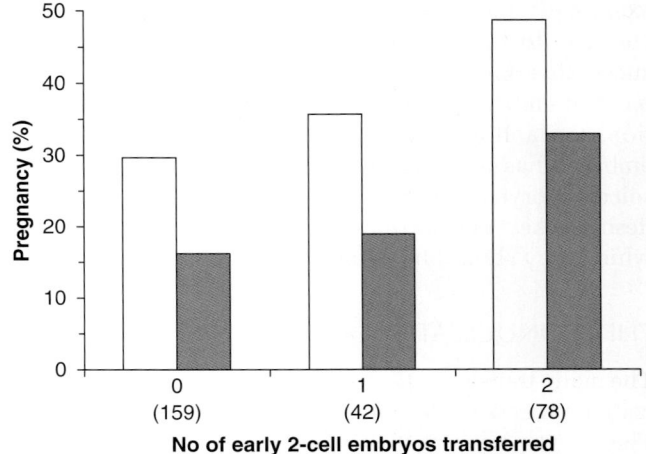

Figure 18.2 The percentage of clinical pregnancies (light columns) and implantation rate (dark columns) in relation to whether patients had 0, 1, or 2 early cleavage embryos transferred. The numbers in parentheses indicate the number of cycles per group.

of early cleaving (50%) rather than non-early cleaving (26.4%) embryos. The embryos that cleave early to the two-cell stage have also been reported to have a significantly higher blastocyst formation rate (36,37). It is also interesting to note that, in the embryo scoring system described by Scott and Smith (23), embryos that had already cleaved to the 2-cell stage by 25 to 26-hour post insemination were assigned an additional score of 10. This score for early cleavage is heavily weighted when one considers that the high quality embryos were judged to be those scoring >15, that is, to score as high quality the embryo had to have cleaved early.

Recently a large data set has been reported examining the sequential growth of 4042 embryos individually cultured from day 1 to days 5–6 (37). Pronuclear morphology on day 1, and early cleavage, cell number, and fragmentation rate on day 2 were evaluated for each zygote. Interestingly, early cleavage and cell number on day 2 were the most powerful parameters to predict the development of a good morphology blastocyst at day 5. This is also supported by the real-time imaging data of Wong et al. (25) and Meseguer et al. (38).

DEVELOPMENT TO THE BLASTOCYST STAGE

It is now becoming clear that success rates after blastocyst transfer compared with cleavage stage are improved, even when controlling for age (39). The commercial availability of sequential culture media systems has led to the routine use of blastocyst culture in many IVF clinics. The type of blastocyst obtained is, however, of critical importance. As with the scoring of embryos during the cleavage stages, time and morphology play an important part in selecting the best blastocyst. The scoring assessment for blastocysts devised by Gardner and Schoolcraft (40) is based on the expansion state of the blastocyst and on the consistency of the inner cell mass and trophectoderm cells (Fig. 18.3). Examples of high

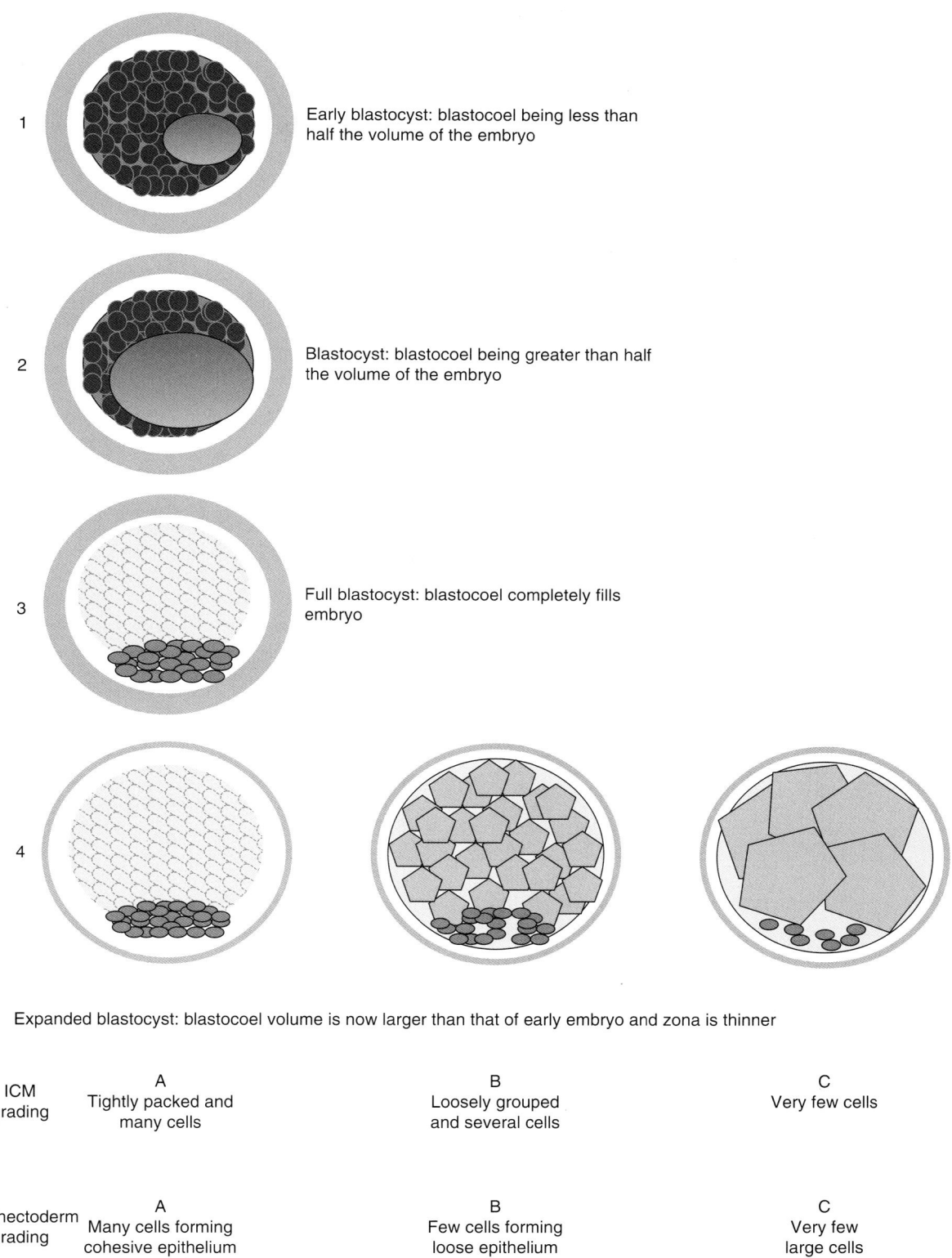

Figure 18.3 The blastocyst grading system. *Source*: Modified from Gardner and Schoolcraft (40).

quality blastocysts are shown in Figure 18.4. Using such a grading system it was determined that when two high scoring blastocysts (>3 AA), i.e. an expanded blastocoel with compacted inner cell mass and cohesive trophectoderm epithelium, are transferred a clinical pregnancy and implantation rate of >80% and 69% can be attained (41). When two blastocysts not achieving these scores (<3 AA) are transferred the clinical pregnancy and implantation rate are significantly lower, 50% and 33%(42). Although reduced from the values obtained with top scoring blastocysts, it is evident that early blastocysts on day 5 still have high developmental potential.

The time of blastocyst formation is also crucial. When cases were compared where only day 5 and 6 frozen blastocysts were transferred to those frozen on or after day 7 and transferred, the pregnancy rates were 7/18 (38.9%)

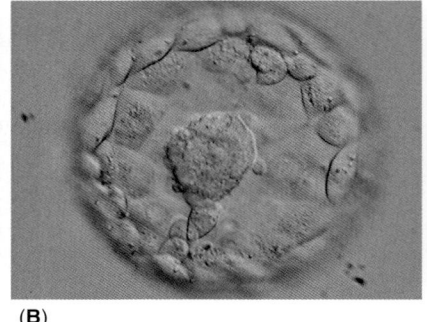
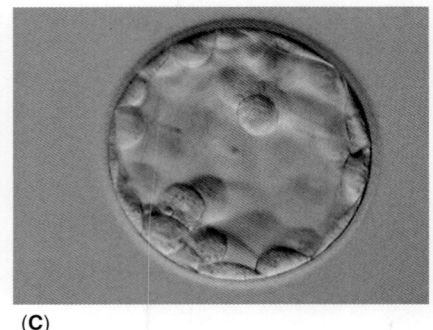

(A) (B) (C)

Figure 18.4 Day 5 human blastocysts. Scores based on the grading system reported by Gardner and Schoolcraft (40). Blastocysts in (**A**) and (**B**) would both score 4 AA, the embryo in (**C**) would only score 4CA due to the apparent absence of an inner cell mass, in spite of the development of an excellent trophectoderm.

and 1/16 (6.2%), respectively (43). In these cases, expanded blastocysts with a definable inner cell mass and trophectoderm were frozen. These results show that even though blastocysts can be obtained, a crucial factor is when they form blastocysts. When taking this into account, the best blastocysts would be those that develop by day 5. Selecting the fastest blastocysts had been proposed to create a bias in sex selection, as Menezo et al. (44) reported that blastocysts transferred after development in co-culture gave rise to the birth of more male offspring. Milki et al. (45) also reported that combined data from the literature show a male-to-female ratio percentage of 57.3:42.7 in blastocyst transfer compared with that of 51.2:48.8 in day 3-ET (P = 0.001). Recently, the Australian and New Zealand registry was used to show that blastocyst culture might also skew the male outcome to 54.1% (46). Other evidence also now indicates that faster growing blastocysts could be preferentially male (47).

A STRATEGY FOR SELECTING THE BEST EMBRYO BY MORPHOLOGY

The above selection criteria have all shown that they generate some benefit in identifying individual embryos that have a high viability.

How do we implement a strategy for selecting a single embryo when we have many to choose from? A multiple-step scoring system that encompasses all the above criteria would allow us to reach this goal. The use of sequential scoring systems has been shown to be beneficial by a number of authors (27,36,48). Here, we propose the following plan for sequential embryo assessment:

18–19 Hours Post Insemination/ICSI: (Fig. 18.1)

The pronuclei are examined for the following:

1. Symmetry
2. The presence of even numbers of NPB
3. The positioning of the polar bodies

25–26 Hours Post Insemination/ICSI: (Fig. 18.5)

1. Embryos that have already cleaved to the two-cell stage
2. Zygotes that have progressed to nuclear membrane breakdown

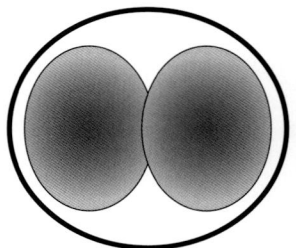

25–26 hr postinsemination/injection–embryo should be at the 2-cell stage with equal blastomeres and no fragmentation

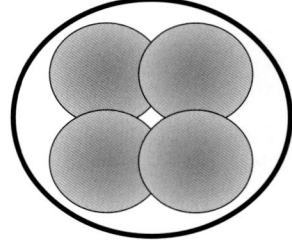

42–44 hr postinsemination/injection–embryo should have 4 or more blastomeres and less than 20% fragmentation

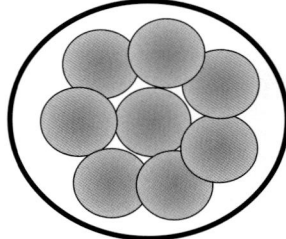

66–68 hr postinsemination/injection–embryo should have 8 or more blastomeres and less than 20% fragmentation

Figure 18.5 Ideal features of embryos scored at 25–26 hours, 42–44 hours, and 66–68 hours post insemination/intracytoplasmic sperm injection (ICSI). For further details on the scoring criteria see Sakkas et al. (32), Shoukir et al. (31), and Van Royen et al. (27).

42–44 hours Post Insemination/ICSI: (Fig. 18.5)

1. Number of blastomeres should be greater or equal to 4
2. Fragmentation of less than 20%
3. No multinucleated blastomeres

66–68 Hours Post Insemination/ICSI: (Fig. 18.5)

1. Number of blastomeres should be greater or equal to 8
2. Fragmentation of less than 20%
3. No multinucleated blastomeres

106–108 Hours Post Insemination/ICSI: (Figs. 18.3 and 18.4)

1. The blastocelic cavity should be full.
2. Inner cell mass should be numerous and tightly packed.
3. Trophectodermal cells should be numerous and cohesive.

Which of the above criteria would be the most important? To select the best embryos we could envisage a fluid selection process that would mark embryos as they develop. The above criteria would therefore be seen as ideal hurdles of development. At every step an embryo would be given a positive mark when it reached the ideal criteria of a certain stage. It would, however, be possible that an embryo may not pass one step, but would pass the hurdle at a following step. The embryo or embryos attaining the best criteria at each step would therefore be the ones that would be selected for transfer. For example, if we are attempting to transfer a single embryo to a patient the following scenario could be envisaged. An embryo may not pass any of the earlier hurdles but still form a high grade blastocyst on day 5. If this were the most successful of the cohort of embryos then this would be the one selected. However, if six blastocysts were observed on day 5, all of equally high grade, then the blastocyst that had achieved the most positive scores at each of the previous hurdles could be transferred. Furthermore, patients who have low numbers of embryos, and will have transfer on day 2 or 3, could be assessed using the initial criteria and the embryo that passed the initial hurdles would be selected. A proposed schedule of embryo selection is given in Fig. 18.6. It is important to note that to date the strongest criteria of selection appear to be the selection of a high-quality blastocyst on day 5 of development (37,41).

The practical issues for performing such a selection process would be that embryos would need to be cultured in individual drops. This may remove any necessary benefits of culturing embryos in groups (49–51). A further practical issue is that embryos will need to be observed more often; however, using drop culture systems under oil do allay this. The extra observations, if performed under a controlled heated and gassed climate, should not be detrimental to the embryo. In prolonged culture, pronuclear assessment, change over into new media on day 3 and assessment of the blastocyst is already performed. The extra assessment periods would be the check of early cleaving two-cell embryos and assessment of embryos on day 2. Optional observations could include that of the polar body placement, as described by Garello et al. (22). These assessment criteria involve photography, followed by calculation from the photograph, which would involve a further manipulation of the zygote once the polar body displacement has been calculated. A further observation would be to determine the degree of blastulation on the afternoon of day 4, this reflecting the speed at which a given embryo is developing. Recent evidence has indicated some benefit from observations and transfer on day 4 (52).

The move to commercialize real-time imaging of embryos has now placed the above sequential assessment procedure closer to a practical reality, removing any concerns related to constant visualization of the embryos away from the incubator (25,38). The further development of this type of imaging system is covered in chapter 19 by Basile and colleagues.

So it is evident that with improved culture conditions, together with suitable grading systems, it is possible to dramatically increase implantation rates and therefore decrease the number of embryos transferred. However, this approach raises two issues; if the laboratory in question is not performing blastocyst transfer, then it cannot rely on advanced grading systems, and second, morphology will only tell us a limited amount about the physiological status of the embryo. The rest of this chapter is, therefore, devoted to the application of novel tests of embryonic function. It is assumed that such tests must be noninvasive for the adoption in clinical use. Therefore, methods that can be considered as semi-invasive, that is, those that involve embryo biopsy prior to cell analysis, are not considered here.

BEYOND EMBRYO MORPHOLOGY: THE NONINVASIVE QUANTIFICATION OF NUTRIENT UTILISATION AND THE METABOLOME

The inherent ease for the laboratory to assess various morphological markers makes it the preferred assessment technique to transfer embryos. Even with the adoption of more complex forms of analysis it will still remain as one of the tools we have in our armory for assessment. However, a number of quantitative techniques are now being optimized which can monitor the uptake of specific nutrients by the embryo from the surrounding medium, and to detect the secretion of specific metabolites and factors into the medium (Fig. 18.7). To measure such changes in culture media the noninvasive assessment tools must fulfill a number of criteria so that they can be applicable in IVF clinics.

A technical problem to performing these types of measurements in clinical IVF has always been the ability to measure the change

1. without damaging the embryo
2. quickly
3. consistently and accurately

The analysis of metabolite levels within spent embryo culture media fulfills the above criteria, and is being developed to augment the analysis of embryo morphology as a means of embryo selection. Three approaches are currently being evaluated; analysis of carbohydrate utilization, the turnover of amino acids, and the analysis of the embryonic metabolome. The first two approaches could be considered analysis of the activity of specific metabolic pathways, whereas analysis of the metabolome should be considered as the systematic analysis of the inventory of metabolites that represent the functional phenotype at the cellular level. Depending upon the

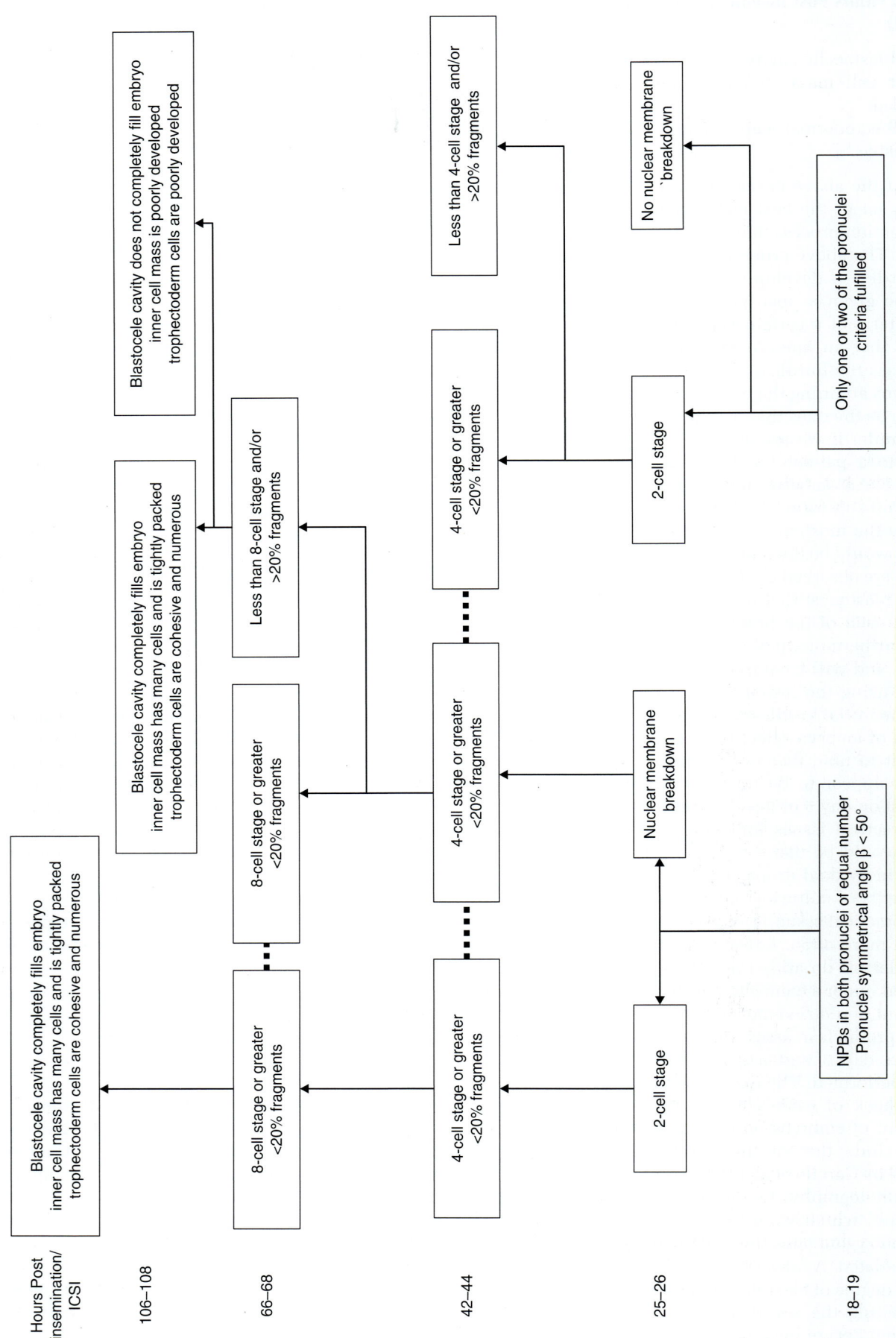

Figure 18.6 A strategy for the sequential analysis of embryo development with the aim of selecting a single embryo for transfer.

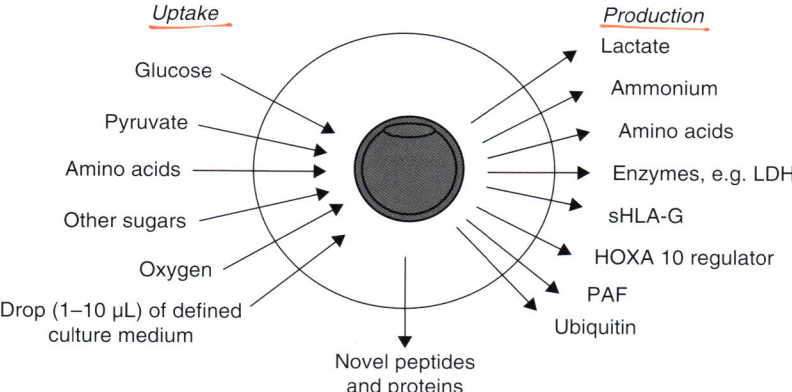

Figure 18.7 Noninvasive analysis of human embryo nutrient consumption and metabolite/factor production. Individual blastocysts are incubated in 1.0 to 10.0 μl volumes of the defined medium. Serial or end point samples of the medium can then be removed for analysis. An indirect measurement of metabolic pathways, that is, glycolysis and transamination can be obtained by measuring specific nutrients in combination, such as glucose uptake and lactate production, or amino acid turn over with ammonium production.

technology employed to analyze the metabolome, one does not necessarily obtain identification of specific metabolites, but rather one creates an algorithm that relates to cell function.

ANALYSIS OF CARBOHYDRATE UTILIZATION

A relationship between metabolic activity and embryo development and viability has been established over several decades (53). As early as 1970, Menke and McLaren revealed that mouse blastocysts, developed in basic culture conditions, lost their ability to oxidize glucose (54). This initial observation was followed by several studies that elucidated changes in embryo metabolism associated with loss of developmental capacity in vitro (reviewed by Ref. (55)). In 1980, Renard et al. (56) observed that day-10 cattle blastocysts which had an elevated glucose uptake developed better, both in culture and in vivo after transfer than those blastocysts with a glucose uptake below this value. In 1987, using the relatively new technique of noninvasive microfluorescence, Gardner and Leese (57) measured glucose uptake by individual day-4 mouse blastocysts prior to transfer to recipient females. The embryos that went to term had a significantly higher glucose uptake in culture than those embryos that failed to develop after transfer. This work was then built on by Lane and Gardner (58), who showed that the glycolytic rate of mouse blastocysts could be used to select embryos for transfer prospectively. Morphologically identical mouse blastocysts with equivalent diameters were identified using metabolic criteria as "viable" prior to transfer and had a fetal development of 80%. In contrast, those embryos that exhibited an abnormal metabolic profile (compared to in vivo developed controls) developed at a rate of only 6%. Clearly such data provide dramatic evidence that metabolic function is linked to embryo viability (Figs 18.8 and 18.9).

Analysis of the relationship between human embryo nutrition and subsequent development in vitro (59,60) was undertaken by Gardner et al. (59). It was determined that glucose consumption on day 4 by human embryos was twice as high in those embryos that went on to form blastocysts. Subsequently, Gardner and colleagues (61) have gone on to confirm a positive relationship between glucose uptake and human embryo viability on day 4 and day 5 of development (Fig. 18.10). Furthermore, the data generated indicate that differences in nutrient utilization differ between male and female embryos, a phenomenon previously documented in other mammalian species (62,63).

ANALYSIS OF AMINO ACID UTILIZATION

In a study on amino acid turnover by human embryos, Houghton et al. (60) determined that alanine release into the surrounding medium on day 2 and day 3 was the highest in those embryos that did not form blastocysts. Therefore, assessing metabolic activity and metabolic normality may prove to be a feasible way to determine human embryonic "health." To this end, Brison et al. (64) have reported that changes in concentration of amino acids in the spent medium of human zygotes cultured for 24 hours in an embryo culture medium containing a mixture of amino acids using high performance liquid chromatography. They found that asparagine, glycine, and leucine utilized in the 24 hours following fertilization were all significantly associated with clinical pregnancy and live birth. Recent work has also revealed an association with aneuploidy and embryonic sex with amino acid turnover (65). Ongoing studies in this area will help identify the group of amino acids at each stage of development whose usage is linked with subsequent viability.

OTHER SPECIFIC FACTORS

Other techniques have also been reported to measure metabolic parameters in culture media; however, they have yet to be tested in a clinical IVF setting. These include the self-referencing electrophysiological technique, which is a noninvasive measurement of the physiology of individual cells and monitors the movement of ions and molecules between the cell and the

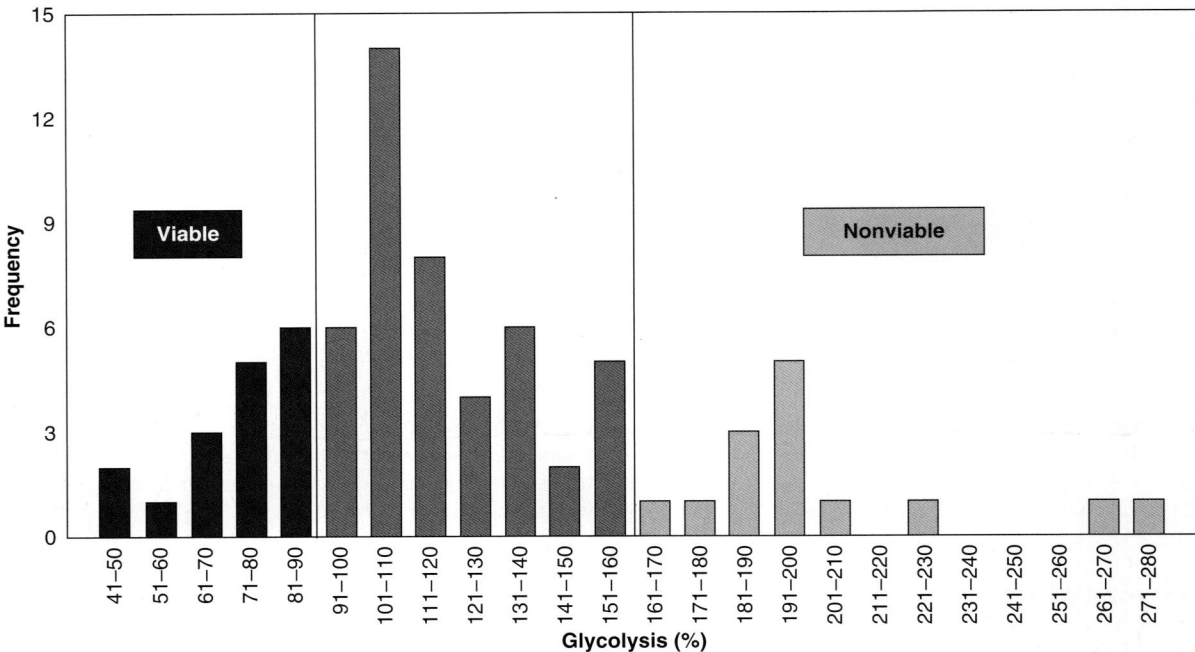

Figure 18.8 Distribution of glycolytic activity in a population of 79 morphologically similar mouse blastocysts cultured in medium DM1. The lowest 15% of glycolytic activity (<88%) was considered viable, while the highest 15% of the range (>160%) was deemed nonviable. *Source*: Adapted from Ref. 58.

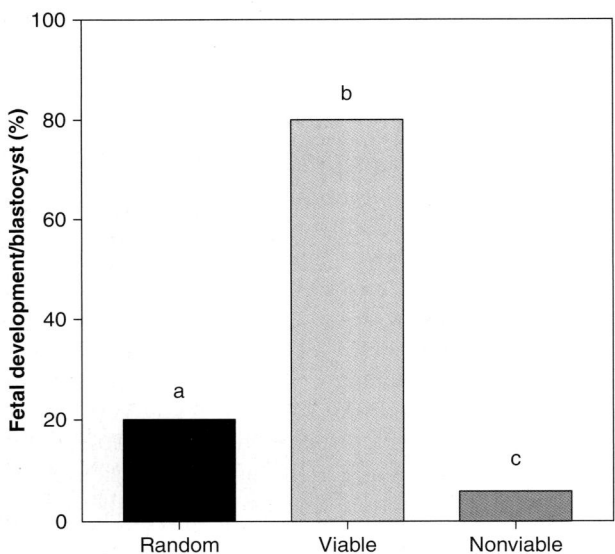

Figure 18.9 Fetal development of mouse blastocysts selected for transfer using glycolytic activity as a biochemical marker. "Viable" blastocysts were classified as those with a glycolytic rate close to in vivo developed blastocysts (<88%), while "Nonviable" blastocysts had a glycolytic rate in the highest 15% of the distribution (<160%). On each day of the experiment, a few blastocysts were selected and transferred at random, along with those selected as either viable or nonviable. [a–c]Different superscripts indicate significantly different populations ($P < 0.01$). *Source*: Adapted from Ref. 58.

surrounding media (66,67). One technique that is of the above mentioned mode is that which noninvasively measures oxygen consumption of developing embryos. Interestingly, although this technology has been shown to correlate with bovine blastocyst development it was less successful in predicting mouse embryo development (68,69).

A number of studies have also investigated the assessment of secreted factors in the embryo culture media (Fig. 18.7) and correlated them with better embryo development and pregnancy rates. One such factor is soluble human leukocyte antigen G (HLA-G) (70,71) which is believed to protect the developing embryo from destruction by the maternal immune response. Soluble HLA-G has been found in the media surrounding the early embryo and a number of papers have also reported that its presence correlates with the improved pregnancy potential of an embryo (72–74). Recently, some studies have raised some serious concerns regarding the use of HLA-G production as a marker of further developmental potential (75–77) and prospective clinical trials are needed to further evaluate this parameter. Included, in the studies examining secretion of factors in the media by embryos are numerous papers examining the secretion of platelet activating factor (PAF). The clinical utility of PAF in an IVF setting has also yet to be stringently examined (see review by O'Neill (78)). Another indirect assay of soluble markers that may be present in embryo culture media was that described by Sakkas et al. (79) where it was determined that cell-free media from human embryos cultured to the blastocyst stage contained a soluble molecule that induced HOXA10 expression in an endometrial epithelial cell line (Ishikawa). More recently, preimplantation factor (PIF) has been reported to provide some indication of embryo viability when measured and to possibly improve embryo quality when placed in culture media (80). Finally, a more direct analysis of protein markers in embryo culture media has been shown by Katz-Jaffe et al.

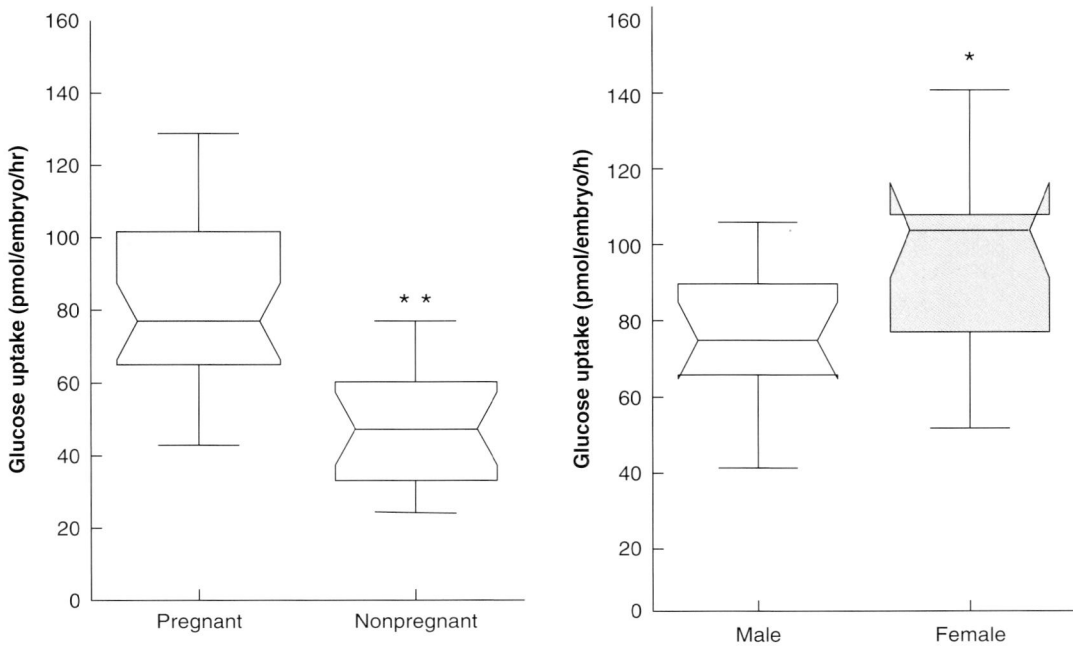

Figure 18.10 Relationship between glucose consumption on day 4 of development and human embryo viability and embryo sex. (**A**) Glucose uptake on day 4 of embryonic development and pregnancy outcome (positive fetal heartbeat). Notches represent the confidence interval of the median, the depth of the box represents the interquartile range (50% of the data), and whiskers represent the 5% and 95% quartiles. The line across the box is the median glucose consumption. **, significantly different from pregnant ($P < 0.01$). (**B**) Glucose uptake by male and female embryos on day 4 of development. Notches represent the confidence interval of the median; the depth of the box represents the interquartile range (50% of the data); whiskers represent the 5% and 95% quartiles. The line across the box is the median glucose consumption. *, significantly different from male embryos ($P < 0.05$). *Source*: Adapted from Ref. 85.

(81,82), using proteomic based technology. They found differential protein expression profiles between early and expanded blastocysts, as well as between developing blastocysts and degenerate embryos.

ANALYSIS OF METABOLOMICS

A new and emerging technology which may allow us in the future to measure factors in embryo culture media is metabolomics. The complete array of small-molecule metabolites that are found within a biological system constitutes the metabolome and reflects the functional phenotype (83). Metabolomics is the systematic study of this dynamic inventory of metabolites, as small molecular biomarkers, representing the functional phenotype in a biological system. Using various forms of spectral and analytical approaches, metabolomics attempts to determine metabolites associated with physiologic and pathologic states (84). Metabolic studies of embryos indicated that embryos that result in pregnancy are different in their metabolomic profile compared to those that do not lead to pregnancies (85). Investigation of the metabolome of embryos, as detected in the culture media they grow in, using targeted spectroscopic analysis and bioinformatics may therefore divulge these differences. In an initial proof of principle study, Seli et al. (85) established that these differences are detectable in the culture media using both Raman and near infrared (NIR) spectroscopy. Briefly a statistical formula was used to assign a relative "embryo viability score"—equating to embryo reproductive potential—and it was found that this score correlated to positive or negative implantation outcomes. Interestingly when human embryos of similar morphology were examined using the same NIR spectral profile their viability scores varied remarkably in relation to morphology indicating that the metabolome of embryos that look similar differ significantly (86,87). This observation is in agreement with the study of Katz-Jaffe et al. (81,88), who revealed that the proteome of individual human blastocysts of the same grade differed between embryos, again indicating that embryo morphology is not completely linked to its physiology.

Although a series of preliminary studies (86,87,89–91) showed a benefit of this technique they were largely based on retrospective studies and performed in a single research laboratory as distinct from a real clinical setting. Recently a number of in-house clinical studies have been reported using either a prototype or commercial version of the NIR system from Molecular Biometrics, Inc., Norwood, MA showing inconsistent results (Table 18.1). The largest of these studies were performed as randomized clinical trials after SET. All studies compared standard morphological techniques for embryo selection versus using the NIR system to rank embryos within a cohort that had good morphology and were being selected for either transfer or cryopreservation. In the Gothenburg study (92) both day 2 and day 5 SETs were included. Although not significant, the results indicated a possible benefit of embryo selection through addition of NIR on day 2 transfer. However, it failed to show any benefit for

Table 18.1 A Summary of Randomized Clinical Studies Examining the Use of Metabolomics to Assess the Cohort of Good Morphology Embryos in Patients (Morphology Plus Viametrics Using Near Infra Red Versus the Selection of Embryos Using Morphology Alone)

Type of NIR instrument	Study type		Morphology	Morphology plus viametrics (NIR)	Improvement in outcome
Prototype	SET	IR	Day 2: 22/83 (26.5%)	Day 2:27/87 (31.0%)	Yes
Hardarson et al. (92)			Day 5: 36/80 (45.0%)	Day 5: 30/77 (39.0%)	No
Prototype	SET	CPR	Day 3: 68/163 (41.7%)	Day 3:61/146 (41.8%)	No
Vergouw (96)					
Commercial Economou et al. (97)	DET	CPR	8/28 (29%)	16/28 (57%)	Yes
Commercial Sfontouris et al. (98)	MET	CPR	41/86 (47.7%)	21/39 (53.9%)	Yes
		IR	66/257 (25.7%)	35/102 (34.3%)	

Abbreviations: CPR, clinical pregnancy rate; DET, double embryo transfer; IR, implantation rate; MET, multiple embryo transfer; SET, single embryo transfer; NIR, near infra red.

selection of day 5 SET. Interestingly, the benefits of selecting a single good quality blastocyst on day 5 have also been found to be beneficial in many other studies (93).

One of the underlying problems encountered in the NIR system was that the threshold of signal distinguishing between a viable and nonviable embryo was susceptible to signal noise. NIR spectroscopy systems and the algorithms generated from them can create models that inadvertently conceal problems in a particular platform. In doing so a method that has been established and cross-validated on a larger scale, can still be problematic as the variation can still lie within the technical platform itself. The commercial version of the NIR instrument has recently been withdrawn due to the wide variability in performance between clinics. This is not dissimilar to the situation faced by aneuploidy screening of embryos, whereby chromosomal screening of preimplantation embryos has always thought to be a strong concept. However, using FISH has proved to be inadequate (94) while it now appears that modern comprehensive screening techniques are providing more consistent results (95).

It is beyond question that markers do exist in the spent embryo culture media indicative of viability. The major benefits of a noninvasive type of technology is the fact that the technology can be used on spent media and the time taken to assess the samples is very short, making it possible to perform the analysis just prior to ET. So far NIR spectroscopy, when tested in stringent clinical trials, does not appear to consistently improve the chance of selecting a single embryo for a viable pregnancy and the NIR technology appears to need further development before being used as an objective marker of embryo viability. Therefore, although NIR met the first two key criteria necessary to be used routinely in a clinical IVF it currently fails to consistently meet the final criterion.

SUMMARY

Analysis of embryo morphology and the development of suitable grading systems have greatly assisted in the selection of human embryos for transfer. However, it is proposed that in the near future embryo selection will also be significantly aided by the noninvasive analysis of embryo physiology and function, using approaches that better quantify embryo metabolism. The addition of such technologies will be of immense value in helping both clinicians and embryologists to more confidently select the most viable embryos within a cohort, helping the move to single embryo transfers.

REFERENCES

1. De MJ, Goossens V, Bhattacharya S, et al. Assisted reproductive technology in Europe, 2006: Results generated from European registers by ESHRE. Hum Reprod 2010; 258: 1851–62.
2. Society for Assisted Reproduction Technology (SART) data. 2006. [Available from: https://www.sartcorsonline.com/rptCSR_PublicMultYear.aspx?ClinicPKID=0]
3. The Australia and New Zealand Assisted Reproduction Database (ANZARD) data. 2006. [Available from: http://www.preru.unsw.edu.au/PRERUWeb.nsf/resources/ART_2005_06/$file/art12.pdf]
4. Nyboe AA, Goossens V, Bhattacharya S, et al. Assisted reproductive technology and intrauterine inseminations in Europe, 2005: results generated from European registers by ESHRE: ESHRE. The European IVF Monitoring Programme (EIM), for the European Society of Human Reproduction and Embryology (ESHRE). Hum Reprod 2009; 24: 1267–87.
5. Society for Assisted Reproduction Technology (SART) data. 2009. [Available from: https://www.sartcorsonline.com/rptCSR_PublicMultYear.aspx?ClinicPKID=0]
6. Adashi EY, Barri PN, Berkowitz R, et al. Infertility therapy-associated multiple pregnancies (births): An ongoing epidemic. Reprod Biomed Online 2003; 7: 515–42.
7. Ledger WL, Anumba D, Marlow N, Thomas CM, Wilson EC. The costs to the NHS of multiple births after IVF treatment in the UK. BJOG 2006; 113: 21–5.
8. Inge GB, Brinsden PR, Elder KT. Oocyte number per live birth in IVF: were Steptoe and Edwards less wasteful? Hum Reprod 2005; 20: 588–92.
9. Patrizio P, Sakkas D. From oocyte to baby: a clinical evaluation of the biological efficiency of in vitro fertilization. Fertil Steril 2009; 91: 1061–6.
10. Cummins J, Breen T, Harrison K, et al. A formula for scoring human embryo growth rates in in vitro fertilization: its value in predicting pregnancy and in comparison with

visual estimates of embryo quality. J In Vitro Fert Embryo Transf 1986; 3: 284–95.
11. Edwards R, Fishel S, Cohen J. Factors influencing the success of in vitro fertilization for alleviating human infertility. J In Vitro Fert Embryo Transf 1984; 1: 3–23.
12. De Neubourg D, Gerris J. Single embryo transfer-state of the art. Reprod Biomed Online 2003; 7: 615–22.
13. Sakkas D. Evaluation of Embryo Quality. In: Gardner DK, Weissman A, Howles CM, Shoham Z, eds. Textbook of Reproductive Techniques: Laboratory and Clinical Perspectives. London: Martin Dunitz Press, 2001; 223–32.
14. Sakkas D, Gardner DK. Noninvasive methods to assess embryo quality. Curr Opin Obstet Gynecol 2005; 17: 283–8.
15. Gardner DK, Surrey E, Minjarez D, et al. Single blastocyst transfer: a prospective randomized trial. Fertil Steril 2004; 81: 551–5.
16. Braude P, Bolton V, Moore S. Human gene expression first occurs between the four and eight cell stages of preimplantation development. Nature 1988; 332: 459–61.
17. Tesarik J, Greco E. The probability of abnormal preimplantation development can be predicted by a single static observation on pronuclear stage morphology. Human Reprod 1999; 14: 318–23.
18. Scott L, Alvero R, Leondires M, Miller B. The morphology of human pronuclear embryos is positively related to blastocyst development and implantation. Hum Reprod 2000; 15: 2394–403.
19. Gardner R. The early blastocyst is bilaterally symmetrical and its axis of symmetry is aligned with the animal-vegetal axis of the zygote in mouse. Development 1997; 124: 289–301.
20. Antczak M, Van Blerkom J. Oocyte influences on early development: the regulatory proteins leptin and STAT3 are polarized in mouse and human oocytes and differentially distributed within the cells of the preimplantation stage embryo. Mol Hum Reprod 1997; 3: 1067–86.
21. Antczak M, Van Blerkom J. Temporal and spatial aspects of fragmentation in early human embryos: possible effects on developmental competence and association with the differential elimination of regulatory proteins from polarized domains. Hum Reprod 1999; 14: 429–47.
22. Garello C, Baker H, Rai J, et al. Pronuclear orientation, polar body placement, and embryo quality after intracytoplasmic sperm injection and in-vitro fertilization: further evidence for polarity in human oocytes? Hum Reprod 1999; 14: 2588–95.
23. Scott LA, Smith S. The successful use of pronuclear embryo transfers the day following oocyte retrieval. Hum Reprod 1998; 13: 1003–13.
24. Scott L. Pronuclear scoring as a predictor of embryo development. Reprod Biomed Online 2003; 6: 201–14.
25. Wong CC, Loewke KE, Bossert NL, et al. Non-invasive imaging of human embryos before embryonic genome activation predicts development to the blastocyst stage. Nat Biotechnol 2010; 28: 1115–21.
26. Gerris J, De Neubourg D, Mangelschots K, et al. Prevention of twin pregnancy after in-vitro fertilization or intracytoplasmic sperm injection based on strict embryo criteria: a prospective randomized clinical trial. Hum Reprod 1999; 14: 2581–7.
27. Van Royen E, Mangelschots K, De Neubourg D, et al. Characterization of a top quality embryo, a step towards single-embryo transfer. Hum Reprod 1999; 14: 2345–9.
28. De Neubourg D, Gerris J, Mangelschots K, et al. Single top quality embryo transfer as a model for prediction of early pregnancy outcome. Hum Reprod 2004; 19: 1476–9.
29. Van Royen E, Mangelschots K, Vercruyssen M, et al. Multinucleation in cleavage stage embryos. Hum Reprod 2003; 18: 1062–9.
30. Bavister B. Culture of preimplantation embryos: facts and artefacts. Hum Reprod Update 1995; 1: 91–148.
31. Shoukir Y, Campana A, Farley T, Sakkas D. Early cleavage of in-vitro fertilized human embryos to the 2-cell stage: a novel indicator of embryo quality and viability. Hum Reprod 1997; 12: 1531–6.
32. Sakkas D, Shoukir Y, Chardonnens D, Bianchi PG, Campana A. Early cleavage of human embryos to the two-cell stage after intracytoplasmic sperm injection as an indicator of embryo viability. Hum Reprod 1998; 13: 182–7.
33. Sakkas D, Percival G, D'Arcy Y, Sharif K, Afnan M. Assessment of early cleaving in vitro fertilized human embryos at the 2-cell stage before transfer improves embryo selection. Fertil Steril 2001; 76: 1150–6.
34. Salumets A, Hyden-Granskog C, Makinen S, et al. Early cleavage predicts the viability of human embryos in elective single embryo transfer procedures. Hum Reprod 2003; 18: 821–5.
35. Van Montfoort AP, Dumoulin JC, Kester AD, Evers JL. Early cleavage is a valuable addition to existing embryo selection parameters: a study using single embryo transfers. Hum Reprod 2004; 19: 2103–8.
36. Neuber E, Rinaudo P, Trimarchi JR, Sakkas D. Sequential assessment of individually cultured human embryos as an indicator of subsequent good quality blastocyst development. Hum Reprod 2003; 18: 1307–12.
37. Guerif F, Le Gouge A, Giraudeau B, et al. Limited value of morphological assessment at days 1 and 2 to predict blastocyst development potential: a prospective study based on 4042 embryos. Hum Reprod 2007; 22: 1973–81.
38. Meseguer M, Herrero J, Tejera A, et al. The use of morphokinetics as a predictor of embryo implantation. Hum Reprod 2011; 26: 2658–71.
39. Zander-Fox DL, Tremellen K, Lane M. Single blastocyst embryo transfer maintains comparable pregnancy rates to double cleavage-stage embryo transfer but results in healthier pregnancy outcomes. Aust NZ J Obstet Gynaecol 2011; 51: 406–10.
40. Gardner DK, Schoolcraft WB. In vitro culture of human blastocysts. In: Jansen R, Mortimer D, eds. Towards Reproductive Certainty: Infertility and Genetics Beyond. Carnforth: Parthenon Press, 1999: 378.
41. Gardner DK, Lane M, Stevens J, Schlenker T, Schoolcraft WB. Blastocyst score affects implantation and pregnancy outcome: towards a single blastocyst transfer. Fertil Steril 2000; 73: 1155–8.
42. Gardner DK, Stevens J, Sheehan CB, Schoolcraft WB. Morphological assessment of the human blastocyst. In: Elder KT, Cohen J, eds. Analysis of the Human Embryo. London, Informa Healthcare 2007: 79–87.
43. Shoukir Y, Chardonnens D, Campana A, Bischof P, Sakkas D. The rate of development and time of transfer play different roles in influencing the viability of human blastocysts. Hum Reprod 1998; 13: 676–81.
44. Menezo YJ, Chouteau J, Torello J, Girard A, Veiga A. Birth weight and sex ratio after transfer at the blastocyst

stage in humans [see comments]. Fertil Steril 1999; 72: 221–4.
45. Milki AA, Jun SH, Hinckley MD, et al. Comparison of the sex ratio with blastocyst transfer and cleavage stage transfer. J Assist Reprod Genet 2003; 20: 323–6.
46. Dean JH, Chapman MG, Sullivan EA. The effect on human sex ratio at birth by assisted reproductive technology (ART) procedures an assessment of babies born following single embryo transfers, Australia and New Zealand, 2002–2006. BJOG 2010; 117: 1628–34.
47. Alfarawati S, Fragouli E, Colls P, et al. The relationship between blastocyst morphology, chromosomal abnormality, and embryo gender. Fertil Steril 2011; 95: 520–4.
48. Fisch JD, Rodriguez H, Ross R, Overby G, Sher G. The Graduated Embryo Score (GES) predicts blastocyst formation and pregnancy rate from cleavage-stage embryos. Hum Reprod 2001; 16: 1970–5.
49. Wiley LM, Yamami S, Van Muyden D. Effect of potassium concentration, type of protein supplement, and embryo density on mouse preimplantation development in vitro. Fertil Steril 1986; 45: 111–19.
50. Lane M, Gardner DK. Effect of incubation volume and embryo density on the development and viability of mouse embryos in vitro. Hum Reprod 1992; 7: 558–62.
51. Gardner DK, Lane M, Spitzer A, Batt PA. Enhanced rates of cleavage and development for sheep zygotes cultured to the blastocyst stage in vitro in the absence of serum and somatic cells: amino acids, vitamins, and culturing embryos in groups stimulate development. Biol Reprod 1994; 50: 390–400.
52. Feil D, Henshaw RC, Lane M. Day 4 embryo selection is equal to Day 5 using a new embryo scoring system validated in single embryo transfers. Hum Reprod 2008; 23: 1505–10.
53. Bowman P, McLaren A. Viability and growth of mouse embryos after in vitro culture and fusion. J Embryol Exp Morphol 1970; 23: 693–704.
54. Menke TM, McLaren A. Mouse blastocysts grown in vivo and in vitro: carbon dioxide production and trophoblast outgrowth. J Reprod Fertil 1970; 23: 117–27.
55. Gardner DK. Changes in requirements and utilization of nutrients during mammalian preimplantation embryo development and their significance in embryo culture. Theriogenology 1998; 49: 83–102.
56. Renard JP, Philippon A, Menezo Y. In-vitro uptake of glucose by bovine blastocysts. J Reprod Fertil 1980; 58: 161–4.
57. Gardner DK, Leese HJ. Assessment of embryo viability prior to transfer by the noninvasive measurement of glucose uptake. J Exp Zool 1987; 242: 103–5.
58. Lane M, Gardner DK. Selection of viable mouse blastocysts prior to transfer using a metabolic criterion. Hum Reprod 1996; 11: 1975–8.
59. Gardner DK, Lane M, Stevens J, Schoolcraft WB. Noninvasive assessment of human embryo nutrient consumption as a measure of developmental potential. Fertility & Sterility 2001; 76: 1175–80.
60. Houghton FD, Hawkhead JA, Humpherson PG, et al. Non-invasive amino acid turnover predicts human embryo developmental capacity. Hum Reprod 2002; 17: 999–1005.
61. Gardner DK, Wale PL, Collins R, Lane M. Glucose consumption of single post-compaction human embryos is predictive of embryo sex and live birth outcome. Hum Reprod 2011; 26: 1981–6.
62. Gardner DK, Larman MG, Thouas GA. Sex-related physiology of the preimplantation embryo. Mol Hum Reprod 2010; 16: 539–47.
63. Sturmey RG, Bermejo-Alvarez P, Gutierrez-Adan A, et al. Amino acid metabolism of bovine blastocysts: a biomarker of sex and viability. Mol Reprod Dev 2010; 77: 285–96.
64. Brison DR, Houghton FD, Falconer D, et al. Identification of viable embryos in IVF by non-invasive measurement of amino acid turnover. Hum Reprod 2004; 19: 2319–24.
65. Picton HM, Elder K, Houghton FD, et al. Association between amino acid turnover and chromosome aneuploidy during human preimplantation embryo development in vitro. Mol Hum Reprod 2010; 16: 557–69.
66. Trimarchi JR, Liu L, Porterfield DM, Smith PJ, Keefe DL. A non-invasive method for measuring preimplantation embryo physiology. Zygote 2000; 8: 15–24.
67. Trimarchi JR, Liu L, Smith PJ, Keefe DL. Noninvasive measurement of potassium efflux as an early indicator of cell death in mouse embryos. Biol Reprod 2000; 63: 851–7.
68. Ottosen LD, Hindkjaer J, Lindenberg S, Ingerslev HJ. Murine pre-embryo oxygen consumption and developmental competence. J Assist Reprod Genet 2007; 24: 359–65.
69. Lopes AS, Larsen LH, Ramsing N, et al. Respiration rates of individual bovine in vitro-produced embryos measured with a novel, non-invasive and highly sensitive microsensor system. Reproduction 2005; 130: 669–79.
70. Kovats S, Main EK, Librach C, et al. A class I antigen, HLA-G, expressed in human trophoblasts. Science 1990; 248: 220–3.
71. Jurisicova A, Casper RF, MacLusky NJ, Mills GB, Librach CL. HLA-G expression during preimplantation human embryo development. Proc Natl Acad Sci USA 1996; 93: 161–5.
72. Noci I, Fuzzi B, Rizzo R, et al. Embryonic soluble HLA-G as a marker of developmental potential in embryos. Hum Reprod 2005; 20: 138–46.
73. Sher G, Keskintepe L, Nouriani M, Roussev R, Batzofin J. Expression of sHLA-G in supernatants of individually cultured 46-h embryos: a potentially valuable indicator of 'embryo competency' and IVF outcome. Reprod Biomed Online 2004; 9: 74–8.
74. Yie SM, Balakier H, Motamedi G, Librach CL. Secretion of human leukocyte antigen-G by human embryos is associated with a higher in vitro fertilization pregnancy rate. Fertil Steril 2005; 83: 30–6.
75. Menezo Y, Elder K, Viville S. Soluble HLA-G release by the human embryo: an interesting artefact? Reprod Biomed Online 2006; 13: 763–4.
76. Sageshima N, Shobu T, Awai K, et al. Soluble HLA-G is absent from human embryo cultures: a reassessment of sHLA-G detection methods. J Reprod Immunol 2007; 75: 11–22.
77. Sargent I, Swales A, Ledee N, Kozma N, Tabiasco J. Le Bouteiller P. sHLA-G production by human IVF embryos: can it be measured reliably? J Reprod Immunol 2007; 75: 128–32.
78. O'Neill C. The role of paf in embryo physiology. Hum Reprod Update 2005; 11: 215–28.

79. Sakkas D, Lu C, Zulfikaroglu E, Neuber E, Taylor HS. A soluble molecule secreted by human blastocysts modulates regulation of H0XA10 expression in an epithelial endometrial cell line. Fertil Steril 2003; 80: 1169–74.
80. Stamatkin CW, Roussev RG, Stout M, et al. PreImplantation Factor (PIF) correlates with early mammalian embryo development-bovine and murine models. Reprod Biol Endocrinol 2011; 9: 63.
81. Katz-Jaffe MG, Gardner DK, Schoolcraft WB. Proteomic analysis of individual human embryos to identify novel biomarkers of development and viability. Fertil Steril 2006; 85: 101–7.
82. Katz-Jaffe MG, McReynolds S, Gardner DK, Schoolcraft WB. The role of proteomics in defining the human embryonic secretome. Mol Hum Reprod 2009; 15: 271–7.
83. Nicholson JK, Connelly J, Lindon JC, Holmes E. Metabonomics: a platform for studying drug toxicity and gene function. Nat Rev Drug Discov 2002; 1: 153–61.
84. Ellis DI, Goodacre R. Metabolic fingerprinting in disease diagnosis: biomedical applications of infrared and Raman spectroscopy. Analyst 2006; 131: 875–85.
85. Seli E, Sakkas D, Scott R, et al. Non-invasive metabolomic profiling of embryo culture media using Raman and near infrared spectroscopy correlates with reproductive potential of embryos in women undergoing in vitro fertilization. Fertil Steril 2007; 88: 1350–7.
86. Seli E, Vergouw CG, Morita H, et al. Noninvasive metabolomic profiling as an adjunct to morphology for noninvasive embryo assessment in women undergoing single embryo transfer. Fertil Steril 2010; 94: 535–42.
87. Vergouw CG, Botros LL, Roos P, et al. Metabolomic profiling by near-infrared spectroscopy as a tool to assess embryo viability: a novel, non-invasive method for embryo selection. Hum Reprod 2008; 23: 1499–504.
88. Katz-Jaffe MG, Schoolcraft WB, Gardner DK. Analysis of protein expression (secretome) by human and mouse preimplantation embryos. Fertil Steril 2006; 86: 678–85.
89. Scott R, Seli E, Miller K, et al. Noninvasive metabolomic profiling of human embryo culture media using Raman spectroscopy predicts embryonic reproductive potential: a prospective blinded pilot study. Fertil Steril 2008; 90: 77–83.
90. Seli E, Bruce C, Botros L, et al. Receiver operating characteristic (ROC) analysis of day 5 morphology grading and metabolomic Viability Score on predicting implantation outcome. J Assist Reprod Genet 2011; 28: 137–44.
91. Ahlstrom A, Wikland M, Rogberg L, et al. Cross-validation and predictive value of near-infrared spectroscopy algorithms for day-5 blastocyst transfer. Reprod Biomed Online 2011; 22: 477–84.
92. Hardarson T, Ahlstrom A, Rogberg L, et al. Non-invasive metabolomic profiling of Day 2 and 5 embryo culture media: a prospective randomized trial. Hum Reprod 2012; 27: 89–96.
93. Blake DA, Farquhar CM, Johnson N, Proctor M. Cleavage stage versus blastocyst stage embryo transfer in assisted conception. Cochrane Database Syst Rev 2007; 4: CD002118.
94. Mastenbroek S, Twisk M, van Echten-Arends J, et al. In vitro fertilization with preimplantation genetic screening. N Engl J Med 2007; 357: 9–17.
95. Wells D, Alfarawati S, Fragouli E. Use of comprehensive chromosomal screening for embryo assessment: microarrays and CGH. Mol Hum Reprod 2008; 14: 703–10.
96. Vergouw CG. Metabolomic profiling of culture media by NIR spectroscopy as an adjunct to morphologyfor selection of a single Day 3 embryo to transfer: a double blind randomised trial; Human Reprod (in press).
97. Economou K, Davies S, Argyrou M, et al. Selection of embryos with the best reproductive potential according to their metabolomics profile using near infrared spectroscopy: a prospective randomized study. Hum. Reprod 2011; 26(Suppl 1): 679–90.
98. Sfontouris I, Lainas G, Sakkas D, et al. Assessment of embryo selection using non-invasive metabolomic analysis as an adjunct to morphology indicates improvement in implantation with fetal cardiac activity rates. Hum.Reprod 2011; 26(Suppl 1): i86.

19

Evaluation of embryo quality: Time-lapse imaging to assess embryo morphokinesis

Natalia Basile, Juan García-Velasco, and Marcos Meseguer

INTRODUCTION

In the past 20 years, advances in assisted reproduction have resulted in over a million babies born worldwide. Pregnancy rates have doubled, while at the same time we have managed to reduce the number of embryos transferred, reflecting major advances in laboratory procedures. From a clinical point of view two major achievements are worth mentioning: first, physicians have learned to handle the stimulation drugs, more pure, more powerful, and more comfortable to the patient; second, an increased knowledge of the pathophysiology of ovarian hyperstimulation syndrome has made the frequency of this syndrome almost anecdotal. On the other hand, concerns about the "epidemic" of multiple gestations have raised awareness of the risks associated not only to the mother (gestational diabetes, hypertension, and anemia) but also for the babies: extreme prematurity, low birth weight, children with neurological damage, etc., not to mention the psychological burden and suffering for the parents and the tremendous health costs that it entails.

In some countries legislation has supported the transfer of a single embryo in cases of good prognosis. In other countries, the law establishes an upper limit, leaving it up to the physician's discretion the number of embryos to transfer. Consequently there is an urgent demand to develop more accurate methods to choose the one embryo with the highest implantation potential for transfer. Improvements in the media and culture conditions (clean air, heated surfaces, triple gas incubators, etc.) are reflected in the good quality of the embryos grown in the laboratory. But much more remains to be done with respect to the selection procedure.

Information obtained from microscopic observations have contributed significantly to the great success of in vitro fertilization (IVF); however, it is becoming more challenging to identify embryos with the highest implantation potential due to the static and notoriously subjective character of this type of morphological evaluation. In order to choose the best embryo for transfer, noninvasive embryo quality markers are being sought to improve IVF success (chap. 18 by Sakkas and Gardner).

The study of embryo kinetics through time-lapse technology has given rise to new markers for embryo selection and represents a new and exciting powerful tool for viewing cellular activity and embryogenesis in a coherent, uninterrupted manner, otherwise not available through the standard methods of embryo evaluation.

TIME-LAPSE IMAGING: APPLICATIONS IN EMBRYOLOGY

The study of cell movement has been considered a fundamental step in understanding the dynamic nature of the cells. In the past 25 years, cell biology has benefited from the achievements in image analysis technology. During the 1980s, the use of analog videos greatly expanded the use of the microscope as an analytical tool (1,2) and most recently, analog systems have been replaced by digital ones (3,4). As previously mentioned most of the methods used to evaluate embryo viability are subjective and based on morphological observations. Classification systems based solely on qualitative criteria can be a major cause of "inter-observer" and "intra-observer" variations. Such variations could alter the expected quality of the embryos transferred as well as the number transferred, as both of which can directly impact the success of the IVF program (5). Evaluations based on image analysis systems add objectivity to the process of embryo selection. However, the automatic recognition of embryonic traits can be problematic depending on the quality of the image, the morphological differences depending on the developmental stage, the volume of the analyzed data, and the position and transparency of the embryo. Thanks to the development of bioinformatics, new programs that allow the automatic analysis of the images obtained under the microscope have been created. These programs also allow the quantitative assessment of key aspects of embryo development and morphology and the storage of the data related to these determinations. These data can then be used to improve our knowledge on early embryonic development and lead to morphological classification systems that are more objective and potentially more sophisticated.

In contrast to the daily evaluations routinely performed in the IVF laboratory, image analysis systems offer a series of benefits that include not only the precise determinations of cell divisions but a closer monitoring of morphological events such as the formation and reabsorption of fragments, (6–8) the initiation of compaction, and the appearance of the blastocele cavity. It prevents incorrect interpretations of certain phenomena such as confusing a large fragment with a cell at any given time, missing multinucleation, and categorizing a zygote as a two pronucleate (2PN) when a third pronucleate had been present at some point in time. It is typical in embryology to study the level of fragmentation, whose appearance is common in early embryonic development. The estimation of the percentage and size of fragments during early stages of embryo development forms part of many schemes of embryo classification. It has been proposed that specific patterns of fragment distribution, in space and time, are more closely related to the embryo competence than the fragmentation itself (9). In IVF cycles it is difficult to distinguish between acute or progressive fragmentation considering that the embryos are assessed only once a day. This highlights the importance of time-lapse technology, especially taking into consideration the results of different studies that provide new insights about the morphodynamics of fragmentation and show that this phenomenon is not stationary (6–8,10).

Time-lapse technology has been used for decades, especially in the research area (11–13) but technical and financial complications have hindered its implementation. Three possible solutions are offered nowadays:

1. To build an incubator around a commercially available microscope (7,14) (Stage-top Incubator, Tokai-hit, Japan)
2. To insert a microscope inside a commercially available incubator (6,15,16) (Primo Vision®, Cryo Innovations Ltd., Budapest, Hungary; EmbryoGuard®, IMT Ltd., Israel)
3. To have all the items integrated in a single equipment (17,18) (EmbryoScope™, Unisense Fertilitech, Denmark; Live-Cell incubator, Sanyo, Japan; BioStation®, Nikon, Japan)

However, the automatic analysis of embryo images represents several challenges for the scientific community. First, most of the morphological features analyzed are not perceived correctly the first time and adjustments, usually related to the focus of the microscope, are needed; we must remember that an embryo is three dimensional and that some structures that are clearly visible on one plane can disappear in the next one. Therefore, an image analysis system should include the possibility of taking images from different planes of the embryo in order to be reliable.

Although published studies describe some progress in the use of image analysis technology on embryo development, (19–21) the overall quantity of available material is scarce, even though there is increasing data supporting that a sequential embryo assessment method, derived from multiple independent evaluations, is the best guide for assessing the potential of an embryo (22). The new generation of systems that combine microscope and incubator offers the possibility to describe morphological characteristics without removing the embryos from the optimal conditions of gas and temperature and thus reducing the environmental stress experienced by the embryo.

The use of image analysis technology saves time to the embryologist and offers the availability of a 24-hour continuous observation. Furthermore, it has the potential to improve the effectiveness of IVF cycles, reducing costs and increasing the ability to identify embryos with higher viability. Progress in this scientific field can become very important when implementing a policy of single embryo transfer considering that it offers the embryologist a system for decision making that is more powerful and that it is based not only on the real-time status of the embryo but in a more authentic and dynamic view of the entire process of the embryonic development. The study of development of preimplantation embryos by time-lapse technology can reveal the importance of certain factors that have some predictive value of embryo competence, such as the kinetics of development and the intracellular dynamics.

KINETICS OF DEVELOPMENT AND INTRACELLULAR DYNAMICS

The selection of embryos on the day of transfer is based on morphological criteria strongly established in the daily work of an IVF laboratory. However, the study of cellular activity during the early stages of embryonic development provides additional information that can later be used in the selection process. We know that the time between fertilization and the first cleavage is an objective parameter that can easily be determined with certain predictive value of embryo viability (23,24). Although the correlation between the number of cells and the embryo's developmental stage has been widely described, the assessment of early cleavage and its importance in embryo selection procedures is relatively recent.

The mechanisms underlying the link between the first division and the future embryo development have not been described but several explanations have been proposed:

- The transition from one fertilized egg to a two-cell embryo depends on a highly regulated sequence of cellular processes that start with transient increases in intracellular calcium concentrations induced by the sperm's entry (25).
- Fidelity in DNA replication: the duration of the first S phase of the cell cycle appears to influence the formation of the blastocyst; a long S phase combined with a short G1 phase in the case of bovine embryos (26) or a short G2 phase in mouse embryos (27) improves the rates of blastocyst development. It is reasonable to think that zygotes with a shortened S phase are predisposed to an incomplete replication and/or aberrant

DNA, which is not compatible with a normal development to the blastocyst stage and may impose a delay in G2 and M phases by activating a control point of the cell cycle at the level of DNA replication.
- Oocyte maturation: in relation to the capacity acquired by the oocyte to respond to calcium stimulus following sperm's entry. Transient increases in calcium are essential for cortical granule release, completion of meiosis, and pronuclear formation, (28) thus oocyte maturation is considered an important factor in determining the time of first cleavage (29).
- Inherent characteristics of gametes: the presence of mouse Ped gene (30) as well as human leukocyte antigen-F (HLA-F) (31) and HLA-G (32) in humans.

Human Models

Current knowledge related to the first cell cycle in human zygotes is based on observations made both in IVF and intracytoplasmic sperm injection (ICSI) cycles. Following the sperm's entry, oocyte metabolism intensifies, the second meiotic division is completed, and the second polar body (CP) is extruded, which marks the beginning of the G1 phase of the first cell cycle. (33) Despite the observed variations in the duration and characteristics of the first cell cycle, we can draw the following general conclusions (34–36):

1. G1 phase begins with the appearance of the second polar body and the completion of the second meiotic division. Pronuclei appear which are visible under light microscope after seven to eight hours postinsemination/injection (hpi). Most of the zygotes enter G1 about 3 hpi and complete G1 around 14 hpi, especially the zygotes derived from ICSI.
2. DNA synthesis (S phase) is initiated at 8–14 hpi and completed at 14–24 hpi.
3. Early zygotes enter the G2 phase around 12 hpi and late zygotes around 30–31 hpi. G2 phase takes five to six hours approximately.
4. The duration of M phase is relatively constant (3 hours) and takes place between the disappearance of the pronuclei and the first division of the zygote. Most of the zygotes enter M phase between 24 and 30 hpi and complete their first cell cycle between 27 and 33 hpi.

The phenomenon of early cleavage and its impact on pregnancy rates was first studied by Edwards (37). Subsequently numerous studies have been published in which the common idea is that the transfer of embryos with early cleavage improves pregnancy and implantation rates. Shoukir (23) was the first to demonstrate that the transfer of embryos that had completed their first division by 25 hpi after conventional IVF, significantly improved pregnancy and implantation rates compared with those embryos that had not yet divided. Later Sakkas (24) obtained the same results but with embryos derived from ICSI cycles where fertilization times are more defined. A noteworthy aspect is that in Shoukair's study, the percentage of early cleavage embryos is lower than that in the study by Sakkas. Still, both studies demonstrate the utility of the "early cleavage" as an indicator of embryo viability as predictor of pregnancy. The fact that early embryos have a higher percentage of viability, despite the insemination method utilized, rules out the effect of the time of fertilization but supports the possible involvement of intrinsic factors from the oocyte/embryo in the manifestation of this phenomenon.

Most early cleavage studies compared cycles where at least one early-cleavage embryo was transferred with data from cycles where no early-cleavage embryos were transferred (23,24,38,39) which makes it rather difficult to know which embryo has implanted. To solve this issue, some research groups have focused on homogeneous transfers where all the embryos transferred fall in a single category; (40–45) these studies clearly demonstrate an increase in pregnancy and implantation rates for early cleavage embryos. It is worth mentioning the studies by Van Montfoort (42) and Salumets (44) where single embryo transfers were performed representing a good opportunity to examine the effect of early cleavage on embryo viability and implantation potential.

Based on the association between early cleavage and pregnancy and implantation rates a correlation between early cleavage and blastocyst developmental potential has been observed. Fenwick (46) has demonstrated that early cleavage embryos have better blastocyst formation rates but wonders whether this is really a function of the time of the first cleavage or it is a reflection of an increased competence of the embryo cohort. Therefore, we can assume that the study of the kinetics of development helps to discriminate between embryos of similar characteristics enhancing the differences between them. However, due to the characteristics of the current culture systems, the monitoring of the embryo development has to be intermittent and we can end up losing accuracy in the results related to embryo divisions. Embryo observation linked to arbitrary times can be quite misleading when categorizing the cell stage and timing of development (47). With the introduction of time-lapse and digital image analysis, we can not only get a full picture of the embryo development but also determine with precision the time of each cleavage and the time of any intracellular phenomenon surrounding fertilization.

TIME-LAPSE STUDIES

The first experiments in which time-lapse technology was introduced to study the kinetics of human embryonic development were aimed at validating the clinical utility of the system as an incubator (10,48–51).

Initial studies by Meseguer et al. (unpublished) compare biochemical pregnancy rates (BPRs) and clinical pregnancy rates (CPRs) between cycles incubated in the EmbryoScope (Unisense Fertilitech, Denmark) (ESD) and in a standard incubator (SI) in a retrospective match

Table 19.1 Variables Compared Between Patients Whose Embryos Were Cultured in the ESD or SI

Analyzed variables	SI	ESD	P value	Statistic test
N	279	77		
Mean Age	34.5 ± 3.6	34.2 ± 3.7	0.5	Student's t-test
Mean no. of oocytes retrieved	11.1	11.7	0.17	Mann–Whitney U-test
No. of transfers: 1 embryo	65 (23%)	20 (26%)	0.65	Fisher
No. of transfers: 2 embryos	197 (71%)	53 (69%)	0.78	Fisher
No. of transfers: 3 embryos	17 (6%)	4 (5%)	1	Fisher
Abortion (%)	33 (12%)	11 (14%)	0.56	Fisher
Mean FSH dose (pg/mL)	1777	1713	0.30	Mann–Whitney U-test
Mean LH dose (pg/mL)	161	108	0.19	Mann–Whitney U-test
Mean high-quality embryos	3.57	3.9	0.15	Student's t-test

Abbreviations: ESD, EmbryoScope (Unisense Fertilitech); FSH, follicle-stimulating hormone; LH, luteinizing hormone; SI, standard incubator.

Table 19.2 Results for ICSI Cycles Between ESD and SI

Analyzed variable	SI	ESD	P value	Statistic test
BPR	165 (59%)	49 (64%)	0.51	Fisher
CPR	138 (49%)	42 (55%)	0.44	Fisher

Abbreviations: BPR, Biochemical pregnancy rate; CPR, clinical pregnancy rate; ESD, EmbryoScope (Unisense Fertilitech); ICSI, intracytoplasmic sperm injection; SI, standard incubator.

cohort study. Table 19.1 shows the details of this comparative study.

No significant differences were observed for any of the variables studied between the two groups considered (P > 0.05). This demonstrates the homogeneity of both groups and allows us to make a reliable comparison of the BPRs and CPRs obtained with both types of incubators as observed in Table 19.2.

The table shows that the BPR for ESD was 64% and for SI 59%, with a P-value of 0.51. With respect to the CPR, a 55% was obtained for ESD and 49% for SI, with a P-value of 0.44. No significant differences are observed for ICSI cycles performed in both incubators. However, it is observed in the Figure 19.1 that both the BPR and the CPR values are slightly higher in ESD than in the SI (not significant).

Continuing to validate time-lapse technology for clinical use Cruz et al. (17) compared the blastocyst formation rate and the percentage of useful embryos (transferred + frozen) in a prospective study in which oocytes from the same patient were randomly split between an SI and the ESD (Unisense-Fertilitech, Denmark) after ICSI. No significant differences were observed for any of the variables studied (ESD vs. SI) Table 19.3.

According to the guidelines of the Spanish Association of Reproductive Biology (ASEBIR) (52) embryos are classified from A to D depending on their quality. In the same study by Cruz et al. (17) embryo quality was also analyzed and no differences were observed inside and outside of the EmbryoScope (Fig. 19.2).

Once the time-lapse technology is validated as an incubation system, further studies were aimed at determining specific time for kinetics parameters such as the first and second cleavage and for events related to intracellular dynamics including the extrusion of the second polar body, the appearance/disappearance of the pronuclei and the apposition and syngamy of the pronuclei. Table 19.4 shows the average times in hours for every cell division between two and eight cells and the average time for the appearance of morula and blastocysts in over a thousand embryos analyzed.

TIME-LAPSE IMAGING AS A SELECTION TOOL

Correlation Between Embryo Implantation and Variables Measured by Time-Lapse Analysis

The analysis of videos generated from 159 human embryos incubated with a time-lapse system allowed us to determine the time ranges for certain embryonic events as presented in (Table 19.5).

Of the 159 embryos included in this experiment 35 were implanted (group 1) and 124 were not implanted (group 2). For both groups the time of appearance and disappearance of the PN and the timing of the first (2 cells), second (3 cells), and third (4 cells) embryo cleavage were studied. The following figures represent the time distribution for each embryonic event according to implantation (0% vs. 100%):

- PN appearance (Fig. 19.3).
- Disappearance of pronuclei (Fig. 19.4).

The time distribution appears to be similar for PN appearance in both groups (between 5 and 17 hours after ICSI). However, group 2 includes two embryos with PN appearing too late (more than 24 hours). As observed in

Table 19.3 Blastocyst Rate and Proportion of Transferred and Frozen Embryos Incubated in the Embryoscope

	Blastocyst	CI 95%	Frozen	CI 95%	Transferred	CI 95%
ESD (n = 238)	54.8 (n = 130)	47.5–62.1	7.6 (n = 18)	2.8–12.4	21.0 (n = 50)	15.9–26.9
SI (n = 240)	50.6 (n = 121)	44.3–56.9	10.9 (n = 26)	7–14.8	24.1 (n = 58)	18.7–29.5
P value	Not significant (NS)		NS		NS	

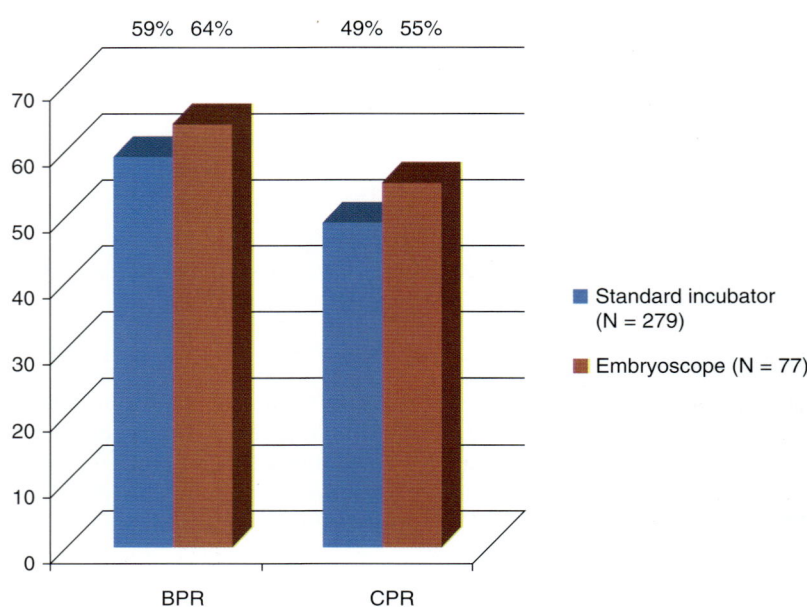

Figure 19.1 Biochemical pregnancy rate (BPR) and clinical pregnancy rate (CPR) obtained for both incubators.

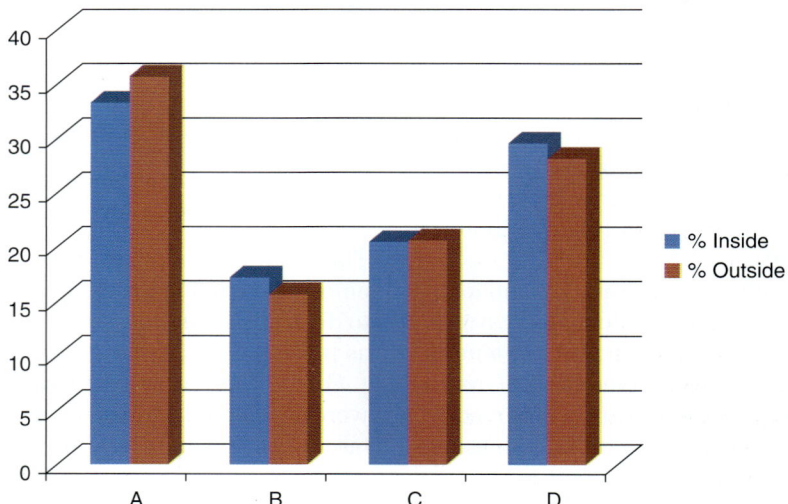

Figure 19.2 The embryo quality inside and outside of the EmbryoScope.

Figure 19.3, the majority of the implanted embryos had formed PN at 15 hours after ICSI, although in an isolated case, this time was extended to 20 hours. These results are in agreement with the 2008 guidelines by ASEBIR to observe the PN between 16 and 19 hours post insemination since PN disappearance starts at 20 hours. Furthermore, these results would also agree with those by Fancsovits et al. (53) who proposed early PN disappearance (between 22 and 25 hours) as a good indicator of embryo viability. Figure 19.4 shows that a large number of implanted embryos had their PN disappeared in this time range and that it could even be extended from 20 to 25 hours post microinjection. Moreover, Figure 19.4 shows (marked with red circle) that if the PN disappears too late (between 28 and 35 hours after ICSI) embryos do not implant.

Table 19.4 Precise Definition of Exact Imings (n = 1340)

Variable	Media	CI 95%		Minimum	Maximum
		Lower limit	Upper limit		
t2	26.10	25.47	26.73	20.40	35.56
t3	36.27	35.35	37.19	24.08	44.45
t4	38.02	37.05	38.99	24.74	48.23
t5	48.95	47.56	50.33	35.64	64.44
t6	52.05	50.78	53.32	39.55	66.41
t7	54.39	53.01	55.77	39.55	69.75
t8	58.41	56.82	60.01	39.55	73.08
Morula	85.61	84.80	86.42	70.22	99.65
Blastocyst	97.68	96.65	98.71	79.94	115.65

Table 19.5 Time Ranges for PN Appearance and Disappearance, 1st, 2nd, and 3rd Cleavage of Human Embryos

Variable	Time range (hr)		Mean (hr)
	Minimum	Maximum	
Pronucleate (PN) appearance	5.8	29.4	9.9
PN disappearance	17.7	37.5	23.7
First cleavage	19.9	40.5	26.7
Second cleavage	23.2	64.7	37.8
Third cleavage	25.34	63.87	39.3

- First embryonic division (Figs. 19.5 and 19.6).
  Embryos that initiated the first cleavage too late (>32 hours) failed to implant except for one embryo that divided for the first time at 37 hours but nevertheless presented normal kinetics on day 2 and day 3.
- Second and third embryonic division (Fig. 19.7).

Embryos that initiated the second cleavage too early or too late (>41 hours or <27 hours) failed to implant. Similar results were observed for the third cleavage (>43 hours or <29 hours). We should note that the second embryo cleavage is a synchronous event that involves two cells dividing at the same time. However, asynchrony is observed in numerous occasions allowing us to distinguish between a three-cell and a four-cell embryo. This asynchrony may take from a few minutes to hours and later on we will see that calculating this time may serve as a marker to select embryos with higher implantation rates.

In summary these results allow us to present the following profile for implanting embryos:

1. Embryos in which the appearance of PN occurs early (between 5 and 17 hours post ICSI), the disappearance of PN will also occur early (between 20 and 25 hours post ICSI).
2. The first cleavage (2 cells) should occur before 32 hours and the second and third cleavage (3–4 cells) before 43 hours post microinjection.

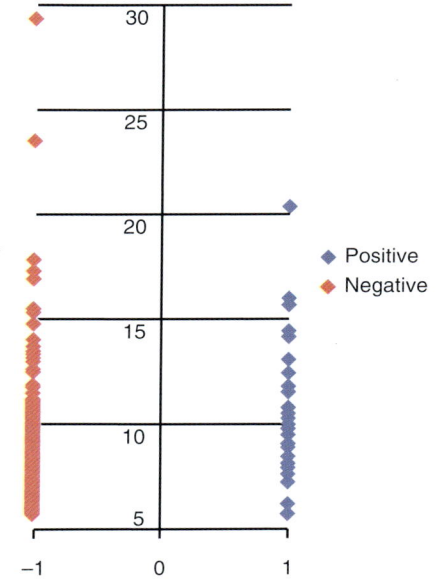

Figure 19.3 Time distribution for PN appearance in human embryos. The vertical axis indicates the time (in hours). Red = 0% implantation (no embryo implanted); blue = 100% implantation (all embryos implanted).

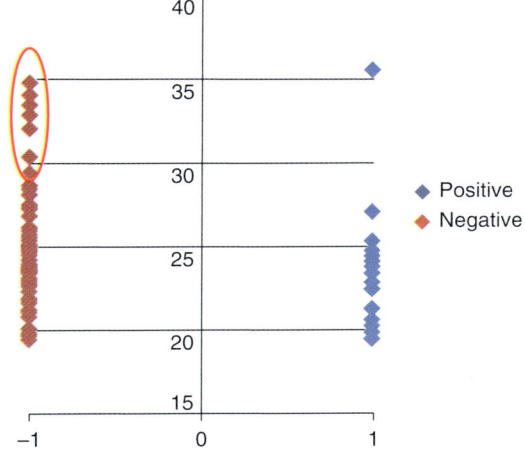

Figure 19.4 Time distribution for PN disappearance in human embryos. The vertical axis indicates the time (in hours). Red = 0% implantation (no embryo implanted); blue = 100% implantation (all embryos implanted).

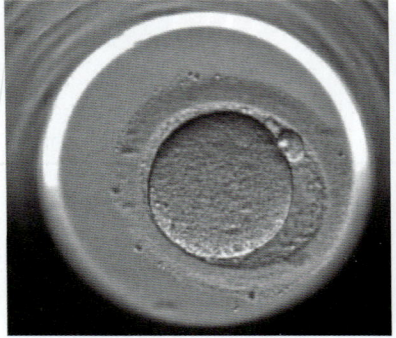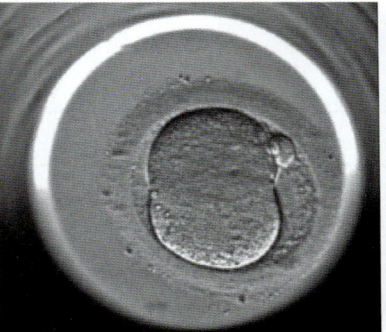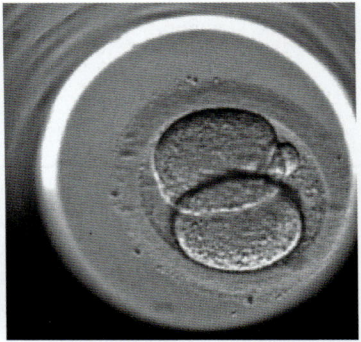

Figure 19.5 The first embryonic division. A single-cell zygote divides into two daughter cells.

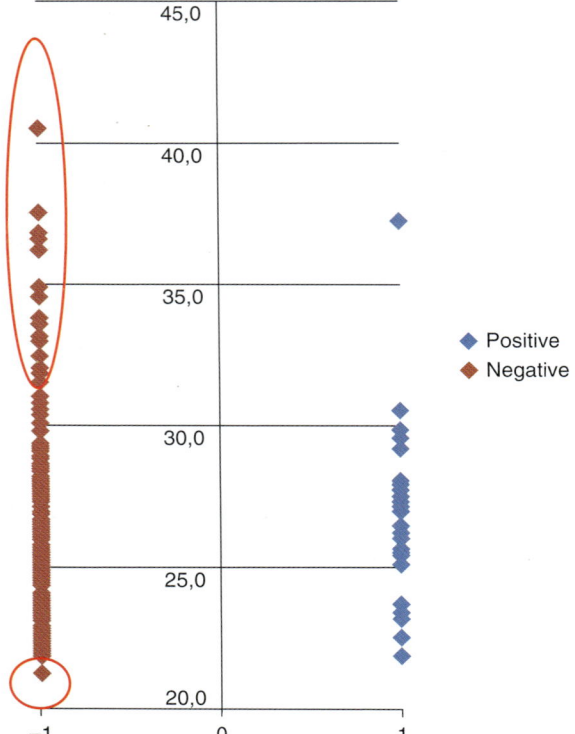

Figure 19.6 Time distribution for the first cleavage in human embryos. The vertical axis indicates the time (in hours). Red = 0% implantation (no embryo implanted); blue = 100% implantation (all embryos implanted).

Mean averages for each embryo events were analyzed. Table 19.5 presents the mean time for onset and disappearance of the PN and for the first, second, and third embryo cleavages (hours after ICSI) according to implantation (0% vs. 100%) (Table 19.6).

Establishing Kinetic Markers

Based on the previous observations through time lapse in human embryos we continued analyzing kinetic variables in order to establish new markers for embryo selection. When comparing mean values for each event (Table 19.5) significant differences (P-value <0.05, Student's t-test) were observed between groups 1 and 2. More specifically, the mean values for all variables were lower for all the embryos in group 1 (100% implantation) compared with the embryos in group 2 (0% penetration).

This would suggest that implanted embryos have a higher division rate than nonimplanted ones or, in other words, nonimplanting embryos have a tendency to divide later. Considering that the mean is not an informative indicator of implantation (since the differences are very small), a better way to analyze differences between implanting and nonimplanting embryos will be to divide the initial samples in quartiles and to establish optimal ranges for each embryo event. In a recent study by Meseguer et al. (18) optimal ranges were proposed for certain variables based on the analysis of 247 transferred embryos that were cultured in a time-lapse system. The following figures describe optimal ranges for PN appearance, time to two cells (t2), three cells (t3), and 5 cells (t5) (Fig. 19.8).

As the limits for the ranges were defined as quartiles, each column represents the same number of transferred embryos with known implantation outcomes. For all cleavage times there is a significant difference in implantation rate between embryos within the optimal range as opposed to those outside the range. However, it should be noted that this difference in implantation rates increases with successive cell divisions. For t2 the difference in implantation rate is 12%, for t3 is 21%, and for t5 it reaches to 24%. The implantation of embryos with a t5 within the optimal range is 2.6 times the implantation rate for embryos outside this range. Therefore, selection based on the timing of cleavage to the five-cell stage provides the best single criteria to select embryos with improved implantation potential.

Two other variables were considered in this study. The first one, defined as the second cell cycle (cc2), represents the time from the division to a two-blastomere embryo until the time to the division to a three-blastomere embryo (cc2 = t3–t2 represents the duration of the period as two-blastomere embryo). The second one, defined as s2, represents the duration of the transition from a two-blastomere embryo to a four-blastomere embryo (s2 = t4–t3 represents the duration of the period as a three-blastomere embryo). Figure 19.9 describes the different variables included in the study.

For both, the duration of the second cell cycle (cc2) and the synchrony from two-cell stage to four-cell stage

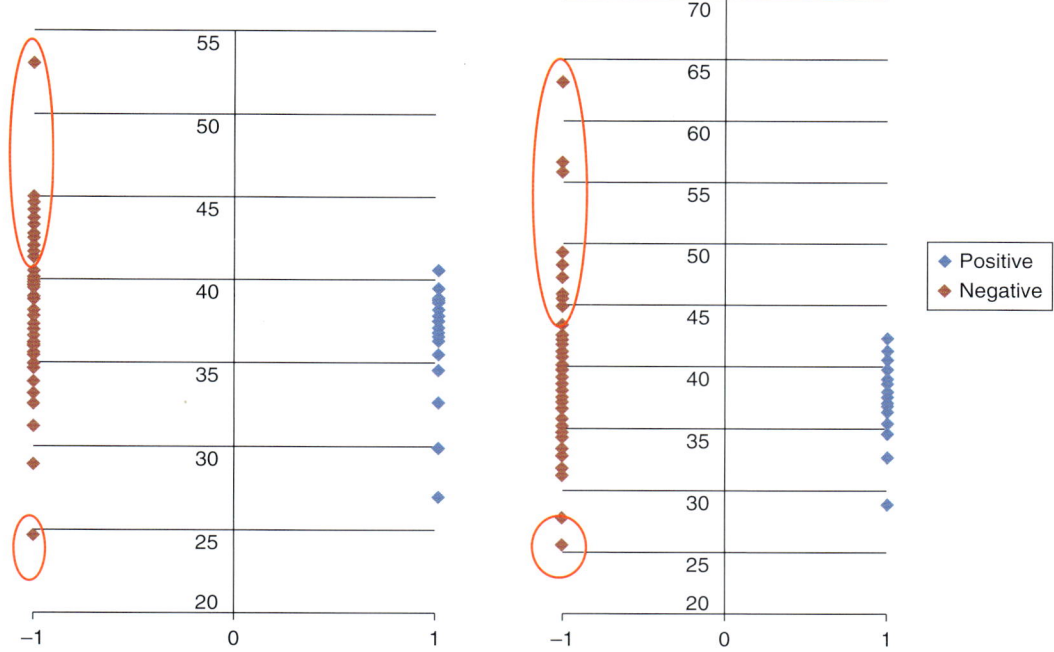

Figure 19.7 Time distribution for the second (*left*) and third (*right*) cleavage in human embryos. The vertical axis indicates the time (in hours). Red = 0% implantation (no embryo implanted); blue = 100% implantation (all embryos implanted).

Table 19.6 Mean Averages for Each Embryo Event According to Implantation (100% Vs. 0%)

Variable	Mean (hr)
PN Appearance	
Implanted	9.38
Not implanted	9.99
PN Disappearance	
Implanted	23.02
Not implanted	24.82
First Cleavage	
Implanted	25.9
Not implanted	26.6
Second Cleavage	
Implanted	37.1
Not implanted	38.27
Third Cleavage	
Implanted	37.5
Not implanted	39.8

(s2) we found that embryos falling within optimal ranges had a significantly higher implantation rate than those outside of the range (Fig. 19.10).

Another aspect worth mentioning is the possible correlation between implantation rates and certain morphological events that can only be determined through time-lapse analysis. Three different morphological events have been correlated with poor implantation potential: (18)

1. Direct cleavage from zygote to three-blastomere embryo, defined as: cc2 = t3–t2 < 5 hours.
2. Uneven blastomere size at the two-cell stage during the interphase where the nuclei are visible
3. Multinucleation at the four-cell stage during the interphase where the nuclei are visible

Given the low implantation rates (4/48 embryos studied = 8%) for embryos presenting any of these features it has been suggested using the above listed observations as exclusion criteria for embryo selection.

CONCLUSIONS

The increasing pressure to reduce the number of embryos transferred to the uterus leads to the development of new strategies aimed to optimize the predictive power of embryo viability. Studies comparing pregnancy and implantation rates depending on whether embryos are transferred at the cleavage stage and/or blastocyst stage are confusing considering that some studies promote the transfer of embryos on day 5 of culture (54–56) while others find no difference (57,58). Alternative strategies suggest embryo selection based on pronuclear morphology, (59,60) or early cleavage times (34,61,62) and much of the past research has focused on exploring the utility of these determinations as possible markers of embryo competence. Alternatively, Cummings (63) confirms the efficacy of combining a subjective score of embryo quality with the rate of development in culture to predict a possible pregnancy. Other studies have also found advantages in combining both, morphological and developmental assessment stressing the importance of selecting a critical point for maximizing the differences between embryos (23). In the search for new markers for clinical use, the relationship between the kinetics of cleavage and the subsequent blastocyst formation rate becomes a valid alternative as an early approximation

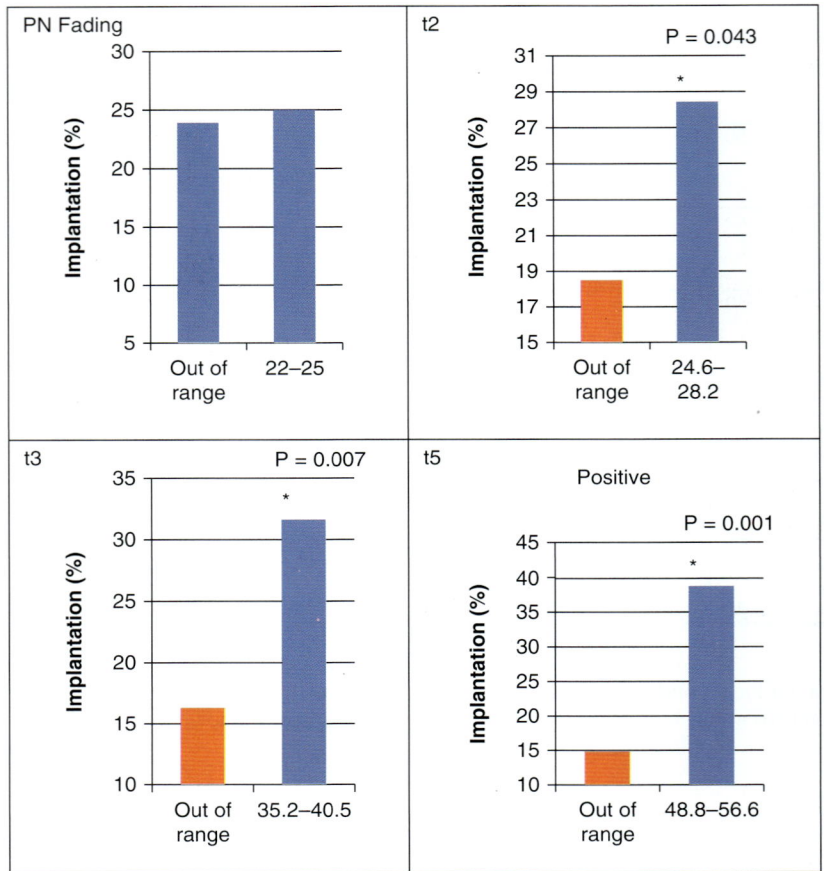

Figure 19.8 Optimal ranges for PN fading, T2, T3, and T5.

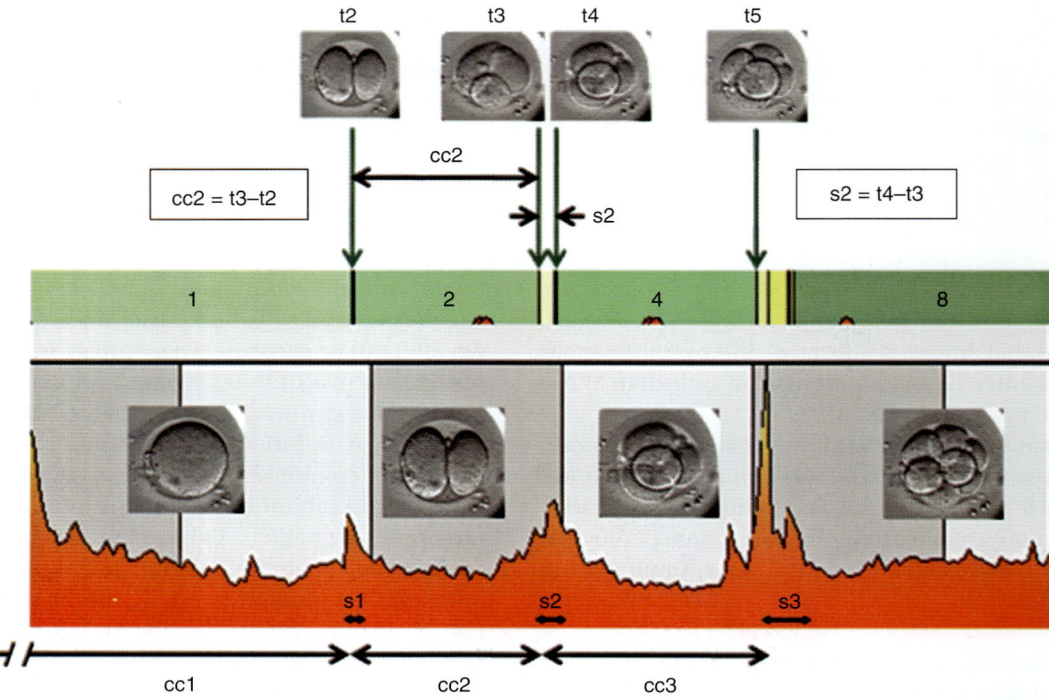

Figure 19.9 A graphic representation of the considered embryo developmental events t2, t3, t4, t5, cc2 = t3−t2 and s2 = t4−t3. Times were measured in hours post intracytoplasmic sperm injection. *Source*: Adapted from Ref. 18.

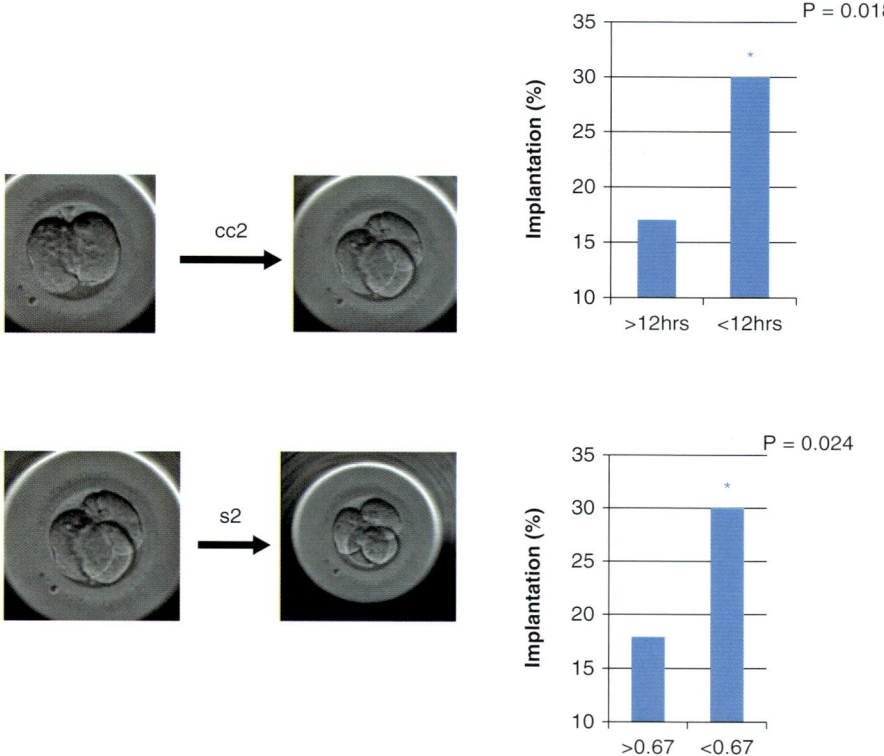

Figure 19.10 Optimal ranges for the interval limits cc2 and s2.

method for the selection of embryos with higher implantation potential. The importance of establishing the chronology in development has been previously described in the animal model which shows that the embryos that divide earlier for the first time are more likely to develop into blastocysts and have a higher percentage of viability at the time of transfer (13,64,65).

Noninvasive analysis of embryo development based on time-lapse imaging is useful not only to understand the morphological events associated with fertilization but also to evaluate the physiological importance of these events during the early stages of embryonic development. So far, most of the human embryo research on morphokinetic development has been based on the small number of samples generated under diverse experimental conditions (10,33,49,51,66). The majority of the studies that involve imaging have been limited to measurements of early development, such as pronuclear formation and fusion, and time of the first cleavage (10,35,46,67). More recent studies aimed to overcome these limitations have correlated imaging profiles and molecular data throughout development from the zygote to the blastocyst stage (66) and have proposed new specific markers for later stages of embryo development that can predict implantation. (18) Recently, the first pregnancy resulting from the selection of a single blastocyst through time-lapse analysis was reported (15). It was the first time that the development of multiple embryos was monitored and a blastocyst was selected based on division times. In summary, routine time-lapse monitoring of embryo development in a clinical setting provides novel information about developmental parameters that differ between implanting and nonimplanting embryos allowing us to identify embryos with a higher implantation potential.

REFERENCES

1. Inoué S. Video Microscopy. New York: Plenum Press, 1986.
2. Salmon ED. VE-DIC light microscopy and the discovery of kinesin. Trends Cell Biol 1995; 5: 154–8.
3. Inoué S, Spring K. Video Microscopy. 2nd edn. New York: Plenum Press, 1997.
4. Sluder G, Wolf D. Digital microscopy: a second edition of video microscopy. Methods Cell Biol 2003; 72: 1–523.
5. Bendus AEB, Mayer JF, Shipley SK, Catherino WH. Interobserver and intraobserver variation in day 3 embryo grading. Fertil Steril 2006; 86: 1608–15.
6. Pribenzsky C, Losonczi E, Molnár M, et al. Prediction of in vitro developmental competence of early cleavage-stage mouse embryos with compact time-lapse equipment. RBM Online 2010; 20: 371–9.
7. Hardarson T, Löfmann C, Coull G, et al. Internalization of cellular fragments in a human embryo: time-lapse recordings. RBM Online 2002; 5: 36–8.
8. Van Blerkom J, Davis P, Alexander S. A microscopic and biochemical study of fragmentation phenotypes in stage-appropriate human embryos. Hum Reprod 2001; 16: 719–29.
9. Alikani M, Cohen J, Tomkin G, et al. Human embryo fragmentation in vitro and its implications for pregnancy and implantation. Fertil Steril 1999; 71: 836–42.
10. Lemmen JG, Agerholm I, Ziebe S. Kinetic markers of human embryo quality using time-lapse recordings of IVF/ICSI fertilized oocytes. RBM Online 2008; 17: 385–91.

11. Cole RJ. Cinemicrographic observations on the trophoblast and zona pellucida of the mouse blastocyst. J Embryol Exp Morph 1967; 17: 481–90.
12. Massip A, Mulnard J. Time-lapse cinematographic analysis of hatching of normal and frozen-thawed cow blastocysts. J Reprod Fertil 1980; 58: 475–8.
13. Grissart B, Massip A, Dessy F. Cinematographic analysis of bovine embryo development in serum-free oviduct-conditioned medium. J Reprod Fertil 1994; 101: 257–64.
14. Holm P, Booth PJ, Callesen H. Kinetics of early in vitro development of bovine in vivo- and in vitro-derived zygotes produced and/or cultured in chemically defined or serum containing media. Reproduction 2002; 123: 553–65.
15. Pribenszky C, Mátyás S, Kovács P, et al. Pregnancy achieved by transfer of a single blastocyst selected by time-lapse monitoring. RBM Online 2010; 21: 533–6.
16. Arav A, Aroyo A, Yavin S, Roth Z. Prediction of embryonic developmental competence by time-lapse observation and "shortest-half" analysis. RBM Online 2008; 17: 669–75.
17. Cruz M, Gadea B, Garrido N, et al. Embryo quality, blastocyst and ongoing pregnancy rates in oocyte donation patients whose embryos were monitored by time-lapse imaging. J Assist Reprod Genet 2011; 28: 569–73.
18. Meseguer M, Herrero J, Tejera A. The use of morphokinetics as a predictor of embryo implantation. Hum Reprod 2011; 26: 2658–71.
19. Hnida C, Engenheiro E, Ziebe S. Computer-controlled, multilevel, morphometric analysis of blastomere size as biomarker of fragmentation and multinuclearity in human embryos. Hum Reprod 2004; 19: 288–93.
20. Angerholm I.E, Hnida C, Cruger D.G, et al. Nuclei size in relation to nuclear status and aneuploidy rate for chromosomes in donates four cells embryos. J Assist Reprod Genet 2008; 25: 95–102.
21. Beuachat A, Thevenaz P, Unser M, et al. Quantitative morphometrical characterization of human pronuclear zygotes. Hum Reprod 2008; 23: 1983–192.
22. Neuber E, Mahutte NG, Arici A, Sakkas D. Sequential embryo assessment out performs investigator-driven morphological assessment at selecting a good quality blastocyst. Fertil Steril 2006; 85: 794–6.
23. Shoukir Y, Campana A, Farley T, Sakkas D. Early cleavage of in-vitro fertilized human embryos to the 2-cell stage: a novel indicator of embryo quality and viability. Hum Reprod 1997; 12: 1531–6.
24. Sakkas D, Shoukir Y, Chardonnens D, et al. Early cleavage of human embryos to the two-cell stage after intracytoplasmic sperm injection as an indicator of embryo viability. Hum Reprod 1998; 13: 182–7.
25. Kline D, Kline JT. Repetitive calcium transients and the role of calcium exocytosis and cell cycle activation in the mouse egg. Dev Biol 1992; 149: 80–9.
26. Comizzoli P, Marquant-Le Guienne B, Heyman Y, Renard JP. Onset of the first S-phase is determined by a paternal effect during the G1-phase in the bovine zygotes. Biol Reprod 2000; 62: 1677–84.
27. Schabronath J, Gartner K. Paternal influence on timing of pronuclear DNA synthesis in naturally ovulated and fertilized mouse eggs. Biol Reprod 1988; 38: 744–9.
28. Schultz RM, Kopf GS. Molecular basis of mammalian egg activation. Curr Topics Dev Biol 1995; 30: 21–62.
29. Herbert M, Gillespie JI, Murdoch AP. Development of calcium signaling mechanisms during maturation of human oocytes. Mol Hum Reprod 1997; 3: 965–73.
30. Goldbard SB, Warner CM. Genes affect the timing of early mouse embryo development. Biol Reprod 1982; 27: 419–24.
31. Stroynowsky I. Molecules related to class-I major histocompatibility complex antigens. Annu Rev Immunol 1990; 8: 501–30.
32. Jurisicova A, Casper RF, MacLusky NJ, et al. HLA-G expression during preimplantation human embryo development. Proc Natl Acad Sci USA 1996; 93: 161–5.
33. Palermo G, Joris H, Devroey P, Van Steirteghem AC. Pregnancies after intracytoplasmic injection of single spermatozoon into an oocyte. Lancet 1992; 340: 17–18.
34. Payne D, Flaherty SP, Barry MF, Matthews CD. Preliminary observations on polar body extrusion and pronuclear formation in human oocytes using time-lapse video cinematography. Hum Reprod 1997; 12: 532–41.
35. Nagy ZP, Liu J, Joris H, et al. Time-course of oocyte activation, pronucleus formation and cleavage in human oocytes fertilized by intracytoplasmic sperm injection. Hum Reprod 1994; 9: 1743–8.
36. Plachot M. Fertilization. Hum Reprod 2000; 15(Suppl 4): 19–30.
37. Edwards RG, Fishel SB, Cohen J, et al. Factors influencing the success of in vitro fertilization for alleviating human infertility. J In Vitro Fert Embryo Trans 1984; 1: 3–23.
38. Bos-Mikich A, Mattos AL, Ferrari AN. Early cleavage of human embryos: an effective method for predicting successful IVF/ICSI outcome. Hum rerpod 2001; 16: 2658–61.
39. Neuber E, Rinaudo P, Trimarchi JR, Sakkas D. Sequential assessment of individually cultured human embryos as an indicator of subsequent good quality blastocyst development. Hum Reprod 2003; 18: 1307–12.
40. Sakkas D, Percival G, Doarcy Y, et al. Assessment of early clearing in Vitro fertilized human embryos at the 2-cell stage before transfer improves embryo selection. Fertil Steril 2001; 76: 1150–6.
41. Wharf E, Dimitrakopulos A, Khalaf Y, Pickering S. Early embryo development is an indicator of implantation potential. RBM Online 2004; 2: 212–18.
42. Van Montfoort AP, Dumoulin JC, Kester AD, Evers JL. Early cleavage is a valuable addition to existing embryo selection parameters: a study using single embryo transfers. Hum Reprod 2004; 19: 2103–8.
43. Lundin K, Bergh C, Hardarson T. Early embryo cleavage is a strong indicator of embryo quality in human IVF. Hum Reprod 2001; 16: 2652–7.
44. Salumets A, Hyden-Granskog C, Mäkinen S, et al. Early cleavage predicts the viability of human embryos in elective single embryo transfers procedures. Hum Reprod 2003; 18: 821–5.
45. Tsai YC, Chung MT, Sung YH, et al. Clinical value of early cleavage embryo. INnt. J Gynaecol Obstet 2002; 76: 293–7.
46. Fenwick J, Platteau P, Murdoch AP, Herbert M. Time from insemination to first cleavage predicts developmental competence of human preimplantation embryos in vitro. Hum Reprod 2002; 17: 407–12.
47. Bavister BD. Culture of preimplantation embryos: facts and artifacts. Hum Reprod Update 1995; 1: 91–148.

48. Mio Y. Morphological analysis of human embryonic development using time-lapse cinematography. J Mamm Ova Res 2006; 23: 27–35.
49. Mio Y, Maeda K. Time-lapse cinematography of dynamic changes occurring during in vitro development of human embryos. Am J Obstet Gynecol 2008; 199: 660.e1–660.e5.
50. Mio Y. The beginning of human life under time-lapse cinematography. Periodicum Biologorum 2009; 111: 323–7.
51. Nakahara T, Iwase A, Goto M, et al. Evaluation of the safety of time-lapse observations for human embryos. J Assit Reprod Genet 2010; 27: 93–6.
52. ASEBIR 2008. Cuadernos de embriología clínica. Criterios ASEBIR de valoración morfológica de oocitos, embriones tempranos y blastocistos humanos. 2° Ed
53. Fancsovits P, Laszlone MS, Zoltan F, et al. Early pronuclear breakdown is a good indicator of embryo quality and viability. Fertil Steril 2005; 84: 881–7.
54. Milki AA, Hinckley M, Fisch J, Dasig D, Behr B. Comparison of blastocyst transfer with day 3 embryo transfer in similar patient populations. Fertil Steril 2000; 73: 126–9.
55. Gardner DK, Schoolcraft WB, Wagley L, et al. A prospective randomized trial of blastocyst culture and transfer in in-vitro fertilization. Hum Reprod 1998; 13: 3434–40.
56. Marek D, Langley M, Gardner DK, et al. Introduction of blastocyst culture and transfer for all patients in an in vitro fertilization program. Fertil Steril 1999; 73: 1035–40.
57. Coskun S, Hollanders J, Al-Hassan S, et al. Day 5 versus day 3 embryo transfer: a controlled randomized trial. Hum Reprod 2000; 15: 1947–52.
58. Huisman GJ, Fauser BC, Eijkemans MJ, Pieters MH. Implantation rates after in vitro fertilization and transfer of a maximum of two embryos that have undergone three to five days in culture. Fertil Steril 2000; 73: 117–22.
59. Scott L, Alvero R, Leondires M, Miller B. Morphology of human pronuclear embryo is positively related to blasotcyst development. Hum Reprod 2000; 15: 2394–403.
60. Tesarik J, Greco E. The probability of abnormal preimplantation development can be predicted by a single static observation on pronuclear stage morphology. Hum Reprod 1999; 14: 1318–23.
61. Nagy ZP, Janssenswillen C, Janssesns R, et al. Timing of oocyte activation, pronucleus formation, and cleavage in humans after intracytoplasmic sperm injection (ICSI) with testicular spermatozoa and after ICSI or in-vitro fertilization on sibling oocytes with ejaculated spermatozoa. Hum Reprod 1998; 13: 1060–612.
62. Capmany G, Taylor A, Braude PR, Bolton VN. Timing of pronuclear formation, DNA synthesis and cleavage in the human 1-cell embryo. Mol Hum Reprod 1996; 2: 299–306.
63. Cummings JM, Breen TM, Harrison KL. A formula for scoring human embryo growth rates in in vitro fertilization: its values in predicting pregnancy and in comparison with visual estimates of embryo quality. J In Vitro Fert Embryo Transf 1986; 3: 284–95.
64. MacLaren A, Bowman P. Genetic effects on the timing of early development in the mouse. J Embryol Exp Morph 1973; 30: 491–8.
65. Lonergan P, Khatir H, Piumi F, et al. Effect of time interval from insemination to first cleavage on the developmental characteristics, sex ratio and pregnancy rate after transfer of bovine embryos. J Reprod Fertil 1999; 117: 159–67.
66. Wong CC, Loewke KE, Bossert NL, et al. Non-invasive imaging of human embryos before embryonic genome activation predicts development to the blastocyst stage. Nat Biotechnol 2010; 28: 1115–21.
67. Lundin K, Bergh C, Hardarson T. Early embryo cleavage is a strong indicator of embryo quality in human IVF. Hum Reprod 2001; 16: 2652–7.

20

Evaluation of embryo quality: Proteomic strategies

Mandy Katz-Jaffe

INTRODUCTION

Unlike the human genome that is relatively fixed and steady throughout the human body, the human proteome (PROTE in complement to the GENOME) is by several orders of magnitude, more complex, diverse, and dynamic. Any single gene can produce a heterogeneous population of proteins that can be further modified by post-translational modifications such as phosphorylation. The result is a human proteome estimated at considerably over a million proteins to only ~25,000 human genes (1). Several studies have indicated that the genome's transcriptome (mRNA expression levels) does not necessarily predict the abundance or functional activity of proteins (2,3). Rather, it is the human proteome that significantly contributes to physiological homeostasis in any cell or tissue (4). Various biological conditions including age, gender, diet, life style, medication, and disease, among others, directly impact the composition of the human proteome in any particular cell or tissue generating a unique proteomic signature (5). The characterization of protein signatures during embryonic development has the potential to address a variety of unresolved topics, with the ultimate goal to expand our knowledge of embryonic cellular processes and the evolution of viability assays.

Relatively little is known regarding the proteome of the human preimplantation embryo, in particular, the protein production of the blastocyst just prior to implantation. The task begins with identifying the proteins expressed, including those proteins changing in response to internal and external stimuli. These individual proteins can then be quantified and characterized, at the same time examining their interactions during embryonic development. In order to elucidate embryonic cellular architecture and function, a detailed understanding of the complexity at the protein level is essential. Of particular interest is the cell surface proteome as it may pinpoint key molecules associated with implantation, including cell surface receptors as well as the protein–protein interactions occurring between the developing embryo and the surrounding maternal environment.

Zeptoproteomics is the term that has been coined to define proteomic technology optimized to analyze protein expression in a limited number of cells (6). The preimplantation embryonic stage represents the most difficult challenge for zeptoproteomics with the combined effect of limited numbers of cells and minimal protein expression, resulting in extremely low levels of total protein available for analysis, only 27 ng of protein in a single mouse embryo (7).

THE EMBRYONIC PROTEOME

Two-dimensional polyacrylamide gel electrophoresis (2D-PAGE) is at present the standard technique for separation of total protein. This technology separates proteins in the horizontal dimension by isoelectric focusing (a pH gradient range of typically 3–10), and in the vertical dimension by molecular weight in a polyacrylamide gel gradient (8). The 2D-PAGE method is efficient at differential protein quantitation and detecting post-translational modifications with starting amounts of total protein isolated from typically 10^6 cells. Limitations to this technology include a long processing time, weak detection of low concentration proteins, and the inability to capture or resolve very acidic or basic proteins, membrane proteins, as well as very small or large molecular weight proteins (8).

Protein databases involving 2D-PAGE that represent the entire mouse preimplantation period from fertilization to the blastocyst stage have been constructed to provide a means to study protein synthesis and characterize protein changes (9,10). The 2D-PAGE was performed through the analysis of radiolabeled proteins after embryos were exposed to one- to three- hour incubation in a high concentration of radiolabeled amino acids. After protein resolution, spots were detected by fluorography and a software program assembled the images into protein databases (9). A comparison of the proteins between the eight-cell mouse embryo and the fully expanded mouse blastocyst database identified a total of 43 spots, approximately 3% of all total spots, which were only detected at the eight-cell stage and 75 spots identified solely at the blastocyst stage (10).

The 2D-PAGE technique in the field of embryology has been limited due to the requirement for larger amounts of starting template as well as the lack of robustness and degree of labor intensity. Consequently, protein-based studies have concentrated on identifying and localizing individual proteins by western blot analysis. Two insulin-responsive glucose transporter isoforms (GLUT4 and GLUT8) and the insulin receptor proteins were confirmed by western blot analysis as being present in rabbit blastocysts (11). Another study observed the expression of stress-activated protein kinase/Jun N-terminal kinase (SAPK/JNK) phospho proteins and p38 mitogen-activated protein kinases (MAPKs) by western blotting from groups of over 100 mice embryos (12). A limitation of this approach is that proteins do not function individually, but within pathways, thus the analysis of the embryonic proteome as a whole is critical.

Mass spectrometry (MS) has rapidly become the key technology in proteomics, allowing for rapid identification and quantitation of proteins including low expression proteins. An array of templates can be applied including tissues, cells, and biological fluids. MS involves an ion source for the production of charged species in the gas phase, and the analyzer, which separates ions by their mass-to-charge (m/z) ratio. The commonly used ionization methods include electrospray ionization, matrix-assisted laser desorption/ionization (MALDI), and surface-enhanced laser desorption/ionization (SELDI) and are most commonly coupled to time-of-flight (TOF), ion trap, or quadrupole analyzers. Post-translational modifications are also identifiable since the modification will change the mass-to-charge ratio of a protein. Protein identification can then be performed by protease digestion to generate specific fragments from well-characterized cleavage products. These fragments are identifiable following tandem MS analysis and protein database searching (13).

A comprehensive proteomics approach has been applied to study the mammalian oocyte; however, in these studies the starting template is still considerable. In one study, approximately 200 porcine oocytes were used to separate and visualize proteins of interest by 2D-PAGE, with an even larger starting template used for peptide profiling by MALDI TOF MS and peptide sequencing by liquid chromatography-tandem MS (14). More recently, Vitale et al. (15) used 2D-PAGE and MS to identify differentially expressed proteins during murine oocyte maturation; 500 GV and MII oocytes were extracted and resolved on 2D gels stained with silver. A total of 12 proteins were observed to be differentially expressed between the GV and MII stages. These proteins were then characterized by MS with the identification of nucleoplasmin 2 (Npm2), an oocyte-restricted protein (15). Another study investigated mature mouse cumulus–oocyte complexes identifying 156 individual proteins following 2D-PAGE and MS. Several protein families were discovered which may play important roles in ovarian follicular development (16).

With further advances in proteomic technologies, the identification and quantitation of very small quantities of proteins has become more of a reality. SELDI-TOF MS involves the application of small sample volumes (µL range) and enables detection of both the low- and higher-molecular-weight proteins with the optimal range for the technology at <20 kDa. The sensitivity is stated to be in the picomole to femtomole range, making proteomic profiling of diverse and limited biological samples possible. This technology is also capable of studying samples based on activated surfaces for preselection including hydrophobic interaction; anion or cation exchange and metal affinity capture (17). Bound proteins are laser activated thereby liberating gaseous ions by desorption/ionization. The time of flight tube is under a vacuum which causes smaller ions to travel faster toward the detector, thereby, allowing for a separation of these ions according to mass-to-charge ratio. The technology has been applied to a variety of biological sources including serum (18) and cell lysates (19), with specific focus on oncoproteomics and the early detection, metastatic ability, and therapeutic outcome of an assortment of different cancers through associated biomarkers (20). Biomarkers can be defined as candidate proteins or peptides that are either down- or upregulated in response to different physiological states. Pregnancy-related problems have also been the subject of SELDI-TOF MS studies searching for early detection of conditions including ectopic pregnancy (21) and neonatal sepsis (22). Some concerns regarding this technology involve the dynamic and sensitive nature of the proteome to variables during sample collection, handling, processing, and storage as well as peaks prejudiced by MS calibration and instrument drift (23).

The development of a zeptoproteomics approach using SELDI-TOF MS has led to the characterization of protein profiles representing individual murine and human embryos across all stages of preimplantation development (24,25). Due to the multifactorial nature of mammalian embryonic development, panels of proteins specific to each of the individual stages were successfully identified allowing for the possibility of utilizing these panels to accurately gauge the level of perturbation of a biological system and effectively diagnose developmental competence (Fig. 20.1) (24). The individual human embryonic proteome demonstrated that human blastocysts with similar morphology do not typically have identical protein signatures (25). This finding is consistent with the observations that human blastocysts from the same patient with similar morphologies vary greatly in their metabolic fingerprint (26). Furthermore, specific blastocyst developmental stages displayed differential protein expression profiles as shown by the significant up- and downregulation of biomarkers in expanded blastocysts compared with early blastocysts (25). Taken as a whole, human blastocyst morphology could be recognized according to specific individual protein signatures with significant differences in protein expression related to specific blastocyst developmental time points and/or degeneration. (Fig. 20.2) (25). A panel of upregulated biomarkers distinguished arrested embryos from developing blastocysts (Fig. 20.3). Candidate identification implicated

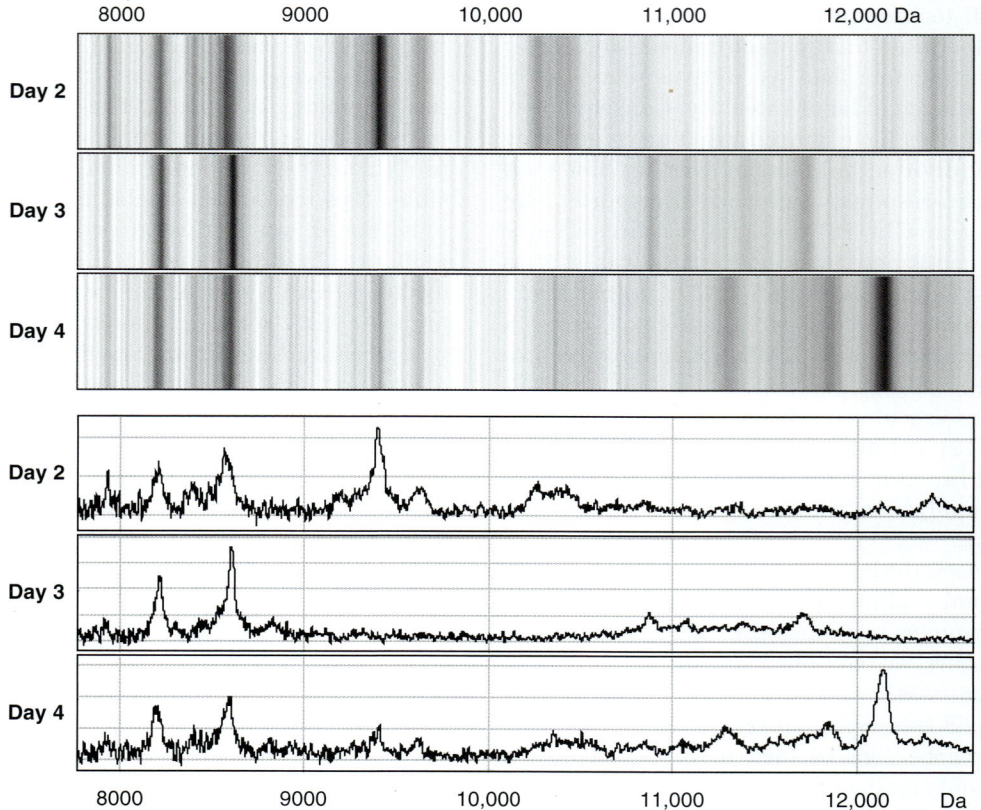

Figure 20.1 Protein profiling signatures across preimplantation embryonic development in the mass-to-charge range from 8000 to 12,000 Da. Data are shown as the original spectra and gel view 24.

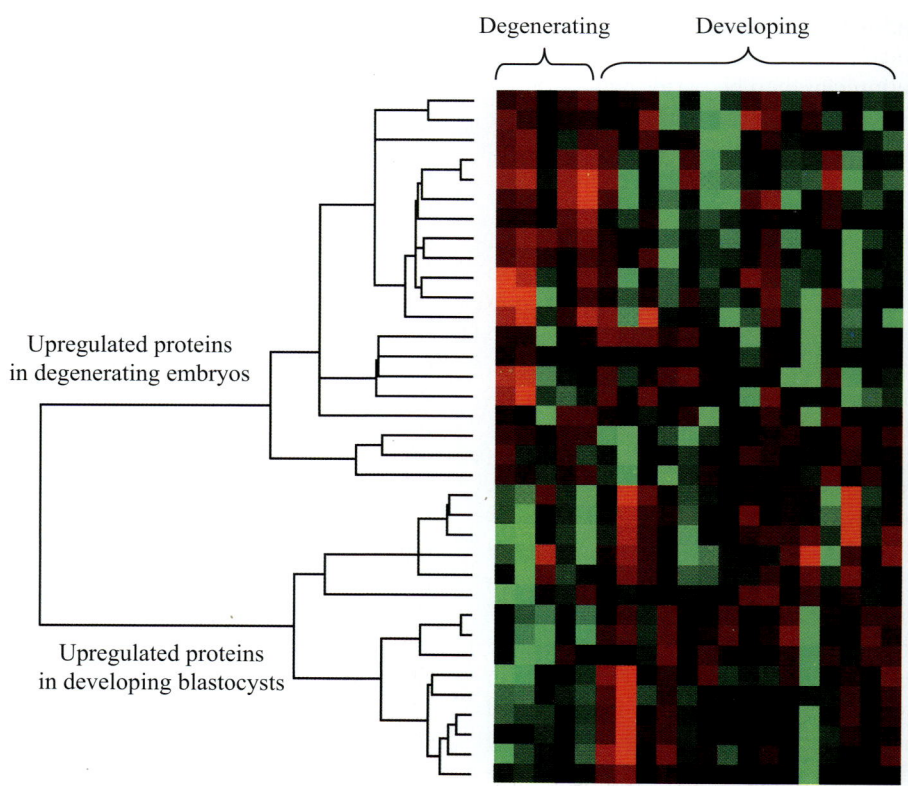

Figure 20.2 A heat map segregating developing human blastocysts and degenerate human embryos according to protein signatures. Each column of squares represents an individual human embryo, while each row of squares represents an individual protein profile. Clustering analysis facilitates the grouping of similar protein expression profiles. Two major clusters were classified as shown on the left of the heat map. The top cluster identified proteins that are upregulated (red) in degenerating embryos, while the bottom cluster identified proteins that are upregulated (red) in developing blastocysts. Red, upregulated proteins; green, downregulated proteins 25.

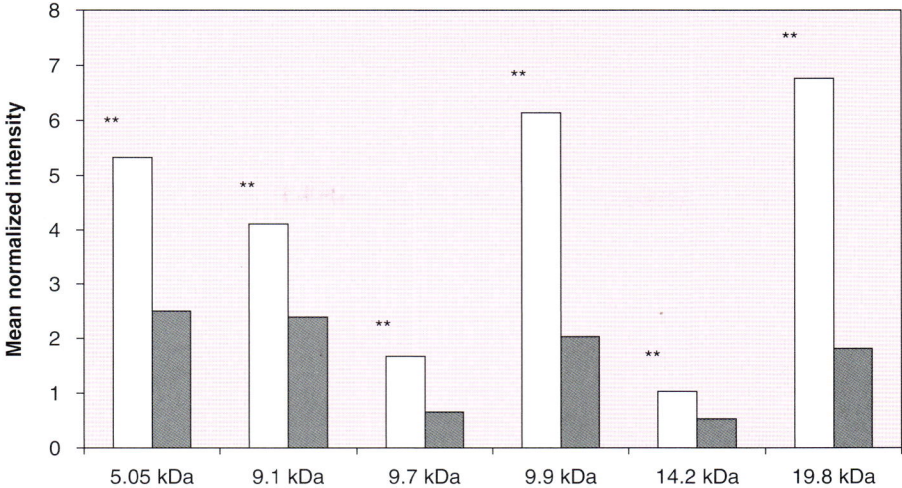

Figure 20.3 Negatively charged proteins showing significant differential expression related to blastocyst morphology. Open bars, degenerating embryos; solid bars, developing blastocysts. **Significantly different from developing blastocysts ($P < 0.01$) 25.

both apoptotic and growth inhibiting pathways (25). It is also probable that some of these differential proteins or peptides are secreted by the embryo reflecting a signature of developmental competence.

THE EMBRYONIC SECRETOME

With the knowledge that blastocyst morphology could be recognized according to specific protein expression (25), it is proposed that developmentally viable embryos will also possess a unique proteome profile with some of these expressed proteins secreted into the surrounding environment (secretome). Analysis of the embryonic proteome, as described in the previous section, represents a destructive approach. On the other hand, analysis of the embryonic secretome is a noninvasive method suitable for clinical application.

Currently, the selection of embryos for transfer is based on morphological indices (27). Though successful, the field of assisted reproductive technique would benefit from more quantitative and noninvasive methods of viability determination to run alongside morphological assessment. These quantitative methods hold the promise of improving in vitro fertilization (IVF) success rates as well as optimizing single embryo transfer (28). There have been several studies that have shown the existence of soluble factors secreted by human embryos that could impact either or both developmental competence and implantation. The initial studies of the human embryonic secretome involved targeted analysis of individual proteins and molecules. The soluble factor, 1-o-alkyl-2-acetyl-sn-glycero-3-phosphocholine (PAF), has been identified as one of the first targeted molecules. PAF was shown to be produced and secreted by mammalian embryos during preimplantation development (29). Secreted PAF could be working in an autocrine fashion as a survival factor, as well as influencing maternal physiology alterations including platelet activation and immune function (29).

Leptin, a 16 kDa, small pleiotropic peptide, was also observed to be secreted by human blastocysts during the interaction between the embryo and endometrial epithelial cells (EECs) (30). In this study, competent human blastocysts secreted higher leptin concentrations into the surrounding medium than arrested embryos. Leptin has been hypothesized to interact with leptin receptors in the maternal endometrium during the window of implantation (31).

In another study by Sakkas et al. (32) a soluble molecule secreted by human blastocysts that modulates regulation of HOXA10 expression in an epithelial endometrial cell line was identified (32). This form of reciprocal embryo–endometrial interaction could transform the local uterine environment directly impacting the implantation process. More recently, the presence of soluble human leukocyte antigen G (sHLA-G) in embryo spent culture media has been linked to successful pregnancy outcome and suggested as a noninvasive marker to predict embryo quality and implantation success, especially when used in conjunction with current morphological embryo assessment methods. These results, however, have not been absolute with pregnancies established from sHLA-G negative embryos (33,34) as well as data revealing the inability to measure sHLA-G production in some supernatants (35).

It is more than likely that the multifactorial nature of embryonic development will dictate a panel of molecules to assess developmental competence and/or implantation potential than just the single variable. The SELDI-TOF MS analysis of proteins in the secretome of mammalian embryos throughout preimplantation development highlighted distinctive protein signatures at each 24-hour developmental stage (Table 20.1) (36). These signatures uniquely identified an embryo, independent of morphology. Comparison of mouse and human secretomes across preimplantation development revealed similar patterns and little differences between species (36).

Subsequent analysis revealed protein expression only at specific 24-hour developmental time points, while

Table 20.1 Each Stage of Mammalian Embryonic Development Revealing a Panel of Significant Biomarkers That Were Detected Only in the Drops of Spent IVF Culture Media at Specific Stages of Development ($P < 0.05$) (36)

Stage of embryonic development	No. of proteins/biomarkers	Description of events
Day 1–2	~20 candidate peaks	Maternal control of early embryonic development
Day 2–3	~20 candidate peaks	Embryonic genome activated
Day 3–4	~20 candidate peaks	Embryonic proteins translated
Day 4–5	~20 candidate peaks	Initiation of blastocyst implantation

other proteins were observed through several embryonic stages, particularly occurring either before or after the activation of the embryonic genome (36). Examples are shown in Figure 20.4; the light gray boxes highlight the profile of several biomarkers only secreted during the first 24 hours from day 1 to day 2 of mouse embryonic development ($P < 0.05$). Other biomarkers were observed to be secreted at all stages of embryonic development with increasing expression toward the blastocyst stage as shown in Figure 20.4 (dark gray box; $P < 0.05$). In addition, the expression of numerous biomarkers was only observed after the activation of the embryonic genome (Fig. 20.4; black boxes). The transition from maternal inherited transcripts and proteins to the activation of the embryonic genome and the expression of key embryonic proteins must occur for continued embryonic development (37). Thus, embryos with a correctly activated embryonic genome, and hence, a fully functional embryonic proteome may have a higher potential of developmental competence.

Secretome analysis on day 5 was directly correlated with continuing blastocyst development, including the identification of differentially expressed biomarkers. The profile of an 8.5 kDa protein that was secreted every 24 hours from day 2 to day 5 of human embryonic development, with significantly increasing intensity toward the blastocyst stage, was also directly associated with ongoing development (Fig. 20.5). The near lack of expression of this 8.5 kDa protein/biomarker from degenerating embryos, in conjunction with its high expression from developing blastocysts, potentially indicates an association between this biomarker and ongoing blastocyst development (Fig. 20.5; $P < 0.05$) (36). Initial identification of this 8.5 kDa biomarker involving reverse phase chromatography, SDS-PAGE, trypsin digest, tandem MS, and database peptide sequence searching indicated that the best candidate was ubiquitin. Ubiquitin is a component of the ubiquitin-dependent proteasome system that is involved in a number of physiological processes including proliferation and apoptosis. Secreted ubiquitin has been shown to be upregulated in body fluids in certain disease states providing evidence for an increase in protein turnover (38,39). In addition, ubiquitin has been implicated to play a crucial role during mammalian implantation by directing the activities and turnover of key signaling molecules (40).

Protein microarrays have also been utilized to generate human secretome protein profiles (41). In a retrospective study, 120 antibody targets were used to compare implanted versus nonimplanted blastocyst conditioned media. Due to the requirement of at least 10 pg/mL of protein, samples were pooled following single embryo transfer following classification of pregnancy outcome. An increased expression of the soluble TNF receptor 1 and IL-10, and the decreased expression of MSP-alpha, SCF, CXCL13, TRAILR3, and MIP-1beta were observed in the conditioned media compared with control media (41). In addition, the presence of two significantly decreased proteins, CXCL13 and GM-CSF, were observed in the pooled implanted blastocyst conditioned media compared with nonimplantation. These results reflect the findings of other studies showing that GM-CSF may promote embryo development and implantation when present in both human and mice blastocyst culture media (42).

In a follow-up study conducted by the same lab the protein secretome profiles of an EEC co-culture system were compared with a sequential microdrop culture media system revealing differential protein secretome profiles (43). Several molecules were increased in the EEC co-culture profile including IL-6, PLGF, and BCL (CXCL13), while other proteins such as FGF-4, IL-12p40, VEGF, and uPAR were decreased (consumed). Interleukin-6 (IL-6) was the most secreted protein by the EEC co-culture system and in subsequent experiments using an IL-6 ELISA assay, the sequential culture media secretome of viable blastocysts displayed an increased uptake compared with nonimplanting blastocysts, suggesting a potential role for IL-6 in blastocyst development and implantation (43).

An essential requirement for healthy embryo and fetal development is the presence of all 23 pairs of human chromosomes (euploidy). Typically embryos produced from these aneuploid embryos (incorrect number of chromosomes) have little potential of forming a viable pregnancy. Indeed, over 60% of first trimester miscarriages are associated with chromosomal aneuploidy (44). To date only invasive biopsy techniques that potentially could compromise outcome, are able to screen for chromosomal aneuploidies in IVF embryos.

Using a liquid chromatography MS/MS platform, the protein secretome profile of pooled euploid blastocysts was notably different from the protein secretome profile of pooled aneuploid blastocysts (45). Nine potential candidate biomarkers characteristically classified chromosome aneuploidy with the most significant differentially expressed protein, lipocalin-1. Lipocalin-1 was shown to be increased in expression in the aneuploid protein

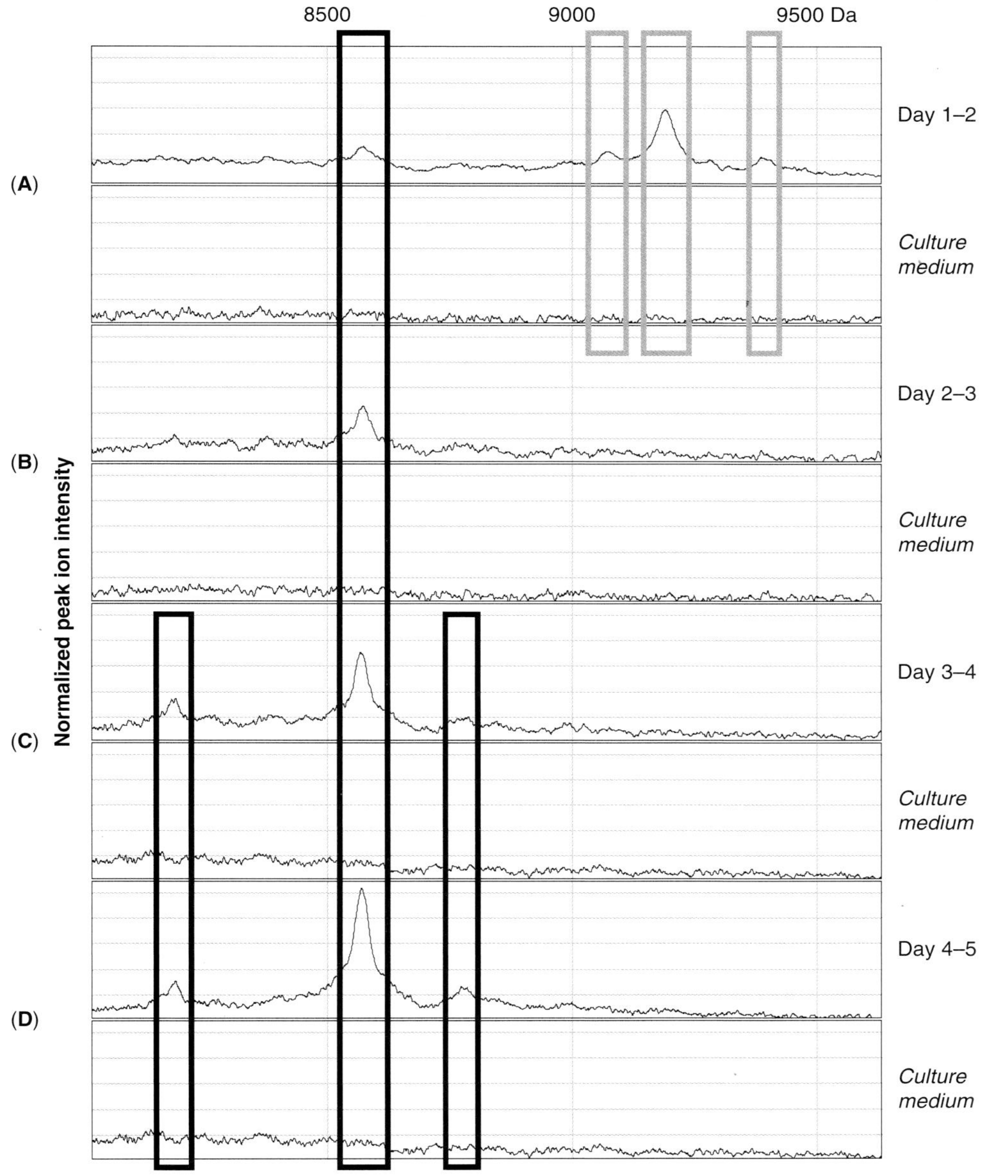

EVALUATION OF EMBRYO QUALITY: PROTEOMIC STRATEGIES   271

Figure 20.4 Protein profiles enhan-ced around the 7–10 kDa range for the secretome of each individual stage of mouse embryonic development. The bottom profiles for each 24 hours are from the control drops of media cultured under exact incubation conditions without embryos: (**A**) day 1–2; (**B**) day 2–3; (**C**) day 3–4; (**D**) day 4–5. Dark gray boxes display protein expression across all developmental stages. Light gray boxes highlight day 1–2 maternal protein expression, while black boxes indicate protein expression after the activation of the embryonic genome 36.

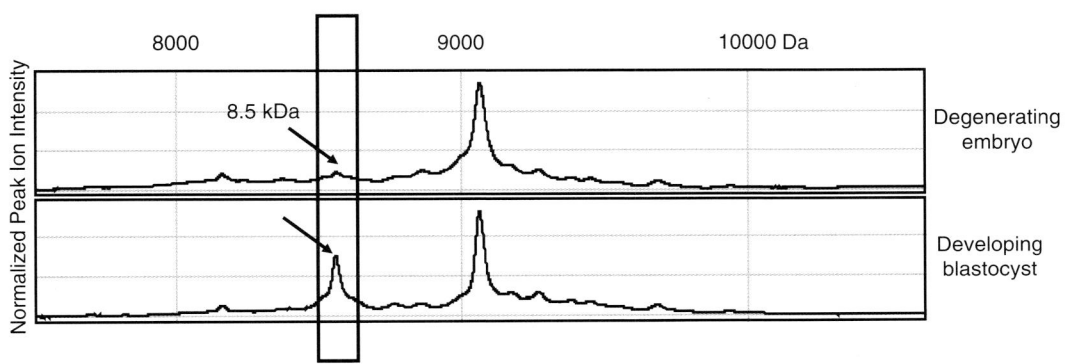

Figure 20.5 The expression of this 8.5 kDa protein/biomarker appears to be directly associated with ongoing blastocyst development. Black box highlights differences in protein expression across morphological different day 5 embryos 36.

secretome and was confirmed with individual samples with a commercially available lipocalin-1 ELISA kit (USCN Life Science, Inc. Wuhan, China) (Fig. 20.6). Further MS/MS experiments that included the analysis of the secretome from euploid blastocysts resulting in negative implantation showed the same expression profile of lipocalin-1 as spent IVF culture media from euploid blastocyst resulting in pregnancy (45). This suggests that the altered expression levels of lipocalin-1 are related to aneuploidy and not to failed implantation revealing its potential as a biomarker for noninvasive aneuploidy screening. In these experiments protein secretome analysis clearly discriminated between euploid and aneuploid blastocysts (45).

Protein identification and association of biomarkers with embryonic developmental competence, IVF outcome and chromosome constitution are ongoing. Such data will provide insight into the unique molecular events occurring during embryonic development including revealing some of the complex dialogue between the developing embryo and its maternal environment. This research could also translate into a cost-effective and reproducible assay for assessment of human embryonic viability. From a clinical perspective, noninvasive quantification of human embryonic viability incorporating chromosome screening may lead to routine single embryo transfers, a reduction in pregnancy losses and increased singleton deliveries.

PROTOCOL FOR INDIVIDUAL EMBRYONIC PROTEIN SECRETOME PROFILING

Ion Exchange Chromatography

Protein chips are washed several times with appropriate binding buffer (Bio-Rad Technologies, Hercules, CA, USA). Spent media are spotted onto protein chips and incubated in a humid chamber at room temperature for 30–60 minutes depending on the type of protein chip. Any unbound sample is then discarded and each spot washed a further three times with binding buffer and twice with MQ-H_2O for the removal of salts and detergents. Sinapinic acid, an energy absorbing molecule (Bio-Rad Technologies), prepared as a saturated solution in 50% acetonitrile/0.5% trifluoroacetic acid, is applied twice in 1 µL aliquots and allowed to air-dry prior to MS analysis.

SELDI-Time of Flight MS

Time of flight data are collected for low-molecular-weight peptides and proteins <20,000 Da at a lower laser intensity averaging 530 laser shots per spot. High-molecular-weight proteins >20,000 Da are collected using a higher laser intensity averaging 530 laser shots per spot. Spectra are generated by Express® Software, Bio-Rad Technologies. Mass accuracy is calibrated with the all-in-one peptide molecular mass standard for the mass range of <20 kDa and with the all-in-one protein molecular mass standard for the mass range of 10–300 kDa (Bio-Rad Technologies).

Statistical Analysis

Protein profiles are normalized to the total ion current and peaks with a signal-to-noise ratio higher than 6 are selected for statistical analysis. Hierarchical clustering is performed to group samples with similar protein expression profiles. Univariate statistical analysis of the peak masses and relative intensity values is performed by the Mann–Whitney nonparametric test (Express Software; Bio-Rad Technologies). To test reproducibility, one sample is analyzed in triplicate and the coefficient of variance of individual peaks in the replicate spectra is calculated by dividing the SD by the mean peak height multiplied by 100%.

CONCLUSIONS AND FUTURE PERSPECTIVES

Recent advances in zeptoproteomics have initiated new studies to characterize the proteins expressed, as well as secreted, by the mammalian embryo during all stages of preimplantation development. This information has the potential to provide insight into the cellular function and biological processes during embryonic development and the implantation process. In addition, this technology could be of value in the development of noninvasive viability assays that in conjunction with current morphologically based selection methods and perhaps other "omics" technologies may increase IVF success rates while reducing the number of embryos transferred.

Looking toward the future of zeptoproteomics and the diagnostic capabilities of detecting and quantifying low-abundant biomarkers in complex biological systems, several platforms show promise. The first is protein microarray technology, with the advantage of offering confirmatory and complementary information to mRNA expression studies. However, there are several hurdles to

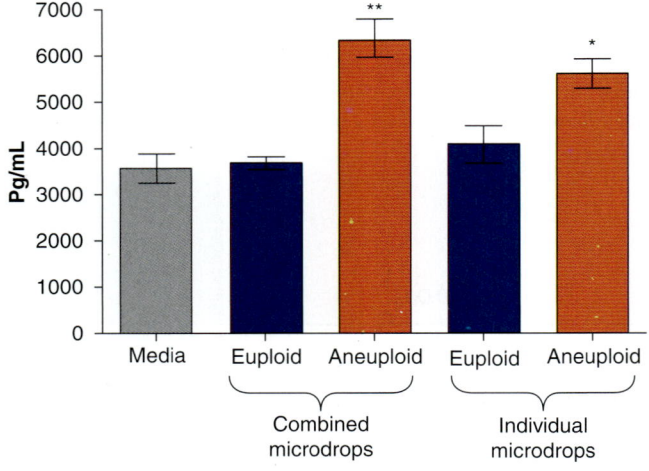

Figure 20.6 Lipocalin-1 concentration in the human embryonic protein secretome was measured by ELISA and statistically analyzed by a Student's t-test. Control media (n = 5); combined microdrops from euploid (n = 12) and aneuploid (n = 12) blastocysts (**$P < 0.01$); individual microdrops from euploid (n = 4) and aneuploid (n = 4) blastocyst (*$P < 0.05$). Control media, gray bar; euploid secretome, blue bars; aneuploid secretome, red bars 45.

overcome including the high cost of microarrays, dependence on the existence of antibodies, and problems with non-specific interactions (46). Another platform is 2D-capillary electrophoresis. A proof of principle study demonstrated the ability to separate and detect proteins from single mouse zygotes. The protein signature was produced by separation according to molecular weight in the first dimension capillary sieving electrophoresis followed by separation by micellar electrokinetic capillary chromatography (47).

The emergence of nanotechnologies will also be fundamental to the detection of low-abundant biomarkers in complex biological systems. Advances incorporating nanofluidics, nanoparticles, and nanostructures promise microscopic volume liquid handling and the monitoring of concentration changes that have never before been detectable, as well as the potential for separation- and label-free protein analysis (48). The advent of the field of nanoproteomics will offer exciting opportunities to discover diagnostic biomarkers of preimplantation embryonic development and viability.

REFERENCES

1. Kenyon GL, DeMarini DM, Fuchs E, et al. Defining the mandate of proteomics in the post-genomics era: workshop Report. Mol Cell Proteomics 2002; 1: 763–80.
2. Gygi SP, Rochon Y, Franza BR, Aebersold R. Correlation between protein and mRNA abundance in yeast. Mol Cell Biol 1999; 19: 1720–30.
3. Wulfkuhle JD, Liotta LA, Petricoin EF. Proteomic applications for the early detection of cancer. Nat Rev Cancer 2003; 3: 267–75.
4. Espina V, Dettloff KA, Cowherd S, Petricoin EF, Liotta LA. Use of proteomic analysis to monitor responses to biological therapies. Expert Opin Biol Ther 2004; 4: 83–93.
5. Petricoin EF, Liotta LA. Clinical applications of proteomics. J Nutr 2003; 133: 2476S–84S.
6. Hachey DL, Chaurand P. Proteomics in reproductive medicine: the technology for separation and identification of proteins. J Reprod Immunol 2004; 63: 61–73.
7. Brinster RL. Protein content of the mouse embryo during the first five days of development. J Reprod Fertil 1967; 13: 413–20.
8. Patton WF. Detection technologies in proteome analysis. J Chromatogr B Analyt Technol Life Sci 2002; 771: 3–31.
9. Latham KE, Garrels JI, Chang C, Solter D. Analysis of embryonic mouse development: construction of a high-resolution, two-dimensional gel protein database. Appl Theor Electroph 1992; 2: 163–70.
10. Shi CZ, Collins HW, Garside WT, et al. Protein databases for compacted eight-cell and blastocyst-stage mouse embryos. Mol Reprod Develop 1994; 37: 34–47.
11. Navarette Santos A, Tonack S, Kirstein M, Kietz S, Fischer B. Two insulin-responsive glucose transporter isoforms and the insulin receptor are developmentally expressed in rabbit preimplantation embryos. Reproduction 2004; 128: 503–16.
12. Wang HM, Zhang X, Qian D, et al. Effect of ubiquitin-proteasome pathway on mouse blastocyst implantation and expression of matrix metalloproteinases-2 and -9. BOR 2004; 70: 481–7.
13. Liebler DC. Introduction to Proteomics: Tools for the New Biology. Totowa, New Jersey: Humana Press, 2002.
14. Ellederova Z, Halada P, Man P, et al. Protein patterns of pig oocytes during in vitro maturation. BOR 2004; 71: 1533–9.
15. Vitale AM, Calvert ME, Mallavarapu M, et al. Proteomic profiling of murine oocyte maturation. Mol Reprod Dev 2006; 74: 608–16.
16. Meng Y, Liu XH, Ma X, et al. The protein profile of mouse mature cumulus-oocyte complex. Biochim Biophys Acta 2007; 1774: 1477–90.
17. Seibert V, Wiesner A, Buschmann T, Meuer J. Surface-enhanced laser desorption ionization time-of-flight mass spectrometry (SELDI TOF-MS) and ProteinChip technology in proteomics research. Pathol Res Pract 2004; 200: 83–94.
18. Cazares LH, Diaz JI, Drake RR, Semmes OJ. MALDI/SELDI protein profiling of serum for the identification of cancer biomarkers. Methods Mol Biol 2007; 428: 125–40.
19. Jansen C, Hebeda KM, Linkels M, et al. Protein profiling of B-cell lymphomas using tissue biopsies: a potential tool for small samples in pathology. Cell Oncol 2008; 30: 27–38.
20. Cho WC. Contribution of oncoproteomics to cancer biomarker discovery. Mol Cancer 2007; 6: 25.
21. Gerton GL, Fan XJ, Chittams J, et al. A serum proteomics approach to the diagnosis of ectopic pregnancy. Ann N Y Acad Sci 2004; 1022: 306–16.
22. Buhimschi CS, Bhandari V, Hamar BD, et al. Proteomic profiling of the amniotic fluid to detect inflammation, infection and neonatal sepsis. PLoS Med 2007; 4: e18.
23. Poon TC. Opportunities and limitations of SELDI-TOF-MS in biomedical research: practical advices. Expert Rev Proteomics 2007; 4: 51–65.
24. Katz-Jaffe MG, Linck DW, Schoolcraft WB, Gardner DK. A proteomic analysis of mammalian preimplantation embryonic development. Reproduction 2005; 130: 899–905.
25. Katz-Jaffe MG, Gardner DK, Schoolcraft WB. Proteomic analysis of individual human embryos to identify novel biomarkers of development and viability. Fertil Steril 2006; 85: 101–7.
26. Gardner DK, Lane M, Stevens J, Schoolcraft WB. Noninvasive assessment of human embryo nutrient consumption as a measure of developmental potential. Fertil Steril 2001; 76: 1175–80.
27. Ebner T, Moser M, Sommergruber M, Tews G. Selection based on morphological assessment of oocytes and embryos at different stages of preimplantation development: a review. Hum Reprod Update 2003; 9: 251–62.
28. Sakkas D, Gardner DK. Noninvasive methods to assess embryo quality. Curr Opin Obstet Gynecol 2005; 17: 283–8.
29. O'Neill C. The role of paf in embryo physiology. Hum Reprod Update 2005; 11: 215–28.
30. Gonzalez RR, Caballero-Campo P, Jasper M, et al. Leptin and leptin receptor are expressed in the human endometrium and endometrial leptin secretion is regulated by the human blastocyst. J Clin Endocrinol Metab 2000; 85: 4883–8.
31. Cervero A, Horcajadas JA, Dominguez F, Pellicer A, Simon C. Leptin system in embryo development and implantation: a protein in search of a function. Reprod Biomed Online 2005; 10: 217–23.

32. Sakkas D, Lu C, Zulfikaroglu E, Neuber E, Taylor HS. A soluble molecule secreted by human blastocysts modulates regulation of HOXA10 expression in an epithelial endometrial cell line. Fertil Steril 2003; 80: 1169–74.
33. Noci I, Fuzzi B, Rizzo R, et al. Embryonic soluble HLA-G as a marker of developmental potential in embryos. Hum Reprod 2005; 20: 138–46.
34. Fisch JD, Keskintepe L, Ginsburg M, Adamowicz M, Sher G. Graduated embryo score and soluble human leukocyte antigen-G expression improve assisted reproductive technology outcomes and suggest a basis for elective single-embryo transfer. Fertil Steril 2007; 87: 757–63.
35. Sargent I, Swales A, Ledee N, et al. SHLA-G production by human IVF embryos: can it be measured reliably? J Reprod Immunol 2007; 75: 128–32.
36. Katz-Jaffe MG, Schoolcraft WB, Gardner DK. Quantification of protein expression (secretome) by human and mouse preimplantation embryos. Fertil Steril 2006; 86: 678–85.
37. Telford NA, Watson AJ, Schultz GA. Transition from maternal to embryonic control in early mammalian development: a comparison of several species. Mol Reprod Dev 1990; 26: 90–100.
38. Delbosc S, Haloui M, Louedec L. Proteomic analysis permits the identification of new biomarkers of arterial wall remodeling in hypertension. Mol Med 2008; 14: 383–94.
39. Sandoval JA, Hoelz DJ, Woodruff HA, et al. Novel peptides secreted from human neuroblastoma: useful clinical tools? J Pediatr Surg 2006; 41: 245–51.
40. Wang Y, Puscheck EE, Lewis JJ, et al. Increases in phosphorylation of SAPK/JNK and p38MAPK correlate negatively with mouse embryo development after culture in different media. Fertil Steril 2005; 83: 1144–54.
41. Dominguez F, Gadea B, Esteban FJ, et al. Comparative protein-profile analysis of implanted versus non-implanted human blastocysts. Hum Reprod 2008; 23: 1993–2000.
42. Robertson SA. GM-CSF regulation of embryo development and pregnancy. Cytokine Growth Factor Rev 2007; 18: 287–98.
43. Dominguez F, Gadea B, Mercader A, et al. Embryologic outcome and secretome profile of implanted blastocysts obtained after coculture in human endometrial epithelial cells versus the sequential system. Fertil Steril 2010; 93: 774–82.
44. Martinez MC, Mendez C, Ferro J, et al. Cytogenetic analysis of early nonviable pregnancies after assisted reproduction treatment. Fertil Steril 2010; 93: 289–92.
45. McReynolds S, Vanderlinden L, Stevens J, et al. Lipocalin-1 a potential marker for non-invasive aneuploidy screening. Fertil Steril 2011; 95: 2631–3.
46. Spisak S, Tulassay Z, Molnar B, Guttman A. Protein microchips in biomedicine and biomarker discovery. Electrophoresis 2007; 28: 4261–73.
47. Harwood MM, Christians ES, Fazal MA, Dovichi NJ. Single-cell protein analysis of a single mouse embryo by two-dimensional capillary electrophoresis. J Chromatography A 2006; 1130: 190–4.
48. Marko NF, Weil RJ, Toms SA. Nanotechnology in proteomics. Expert Rev Proteomics 2007; 4: 617–26.

21

The human oocyte: Controlled rate cooling

Andrea Borini and Veronica Bianchi

INTRODUCTION

Cells can be stored at low temperatures such as −196°C for unlimited time; the real challenge is their survival after returning to physiological conditions. One of the main issues in achieving the goal is the intracellular freeze that has to be overcome to increase survival. Mazur in 1984 (1) described equations that have been developed to analyze the kinetics of cellular water loss and permit one to predict the likelihood of intracellular freezing as a function of cooling rate.

In 1983 for the first time, live pregnancies were obtained using cryopreserved human embryos (2). This new procedure influenced the world of in vitro fertilization (IVF) leading to new options for the patients. Multiple pregnancies were reduced and repeated stimulations were not necessary thanks to embryo freezing. Nevertheless over time this technique led to several issues mainly concerned with moral and legal aspects. However, the ability to freeze embryos shed a light on the possibility to cryopreserve eggs as well even though the cellular composition between oocyte and embryos is very different. The human oocyte is one of the largest cells of the body and its cytoplasm contains a high amount of water. This characteristic can induce damages in the ultra structures of the cell caused by ice crystal formation during the transition of water into ice. To overcome this issue, protocols developed up to now include a progressive dehydration of eggs before and during the cooling phase to reduce ice crystal formation.

The mouse was the first model in which egg freezing gave results around 30 years ago (3); here the mouse cell could survive well below temperature due to its reduced size and content of water. On the contrary, the first pregnancy in the human was achieved only in 1986 (4) and afterward just a sporadic success has been reported due to technical issues.

A considerably important step forward has been made in Italy after the introduction of a very restrictive law, which had forbidden embryo freezing and allowed to inseminate just three eggs for fresh embryo transfer. At that point freezing the remaining oocytes represented the best way to optimize the stimulation cycles. In fact, by preserving supernumerary oocytes it is possible to avoid extra embryo freezing and, at the same time, avert repeated ovarian stimulations. There are several other benefits associated with the cryopreservation of oocytes: it represents an important chance not only for women at risk of losing their fertility due to malignant disease or premature ovarian failure but also for women who choose to postpone motherhood for personal or professional reasons. The possibility to cryopreserve oocyte as a routine IVF procedure is an important option to maximize egg donation, avoiding donor/recipient synchronization and making quarantine of specimens possible. Last but not least, egg freezing helps bypass any potential conflicts associated with legal ownership of cryopreserved embryos in the event of divorce.

For several years, the unique nature of the human oocyte together with the lack of cryobiological data posed several concerns around this technique so, egg freezing has been considered for a long period as an experimental procedure. Things started to change after the introduction of intracytoplasmic sperm injection (ICSI) as the elective technique for the insemination of thawed oocytes. In this way, at least, fertilization problems were mostly overcome. In fact, together with the survival rate, insemination of thawed eggs was a problem due to the premature release of cortical granules and the phenomenon known as zona hardening (5) that limited the fertilization with standard IVF.

BIOPHYSICS OF CONTROLLED RATE COOLING

The unique nature of the human oocyte is mainly responsible for the low survival after thawing.

To improve the outcome different protocols have been developed with the aim of reducing intracellular ice crystal formation. To do so, it is necessary to reach a sufficient dehydration thanks to specific molecules called cryoprotectant agents (CPAs) that can be differently mixed in order to maximize the outcome.

These compounds can be divided into two groups according to their proprieties:

1. Permeating agents such as glycerol, dimethyl sulfoxide (DMSO), ethylene glycol (EG), and (1,2) propanediol (PROH). They all have a low molecular weight and can penetrate the lipid bilayer of the cell but slower than water.

2. Nonpermeating agents such as sugars and other macromolecules (ficoll, raffinose, as well as proteins and lipoproteins). They have a high molecular weight so they remain in the extracellular solution.

The basic task of the CPAs is to reduce possible damages due to ice crystal formation inside the cell. At the same time they play a role in protective effects thanks to their ability to create hydrogen bond achieving high aqueous solubility. In fact, during slow cooling, when the cells are very dehydrated and surrounded by concentrated salts, the cryoprotectants appear to reduce possible damages caused by this osmotic milieu.

In slow freezing protocols before cooling the cell to subzero temperatures, a two-step dehydration is normally carried out. In the first step, concentrations of permeating CPAs (1.0–1.5 mol/L) are utilized to remove water from the cell preventing ice formation. The most widely used cryoprotectants in this phase are propanediol (PROH), dimethyl sulfoxide (Me2SO), or EG. The presence of CPA in the extracellular media creates an osmotic gradient which draws water out of the cell. The oocyte dehydrates and shrinks then it returns to near the original volume as the cryoprotectant enters the cell replacing the water. This causes a double flux across the membrane (the water exits the cell while the CPA enters) that influences both the intracellular solute concentration and the cell volume Fig. 21.1.

The extent of shrinkage and swelling can cause damage or even cell death because of the osmotic stress acting on the oocyte membrane. To minimize this phenomenon in the second phase of dehydration a nonpermeating molecule is usually added to the mixture. Sucrose is the most commonly used but also trehalose and choline have been applied successfully (6–8).

This new agent creates a second-phase dehydration in which the shrinkage rate is faster with a higher reduction of the cell volume before freezing. This phenomenon decreases, further on, the likelihood of intracellular ice crystal formation. Afterward, the cell is cooled down to subzero temperatures slowly (around −2°C/min) to avoid possible shock. Once the sample temperature has been lowered to −6 to −8°C (just below the equilibrium freezing point of the mixture), ice nucleation is induced by touching the straws with precooled forceps. This procedure, known as seeding, allows the conversion of extracellular water into ice. In most slow cooling protocols for embryos and oocytes it is necessary to induce ice formation in the external solution manually, because this prevents super cooling and starts the dehydration process. After seeding at one point, ice spreads throughout the entire solution. When solutions are seeded at 5–7°C, ice crystals do not enter the cell because of the marginally higher osmolarity (lower freezing point) of their intracellular environment. Following the seeding, the concentration of the solutes in the non-frozen fraction gradually

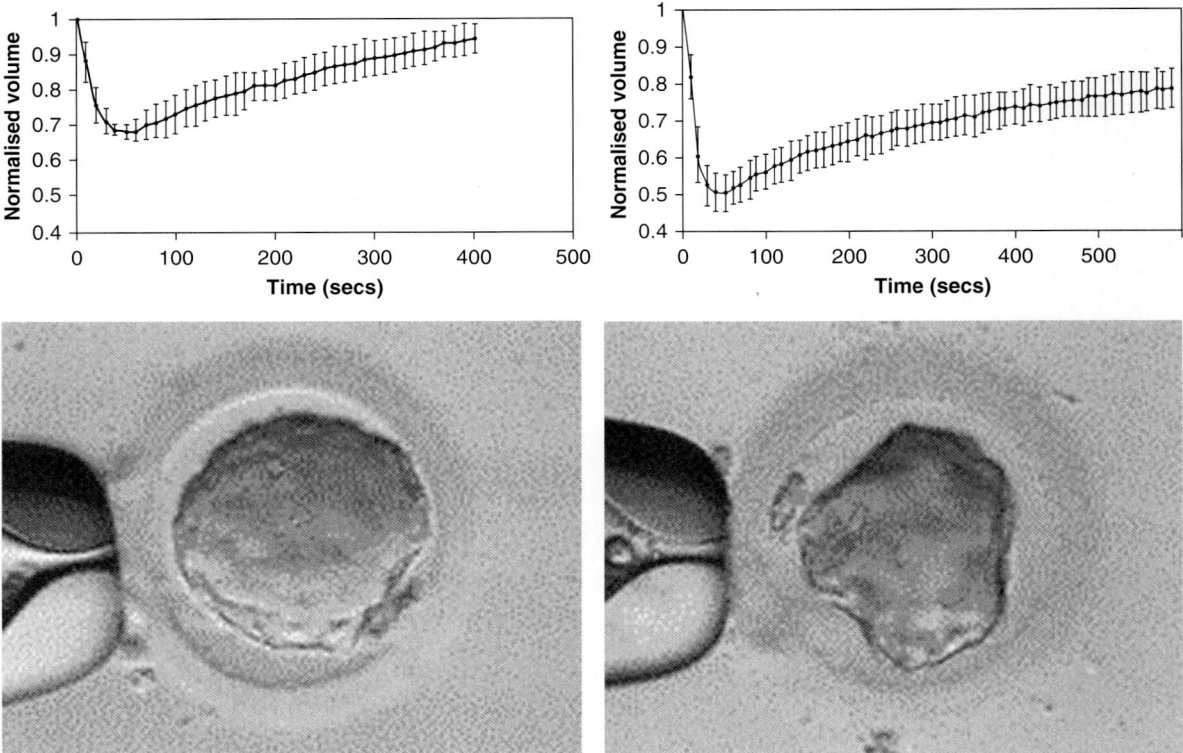

Figure 21.1 Mean ± SD normalized volume of human oocytes during exposure to 1.5 mol/L propanediol (9) (*left*) or ethylene glycol (11) (*right*) at 25°C. The magnitude and kinetics of volume changes are dictated by the relative oolemma permeability to water and cryoprotective agent (CPA). Low permeability to CPA and, consequently, more pronounced volume reduction may cause major transient perturbations of the original spherical shape (*right*).

increases as water is incorporated into the extracellular ice crystals. The increasing concentration in the solutes generates an osmotic gradient across the cell membrane, which draws more water out causing the cell to dehydrate. By lowering very slowly the temperature, nearly all of the water can be removed from the cell without ice crystal formation and, at the same time, damages caused by the extracellular solute concentration can be minimized. At this point the samples can be plunged directly in liquid nitrogen.

The rewarming phase is usually fast in order to avoid intracellular small crystals to reach a size that can be detrimental for the cell organelles. Cell rehydration is usually performed by a stepwise dilution of the intracellular CPA present in the freezing media together with a high concentration of the extracellular CPA, such as sugar which acts as osmotic buffer. This phenomenon reduces the flux of water toward the membrane during the thawing phase thus avoiding swelling or bursting of the egg. The analysis of cell volume changes during the freezing–thawing procedures is important to evaluate different CPAs and, eventually new approaches to improve freezing protocols. An optimal exposure should aim at minimizing osmotic stress while avoiding chemical toxicity and allow sufficient permeation and dehydration to achieve protection from freezing injury.

Paynter et al. (9,10) tried to evaluate the osmotic response by monitoring the oocytes for 10 minutes during a two-step addition of the permeating cryoprotectant PROH (0.75 M and 1.5 M PROH). Following this, the oocyte osmotic response to 1.5 M PROH and 0.2 M or 0.3 M sucrose was measured. Each oocyte shrank during the first exposure to the cryoprotectant (0.75 M PROH) as water left the cell and then gradually re-expanded as cryoprotectant entered; this process lasted around 20 minutes. The same happened during the second exposure to an increased cryoprotectant concentration (1.5 M PROH) and, in the 1.5 M PROH plus sucrose solution the shrinkage rate was higher with a reduction of cell volume before freezing to avoid intracellular ice crystal formation.

Experiments with EG were carried out in a similar fashion (11), during EG exposure oocytes underwent an abrupt 50% volume reduction and a complete recovery of the initial volume was not observed. Survival rates after freezing with EG were lower than with PROH (51.6% vs. 71.5%, respectively, $P < 0.05$). The frequencies of normal spindle configuration were lower in frozen EG and frozen PROH oocytes compared with fresh controls (53.8%, 50.9%, and 66.7%, respectively, $P < 0.05$).

Selection of the right mixture together with optimal exposure times is mandatory to have a good recovery during slow freezing procedures.

OOCYTE SELECTION

Oocyte selection prior to freeze represents a difficult task for the embryologist. Beside evident cytoplasm anomalies (a large first polar body, macro cytoplasm, and perivitelline space debris) it is difficult to select which morphological features may affect the outcome. Moreover, post-thaw survival is not always synonymous with viability. Unfortunately, methods to assess the quality of the oocytes are usually invasive and thus nonconservative. In addition to surviving the cryopreservation, the oocyte needs to maintain competence to fertilize and develop into a viable embryo to be able to result in a pregnancy. Nevertheless, it has been widely demonstrated that, low temperatures during freezing may induce alteration to the cell substructures, especially due to the unique nature of the metaphase II oocyte.

At this stage the chromosomes are in strict relation to the meiotic spindle which is responsible of chromosome segregation during the extrusion of the second polar body.

This structure is made of microtubules that can disassemble and reassemble under certain conditions. It has been assessed, in the mouse and in the human that even a transient decrease in the temperature might lead to a depolymerization of the spindle. Nevertheless, the return to normal conditions shows that the spindle is able to significantly reassemble (12–14).

During slow freezing, the egg undergoes a drastic change in temperature that can be detrimental for the spindle leading to an increase in aneuploidy; on the other hand, CPAs play an important role in protecting the spindle.

Unfortunately, in order to have accurate information, cytogenetic or confocal analyses should be performed on oocytes after thawing with the consequent loss of viability. An acceptable alternative to visualize the recovery of the meiotic spindle is the Polscope which is a microscopy optical system that allows the observation of highly ordered subcellular structures, such as the spindle, through polarized light (15). Microtubules are responsible for spindle birefringence and their density is measured by the retardance. Polscope offers the advantage of being noninvasive thus preserving egg viability; for this reason it is used as a potential tool for oocyte selection, considering that not all the oocytes showing an extruded polar body and actually mature.

This system can also be used to evaluate spindle recovery after thawing in order to select the best oocytes to inject. Several authors used different slow freezing protocols and try to visualize the reappearance of the spindle after rewarming. Rienzi et al. (16) used a 1.5 M PROH plus 0.1 M sucrose mixture and showed a recovery in 37% of the oocytes immediately after thawing and after a transient disappearance the spindle was present in all the eggs survived within three hours of incubation at 37°C. Similar data were published by Bianchi et al. (17) using a comparable freezing protocol with higher sucrose concentration (0.3 M). Immediately after thawing, only 22.9% of oocytes showed a weak birefringence signal, while only 1.2% of oocytes displayed a high signal. After three hours' culture 49.4% of the oocytes showed a weak birefringence while 18.1% a high intensity signal. There was a statistically significant increase in signal restoration after three hours of culture ($P < 0.001$). Sereni et al. (18), studying a larger cohort of eggs, demonstrated a 90% of signal restoration after one hour of culture. The authors stated that post-thaw culture could be considerably shortened to one hour. Furthermore, they speculated that a

Table 21.1 The Oocyte Cryopreservation Outcome Generated in Three Different Studies Adopting the Same Freezing Protocol (24)

	Borini et al. (46)	Levi setti et al. (47)	De santis et al. (48)
Patients	146	120	66
Thaws	201	159	68
Oocytes:			
Thawed	927	1087	396
Survived (%)	687 (74)	760 (69)	282 (71.2)
Microinjected	589	687	194
2PN	448 (76)	464 (67)	156 (80.4)
Embryos:			
Cleaved	404 (90)	413 (89)	142 (91)
Mean transferred	2.1 ± 0.8		
Pregnancies (% per ET)	18 (9.7)	18 (12.4)	6 (9.5)
Implantations (%)	21 (5.2)	19 (5.7)	7 (5.7)
Implantation efficiency per thawed oocyte	2.6%	1.9%	2.6%

Abbreviations: 2PN, two pronuclei; ET, embryo transfer.

short culture time could be beneficial to the whole cryopreservation procedure, making less likely the risk of aging in vitro which, on the contrary, may occur after thawing, when oocytes are incubated for longer periods in preparation for insemination.

A further confirmation was obtained by confocal microscopy (19) where fresh control oocytes were compared with frozen eggs fixed at different times after thawing (0, 1, 2, and 3 hours). All the control oocytes (100.0%) displayed normal bipolar spindles. Directly after thawing at T = 0 it was observed a significant reduction of oocytes with bipolar spindles (59.1%) while after one hour of culture (T1) 85.7% regained bipolar spindles. Oocytes cultured for longer (2 or 3 hours) displayed 73.7% and 72.7% bipolar spindles, respectively.

Unfortunately, Coticchio et al. (20) demonstrated that Polscope is useful for showing the presence and the dynamic of the spindle, but the morphometric evaluation of the spindle through the Polscope is not consistent with confocal analysis

REPRODUCIBILITY

One of the advantages of the slow freezing technique is the high degree of reproducibility. This is extremely important since in any laboratories different operators with different skills should be able to reproduce comparable outcomes. This may include different aspects, like the accuracy of making homemade solutions or also the ability to provide strict adherence to the protocol. For these reasons all the procedures should be written by a laboratory director not to leave room for personal interpretation. The storage devices are important as well; in the slow freezing standard plastic straws are usually employed for the cryopreservation of oocytes and embryos; this limits fluctuation between different procedures. Generally differences in size, volume, and wall thickness between various devices may influence the transmission of heat and potentially affect the freezing–thawing process. For this reason, the volume of the freezing mixture loaded into straws should be standardized.

Almost all the slow freezing protocols generally required a longer operational time than other techniques (i.e., vitrification) so different manual skills can have a lower influence on the outcome. In fact, incubation times either in the freezing or in the thawing procedure range from 5 to 15 minutes instead of few minutes or seconds. Moreover, slow freezing has been applied to embryo cryopreservation for several years; consequently, laboratories with experience in performing embryo cryopreservation would take a shorter time to reach an optimal performance with egg slow cooling.

Another important aspect is related to the temperature. It is well known that lower supra-zero temperatures reduce the toxicity of cryoprotectants but, at the same time may be detrimental for cell membrane and cytoskeleton. Therefore, the temperature at which dehydration/rehydration solutions are utilized should be precisely regulated. In controlled rate freezing, thanks to the automated machine, the decrease in temperature is finely monitored and recorded. Cooling rates during water to ice transition are slow (−0.3°C/min) and protracted for over 70 minutes, conditions which are believed to ensure good consistency. An example of this protocol reproducibility is provided by the comparison of three studies that were carried out with a large number of patients, using the same slow freezing method (Table 21.1). From these data it is possible to observe that survival, fertilization, cleavage, and implantation rates were rather similar, despite the fact that the three studies were conducted in different centers.

SURVIVAL AND INSEMINATION OF FROZEN–THAWED OOCYTE

The controlled rate cooling procedure is based on a slow decreasing temperature rate. Several mathematical analyses have been made to define an optimal curve applicable to oocytes in order to balance the need to obtain a sufficient dehydration and the likelihood of ice crystal formation.

At the very beginning the slow cryopreservation protocol applied worldwide was the same used for embryos (21). Cryopreservation solutions consisted of a mixture of PROH (1.5M) and sucrose (0.1M) which was a good recipe for embryo freezing but did not give good outcomes with oocytes (22,23).

The difference is probably due to the insufficient dehydration of the oocytes that was not optimal with such a lower concentration of sucrose. Generally eggs are incubated for 10 minutes in a 1.5 M PROH solution with 20% protein supplement during the equilibration phase; during this period the PROH enters the cell and the water exits. During the second step (1.5 M PROH plus sucrose) the increased dehydration is proportional to the amount of sucrose contained in the solution. Fabbri et al. (24) proved that when the amount of sugar was increased, the loss of water from the oocyte also was higher. The survival rate was significantly improved with this modification to the protocol.

Recently Bianchi et al. (25) tried to modulate sucrose concentration during freezing–thawing in order to optimize the dehydration–rehydration conditions avoiding excess of shrinkage. In previous osmotic response experiments (10), it emerged that after around three minutes of exposure to 1.5M PROH in the presence of 0.3 M sucrose, oocyte volume decreases rapidly, reaching values below the 30% threshold excursion, which may be detrimental to cell viability. With a reduced sucrose concentration (0.2 M) the 30% volume change is not reached until after 10 minutes of exposure. Therefore, dehydration may be achieved slower and less traumatically. The steps of this protocol based on a freezing solution containing 0.2 M sucrose and thawing solutions made with 0.3 M sucrose are described in Table 21.2.

Besides using the combination of PROH and sucrose other approaches have been studied to overcome the accumulation of solutes during extracellular ice formation which is believed to affect the stability of the oolemma and the intracellular membranes. Stachecki et al. (8) tried, in the mouse model, to replace sodium with equimolar amounts of choline that does not diffuse through the membrane and should be less toxic. Results were encouraging showing an increase in the rates of survival, fertilization, and preimplantation development. More recently, low-sodium media have been used on human oocytes; nevertheless, despite the encouraging survival rate reported initially, studies involving larger number of patients have not been reported.

In a clinical study, Boldt et al. (26) used choline plus 0.3M sucrose but survival rates were disappointing irrespective of the adoption of phosphate-buffered saline (PBS) or HEPES as pH buffers. Other authors have tested the effect of sodium-depleted media on the cryopreservation of human oocytes (27,28). In all these cases, survival rates remained rather low, generally below 62%, not confirming the beneficial effect of choline.

Table 21.2 Schematic Description of a Slow Cooling Rate Protocol Involving the Use of 0.2 and 0.3 mol/L Sucrose for (A) Dehydration and (D) Rehydration, Respectively. Solutions are Prepared in PBS Media and Supplemented with 10 mg/mL of Human Serum Albumin

A Dehydration

Solution	Time	Temperature
1.5 mol/L PROH	10 min	24°C
1.5 mol/L PROH, 0.2 mol/L sucrose	5 min	24°C

B Controlled Rate Cooling

Ramp	Thermal Interval
1	+20 to −8°C, −2.0°C/min
2	−8°C, hold for 10 min. Seed at about 30% of ramp
3	−8°C to −30°C, −0.3°C/min
4	−30°C to −150°C, −50.0°C/min
5	−150°C, hold for 10 min, then plunge into LN_2

C Thawing

Time	Temperature
30 sec	24°C
40 sec	30°C, water bath

D Rehydration

Solution	Time	Temperature
1.0 mol/l PrOH, 0.3 mol/l sucrose	5 min	24°C
0.5 mol/l PrOH, 0.3 mol/l sucrose	5 min	24°C
0.3 mol/l sucrose	10 min	24°C
Buffer	10 min	24°C

Abbreviations: LN_2, liquid nitrogen; PROH, propanediol.

TIMING OF FREEZING AND INSEMINATION

During the routine procedure in the laboratory the oocytes are cultured for several hours following the retrieval before being inseminated. The approximate interval is around 40 hours after human chorionic gonadotropin (hCG) administration; this is actually about the time required for the oocytes to undergo a nuclear and cytoplasmic maturation. Normally in vivo this process occurred within the follicle unit; once the oocyte is separated from the follicular fluid mainly the cytoplasmic maturation may be compromised. One of the concerns related to egg cryopreservation is the likelihood of creating a discontinuity in oocyte life during the critical period between the recovery and fertilization. The right time in which oocyte should be frozen is still under debate; Parmigiani et al. (29) in a clinical retrospective study involving 75 patients and 93 oocyte thawings achieved a significantly improved embryo quality and clinical outcome when oocyte cryopreservation was performed within two hours from the retrieval.

These results were later confirmed by Lappi et al. (30) in a retrospective study on 311 thawing cycles using a slow freezing protocol with 1.5 M PROH and 0.3 M sucrose. Patients involved in the study were less than 40 years old. Oocytes frozen within 40 hours from the hCG injection showed significantly higher pregnancy and implantation rates compared with eggs cryopreserved more then 40 hours after the hCG administration (22% vs. 12% pregnancy/transfer with $P < 0.05$ and 13% vs. 7% implantation with $P < 0.05$). No difference was found in the time between end of thawing and micro injection. According to these results, the timing of oocyte cryopreservation seems to play a key role in determining the clinical outcome after thawing. In particular, the hour post-hCG at which freezing is performed is very important in determining the developmental potential of oocytes from frozen cycles. Conversely, while using a different sucrose concentration in the freezing–thawing media (23) this difference was not observed. In a recent study (31) on 325 patients (under 35 years of age) and 375 thawing cycles it was evidenced that the time before freezing does not compromise the final outcome. Instead, a more important role is played by the after-thawing culture time. This result can probably be associated with the protective effect that cumulus cells exert on the oocyte limiting its aging thus, denuded oocytes might be more sensitive to damage. Consequently it is suggested to inject the oocytes within two hours after the end of the thawing procedure.

A non-invasive tool that can be useful to determine the right time to freeze and microinject the eggs after thawing is the Polscope. This system is useful since it allows the visualization of the spindle. Visualization of meiotic spindle occurs more frequently when made at least 38 hours after administration of hCG than when this analysis is performed first (81.5% vs. 61.6%) (32). This can be explained by the fact that oocytes with an extruded polar body may be in a phase that precedes the meiotic metaphase II (telophase I or prometaphase II). Therefore, assessment of oocytes with polarized light can be used prior to cryopreservation to check their proper meiotic stage. The help of the polarized light should increase the effectiveness of freezing and, at the same time can help to improve standardization of the technique. Moreover the Polscope is a noninvasive method and thus it can preserve oocyte viability while allowing repeated observations over time. In the literature there is a general agreement about the correlation between the spindle and fertilization rates during IVF (33,34) or embryo development potential (35).

Not much information is, instead, available about the time frame needed between the end of thawing and the injection. This time generally is about three to four hours but, even though still under debate, it seems that approximately one to two hours should allow a good recovery of the oocytes. The few hours' time is needed for the culture to obtain the correct spindle reorganization after thawing. Nevertheless, in many studies, the duration of this recovery period is not reported.

Confocal microscopy confirmed that the overall structure of the meiotic spindle can be restored after cryopreservation (19). Stachecki et al., (36) using choline (as a substitute for sodium) and a 0.2 M sucrose concentration, observed that the frequency of oocytes with a normal shaped spindle and an array of regular chromosomes were not statistically different between fresh and thawed states (76.7% vs. 69.7% and 76.7% vs. 71.2%, respectively).

More recently another study (37) used slow freezing and a mixture of 1.5 M PROH plus different sucrose concentrations (either 0.1 M or 0.3 M) and revealed that while in the fresh control group 73.1% of oocytes displayed a normal bipolar spindle with equatorial aligned chromosomes the organization of chromatin and spindle was significantly affected (50.8%) after cryopreservation with the lowest concentration of sucrose. These parameters instead remained unchanged (69.7%) with 0.3 M sucrose. It is evident that cryopreservation can induce damage in oocytes but these alterations are acceptable using higher sucrose concentration. The higher dehydration reached with a 0.3 M sucrose limits the amount of intracellular water preventing ice crystal formation. As a consequence the spindle is probably better preserved. Unfortunately not a lot is known on the actual mechanism of depolymerization of the spindle during freezing and thawing. In order to figure out the right time for the microinjection after thawing it is important to balance carefully the recovery time that oocytes need in order to restore the meiotic spindle with oocyte aging, which must be avoided. This phenomenon consists of disorders of some oocytes key factors (cell cycle kinase, intracellular calcium, cytoskeleton, etc.) that are apparently still compatible with a normal fertilization, but, if compromised, can lead to lower implantation rates (38). Other structures may undergo important modifications during the freezing–thawing procedures (cortical granules, mitochondria, or Golgi apparatus) but very little information is available. One recent study focused on the ultrastructural features in cryopreserved oocytes (39) showing differences in the mitochondria setting. In fresh samples mitochondria had a regular shape with few short cristae, whereas in the frozen–thawed group a high percentage of oocytes (72%) showed a variable and, in some cases, a very high fraction of mitochondria with decreased electron density of the matrix or ruptures of the outer and inner membranes. Moreover in those oocytes, the mitochondrial damage was associated with SER swelling.

OOCYTE PREPARATION FOR FREEZING

Just after the retrieval, cumulus–corona complexes consist of an oocyte and somatic cells with a highly hydrated extracellular matrix. The presence of the cumulus might influence the exchange of water and CPAs during dehydration and rehydration of the oocytes, and then ultimately has an effect on the cryopreservation procedure. Very few studies are available in the literature about the influence of the cumulus on the freezing outcome. One of the first papers was published by Gook et al. (40) where oocytes with intact cumulus or totally decumulated were frozen using the protocol initially described by Lassalle for embryo cryopreservation (21). A higher survival rate was observed in the group without cumulus compared with the cumulus-enclosed complexes (69% vs. 48%, respectively). Conversely these preliminary data were not confirmed by Fabbri et al. (24). The author compared the survival rates in oocytes frozen after complete denudation or partial mechanical removal of the cumulus. Regardless of the concentration of sucrose in the freezing mixture (0.1, 0.2, or 0.3 M) the survival rates were comparable between the two groups of oocytes (39% vs. 31%, 58% vs. 60%, and 83% vs. 81%, respectively), suggesting that the removal or retention of part of the cumulus is irrelevant to the viability of oocytes after thawing. More recently, Kuwayama et al. (41) showed that using vitrification procedure the survival rate was higher in oocytes frozen with the cumulus rather than without (75.8% vs. 30%, respectively). However, the very low number of oocytes included in the groups (33 and 10 eggs) did not allow any conclusions. Therefore, the evidence of the possible effect of the presence of cumulus on the viability of the thawed oocytes remains controversial. In the absence of a clear beneficial effect, the complete removal of cumulus–corona complex before freezing is recommended since the differences in the amount of left cumulus cells prior to freezing will introduce a source of variability that can affect the standardization of the cryopreservation. Moreover, the presence of the cumulus cells does not allow a clear assessment of the nuclear meiotic state of oocytes.

DEVELOPMENTAL PERFORMANCE OF FROZEN–THAWED OOCYTES

The final parameter to be considered in order to validate a particular technique is the live birth rate that, as pregnancy depends on the embryo intrinsic viability. Several information are available in the literature about the relation between different freezing conditions and the embryo's ability to resume the mitotic cycle. This factor can help predicting the implantation potential of frozen–thawed embryos (42,43). On the contrary a little is known about the early developmental competence of embryos coming from frozen eggs; possible deleterious effects of oocyte cryopreservation can already appear during preimplantation development. In a previous study (44) we compared the frequency of early cleavage, cell number, and degree of fragmentation in embryos derived from sibling fresh and frozen–thawed oocytes of patients undergoing IVF treatment to evidenced possible differences.

The slow freezing protocol used in this first approach was based on a 1.5 M PROH and 0.3 M sucrose mixture (24) and ICSI was used as elective insemination technique. Despite the same rate of fertilization 59% of fresh zygotes showed early cleavage while in the frozen–thawed sibling that happened just in 7.1% of cases. A statistical significance was evidenced ($P < 0.001$).

Moreover, despite the overall cleavage rate at transfer being similar in the two groups, fresh embryos appeared to cleave with a faster rate, only 39% were at the two-cell stage while in the frozen–thawed group the majority of cleaved embryos (61%) were at the two-cell stage. These data are consistent with the hypothesis that to some extent the implantation potential of embryos developing from frozen oocytes may be affected by freezing with high sucrose concentration (45). It has been evidenced by different authors that high cleavage rates is not necessarily related to a high implantation potential (46–48). In these publications high rates of cleavage (90–93%) resulted in scarce implantation rates (5–6%).

Conversely when our group (49) compared the developmental ability of embryos derived from sibling fresh and frozen–thawed oocytes using a modified slow cooling protocol involving 1.5 M PROH and differential sucrose concentrations in freezing (0.2 M) and thawing (0.3 M) solutions the outcome was different. Embryos from fresh and frozen oocytes were assessed by comparing the frequencies of fertilization, cleavage, and the number of blastomeres at (42–44) after microinjection.

In 85 fresh cycles, 244 oocytes were inseminated while in 104 frozen cycles, 357 out of 525 oocytes survived after thawing (68%) and 248 were microinjected. Normal fertilization was high in both fresh and frozen groups (81.9% and 81.4%, respectively). Cleavage rate was 96.5% and 93.1% in fresh and frozen oocytes, respectively. The frequencies of two-, three-, four-, more than four-cell embryos were also statistically similar. In particular, the rate of four-cell embryos was 47.0% and 47.2% in fresh and frozen groups, respectively. The overall implantation rate of embryos developed from frozen oocytes was 15.7%, while this frequency increased to 26.9% in cases in which at least two 4-cell embryos were transferred. Following cryopreservation the early developmental ability of frozen–thawed oocytes does not appear affected in comparison to the one of sibling non-frozen oocytes. These results overlapped perfectly the clinical outcomes observed using this slow freezing protocol (25). Moreover, from these preliminary studies it is possible to affirm that the timing of the first cleavage gives some understandings of the implantation potential of embryos coming from cryopreserved eggs.

CLINICAL EFFICIENCY OF OOCYTE CRYOPRESERVATION

In the last decade a renewed interest in oocyte freezing gave rise to several studies aimed at improving protocols and techniques to make this option reliable. Since the first pregnancy dating back to 1986 (4), several steps forward have been made (50,51) leading to numerous publications (46–48).

Slow freezing method was the first applied to oocyte cryopreservation exactly as it has been conceived by Lassale et al. (21) for embryo freezing. The freezing mixture, the exposure time, and the temperature curve were the same. Unfortunately, the results were not comparable with the embryo outcomes. The main problem was related to the low oocyte survival; the poor recovery did not guarantee any kind of embryo selection. Our group in 2004 (23) published clinical data on 68 patients and actually the survival rate was just 37%. The same was for the fertilization rate (45.4%) while, instead, cleavage and pregnancy per patient rates were quite high (86.3% and 22%, respectively).

The turning point arrived in 2001 with the increase in sucrose concentration introduced by Fabbri et al. (24) that drastically improved the survival rate and thus the possibility to have more oocytes to inject and a cohort of embryos among to choose. The reported post-thaw recovery was directly related to the amount of sugar used in the freezing solutions ranging from 34% with 0.1 M sucrose up to 82% when the concentration was increased to 0.3 M. The exposure times were maintained unchanged so was the lowering temperature curve and, consequently, the increase in the survival could be directly correlated to a higher dehydration of the oocyte. The reduced amount of water inside the cell avoided ice crystal formation improving the post-thaw recovery. The limit of this study was related to the absence of clinical data so it was not possible to assess the real outcome in terms of pregnancy or live birth rates.

These data were later confirmed by several authors, but the worldwide results were often related to a small number of patients since the procedure was considered experimental (52–54).

Later on, due to the change in the Italian law (40/2004), oocyte cryopreservation became an important tool in the IVF routine. In fact, since just three eggs could be inseminated and embryo freezing was not allowed, oocyte cryopreservation was the only option available to avoid repeated stimulation cycles. As a consequence, several reports have been published since then. One of the first was by our group in 2006 (46) on 146 patients. Out of 927 oocytes included the survival rate was good (74.1%) confirming the hypothesis that a higher sucrose concentration can improve the recovery. Nevertheless, the implantation was very low (around 5%) suggesting that something could be compromised by this excessive dehydration.

Other reports (46–48) confirmed our results; high survival rates were reported (ranging from 65% to almost 80%) but the implantation was in all cases around 5% (Table 21.3). Boltd et al., (26) using a sodium-depleted and HEPES-buffered freezing media reported a lower survival rate (59.5%) but high implantation (15.9%). Unfortunately these data only included (23) patients and did not have any control group. In the same year De Santis et al. (48) compared different outcomes using either 0.1 M or 0.3 M sucrose concentration; the survival was, as expected, significantly improved using 0.3 M sucrose but pregnancy and implantation rates were higher using 0.1 M sucrose.

In 2007 our group (25) modified the freezing protocol in order to balance the need to have a high survival recovery but, at the same time, to achieve an acceptable pregnancy and implantation rates. Freezing and thawing solutions used different sugar concentrations; during the cryopreservation a mixture of 1.5 M PROH and 0.2 M sucrose was utilized in order to limit the oocyte shrinkage but a higher sucrose concentration (0.3 M) was used during thawing to better balance the rehydration.

This combination resulted in a high survival (76.0%) without compromising the pregnancy/transfer and the implantation (21.2% and 13.4%, respectively). Besides the row data about oocyte cryopreservation itself it is interesting to observe the contribution of egg freezing in raising the cumulative pregnancy rate (55). This technique can actually add value in countries with a restrictive law. The cumulative pregnancy rate obtained with transfer of fresh embryos and embryos coming form frozen thawed eggs was 47.5%.

In 2010 Borini et al. (56) published a multicenter study with the outcome of egg freezing in Italy after the application of the law. The protocol used a two-step PROH–sucrose-based solution and, out of 2046 patients the overall survival rate was 55.8%. An overall pregnancy rate above 14% was achieved with a good degree of reproducibility in all the clinics. Another important aspect, besides the outcome, is the follow-up of the babies born from egg freezing. Noyes et al. (57) collected results from (58) reports ((43) using slow freeze, 12 vitrification and three both methods) between 1986 and 2008. The number of babies born was almost the same using slow freezing and vitrification (308 from slow freezing and 289 from vitrification and 12 from a combination of both protocols). The rate of single pregnancy was 81% compared to 19% for multiples. Moreover, the overall rate of birth anomalies has been reported to be eight: three ventricular septal cardiac defects, one choanal atresia, one biliary atresia, one Rubinstein–Taybi syndrome, one clubfoot, and one skin hemangioma. Fortunately, the offspring arising from frozen eggs have no significant difference in

Table 21.3 Recently Reported Rates of Survival, Fertilization, Cleavage, and Implantation Following Oocyte Cryopreservation

Reference	Method	No. of thawed oocytes	Survival (%)	2PN (%)	Cleavage (%)	Implantation (%)
Borini et al. (46)	PROH /0.3–0.3 mmol/L sucrose	927	74.1	76.1	90.2	5.2
Boldt et al. (26)	PROH /Na-depleted	190	59.5	67.9	n.r.	15.9
Chamayou et al. (45)	PROH /0.3–0.3 mmol/L sucrose	337	78.0	67.9	77.3	5.6
Levi Setti et al. (47)	PROH /0.3–0.3 mmol/L sucrose	1087	69	67.5	89.1	5.7
Bianchi et al. (25)	PROH /0.2–0.3 mmol/L sucrose	325	75.1	77.3	93.0	16.7
De Santis et al. (48)	PROH /0.3–0.3 mmol/L sucrose	396	71.2	80.4	91.0	5.7

Abbreviations: 2PN, two pronuclei; PROH, propanediol; n.r., not recorded.

abnormalities compared with naturally conceived children. Consequently it has been proposed to remove the "experimental" label from oocyte cryopreservation (58) and consider this technique as a routine procedure applicable in IVF laboratories.

SUMMARY

Oocyte freezing has been considered as an experimental procedure for decades while it would be an important tool to use in IVF routine. In fact, a safe and efficient program would be of substantial benefit for infertile patients and also for women at risk of losing their fertility due to radio- or chemotherapy treatments. Moreover, egg cryopreservation could replace embryo freezing which instead involves important legal and ethical drawbacks.

After the initial disappointment due to the low survival rate diverse methods have been developed raising the post-thaw recovery. The fertilization and cleavage performance of frozen eggs are now not so different from the fresh sibling oocytes, even though not a lot is known about the early implantation potential. Worldwide there is an increased interest in analyzing intrinsic factors connected to the ability of these eggs to give a live birth. What is clear up to now is that certain oocyte cryopreservation protocols may affect cell division and is thus being associated with low implantation rate. Other freezing methods, instead, seem not to affect the postimplantation development and are going to be used in laboratories as an alternative to embryo freezing.

It would be very important to have randomized studies that underline any possible differences between various technical approaches and also to obtain more data on the cumulative pregnancy rate and on the long-term follow-up of the babies born thanks to egg freezing. At the moment, as in the previous edition of this book, we still miss a large randomized prospective study.

REFERENCES

1. Mazur P. Equilibrium, quasiequilibriurn, and non-equilibriurn freezing of mammalian embryos. Cell Biophysiol 1990; 17: 53.
2. Trounson A, Mohr L. Human pregnancy following cryopreservation, thawing and transfer of an eight cell embryo. Nature 1983; 305: 707–9.
3. Wittingham DG. Fertilization in vitro and developmental to term of unfertilized mouse oocytes previously stored at −196°C. J Reprod Fertil 1977; 49: 89–94.
4. Chen C. Pregnancies after human oocyte cryopreservation. Lancet 1986; 1: 884–6.
5. Gook DA, Schiewe MC, Osborn SM, et al. Intracytoplasmic sperm injection and embryo development of human oocytes cryopreserved using 1,2-propanediol. Hum Reprod 1995; 10: 2637–41.
6. Eroglu A, Toner M, Toth T. Beneficial effect of microinjected trehalose on the cryosurvival of human oocytes. Fertil Steril 2002; 77: 152–8.
7. Wright D, Eroglu A, Toner M, Toth T. Use of sugar in cryopreservation of human oocytes. Reprod Biomed Online 2004; 9: 179–86.
8. Stachecki J, Cohen J, Willadsen S. Cryopreservation of unfertilized mouse oocytes: The effect of replacing sodium with choline in the freezing medium. Cryobiology 1998; 37: 346–54.
9. Paynter SJ, O'Neil L, Fuller BJ, Shaw RW. Membrane permeability of human oocytes in the presence of the cryoprotectant propane-1,2-diol. Fertil Steril 2001; 75: 532–8.
10. Paynter SJ, Borini A, Bianchi V, et al. Volume changes of mature human oocytes on exposure to cryoprotectant solutions used in slow cooling procedures. Hum Reprod 2005; 20: 1194–8.
11. De Santis L, Coticchio G, Paynter S, et al. Permeability of human oocytes to ethylene glycol and their survival and spindle configurations after slow cooling cryopreservation. Hum Reprod 2007; 22: 2776–83.
12. Pickering SJ, Braude PR, Johnson MH, et al. Transient cooling to room temperature can cause irreversible disruption of the meiotic spindle in the human oocyte. Fertil Steril 1990; 54: 102–8.
13. Zenzes MT, Bielecki R, Casper RF, Leibo SP. Effects of chilling to 0 degrees C on the morphology of meiotic spindles in human metaphase II oocytes. Fertil Steril 2001; 75: 769–77.
14. Pickering SJ, Johnson MH. The influence of cooling on the organization of the meiotic spindle of the mouse oocyte. Hum Reprod 1987; 2: 207–16.
15. Sato H, Ellis GW, Inouè S. Microtubular origin of mitotic spindle from birefringence: Demonstration of the applicability of Wiener's equation. J Cell Biol 1975; 67: 501–17.
16. Rienzi L, Martinez F, Ubaldi F, et al. Polscope analysis of meiotic spindle changes in living metaphase II human oocytes during the freezing and thawing procedures. Hum Reprod 2004; 19: 655–9.
17. Bianchi V, Coticchio G, Fava L, et al. Meiotic spindle imaging in human oocytes frozen with a slow freezing procedure involving high sucrose concentration. Hum Reprod 2005; 20:1078–83.
18. Sereni E, Sciajno R, Fava L, et al. A PolScope evaluation of meiotic spindle dynamics in frozen-thaw oocytes. Reprod Biomed Online 2009; 19: 191–7.
19. Bromfield JJ, Coticchio G, Hutt K, et al. Meiotic spindle dynamics in human oocytes following slow-cooling cryopreservation. Hum Reprod 2009; 24: 2114–23.
20. Coticchio G, Sciajno R, Hutt K, et al. Comparative analysis of the metaphase II spindle of human oocytes through polarized light and high-performance confocal microscopy. Fertil Steril 2010; 93: 2056–64.
21. Lassalle B, Testart J, Renard JP. Human embryo features that influence the success of cryopreservation with the use of 1,2 propanediol. Fertil Steril 1985; 44: 645–51.
22. Tucker M, Wright G, Morton P, et al. Preliminary experience with human oocyte cryopreservation using 1,2-propanediol and sucrose. Hum Reprod 1996; 11: 1513–15.
23. Borini A, Bonu MA, Coticchio G, et al. Pregnancies and births after oocyte cryopreservation. Fertil Steril 2004; 82: 601–5.
24. Fabbri R, Porcu E, Marsella T, et al. Human oocyte cryopreservation: New perspectives regarding oocyte survival. Hum Reprod 2001; 16: 411–16.
25. Bianchi V, Coticchio G, Distratis V, et al. Differential sucrose concentration during dehydration (0.2 mol/L) and rehydration (0.3 mol/L) increases the implantation

26. Boldt J, Tidswell N, Sayers A, et al. Human oocyte cryopreservation: 5-year experience with a sodium-depleted slow freezing method. Reprod Biomed Online 2006; 13: 96–100.
27. Quintans CJ, Donaldson MJ, Bertolino MV, Pasqualini RS. Birth of two babies using oocytes that were cryopreserved in a choline-based freezing medium. Human Reprod (Oxford, England) 2002; 17: 3149–52.
28. Petracco A, Azambuja R, Okada L, et al. Comparison of embryo quality between sibling embryos originating from frozen or fresh oocytes. Reprod Biomed Online 2006; 13: 497–503.
29. Parmigiani L, Cognigni GE, Bernardi S, et al. Freezing within 2 h from oocytes retrieval increases the efficiency of human oocyte cryopreservation when using slow freezing/rapid protocol with high sucrose concentration. Hum Reprod 2008; 23: 1771–7.
30. Lappi M, Magli MC, Muzzonigro F, et al. Early time of freezing affects the clinical outcome of oocyte cryopreservation. Hum Reprod 2009; 24(Suppl 1): 90.
31. Bianchi V, Lappi M, Bonu MA, Borini A. Elapsing time: a variable to consider in oocyte cryopreservation. Hum Reprod 2011; 26(Suppl 1): 197.
32. Cohen Y, Malcov M, Schwartz T, et al. Spindle imaging: a new marker for optimal timing of ICSI? Hum Reprod 2004; 19: 649–54.
33. Wang WH, Meng L, Hackett RJ, Keefe DL. Developmental ability of human oocytes with or without birefringent spindles imaged by Polscope before insemination. Hum Reprod 2001; 16: 1464–8.
34. De Santis L, Cino I, Rabelotti E, et al. Polar body morphology and spindle imaging as predictors of oocyte quality. Reprod Biomed Online 2005; 11: 36–42.
35. Madaschi C, Carvalho de et al. Spindle imaging: a marker for embryo development and implantation. Fertil Steril 2008; 90: 194–8.
36. Stachecki JJ, Munne S, Cohen J. Spindle organization after cryopreservation of mouse, human, and bovine oocytes. Reprod Biomed Online 2004; 8: 664–72.
37. Coticchio G, De Santis L, Rossi G, et al. Sucrose concentration influences the rate of human oocytes with normal spindle and chromosome configurations after slow-cooling cryopreservation. Hum Reprod 2006; 21: 1771–6.
38. Ducibella T. Biochemical and cellular insights into the temporal window of normal fertilization. Theriogenology 1998; 49:53–65.
39. Gualtieri R, Iaccarino M, Mollo V, et al. Slow cooling of human oocytes: ultrastructural injuries and apoptotic status. Fertil Steril 2009; 91: 1023–34.
40. Gook DA, Osborn SM, Johnston WI. Cryopreservation of mouse and human oocytes using 1,2-propanediol and the configuration of the meiotic spindle. Hum Reprod 1993; 8: 1101–9.
41. Kuwayama M, Vajta G, Kato O, Leibo SP. Highly efficient vitrification method for cryopreservation of human oocytes. Reprod Biomed Online 2005; 11: 300–8.
42. Edgar DH, Archer J, Bourne H. The application and impact of cryopreservation of early cleavage stage embryos in assisted reproduction. Hum Fertil (Camb) 2005; 8: 225–30.
43. Gabrielsen A, Fedder J, Agerholm I. Parameters predicting the implantation rate of thawed IVF/ICSI embryos: a retrospective study. Reprod Biomed Online 2006; 12: 70–6.
44. Bianchi V, Coticchio G, Distratis V, et al. Early cleavage delay in cryopreserved human oocytes. 2005; 20(Suppl 1): i54.
45. Chamayou S, Alecci C, Ragolia C, et al. Comparison of in-vitro outcomes from cryopreserved oocytes and sibling fresh oocytes. Reprod Biomed Online 2006; 12: 730–6.
46. i Borini A, Sciajno R, Bianchet al. Clinical outcome of oocyte cryopreservation after slow cooling with a protocol utilizing a high sucrose concentration. Hum Reprod 2006; 21: 512–17.
47. Levi Setti PE, Albani E, et al. Cryopreservation of supernumerary oocytes in IVF/ICSI cycles. Hum Reprod 2006; 21: 370–5.
48. De Santis L, Cino I, Rabellotti E, et al. Oocyte cryopreservation: clinical outcome of slow-cooling protocols differing in sucrose concentration. Reprod Biomed Online 2007; 14: 57–63.
49. Coticchio G, Di Stratis V, Bianchi V, et al. Fertilization and early developmental ability of cryopreserved human oocytes is not affected compared to sibling fresh oocytes. Fertil Steril 2007; 88(Suppl 1): 340.
50. Porcu E, Fabbri R, Seracchioli R, et al. Pregnancy of a healthy female after intracytoplasmic sperm injection of crypreserved human oocyte. Fertil Steril 1997; 68: 724–6.
51. Borini A, Bafaro MG, Bonu MA, et al. Pregnancies after oocyte freezing and thawings: preliminary data. Hum Reprod 1998; 13(Suppl): 124–5.
52. Li X-H, Chen S-U, Zhang X, et al. Cryopreserved oocyte in infertile couples undergoing assisted reproductive technology could be an important source of oocyte donation: a clinical report of successful pregnancies. Hum Reprod 2005; 20: 3390–4.
53. Fosas N, Marina F, Torres PJ, et al. The births of five Spanish babies from cryopreserved donated oocytes. Hum Reprod 2003; 18: 1417–21.
54. Tjer GC, Chiu TT, Cheung LP, et al. Birth of a healthy baby after transfer of blastocysts derived from cryopreserved human oocytes fertilized with frozen spermatozoa. Fertil Steril 2005; 83: 1547–9.
55. Borini A, Lagalla C, Bonu MA, et al. Cumulative pregnancy rates resulting from the use of fresh and frozen oocytes: 7 years' experience. Reprod Biomed Online 2006; 12: 481–6.
56. Borini A, Levi Setti PE, Anserini P, et al. Multicentric observational study on slow-cooling oocyte cryopreservation: Clinical outcome. Fertil Steril 2010; 94: 1662–8.
57. Noyes N, Porcu E, Borini A. Over 900 oocyte cryopreservation babies born with no apparent increase in congenital anomalies. Reprod Biomed Online 2009; 18: 769–76.
58. Noyes N, Boldt J, Nagy P. Oocyte cryopreservation: Is it time to remove its experimental label? J Assist Repro Genet 2010; 27: 69–7.

22

The human oocyte: Vitrification

Masashige Kuwayama

INTRODUCTION

The past 50 years have yielded impressive breakthroughs in cryopreservation as applied to the discipline of reproductive biology. Techniques were usually derived initially in experimental and domestic animals, and subsequently applied to humans. The first successes in freezing cells were achieved with spermatozoa (1), and were followed by successful cryopreservation of preimplantation embryos at different stages of development (2–4). Since the first report in 1972 of cryopreservation of mammalian embryos resulting in the birth of live offspring (2), attempts to cryopreserve human oocytes, similar to the results with oocytes of domestic animals, mostly failed for many years. However, the development of an ultra-rapid vitrification method now means that oocytes can be cryopreserved with little loss of their viability and such oocytes may be used clinically (5).

The reasons to cryopreserve human oocytes are widely known and were summarized recently (6). Common indications for this procedure include diseases and their treatments, that is, to preserve the reproductive competence of young cancer patients who need irradiation of the pelvic region or chemotherapy, or who require surgical intervention before or during their reproductive age that may involve removal of ovaries. Problems resulting from ovarian malfunction include premature menopause, ovarian hyperstimulation syndrome, or poor response to ovarian stimulation. Legal, ethical, social, and practical problems may also require oocyte cryopreservation. For example, many countries restrict or prohibit embryo cryopreservation; women may wish to delay motherhood for various reasons, such as career priorities; and there may be no semen available after a successful oocyte retrieval.

However, as discussed in detail recently (6), in broader terms oocyte cryopreservation is also needed to compensate for the unique situation of women with respect to reproduction. As in most mammalian species, women suffer more and sacrifice more for their offspring both physically and emotionally. Yet a woman's reproductive capability is restricted in terms of quantity and duration. Men produce millions of sperm in a single ejaculation, while women ovulate only one or two mature oocytes every 28 days. From the time that he reaches puberty, a man's reproductive capability is almost unlimited, while that of a woman (discounting special treatments) is limited to a period of just 15–20 years. Assisted reproductive techniques did not eliminate this difference. In fact, with the introduction of the procedure of intracytoplasmic sperm injection (ICSI) and successful cryopreservation of sperm, the gap has widened considerably. Apart from the practical goals, our moral duty is to help develop an efficient and safe oocyte cryopreservation method to enhance the reproductive capability of women.

Unfortunately, the task is rather demanding. Although the first pregnancy from cryopreserved oocyte was achieved more than 20 years ago (7), advances until recently were very slow. Generally, inefficiency and lack of consistency were the two main problems (8). Oocytes are unique cells. Their large size, spherical shape, single cell number, and general fragility explain many of the difficulties that occur during cryopreservation.

Oocytes are often described as the largest cells of the mammalian body. Cell volume is known to be a principal parameter that determines the likelihood of success when a cell is cryopreserved. Viruses and bacteria may survive deep freezing without any special treatment, such as use of cryoprotectants or controlled rate cooling. The resistance of microorganisms to damage from freezing may also be the source of potential problems in embryology. Freezing of fibroblasts or epidermal cells is usually an easy and efficient routine task in tissue culture laboratories, and does not need any special instruments. Sperm cryopreservation can be efficiently performed with the use of a controlled-rate freezer. Early cleavage-stage embryos with individual blastomeres having 50% to as little as 10% of the original size of oocytes survive traditional slow-rate freezing very well, and their developmental competence is usually well preserved. Preantral and primary follicles can also be frozen successfully, in contrast to the large, fully developed, metaphase II-stage (MII) oocytes.

The near-spherical shape of the oocyte does not confer an advantage from the point of view of cryopreservation. During equilibration and dilution before and after cooling and warming, permeable cryoprotectants must be distributed rapidly and uniformly throughout the ooplasm. A large spherical object, such as an oocyte, has the lowest surface area and volume ratio of any geometric shape. An irregular object, such as a fibroblast or lymphocyte, has a much larger surface area and volume ratio and will equilibrate osmotically much faster than an oocyte.

The one-cell stage of an oocyte also severely limits options, as there is no margin for error. The single cell survives OR it does not. Multicellular embryos may survive and develop even if more than 50% of their cells are damaged. (This fact is clearly demonstrated by successful births resulting from bisected embryos of domestic animals.)

However, apart from the size, shape, and cell number, other factors may also play an important role in limiting successful oocyte cryopreservation. Germinal vesicle (GV) stage oocytes and fertilized zygotes have almost exactly the same characteristics. However, zygotes are considerably more resistant to cryoinjuries while GV-stage oocytes are even more sensitive than MII-stage oocytes. Factors that are known to influence their sensitivity include chilling injury, serious deformation of shape during exposure to and/or removal of cryoprotectants, and hardening of the zona pellucida.

Chilling injury is probably one of the least understood types of injuries during cryopreservation, involving damage of lipid droplets, lipid-rich membranes, and microtubules. The temperature zone at which such injury occurs is rather high, between +15° (in some biological objects +20) and −5°C (9). The damage to lipids is irreversible and causes death of the oocytes. Compared with other species, the lipid content of human oocytes is relatively low. Yet, their sensitivity to chilling is still considerable, caused probably by membrane damage and depolymerization of microtubules, with all of the subsequent consequences, including misalignment of chromosomes and aneuploidy (10–14); however, the latter effect may be less detrimental than the earlier supposed effect (15). Chilling damage of membranes in human mature oocytes seems to be much more serious than at later developmental stages, for example, zygotes, a possible cause for the well-known stage-dependent sensitivity (16).

As a result of osmotic effects, serious deformation of the shape may occur when oocytes are exposed to cryoprotectant solutions. However, in spite of the somewhat peculiar morphology that oocytes may exhibit during exposure to cryoprotectants, they do seem to tolerate these deformations rather well. Careful addition of cryoprotectants may minimize deleterious effects of such morphological alterations. An alternative strategy, such as addition of cytoskeleton relaxants used with porcine embryos (17), may not be required in the human counterparts. On the other hand, during the removal of the cryoprotectant, the spherical shape of the oocyte may allow only a minimal expansion; accordingly, the inrushing water may disrupt the cell membrane.

VITRIFICATION VS. TRADITIONAL FREEZING

During the past two decades, two major strategies for cryopreservation of oocytes and embryos in mammalian species have been developed (18). Traditional slow-rate freezing establishes a delicate balance between various sources of injuries, while the principal goal of vitrification is to eliminate ice crystal formation entirely in the whole solution containing the embryos and oocytes. To achieve this ice-free glass-like solidification of solutions, which may also be defined as an extremely increased viscosity, high cryoprotectant concentrations and/or very high cooling rates are required. To decrease the potential osmotic and toxic damage caused by cryoprotectants, recent vitrification methods have focused on increasing the cooling and warming rates (19–22). Most successful vitrification methods are based on use of extremely small volumes of solution containing the specimens and direct contact between this solution and liquid nitrogen.

One of these approaches, the minimum drop size method was first applied by Arav (23), and further modified by Hamawaki et al. (24). Based on these earlier results, a novel method, called the Cryotop vitrification technique, was developed for cryopreservation of oocytes and embryos (25). The Cryotop has been used successfully to cryopreserve embryos from a wide variety of mammalian species, and has resulted in a considerable increase in the overall efficiency of cryopreservation of human oocytes and embryos (26–29).

USE OF THE CRYOTOP VITRIFICATION METHOD TO CRYOPRESERVE HUMAN MII-PHASE OOCYTES

The following is a description of the steps that should be followed carefully to utilize the Cryotop method to its full capability.

Timing

Oocytes should be vitrified between one and six hours after ovum pick-up, and immediately after denudation (cumulus cell removal). ICSI can be performed within two to four hours after the oocytes have been warmed. This short time of culture is required to allow the oocytes to recover the plasticity of their membranes during the puncture by the ICSI needle.

Device

The Cryotop consists of a 0.4 mm wide, 20 mm long, and 0.1 mm thick flexible filmstrip attached to a rigid plastic handle (Fig. 22.1). To protect the filmstrip and the sample cryopreserved on it, a 30 mm long transparent plastic cap is also provided to cover this part during storage in liquid nitrogen. The device is sterilized and should be handled under aseptic conditions and only for one cycle of vitrification.

Solutions

Media for all phases of vitrification are listed in Table 22.1.

Working Environment and Preparation Steps

The vitrification procedure has to be performed in a well-ventilated laboratory at room temperature of 25–27°C.

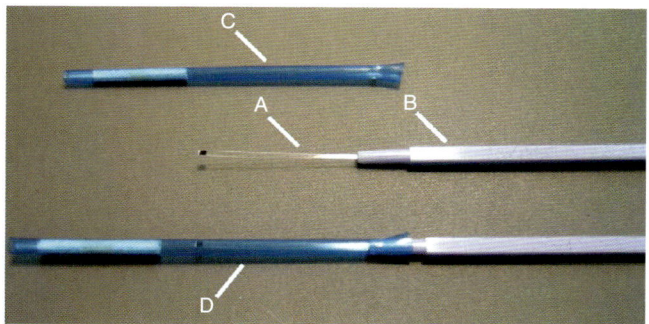

Figure 22.1 The Cryotop vitrification device. The polypropylene strip (**A**) is attached to a rigid plastic handle (**B**). After vitrification, a plastic cover (**C**) is attached to protect strip during storage in liquid nitrogen (**D**).

Table 22.1 Solutions Used for Cryotop Vitrification

Name	Basic medium	Permeable cryoprotectants	Nonpermeable cryoprotectants
Washing solution	M199 + 1% SSS	–	–
Equilibration solution	M199 + 1% SSS	7.5% EG, 7.5% DMSO	–
Vitrification solution	M199 + 1% SSS	15% EG, 15% DMSO	0.5 M sucrose
Thawing solution	M199 + 1% SSS	–	1.0 M sucrose
Dilution solution	M199 + 1% SSS	–	0.5 M sucrose

Abbreviations: DMSO, dimethyl sulfoxide; EG, ethylene glycol; M199, HEPES-buffered TCM 199 medium: SSS, synthetic serum substitute (Irvine Scientific, Santa Ana, California, USA). All chemicals except for otherwise indicated are derived from Sigma Chemical Co. (St Louis, Missouri, USA).

Because all equilibration and dilution parameters described below are adjusted for this temperature, it is very important to warm media that have been stored in the refrigerator to 25–27°C. This is easily achieved by placing all the solutions and vials on a clean bench for more than one hour, preferably inside a laminar-flow hood. The only exception is the thawing solution (TS) that should be warmed to 37°C to obtain the highest warming rate of the vitrified oocytes. Note that the basic solution contains HEPES buffer as well as bicarbonate buffer, and has been adjusted to maintain the appropriate pH even when exposed to air. Therefore, a carbon dioxide incubator is not required for warming of solutions in closed vials.

Additional Tools

Vitrification has to be performed in a 300 µL volume 3-well plate (Vitri-Plate, CryoTec Lab., Buenos Aires, Argentina) (Fig. 22.3). To obtain the optimum gradual change of osmolality of the extracellular solutions for the best post-thaw survival of the oocytes, it is very important that precise proportions of the volume of each solution and transferred solution be used. For practical reasons, a relatively small, thick-walled Styrofoam box (approximately 250 × 150 × 200 cm for length, width, and height) with a minimum of 3 cm thick walls and bottom is suggested, preferably with an appropriate Styrofoam cover. The box should be placed on a stable surface within easy reach but with little risk of accidentally spilling or pouring off the liquid nitrogen. All safety instructions related to work with liquid nitrogen should be strictly followed. Points for selection of optimal sources and possible pretreatment of liquid nitrogen will be discussed later. The Styrofoam box should also contain plastic racks for temporary storage of the device.

Cryotop vitrification requires adept handling of oocytes and embryos. For vitrification and warming, a relatively simple stereomicroscope equipped with a zoom lens and capable of providing sharp, contrast images is appropriate. Except for special purposes, there is no need for an upright or inverted compound microscope or for fluorescent equipment. There is no need to restrict illumination if light sources are filtered for UV lights. Use microscope lights only when required.

Equilibration and Cooling

Gently mix vials of prewarmed equilibration solution (ES) and vitrification solution (VS) (one vial of each). Pour 300 µL of ES into well 1, and 300 µL of VS into wells 2 and 3 in the proper three-well plate.

Before starting the vitrification procedure, check the quality and perivitelline space of the oocytes, and compare it with the thickness of the zona pellucida, and record any characteristics that might affect oocyte survival. The equilibration and vitrification procedure consists of the following steps (Fig. 22.2).

1. Place the oocytes in the center of the surface of ES. The oocytes will begin to contract osmotically and they will sink by their own density to the bottom of the well.
2. Contraction of the oocytes should occur at the latest within 90 seconds after placing them into the ES. Wait for 12 minutes and observe the recovery of the oocytes. If full re-expansion of oocytes occurs (the perivitelline space should be the same as before equilibration), oocytes should be picked up for the next step. If the volumetric recovery of the oocytes is incomplete, continue the equilibration until 15 minutes altogether. The recovery period can be used to prepare the liquid nitrogen container and to label the Cryotops (Fig. 22.3).
3. Pick up oocytes with the pipette, and expel the oocytes at the middle depth of VS1 with ES. Oocytes will immediately float to the surface of VS1. Expel and wash the inside of the pipette with fresh VS, and

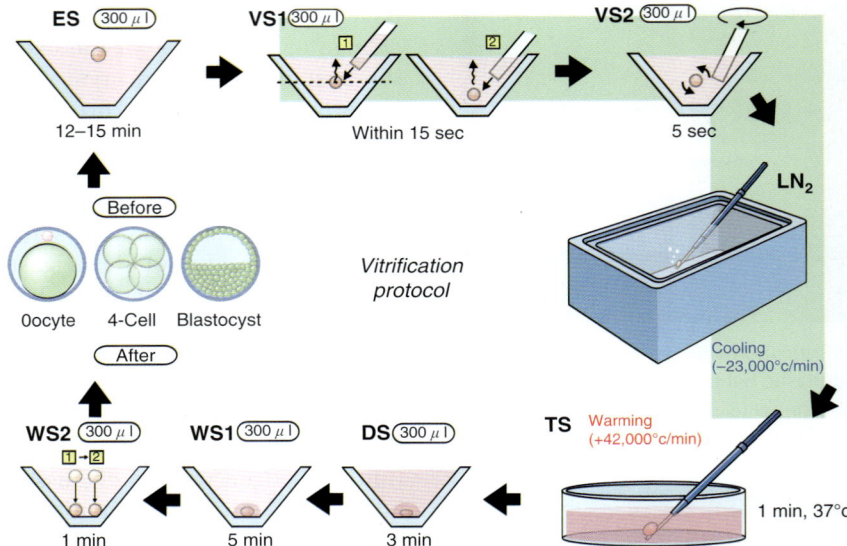

Figure 22.2 Protocol of oocyte vitrification.

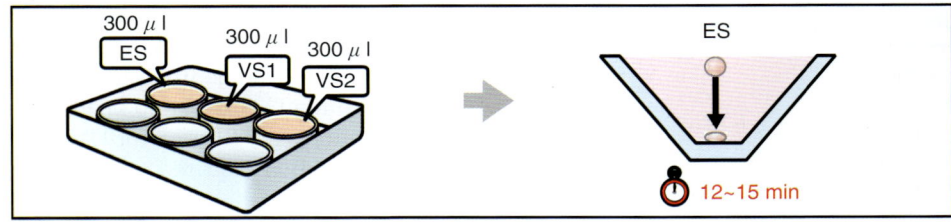

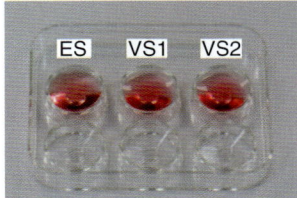

Figure 22.3 Preparation of plate for vitrification and equilibration procedure. See text for details. *Abbreviations*: ES, equilibration solution; VS, vitrification solution.

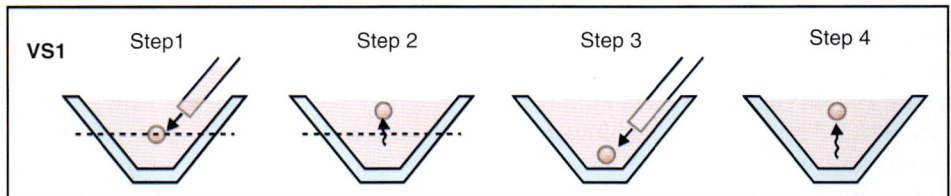

Figure 22.4 Vitrification solution equilibration procedure 1 (VS1) See text for details.

pick up the oocytes and expel them again at the bottom of VS. The oocytes will slowly float to the surface again. Ten seconds after the second rinse, expel and wash the inside of the pipette with fresh VS, and aspirate the oocytes at the top inside of pipette to move to VS2 (Fig. 22.4).

4. Expel the oocytes into the middle depth of VS2. Expel and aspirate fresh VS from the edge of surface, and expel it outside of the well. Aspirate fresh VS2 again from the surface. Blow out VS from the pipette and mix the solution around the oocyte to disperse the remainder of the previous solution (Fig. 22.5). Expel and wash the inside of the pipette with fresh VS, and aspirate the oocytes at the top inside of the pipette to put the oocytes on to the Cryotop.

5. Pick up the oocytes with the pipette in the smallest possible amount of solution and place them on the strip of the Cryotop near the black mark. Excess medium must be completely avoided or removed with the pipette after expelling the oocytes. If there

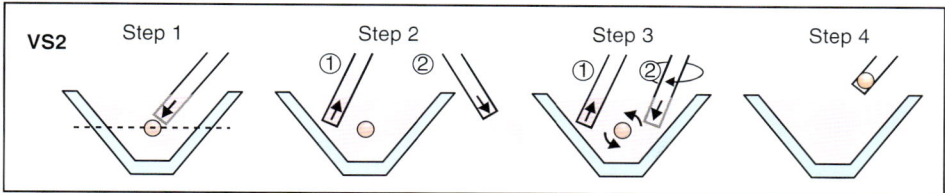

Figure. 22.5 Vitrification solution equilibration procedure 2 (VS2). See text for details.

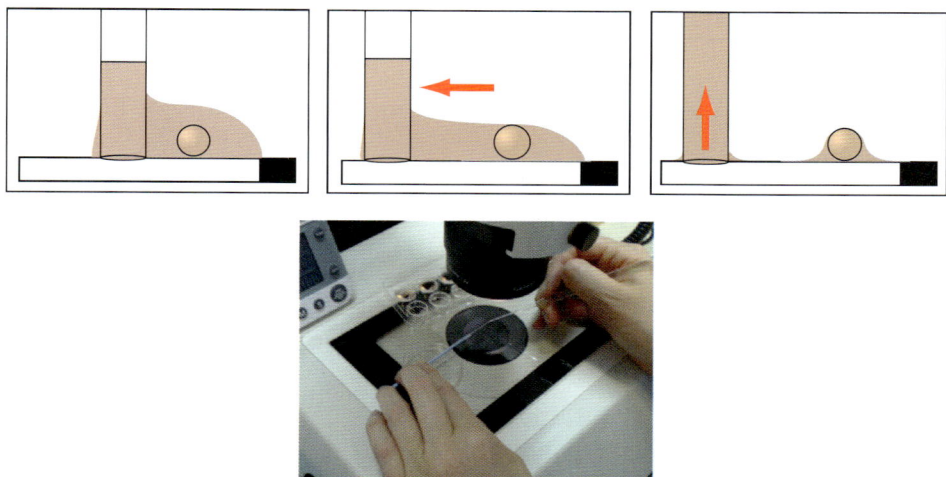

Figure 22.6 Arrangement of the oocyte on the filmstrip of the Cryotop. (How to minimize the vitrification solution containing oocyte on Cryotop before submerging in liquid nitrogen.)

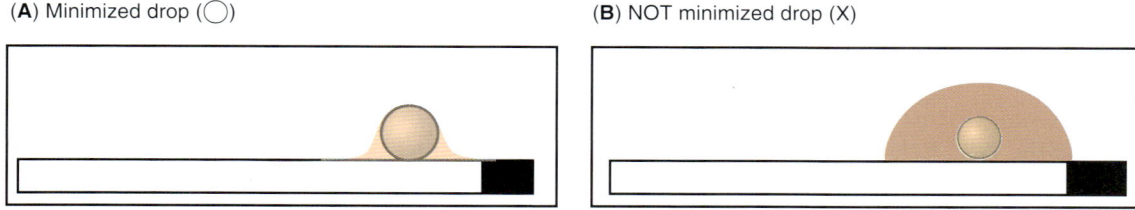

Figure 22.7 Minimized vitrification solution drop containing oocytes on Cryotop. (**A**) Minimized drop (○). (**B**) NOT minimized drop (X).

is too much medium, just remove it by using the pipette; medium will enter the pipette by capillarity (Figs. 22.6 and 22.7).

6. Immerse the Cryotop directly into the liquid nitrogen in the Styrofoam box and rapidly stir the Cryotop in the liquid nitrogen to obtain the maximum cooling rate (23,000°C/min). While keeping the Cryotop submerged in liquid nitrogen, cover the strip of the Cryotop with the plastic cap using tweezers.

Warming and Dilution

An unopened vial of TS and one Petri dish marked with TS should be prewarmed to 37°C in an incubator for at least one hour. All other solutions should be kept at room temperature, that is, 25–27°C.

Gently mix prewarmed DS and WS vials with an up-and-down movement. Pour 300 μL of DS into well 1, and 300 μL of WS into wells 2 and 3 in the proper three-well plate. Use the same procedure for the WS. However, prepare the dish just before the thawing to maintain its temperature to obtain the required warming rate (42,000°C/min).

The warming and dilution procedures consist of the following steps (dilution is also shown in Fig. 22.8):

1. Using tweezers, remove the plastic cap of the Cryotop while it is still submerged in liquid nitrogen. This manipulation can be performed easily if the Styrofoam box is filled almost entirely with liquid nitrogen. The container should be positioned close to the microscope to avoid delay when transferring the Cryotop. The microscope should be focused at the center of the WS dish with low magnification.

2. Hold the Cryotop and look for the black mark while maintaining the tip submerged in liquid nitrogen. Remove the Cryotop with a rapid movement from the

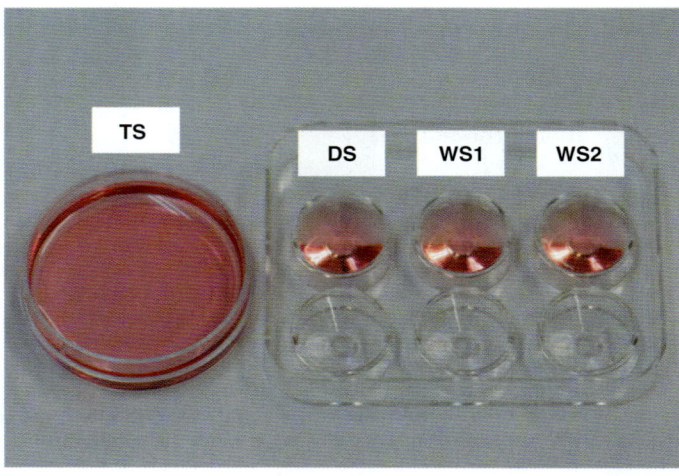

Figure 22.8 Preparation of the plate for thawing and thawing procedure. See text for details. *Abbreviations*: DS, dilution solution; TS, thawing solution; VS, vitrification solution; WS, washing solution.

liquid nitrogen and place the tip immediately into the middle of the WS plate.

3. Find the oocytes adjusting the focus on the black mark of the Cryotop sheet. One minute after immersing into TS, while keeping the Cryotop sheet in the middle of TS, oocytes will separate themselves from the Cryotop sheet and will begin to float. Follow all movements of the oocytes continuously, as they become transparent at this phase of the procedure and it is easy to lose them. Later, they will regain their normal appearance.

4. After 60 seconds total, gently pick up the oocytes into the capillary and also aspirate an additional 2 mm-long TS column to the end of the capillary. Transfer the capillary into the DS dish and expel the contents gently in the bottom: first the WS media, allowing it to form a small "mountain" of fluid, then the oocytes on the top of this mountain. Just do nothing. Wait for three minutes.

5. Subsequently, the same method of transfer should be applied but with different solutions: oocytes will be placed on the top of the mountain formed from DS medium in the WS1 dish for five minutes, without any stirring or mixing of the media.

6. After 5 minutes, place oocytes onto the surface of WS2 plate and wait for an additional 5 minutes.

7. Finally, oocytes are transferred into the culture dish and their morphology is examined under the stereomicroscope. ICSI can be performed after a recovery period of at least two hours.

THE DANGER OF LIQUID NITROGEN-MEDIATED DISEASE TRANSMISSION

Safety issues regarding open methods of vitrification have been discussed recently in detail (5,18,30). Liquid nitrogen may become contaminated with pathogenic agents and can transmit these agents to other samples stored in the same tank of liquid nitrogen. Under experimental conditions, transmission has also been demonstrated between embryological samples (31,32). Although no disease transmission related to liquid nitrogen-mediated contamination and embryo transfer has been reported for humans or animals during the past 30 years, a theoretical danger exists and should be minimized with rational measures. According to most observations, hermetical isolation of samples from liquid nitrogen or medium during cooling and thawing considerably decreases cooling and warming rates and, as a consequence, also reduces survival of oocytes. One reasonable solution to this problem is to separate cooling and thawing of oocytes from their storage. Cooling can be performed in liquid nitrogen that is directly provided from the factory, has not been in contact with any other biological samples, and has been filtered before use (33,34). For storage, samples may be sealed into a pre-cooled, hermetically isolated container, for example, 1 mL diameter CBS straw (IMV, L'Aigle, France). An analog of the system has been used for open pulled straw (OPS) vitrification (32) and the required instrument is commercially available (Vit-Set, Minitüb, Landshut, Germany) (30). At warming, the end of the 1 mL straw may be cut with sterile scissors while the rest of the straw is still submerged in liquid nitrogen, and the Cryotop can be quickly removed with a narrow forceps for immersion into the proper medium. However, high post-warm survival rates of oocytes have not been obtained in these partially closed or fully closed systems, possibly because of the lower cooling and warming rates than those in ultra-rapid vitrification. The fact is that no viral transmission problems have occurred after more than 500,000 cases of clinical applications of the Cryotop method for 11 years. This provides the best practical evidence for the safety of this method with respect to possible liquid nitrogen-mediated disease transmission.

RESULTS ACHIEVED WITH CRYOTOP VITRIFICATION OF HUMAN OOCYTES

The first baby born after human oocyte vitrification was achieved with the OPS technique (35). However, the survival rate was not too high and no replicate results were reported. This is similar to the first success of human oocyte freezing in 1986 (7). The OPS method may briefly expose the VS to liquid nitrogen, and it contains more than 1 μL volume of VS, which may cause a lower cooling rate. Nevertheless, this technique does work very well for mammalian embryos, even if less well for oocytes.

Before being cryopreserved, the potential development rate of oocytes is 100%. If some oocytes undergo serious damage during cryopreservation, those oocytes die, resulting in a lower overall survival rate. A lower survival rate is an evidence of increasing damage caused by cryopreservation. Therefore, especially in clinical applications of vitrification, it is very important that the highest survival be attained not only for the efficiency of the treatment but also to assure the likelihood of producing normal, healthy babies. Such high post-warm survival of oocytes can be obtained using an ultra-rapid vitrification method.

After the first successful report of oocyte vitrification with the Cryotop vitrification method in 2000 (25), the protocol has gradually become used around the world, being adapted for various clinical needs in each country.

In Japan, using this method, 91% post-thaw survival rate, 90% fertilization and 50% blastocyst formation rate after ICSI and in vitro culture were first reported (27). After embryo transfer, a pregnancy rate of 41% was achieved. The ultimate birth rate of those embryos that implanted was 83%. A total of 20 healthy babies were delivered in that clinical trial. This ultra-rapid vitrification method has been used to establish the first oocyte bank for unmarried cancer patients in 2001. More than 600 oocytes from 112 patients have been cryopreserved for their future IVF treatment use.

In the United States, Katayama et al. (26) repeatedly used the Cryotop method and achieved a post-thaw survival rate for oocytes of 97%, and they obtained the first live baby from a vitrified oocyte in the United States. They also established an oocyte bank for unmarried cancer patients and also for healthy women for social reasons in 2003.

In Spain, Cobo et al. (34) reported that the survival rate of 231 oocytes that were thawed after vitrification was 97%; the respective fertilization, cleavage, and blastocyst rates were 76%, 94%, and 49%. Embryo transfer performed on 23 patients resulted in a 65% pregnancy rate, although with a miscarriage rate of 20%. The Spanish team is the largest IVF unit in Europe and has used oocyte vitrification for an egg donation program (36). More than 1000 healthy babies have been born from oocytes that were vitrified by this team alone.

In Italy, embryo preservation has not been permitted and the number of oocytes that may be used for insemination has been limited to a maximum of three for a long time. Therefore, there has been a clear need for a reliable oocyte cryopreservation technique. The Cryotop method was introduced in Italy in 2006, and rather quickly became widely used in response to patients' needs. Of 330 oocytes, Antinori et al. (37) achieved a post-thaw survival rate of 99%, a fertilization rate of 93%, and a pregnancy rate of 33%. The method has been adopted for routine application in IVF treatment. In addition, analogous high rates of post-thaw survival of oocytes after vitrification have also been attained in Mexico and Colombia. More than 2000 babies have been delivered ((38); Dr Ruvalcaba, pers. commun.).

As a result of personal communication with colleagues in several countries, I estimate that more than 30,000 oocytes have been cryopreserved by the Cryotop method, and more than 3000 healthy babies have been delivered thus far. The fact that such results have been reported by several independent clinical groups in different countries with no direct or commercial connection for the past decade may indicate that a reliable clinical procedure to cryopreserve human oocytes has been obtained.

CONCLUSION

Cryopreservation of oocytes is regarded as one of the most demanding tasks of human assisted reproduction. With scrupulous attention to numerous details and proper application of the latest vitrification techniques, efficiency of the procedure has been substantially improved. The Cryotop vitrification method has resulted in high rates of survival, fertilization, pregnancy, and births, comparable to those achieved with nonvitrified control oocytes. The technique can be useful in diverse situations where oocyte storage is required or considered.

ACKNOWLEDGMENTS

The author is very grateful to Prof. Stanley Leibo for the critical reading of the manuscript and to Dr Noriko Kagawa for her excellent support of the work.

REFERENCES

1. Polge C, Smith AY, Parkes AS. Revival of spermatozoa after vitrification and dehydration at low temperatures. Nature (London) 1949; 164: 666.
2. Whittingham DG, Leibo SP, Mazur P. Survival of mouse embryos frozen to −196°C and -269°C. Science 1972; 178: 411–14.
3. Wilmut I. The effect of cooling rate, warming rate, cryoprotective agent and stage of development on survival of mouse embryos during freezing and thawing. Life Sci 1972; 11: 1071–9.
4. Trounson A, Mohr L. Human pregnancy following cryopreservation, thawing, and transfer of an eight-cell embryo. Nature 1983; 305: 707–9.
5. Kuwayama M. Highly efficient vitrification for cryopreservation of human oocytes and embryos: the Cryotop method. Theriogenology 2007; 67: 73–80.
6. Kuwayama M, Cobo A, Vajta G. Vitrification of oocytes: general considerations and the use of the Cryotop method. In: Tucker MJ, Liebermann J, eds. Vitrification in Assisted Reproduction. London: Informa Healthcare, 2008: 119–28.
7. Chen C. Pregnancy after human oocyte cryopreservation. Lancet 1986; 1: 884–6.
8. Liebermann J, Tucker MJ. Comparison of vitrification and conventional cryopreservation of day 5 and day 6 blastocysts during clinical application. Fertil Sterill 2006; 86: 20–6.
9. Leibo SP, Martino A, Kobayashi S, Pollard JW. Stage-dependent sensitivity of oocytes and embryos to low temperatures. Anim Reprod Sci 1996; 42: 45–53.
10. Magistrini M, Szollosi D. Effects of cold and of isopropyl N-phenylcarbamate on the second meiotic spindle of mouse oocytes. Eur J Cell Biol 1980; 22: 699–707.
11. Sathananthan AH, Ng SC, Trounson AO, et al. The effects of ultrarapid freezing on meiotic and mitotic spindles of oocytes and embryos. Gam Res 1998; 21: 385–401.
12. Pickering SJ, Braude PR, Johnson MH, Cant A, Currie J. Transient cooling to room temperature can cause irreversible disruption of the meiotic spindle in the human oocyte. Fertil Steril 1990; 54: 102–8.
13. Fabbri R, Porcu E, Marsella T, et al. Human oocyte cryopreservation: new perspectives regarding oocyte survival. Hum Reprod 2001; 16: 411–16.
14. Stachecki JJ, Munne S, Cohen J. Spindle organization after cryopreservation of mouse, human, and bovine oocytes. Reprod BioMed Online 2004; 8: 664–72.
15. Stachecki JJ, Munne S, Cohen J. Spindle organization after cryopreservation of mouse, human, and bovine oocytes. Reprod BioMed Online 2004; 8: 664–72.
16. Ghetler Y, Yavin S, Shalgi R, Arav A. The effect of chilling on membrane lipid phase transition in human oocytes and zygotes. Hum Reprod 2005; 20: 3385–9.
17. Dobrinsky JR, Pursel VG, Long CR, Johnson LA. Birth of piglets after transfer of embryos cryopreserved by cytoskeletal stabilization and vitrification. Biol Reprod 2000; 62: 564–70.
18. Vajta G, Nagy PZ. Are programmable freezers still needed in the embryo laboratory? Review on vitrification. Reprod Biomed Online 2006; 12: 779–96.
19. Martino A, Songsasen N, Leibo SP. Development into blastocysts of bovine oocytes cryopreserved by ultrarapid cooling. Biol Reprod 1996; 54: 1059–69.
20. Vajta G, Holm P, Kuwayama M, et al. Open pulled straw (OPS) vitrification: a new way to reduce cryoinjuries of bovine ova and embryos. Mol Reprod Dev 1998; 51: 53–8.
21. Lane M, Schoolcraft WB, Gardner DK. Vitrification of mouse and human blastocysts using a novel cryoloop container-less technique. Fertil Steril 1999; 72: 1073–8.
22. Lane M, Bavister BD, Lyons EA, Forest KT. Containerless vitrification of mammalian oocytes and embryos. Nature Biotechnol 2001; 17: 1234–6.
23. Arav A. Vitrification of oocytes and embryos. In: Lauria A, Gandolfi F, eds. New Trends in Embryo Transfer. Cambridge, UK: Portland Press, 1992: 255–64.
24. Hamawaki A, Kuwayama M, Hamano S. Minimum volume cooling method for bovine blastocyst vitrification. Theriogenology 1999; 51: 165.
25. Kuwayama M, Kato O. All-round vitrification method for human oocytes and embryos. J Assist Reprod Genet 2000; 17: 477.
26. Katayama P, Stehlik J, Kuwayama M, Kato O, Stehlik E. High survival rate of vitrified human oocytes results in clinical pregnancy. Fertil Steril 2003; 80: 223–4.
27. Kuwayama M, Vajta G, Kato O, Leibo S. Highly efficient vitrification method for cryopreservation of human oocytes. Reprod Biomed Online 2005; 11: 300–8.
28. Kuwayama M, Vajta G, Ieda S, Kato O. Vitrification of human embryos using the CryoTip™ method. Reprod Biomed Online 2005; 11: 608–14.
29. Kuwayama M, Leibo S. Cryopreservation of human embryos and oocytes. J Mamm Ova Res 2010; 25: 79–86.
30. Vajta G, Kuwayama M, Vanderzwalmen P. Disadvantages and benefits of vitrification. In: Tucker MJ, Liebermann J, eds. Vitrification in Assisted Reproduction. London: Informa Healthcare, 2008: 33–44.
31. Bielanski A, Nadin-Davis S, Sapp T, Lutze-Wallace C. Viral contamination of embryos cryopreserved in liquid nitrogen. Cryobiology 2000; 40: 110–16.
32. Bielanski A, Bergeron H, Lau PC, Devenish J. Microbial contamination of embryos and semen during long-term banking in liquid nitrogen. Cryobiology 2003; 46: 146–52.
33. Vajta G, Lewis IM, Kuwayama M, Greve T, Callesen H. Sterile application of the Open Pulled Straw (OPS) vitrification method. Cryo Lett 1998; 19: 389–92.
34. Cobo A, Kuwayama M, Pérez S, et al. Comparison of concomitant outcome achieved with fresh and cryopreserved donor oocytes vitrified by the Cryotop method. Fertil Steril 2008; 89: 1657–64.
35. Kuleshova L, Gianaroli L, Magli C, Trounson A. Birth following vitrification of a small number of human oocytes. Hum Reprod 1999; 14: 3077–9.
36. Cobo A, Remohi J, Chang CC, Nagy ZP. Oocyte cryopreservation for donor egg banking. Reprod Biomed Online 2011; 11: 300–8.
37. Antinori M, Licata E, Dani G, et al. Cryotop vitrification of human oocytes results in high survival rate and healthy deliveries. Reprod Biomed Online 2007; 14: 72–9.
38. Lucena E, Bernal DP, Lucena C, et al. Successful ongoing pregnancies after vitrification of oocytes. Fertil Steril 2006; 85: 108–11.

23

The human embryo: Slow freezing*

Nikica Zaninovic, Richard Bodine, Robert N. Clarke, Sam Jones, Ye Zhen, and Lucinda L. Veeck Gosden

*This chapter was originally written by Lucinda L. Veeck Gosden; it has been revised and updated by Nikica Zaninovic for this book.

OVERVIEW

Since the birth of the first in vitro fertilization (IVF) baby in 1979, there have been numerous advances in the field of assisted reproductive technique (ART), including improvements in hormonal stimulation regimens, the formulation of optimal embryo culture media, and refinements in embryo replacement techniques. As a result, it has become a common occurrence in many ART programs to have patients with large numbers of good-quality embryos or blastocysts available for transfer. In addition, there are times when patients with certain medical conditions may need to freeze all conceptuses in lieu of transfer. Thus, the need for an adequate embryo cryopreservation program in most centers has evolved from one of luxury to one of necessity.

Until the mid-1990s, the number of ART centers performing cryopreservation and the pregnancy results following the transfer of cryopreserved–thawed conceptuses were relatively low. By way of comparison, as early as 1989, Fugger (1) reported results from 25 IVF member institutions of the Society of Assisted Reproductive Technique (SART) with cryopreservation experience. In these centers, the total number of cleaved embryos and blastocysts frozen was 4460 and 341, respectively. The average clinical pregnancy rate per transfer was 13.4%. In contrast, 1999 results reported by the SART registry from 348 ART programs in the United States performing cryopreservation indicated that over 12,000 cryo–thaw cycles were initiated resulting in an overall clinical pregnancy rate per transfer of 24.1% and a delivery rate per transfer of 18.6% (2). While these percentages are far lower than those reported for fresh IVF cycles (38.0% and 31.6%, respectively), many centers today experience higher cryopreservation/thaw success rates, almost equivalent to their fresh counterparts. Indeed, advances in these techniques, procedures, and cryoprotective media have made cryopreservation an important adjunct treatment for many ART patients. This is reflected in a 1999 report from Hoffman et al. (3), who estimated that nearly 400,000 embryos were frozen and stored in ART centers in the United States. This number today is most likely much higher. SART data for 2009 (www.sart.org) revealed that over 20,000 frozen embryo transfers (FETs) were performed in the United States with an overall delivery rate per transfer of 27.4% across all age groups. Interestingly, there was a trend of higher delivery rate in FET cycles compared with the fresh cycles in patents over 40 years old. This can be a reflection of the good prognosis patients in FET groups who have embryos frozen and "younger" age of the embryos at the time of freezing.

Before cryopreservation methods were common in human ART practice, a patient with multiple oocytes harvested had few options for optimizing her IVF attempt, and most of these options resulted in either clinical or ethical dilemmas. Patients would sometimes choose to only inseminate the number of oocytes equal to the number of embryos they were willing to transfer. Since there was no guarantee of 100% fertilization and some embryos would surely be of poor quality, suboptimal transfers were commonplace in these situations. Alternatively, patients choosing to inseminate all available oocytes were often faced with the possibility of having to discard or donate potentially viable conceptuses after transfer.

Since the birth of the first child following the transfer of a cryopreserved human embryo in 1983 (4) and human blastocyst in 1985 (5), much work has been performed by embryologists, clinicians, and animal researchers to optimize methods for freezing and thawing human conceptuses. These studies have focused primarily on methods and/or identification of clinical or laboratory variables which affect potential clinical outcome following cryopreservation. Method studies have focused on the formulation of cryopreservation media (including type and concentration of cryoprotectant and the addition of dehydrating agents), cryopreservation equipment, and post-thaw culture conditions. Clinical cryopreservation reports have attempted to identify factors that affect cryopreservation/thawing success and outcome, including patient age, stimulation regimens, embryo quality considerations, timing of thawed conceptus transfer, and the methods for endometrial preparation for transfer.

It is safe to say that, in general, patient variables that affect clinical outcome of fresh cycles will similarly alter the success of cryopreserved cycles. Similar to fresh cycles, advanced patient age has a negative effect on pregnancy rate following the transfer of thawed conceptuses (6,7). In addition, Toner and Veeck (8) found basal follicle-stimulating hormone levels and age to affect embryo cryopreservation outcome. It is well accepted that the transfer of good-quality fresh embryos results in higher pregnancy rates than the transfer of morphologically poor or developmentally delayed ones. Similarly, the transfer of good-quality frozen and thawed conceptuses results in more optimal clinical outcomes (6,9–11). There appears to be no effect of patient stimulation regimen on subsequent clinical outcome following cryopreservation (12).

There are conflicting reports on the effect of other clinical factors on cryopreservation success, including the role of intracytoplasmic sperm injection (ICSI), the method of endometrial preparation, and the timing of transfer. While Oehninger et al. (12) reported no difference between ICSI or inseminated frozen–thawed embryos in terms of survival or subsequent clinical pregnancy rates, another report (13) demonstrated higher post-thaw mortality and pregnancy losses in ICSI frozen–thawed embryos. Similarly, Oehninger et al. (12) reported no difference between natural or programmed replacement thaw cycles, while Loh and Leong (14) found endometrial preparation to be the most important factor in determining post-thaw clinical success. In the Cornell ART Program, we have found neither the method of fertilization nor that of endometrial preparation to be critical factors in subsequent post-thaw clinical success.

Much of the improved success in clinical outcome of thawed human cycles can be traced to overall improvements in embryo culture conditions which have resulted in better-quality fresh embryos and blastocysts available for cryopreservation. Formulation of improved culture media and more optimal culture conditions over recent years have contributed to higher clinical success rates for fresh and frozen conceptuses. Many of these improvements have stemmed from earlier animal experiments, including the use of ultra-microfluorometry in determining very subtle changes in mouse embryo metabolism during embryo culture (15). In 2002, Lane et al. (16) showed that the addition of ascorbate to mouse embryo culture media resulted in lower hydrogen peroxide accumulation and increased the development of the inner cell mass of resulting blastocysts. It still remains unclear whether these types of medium additives prove beneficial to the culture of human fresh and frozen conceptuses.

The type of cryoprotectant and the use of dehydrating agents such as sucrose are important considerations in a cryopreservation program. Most ART centers are using either 1,2 propanediol (PROH) or dimethyl sulfoxide (DMSO) as the cryoprotectant of choice for embryos, while glycerol is routinely used when freezing human blastocysts. Sucrose has been added in many cases to both systems to aid in cellular dehydration and reduce osmotic shock. Method of cooling (slow freezing vs. vitrification) is also an important consideration. The majority of ART laboratories are using slow-cooling methods for freezing human conceptuses, based on the original work of Testart (17,18) while most of the human blastocyst freezing protocols have evolved from the earlier work of Menezo (19,20). Many laboratories have modified these original protocols over the years, and some have found that very subtle changes in freezing procedures can improve post-thaw results. Recently, Gardner et al. (21) showed that changing the starting temperature and cooling rate in a slow-freezing protocol significantly increased human blastocyst post-thaw viability. Rapid-freezing techniques (vitrification) have gained popularity recently (22–26). During slow freezing, embryos are exposed to the low concentration of cryoprotectants at a controlled rate of freezing, avoiding intracellular ice crystal formation. On the contrary, during vitrification, embryos are exposed to high concentration of cryoprotectants and directly immersed into liquid nitrogen, solidifying the embryo without ice crystal formations. The feasibility of using vitrification for embryo freezing of all developmental stages has been shown recently (26). With comparable or even better survival rates and pregnancies, vitrification has become a more attractive method than slow freezing as it does not require expensive equipment and is not time-consuming. The main concern is the potential toxic effect of high concentrations of the cryoprotectants and the potential risk of cross-contamination via direct exposure to the liquid nitrogen (26,27).

METHODS

The primary goal in establishing an appropriate freezing protocol is to do as little damage as possible while exposing specimens to nonphysiologic ultra-low temperatures. Popular protocols essentially *freeze-dry* or dehydrate blastocysts to prevent intracellular ice from forming.

The formation of intracellular ice crystals can mechanically damage specimens by disrupting and displacing organelles, or slicing through membranes. This is why freezing techniques use cryoprotective agents and control ice formation at critical temperatures. It has been shown that when human cells are placed into a medium that contains an intracellular cryoprotective agent, intracellular water readily exits the cell as a result of the higher extracellular concentration of cryoprotectant. This causes some cell shrinkage until osmotic equilibrium is reached by the slower diffusion of the cryoprotectant into the cell. Once equilibrium is reached, the cell resumes a normal appearance. The rate of permeation of cryoprotectant and water is dependent on temperature; equilibrium is achieved faster at higher temperatures. However, some cryoprotectants like DMSO are toxic at elevated concentrations and must be used at lower temperatures to reduce adverse effects.

Cryoprotectants are also beneficial in their ability to lower the freezing point of a solution. Solutions may remain unfrozen at −5°C to −15°C because of *super cooling* (cooling to well below the freezing point without extracellular ice formation). When solutions turn supercool, cells do not dehydrate appropriately since there is no increase in osmotic pressure from the formation of extracellular ice crystals. To prevent super-cooling, an ice crystal is introduced in a controlled fashion in the process called *seeding*. This contributes to intracellular dehydration as water leaves the cell to achieve equilibrium with the extracellular environment. If the rate of cooling is too rapid, water cannot pass quickly enough from the cell, and as temperature continues to drop, it reaches a point when the intracellular solute concentration is not high enough to prevent the formation of ice crystals.

Membrane permeability by cryoprotectants varies between developmental stages. While DMSO and 1,2 propanediol (PROH) are frequently used for freezing early cleavage-stage embryos, glycerol is commonly used for blastocysts. All three intracellular agents have fairly small molecules that permeate cell membranes easily. In addition to these, there are several extracellular substances that help dehydrate and protect cells. The most frequently used is sucrose, which possesses large, non-permeating molecules and exerts an osmotic effect to aid in accelerated cell dehydration. Sucrose cannot be used alone but is often used in conjunction with standard permeating, intracellular cryoprotectants.

Most embryo-freezing protocols used today are based loosely on the original work from the mid-1980s by Jacques Testart and his colleagues (17,18). On the other hand, most blastocyst-freezing protocols have evolved from the published work of Yves Ménézo (19,20). Cornell methods utilize PROH for embryo stages, and glycerol for blastocysts; sucrose aids cell dehydration. All specimens have been frozen in sterile cryovials within a cryoprotectant medium volume of 0.3 mL. A Planer Series III biological freezer (Kryo10–1.7, TS Scientific, Perkasie, Pennsylvania, USA) is utilized. The Cornell protocols have been amended from the early published work in several ways to fit our current needs. Modifications include (*i*) the base medium is a phase I sequential formulation, modified by HEPES buffers; (*ii*) extra macromolecules (protein) are added in the form of 30% Plasmanate (Telecris, Research Triangle Park, North Carolina, USA); and (*iii*) for blastocysts, the freezing cryoprotectant concentration is elevated to 10% and additional dilutions are included for the thawing process.

Embryo Freezing

Embryos are exposed to increasing concentrations of cryoprotective medium at room temperature: 0.5 M/L PROH for five minutes, 1.0 M/L PROH for five minutes, 1.5 M/L PROH for 10 minutes, and 1.5 M/L PROH/0.2 M sucrose for 10 seconds. They are then loaded into cryovials containing 1.5 M/L PROH/0.2 M sucrose. Cryovials are equilibrated for 15 minutes at room temperature before being cooled at a rate of −2.0°C/min until −7.0°C. They are held for five minutes, manual seeding is performed, and they are held for an additional five minutes. Cooling is continued at a rate of −0.3°C/min until −30°C. Cryovials are then plunged into liquid nitrogen.

Embryo Thawing

Cryovials are warmed in a 3°C water bath for 30–90 seconds and then held for five minutes at room temperature before embryos are removed. Embryos are taken through decreasing concentrations of cryoprotective medium: 1.0 M/L PROH/0.2 M sucrose for three minutes, 0.75 M/L PROH/0.2 M sucrose for three minutes, 0.5 M/L PROH/0.2 M sucrose for three minutes, 0.25 M/L PROH/0.2 M sucrose for three minutes, and (no PROH/0.2 M sucrose for three minutes. Specimens are then washed thoroughly and incubated until intrauterine transfer.

Blastocyst Freezing (7)

Blastocysts are exposed to two concentrations of cryoprotective medium at room temperature: 5% glycerol solution for 10 minutes and 10% glycerol/0.2 M/L sucrose solution for 10 minutes. They are then loaded into cryovials and cooled at a rate of −2.0°C/min until −7.0°C. Cryovials are held for five minutes, manual seeding is performed, and they are held for another 10 minutes. Cooling is continued at −0.3°C/min until −38°C. Cryovials are then plunged into liquid nitrogen.

Blastocyst Thawing (7)

Cryovials are thawed at room temperature for 60 seconds before being warmed in a 30°C water bath for 30–90 seconds (until all ice is removed). Blastocysts are removed from the cryovials and taken through decreasing concentrations of cryoprotective medium: 10% glycerol + 0.4 M/L sucrose for 30 seconds, 5% glycerol + 0.4 M/L sucrose solution for three minutes, 0.4 M/L sucrose solution (no glycerol) for three minutes, 0.2 M/L sucrose solution (no glycerol) for 2 minutes, and 0.1 M/L sucrose solution (no glycerol) for 1 minutes. Specimens are then washed thoroughly and incubated until transfer. Blastocysts frozen on day 5 are incubated overnight; blastocysts frozen on day 6 are transferred the same day as thawing.

REPLACEMENT STRATEGIES IN CORNELL (7)

At Cornell, frozen–thawed conceptuses are replaced in either natural or programmed cycles. Natural cycles are not supplemented with progesterone unless there is an overwhelming reason to do so, and all women are treated in a prophylactic manner for four days with antibiotics and corticosteroids.

Natural Cycle Replacement (Used in Ovulatory Cycles with Normal Concentrations of Luteal Phase Progesterone)

Supplemental progesterone is not administered unless medically indicated or unless the patient experienced a previous pregnancy failure using a nonsupplemented protocol. If administered, 200 mg micronized progesterone is given vaginally b.i.d. or t.i.d. and continued until a negative pregnancy test 14 days after replacement or through week 12 if pregnant (weaned down starting weeks 9–10). Medrol (16 mg/day) and tetracycline (250 mg, q.i.d.) are administered two days prior to embryo transfer.

Cleavage embryos are thawed one day after ovulation (two days after luteinizing hormone (LH) peak and/or a day after estradiol dip) and transferred on the day of thawing.

Blastocysts are thawed four days after the LH peak and transferred on the following day (day 5 blastocysts) or thawed five days after LH peak and transferred on the same day (day 6 blastocysts).

Programmed Cycle Replacement (Adequate Suppression Confirmed on Day 2 of Cycle)

Luteal suppression is accomplished using 0.2 mg gonadotropin-releasing hormone agonist (GnRHa). This dosage is reduced to 0.1 mg starting on the predetermined day 1 of the cycle and maintained until day 15.

Transdermal estrogen patches (Climara, 0.1 mg patch) are administered as follows: days 1–4, 0.1 mg every other day; days 5–8, 0.2 mg every other day; days 9–10, 0.3 mg every other day (depending on estradiol concentrations); days 11–14, 0.4 mg every other day; days 15+, 0.2 mg (two patches every other day, seven weeks).

Progesterone (50 mg i.m.) is administered beginning on day 15 through 12 weeks' gestation (weaned down starting week 9–10, depending on serum concentrations). Medrol (16 mg/day) and tetracycline (250 mg, q.i.d.) are administered two days prior to transfer. Embryos are thawed on day 17 and transferred the same day; blastocysts frozen on day 5 are thawed on day 19 and transferred the following day; blastocysts frozen on day 6 are thawed on day 20 and transferred the same day.

RESULTS

Embryos

Embryos freeze well and implant at acceptable rates after thaw and transfer. Almost any embryo stage specimen can be frozen successfully, from one-cell to blastocyst. Retrospective analysis of the last 10 years at Cornell freezing program showed 2PN (one-cell) survival rate of 66% (921 thawed); cleavage-stage embryos (day 2 or 3) of 76% (920 thawed); and blastocysts of 79% (4919 thawed). One-cell freezing is primarily indicated for patients with fertility preservation where a high number of zygotes are frozen. The drawbacks of this freezing stage are the unknown growth and quality of the embryos (28).

Freezing of cleavage stage embryos is fairly convenient because there are no urgent timing considerations. In addition, information is known about both morphology and growth rate, allowing the selection of potentially viable conceptuses for either fresh transfer or storage. It has become extremely common in the last decade to choose embryos with the best morphology for fresh transfer and to freeze others with acceptable morphology only after fresh selection has been made.

Sometimes survival after thaw is difficult to evaluate because not all blastomeres endure the rigors of freezing and thawing. Dying blastomeres may be present among living ones, but these can be removed easily by aspirating them out through an artificial hole in the zona pellucida. Generally, an embryo possessing >50% viable blastomeres upon thaw is considered a survivor (Figs. 23.1–23.6).

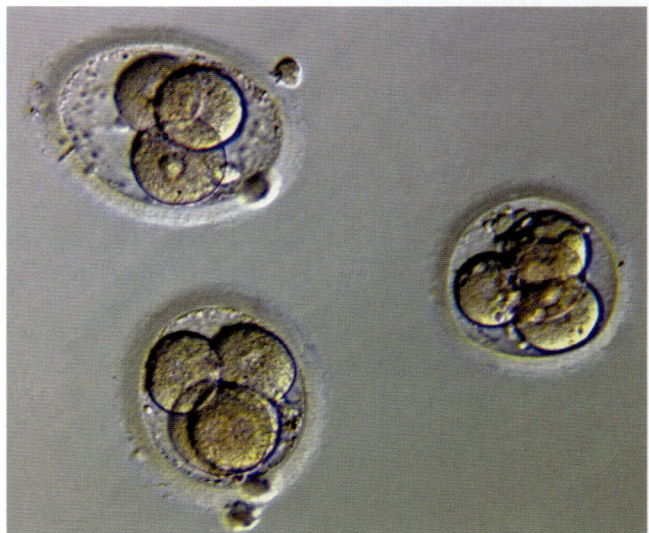

Figure 23.1 Three embryos that were frozen longer than 5 years. Upon thawing, two of the three were completely intact (lower and right). The third displayed three surviving blastomeres of a total of four. The degenerative blastomere was removed through micromanipulative procedures. Following the transfer of these three conceptuses to a 42-year-old woman who had conceived in her fresh cycle, implantation failed to occur.

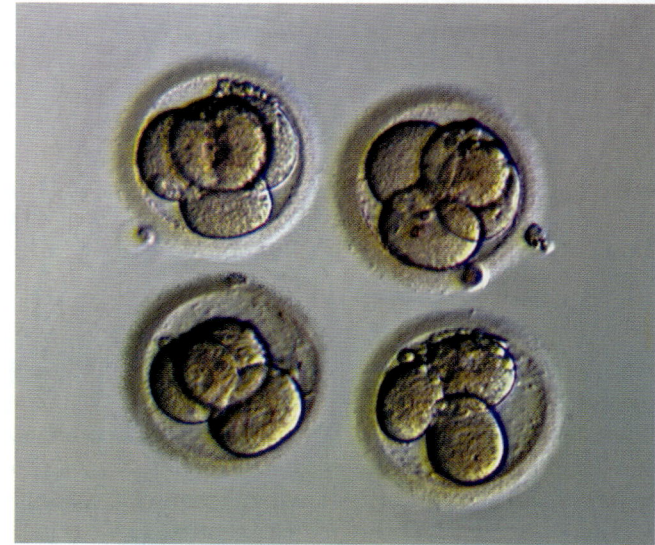

Figure 23.2 In this example, two of four embryos, stored for 861 days, survived thawing with all blastomeres intact. The remaining two conceptuses lost a single blastomere during the process. Degenerative cells were removed before intrauterine transfer to a 35-year-old woman. A singleton pregnancy was established and a healthy male child was delivered.

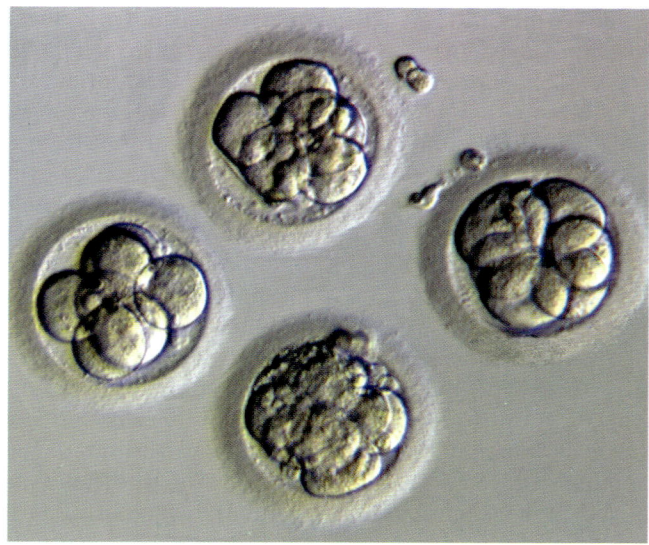

Figure 23.3 Four embryos photographed on day 3 after harvest, just before freezing was carried out.

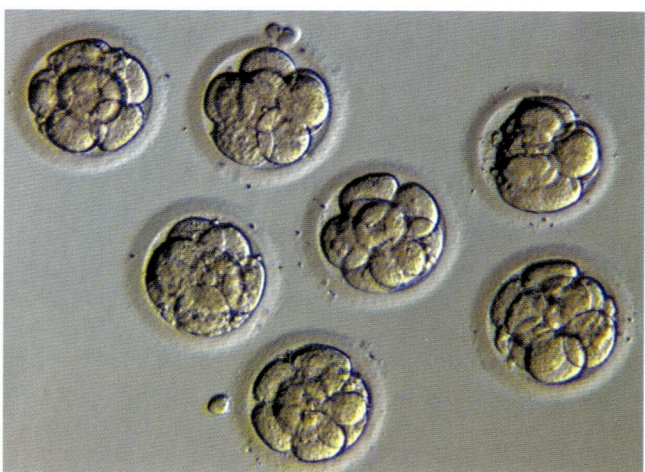

Figure 23.5 Seven healthy-appearing conceptuses photographed before freezing on day 3 after harvest.

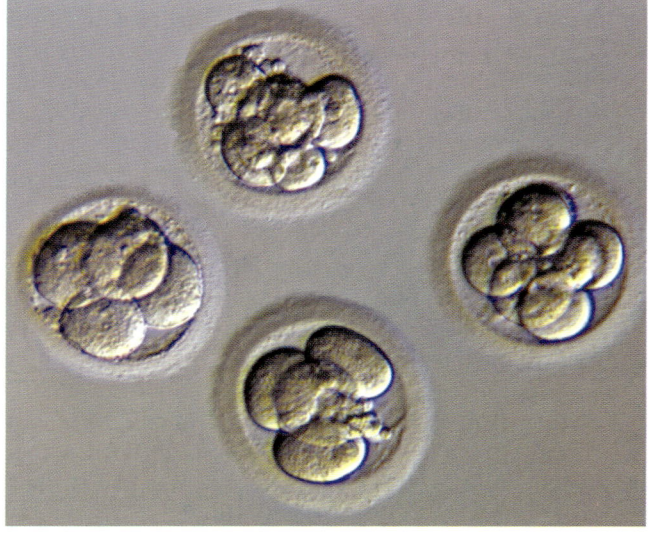

Figure 23.4 The same four embryos as in Figure 23.3 photographed a few hours after thawing 68 days later. Two of these had degenerative blastomeres and fragments removed before the photograph was taken. The 37-year-old patient became pregnant after the transfer of these conceptuses, with two sacs and one fetal heart by ultrasound. A healthy female child was delivered.

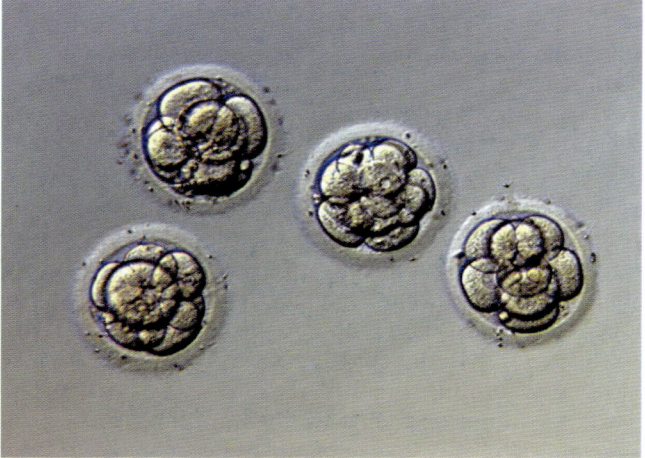

Figure 23.6 Upon thawing four of the conceptuses shown in Figure 23.5 after 122 days, all survived.

There is no convincing evidence to suggest that the loss of one or two blastomeres is detrimental to eight-celled human or mouse embryos (29–31) Nonetheless, it has been reported that fully intact embryos demonstrate higher implantation rates than do partially intact ones (32).

Blastocysts

The advantage of blastocyst freezing over the cleavage-stage embryos is embryo selection in culture resulting in high-grade-quality embryos that are frozen. Blastocysts comprise of many cells so the loss of a few cells during freezing and thawing will not compromise the integrity of the entire specimen. This may be one reason why blastocysts have been frozen and thawed so successfully over the years in domestic animals for both research and commercial purposes. Blastocyst cryopreservation in the human was first reported by Cohen et al. (5), who used glycerol in a series of 10 increasing concentrations. Following that initial report, blastocyst freezing was only occasionally incorporated into clinical protocols because of the difficulties involved with maintaining high rates of blastocyst development in vitro.

Through the 1990s, reports of clinical pregnancy after blastocyst thaw fell in the range of 10–30% per transfer (33), percentages not significantly better than results with earlier stages. Although several groups reported freezing blastocysts quite successfully, early attempts often relied on co-culture systems to support embryo growth (19,34,35). Today, the availability of sequential media has led to a dramatic increase in the practice of blastocyst freezing, and pregnancy rates well over 50% have been reported following the replacement of thawed blastocysts (7).

Few reports have been published detailing the efficiency of blastocyst freezing after culture in sequential media. Langley et al. describe a comparison of thawed day 3 embryos versus blastocysts during a 30-month period (36). In this study, the survival rate was higher for blastocysts and the implantation rate was doubled (21.9% vs. 10.1%, 72 blastocyst cycles). In 2002, Behr et al. reported a 36% clinical pregnancy rate and 16% implantation rate for thawed blastocysts from 64 cycles (37). Nonetheless, the Cornell program has benefited greatly from the adoption of blastocyst freezing protocols (Table 23.1) (7). While acceptable clinical pregnancy rates of nearly 40% have been realized after freezing and thawing cleavage-stage embryos, much higher rates have been established using blastocysts (59%) without any concomitant drop in the number or proportion of patients having conceptuses frozen. Reviewing the last 10 years, nearly one in five women under the age of 40 has had blastocysts frozen after undergoing day 3 transfers, and 60% of women undergoing day 5 transfers have had at least one blastocyst cryopreserved on day 5 or day 6. Well above 12,000 blastocysts have been frozen in over 15 years, though less than 50% have been thawed since so many of the patients involved have not returned for a FET after becoming pregnant from their fresh cycles.

Most of the blastocysts frozen in the Cornell program are generated following the fresh transfer of day 3 conceptuses. After intrauterine transfer, remaining viable embryos are examined each day for two or three additional days to evaluate their suitability for freezing. This has been termed the post-transfer observation period. Blastocysts forming on either day 5 or day 6 are cryopreserved for future use. Only rarely and under special circumstances have day 7 conceptuses been frozen.

The survival rate for thawed blastocysts has been very stable at 76%. Clinical pregnancy per cycle with only blastocysts thawed and replaced is 59%; the delivery rate was 50% and the implantation rate was 39.8% (7). These outcomes are quite high for FET and are probably the result of the selection of good-quality blastocysts for freezing. Retrospective analysis of blastocyst grade at transfer and pregnancy outcome reveal that "good" quality blastocysts (grade A or B for ICM and/or trophectoderm) (7) had a higher pregnancy rate than "fair" or "poor" blastocysts (grade C). In addition, FET using morula resulted in fewer pregnancies than if blastocysts had been transferred. Pregnancy rates are not different whether blastocysts are replaced in either natural or programmed cycles (61% vs. 56%) (7). Furthermore, pregnancy rates with blastocysts are dependent on maternal age; 7/20 women (35%) over the age of 41 have established clinical pregnancies; although their miscarriage rate is more than double that observed for younger women (57%).

It is generally assumed that blastocysts that develop in a timely manner in vitro are of better quality than those that develop more slowly. However, this study and an earlier retrospective analysis of blastocyst thaw outcomes from our program demonstrate otherwise. In 154 consecutive patients returning for thawed blastocysts, 60 patients received a transfer of day 5 frozen–thawed blastocysts and 94 patients underwent transfer with day 6 blastocysts. No significant differences were observed between groups for patient age, blastocyst survival rates, the average number of blastocysts replaced, morphology of thawed blastocysts, clinical pregnancy rates, ongoing pregnancy rates, or implantation rates (7). These findings are identical to those presented in an earlier study from this center (38) and others (11,37).

While it is intuitive to assume that embryos reaching the blastocyst stage faster (day 5) might be "healthier" than their day 6 counterparts, these data suggest that the rate of development may not be crucial to subsequent post-thaw success. At Cornell, blastocysts implanted equally well in FET cycles when frozen on day 5 or day 6 (38% vs. 39%, respectively) (7). Surprisingly, this is in direct conflict to reports of fresh transfer using day 5 and day 6 blastocysts, where pregnancy has been observed to be significantly lower with slower-growing day 6 conceptuses (39). One of the reasons for equally successful pregnancy rates with day 5 or day 6 blastocysts is better synchronization between uterus and blastocyst, where embryos are generally replaced 1–2 days earlier compared with the fresh IVF cycle. In contrast to our work, Marek carried out a study comparing outcomes from 127 thawed blastocyst cycles where blastocysts were frozen on day 5 or day 6 (40). Survival rates post-thaw were good for both groups, but the clinical pregnancy rate per thaw (50% vs. 29%, respectively), ongoing pregnancy rate per thaw (43% vs. 23%), and implantation rate (34% vs. 15%) were all significantly higher for day 5 blastocysts.

We, like others, observed that blastocysts with a high probability of survival after thaw acted as perfect osmometers, shrinking, re-expanding, and swelling in accordance with their osmotic environment (Figs. 23.13, 23.14) (41). One uneasy task immediately after thawing was to determine that a blastocyst had indeed survived since it often presented a contracted state for up to several hours after reincubation in culture medium (Fig. 23.14). It has been our experience that blastocysts that shrink appropriately in response to cryoprotective agents and exhibit contracted, healthy-appearing cells after thaw do quite well in their ability to survive the rigors of freezing and thawing (Figs. 23.7–23.12).

Table 23.1 Pregnancy and Implantation by Stage of Development[a]

Stage transferred	Clinical pregnancies/ transfer (%)	Implanted/no. transferred (%)
Embryos only	173/444 (39.0)[b]	262/1645 (15.9)[d]
Blastocysts only	125/211 (59.2)[c]	170/440 (38.6)[e]

$P < 0.05$ in favor of blastocysts for comparisons b versus c, d versus e.
[a]Embryos frozen from January 1995 to March 2002; blastocysts frozen from July 2000 to June 2003 (7).

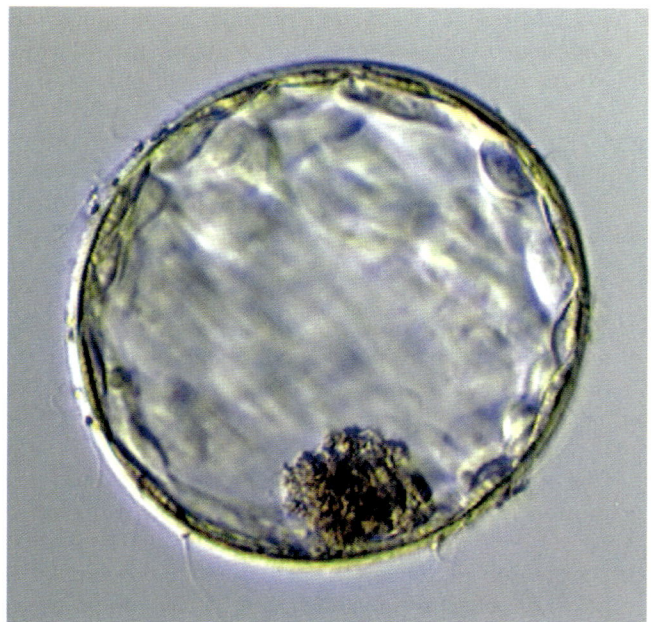

Figure 23.7 Nonviable inner cell mass despite blastocele reexpansion after the thaw.

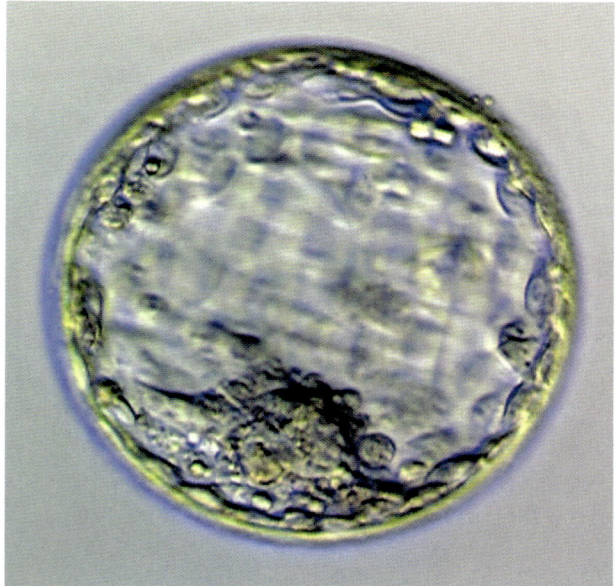

Figure 23.9 Same blastocyst as in Figure 23.8 after thawing 56 days later; most cells appear viable. This blastocyst was transferred, implanted, and a healthy female child was delivered. Note here that the blastocyst was thawed almost one full day before replacement and that the trophectoderm appears quite different after prolonged culture, being made up of many more cells.

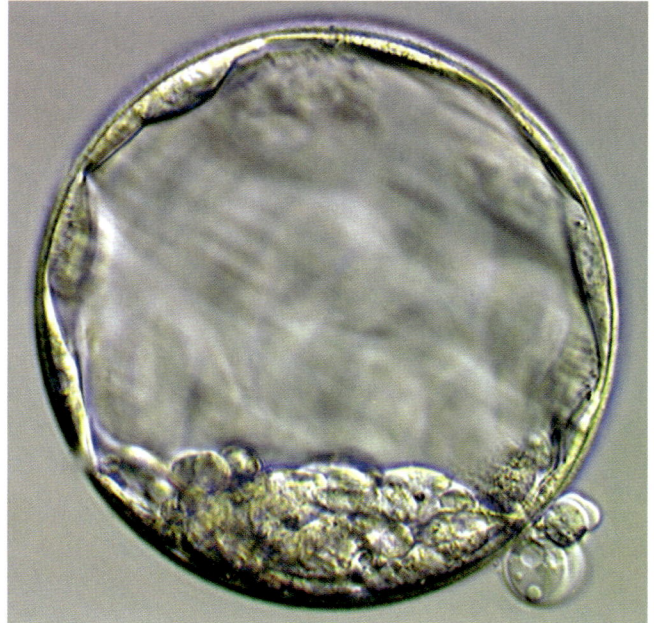

Figure 23.8 Expanded blastocyst immediately before freezing; inner cell mass is large and trophectoderm is sparse.

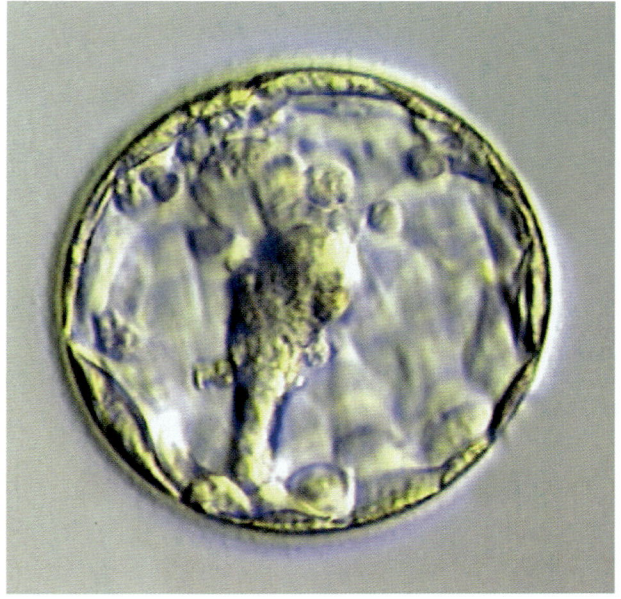

Figure 23.10 Blastocyst known to have implanted after freeze, thaw, and transfer. After cryostorage for 57 days, this blastocyst was thawed and led to the birth of a healthy female child.

Calculating Pregnancy Potential from Embryo and Blastocyst Stages

Of the many tribulations associated with running a cryopreservation program, one of the most frustrating is that embryologists cannot reap the fruits of their labor (pregnancy after thawing) until months or years have passed. It is common for patients to wait for some time before returning for a thaw attempt after a negative fresh cycle, or to delay two or more years after the birth of a child. This situation gives rise to special problems in tracking results during a given freezing period and makes it difficult to identify the efficiency of a new protocol.

There are three common ways to analyze freezing/thawing results:

1. calculating pregnancy rate per thaw attempt,
2. calculating pregnancy rate per cycle with transfer of thawed conceptuses, or

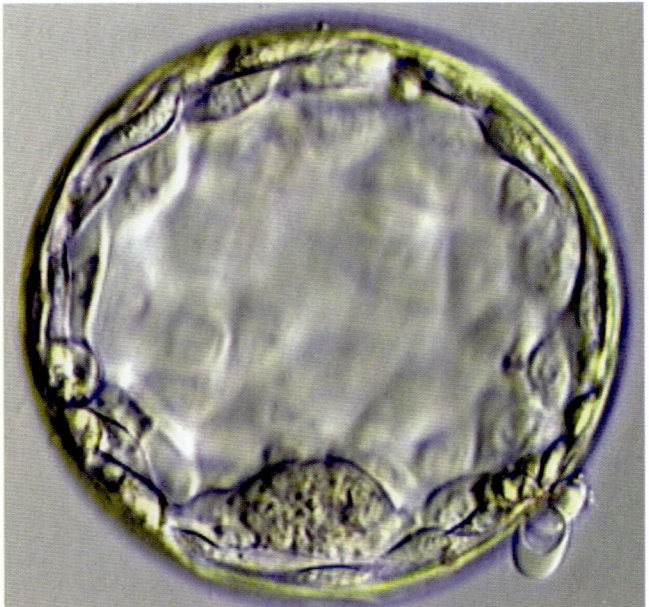

Figure 23.11 Blastocyst known to have implanted after freeze, thaw, and transfer. After cryostorage for 57 days, this blastocyst was thawed and led to the birth of a healthy female child.

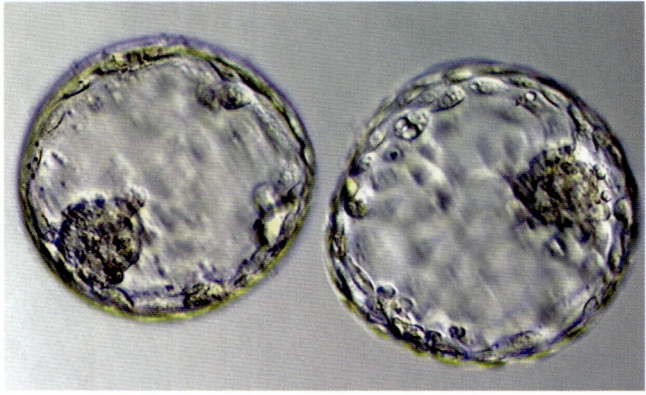

Figure 23.12 Two blastocysts known to have implanted after freeze, thaw, and transfer. After cryostorage for 84 days, two healthy male children were subsequently delivered.

3. calculating an *augmented* pregnancy rate per cycle with freezing based on fresh pregnancy plus thawed pregnancy. This last method has been discussed in detail in numerous publications (7,28,42–45).

In the last analysis, *augmented* pregnancy rate refers to the actual cumulative pregnancy rate achieved by patients upon combining pregnancies established from both fresh and thawed transfers:

1. The *base* fresh pregnancy rate is defined as the number of clinical pregnancies established after the transfer of noncryopreserved embryos over the number of noncryopreserved (fresh) transfer cycles, that is, $(250/500) \times 100 = 50\%$.
2. The *augmented* pregnancy rate is defined as the actual number of clinical pregnancies generated by the transfer of noncryopreserved embryos *plus* the actual number of clinical pregnancies generated by the transfer of thawed embryos in cycles failing to become pregnant with fresh transfer, over the number of transfer cycles, that is, $(250 + 125/500) \times 100 = 75\%$.
3. A *projected* augmented pregnancy rate can be defined as the actual number of clinical pregnancies generated by the transfer of noncryopreserved embryos *plus* the actual number of clinical pregnancies generated by the transfer of thawed embryos in cycles failing to become pregnant with fresh transfer, *plus* the number of clinical pregnancies expected from the potential transfer of conceptuses still in cryostorage for patients not yet pregnant from fresh or thawed attempts (this last calculation uses the thawed pregnancy rate established to date) over the total number of cycles with a transfer, that is, $(250 + 125 + 25/500) \times 100 = 80\%$. The validity of reporting this last *projected* cumulative pregnancy rate is open to criticism because of its reliance on past performance and assumptions that future results will be similar.

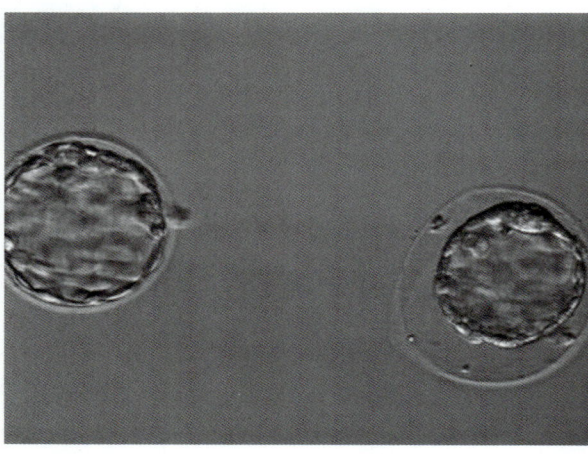

(A)

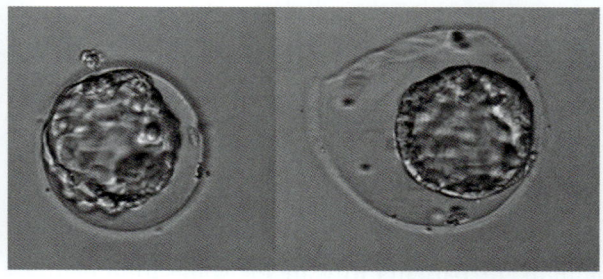

(B)

Figure 23.13 Two blastocysts during the process of freezing: (**A**) 5% glycerol; (**B**) 10% glycerol + 0.2 M sucrose. Blastocele shrinkage and collapse is evident during cryoprotectants dilutions.

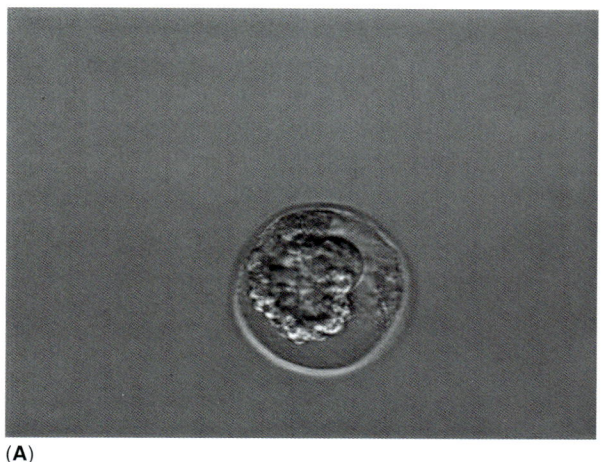 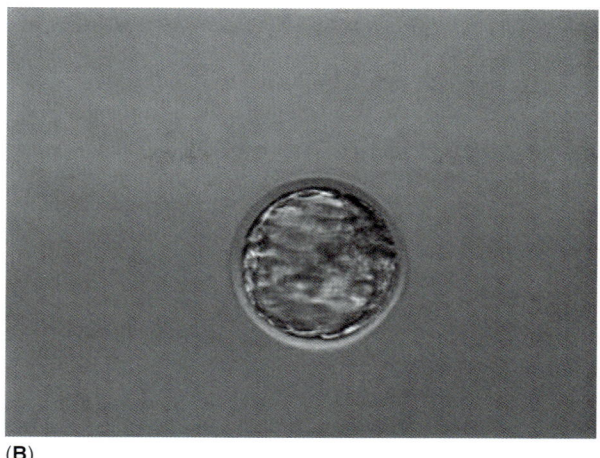

Figure 23.14 Blastocyst after thaw. (**A**) Blastocyst is collapsed and contracted immediately after thaw. (**B**) After 3 hours, blastocyst reexpands and resumes normal morphology.

Table 23.2 Cumulative Pregnancies from January 1995 to March 2003

	Embryos only frozen (%)	Blastocysts only frozen (%)
Fresh *base* clinical pregnancies/transfer	69.3	71.8
True *augmented* cumulative	73.9	81.5
Projected *total* cumulative	74.6[a]	87.1[a]

[a]$P < 0.0001$.
Blastocyst data from Veeck et al. (7).

Using the augmented pregnancy model described here, Cornell results are shown in Table 23.2 where blastocysts appear to be an optimal stage for freezing.

Slow Freezing Vs. Vitrification

Slow freezing of 2PN zygotes (one-cell) has been a well-established method for embryo preservation (28,46). Some reports indicate higher survival and pregnancy with 2PN stages than with cleavage stage embryos (28,46,47). On the other hand, successful vitrification of pronuclear oocytes was reported (48,49) with higher survival and pregnancy rates of the vitrified specimens as compared with slow frozen ones (50–52).

Several studies of cleavage-stage vitrification have been reported with high survival (>80%) and pregnancy rates (53–55). In a large comparative study from Kuwayama et al. (50) comparing slow freezing and vitrification of cleavage embryos, survival and pregnancy rates were comparable between techniques. Other groups report higher rates using vitrification over slow freezing (54–58).

Cornell demonstrated high survival and pregnancy rates using slow freezing of blastocysts (7). The first pregnancy using vitrified human blastocyst was reported in 2000 (59). Soon after, many reports indicated high survival and increased pregnancy rates following transfer of vitrified blastocysts (50,53).

In a recent review from Kolibianakis et al. (60) looking at randomized controlled trials between slow freeze and vitrification methods, they concluded that vitrification is apparently associated with a higher survival rate in cleavage embryos and blastocysts, but may not be always associated with better outcome, especially in experienced groups where slow freezing still presents the gold standard for cryopreservation. Direct comparison between groups is difficult since different levels of experience, different stimulation regimes, culture conditions, and cryo methods have been used. For this reason it is advised that laboratories perform their own comparison and choose the method most suitable to them.

Children Born Following Cryopreservation and Thawing

Cryopreservation has no apparent negative impact on perinatal outcome and does not appear to affect adversely the growth or health of children during infancy or early childhood (61–63). Furthermore, the available data do not indicate an elevation in congenital malformations for children born after freeze–thaw procedures (64–67). Reviewing data from our institution, we did not observe an increase in abnormalities in children born after FET compared with fresh IVF (0.5% in FET compared with <3% in fresh). While it remains unclear if freezing poses long-term risks to children so conceived, there is no direct evidence thus far to raise concern.

GENERAL CONSIDERATIONS

Before beginning a cryopreservation program in an ART setting, a few general considerations should be taken into account. First and foremost is the adequate training of personnel by an experienced embryologist who is skilled and fully versed in cryopreservation techniques. Whenever possible it is also a good idea to have a back-up biological freezer. This will prevent loss of specimens in the unfortunate event a machine malfunctions. Furthermore, in today's busy laboratory, it is not uncommon to undertake day 1, day 3, and day 5 freezes all in the same day.

It is important to have at least one back-up source for liquid nitrogen delivery. If for some reason a primary source fails (faulty valve or level indicator) or one experiences delivery problems from the vendor, it is a good idea to have an alternative option.

An emergency power supply system is also a serious consideration. The need for an expensive backup power supply may depend on the facility (some buildings have backup power sources built in) and the reliability of the local power company. For most laboratories it is wise to invest in an uninterrupted power supply system that sits next to the biological freezer(s). One of the more mundane but essential tasks in running a cryopreservation program is the scheduling of daily inspection and documentation of liquid nitrogen levels in the storage tanks. These inspections should be carried out two to three times a week at regular intervals. It is also important, and in most IVF programs mandatory, to install alarm systems to monitor the levels of liquid nitrogen in storage tanks. If liquid nitrogen levels drop dangerously during off hours, the system should be able to alert a predefined list of people by phone or beeper. It is also a good idea to have at least one empty, fully charged tank ready in case of such an emergency.

Quality Control Issues

A good quality control program is essential to every aspect of ART, and cryopreservation is no exception.

Preventive Maintenance

A good preventive maintenance schedule is essential. We recommend having a specialist examine each biological freezer and perform recalibration procedures twice a year.

Testing of Freezing and Thawing Solutions

Each new batch of culture medium, whether prepared in-house or purchased from outside, must pass rigid quality control testing. This is achieved by means of endotoxin testing, a human sperm survival bioassay, and a mouse embryo bioassay. Any problematic batch of medium, any medium component, or any lot of plasticware is immediately discarded and replaced.

Endotoxin Testing and Interpretation

Bacterial endotoxins are common contaminants of materials and solutions used in culture. A sensitive assay to quantitate endotoxin contamination levels is necessary. Evidence suggests that endotoxins may be responsible for much of the variability in cell culture that is often associated with changes in batch or formulation of media. The ubiquitous gram-negative bacteria that produce these endotoxins can and do contaminate a variety of materials used to cultivate cells in vitro. A sample of each culture medium is sent to an independent testing center each week. For our purposes, only values <0.03 EU are acceptable when using the Limulus amebocyte lysate assay.

Human Sperm Survival Assay

Each batch of culture medium is tested using human sperm (the same donor is used for each assay). The sperm sample is split into as many fractions as the number of assays to be performed, and prepared using a culture medium lot currently in use (control) and the new lot to be tested (test). A 24-hour and 48-hour motility and progression assessment is performed on a sample prepared by standard swim-up procedures. A motility of >70% and a progression of >40% type "a" motility is considered acceptable. A comparison should be made between the control sample and the test sample; any significant difference between the two should be interpreted as problematic.

Mouse Embryo Bioassay

The in vitro development of mouse one-cell or two-cell embryos to the hatched blastocyst stage has traditionally been used as a quality control system in IVF laboratories. Based on a large body of evidence, we believe this test to be less reliable than the human sperm survival assay and the results unrelated to the pattern of development of human embryos in vitro. Mouse embryos easily reach the blastocyst stage in the presence or absence of exogenous protein and the great majority of these blastocysts hatch when provided with protein. Slight variations in culture media composition or minute amounts of endotoxin do not appear to affect the rate of blastocyst formation or hatching. To increase the specificity of the mouse assay, one-cell embryos can be used with protein supplementation only in phase 1 of the sequential medium and in phase 2 without protein. Results of >80% mouse blastocyst rate are expected.

Logging Seeding Temperatures

It is important to keep a log of seeding temperatures for each individual freezing run. Tracking these values help to alert personnel if the machine's seeding temperature begins to drift out of an acceptable range.

COMPLICATIONS

Trouble Shooting Procedures (i.e., "What if...")

What If the Source Liquid Nitrogen Tank Empties or Malfunctions During a Freezing Run?

If the liquid nitrogen source tank runs dry or does not possess adequate pressure to supply the freezing unit, most biological freezers will sound an alarm. On our Planer unit (K10–1.7), an audible alarm is triggered and the display panel flashes "control deviation." The first thing one should do is examine the display to determine whether the chamber temperature is beginning to rise and check the plotted temperature graph. If the unit is not receiving liquid nitrogen, the bursts of sound normally heard as liquid nitrogen rushes into the chamber will sound quite different. If the temperature is rising or the unit sounds much different, first inspect the feed tank. If it is empty, change it immediately. The Planer will automatically adjust and bring the chamber to its proper temperature once the flow of liquid nitrogen is restored. If the tank is full, check the pressure gauge. It's possible that the safety valve that allows excess pressure to escape will become frozen in the open position. Once the pressure drops too low, the tank will not be able to feed the unit. In this case, again, change the tank immediately. One may be able to thaw the stuck valve by applying hot water, but all malfunctions should be documented and reported.

What If an Embryo Cannot Be Located After Thawing a Cryovial or Straw?

Thoroughly re-examine the contents of the freezing vessel. Pay special attention to any small bubbles floating on the surface as embryos may become attached. If the specimen still cannot be visualized, flush the straw or fill the empty cryovial with a medium kept at room temperature. It is preferable to flush with the medium which is used for the first thawing dilution. Withdraw the contents using the pipette, transfer contents to a fresh Petri dish, and check for the missing specimen. If this fails, one can try half-filling the cryovial, capping it, and gently agitating. More aggressive agitation follows if the embryo is still not located. Doing so may release an embryo stuck to its inner walls.

After Loading an Embryo into a Cryovial, What Should One Do If It Cannot Be Visualized Under the Stereomicroscope?

First, try flicking the cryovial gently with a finger to set its contents in motion. This should enable easier visualization of the embryo. If this is unsuccessful, examine the inner walls of the cryovial for small medium droplets—occasionally, if the embryo is too close to the opening of the pipette and the inner wall is touched with the tip, the embryo will be dislodged along with a droplet of the media. If the embryo is located on the inner wall, it may be washed off or picked up with the pipette, or the cryovial can be filled and emptied. Should none of these methods be successful for locating the embryo, be sure to visually check the walls of the loading pipette.

What If One Loses Track of an Embryo as It is Moved Through Freezing or Thawing Dilutions?

Tapping the side of the vessel and adjusting the contrast on the stereomicroscope may assist visualization. Examine any bubbles that might be in the vessel and rinse and check the pipette. It is also helpful to ask another experienced embryologist to examine the materials. If all else fails, draw the entire contents of the dish/well into a fresh pipette and transfer to a large Petri dish for examination.

Exploding Cryovials

During the freezing process the o-ring that sits between the cryovial and the cap shrinks, becomes rigid, and may cause the seal to loosen. Under these circumstances, a slight vacuum is formed within the cryovial that allows air or liquid nitrogen vapor to enter. As the cryovial is warmed during a subsequent thaw, the o-ring expands and become more malleable, creating a tighter seal. The cold air/vapor within the vial begins to expand with the rising temperature. If the pressure inside the vial becomes too great for the o-ring to contain, the vial may expel a burst of air. If this happens while the vial is sitting in a rack waiting to be examined, it may "jump" out of the rack allowing the medium inside the vial to splash around and make the embryo much more difficult to locate. One way to avoid this situation is to loosen the cap of the vial immediately after it has been thawed. This should release any built-up pressure inside the vial without disrupting its contents.

Tips for Success

Preparing Media: Appropriate Delivery of Cryoprotective Solutions

It is important to ensure that the appropriate volume of cryoprotectant is delivered to freezing and thawing media made on-site. Failing to prepare solutions properly can result in reduced survival and pregnancy rates after thawing. Cryoprotectants, especially glycerol, are very viscous and tend to adhere to the inside and outside walls of the delivery pipette. In order to ensure that all the cryoprotectant solution is delivered to the medium one must rinse the pipette repeatedly. Even a relatively small reduction in the amount of cryoprotectant can influence the success of a frozen/thawed cycle.

Moving Through Dilutions

When moving from one dilution to another, aspirate an appropriate volume of medium into the pipette before picking the conceptus in an effort to avoid creating bubbles, but not so much as to interfere with the dilution concentrations. Make sure to wash the conceptus several times in each new dilution. This also applies when moving thawed embryos into fresh culture media. Washing them in a few different droplets before placing them in a clean, fresh droplet will help ensure that most of the cryoprotectant has been removed.

Safety: Cryopreserving Multiple Patients Simultaneously

When cryopreserving multiple patients it is best to prepare a separate rack for each. Each rack holds one patient's dilutions, culture dishes, and cryovials. This helps ensure that samples stay separated and will make multiple freezes more manageable. Never place culture dishes or dilutions from different patients on the microscope's stage simultaneously. During each step in the process one should verify a patient's name with another embryologist.

SUMMARY

Most highly successful ART centers in the United States and around the world offer as part of their treatment services a well-organized and successful cryopreservation program. Organization and success are most often reflected in a high overall cumulative pregnancy rate, which takes into account both fresh and frozen–thawed pregnancies per cycle (7,68). While the benefits of such a program to the ART patient are obvious, there are other smaller groups of patients who also benefit greatly from cryopreservation. Patients at risk for ovarian hyperstimulation can have all of their conceptuses frozen, which greatly reduces their risk of severe clinical symptoms should they become pregnant (69,70). In addition, patients with cancer can opt for IVF followed by cryopreservation to preserve fertility (71,72).

Final consideration must be given to the reduction of costs associated with FET compared with fresh cycles (73). As medical costs escalate and costs associated with newborn care increase, particularly in cases of multiple births, cryopreservation offers a valuable and less expensive alternative for ART patients. Using embryo and blastocyst freezing, patients can choose to reduce the number of embryos transferred during a fresh cycle, thus reducing their chances and risks of multiple pregnancies. Adding to this benefit, the overall costs of a thaw cycle are considerably lower than a fresh cycle in that cryo–thaw patients do not usually incur extensive hospital, clinical, and laboratory fees. For these reasons, the addition of cryopreservation as an alternative for ART patients in today's world has become of primary importance.

The value of cryopreserving embryos and blastocysts for future thaw and transfer is an important consideration of every IVF program. The convergence of two factors, a higher pregnancy rate and a lower multiple gestation rate, can be managed effectively through the establishment of a successful cryopreservation program.

REFERENCES

1. Fugger EF. Clinical status of human embryo cryopreservation in the United States of America. Fertil Steril 1989; 52: 986–90.
2. The Society for Assisted Reproductive Technology, American Society for Reproductive Medicine, Assisted Reproductive Technology in the United States: 1999 results generated from the American Society for Reproductive Medicine/Society for Assisted Reproductive Technology Registry. Fertil Steril 2002; 78: 918–31.
3. Hoffman DI, Zellman GL, Fair CC, et al. Cryopreserved embryos in the United States and their availability for research. Fertil Steril 2003; 79: 1063–9.
4. Trounson A, Mohr L. Human pregnancy following cryopreservation, thawing and transfer of an eight-cell embryo. Nature 1983; 305: 707–9.
5. Cohen J, Simons RF, Edwards RG, Fehilly CB, Fishel SB. Pregnancies following the frozen storage of expanding human blastocysts. J In Vitro Fert Embryo Transf 1985; 2: 59–64.
6. Karlstrom PO, Bergh T, Forsberg AS, Sandkvist U, Wikland M. Prognostic factors for the success rate of embryo freezing. Hum Reprod 1997; 12: 1263–6.
7. Veeck LL, Bodine R, Clarke RN, et al. High pregnancy rates can be achieved after freezing and thawing human blastocysts. Fertil Steril 2004; 82: 1418–27.
8. Toner JP, Veeck LL, Muasher SJ. Basal follicle-stimulating hormone level and age affect the chance for and outcome of pre-embryo cryopreservation. Fertil Steril 1993; 59: 664–7.
9. Mandelbaum J, Junca AM, Plachot M, et al. Human embryo cryopreservation, extrinsic and intrinsic parameters of success. Hum Reprod 1987; 2: 709–15.
10. Schalkoff ME, Oskowitz SP, Powers RD. A multifactorial analysis of the pregnancy outcome in a successful embryo cryopreservation program. Fertil Steril 1993; 59: 1070–4.
11. Shoukir Y, Chardonnens D, Campana A, Bischof P, Sakkas D. The rate of development and time of transfer play different roles in influencing the viability of human blastocysts. Hum Reprod 1998; 13: 676–81.
12. Oehninger S, Mayer J, Muasher S. Impact of different clinical variables on pregnancy outcome following embryo cryopreservation. Mol Cell Endocrinol 2000; 169: 73–7.
13. Van den Abbeel E, Camus M, Joris H, Van Steirteghem A. Embryo freezing after intracytoplasmic sperm injection. Mol Cell Endocrinol 2000; 169: 49–54.
14. Loh SK, Leong NK. Factors affecting success in an embryo cryopreservation programme. Ann Acad Med Singapore 1999; 28: 260–5.
15. Gardner DK, Leese HJ. Assessment of embryo viability prior to transfer by the noninvasive measurement of glucose uptake. J Exp Zool 1987; 242: 103–5.
16. Lane M, Maybach JM, Gardner DK. Addition of ascorbate during cryopreservation stimulates subsequent embryo development. Hum Reprod 2002; 17: 2686–93.
17. Testart J, Lassalle B, Belaisch-Allart J, et al. High pregnancy rate after early human embryo freezing. Fertil Steril 1986; 46: 268–72.
18. Testart J, Lassalle B, Belaisch-Allart J, Forman R, Frydman R. Cryopreservation does not affect future of human fertilised eggs. Lancet 1986; 2: 569.
19. Menezo Y, Nicollet B, Herbaut N, Andre D. Freezing cocultured human blastocysts. Fertil Steril 1992; 58: 977–80.
20. Menezo YJ, Nicollet B, Dumont M, Hazout A, Janny L. Factors affecting human blastocyst formation in vitro and freezing at the blastocyst stage. Acta Eur Fertil 1993; 24: 207–13.
21. Gardner DK, Lane M, Stevens J, Schoolcraft WB. Changing the start temperature and cooling rate in a slow-freezing protocol increases human blastocyst viability. Fertil Steril 2003; 79: 407–10.
22. Choi DH, Chung HM, Lim JM, et al. Pregnancy and delivery of healthy infants developed from vitrified blastocysts in an IVF-ET program. Fertil Steril 2000; 74: 838–9.
23. Yokota Y, Sato S, Yokota M, et al. Successful pregnancy following blastocyst vitrification: case report. Hum Reprod 2000; 15: 1802–3.
24. Yokota Y, Sato S, Yokota M, Yokota H, Araki Y. Birth of a healthy baby following vitrification of human blastocysts. Fertil Steril 2001; 75: 1027–9.
25. Mukaida T, Nakamura S, Tomiyama T, et al. Successful birth after transfer of vitrified human blastocysts with use of a cryoloop containerless technique. Fertil Steril 2001; 76: 618–20.
26. Granne I, Child T, Hartshorne G. Embryo cryopreservation: evidence for practice. British Fertility Society. Hum Fertil (Camb) 2008; 11: 159–72.
27. Pomeroy KO, Harris S, Conaghan J, et al. Storage of cryopreserved reproductive tissues: evidence that

cross-contamination of infectious agents is a negligible risk. Fertil Steril 2010; 94: 1181–8.
28. Veeck LL, Amundson CH, Brothman LJ, et al. Significantly enhanced pregnancy rates per cycle through cryopreservation and thaw of pronuclear stage oocytes. Fertil Steril 1993; 59: 1202–7.
29. Veiga A, Calderon G, Barri PN, Coroleu B. Pregnancy after the replacement of a frozen-thawed embryo with less than 50% intact blastomeres. Hum Reprod 1987; 2: 321–3.
30. Hartshorne GM, Elder K, Crow J, Dyson H, Edwards RG. The influence of in-vitro development upon post-thaw survival and implantation of cryopreserved human blastocysts. Hum Reprod 1991; 6: 136–41.
31. Rulicke T, Autenried P. Potential of two-cell mouse embryos to develop to term despite partial damage after cryopreservation. Lab Anim 1995; 29: 320–6.
32. Van den Abbeel E, Camus M, Van Waesberghe L, Devroey P, Van Steirteghem AC. Viability of partially damaged human embryos after cryopreservation. Hum Reprod 1997; 12: 2006–10.
33. Kaufman RA, Menezo Y, Hazout A, et al. Cocultured blastocyst cryopreservation: experience of more than 500 transfer cycles. Fertil Steril 1995; 64: 1125–9.
34. Freitas S, Le Gal F, Dzik A, et al. Value of cryopreservation of human embryos during the blastocyst stage. Contracept Fertil Sex 1994; 22: 396–401.
35. Menezo YJ, Ben Khalifa M. Cytogenetic and cryobiology of human cocultured embryos: a 3-year experience. J Assist Reprod Genet 1995; 12: 35–40.
36. Langley MT, Marek DM, Gardner DK, Doody KM, Doody KJ. Extended embryo culture in human assisted reproduction treatments. Hum Reprod 2001; 16: 902–8.
37. Behr B, Gebhardt J, Lyon J, Milki AA. Factors relating to a successful cryopreserved blastocyst transfer program. Fertil Steril 2002; 77: 697–9.
38. Clarke RN, Bodine R, Zaninovic N. A comparison of post-thaw survival and pregnancy rates in day 5 and 6 frozen-thawed human blastocysts. Oral presentation for the 58th Annual Meeting of the American Society for Reproductive Medicine. Seattle, WA, 2002; 78(Suppl): 1001; S12.
39. Shapiro BS, Richter KS, Harris DC, Daneshmand ST. A comparison of day 5 and day 6 blastocyst transfers. Fertil Steril 2001; 75: 1126–30.
40. Marek DM, Langley MT, McKean C, et al. Frozen embryo transfer FET of day 5 blastocyst embryos compared to transfer of day 6 blastocyst embryos. Fertil Steril 2000; 74: S52–3.
41. Kaidi S, Donnay I, Lambert P, Dessy F, Massip A. Osmotic behavior of in vitro produced bovine blastocysts in cryoprotectant solutions as a potential predictive test of survival. Cryobiology 2000; 41: 106–15.
42. Jones HW Jr, Veeck LL, Muasher SJ. Cryopreservation: the problem of evaluation. Hum Reprod 1995; 10: 2136–8.
43. Jones HW Jr, Jones D, Kolm P. Cryopreservation: a simplified method of evaluation. Hum Reprod 1997; 12: 548–53.
44. Jones HW Jr, Out HJ, Hoomans EH, Driessen SG, Coelingh Bennink HJ. Cryopreservation: the practicalities of evaluation. Hum Reprod 1997; 12: 1522–4.
45. Schnorr JA, Muasher SJ, Jones HW Jr. Evaluation of the clinical efficacy of embryo cryopreservation. Mol Cell Endocrinol 2000; 169: 85–9.
46. Damario MA, Hammitt DG, Session DR, Dumesic DA. Embryo cryopreservation at the pronuclear stage and efficient embryo use optimizes the chance for a liveborn infant from a single oocyte retrieval. Fertil Steril 2000; 73: 767–73.
47. Salumets A, Tuuri T, Mäkinen S, et al. Effect of developmental stage of embryo at freezing on pregnancy outcome of frozen-thawed embryo transfer. Hum Reprod 2003; 18: 1890–5.
48. Park SP, Kim EY, Oh JH, et al. Ultra-rapid freezing of human multipronuclear zygotes using electron microscope grids. Hum Reprod 2000; 15: 1787–90.
49. Jelinkova L, Selman HA, Arav A, et al. Twin pregnancy after vitrification of 2-pronuclei human embryos. Fertil Steril 2002; 77: 412–14.
50. Kuwayama M, Vajta G, Ieda S, Kato O. Comparison of open and closed methods for vitrification of human embryos and the elimination of potential contamination. Reprod Biomed Online 2005; 11: 608–14.
51. Griesinger G, Berndt H, Schultz L, Depenbusch M, Schultze-Mosgau A. Cumulative live birth rates after GnRH-agonist triggering of final oocyte maturation in patients at risk of OHSS: a prospective, clinical cohort study. Eur J Obstet Gynecol Reprod Biol 2010; 149: 190–4.
52. Al-Hasani S, Ozmen B, Koutlaki N, et al. Three years of routine vitrification of human zygotes: is it still fair to advocate slow-rate freezing? Reprod Biomed Online 2007; 14: 288–93.
53. Son WY, Tan SL. Comparison between slow freezing and vitrification for human embryos. Expert Rev Med Devices 2009; 6: 1–7.
54. Rama Raju GA, Haranath GB, Krishna KM, Prakash GJ, Madan K. Vitrification of human 8-cell embryos, a modified protocol for better pregnancy rates. Reprod Biomed Online 2005; 11: 434–7.
55. Balaban B, Urman B, Ata B, et al. A randomized controlled study of human Day 3 embryo cryopreservation by slow freezing or vitrification: vitrification is associated with higher survival, metabolism and blastocyst formation. Hum Reprod 2008; 23: 1976–82.
56. Loutradi KE, Kolibianakis EM, Venetis CA, et al. Cryopreservation of human embryos by vitrification or slow freezing: a systematic review and meta-analysis. Fertil Steril 2008; 90: 186–93.
57. Herrero L, Martínez M, Garcia-Velasco JA. Current status of human oocyte and embryo cryopreservation. Curr Opin Obstet Gynecol 2011; 23: 245–50.
58. Capalbo A, Rienzi L, Buccheri M, et al. The worldwide frozen embryo reservoir: methodologies to achieve optimal results. Ann N Y Acad Sci 2011; 1221: 32–9.
59. Yokota Y, Sato S, Yokota M, et al. Successful pregnancy following blastocyst vitrification: case report. Hum Reprod 2000; 15: 1802–3.
60. Kolibianakis EM, Venetis CA, Tarlatzis BC. Cryopreservation of human embryos by vitrification or slow freezing: which one is better? Curr Opin Obstet Gynecol 2009; 21: 270–4.
61. Wennerholm UB, Albertsson-Wikland K, Bergh C, et al. Postnatal growth and health in children born after cryopreservation as embryos. Lancet 1998; 351: 1085–90.
62. Wikland M, Hardarson T, Hillensjö T, et al. Obstetric outcomes after transfer of vitrified blastocysts. Hum Reprod 2010; 25: 1699–707.

63. Liebermann J, Tucker MJ. Comparison of vitrification and conventional cryopreservation of day 5 and day 6 blastocysts during clinical application. Fertil Steril 2006; 86: 20–6.
64. Wada I, Macnamee MC, Wick K, Bradfield JM, Brinsden PR. Birth characteristics and perinatal outcome of babies conceived from cryopreserved embryos. Hum Reprod 1994; 9: 543–6.
65. Tarlatzis BC, Grimbizis G. Pregnancy and child outcome after assisted reproduction techniques. Hum Reprod 1999; 14(Suppl 1): 231–42.
66. Wennerholm WB. Cryopreservation of embryos and oocytes: obstetric outcome and health in children. Hum Reprod 2000; 15(Suppl 5): 18–25.
67. Wennerholm UB, Söderström-Anttila V, Bergh C, et al. Children born after cryopreservation of embryos or oocytes: a systematic review of outcome data. Hum Reprod 2009; 24: 2158–72.
68. Veeck LL. Does the developmental stage at freeze impact on clinical results post-thaw? Reprod Biomed Online 2003; 6: 367–74.
69. Pattinson HA, Hignett M, Dunphy BC, Fleetham JA. Outcome of thaw embryo transfer after cryopreservation of all embryos in patients at risk of ovarian hyperstimulation syndrome. Fertil Steril 1994; 6: 1192–6.
70. Queenan JT Jr. Embryo freezing to prevent ovarian hyperstimulation syndrome. Mol Cell Endocrinol 2000; 169: 79–83.
71. Brown JR, Modell E, Obasaju M, King YK. Natural cycle in-vitro fertilization with embryo cryopreservation prior to chemotherapy for carcinoma of the breast. Hum Reprod 1996; 11: 197–9.
72. Oktay K, Buyuk E, Davis O, et al. Fertility preservation in breast cancer patients: IVF and embryo cryopreservation after ovarian stimulation with tamoxifen. Hum Reprod 2003; 18: 90–5.
73. Van Voorhis BJ, Syrop CH, Allen BD, Sparks AE, Stovall DW. The efficacy and cost effectiveness of embryo cryopreservation compared with other assisted reproductive techniques. Fertil Steril 1995; 64: 647–50.

24

The human embryo: Vitrification

Zsolt Peter Nagy, Ching-Chien Chang, and Gábor Vajta

INTRODUCTION

Decades ago, most assisted reproductive techniques including in vitro fertilization (IVF) and cryopreservation of embryos by traditional freezing were applied to humans almost immediately after the first successes in some experimental or domestic species (Table 24.1). However, there are some techniques, where efforts to adopt a new approach were insufficient and sporadic, consequently the practical application has been considerably delayed. Vitrification belongs to the latter group. Reasons of this delay may include the fact that cryopreservation of zygote, cleavage- and, blastocyst-stage human embryos was more or less resolved by traditional freezing; vitrification has and still uses a seemingly very primitive manual technology compared with the fascinating automatic traditional freezers and standardized, ready to use media. High concentrations of cryoprotectants required to vitrification discouraged potential users.

A few years ago scientists began to apply the technique with mass production of results of applicability of vitrification in human fields. However, additional years were still required to get the approach acknowledged, to develop commercially available tools and kits, and to teach both distributors and consumers about the benefit of vitrification. Eventually, the overwhelming comparative evidence made clear to almost everybody that in all developmental stages, vitrification produces better survival and more competent oocytes/embryos than traditional freezing. Today, the rapidly increasing interest toward vitrification creates novel problems such as diversity of tools and media, lack of information regarding ingredients, insufficient teaching, and suboptimal application. Legal concerns on bio safety issues have also emerged, although no scientific proof exists about the magnitude or existence of danger.

In this chapter, we summarize and compare the basic features of traditional freezing and vitrification, explain some special features of vitrification, and provide data about the efficiency of vitrification for cryopreservation of human preimplantation-stage embryos at different developmental stages. Additionally, factors hampering the more rapid spreading and more efficient practical application of vitrification in human embryology will also be discussed.

For terms and definitions, we accept and use the excellent review and suggestions of Shaw and Jones (1). For the basic principles of cryobiology we refer earlier reviews (2–5).

MAIN CRYOPRESERVATION APPROACHES

In approximately a decade after the first successes with cryopreservation of mammalian embryos, (6–10) the first human pregnancies were achieved (11,12). All these works have been performed with traditional slow freezing. Vitrification was first applied for cryopreservation of mammalian embryos in 1985 (13) but regarded as a curiosity and experimental procedure for almost a decade, when practical application has been started in domestic animal embryology and sporadic approaches in humans. Competitive vitrification strategies for human embryo and oocyte cryopreservation have only been developed around a decade ago.

The strategies of the two cryopreservation approaches are basically different. So far the most important source of damage at cryopreservation is ice crystal formation. To minimize this injury, application of various chemicals (cryoprotectants) is required, which, unfortunately, may also induce various injuries including toxic and osmotic damages.

Traditional slow-rate freezing creates a delicate balance between these factors. Embryos are typically exposed to 1 to 2 mol/L solutions of permeable and (less concentrated, if any) nonpermeable cryoprotectants, then loaded into a 0.25 mL straw, sealed, and cooled to −6°C relatively rapidly, by placing the straws into a controlled-rate freezer. With the given cryoprotectant concentration, no spontaneous ice formation occurs at this temperature; however, ice nucleation can be induced by "seeding," that is, touching the straw with a forceps that has been previously immersed into liquid nitrogen. This seeding is performed far from the embryo, and during the subsequent steps, this ice grows stepwise toward the embryo. The controlled-rate freezer is adjusted to make a very slow cooling (usually 0.3°C/min, to around −30°C, then the straws are immersed into liquid nitrogen for a final cooling and storage. In slow freezing, the toxic and osmotic damages caused by the relatively low concentration of cryoprotectant solutions may not be too serious.

Table 24.1 Various Vitrification Techniques in Embryology

System	Reference
Direct dropping into liquid nitrogen	Landa and Tepla (63)
Electron microscopic grids	Martino et al. (23)
Open-pulled straw (OPS)	Vajta et al. (70)
Glass micropipettes	Kong et al. (195)
Super-finely pulled OPS	Isachenko et al. (196)
Gel-loading tips	Tominaga and Hanada (197)
Sterile stripper tip	Kuleshova and Lopata (106)
Flexipet denuding pipette	Liebermann et al. (198)
Fine diameter plastic micropipette	Cremades et al. (199)
100 μL pipetting tip	Hredzak et al. (200)
Closed-pulled straw	Chen et al. (201)
Sealed OPS	Lopez-Bejar and Lopez-Gatius (202)
Cryotip	Kuwayama et al. (61)
Cryoloop	Lane et al. (78)
Nylon mesh	Matsumoto et al. (84)
Minimum drop size	Arav (203)
Minimum volume cooling	Hamawaki et al. (86)
Hemi-straw system	Vanderzwalmen et al. (87)
Cryotop	Kuwayama et al. (60)
VitMaster	Arav et al. (72)
Solid surface vitrification	Dinnyes et al. (95)

Sources: Adapted from Ref. 204. Courtesy of Reproductive Healthcare Ltd, Cambridge, UK.

However, this concentration is insufficient to avoid ice crystal formation; therefore an additional manipulation is required to minimize the damage. It is the slow cooling and seeding that result in controlled growth of ice in the extracellular solution; consequently, a considerable increase of the concentration of ions, macromolecules, and other components, including cryoprotectants, occurs in the remaining fluid. The slow rate of the procedure allows solution exchange between the extracellular and intracellular fluids without serious osmotic effects and deformation of the cells (this fact is reflected in the other name of the procedure: equilibrium freezing; (14).

The strategy of vitrification is much more radical. The main purpose (according to the cryobiological definition) is the complete elimination of ice formation in the whole solution the sample is cooled in. Evidently, this can only be performed with the use of high cryoprotectant concentration that may theoretically induce serious toxic and osmotic damages. A huge variety of cryoprotectants were tested so far, and although no consensus has been achieved yet regarding the best components, combinations, and concentrations, some principles have already been obtained (see later in text). Cell shrinkage caused by nonpermeable cryoprotectants and the incomplete penetration of permeable components may cause a relative increase of intracellular concentration of macromolecules that is enough to hamper intracellular ice formation. Accordingly, vitrification belongs to the group of nonequilibrium cryopreservation methods.

Another possibility to minimize the chance of ice formation during vitrification is to increase the cooling and warming rates. The higher the cooling rate, the lower the required cryoprotectant concentration is, and vice versa. Eventually, even the radical approach of vitrification has to establish a delicate balance, as it requires (*i*) establishment of a safe system for maximal and reliable cooling (and warming) rates while avoiding consequent damage including fracture of the zona pellucida or the cells and (*ii*) elimination or minimization of the toxic and osmotic effects of high cryoprotectant concentrations needed to obtain and maintain the glass-like solidification.

There is, however, a small, poorly defined group of cryopreservation techniques that shares some features with both vitrification and slow rate freezing. In this method, cryoprotectant concentrations are insufficient to establish vitrification (7,15–17). This approach has been established entirely empirically, and does not meet any supposed requirements of cryopreservation in embryology. Although ice is formed in the solution, under certain (and sometimes unpredictable) conditions embryos survive and develop further (18,19). However, the lack of control may result in inconsistent survival and developmental rates. On the other hand, some of the early experiments characterized as rapid freezing were in fact vitrification (20,21).

INJURY AND PREVENTION DURING CRYOPRESERVATION

Exposition to deep subzero temperatures is a situation mammalian cells never meet under physiological circumstances. The injury may occur at all phases of the procedure.

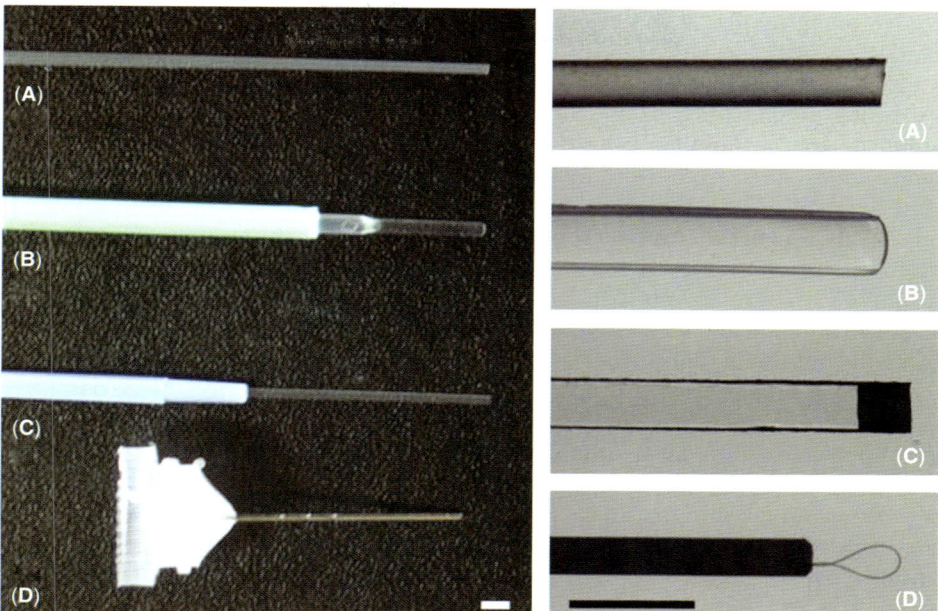

Figure 24.1 Examples for commercially available tools used as carriers for high-speed vitrification. (**A**) Open pulled straw (Minitüb, Landshut, Germany); (**B**) McGill Cryoleaf (MediCult, Jyllinge, Denmark); (**C**) Cryotop (Kitazato, Tokyo, Japan); (**D**) Cryoloop (Hampton Research, Aliso Viejo, California, USA). Bars represent 2 mm.

During cooling, different types of damage may occur when embryos pass through three overlapping temperature zones.

1. At relatively high temperatures between +15 and −5°C, the chilling injury is the major factor, damaging predominantly the cytoplasmic lipid droplets and microtubules including the meiotic spindle (22–24). While the latter damage may be reversible, the former is always irreversible and contributes to the death of cryopreserved lipid-rich oocytes and embryos of some species.
2. Between −5 and −80°C, extracellular or, predominantly, intracellular ice crystal formation is the main source of injury.
3. Temperatures between −50 and −150°C can cause fracture damage to the zona pellucida or the cytoplasm (25) which are postulated to occur (although the mechanism and the actual temperature of occurrence is not entirely defined). However, it is unlikely that zona fracture could occur as a simple consequence of osmotic stress, as suggested by Smith and Silva (4).

Storage below 150°C (typically in liquid nitrogen, at 196°C) is probably the least dangerous phase of the cryopreservation procedure.

Importantly, accidental warming is probably the most frequent form of injury. The effect of background irradiation seems to be less harmful than supposed, and is not a significant source for DNA injury in a realistic time interval, that is years, decades, or even centuries (26). There is increasing and plausible concern regarding possible disease transmission between the stored samples mediated by the liquid nitrogen, although at this time there are no reported cases in literature involving embryos.

At warming, the same types of injuries may occur as at cooling, obviously in inverse order.

Apart from these processes, there are some partially understood injuries including damage of intracellular organelles, cytoskeleton and cell-to-cell contacts (27,28).

All embryos subject to cryopreservation may suffer a considerable damage during cooling and warming. Fortunately, they also have a remarkable, sometimes surprising ability to repair fully or partially this damage, and in the best case to continue normal development. All cryopreservation methods try to decrease the damage and facilitate the regeneration process.

Cryoprotectants are a diverse group of simple or complex, permeable or nonpermeable, organic or inorganic compounds with two common features: they are water-soluble and they protect the cells from cryoinjuries. The range is wide, expanding from well-known simple organic solvents such as ethanol to the complex, partially known substances as serum or egg yolk. Permeable cryoprotectants enter the cells and minimize ice formation with various mechanisms depending on their structure and chemical activity, while nonpermeable cryoprotectants remain outside the cells and minimize ice formation by removing water from the cells by osmotic effect. However, there are certain overlaps between the two groups especially in vitrification methods, where the usually applied short exposition to the concentrated, theoretically permeable components do not allow full equilibrium, therefore part of the effect of permeable cryoprotectants is dehydration, as well. Additionally, both permeable and nonpermeable components may have some other specific cryoprotectant effects, for example stabilization of cell membranes, the meiotic spindle, or other cellular structures (29). Unfortunately, most cryoprotectants have some negative effects, including toxicity and, obviously, osmotic effect. Toxicity is usually in direct correlation with the concentration of the substance, temperature, and the time of exposure while the osmotic effect is mostly proportional to the concentration. In case of permeable or partially permeable cryoprotectants, the osmotic effect can be minimized by slow, stepwise addition and removal during equilibration and dilution, respectively. The mechanism and reasons for damage during cryopreservation as well as the precise protective mechanisms of cryoprotectants are poorly understood at present. Morphological observations of the intracellular structures during the actual phase of cooling (especially at subzero temperatures) are difficult, functional analysis of specific processes at a given moment is almost impossible. The most frequently applied approaches are to investigate the effect of cryoprotectants without cooling and warming, or make retrospective conclusions based on the damage that can be observed after warming. However, the effects of a given cryoprotectant may substantially differ at physiological and at low temperatures; thus, the retrospective analysis of damage may result in faulty conclusions. Considering these uncertainties, it is not surprising that a vast majority of existing cryopreservation techniques were established empirically, based on rough morphological changes observed under a stereomicroscope, and justified by the outcome, that is in vitro and in vivo survival. This is valid for the development and perfection of the vitrification technique as well as for the slow freezing technology. It is just very recent development that using highly sophisticated diagnostics would help to assess freezing conditions; such as using protein expression to detect gene expression (30).

VITRIFICATION

Cryoprotectants

No cryoprotectants exclusively designed or used for vitrification have been developed yet. However, some components and combinations [e.g., ethylene glycol, dimethyl sulfoxide (DMSO), and sucrose] are typically used for vitrification purposes, and the concentration of specific components is significantly higher at vitrification than in traditional or rapid freezing.

The most common permeable components are ethylene glycol, propylene glycol, acetamide, glycerol, raffinose, and DMSO were tested in various combinations (3,31). Due to the low toxicity, high permeability, and excellent ice-blocking ability ethylene glycol is an almost indispensable component of all cryoprotectant solutions. However, a common strategy to decrease the specific toxicity of any one cryoprotectant is to use the mixture of two permeable cryoprotectants, that is, mixture of ethylene glycol and either DMSO or propylene glycol, or less typically other components. Eventually the mixture of ethylene glycol and DMSO appears to be used frequently (32,33). According to some studies, the permeability of this mixture is higher than that of the individual components (34). It should be noted that the earlier concerns regarding the genotoxicity and cytotoxicity of DMSO have been dismissed (35,36).

Commonly used nonpermeable cryoprotectants include mono- and disaccharides, sucrose, trehalose, glucose, and galactose (37–39). Recently, sucrose has become an almost standard component of vitrification mixtures. This is true, even though nearly all comparative investigations proved the superiority of trehalose. Sucrose as well as other sugars may not have any toxic effects at low temperatures, but may compromise embryo survival when applied extensively to counterbalance embryo swelling after warming (40–42), although this effect has not always been demonstrated (43). Several polymers were also suggested for the purpose, including polyvinyl pyrrolidine, polyethylene glycol, Ficoll, dextran, and polyvinyl alcohol (44–49). However, from this group the only widely used compound is Ficoll, predominantly in combination with ethylene glycol and sucrose (50). Various forms of protein supplementation have also been used including egg yolk, but its optically dense appearance made the microscopic manipulation rather difficult. High concentrations of sera of different origins as well as serum albumin preparations (51) are common additives. In the bovine model, recombinant albumin and hyaluronan were also effective (52). On the other hand, the use of antifreeze proteins isolated from arctic animals (53–55) has largely been abandoned.

Another practical feature is the stepwise addition of increasing concentrations of cryoprotectants (51,56–58).

After several early attempts the two-step equilibration has become the most commonly used approach, with the first solution containing approximately 50% of the final cryoprotectant concentration. Embryos and oocytes are equilibrated for a relatively long period (5–15, sometimes up to 21 minutes) in the first solution, then for a short period (approximately 1 minute) in the second one (59–61). This approach may increase slightly the toxic effect, but provides a much better protection for the whole cell, and may be especially beneficial in the case of large substance with a low surface and volume ratio including oocytes or early-stage embryos. On the other hand, earlier attempts to cool the concentrated solution to 4°C to decrease toxicity have been found later unnecessary.

Traditional Tools of Cryopreservation Used for Vitrification

Plastic insemination straws or cryovials were used initially for vitrification experiments. These tools were not designed for the special purpose of vitrification, had a thick wall and required a relatively large amount of solution for safe loading. Accordingly, the cooling and warming rates were quite limited (approximately 2500°C/min for straws; (62); and even less for cryovials). This relatively low rate was still hazardous to perform, as direct immersion into liquid nitrogen at cooling, and a transfer to a water bath at warming induced extreme pressure changes in the closed system and frequently led to the collapse or explosion of the straws and loss of the sample.

One of the other consequences of these manipulations was the decreased and inconsistent rates: the temperature of the vapor of liquid nitrogen was variable, depending on many factors, and the definition of "room temperature" laboratory air may mean 5–7°C differences, even at the same place on the same day. Consequently, a minimum 5–7 mol/L cryoprotectant concentration was required, and chilling injury could not be lowered to the level occurring at slow freezing.

Increasing Cooling Rates with New Carrier Tools

Although the increased cooling and warming rate was a well-known possibility to keep the concentration of cryoprotectants as low as possible, and minimize the related toxic and osmotic injuries, this option has remained unexploited for a relatively long period of time. The first purpose-made tools were only produced approximately 15 years ago. Today, however, the contrary is the problem, huge variety of tools (Table 24.1 and Figure 24.1), methods and approaches are available, and without authentic comparative studies, the selection of the best choice is a serious problem for embryologists working in a routine human IVF laboratory.

The most logical way to increase cooling and warming rates is to decrease the volume of the solution that surrounds the sample, and to establish a direct contact between the sample and the liquid nitrogen.

Seemingly the simplest way to accomplish this task is the direct dropping into liquid nitrogen (59,63–65). Unfortunately, to form a drop from a water-based solution requires a relatively large amount of solution (4–6 µL), and the drop does not sink immediately into the liquid nitrogen, because for the initial seconds the drop is surrounded by the vapor that induced by the warm solution, and does not allow the sample to sink.

Accordingly, some carrier tools have been used to push the sample immediately below the level of liquid nitrogen, to serve as a storage device after cooling and to facilitate quick warming, as well. Electron microscopic grids have proved to be of practical value during the proof of principle steps (63,64,66,67). In this system, the size of the drop surrounding the sample was extremely small, as after loading, most of it was removed by placing the grid on a filter membrane. The thermoconductive metal grid also contributed to improve the cooling and warming rates. Surprisingly, the solidified cryoprotectant solution fixed the sample safely to the grid during cooling and storage, and released it easily after warming (68). However, the storage and handling of the tiny grid has been a demanding task.

The first purpose-made tool for vitrification was the open pulled straw (OPS), a modification of a standard 0.25 mL plastic straw, with decreased diameter and wall thickness. This modification enabled loading with the capillary effect, and the minimum volume decreased to approximately 0.5–1 µL, that is, five to ten times smaller than that of the original straw that results in approximately 10-fold increase in the achievable cooling and warming rates, and a 30% decrease of the cryoprotectant concentration required for vitrification. An additional benefit was related to the open system: no explosion of the straws occurred, and the fracture damage (with some precautions) could be entirely eliminated. The OPS has become a widely used approach for ultrarapid vitrification (69–77). According to preliminary experiments, by using recent equilibration and dilution parameters, results achieved with OPS vitrification of human oocytes and embryos are at least as good as with the other, commonly used vitrification tools.

The Cryoloop is another approach using the small volume–direct contact principle. A small nylon loop attached to a holder and equipped with a container. It has been used for cryopreservation in crystallography and is now used widely for oocyte and embryo cryopreservation (78–81). The solution film bridging the hole of the loop is strong enough to hold the oocyte or the embryo, and with this minimal solution volume, the achievable cooling rate may be extremely high, up to an estimated 700,000°C/min (82). Using this tool, safe cryopreservation can be achieved even in the vapor of liquid nitrogen (83,84).

The minimum drop size method of Arav (85) consisting of a small droplet of vitrification solution containing the oocyte or embryo placed on a solid surface that is immersed into liquid nitrogen. The approach was used later with some modifications called the minimum volume cooling (86) or in the hemi-straw system, (87), where the carrier tool was a cut-open straw.

Currently, the most commonly used tool for vitrification of human oocytes and embryos is the Cryotop, an advanced version of the minimum volume cooling technology (61,86). It consists of a flexible transparent plastic film attached to a handle, and also equipped with a protective tube to avoid damages of the film during storage in liquid nitrogen. The sample is loaded on the film, the excess solution is removed, and the film is immersed into the liquid nitrogen. At warming, the Cryotop is quickly removed from the liquid nitrogen, and the film is immersed into the warming medium. This simple system, with appropriate solutions and equilibration parameters triggered an exponential increase of the use of vitrification in human embryology. Since its first introduction, several studies have confirmed its value (88–90). Yet another carrier, Cryolock, similar in its design to Cryotop is gaining more popularity and being used efficiently (91).

Cryopette is probably the first carrier that is designed by aiming to combine the benefit of very low volume solution with the benefit of a closed system. Studies are currently being performed to test the system, but not yet appeared in publications. It is expected that there will be more carriers and systems brought to the market which will try to serve the same purpose: efficient vitrification using minimal volume in a closed system—like the Rapid-I (92). However, it awaits confirmation whether open systems provide superior outcomes and preserve the original physiological cell condition (93).

The flow chart of a typical high-speed vitrification procedure is summarized in Figure 24.2.

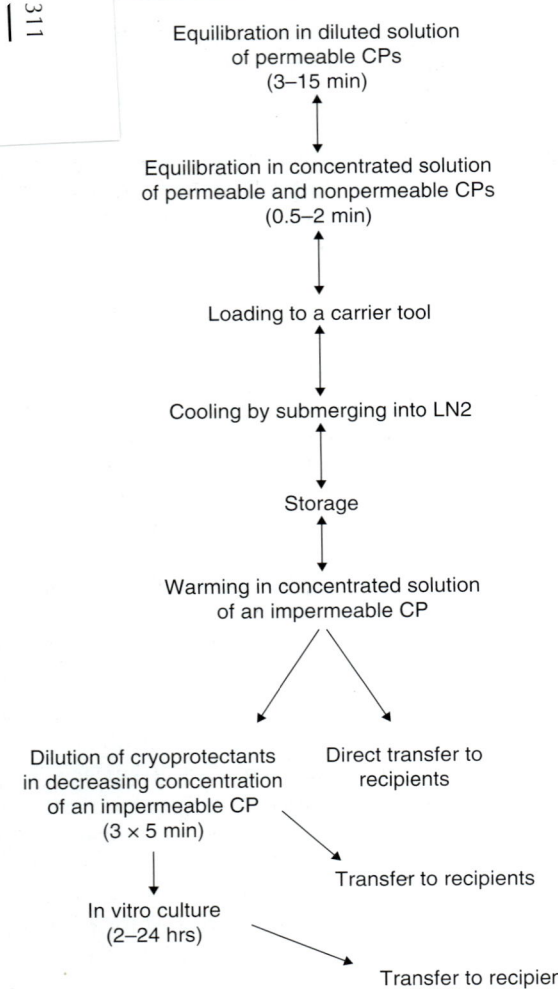

Figure 24.2 Flow chart of a typical high-speed vitrification procedure.

Decreased Vapor Formation for Increased Cooling Rates

One major limitation of the achievable cooling rates around the sample is the vapor that is formed around at immersion. At −196°C, liquid nitrogen is at boiling point, accordingly a submerged warmer item will induce an extensive evaporation around the sample, producing a thermoinsulating coat around the sample and decreasing the achievable cooling rate, especially at the initial moments, when the chilling injury may develop.

One possibility to avoid this phenomenon is to expose liquid nitrogen to a vacuum for several minutes. Part of the liquid nitrogen will evaporate, and the rest will cool down to −203 to −207°C, where it starts to get solidified, that is, slush is formed. As the nitrogen escapes from the fragile boiling zone, the immersed sample creates a minimal evaporation, consequently the cooling rate gets considerably higher (72,73,94).

The other way to eliminate the vapor is the use of precooled metal surfaces instead of the liquid nitrogen for cooling. It can be performed by immersing a metal block into liquid nitrogen (95), or by using a more sophisticated, commercially available version (CMV; CryoLogic, Mulgrave, Victoria, Australia).

The available free comparative data do not provide entirely convincing evidence regarding the superiority of these vapor-minimizing or vapor-free approaches compared with other vitrification procedures.

Transmission of Infectious Agents

One of the concerns regarding the use of vitrification in human embryology is the potential risk of liquid nitrogen-mediated disease transmission. To understand better, we need to consider the following:

1. Semen and embryo collection, processing and cryopreservation protocols are not sterile procedures (96); consequently, the contents of virtually all stored straws and cryovials may be a source of infection.
2. In human embryology, liquid nitrogen may also be contaminated by the surface of straws, cryovials, racks, and other tools that are usually not handled fully aseptically. Accordingly, the presence of infective agents is not strictly related to leaky or open containers.
3. Seemingly sterile containers may not be as safe as supposed. Infection may occur in common straws in slow freezing (through the holes of incomplete sealing or pores of the plastic walls), and most cryovials do not have secure caps. A possible source of infection may also be the inappropriate decontamination of the outer walls of straws before loading and expelling.
4. Liquid nitrogen in storage tanks likely contains a number of commensal and potentially pathogenic environmental microorganisms (96).
5. Cases of liquid nitrogen-mediated transmission of pathogens (97–99) have been documented but never in relation to cryopreserved oocytes or embryos. Disease transfer has occurred only on one occasion, where two leaky bags containing blood samples were stored in the same dewar (97).
6. According to the experiments of Bielanski et al. (100), cross-contamination may also occur during storage between open embryo storage if one of them is artificially infected. However, the volume of the microbes was extremely high, a concentration that may never happen in clinical situation.
7. Not a single case of any disease transmission in ART has been found to be related to liquid nitrogen-mediated cross-contamination, in spite of the enormous amount of human sperm samples, embryos, and oocytes stored worldwide, neither related to traditional, supposedly closed (but very often leaky or inappropriately handled) systems, nor with the open vitrification systems, in spite of the enormous focus on the latter. There is no doubt that closed and properly handled systems should always be preferred, provided the outcome is comparable with the open systems. Results achieved by using closed systems for cleavage-stage human embryos and blastocysts are promising (101–103). A possible solution is to

make cooling in sterilized liquid nitrogen (104,105) and store the samples in precooled, hermetically sealed containers afterwards (70,106). Alternatively, open carriers can also be stored in cryotanks, where instead of liquid the vapor of nitrogen maintains the low storage temperature. There have been a number of studies demonstrating the efficiency of the vapor storage system for vitrified oocytes/embryos using open carriers both in animal and human system (107–109). Concerns may also be raised regarding the applicability of closed systems for other chilling sensitive objects including cattle oocytes and early-stage embryos, porcine blastocysts, or human oocytes (110), regarding not just in vitro survival rates, but in vitro development, pregnancies, and birth of healthy offspring.

Warming

Earlier, Rall (51) has found that high survival of vitrified embryos can be achieved with rather slow warming rates. However, most vitrification methods use rapid warming procedures, and recently it has been demonstrated that warming rates may be even more important than cooling rates (111). Closed systems are usually immersed into water baths, while open systems can be directly submerged into the medium, this way the warming and the first dilution is performed in a single step. The seemingly negligible difference may contribute considerably in the inferior results achieved with some closed systems consisting of a simple plastic or glass tube. After warming in the water bath, the surface has to be decontaminated quickly with a nontoxic but perfectly safe disinfectant, then the tube is cut and the sample is expelled into the appropriate medium. It means a significant delay between the warming and dilution, accordingly the samples in this critical, very fragile phase are exposed for a relatively long period of time (5–10 seconds) to the concentrated cryoprotectants.

Although a slight devitrification (occurrence of ice crystals) may occur, especially when the cryoprotectant level is kept at the minimum level, this transitional change is usually restricted to a part of the embryo-containing medium and most probably does not involve intracellular crystal formation, and consequently does not cause significant harm in the embryos or oocytes (112).

In routine warming protocols of vitrified embryos, the dilution is a multistep procedure with decreasing concentration of osmotic buffers (usually sucrose) to counterbalance the swelling caused by the permeable cryoprotectant that leaves the cells relatively slowly. This delicate multistep dilution procedure seems to be indispensable for human embryos or oocytes, although one-step dilution without significant decrease of in vitro survival was reported in some animal species including cattle (42,57,113), and pig (114). Based on this approach, direct transfer methods after ultra rapid vitrification of embryos resulted in offspring after transfer in cattle (115) and sheep (116).

FACTORS INFLUENCING THE OUTCOME

Species, Genotype

There are well-demonstrated but poorly understood differences in sensitivity to cryoinjuries between different species in mammals. It appears that transparent oocytes and embryos are usually more resistant, while dense dark ones are more fragile, due to the increased lipid content. Accordingly, cryopreservation of light mouse embryos is a relatively easy task, darker bovine embryo is a more difficult task, and the cryopreservation of dense pig embryos is truly a challenge in cryobiology. In parallel with the lighter appearance of the cytoplasm, considerably increased survival rates were detected after both slow freezing (117) and vitrification (118–121). This approach also improves in vitro survival of vitrified porcine blastocysts produced by somatic cell nuclear transfer (121,122).

It should also be noted that apart from the differences between species, in mouse, differences between genotypes in the ability to develop after vitrification were also observed (123).

Developmental Stage

The change in the size and shape of the cells is unprecedented in the first five to six days of mammalian development. A relatively simple spherical shape protected by an acellular outer layer develops to a complicated multicellular structure without external protection. Predictably, the extreme differences in morphology also result in considerable differences in sensitivity to cryoinjuries. Generally, the earlier the development stage (starting from the germinal vesicle stage), the more sensitive oocytes and embryos are. However, although there is only a minimal difference between the size and shape, the immature oocytes are usually more sensitive to cryopreservation than mature (MII phase) oocytes (23,110,124). Membrane permeability related to the type and expression levels of aquaporin at different stages may also explain differences in cryoprotectant protection efficiency and thus differences in survival (125,126). Additionally, a very remarkable difference exists between the chilling sensitivity of unfertilized and fertilized human oocytes. A possible explanation for this phenomenon is the increased chilling sensitivity of membranes: the lipid phase transition at room temperature storage in human germinal vesicle and MII-stage oocytes is 10 times higher than that of human pronuclear embryos (110).

In the human, the survival rates after slow freezing are not significantly different between zygotes, cleavage-stage embryos, and blastocysts (between 75 and 80% for each; (127,128). The complex structure of blastocysts may give rise to additional problems. In humans, mechanical reduction of the blastocele by puncturing or repeated pipetting improved survival and pregnancy rates (129–133). The usual explanation is that the large blastocele may not be protected appropriately from ice crystal formation (129). However, other feasible mechanisms may include the inappropriate dilution of the accumulated cryoprotectants after warming (Vajta, unpublished) or increased protection against cryoinjuries due to stress-induced biochemical changes (134).

In Vivo- Vs. In Vitro-Produced Embryos

In lack of in vivo-derived human embryos, such differences can only be evaluated in domestic and experimental animals (135). In these species, in vivo-produced embryos are more resistant to injuries—including cryoinjuries—than their in vitro fertilized or cloned counterparts. Again, there might be some correlation between the increased lipid content of embryos produced in some in vitro systems. In general, the less morphological difference from the in vivo-counterpart is detectable in the in vivo-produced embryos, the small the expected difference in survival after cryopreservation is (136). Although a total elimination of these differences is still impossible, according to the joint conclusion of many publications, vitrification seems to be especially appropriate to counterbalance this handicap (137).

Evidences in Favor of Vitrification

Domestic, Experimental, and Wild Animals

There is an extensive literature of comparative experiments between slow freezing versus vitrification (some examples may include (78,79,123,138–141). The overwhelming majority of these papers prove the superiority of vitrification for the given purpose. Probably less than 10% did not find significant differences, and, according to our knowledge, no publication stated that results achieved by vitrification were significantly worse than those obtained by slow freezing. Moreover, there are situations where vitrification is uniquely or predominantly suitable to achieve the goal: most of these areas are summarized in Table 24.2.

Human Embryos

In humans, the clinical pregnancy rate from embryo transfer after slow freezing is approximately two-thirds of that from the fresh transfer of embryos (142), although new techniques have recently been introduced to restore (cleavage stage) embryo viability (143,144). The theoretical possibility for improvement is supported by the results obtained in cattle, where the difference is no more than 10–15%.

Until recently, the published sporadic results based on relatively low numbers proved only the feasibility and potential competitiveness, but not the superiority of vitrification in this field (3,20,21,66,67,75,76,80,81,87,129, 130,140,145–157).

In 2005, however, three comparative investigations were published and all the three concluded that vitrification was a more efficient way for cryopreservation of human embryos than slow-rate freezing. Zheng et al. (158) performed an in vitro experiment with biopsied nontransferable human embryos. Three versions of slow freezing were compared with vitrification, and survival rates were the highest after vitrification. Stehlik and colleagues (159) used slow freezing versus Cryotop vitrification for cryopreservation of supernumerary human blastocysts, and observed a significant difference in

Table 24.2 Examples in Mammalian Embryology where First Success in Cryopreservation Achieved by Vitrification

Species, stage, system	Reference
Bovine immature oocytes for IVF	Vieria et al. (205)
Bovine in vitro-matured oocytes for IVF	Martino et al. (206); Vajta et al. (70)
Bovine in vitro-matured oocytes for somatic cell nuclear transfer	Hou et al. (207)
Bovine cytoplasts for embryonic cell nuclear transfer	Booth et al. (208)
Bovine early-stage IVF embryos	Vajta et al. (71); in vitro study
Bovine zona-included blastocysts generated by somatic cell nuclear transfer	French et al. (209)
Bovine zona-free blastocysts generated by somatic cell nuclear transfer	Tecirlioglu et al. (115)
Bovine transgenic blastocysts generated by somatic cell nuclear transfer	French et al. (210)
Ovine zona-included embryos generated by nuclear transfer	Peura et al. (211)
Porcine immature oocytes for ICSI	Fujihira et al. (212); in vitro study
Porcine in vitro-matured oocytes for ICSI	Fujihira et al. (213); in vitro study
Porcine in vivo-derived blastocysts	Kobayashi et al. (214)
Porcine in vivo-derived morulae	Berthelot et al. (215)
Porcine in vitro-produced blastocysts	Men et al. (216); in vitro study
Equine in vivo-matured oocytes	Maclellan et al. (217)
European polecat in vivo-derived morulae and blastocysts	Piltty et al. (218)
Siberian tiger in vivo-derived embryos	Crichton et al. (219); in vitro study
Minke whale immature oocytes for maturation	Iwayama et al. (220); in vitro study

Embryos and oocytes were not treated mechanically or chemically to prepare them for the vitrification. Full-term developments were reported except where otherwise indicated.
Abbreviations: ICSI, intracytoplasmic sperm injection; IVF, in vitro fertilization.
Source: Adapted from Ref. 204; courtesy of Reproductive Healthcare Ltd.

pregnancy rates after 44 transfers (16.7 vs 50% respectively). The largest comparative investigation between the effects of slow freezing and vitrification was published by Kuwayama et al. (61), based on cryopreservation of more than 16,000 human embryos at different stages. Cryotop vitrification was found superior for pronuclear embryo cryopreservation in regard to survival, cleavage, and developmental rates (61). Survival rates of cleavage-stage and blastocyst-stage human embryos were also significantly higher than those after slow freezing. Pregnancy and birth rates after cryopreservation with the two methods were not significantly different (61). More recent comparative studies published in the literature have confirmed that vitrification is clearly more efficient than slow freezing using at different embryonic development stages (160–164). Accordingly, these representative comparisons have proved that vitrification is at least as efficient as slow-rate freezing for cryopreservation of human embryos at all stages (165). Additional to those comparative studies, other, noncomparative studies on the efficiency of vitrification have been published, applying the technique at different stages of preimplantation embryo development including zygote, cleavage, and blastocyst stages (102,132,166–170), including also day 7 successful vitrification (171).

Although several tools (carriers) and kits (vitrification solution kits) are currently available for vitrification, two technologies related to the type of carriers have obtained more attention initially: the OPS, predominantly in the animal field, and the Cryotop for human areas. It should be emphasized, however, that the differences do not necessarily mean an unbreakable frontier. The OPS is more robust and easy to perform even under compromised conditions, while the more delicate Cryotop method may be the choice where extremely high cooling rates are the primary objectives. However, if properly applied, both OPS and Cryotop methods seem to be suitable for the given purposes. A good example to support this statement is that very healthy piglets were born after OPS vitrification and transfer of the extremely sensitive somatic cell cloned blastocyst derived from delipated oocytes (122). As written earlier, there are now several new cryotools/carriers available on the market, which are likely to be tested and used more widely for both embryo and oocyte vitrification.

Updated results obtained at Reproductive Biology Associates, the first IVF clinic in the United States to apply in routine patient care embryo (and oocyte) vitrification using the CryoTop or CryoLock approach, demonstrates equal or better outcomes with vitrification compared with slow freezing in comparable patient population (Table 24.3).

Novel ART Services Based on Vitrification

The extreme high efficiency of vitrification applied on oocytes and embryos provide the possibilities for novel patient services. Oocyte vitrification now can provide the base for fertility preservation for both medical and social reasons (172–175); for donor egg banking (88,90), or for various other clinical conditions, such as hyperstimulation, failure to obtain sperm on the day of oocyte collection or due to moral/ethical reason preferring egg preservation instead of embryo (176,177), cryopreserving excess oocytes aspirated from IUI patients with excess follicles (178).

The highly efficient embryo vitrification has opened up several new possibilities. One of the most important benefits relates to embryo biopsy and PGS/PGD. In the past, survival of embryos after slow-freeze/thaw following embryo biopsy was more than disappointing, strongly limiting the use of biopsy and genetic testing—mainly to be performed on day 3 cleavage stage, or for polar body biopsy (179,180). Applying vitrification, instead of slow freezing, on biopsied embryos has significantly improved survival rates (158); thus this procedure has become a routine when embryos are tested genetically (163). Additionally, now biopsy timing can be shifted from day 3 (or day 0/day 1) to day 5/day 6, when embryos develop to the blastocyst stage, as there is no more need to use these embryos for fresh transfer, as they will survive cryopreservation much better, usually perfectly. Biopsying embryos at the blastocyst stage has several advantages compared with earlier stages, specially to day 3-stage biopsy, as embryos are more resistant to the biopsy procedure, more cells can be removed (genetic testing can be

Table 24.3 Outcomes of Embryo Cryopreservation–Embryo transfer Cycles Comparing Vitrification/Warming with Slow Freezing/Thawing (Including 2PN/Day-3 and Blastocyst-Stage Cryopreserved Embryos)

	Slow freeze	Vitrification	P values
All Thaws (2PN/D3/Blast)			
Thaw–warm cycles	132	468	
Average age	36.1	35.9	Not significant
Embryos thawed–warmed	662	1307	
Embryos thawed–warmed cycle	5.0	2.8	<0.001
Survived	529	1246	
Survival rate	79.9%	95.3%	<0.001
Clinical pregnancy rate	48.5%	59.6%	<0.05
Implantation rate	32.6%	39.0%	<0.01

more reliable); less likely to encounter mosaicism, and embryos will be transferred in a (possibly) more receptive uterine environment, all these factors in combination resulting in very high pregnancy rates (181–183). Pregnancies and live births were reported also when vitrification was repeated on the same embryo at the same (or a different) stage or after oocyte vitrification, or even after involving a trophectoderm biopsy, demonstrating the robustness of the technique (91,183–185). Because of the extreme high success rates obtained with vitrified embryos after biopsy, it seems a logical extension of the thinking, that other patients with different clinical conditions, may also will benefit from the "cryopreserve all" embryos and transfer performed in a "cryo cycle." Rationally, patients at risk for ovarian hyperstimulation can clearly benefit from vitrifying all embryos (170); other studies suggest "cryo-embryos" for women with endometriosis (186), while some may consider applying this idea for all IVF patients, looking for the benefit of a more receptive endometrium in a cryo-cycle for patients who underwent ovarian stimulation (187).

Safety of Vitrification

For a new technique or technology to be fully accepted and applied worldwide, there are two critical points which need to be fulfilled. Efficiency and safety are these points. Vitrification of embryos/oocytes is now has been clearly demonstrated to provide extreme high efficiency providing outcomes similar to those achieved by using fresh oocyte/embryo; however, safety is a point yet to be proven beyond any doubt. Though, preliminary outcomes on live birth data (mainly gathered after oocyte vitrification) do not indicate any alarming or unexpected results or trends (166,183,185,188–192), further collection of live birth outcome data is required. It would be most prudent, if national or international IVF societies would organize the needed data collection through registry (or registries). Only a multicenter effort where most IVF clinics participate would be able to provide sufficient amount of data in a reasonable period of time.

CONCLUSIONS

Vitrification as an approach to cryopreserve human embryos or oocytes has achieved a remarkable success. With just a very few publications on clinical results and applications, today there are dozens of papers demonstrating the efficient use of embryo/oocyte vitrification in human assisted reproduction, and there are hundreds, or more likely thousands, of IVF clinics that have switched from slow freezing to vitrification. This extraordinary achievement would not have been possible without the constant dedication and hard work of the few early pioneers, mainly coming from the field of veterinary medicine. It has been both with support and constraint to see this technology prevail. Yves Ménézo (193) stated that the impact of vitrification, especially when ethylene glycol is used, has to be carefully evaluated before its use on a large scale. Ethylene glycol and its metabolites can be toxic at a very low concentration (cited literature: (194). Regarding toxicity as a concern, the result of combined application of different approaches to minimize the toxicity, the concentration of ethylene glycol can be as low as 15% (2.2 mol/L), and is applied for a very short period before and after deep cooling. This concentration is similar to that used at industrial level for traditional slow freezing of cattle embryos, where no increase of developmental abnormalities or other toxic effects has been reported so far. The now large number of studies clearly demonstrates the high efficiency of vitrification for embryo (and oocyte) cryopreservation. On the safety of vitrification, any currently available data do not indicate a higher incidence of malformation—which is reassuring, but obviously needed to be confirmed on a much larger scale.

The overwhelming majority of the studies/publications support the application of vitrification by emphasizing its advantages: the simple, inexpensive, and rapid procedure leading to higher survival and developmental rates than those achievable with alternative methods. Concerns regarding disease transmission are theoretically justified, but safer methods are now available to mitigate this risk. Convincing results like the emerging breakthrough in human oocyte vitrification and the excellent (and improved) results on embryo cryopreservation may help to eliminate these obstacles and the remaining concerns. Recently achieved results using vitrification seem to convince more and more professionals about the advantage of the technique, reflected by the increasing number of publications and also by the number of introduced (or soon to be introduced) commercial kits for vitrification.

In the future, standardization should be attempted after comparing different protocols of vitrification, which also should be adjusted to the different stages of embryo development.

EMBRYO/BLASTOCYST VITRIFICATION PROTOCOL

Vitrification

Materials

- *Equilibration Solution:* ES is a HEPES-buffered medium, 7.5% (v/v) of each DMSO and ethylene glycol, and 20% (v/v) Serum Protein Substitute.
- *Vitrification Solution:* VS is a HEPES-buffered medium, 15% (v/v) of each DMSO and ethylene glycol, and 20% (v/v) Serum Protein Substitute and 0.5 M sucrose.

Cryolock Biodiseño Ltda.; Bogotá D.C; Columbia.

Procedure

1. Bring one vial of each ES and VS to room temperature (20–27 °C) for at least 30 minutes prior to freezing embryos.
2. Fill the liquid nitrogen reservoir with liquid nitrogen.

3. Determine the number of embryos to be vitrified.
4. Label each Cryolock with necessary information.
5. Prepare a 4-well dish with 1.0 mL ES and 1.0 mL VS in each well.
6. Transfer the embryos to ES for 15 minutes.
7. Transfer the embryos to VS for 1 minute.
8. Load the embryos onto the Cryolock with a minimal volume.
9. Plunge the Cryolock into liquid nitrogen (cooling at a rate of −12,000°C/min).
10. Move the plunged Cryolock to the liquid nitrogen freezer for long-term storage.

Warming

Materials

- *Thawing Solution:* TS is a HEPES-buffered medium, 1.0 M sucrose and 20% (v/v) Serum Protein Substitute.
- *Dilution Solution:* DS is a HEPES-buffered medium, 0.5 M sucrose and 20% (v/v) Serum Protein Substitute.
- *Washing Solution:* WS is a HEPES-buffered medium and 20% (v/v) Serum Protein Substitute.

Procedure

1. Bring one vial of each TS, DS, and WS to room temperature (20–27 °C) for at least 30 minutes prior to thawing embryos.
2. Fill the liquid nitrogen reservoir with liquid nitrogen.
3. Determine the number of embryos to be thawed.
4. Take the Cryolock out of the liquid nitrogen and quickly transfer the embryos into TS (3 mL at 37°C), where they should stay for 1 minute.
5. Transfer the embryos into 1.0 mL DS for 3 minutes at RT.
6. Transfer the embryos into 1.0 mL WS for 10 minutes at RT.
7. Transfer the embryos into pre-equilibrated culture medium.

The same protocol and handling applies to all stages of embryos, including zygote, cleavage-stage and blastocyst-stage embryos. Blastocyst-stage embryos (especially well-expanded blastocyst) may be collapsed artificially (for instance, using a laser shot) prior to cryopreservation.

REFERENCES

1. Shaw JM, Jones GM. Terminology associated with vitrification and other cryopreservation procedures for oocytes and embryos. Hum Reprod Update 2003; 9: 583–605.
2. Fuller B, Paynter S. Fundamentals of cryobiology in reproductive medicine. Reprod Biomed Online 2004; 9: 680–91.
3. Kasai M, Mukaida T. Cryopreservation of animal and human embryos by vitrification. Reprod Biomed Online 2004; 9: 164–70.
4. Smith GD, Silva ESCA. Developmental consequences of cryopreservation of mammalian oocytes and embryos. Reprod Biomed Online 2004; 9: 171–8.
5. Stachecki JJ, Cohen J. An overview of oocyte cryopreservation. Reprod Biomed Online 2004; 9: 152–63.
6. Whittingham DG, Leibo SP, Mazur P. Survival of mouse embryos frozen to −196 degrees and −269 degrees C. Science 1972; 178: 411–14.
7. Wilmut I. The effect of cooling rate, warming rate, cryoprotective agent and stage of development on survival of mouse embryos during freezing and thawing. Life Sci II 1972; 11: 1071–9.
8. Wilmut I, Rowson LE. Experiments on the low-temperature preservation of cow embryos. Vet Rec 1973; 92: 686–90.
9. Bank H, Maurer RR. Survival of frozen rabbit embryos. Exp Cell Res 1974; 89: 188–96.
10. Willadsen SM, Polge C, Rowson LE, Moor RM. Deep freezing of sheep embryos. J Reprod Fertil 1976; 46: 151–4.
11. Trounson A, Mohr L. Human pregnancy following cryopreservation, thawing and transfer of an eight-cell embryo. Nature 1983; 305: 707–9.
12. Zeilmaker GH, Alberda AT, van Gent I, Rijkmans CM, Drogendijk AC. Two pregnancies following transfer of intact frozen-thawed embryos. Fertil Steril 1984; 42: 293–6.
13. Rall WF, Fahy GM. Ice-free cryopreservation of mouse embryos at-196 degrees C by vitrification. Nature 1985; 313: 573–5.
14. Mazur P. Equilibrium, quasi-equilibrium, and non-equilibrium freezing of mammalian embryos. Cell Biophys 1990; 17: 53–92.
15. Leibo SP, McGrath JJ, Cravalho EG. Microscopic observation of intracellular ice formation in unfertilized mouse ova as a function of cooling rate. Cryobiology 1978; 15: 257–71.
16. Kasai M, Niwa K, Iritani A. Survival of mouse embryos frozen and thawed rapidly. J Reprod Fertil 1980; 59: 51–6.
17. Wood MJ, Farrant J. Preservation of mouse embryos by two-step freezing. Cryobiology 1980; 17: 178–80.
18. Trounson A, Peura A, Kirby C. Ultrarapid freezing: A new low-cost and effective method of embryo cryopreservation. Fertil Steril 1987; 48: 843–50.
19. Shaw JM, Diotallevi L, Trounson A. Ultrarapid embryo freezing: Effect of dissolved gas and pH of the freezing solutions and straw irradiation. Hum Reprod 1988; 3: 905–8.
20. Barg PE, Barad DH, Feichtinger W. Ultrarapid freezing (URF) of mouse and human preembryos: A modified approach. J In Vitro Fert Embryo Transf 1990; 7: 355–7.
21. Feichtinger W, Hochfellner C, Ferstl U. Clinical experience with ultra-rapid freezing of embryos. Hum Reprod 1991; 6: 735–6.
22. Aman RR, Parks JE. Effects of cooling and rewarming on the meiotic spindle and chromosomes of in vitro-matured bovine oocytes. Biol Reprod 1994; 50: 103–10.
23. Martino A, Pollard JW, Leibo SP. Effect of chilling bovine oocytes on their developmental competence. Mol Reprod Dev 1996; 45: 503–12.
24. Zenzes MT, Bielecki R, Casper RF, Leibo SP. Effects of chilling to 0 degrees C on the morphology of meiotic spindles in human metaphase II oocytes. Fertil Steril 2001; 75: 769–77.
25. Rall WF, Meyer TK. Zona fracture damage and its avoidance during the cryopreservation of mammalian embryos. Theriogenology 1989; 31: 683–92.

26. Rall WF. Cryopreservation of mammalian embryos, gametes and ovarian tissues. Current issues and progress. In: Wolf DP, Zelinski-Wooten M, eds. Assisted Fertilization and Nuclear Transfer in Mammals. Totowa, NJ: HUmana Press, 2001: 173–87.
27. Vincent C, Johnson MH. Cooling, cryoprotectants, and the cytoskeleton of the mammalian oocyte. Oxf Rev Reprod Biol 1992; 14: 73–100.
28. Massip AP, Mermillod Dinnyes A. Morphology and biochemistry of in-vitro produced bovine embryos: Implications for their cryopreservation. Hum Reprod 1995; 10: 3004–11.
29. Chang CC, Sung LY, Lin CJ, et al. The oocyte spindle is preserved by 1,2-propanediol during slow freezing. Fertil Steril 2010; 93: 1430–9.
30. Gardner DK, Sheehan CB, Rienzi L, Katz-Jaffe M, Larman MG. Analysis of oocyte physiology to improve cryopreservation procedures. Theriogenology 2007; 67: 64–72.
31. dela Pena EC, Takahashi Y, Atabay EC, Katagiri S, Nagano M. Vitrification of mouse oocytes in ethylene glycol-raffinose solution: Effects of preexposure to ethylene glycol or raffinose on oocyte viability. Cryobiology 2001; 42: 103–11.
32. Ishimori H, Takahashi Y, Kanagawa H. Factors affecting survival of mouse blastocysts vitrified by a mixture of ethylene glycol and dimethyl sulfoxide. Theriogenology 1992; 38: 1175–85.
33. Ishimori H, Saeki K, Inai M, et al. Vitrification of bovine embryos in a mixture of ethylene glycol and dimethyl sulfoxide. Theriogenology 1993; 40: 427–33.
34. Vicente JS, Garcia-Ximenez F. Osmotic and cryoprotective effects of a mixture of DMSO and ethylene glycol on rabbit morulae. Theriogenology 1994; 42: 1205–15.
35. Aye M, Di Giorgio C, De Mo M, et al. Assessment of the genotoxicity of three cryoprotectants used for human oocyte vitrification: Dimethyl sulfoxide, ethylene glycol and propylene glycol. Food Chem Toxicol 2010; 48: 1905–12.
36. Lawson AH, Ahmad Sambanis A. Cytotoxicity effects of cryoprotectants as single-component and cocktail vitrification solutions. Cryobiology 2011; 62: 115–22.
37. Ali J, Shelton JN. Design of vitrification solutions for the cryopreservation of embryos. J Reprod Fertil 1993; 99: 471–7.
38. Kasai M. Cryopreservation of mammalian embryos. Mol Biotechnol 1997; 7: 173–9.
39. Wright DL, Eroglu A, Toner M, Toth TL. Use of sugars in cryopreserving human oocytes. Reprod Biomed Online 2004; 9: 179–86.
40. Kasai M. Nonfreezing technique for short-term storage of mouse embryos. J In Vitro Fert Embryo Transf 1986; 3: 10–14.
41. Kasai M, Nishimori M, Zhu SE, Sakurai T, Machida T. Survival of mouse morulae vitrified in an ethylene glycol-based solution after exposure to the solution at various temperatures. Biol Reprod 1992; 47: 1134–9.
42. Vajta G, Holm P, Greve T, Callesen H. Survival and development of bovine blastocysts produced in vitro after assisted hatching, vitrification and in-straw direct rehydration. J Reprod Fertil 1997; 111: 65–70.
43. Kuleshova LL, MacFarlane DR, Trounson AO, Shaw JM. Sugars exert a major influence on the vitrification properties of ethylene glycol-based solutions and have low toxicity to embryos and oocytes. Cryobiology 1999; 38: 119–30.
44. Oda K, Gibbons WE, Leibo SP. Osmotic shock of fertilized mouse ova. J Reprod Fertil 1992; 95: 737–47.
45. Ohboshi S, Fujihara N, Yoshida T, Tomogane H. Usefulness of polyethylene glycol for cryopreservation by vitrification of in vitro-derived bovine blastocysts. Anim Reprod Sci 1997; 48: 27–36.
46. Shaw JM, Kuleshova LL, MacFarlane DR, Trounson AO. Vitrification properties of solutions of ethylene glycol in saline containing PVP, Ficoll, or dextran. Cryobiology 1997; 35: 219–29.
47. Naitana S, Ledda S, Loi P, et al. Polyvinyl alcohol as a defined substitute for serum in vitrification and warming solutions to cryopreserve ovine embryos at different stages of development. Anim Reprod Sci 1997; 48: 247–56.
48. Kuleshova LL, Shaw JM, Trounson AO. Studies on replacing most of the penetrating cryoprotectant by polymers for embryo cryopreservation. Cryobiology 2001; 43: 21–31.
49. Asada M, Ishibashi S, Ikumi S, Fukui Y. Effect of polyvinyl alcohol (PVA) concentration during vitrification of in vitro matured bovine oocytes. Theriogenology 2002; 58: 1199–208.
50. Kasai M, Komi JH, Takakamo A, et al. A simple method for mouse embryo cryopreservation in a low toxicity vitrification solution, without appreciable loss of viability. J Reprod Fertil 1990; 89: 91–7.
51. Rall WF. Factors affecting the survival of mouse embryos cryopreserved by vitrification. Cryobiology 1987; 24: 387–402.
52. Lane M, Maybach JM, Hooper K, Hasler JF, Gardner DK. Cryo-survival and development of bovine blastocysts are enhanced by culture with recombinant albumin and hyaluronan. Mol Reprod Dev 2003; 64: 70–8.
53. Rubinsky B, Arav A, Devries AL. The cryoprotective effect of antifreeze glycopeptides from antarctic fishes. Cryobiology 1992; 29: 69–79.
54. Eto TK, Rubinsky B. Antifreeze glycoproteins increase solution viscosity. Biochem Biophys Res Commun 1993; 197: 927–31.
55. Wowk B, Leitl E, Rasch CM, et al. Vitrification enhancement by synthetic ice blocking agents. Cryobiology 2000; 40: 228–36.
56. Vanderzwalmen P, Touati K, Ectors FJ, et al. Vitrification of bovine blastocysts. Theriogenology 1998; 31: 270.
57. Saha S, Takagi M, Boediono A, Suzuki T. Direct rehydration of in vitro fertilised bovine embryos after vitrification. Vet Rec 1994; 134: 276–7.
58. Szell AZ, Windsor DP. Survival of vitrified sheep embryos in vitro and in vivo. Theriogenology 1994; 42: 881–9.
59. Papis K, Shimizu M, Izaike Y. Factors affecting the survivability of bovine oocytes vitrified in droplets. Theriogenology 2000; 54: 651–8.
60. Kuwayama M, Vajta G, Kato O, Leibo SP. Highly efficient vitrification method for cryopreservation of human oocytes. Reprod Biomed Online 2005; 11: 300–8.
61. Kuwayama M, Vajta G, Ieda S, Kato O. Comparison of open and closed methods for vitrification of human embryos and the elimination of potential contamination. Reprod Biomed Online 2005; 11: 608–14.

62. Palasz AT, Mapletoft RJ. Cryopreservation of mammalian embryos and oocytes: recent advances. Biotechnol Adv 1996; 14: 127–49.
63. Landa V, Tepla O. Cryopreservation of mouse 8-cell embryos in microdrops. Folia Biol (Praha) 1990; 36: 153–8.
64. Riha J. Vitrification of cattle embryos by direct dropping into liquid nitrogen and embryo survival after nonsurgical transfer. Zivoc Viroba 1994; 36: 113–20.
65. Yang BC, Leibo SP. Viability of in vitro-derived bovine zygotes cryopreserved in microdrops. Theriogenology 1999; 51: 178.
66. Choi DH, Chung HM, Lim JM, et al. Pregnancy and delivery of healthy infants developed from vitrified blastocysts in an IVF-ET program. Fertil Steril 2000; 74: 838–9.
67. Cho HJ, Son WY, Yoon SH, Lee SW, Lim JH. An improved protocol for dilution of cryoprotectants from vitrified human blastocysts. Hum Reprod 2002; 17: 2419–22.
68. Son WY, Lee SY, Chang MJ, et al. Pregnancy resulting from transfer of repeat vitrified blastocysts produced by in-vitro matured oocytes in patient with polycystic ovary syndrome. Reprod Biomed Online 2005; 10: 398–401.
69. Vajta G, Holm P, Greve T, Callesen H. Vitrification of porcine embryos using the Open Pulled Straw (OPS) method. Acta Vet Scand 1997; 38: 349–52.
70. Vajta G, Holm P, Kuwayama M, et al. Open Pulled Straw (OPS) vitrification: a new way to reduce cryoinjuries of bovine ova and embryos. Mol Reprod Dev 1998; 51: 53–8.
71. Vajta G, Lewis IM, Kuwayama M, Greve T, Callesen H. Sterile application of the open pulled straw (OPS) vitrification method. Cryo Lett 1998; 19: 389–92.
72. Arav A, Zeron Y, Ocheretny A. A new device and method for vitrification increases the cooling rate and allows successful cryopreservation of bovine oocytes. Theriogenology 2000; 53: 248.
73. Arav A, Yavin S, Zeron Y, et al. New trends in gamete's cryopreservation. Mol Cell Endocrinol 2002; 187: 77–81.
74. Chen SU, Lien YR, Chen HF, et al. Open pulled straws for vitrification of mature mouse oocytes preserve patterns of meiotic spindles and chromosomes better than conventional straws. Human Reprod 2000; 15: 2598–603.
75. El-Danasouri I, Selman H. Successful pregnancies and deliveries after a simple vitrification protocol for day 3 human embryos. Fertil Steril 2001; 76: 400–2.
76. Selman HA, El-Danasouri I. Pregnancies derived from vitrified human zygotes. Fertil Steril 2002; 77: 422–3.
77. Isachenko V, Selman H, Isachenko E, et al. Modified vitrification of human pronuclear oocytes: Efficacy and effect on ultrastructure. Reprod Biomed Online 2003; 7: 211–16.
78. Lane M, Bavister BD, Lyons EA, Forest KT. Containerless vitrification of mammalian oocytes and embryos. Nat Biotechnol 1999; 17: 1234–6.
79. Lane M, Schoolcraft WB, Gardner DK. Vitrification of mouse and human blastocysts using a novel cryoloop container-less technique. Fertil Steril 1999; 72: 1073–8.
80. Mukaida T, Nakamura S, Tomiyama T, et al. Successful birth after transfer of vitrified human blastocysts with use of a cryoloop containerless technique. Fertil Steril 2001; 76: 618–20.
81. Mukaida T, Takahashi K, Kasai M. Blastocyst cryopreservation: Ultrarapid vitrification using cryoloop technique. Reprod Biomed Online 2003; 6: 221–5.
82. Isachenko E, Isachenko V, Katkov II, Dessole S, Nawroth F. Vitrification of mammalian spermatozoa in the absence of cryoprotectants: From past practical difficulties to present success. Reprod Biomed Online 2003; 6: 191–200.
83. Larman MG, Sheehan CB, Gardner DK. Vitrification of mouse pronuclear oocytes with no direct liquid nitrogen contact. Reprod Biomed Online 2006; 12: 66–9.
84. Matsumoto H, Jiang JY, Tanaka T, Sasada H, Sato E. Vitrification of large quantities of immature bovine oocytes using nylon mesh. Cryobiology 2001; 42: 139–44.
85. Arav A, Shehu D, Mattioli M. Osmotic and cytotoxic study of vitrification of immature bovine oocytes. J Reprod Fertil 1993; 99: 353–8.
86. Hamawaki A, Kuwayama M, Hamano S. Minimum volume cooling method for bovine blastocyst vitrification. Theriogenology 1999; 51: 165.
87. Vanderzwalmen P, Bertin G, Debauche CH, Standaart V, Schoysman E. In vitro survival of metaphase II oocytes (MII) and blastocysts after vitrification in an Hemi-straw (HS) system. Fertil Steril 2000; 74: S215–16.
88. Nagy ZP, Chang CC, Shapiro DB, et al. Clinical evaluation of the efficiency of an oocyte donation program using egg cryo-banking. Fertil Steril 2009: 2: 520–6.
89. Chang CC, Shapiro DB, Bernal DP, et al. Human oocyte vitrification: In-vivo and in-vitro maturation outcomes. Reprod Biomed Online 2008; 7: 684–8.
90. Cobo A, Kuwayama M, Perez S, et al. Comparison of concomitant outcome achieved with fresh and cryopreserved donor oocytes vitrified by the Cryotop method. Fertil Steril 2008; 9: 1657–64.
91. Chang CC, Shapiro DB, Bernal DP, et al. Two successful pregnancies obtained following oocyte vitrification and embryo re-vitrification. Reprod Biomed Online 2008; 6: 346–9.
92. Larman MG, Ardner DK. Vitrification of mouse embryos with super-cooled air. Fertil Steril 2011; 95: 1462–6.
93. Bonetti A, Cervi M, Tomei F, et al. Ultrastructural evaluation of human metaphase II oocytes after vitrification: Closed versus open devices. Fertil Steril 2011; 95: 928–35.
94. Huang CC, Lee TH, Chen SU, et al. Successful pregnancy following blastocyst cryopreservation using super-cooling ultra-rapid vitrification. Hum Reprod 2005; 20: 122–8.
95. Dinnyes A, Dai Y, Jiang S, Yang X. High developmental rates of vitrified bovine oocytes following parthenogenetic activation, in vitro fertilization, and somatic cell nuclear transfer. Biol Reprod 2000; 63: 513–18.
96. Bielanski A, Bergeron H, Lau PC, Devenish J. Microbial contamination of embryos and semen during long term banking in liquid nitrogen. Cryobiology 2003; 46: 46–52.
97. Tedder RS, Zuckerman MA, Goldstone AH, et al. Hepatitis B transmission from contaminated cryopreservation tank. Lancet 1995; 346: 137–40.
98. Fountain D, Ralston M, Higgins N, et al. Liquid nitrogen freezers: A potential source of microbial contamination

of hematopoietic stem cell components. Transfusion 1997; 37: 585–91.
99. Berry ED, Dorsa WJ, Siragusa GR, Koohmaraie M. Bacterial cross-contamination of meat during liquid nitrogen immersion freezing. J Food Prot 1998; 61: 1103–8.
100. Bielanski A, Nadin-Davis S, Sapp T, Lutze-Wallace C. Viral contamination of embryos cryopreserved in liquid nitrogen. Cryobiology 2000; 40: 110–16.
101. Liebermann J. Vitrification of human blastocysts: An update. Reprod Biomed Online 2009; 19(Suppl 4): 4328.
102. Vanderzwalmen P, Ectors F, Grobet L, et al. Aseptic vitrification of blastocysts from infertile patients, egg donors and after IVM. Reprod Biomed Online 2009; 19: 700–7.
103. Van Landuyt L, Stoop D, Verheyen G, et al. Outcome of closed blastocyst vitrification in relation to blastocyst quality: Evaluation of 759 warming cycles in a single-embryo transfer policy. Hum Reprod 2011; 26: 527–34.
104. Parmegiani L, Accorsi A, Cognigni GE, et al. Sterilization of liquid nitrogen with ultraviolet irradiation for safe vitrification of human oocytes or embryos. Fertil Steril 2010; 94: 1525–8.
105. Parmegiani L, Cognigni GE, Bernardi S, et al. Efficiency of aseptic open vitrification and hermetical cryostorage of human oocytes. Reprod Biomed Online 2011; 23: 505–12.
106. Kuleshova LL, Lopata A. Vitrification can be more favorable than slow cooling. Fertil Steril 2002; 78: 449–54.
107. Eum JH, Park JK, Lee WS, et al. Long-term liquid nitrogen vapor storage of mouse embryos cryopreserved using vitrification or slow cooling. Fertil Steril 2009; 91: 1928–32.
108. Cobo A, Romero JL, Perez S, et al. Storage of human oocytes in the vapor phase of nitrogen. Fertil Steril 2010; 94: 1903–7.
109. AbdelHafez F, Xu J, Goldberg J, Desai N. Vitrification in open and closed carriers at different cell stages: Assessment of embryo survival, development, DNA integrity and stability during vapor phase storage for transport. BMC Biotechnol 2011; 11: 29.
110. Ghetler Y, Yavin S, Shalgi R, Arav A. The effect of chilling on membrane lipid phase transition in human oocytes and zygotes. Hum Reprod 2005; 20: 3385–9.
111. Mazur P, Seki S. Survival of mouse oocytes after being cooled in a vitrification solution to −196 degrees C at 95 degrees to 70,000 degrees C/min and warmed at 610 degrees to 118,000 degrees C/min: A new paradigm for cryopreservation by vitrification. Cryobiology 2011; 62: 1–7.
112. Shaw JM, Kola I, MacFarlane DR, Trounson AO. An association between chromosomal abnormalities in rapidly frozen 2-cell mouse embryos and the ice-forming properties of the cryoprotective solution. J Reprod Fertil 1991; 91: 9–18.
113. Vajta G, Murphy CN, Machaty Z, et al. In-straw dilution of bovine blastocysts after vitrification with the open-pulled straw method. Vet Rec 1999; 144: 180–1.
114. Cuello C, Gil MA, Parrilla I, et al. In vitro development following one-step dilution of OPS-vitrified porcine blastocysts. Theriogenology 2004; 62: 1144–52.
115. Tecirlioglu RT, French AJ, Lewis IM, et al. Birth of a cloned calf derived from a vitrified hand-made cloned embryo. Reprod Fertil Dev 2003; 15: 361–6.
116. Isachenko V, Alabart JL, Dattena M, et al. New technology for vitrification and field (microscope-free) warming and transfer of small ruminant embryos. Theriogenology 2003; 59: 1209–18.
117. Nagashima H, Kashiwazaki N, Ashman RJ, et al. Removal of cytoplasmic lipid enhances the tolerance of porcine embryos to chilling. Biol Reprod 1994; 51: 618–22.
118. Dobrinsky JR, Nagashima H, Pursel VG, et al. Cryopreservation of swine embryos with reduced lipid content. Theriogenology 1999; 51: 164.
119. Beeb LF, Cameron RD, Blackshaw AW, Higgins A, Nottle MB. Piglets born from centrifuged and vitrified early and peri-hatching blastocysts. Theriogenology 2002; 57: 2155–65.
120. Esaki R, Ueda H, Kurome M, et al. Cryopreservation of porcine embryos derived from in vitro-matured oocytes. Biol Reprod 2004; 71: 432–7.
121. Du Y, Kragh PM, Zhang X, et al. Successful vitrification of parthenofenetic porcine blastocysts produced from delipated in vitro matured oocytes. Reprod Fertil Dev 2006; 18: 153.
122. Li R, Lai L, Wax D, et al. Cloned transgenic swine via in vitro production and cryopreservation. Biol Reprod 2006; 75: 226–30.
123. Dinnyes A, Wallace GA, Rall WF. Effect of genotype on the efficiency of mouse embryo cryopreservation by vitrification or slow freezing methods. Mol Reprod Dev 1995; 40: 429–35.
124. Men H, Monson RL, Rutledge JJ. Effect of meiotic stages and maturation protocols on bovine oocyte's resistance to cryopreservation. Theriogenology 2002; 57: 1095–103.
125. Edashige K, Yamaji Y, Kleinhans FW, Kasai M. Artificial expression of aquaporin-3 improves the survival of mouse oocytes after cryopreservation. Biol Reprod 2003; 68: 87–94.
126. Edashige K, Sakamoto M, Kasai M. Expression of mRNAs of the aquaporin family in mouse oocytes and embryos. Cryobiology 2000; 40: 171–5.
127. Veeck LL. Does the developmental stage at freeze impact on clinical results post-thaw? Reprod Biomed Online 2003; 6: 367–74.
128. Pool TB, Leibo SP. Cryopreservation and assisted human conception. Introduction. Reprod Biomed Online 2004; 9: 132–3.
129. Vanderzwalmen P, Bertin G, Debauche CH, et al. Births after vitrification at morula and blastocyst stages: Effect of artificial reduction of the blastocoelic cavity before vitrification. Hum Reprod 2002; 17: 744–51.
130. Son WY, Yoon SH, Yoon HJ, Lee SM, Lim JH. Pregnancy outcome following transfer of human blastocysts vitrified on electron microscopy grids after induced collapse of the blastocoele. Hum Reprod 2003; 18: 137–9.
131. Hiraoka K, Kinutani M, Kinutani K. Blastocoele collapse by micropipetting prior to vitrification gives excellent survival and pregnancy outcomes for human day 5 and 6 expanded blastocysts. Hum Reprod 2004; 19: 2884–8.

132. Raju GA, Prakash GJ, Krishna KM, Madan K. Vitrification of human early cavitating and deflated expanded blastocysts: Clinical outcome of 474 cycles. J Assist Reprod Genet 2009; 26: 523–9.
133. Iwayama H, Hochi S, Yamashita M. In vitro and in vivo viability of human blastocysts collapsed by laser pulse or osmotic shock prior to vitrification. J Assist Reprod Genet 2011; 28: 355–61.
134. Pribenszky C, Molnar M, Cseh S, Solti L. Improving post-thaw survival of cryopreserved mouse blastocysts by hydrostatic pressure challenge. Anim Reprod Sci 2005; 87: 143–50.
135. Roth TL, Swanson WF, Wildt DE. Developmental competence of domestic cat embryos fertilized in vivo versus in vitro. Biol Reprod 1994; 51: 441–51.
136. Enright BP, Lonergan P, Dinnyes A, et al. Culture of in vitro produced bovine zygotes in vitro vs in vivo: Implications for early embryo development and quality. Theriogenology 2000; 54: 659–73.
137. Rizos D, Ward F, Duffy P, Boland MP, Lonergan P. Consequences of bovine oocyte maturation, fertilization or early embryo development in vitro versus in vivo: Implications for blastocyst yield and blastocyst quality. Mol Reprod Dev 2002; 61: 234–48.
138. Mahmoudzadeh AR, Van Soom A, Bols P, Ysebaert MT, de Kruif A. Optimization of a simple vitrification procedure for bovine embryos produced in vitro: Effect of developmental stage, two-step addition of cryoprotectant and sucrose dilution on embryonic survival. J Reprod Fertil 1995; 103: 33–9.
139. Wurth YA, Reinders JMC, Rall WF, Kruip TH. Developmental potential of in vitro produced bovine embryos following cryopreservation and single-embryo transfer. Theriogenology 1994; 42: 1275–84.
140. Reinders JMC. From embryo to a calf after embryo transfer, a comparison of in vivo and in vitro produced embryos. Theriogenology 1995; 43: 306.
141. Agca Y, Monson RL, Northey DL, et al. Transfer of fresh and cryopreserved IVP bovine embryos: Normal calving, birth weight and gestation lengths. Theriogenology 1998; 50: 147–62.
142. Check JH, Choe JK, Nazari A, Fox F, Swenson K. Fresh embryo transfer is more effective than frozen for donor oocyte recipients but not for donors. Hum Reprod 2001; 16: 1403–8.
143. Nagy ZP, Taylor T, Elliott T, et al. Removal of lysed blastomeres from frozen-thawed embryos improves implantation and pregnancy rates in frozen embryo transfer cycles. Fertil Steril 2005; 84: 1606–12.
144. Elliott TA, Colturato LF, Taylor TH, et al. Lysed cell removal promotes frozen-thawed embryo development. Fertil Steril 2007; 87: 1444–9.
145. Jelinkova L, Selman HA, Arav A, et al. Twin pregnancy after vitrification of 2-pronuclei human embryos. Fertil Steril 2002; 77: 412–14.
146. Vanderzwalmen P, Bertin G, Debauche CH, et al. Vitrification of human blastocysts with the Hemi-Straw carrier: Application of assisted hatching after thawing. Hum Reprod 2003; 18: 1504–11.
147. Vanderzwalmen P, Zech H, Birkenfeld A, et al. Pregnancies after vitrification of human day 5 embryos. Hum Reprod 1997; 12(Suppl): 98.
148. Mukaida T, Wada S, Takahashi K, et al. Vitrification of human embryos based on the assessment of suitable conditions for 8-cell mouse embryos. Hum Reprod 1998; 13: 2874–9.
149. Park SP, Kim EY, Oh JH, et al. Ultra-rapid freezing of human multipronuclear zygotes using electron microscope grids. Hum Reprod 2000; 15: 1787–90.
150. Saito H, Ishida GM, Kaneko T, et al. Application of vitrification to human embryo freezing. Gynecol Obstet Invest 2000; 49: 145–9.
151. Yokota Y, Sato S, Yokota M, et al. Successful pregnancy following blastocyst vitrification: Case report. Hum Reprod 2000; 15: 1802–3.
152. Yokota Y, Sato S, Yokota M, Yokota H, Araki Y. Birth of a healthy baby following vitrification of human blastocysts. Fertil Steril 2001; 75: 1027–9.
153. Liebermann J, Tucker MJ. Effect of carrier system on the yield of human oocytes and embryos as assessed by survival and developmental potential after vitrification. Reproduction 2002; 124: 483–9.
154. Reed ML, Lane M, Gardner DK, Jensen NL, Thompson J. Vitrification of human blastocysts using the cryoloop method: Successful clinical application and birth of offspring. J Assist Reprod Genet 2002; 19: 304–6.
155. Son WY, Yoon SH, Park SJ, et al. Ongoing twin pregnancy after vitrification of blastocysts produced by in-vitro matured oocytes retrieved from a woman with polycystic ovary syndrome: Case report. Hum Reprod 2002; 17: 2963–6.
156. Isachenko V, Montag M, Isachenko E, et al. Aseptic technology of vitrification of human pronuclear oocytes using open-pulled straws. Hum Reprod 2005; 20: 492–6.
157. Liebermann J, Tucker MJ. Vitrifying and warming of human oocytes, embryos, and blastocysts: Vitrification procedures as an alternative to conventional cryopreservation. Methods Mol Biol 2004; 254: 345–64.
158. Zheng WT, Zhuang GL, Zhou CQ, et al. Comparison of the survival of human biopsied embryos after cryopreservation with four different methods using non-transferable embryos. Hum Reprod 2005; 20: 1615–18.
159. Stehlik E, Stehlik J, Katayama KP, et al. Vitrification demonstrates significant improvement versus slow freezing of human blastocysts. Reprod Biomed Online 2005; 11: 53–7.
160. Balaban B, Urman B, Ata B, et al. A randomized controlled study of human Day 3 embryo cryopreservation by slow freezing or vitrification: Vitrification is associated with higher survival, metabolism and blastocyst formation. Hum Reprod 2008; 23: 1976–82.
161. Rezazadeh Valojerdi M, Eftekhari-Yazdi P, Karimian L, Hassani F, Movaghar B. Vitrification versus slow freezing gives excellent survival, post warming embryo morphology and pregnancy outcomes for human cleaved embryos. J Assist Reprod Genet 2009; 26: 347–54.
162. Son WY, Chung JT, Gidoni Y, et al. Comparison of survival rate of cleavage stage embryos produced from in vitro maturation cycles after slow freezing and after vitrification. Fertil Steril 2009; 92: 956–8.
163. Keskintepe L, Sher G, Machnicka A, et al. Vitrification of human embryos subjected to blastomere biopsy for pre-implantation genetic screening produces higher survival and pregnancy rates than slow freezing. J Assist Reprod Genet 2009; 26: 629–35.

164. Wilding MG, Capobianco C, Montanaro N, et al. Human cleavage-stage embryo vitrification is comparable to slow-rate cryopreservation in cycles of assisted reproduction. J Assist Reprod Genet 2010; 27: 549–54.
165. AbdelHafez FF, Desai N, Abou-Setta AM, Falcone T, Goldfarb J. Slow freezing, vitrification and ultra-rapid freezing of human embryos: A systematic review and meta-analysis. Reprod Biomed Online 2010; 20: 209–22.
166. Desai N, Blackmon H, Szeptycki J, Goldfarb J. Cryoloop vitrification of human day 3 cleavage-stage embryos: Post-vitrification development, pregnancy outcomes and live births. Reprod Biomed Online 2007; 14: 208–13.
167. Hong SW, Sepilian V, Chung HM, Kim TJ. Cryopreserved human blastocysts after vitrification result in excellent implantation and clinical pregnancy rates. Fertil Steril 2009; 92: 2062–4.
168. Hiraoka K, Kinutani M, Kinutani K. Vitrification of human hatched blastocysts: A report of 4 cases. J Reprod Med 2007; 52: 413–15.
169. Stachecki JJ, Garrisi J, Sabino S, et al. A new safe, simple and successful vitrification method for bovine and human blastocysts. Reprod Biomed Online 2008; 17: 360–7.
170. Selman H, Brusco GF, Fiorini F, et al. Vitrification is a highly efficient method to cryopreserve human embryos in in vitro fertilization patients at high risk of developing ovarian hyperstimulation syndrome. Fertil Steril 2009; 91(4 Suppl): 1611–13.
171. Hiraoka K, Fuchiwaki M, Hiraoka K, et al. Vitrified human day-7 blastocyst transfer: 11 cases. Reprod Biomed Online 2008; 17: 689–94.
172. Knopman JM, Noyes N, Talebian S, et al. Women with cancer undergoing ART for fertility preservation: A cohort study of their response to exogenous gonadotropins. Fertil Steril 2009; 91(4 Suppl): 1476–8.
173. Grifo JA, Noyes N. Delivery rate using cryopreserved oocytes is comparable to conventional in vitro fertilization using fresh oocytes: Potential fertility preservation for female cancer patients. Fertil Steril 2010; 93: 391–6.
174. Noyes N, Labella PA, Grifo J, Knopman JM. Oocyte cryopreservation as a fertility preservation measure for cancer patients. Reprod Biomed Online 2010; 27: 495–9.
175. Lockwood G. Politics ethics and economics: Oocyte cryopreservation in the UK. Reprod Biomed Online 2003; 6: 151–3.
176. Cobo A, Bellver J, Domingo J, et al. New options in assisted reproduction technology: The Cryotop method of oocyte vitrification. Reprod Biomed Online 2008; 17: 68–72.
177. Nagy ZP, Chang CC, Shapiro DB, et al. The efficacy and safety of human oocyte vitrification. Semin Reprod Med 2009; 27: 450–5.
178. Stoop D, Van Landuyt L, Paquay R, et al. Offering excess oocyte aspiration and vitrification to patients undergoing stimulated artificial insemination cycles can reduce the multiple pregnancy risk and accumulate oocytes for later use. Hum Reprod 2010; 25: 1213–18.
179. Joris H, Van den Abbeel E, Vos AD, Van Steirteghem A. Reduced survival after human embryo biopsy and subsequent cryopreservation. Hum Reprod 1999; 14: 2833–7.
180. Jericho H, Wilton L, Gook DA, Edgar DH. A modified cryopreservation method increases the survival of human biopsied cleavage stage embryos. Hum Reprod 2003; 18: 568–71.
181. Schoolcraft WB, Fragouli E, Stevens J, et al. Clinical application of comprehensive chromosomal screening at the blastocyst stage. Fertil Steril 2010; 94: 1700–6.
182. Fragouli E, Katz-Jaffe M, Alfarawati S, et al. Comprehensive chromosome screening of polar bodies and blastocysts from couples experiencing repeated implantation failure. Fertil Steril 2010; 94: 875–87.
183. Schoolcraft WB, Treff NR, Stevens JM, et al. Live birth outcome with trophectoderm biopsy, blastocyst vitrification, and single-nucleotide polymorphism microarray-based comprehensive chromosome screening in infertile patients. Fertil Steril 2011; 96: 638–40.
184. Oakes MB, Gomes CM, Fioravanti J, et al. A case of oocyte and embryo vitrification resulting in clinical pregnancy. Fertil Steril 2008; 90: 2013.e5–8.
185. Peng W, Zhang J, Shu Y. Live birth after transfer of a twice-vitrified warmed blastocyst that had undergone trophectoderm biopsy. Reprod Biomed Online 2011; 22: 299–302.
186. Mohamed AM, Chouliaras S, Jones CJ, Nardo LG. Live birth rate in fresh and frozen embryo transfer cycles in women with endometriosis. Eur J Obstet Gynecol Reprod Biol 2011; 156: 177–80.
187. Shapiro BS, Daneshmand ST, Garner FC, et al. Evidence of impaired endometrial receptivity after ovarian stimulation for in vitro fertilization: A prospective randomized trial comparing fresh and frozen-thawed embryo transfer in normal responders. Fertil Steril 2011; 96: 344–8.
188. Chian RC, Huang JY, Gilbert L, et al. Obstetric outcomes following vitrification of in vitro and in vivo matured oocytes. Fertil Steril 2009; 91: 2391–8.
189. Noyes N, Porcu V, Borini A. Over 900 oocyte cryopreservation babies born with no apparent increase in congenital anomalies. Reprod Biomed Online 2009; 18: 769–76.
190. Rama Raju GA, Jaya Prakash G, Murali Krishna K, Madan K. Neonatal outcome after vitrified day 3 embryo transfers: a preliminary study. Fertil Steril 2009; 92: 143–8.
191. Shu Y, Peng W, Zhang J. Pregnancy and live birth following the transfer of vitrified-warmed blastocysts derived from zona- and corona-cell-free oocytes. Reprod Biomed Online 2010; 21: 527–32.
192. Wikland M, Hardarson T, Hillensjo T, et al. Obstetric outcomes after transfer of vitrified blastocysts. Hum Reprod 2010; 25: 1699–707.
193. Menezo YJ. Blastocyst freezing. Eur J Obstet Gynecol Reprod Biol 2004; 115(Suppl 1): S12–15.
194. Klug S, Merker HJ, Jackh R. Effects of ethylene glycol and metabolites on in vitro development of rat embryos during organogenesis. Toxicol In Vitro 2001; 15: 635–42.
195. Kong IK, Lee SI, Cho SG, Cho SK, Park CS. Comparison of open pulled straw (OPS) vs glass micropipette (GMP) vitrification in mouse blastocysts. Theriogenology 2000; 53: 1817–26.

196. Isachenko V, Alabart JL, Vajta G. Double cryopreservtion of rat embryos at different developmental stages with identical vitrification protocol: The not properly understood phenomenon. J Reprod Abstr Ser 2000; 26: 10.
197. Tominaga K, Hamada Y. Gel-loading tips as container for vitrification of in vitro-produced bovine embryos. J Reprod Dev 2001; 47: 259–65.
198. Liebermann J, Tucker MJ, Graham JR, et al. Blastocyst development after vitrification of multipronuclear zygotes using the Flexipet denuding pipette. Reprod Biomed Online 2002; 4: 146–50.
199. Cremades N, Sousa M, Silva J, et al. Experimental vitrification of human compacted morulae and early blastocysts using fine diameter plastic micropipettes. Human Reprod 2004; 19: 300–5.
200. Hredzak R, Ostro A, Zdilova V, Toporcerova S, Kacmarik J. Clinical experience with a modified method of human embryo vitrification. Ceska Gynekol 2005; 70: 99–103.
201. Chen SU, Lien YR, Cheng YY, et al. Vitrification of mouse oocytes using closed pulled straws (CPS) achieves a high survival and preserves good patterns of meiotic spindles, compared with conventional straws, open pulled straws (OPS) and grids. Human Reprod 2001; 16: 2350–6.
202. Lopez-Bejar M, Lopez-Gatius F. Nonequilibrium cryopreservation of rabbit embryos using a modified (sealed) open pulled straw procedure. Theriogenology 2002; 58: 1541–52.
203. Arav A. Vitrification of oocytes and embryos. In: Gandolfi F, Lauria A, eds. New Trends in Embryo Transfer. Cambridge: Portland Press, 1992: 255–64.
204. Vajta G, Nagy ZP. Are programmable freezers still needed in the embryo laboratory? Review on vit rification. Reprod Biomed Online 2006; 12: 779–96.
205. Vieira AD, Mezzalira A, Barbieri DP, et al. Calves born after open pulled straw vitrification of immature bovine oocytes. Cryobiology 2002; 45: 91–4.
206. Martino A, Songsasen N, Leibo SP. Development into blastocysts of bovine oocytes cryopreserved by ultrarapid cooling. Biol Reprod 1996; 54: 1059–69.
207. Hou YP, Dai YP, Zhu SE, et al. Bovine oocytes vitrified by the open pulled straw method and used for somatic cell cloning supported development to term. Theriogenology 2005; 64: 1381–91.
208. Booth PJ, Vajta G, Høj A, et al. Full-term development of nuclear transfer calves produced from open-pulled straw (OPS) vitrified cytoplasts: Work in progress. Theriogenology 1999; 51: 999–1006.
209. French AJ, Hall VJ, Korfiatis NT, et al. Viability of cloned bovine embryos following OPS vitrification. Theriogenology 2002; 57: 413.
210. French AJ, Lewis IM, Ruddock NT, et al. Generation of aS1 casein gene transgenic calves by nuclear transfer. Biol Reprod 2003; 68: 240.
211. Peura TT. Hartwich KM, Hamilton HM, Walker SK. No differences in sheep somatic cell nuclear transfer outcomes using serum-starved or actively growing donor granulosa cells. Reprod Fertil Dev 2003; 15: 157–65.
212. Fujihira T, Kishida R, Fukui Y. Developmental capacity of vitrified immature porcine oocytes following ICSI: Effects of cytochalasin B and cryoprotectants. Cryobiology 2004; 49: 286–90.
213. Fujuhira T, Naqai H, Fukui Y. Relationship between equilibration timea and the presence of cumulus cells, and effect of taxol treatment for vitrification of in vitro matured porcine oocytes. Cryobiology 2005; 51: 339–43.
214. Kobayashi S, Takei M, Kano M, Tomita M, Leibo SP. Piglets produced by transfer of vitrified porcine embryos after stepwise dilution of cryoprotectants. Cryobiology 1998; 36: 20–31.
215. Berthelot F, Martinat-Botte F, Perreau C, Terqui M. Birth of piglets after OPS vitrification and transfer of compacted morula stage embryos with intact zona pellucida. Reprod Nutr Dev 2001; 41: 267–72.
216. Men H, Agca Y, Critser ES, Critser JK. Beneficial effects of serum supplementation during in vitro production of porcine embryos on their ability to survive cryopreservation by open pulled straw vitrification. Theriogenology 2005; 64: 1340–9.
217. Maclellan LJ, Carnevale EM, Coutinho da Silva MA, et al. Pregnancies from vitrified equine oocytes collected from super-stimulated and non-stimulated mares. Theriogenology 2002; 58: 911–19.
218. Piltti K, Lindeberg H, Aalto J, Korhonen H. Live cubs born after transfer of OPS vitrified-warmed embryos in the farmed European polecat (Mustela putorius). Theriogenology 2004; 61: 811–20.
219. Crichton EG, Bedows E, Miller-Lindholm AK, et al. Efficacy of porcine gonadotropins for repeated stimulation of ovarian activity for oocyte retrieval and in vitro embryo production and cryopreservation in Siberian tigers (Panthera tigris altaica). Biol Reprod 2003; 68: 105–13.
220. Iwayama H, Hochi S, Kato M, et al. Effects of cryodevice type and donors' sexual maturity on vitrification of minke whale (Balaenoptera bonaerensis) oocytes at germinal vesicle stage. Zygote 2004; 12: 333–8.

25

Severe male factor: Genetic consequences and recommendations for genetic testing

Willy Lissens and Katrien Stouffs

OVERVIEW

Infertility associated with a severe male factor such as oligo-astheno-teratozoospermia (OAT) or azoospermia may be of genetic origin. This means that either the number or the structure of the chromosomes may be aberrant or a gene defect may be at stake. Two major reasons are indicated for genetic investigations in case of male infertility. One reason is to understand more about the possible causes of azoospermia or OAT. Another reason is to be able to offer genetic counseling to the patient, his partner, and his family whenever indicated. The role of genetic counseling in case of infertility has increased since the advent of assisted reproductive technique (ART) in general, and certainly since the introduction of intracytoplasmic sperm injection (ICSI) offering the possibility to men with almost no spermatozoa to have children (1–3). In the clinic, genetic investigations are usually performed when the azoospermia or oligozoospermia is part of a more complex disease or syndrome. Based on the available data today a number of genetic tests should also be performed in case of infertility in an otherwise healthy male. In the majority of such cases it will be sufficient to start with the analysis of the karyotype in peripheral lymphocytes, the search for the presence of a Yq11 deletion on the long arm of the Y chromosome and/or the analysis of the CFTR-gene in couples in which the male partner has congenital bilateral absence of the vas deferens (CBAVD). More specific genetic investigations can be done if indicated.

GENETIC CAUSES OF MALE INFERTILITY

Chromosomal Aberrations

It has been known for over 50 years that the presence of an extra X chromosome in males, resulting in a 47,XXY karyotype, causes Klinefelter syndrome with testicular atrophy and nonobstructive azoospermia as main features (4,5). Since then, many chromosomal studies were performed in series of infertile males, and the conclusions drawn from these studies are that constitutional chromosomal aberrations increase as sperm counts decrease.

From these studies it is also clear that the incidence of numerical sex chromosomal aberrations such as 47,XXY and 47,XYY is proportionally higher in males with azoospermia than in males with oligozoospermia, whereas structural chromosomal aberrations of autosomes such as Robertsonian (Fig. 25.1A) and reciprocal (Fig. 25.1B) translocations are proportionally more frequent in oligozoospermic males (Table 25.1) (6–8).

In azoospermic males it is also possible to find a 46,XX karyotype. In roughly 90% of these Klinefelter-like males the SRY-gene, normally located close to the pseudoautosomal region of the short arm of the Y chromosome is now, due to a crossing-over event during meiosis, present in that same region on one of the X chromosomes (9–11). The SRY-gene referring to the sex-determining region of the Y chromosome has to be expressed to induce the sexual development of an embryo toward a male phenotype (12). In the remaining 10% of XX-males most probably other genes with a function in sexual development are involved. Spermatogenesis seems to be absent in these XX-males whereas in apparently non-mosaic Klinefelter patients a few spermatozoa can be found in testicular tissue. Such spermatozoa have been used in ICSI procedures and healthy as well as a few 47,XXY children have been born (reviewed in Ref. 13).

Microdeletions on the Long Arm of the Y Chromosome (Yq11)

The first azoospermic male patients in whom a deletion in the q11 region of the long arm of the Y chromosome (Yq11) was linked to their infertility were identified through conventional cytogenetic analysis (14). At that time the concept of the azoospermia factor (AZF) region, the region lacking factors (genes) necessary for spermatogenesis due to a deletion, was introduced. Since that time, the structure of the Y chromosome, consisting of the gene-containing euchromatic parts (Yp and Yq11) and the polymorphic heterochromatic parts (Yq12) have been studied in much detail using more sensitive molecular techniques. These have also helped to define the AZF region better. In fact, the AZF region consists of

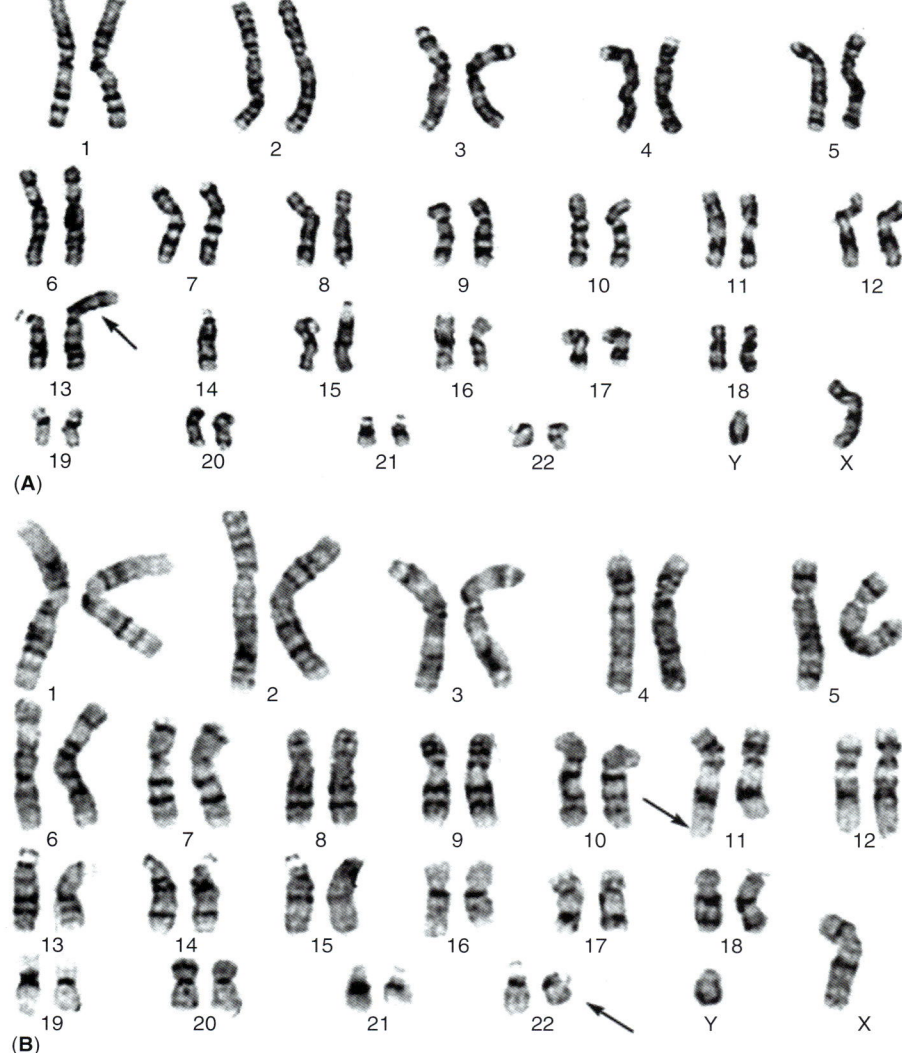

Figure 25.1 (**A**) 45,XY,der(13;14)(q10;q10) karyotype from a phenotypic normal male with a Robertsonian translocation of chromosomes 13 and 14 through centromeric fusion. (**B**) 46,XY,t(11;22)(q24.3;q12) karyotype from phenotypic normal male with a balanced reciprocal translocation of chromosome 11 and 22 with break points in 11q24.3 (↘) and 22q12 (↖).

Table 25.1 Incidence of Chromosomal Aberrations in Infertile Oligozoospermic and Azoospermic Males Compared with Newborns

Aberrations	Infertile males n = 7876	Oligozoospermia n = 1701	Azoospermia n = 1151	Newborns n = 94,465
Autosomes	1.3%	3.0%	1.1%	0.25%
Sex chromosomes	3.8%	1.6%	12.6%	0.14%
Total	5.1%	4.6%	13.7%	0.39%

Source: Summarized from Ref. 6.

three subregions AZFa, AZFb, and AZFc; deletions in these subregions are most of the time not readily detectable by cytogenetic analysis. Almost 100 studies including more than 13,000 infertile males with reduced sperm numbers from azoospermia to oligozoospermia have since been conducted. A prevalence of around 7.4% of Yq microdeletions can be deduced from these studies and again the prevalence is higher in azoospermic (9.7%) than in oligozoospermic (6.0%) males (15). In most patients the deletions span the AZFb and/or AZFc region while in only a small number the AZFa region is deleted. Most deletions occur by intrachromosomal homologous recombination between repeat sequences spread over the Yq11 region (16–18). These repeat sequences are either palindromes consisting of inverted repeat arms or intrachromosomal repetitive sequences. Several genes have been identified in the AZF regions and they are being studied to prove their role in spermatogenesis. It is of course clear that if these microdeletions cause the spermatogenic defect leading to a low to very low sperm count present in the ejaculate or to only a few sperm cells in the testes, these microdeletions will, through the use of ICSI, be transmitted to sons who most probably will be infertile as well (19). However, ICSI children are still too young to evaluate their fertility or their sperm count. In a few exceptional cases, fertility has been described in AZFc-deleted fathers who transmitted the deletion to their now infertile sons (20–22). Age at investigation may play a role as observed in one patient with an AZFc deletion being oligozoospermic and later on azoospermic (23).

CBAVD and Cystic Fibrosis

Men with CBAVD have obstructive azoospermia. Spermatogenesis is usually normal and sperm can be obtained through microsurgical epididymal sperm aspiration, testicular sperm extraction, percutaneous epididymal sperm aspiration, or epididymal or testicular fine needle aspiration. This sperm can be used to fertilize oocytes in vitro through ICSI (2,24). CBAVD was known to be present in 97–99% of male cystic fibrosis (CF) patients. CF is a frequent and by now well-known autosomal recessive disease in the Caucasian population with an incidence of approximately 1/2500. Many patients now surviving into their 30s and 40s suffer from severe lung disease and pancreatic insufficiency. They are often too ill to reproduce although improved survival into adulthood generates interest in reproduction (25,26). The CF transmembrane conductance regulator (CFTR) gene, a gene encoding a protein involved in chloride transport across epithelial membranes, was shown to be responsible for CF due to malfunction of the protein when mutated (27–29).

CBAVD had also been observed in 1–2% of apparently healthy infertile males, and in 6–10% of men with obstructive azoospermia (30). When the CFTR gene was studied in these males, mutations or splice site variants in intron 8 (comprising the so called 5T-variant and the TG dinucleotide repeat upstream of it) interfering with gene expression were found in 80–90% of them (31–36). In the remaining CBAVD patients no link could be found either with aberrant CFTR expression or with any other etiology. However, in these patients CBAVD-associated urinary tract/renal malformations were observed (33,37,38). When performing ICSI with sperm from CBAVD males carrying CFTR mutations, their partners have to be tested for mutations in the same gene since the carrier frequency of CF mutations may be as high as 1/25 in Caucasians. If both partners carry CFTR mutations the risk of having a child with CF is 1/4 or 25% or even 1/2 or 50% (Table 25.2). However, since the incidence and the type of CFTR mutations vary with the ethnic origin as well as with the geographical region, counseling and approach to treatment will have to be adjusted. In high risk situations, prenatal diagnosis or preimplantation genetic diagnosis (PGD) is indicated (see later).

Other Known Genetic Causes of Male Infertility

These males all have a 46,XY normal karyotype. Most of the defects are monogenic and either the specific gene defect is known or a chromosomal locus is known or suggested (39). A number of these rather rare conditions which may be encountered in a fertility clinic have been summarized in Table 25.3. However, the (genetic) cause of male infertility remains unknown in many instances, and probably a large number of genes are involved.

Myotonic dystrophy is a rather common autosomal dominant muscular dystrophy with an incidence of 1/8000. The presence of an expanded CTG-trinucleotide repeat in the DMPK gene interferes with its function (40–43). Symptoms can be very mild such as cataract at an advanced age

Table 25.2 Risk Calculations for a Child with Cystic Fibrosis (CF) or Congenital Bilateral Absence of the Vas Deferens (CBAVD) in a Case of CBAVD

	Male		Female		Risk	
No testing	8/10	×	1/25	×	1/4	= 1/125
Testing female						
Carrier	8/10	×	1	×	1/4	= 1/5
No carrier	8/10	×	1/150	×	1/4	= 1/750
Testing male + female						
Female carrier	CF/CF	×	1	×	1/2	= 1/2
Female no carrier	CF/CF	×	1/150	×	1/2	= 1/300
Female carrier	CF/5T	×	1	×	1/4	= 1/4 (CF)
						= 1/8 (CBAVD)

If the CBAVD patient is not tested for CF mutations, his risk of having at least 1 CF mutation is 8/10; if his partner is not tested and Caucasian, her risk of being a carrier of one CF mutation is 1/25. A carrier has a risk of 1/2 to transmit the mutation. Two carriers have a risk of 1/4 to transmit their mutated gene at the same time. A CBAVD patient with two mutations will always transmit a mutated gene. Risks for CF can be calculated if none of the partners are tested, if only the female partner is tested, if both partners are tested. In high-risk situations preconceptional or preimplantation genetic diagnosis can be offered (91).

Table 25.3 Some Other Known Genetic Causes of Male Infertility

Disease	Frequency	Clinic	Lab tests	Cause	Treatment	Reference
Myotonic dystrophy	1:8000	Male phenotype Myotonia	Normo-/oligospermia LH, FSH normal or ↗ T normal or ↘	AD "CTG" expansion in DMPK gene	ICSI PGD	(40–46)
Kallmann syndrome	1:10,000	Male phenotype Pubertal delay Anosmia	Azoospermia T, FSH, LH ↘ no response to GnRH test	X-linked Abnormal neuronal migration Point mutation in KAL1 gene AR and AD forms exist as well!!	Hormonal substitution	(47–57)
Primary ciliary dyskinesia or Immotile cilia syndrome	1:25,000	Male phenotype	Asthenozoospermia	AR Dynein deficiency Genetic heterogeneity (?)	ICSI	(58–60)
Kennedy disease or Spinal bulbar muscular atrophy	1:50,000	Male (gynecomastia) Muscular atrophy	Oligo-/azoospermia T normal or ↘ LH, FSH ↗	X-linked "CAG" expansion in androgen receptor gene	ICSI or AID	(61,62)

Abbreviations: AD, autosomal dominant; AID, artificial insemination with donor sperm; AR, autosomal recessive; FSH, follicle stimulating hormone; GnRH, gonadotropin-releasing hormone; ICSI, intracytoplasmic sperm injection; LH, luteinizing hormone; PGD, preconceptional/preimplantation genetic diagnosis; T, testosterone.

or very severe, as is the case in the congenital, often lethal, form of the disease. Severity is related to the number of CTG repeats (44). In 60–80% of the male patients testicular tubular atrophy will develop and cause OAT. When such spermatozoa are used to fertilize oocytes, the risk to transmit the disease often in a more severe form due to further expansion of the trinucleotide repeat (called anticipation), is 1/2 or 50%. Prenatal diagnosis or preferentially preimplantation diagnosis should be offered (45,46).

Kallmann syndrome is characterized by hypogonadotropic hypogonadism, due to impaired GnRH secretion, and anosmia. X-linked as well as autosomal-recessive, and autosomal-dominant inheritance exist. The X-linked form of the Kallmann syndrome (KAL1 gene) is the most frequent and the best known one (47). An autosomal dominant form of Kallmann syndrome is caused by mutations in the FGFR1 gene (48). A possible interaction between the gene products of the KAL1 and FGFR1 genes has been suggested as a possible explanation for the higher prevalence of Kallmann syndrome in males than in females (49,50). In addition, mutations in four other genes have been implicated in Kallmann syndrome (51–53). Nevertheless, only about 30% of patients with a clinical diagnosis of Kallmann syndrome have mutations in one of the six genes identified so far (54). The presence of mutations in different genes of some individuals suggests that at least in some patients, a possible digenic mode of inheritance of Kallmann syndrome exists (51,55,56). Hormonal treatment will stimulate spermatogenesis in patients with Kallmann syndrome (57). Genetic counseling is indicated.

Primary ciliary dyskinesia or the immotile cilia syndrome is an autosomal recessive disease presenting with chronic respiratory tract disease, rhinitis, and sinusitis due to immotile cilia. Male patients are usually infertile because of asthenozoospermia (58). If the above symptoms are associated with situs inversus the condition is called the Kartagener syndrome (59,60). Men with this condition can reproduce with the help of ICSI. Genetic counseling is hampered because the possibility for genetic testing is still limited (60). Many genes are probably involved in primary ciliary dyskinesia and Kartagener syndrome. However, if we accept the incidence of 1/25,000, the carrier frequency must be 1/80, which means that the risk of a man to have an affected child is 1/160 (1 × 1/80 × 1/2).

Kennedy's disease or spinal and bulbar muscular atrophy is a neuromuscular disease causing muscular weakness that is associated with testicular atrophy and leads to oligo- or azoospermia. It is an X-linked disease caused by an expanded (CAG) trinucleotide repeat in the transactivation domain of the androgen receptor gene (61,62). If treated with ICSI, again genetic counseling is indicated. Point mutations in the androgen receptor gene resulting in androgen insensitivity through impaired binding of dihydrotestosterone to the receptor will interfere with sexual development. The resulting syndrome is testicular feminization or androgen insensitivity syndrome, causing a female phenotype (63,64). The presenting problem here will not be male infertility. Patients with an autosomal recessive 5-α-reductase deficiency and therefore being unable to synthesize dihydrotestosterone from testosterone may theoretically present at the clinic with azoospermia and pseudohermaphroditism (65,66).

Very rarely patients with other mostly syndrome-associated genetic defects may consult at a male infertility clinic. Up to 80% of patients with *Noonan syndrome* present with oligo- or azoospermia as a result of cryptorchidism (67). The diagnosis is so far based on other symptoms, including a small stature, chest deformity, a rather typical facial dysmorphism, and congenital heart disease. Defects in a gene on chromosome 12q24.1, PTPN11, are responsible for approximately 40% of patients with Noonan syndrome (68). Another six genes involved in Noonan syndrome have been identified; the seven known genes account for around 60% of cases. So, more genes are involved in Noonan syndrome. The autosomal dominant inheritance asks for genetic counseling. Other possible patients may be affected by *Aarskog–Scott* syndrome with acrosomal sperm defects (69,70) or *Beckwith–Wiedemann syndrome* with cryptorchidism (71). Syndromes such as *Bardet–Biedl syndrome* and *Prader–Willi syndrome*, both presenting with hypogonadism are associated with other major symptoms including mental retardation which limit procreation (72–74). Prader–Willi syndrome is an imprinting syndrome resulting from the absence of the expression of the paternal alleles in the 15q11–q13 imprinted region (75–77). Other causes of male infertility include deficiencies in enzymes involved in the synthesis of testosterone (64,66), luteinizing hormone, and luteinizing hormone receptor (78,79).

Defects in energy production by the *mitochondria* have been implicated in male infertility. Mitochondria are the main source of energy production for the cells through the process of oxidative phosphorylation. The synthesis of ATP occurs through the action of 5 enzyme complexes that are encoded by nuclear genes and partly by the small mitochondrial genome that is exclusively maternally inherited. Mitochondrial diseases usually evolve as multisystem disorders mainly affecting the central nervous system and muscle. In addition, these defects in the respiratory function are believed to cause a decline in sperm motility because of ATP depletion that is necessary for flagellar propulsion of the spermatozoa. Reduced sperm motility and resulting male infertility have been well documented in several patients with mitochondrial encephalopathies caused by mitochondrial tRNA point mutations or multiple mtDNA deletions (80).

Globozoospermia is a rare (<0.1%) cause of male infertility. A major characteristic of these round-headed spermatozoa is the malformation or absence of the acrosome (81). So far, at least three genes have been associated with this form of teratozoospermia: SPATA16, PICK1, and deletions encompassing the DPY19L2 gene (82–85). In all of these cases the condition is inherited as an autosomal recessive disease. In another form of morphological abnormal spermatozoa (large-headed multiflagellar polyploid spermatozoa) a condition resulting in male infertility and mainly observed in North-African males, is caused by mutations in the AURKC gene which is involved in chromosomal segregation and cytokinesis (86).

CONSEQUENCES AND RECOMMENDATIONS IN THE CLINIC

Genetic Evaluation of Infertile Males Before ART

A *personal history* from the patient should be taken. In addition, a detailed pedigree should be drawn and completed for miscarriages or children (also deceased) with multiple congenital malformations in first- or second-degree relatives. It is also important to know about infertility in siblings or other family members. This information may suggest a possible chromosomal aberration such as a translocation (Fig. 25.2A) or a monogenic disease like Kallmann syndrome (Fig. 25.2B) or CF (Table 25.2). A thorough inquiry of the proband and his partner may pinpoint other hereditary diseases not necessarily causing infertility but causing morbidity or being lethal to offspring. A complete clinical examination of the proband and his partner is useful to establish a clinical diagnosis of a disease or a syndrome associated with infertility such as Klinefelter syndrome or CF-linked CBAVD. This examination may also reveal other possible hereditary diseases not identified as such before. Since the couple is in that case not aware of a genetic problem they should be counselled before treatment starts. Complementary tests, mainly laboratory investigations will help to confirm a clinical diagnosis. In case of male infertility, the personal history, the clinical examination, a semen analysis, and hormonal tests are sufficient to characterize most of the patients as being

1. infertile in association with other physical or mental problems;
2. infertile but otherwise healthy. These patients can be subdivided into oligozoospermic or eventually OAT males, and in males with obstructive or nonobstructive azoospermia.

Genetic investigations will help to refine the diagnosis, and to counsel the patient/couple accordingly. The above information will help to select the additional tests to be performed. In most cases of male infertility due to severe OAT or nonobstructive azoospermia a peripheral karyotype should be performed, even if the family history is not suggestive of a chromosomal disorder (6–8). In the same patients microdeletions in the AZF regions on Yq11 should be looked for in DNA from peripheral blood. With this genetic test attention should be paid to the techniques used to confirm the presence of a Yq11 deletion. To avoid erroneous results laboratories can now participate in quality control studies (87). The possibility of fertility treatment in couples in whom the male has an AZF deletion is strongly dependent on the type of deletion present (88). Deletions of AZFa or AZFb, or combinations including these regions, have a bad prognosis since no sperm cells will be produced, and ICSI will not be possible. In contrast, spermatozoa can be found in about 70% of patients with a complete deletion of the AZFc region (88). For these patients ICSI will be possible.

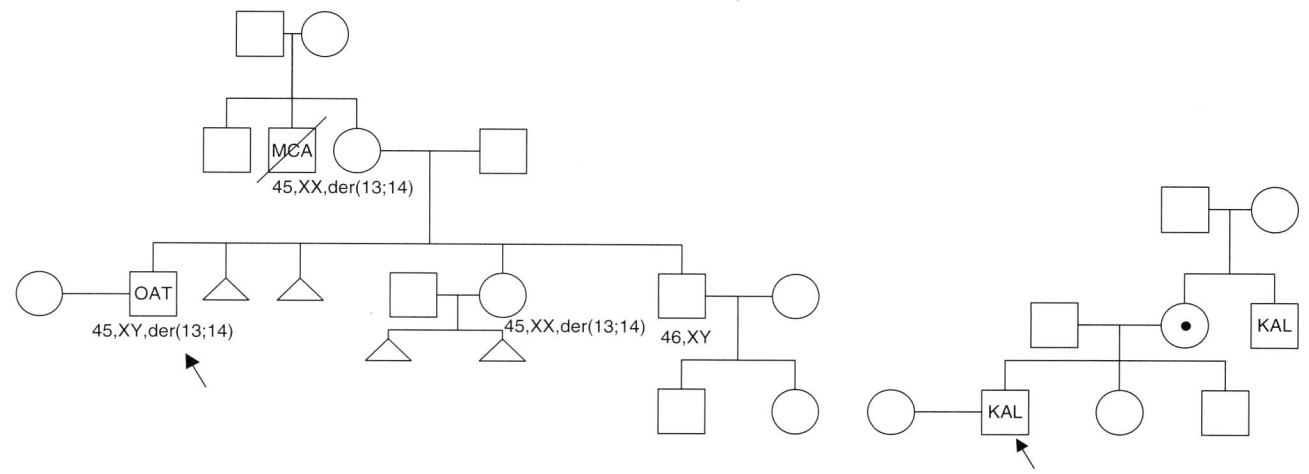

Figure 25.2 (**A**) Segregation of a Robertsonian translocation der(13;14) in a family: its consequences and recommendations. OAT (our proband ⬀) presents with infertility due to oligo-astheno-teratozoospermia (OAT). His sister had two miscarriages (Δ); his brother has two healthy children. His mother had two miscarriages (Δ), lost a brother born with multiple congenital anomalies (MCA), and has a healthy brother without children. This story is suggestive of a chromosomal translocation. The karyotype of OAT points indeed to a Robertson translocation der(13;14) (Fig. 25.1A). His mother and his sister have the same translocation explaining the recurrent miscarriages (Δ). These miscarriages are most probably resulting from a trisomy 14, or a monosomy 13 or 14. The brother of OAT has a normal karyotype which is perfectly possible. The MCA brother of the mother died and had most probably a trisomy 13. OAT should be informed about all the above possible risks in case of pregnancy. In case of ICSI, a preimplantation genetic diagnosis or a prenatal diagnosis should be offered. (**B**) X-linked Kallmann syndrome in a family: its consequences and recommendations. KAL (our proband ⬀) has Kallmann syndrome. The family history fits with an X-linked transmission since the brother of the mother of KAL has the same disease. This means that the mother of KAL must be a carrier ⊙. Her daughter, the sister of our proband has therefore a 50% risk of being a carrier and a 25% risk of having an affected son. Preimplantation or prenatal diagnosis should be discussed. If the wife of KAL becomes pregnant, boys will be healthy and fertile (because they inherit the Y chromosome of their father) while girls will always be carriers.

In men with CBAVD without anomalies of the urogenital tract, mutations in the CFTR gene should be looked for in the patient and, even more important in his partner. At present it is possible to identify 85–90% of the carriers in the Caucasian population (89,90). Depending on whether CFTR mutations have been identified in the male patient and/or his female partner the risk to conceive a child with CF can be calculated (Table 25.2). These figures together with the type of mutations indicate prenatal diagnosis or PGD (26,91,92). More specific tests should be performed if diseases such as Kennedy disease, Kallmann syndrome, myotonic dystrophy, the immotile cilia syndrome, or other syndromes or diseases are suspected. In these cases it is again not only important to establish a correct diagnosis to treat correctly but also to counsel the proband and his family concerning recurrence risks and prenatal or preimplantation diagnosis.

Genetic Testing During ART for Severe Male Infertility

Genetic tests, which can be performed during ART, refer to preconceptional or PGD. They involve the genetic analysis (PGD) of one or two polar bodies before fertilization or the analysis of one or two blastomeres of the 8- to 10-cell embryo in vitro (93–98). The aim is to avoid the birth of a child with a genetic disease. PGD makes conventional prenatal diagnosis, eventually followed by termination of pregnancy, obsolete. PGD is a complex procedure because of the "single cell" genetic diagnosis. It was developed and first applied in the clinic more than 20 years ago (99). Most of the PGDs performed are for CF, myotonic dystrophy, Huntington's disease, and Duchenne muscular dystrophy but many others have been performed for either infertile or fertile couples (95,97). For chromosomal aberrations most PGDs have been done for reciprocal and Robertsonian translocations (100). In general the take-home baby rate is of the same order of magnitude of 20–25% as in the ICSI cycles in general (2,3). A number of PGDs have been performed for Klinefelter patients in whom spermatozoa found in the testes were used to fertilize oocytes (13).

Genetic Evaluation of Pregnancies and Children Conceived Through ICSI Because of Severe Male Infertility

Follow-up studies of pregnancies established and children born after the use of ICSI have been initiated as soon as this new procedure was applied in the clinic. From these still ongoing studies it became clear that the number of major malformations was comparable to the number of major malformations in IVF children and possibly slightly higher than in naturally conceived children. Preliminary results on the psychomotor development of these children are also reassuring (101–108). The "de novo" chromosomal aberrations found at prenatal diagnosis indicate that numerical sex chromosomal anomalies are slightly increased when compared to a large newborn population. If the incidence in the newborn is 0.2%, the incidence in ICSI children is 0.8%. This is a four-fold increase but of course the overall incidence remains low (<1%). Apart from sex chromosome anomalies, de novo balanced translocations also have been observed (106,108). These aberrations occurring in children from men with a normal peripheral karyotype could be related to chromosomal anomalies being present in their sperm but not in their lymphocytes (109–112).

CONTROVERSIES

To Test or Not to Test

Some clinicians claim that now that ICSI is available to alleviate male infertility, it is sufficient to know whether these patients are oligozoospermic or azoospermic. Oligozoospermic and obstructive azoospermic males can be treated immediately and often successfully even if repetitive IVF cycles are necessary (113). Even in case of nonobstructive azoospermia, repeated testicular sperm extraction leads to a high sperm recovery rate that allows ICSI (114). It is probably true that in the majority of the cases a healthy although maybe infertile child will be born. Nevertheless, in a number of cases, for instance in the case of a chromosomal translocation, the treatment will fail and be repeated endlessly or recurrent miscarriages will occur. Furthermore, a few CF children will be born and probably a few other children with genetic disease which could have been avoided. Another option could be to not further use ICSI and leave decisions to nature.

Who to Test?

Among those clinicians who are convinced that genetic tests are useful and among the geneticists performing the tests the main ongoing discussion is in which infertile male patients, karyotypes and Yq deletion tests should be performed. With time many do now agree on performing these genetic tests if the sperm count is below 1 or 5×10^6 spermatozoa/mL. However, chromosomal aberrations as well as Yq microdeletions have been found in patients with more than 5×10^6 spermatozoa/mL, although to a lesser extent (115). Based on a few reports, one can also wonder whether karyotype analysis of the female partners should be performed (116–119). One reason of course to limit the patient population to be tested is that most of these tests are still cumbersome and costly. Prenatal diagnosis through chorionic villus sampling or amniocentesis after ICSI should be discussed with the couple in view of the known increase in sex chromosomal aberrations in the offspring (106,108).

Genetic Testing Vs. Genetic Screening

Genetic screening is different from genetic testing. A screening test is offered to a *"healthy"* population. In that case the persons who are tested have no particular problem but they may be interested to know whether they are carrier of a particular gene mutation to take preventive measures. Examples are screening programs for CF, Tay–Sachs disease, and other diseases common in certain high-risk populations (120–122). Couples may want to know before having children since, if both partners are carrier of such an autosomal recessive gene, the risk of having an affected child is 1/4. Such screening programs are not specific to infertile patients. However, a fertile couple with a 25% recurrence risk may choose to have prenatal diagnosis to prevent the birth of an affected child while if the couple is infertile and can be helped with IVF/ICSI they may choose to have PGD (123).

PGD for Aneuploidy Screening

PGD for aneuploidy screening (preimplantation genetic screening or PGS), a novel approach to select the *"better"* embryos for transfer after IVF/ICSI is at present offered to selected groups of patients. The main indications suggested for PGS are advanced maternal age, repeated implantation failure, repeated miscarriage, and severe male factor infertility. Here, the embryos are biopsied and a variable number of chromosomes, usually 13, 16, 18, 21, 22, X, and Y are enumerated using specific fluorescent in situ hybridization probes. Embryos diploid for the chromosomes tested are then transferred without of course having information on the other chromosomes. The first observations reported that in women over 37 years the IVF success rate increases (124), the rate of miscarriage decreases (125), and the implantation rate per embryo increases (126–128). Since these early times many studies have been performed but little (or no) evidence was found that PGS increases live birth delivery rates. Recent studies focus on the use of polar bodies as the study material, in contrast to blastomeres that were used most of the time before, and other technologies (than FISH) such as comparative genomic hybridization and single nucleotide polymorphism arrays in PGS (129–133). Data are needed to evaluate the possible benefit of these new applications in aneuploidy screening for IVF embryos.

Is ICSI in Case of Severe Male Infertility Safe?

Although the follow-up studies of pregnancies and children born after ICSI are reassuring, still a number of questions remain unanswered, one of them being the concerns in relation to imprinting (105,134–140).

FUTURE FINDINGS

ICSI performed with ejaculated spermatozoa and later on with epididymal and testicular spermatozoa may be considered milestones in infertility treatment for the male patient. Today very few men cannot be helped to have their own child. Research is going on to find other solutions for their fertility problems (141–145). However, some approaches are extremely controversial. ICSI has also triggered basic research in biology and genetics in order to gain more insight in gender development and spermatogenesis. Over the last years many novel genes have been and are being identified. The development of whole genome-scaled techniques (whole exome sequencing, array comparative genomic hybridization) allow a better identification of disease-related abnormalities in known or novel genes (Fig. 25.3). New findings will increase our knowledge and allow more accurate diagnosis and

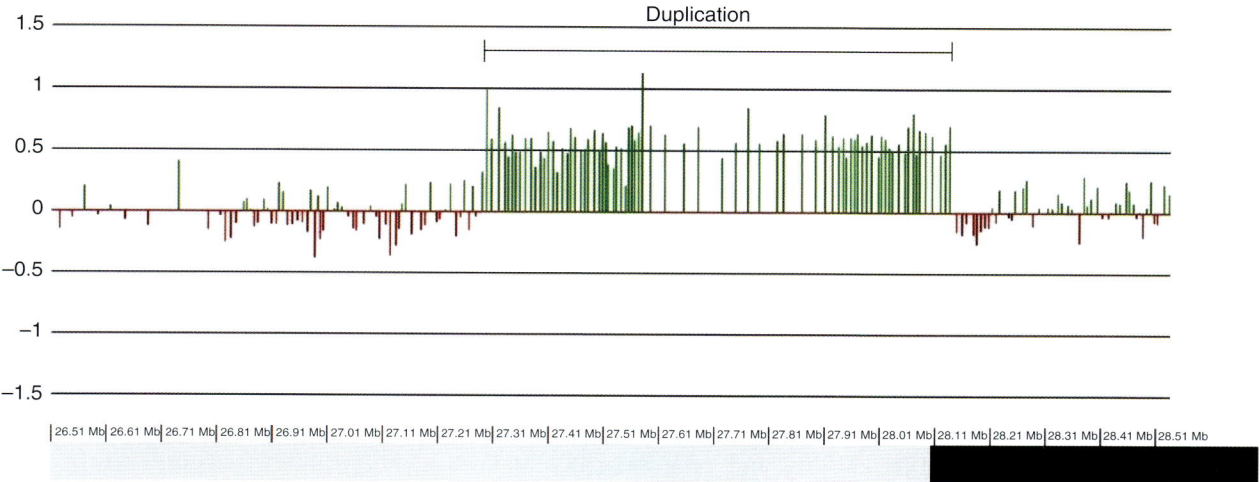

Figure 25.3 Example of a result obtained after array comparative genomic hybridization. The figure shows part of the genome where duplication was detected in an infertile male patient.

counseling, and probably new ways of treatment will become available.

CONCLUSION

In case of severe male infertility, good clinical practice requests genetic evaluation before, during, and after ART in order to properly treat and counsel the proband, the couple and eventually the family. The aim is to inform the patients about possible risks, to improve the success rate of the ART treatment, and to avoid the birth of children affected with a severe genetic disease. Moreover, at present there are still many unknown causes of male infertility. More research, also in the field of genetics, will allow better understanding and defining how great the risks are to transmit infertility or possibly other genetic anomalies to the next generations.

REFERENCES

1. Palermo G, Joris H, Devroey P, et al. Pregnancies after intracytoplasmic injection of single spermatozoon into an oocyte. Lancet 1992; 340: 17–18.
2. Devroey P, Van Steirteghem A. A review of ten years experience of ICSI. Hum Reprod Update 2004; 10: 19–28.
3. The ESHRE Capri Workshop Group. Intracytoplasmic sperm injection (ICSI) in 2006: evidence and evolution. Hum Reprod Update 2007; 13: 515–26.
4. Jacobs PA, Strong JA. A case of human intersexuality having a possible XXY sex-determining mechanism. Nature 1959; 183: 302–3.
5. Forti G, Corona G, Vignozzi L, et al. Klinefelter's syndrome: a clinical and therapeutical update. Sex Dev 2010; 4: 167–9.
6. Van Assche E, Bonduelle M, Tournaye H, et al. Cytogenetics of infertile men. Hum Reprod 1996; 11: 1–26.
7. Yoshida A, Miura K, Shirai M, et al. Cytogenetic survey of 1007 infertile males. Urol Int 1997; 58: 166–76.
8. Martin RH. Cytogenetic determinants of male fertility. Hum Reprod Update 2008; 14: 379–90.
9. Weil D, Wang I, Dietrich A, et al. Highly homologous loci on the X and Y chromosomes are hot-spots for ectopic recombination resulting in XX maleness. Nat Genet 1994; 7: 414–19.
10. Schiebel K, Winkelmann M, Mertz A, et al. Abnormal XY interchange between a novel isolated protein kinase gene, PRKY, and its homologue, PRKX, accounts for one third of all (Y+) XX males and (Y-) XY females. Hum Mol Genet 1997; 6: 1985–9.
11. Vorona E, Zitzmann M, Gromoll J, et al. Clinical, endocrinological, and epigenetic features of the 46, XX male syndrome, compared with 47,XXY Klinefelter patients. J Clin Endocrinol Metab 2007; 92: 3458–65.
12. Sinclair AH, Berta P, Palmer MS, et al. A gene from the human sex-determining region encodes a protein with homology to a conserved DNA-binding motif. Nature 1990; 346: 240–4.
13. Fullerton G, Hamilton M, Maheshwari A. Should non-mosaic Klinefelter syndrome men be labelled as infertile in 2009? Hum Reprod 2010; 25: 588–97.
14. Tiepolo L, Zuffardi O. Localization of factors controlling spermatogenesis in the nonfluorescent position of the human Y chromosome long arm. Hum Genet 1976; 34: 119–24.
15. Massart A, Lissens W, Tournaye H, Stouffs K. Genetic causes of spermatogenic failure. As J Androl 2012; 14: 40–8.
16. Skaletsky H, Kuroda-Kawaguchi T, Minx PJ, et al. The male-specific region of the human Y chromosome is a mosaic of discrete sequence classes. Nature 2003; 423: 825–37.
17. Repping S, Skaletsky H, Lange J, et al. Recombination between palindromes P5 and P1 on the human Y chromosome causes massive deletions and spermatogenic failure. Am J Hum Genet 2002; 71: 906–22.
18. Jobling MA. Copy number variation on the human Y chromosome. Cytogenet Genome Res 2008; 123: 253–62.
19. Silber SH. The Y chromosome in the era of intracytoplasmic sperm injection: a personal view. Fertil Steril 2011; 95: 2439–48.
20. Saut N, Terriou P, Navarro A, et al. The human Y chromosome genes BPY2, CDY1 and DAZ are not

essential for sustained fertility. Mol Hum Reprod 2000; 6: 789–93.
21. Chang PL, Sauer MV, Brown S, et al. Y chromosome microdeletion in a father and his four infertile sons. Hum Reprod 1999; 14: 2689–94.
22. Calogero AE, Garofalo MR, Barone N, et al. Spontaneous transmission from a father to his son of a Y chromosome microdeletion involving the deleted in azoospermia (DAZ) gene. J Endocrinol Invest 2002; 25: 631–4.
23. Girardi SK, Mielnik A, Schlegel PN. Submicroscopic deletions in the Y chromosome of infertile men. Hum Reprod 1997; 12: 1635–41.
24. Sarkar NN. Intracytoplasmic sperm injection: an assisted reproductive technique and its outcome to overcome infertility. J Obstet Gynaecol 2007; 27: 347–53.
25. Sueblinvong V, Whittaker LA. Fertility and pregnancy: common concerns of the aging cystic fibrosis population. Clin Chest Med 2007; 28: 433–43.
26. Keymolen K, Goossens V, De Rycke M, et al. Clinical outcome of preimplantation genetic diagnosis for cystic fibrosis: the Brussels' experience. Eur J Hum Genet 2007; 15: 752–8.
27. Kerem B, Rommens JM, Buchanan JA, et al. Identification of the cystic fibrosis gene: genetic analysis. Science 1989; 245: 1073–80.
28. Riordan JR, Rommens JM, Kerem B, et al. Identification of the cystic fibrosis gene: cloning and characterization of complementary DNA. Science 1989; 245: 1066–73.
29. Rommens JM, Iannuzzi MC, Kerem B, et al. Identification of the cystic fibrosis gene: chromosome walking and jumping. Science 1989; 245: 1059–65.
30. Dubin L, Amelar RD. Etiologic factors in 1294 consecutive cases of male infertility. Fertil Steril 1971; 22: 469–74.
31. Anguiano A, Oates RD, Amos JA, et al. Congenital bilateral absence of the vas deferens. A primarily genital form of cystic fibrosis. J Am Med Ass 1992; 267: 1794–7.
32. Chillon M, Casals T, Mercier B, et al. Mutations in the cystic fibrosis gene in patients with congenital absence of the vas deferens. N Engl J Med 1995; 332: 1475–80.
33. Claustres M. Molecular pathology of the CFTR locus in male infertility. Reprod Biomed Online 2005; 10: 14–41.
34. Cuppens H, Cassiman JJ. CFTR mutations and polymorphisms in male infertility. Int J Androl 2004; 27: 251–6.
35. Lissens W, Mercier B, Tournaye H, et al. Cystic fibrosis and infertility caused by congenital bilateral absence of the vas deferens and related clinical entities. Hum Reprod 1996; 11(Suppl 4): 55–80.
36. Groman JD, Hefferon TW, Casals T, et al. Variation in a repeat sequence determines whether a common variant of the cystic fibrosis transmembrane conductance regulator gene is pathogenic or benign. Am J Hum Genet 2004; 74: 176–9.
37. Dumur V, Gervais R, Rigot JM, et al. Congenital bilateral absence of the vas deferens in absence of cystic fibrosis. Lancet 1995; 345: 200–1.
38. Patrizio P, Zielenski J. Congenital absence of the vas deferens: a mild form of cystic fibrosis. Mol Med Today 1996; 1: 24–31.
39. Lissens W, Liebaers I, Van Steirteghem A. Male infertility. In: Rimoin DL, Connor JM, Pyeritz RE, Korf BC, eds. Emery and Rimoins's Principles and Practice of Medical Genetics. Philadelphia: Churchill Livingstone Elsevier, 2007: 856–74.
40. Aslanidis C, Jansen G, Amemiya C, et al. Cloning of the essential myotonic dystrophy region and mapping of the putative defect. Nature 1992; 355: 548–51.
41. Brook DJ, McCurrach ME, Harley HG, et al. Molecular basis of myotonic dystrophy: expansion of a trinucleotide (CTG) repeat at the 3' end of a transcript encoding a protein kinase family member. Cell 1992; 68: 799–808.
42. Fu HY, Pizzuti A, Fenwick RG, et al. An unstable triplet repeat in a gene related to myotonic muscular dystrophy. Science 1992; 255: 1256–8.
43. Mahadevan M, Tsilfidis C, Sabourin L, et al. Myotonic dystrophy mutation: an unstable CTG repeat in the 3" untranslated region of the gene. Science 1992; 255: 1253–5.
44. Hunter A, Tsilfidis C, Mettler G, et al. The correlation of age of onset with CTG trinucleotide repeat amplification in myotonic dystrophy. J Med Genet 1992; 29: 774–9.
45. Sermon K, De Vos A, Van de Velde H, et al. Fluorescent PCR and automated fragment analysis for the clinical application of preimplantation genetic diagnosis of myotonic dystrophy (Steinert's disease). Mol Hum Reprod 1998; 4: 791–6.
46. Sermon K, Seneca S, De Rycke M, et al. PGD in the lab for triplet repeat diseases – myotonic dystrophy, Huntington's disease and Fragile-X syndrome. Mol Cell Endocrinol 2001; 183(Suppl 1): S77–85.
47. Rugarli EI, Ballabio A. Kallmann syndrome. From genetics to neurobiology. J Am Med Ass 1993; 270: 2713–16.
48. Dodé C, Levilliers J, Dupont JM, et al. Loss-of-function mutations in FGFR1 cause autosomal dominant Kallmann syndrome. Nat Genet 2003; 33: 463–5.
49. Ayari B, Soussi-Yanicostas N. FGFR1 and anosmin-1 underlying genetically distinct forms of Kallmann syndrome are co-expressed and interact in olfactory bulbs. Dev Genes Evol 2007; 217: 169–75.
50. Cadman SM, Kim SH, Hu Y, et al. Molecular pathogenesis of Kallmann's syndrome. Horm Res 2007; 67: 231–42.
51. Dodé C, Teixeira L, Levilliers J, et al. Kallmann syndrome: mutations in the genes encoding prokineticin-2 and prokineticin receptor-2. PloS Genet 2006; 2: 1648–52.
52. Falardeau J, Chung WC, Beenken A, et al. Decreased FGF8 signaling causes deficiency of gonadotropin-releasing hormone in humans and mice. J Clin Invest 2008; 118: 2822–31.
53. Kim HG, Kurth I, Lan F, et al. Mutations in CHD7, encoding a chromatin-remodeling protein, cause idiopathic hypogonadotropic hypogonadism and Kallmann syndrome. Am J Hum Genet 2008; 83: 511–19.
54. Kaplan JD, Bernstein JA, Kwan A, et al. Clues to an early diagnosis of Kallmann syndrome. Am J Med Genet 2010; 152: 2796–801.
55. Pitteloud N, Quinton R, Pearce S, et al. Digenic mutations account for variable phenotypes in idiopathic hypogonadotropic hypogonadism. J Clin Invest 2007; 117: 457–63.

56. Sykiotis GP, Plummer L, Hughes VA, et al. Oligogenic basis of isolated gonadotropin-releasing hormone deficiency. Proc Natl Acad Sci USA 2010; 107: 15140–4.
57. Büchter D, Behre HM, Kliesh S, Nieschlag E. Pulsatile GnRH or human chorionic gonadotropin/human menopausal gonadotropin as effective treatment for men with hypogonatropic hypogonadism: a review of 42 cases. Eur J Endocrinol 1998; 139: 298–303.
58. Cardenas-Rodriguez M, Badano JL. Ciliary Biology: understanding the cellular and genetic basis of human ciliopathies. Am J Med Genet 2009; 151: 263–80.
59. Afzelius BA. Immotile cilia syndrome: past, present, and prospects for the future. Thorax 1998; 53: 894–7.
60. Sutherland MJ, Ware SM. Disorders of left-right asymmetry: heterotaxy and situs inversus. Am J Med Genet 2009; 151: 307–17.
61. Igarashi S, Tanno Y, Onodera O, et al. Strong correlation between the number of CAG repeats in androgen receptor genes and the clinical onset features of spinal and bulbar atrophy. Neurology 1992; 42: 2300–2.
62. Finsterer Perspectives of Kennedy's disease. J Neurol Sci 2010; 298: 1–10.
63. Quigley CA, De Bellis A, Marschke KB, et al. Androgen receptor defects: historical, clinical and molecular perspectives. Endocr Rev 1995; 16: 271–321.
64. Wisniewski AB, Mazur T. 46,XY DSD with female or ambiguous external genitalia at birth due to androgen insensitivity syndrome, 5α-reductase-2 deficiency, or 17-hydroxysteroid dehydrogenase deficiency: a review of quality of life outcomes. Int J Pediatr Endocrinol 2009; 2009: 567430.
65. Sinnecker GH, Hiort O, Dibbelt L, et al. Phenotypic classification of male pseudo hermaphroditism due to steroid 5 α-reductase 2 deficiency. Am J Med Gen 1996; 63: 223–30.
66. Chong CK. Practical approach to steroid 5alpha-reductase type 2 deficiency. Eur J Pediatr 2011; 170: 1–8.
67. Romano A, Allanson J, Dahlgren J, et al. Noonan syndrome: clinical features, diagnosis and management guidelines. Pediatrics 2010; 126: 746–59.
68. Tartaglia M, Mehler EL, Goldberg R, et al. Mutations in PTPN11, encoding the protein tyrosine phosphatase SHP-2, cause Noonan syndrome. Nat Genet 2001; 29: 465–8.
69. Meschede D, Rolf C, Neugebauer DC, et al. Sperm acrosome defects in a patient with Aarskog-Scott syndrome. Am J Med Genet 1996; 66: 340–2.
70. Orrico A, Galli L, Faivre L, et al. Aarskog-Scott syndrome: clinical update and report of nine novel mutations in the FGD1 gene. Am J Med Genet 2010; 152: 313–18.
71. Choufani S, Shuman C, Weksberg R. Beckwith-Wiedemann syndrome. Am J Med Genet 2010; 154C: 343–54.
72. Beales PL, Elcioglu N, Woolf AS, et al. New criteria for improved diagnosis of Bardet-Biedl syndrome: results of a population survey. J Med Genet 1999; 36: 437–46.
73. Cassidy SB. Prader-Willi syndrome. J Med Genet 1997; 34: 917–23.
74. Baker K, Beales PL. Making sense of cilia in disease: the human ciliopathies. Am J Med Genet 2009; 151C: 281–95.
75. Horsthemke B, Dittrich B, Buiting K, et al. Imprinting mutations on human chromosome 15. Hum Mutat 1997; 10: 329–37.
76. Feil R, Khosla S. Genomic imprinting in mammals. Trends Genet 1999; 15: 431–5.
77. Vogels A, Moerman P, Frijns JP, Bogaert GA. Testicular histology in boys with Prader-Willi syndrome: fertile or infertile? J Urol 2008; 180: 1800–4.
78. Weiss J, Axelrod L, Whitcomb RW, et al. Hypogonadism caused by a single amino acid substitution in the β subunit of luteinizing hormone. N Engl J Med 1992; 326: 179–83.
79. Latronico AC, Segaloff DL. Naturally occurring mutations of the luteinizing-hormone receptor: lessons learned about reproductive physiology and G protein-coupled receptors. Am J Hum Genet 1999; 65: 949–58.
80. Rajender S, Rahul P, Mahdi AA. Mitochondria, spermatogenesis and male infertility. Mitochondrion 2010; 10: 419–28.
81. Dam AH, Feenstra I, Westphal JR, et al. Globozoospermia revisited. Hum Reprod Update 2007; 13: 63–75.
82. Dam AH, Koscinski I, Kremer JA, et al. Homozygous mutation in SPATA16 is associated with male infertility in human globozoospermia. Am J Hum Genet 2007; 813–20.
83. Liu G, Shi QW, Lu GX. A newly discovered mutation in PICK1 in a human with globozoospermia. As J Androl 2010; 12: 556–60.
84. Harbuz R, Zouari R, Pierre V, et al. Recurrent deletion of DPY19L2 causes infertility in man by blocking sperm head elongation and acrosome formation. Am J Hum Genet 2011; 88: 351–61.
85. Koscinski I, Ellnati E, Fossard C, et al. DPY19L2 deletion as a major cause of globozoospermia. Am J Hum Genet 2011; 88: 344–50.
86. Dieterich K, Soto Rifo R, Faure AK, et al. Homozygous mutation of AURKC yields large-headed polyploid spermatozoa and causes male infertility. Nat Genet 2007; 39: 661–5.
87. Simoni M, Bakker E, Krausz C. EAA/EMQN best practice guidelines for molecular diagnosis of Y-chromosomal microdeletions. State of the art 2004. Int J Androl 2004; 27: 240–9.
88. Stouffs K, Lissens W, Tournaye H, et al. The choice and outcome of the fertility treatment of 38 couples in whom the male partner has a Yq microdeletion. Hum Reprod 2005; 20: 1887–96.
89. Dequeker E, Stuhrmann M, Morris MA, et al. Best practice guidelines for molecular genetic diagnosis of cystic fibrosis and CFTR-related disorders – updated European recommendations. Eur J Hum Genet 2009; 17: 51–65.
90. World Health Organisation. The molecular genetic epidemiology of cystic fibrosis. Report of a joint meeting of WHO/ECFTN/ICF(M)A/ECFS, 2004. [Available from: www.who.int/genomics/publications/en/]
91. Goossens V, Sermon K, Lissens W, et al. Clinical application of preimplantation genetic diagnosis for cystic fibrosis. Prenat Diagn 2000; 20: 571–81.
92. Dreesen JC, Jacobs LJ, Bras M, et al. Multiplex PCR of polymorphic markers flanking the CFTR gene; a general approach for preimplantation genetic diagnosis of cystic fibrosis. Mol Hum Reprod 2000; 6: 391–6.

93. Braude P, Pickering S, Flinter F, Ogilvie CM. Preimplantation genetic diagnosis. Nat Rev Genet 2002; 3: 941–53.
94. Sermon K, Van Steirteghem A, Liebaers I. Preimplantation genetic diagnosis. Lancet 2004; 363: 1633–41.
95. Geraedts JP, De Wert GM. Preimplantation genetic diagnosis. Clin Genet 2009; 76: 315–25.
96. Harper JC, Sengupta SB. Preimplantation genetic diagnosis: state of the ART 2011. Hum Genet 2011; 131: 175–86.
97. Simpson JL. Preimplantation genetic diagnosis at 20 years. Prenat Diagn 2010; 30: 682–95.
98. Handyside AH. Preimplantion genetic diagnosis after 20 years. Reprod Biomed Online 2010; 21: 280–2.
99. Handyside AH, Kontogianni EH, Hardy K, et al. Pregnancies from biopsied human preimplantation embryos sexed by Y-specific DNA amplification. Nature 1990; 344: 768–70.
100. Harper JC, Coonen E, De Rycke M, et al. ESHRE PGD Consortium data collection X: cycles from January to December 2007 with pregnancy follow-up to October 2008. Hum Reprod 2010; 25: 2685–707.
101. Bonduelle M, Liebaers I, Deketelaere V, et al. Neonatal data on a cohort of 2889 infants born after intracytoplasmic sperm injection (ICSI) (1991–1999) and of 2995 infants born after in vitro fertilization (IVF) (1983–1999). Hum Reprod 2002; 17: 671–94.
102. Bonduelle M, Van Assche E, Joris H, et al. Prenatal testing in ICSI pregnancies: incidence of chromosomal anomalies in 1586 karyotypes and relation to sperm parameters. Hum Reprod 2002; 17: 2600–14.
103. Bonduelle M, Ponjaert I, Van Steirteghem A, et al. Developmental outcome of children born after ICSI compared to children born after IVF at the age of two years. Hum Reprod 2003; 19: 1–9.
104. Leunens L, Celestin-Westreich S, Bonduelle M, Liebaers I, Ponjaert-Kristoffersen I. Cognitive and motor development of 8-year-old children born after ICSI compared to spontanously conceived children. Hum Reprod 2006; 21: 2922–9.
105. Sutcliffe AG, Ludwig M. Outcome of assisted reproduction. Lancet 2007; 370: 351–9.
106. Belva F, De Schrijver F, Tournaye H, et al. Neonatal outcome of 724 children born after ICSI using non-ejaculated sperm. Hum Reprod 2011; 1752–8.
107. De Schepper J, Belva F, Schiettecatte J, et al. Testicular growth and tubular function in prepubertal boys conceived by intracytoplasmic sperm injection. Horm Res 2009; 71: 359–63.
108. Woldringh GH, Besselink DE, Tillema AJ, et al. Karyotyping, congenital anomalies and follow-up of children after intracytoplamic sperm injection with non-ejaculated sperm: a systemic review. Hum Reprod Update 2010; 16: 12–19.
109. Martin RH. Genetics of human sperm. J Assist Reprod Genet 1998; 15: 240–455.
110. Aran B, Blanco J, Vidal F, et al. Screening for abnormalities of chromosomes X, Y, and 18 and for diploidy in spermatozoa from infertile men participating in an in vitro fertilization-intracytoplasmic sperm injection program. Fertil Steril 1999; 72: 696–701.
111. Vegetti W, Van Assche E, Frias A, et al. Correlation between semen parameters and sperm aneuploidy rates investigated by fluorescence in-situ hybridization in infertile men. Hum Reprod 2000; 15: 351–65.
112. Egozcue S, Blanco J, Vendrell JM, et al. Human male infertility: chromosome anomalies, meiotic disorders, abnormal spermatozoa and recurrent abortion. Hum Reprod Update 2000; 6: 93–105.
113. Osmanagaoglu K, Tournaye H, Camus M, et al. Cumulative delivery rates after intracytoplasmic sperm injection: 5 year follow-up of 498 patients. Hum Reprod 1999; 14: 2651–5.
114. Vernaeve V, Verheyen G, Goossens A, et al. How successful is repeat testicular sperm extraction in patients with azoospermia? Hum Reprod 2006; 21: 1551–4.
115. Foresta C, Ferlin A, Gianaroli L, Dallapiccola B. Guidelines for the appropriate use of genetic tests in infertile couples. Eur J Hum Genet 2002: 303–12.
116. Meschede D, Lemcke B, Exeler JR, et al. Chromosome abnormalities in 477 couples undergoing intracytoplasmic sperm injection-prevalence, types, sex distribution and reproductive relevance. Hum Reprod 1998; 13: 576–82.
117. van der Ven K, Peschka B, Montag M, et al. Increased frequency of congenital chromosomal aberrations in female partners of couples undergoing intracytoplasmic sperm injection. Hum Reprod 1998; 13: 48–54.
118. Papanikolaou EG, Vernaeve V, Kolibianakis E, et al. Is chromosome analysis mandatory in the initial investigation of normovulatory women seeking infertility treatment? Hum Reprod 2005; 20: 2899–903.
119. Riccaboni A, Lalatta F, Caliari I, et al. Genetic screening in 2,710 infertile candidate couples for assisted reproductive techniques: results of application of Italian guidelines for the appropriate use of genetic tests. Fertil Steril 2008; 89: 800–8.
120. Vallance H, Ford J. Carrier testing for autosomal-recessive disorders. Crit Rev Clin Lab Sci 2003; 40: 473–97.
121. Kaback MM. Population-based genetic screening for reproductive counseling: the Tay-Sachs disease model. Eur J Pediatr 2000; 159(Suppl 3): 192–5.
122. Gason AA, Sheffield E, Bankier A, et al. Evaluation of a Tay-Sachs disease screening program. Clin Genet 2003; 63: 386–92.
123. Liebaers I, Bonduelle M, Van Assche E, et al. How far should we go with genetic screening in assisted reproduction? In: Kempers RD, Cohen J, Haney AF, eds. "Fertility and Reproductive Medicine. Proceedings of the XVI World Congress on Fertility and Sterility. San Francisco." Amsterdam, The Netherlands: Elseviers Science BV, 1998.
124. Verlinsky Y, Cieslak J, Ivakhnenko V, et al. Prevention of age-related aneuploidies by polar body testing of oocytes. J Assist Reprod Genet 1999; 16: 165–9.
125. Munné S, Magli C, Cohen J, et al. Positive outcome after preimplantation diagnosis of aneuploidy in human embryos. Hum Reprod 1999; 14: 2191–9.
126. Gianaroli L, Magli MC, Ferraretti AP, et al. Preimplantation diagnosis for aneuploidies in patients undergoing in vitro fertilization with a poor prognosis: identification of the categories for what should be proposed. Fertil Steril 1999; 72: 837–44.
127. Staessen C, Platteau P, Van Assche E, et al. Comparison of blastocyst transfer with or without preimplantation genetic diagnosis for aneuploidy screening in couples with advanced maternal age: a prospective randomized controlled trial. Hum Reprod 2004; 19: 2849–58.

128. Mastenbroek S, Twisk M, van Echten-Arends J, et al. In vitro fertilization with preimplantation genetic screening. N Engl J Med 2007; 357: 9–17.
129. Geraedts J, Collins J, Gianarolli L, et al. What next for preimplantation genetic screening? A polar body approach! Hum Reprod 2010; 25: 575–7.
130. Harper J, Coonen E, De Rycke M, et al. What next for preimplantation genetic screening (PGS)? A position statement from the ESHRE PGD Consortium steering committee. Hum Reprod 2010; 25: 821–3.
131. Harper J, Harton G. The use of arrays in preimplantation genetic diagnosis and screening. Fertil Steril 2010; 94: 1173–7.
132. Geraedts J, Montag M, Magli MC, et al. Polar body array CGH for prediction of the status of the corresponding oocyte. Part 1: clinical results. Hum Reprod 2011; 26: 3173–80.
133. Magli MC, Montag M, Köster M, et al. Polar body array CGH for prediction of the status of the corresponding oocyte. Part 2: technical aspects. Hum Reprod 2011; 26: 3181–5.
134. De Rycke M, Liebaers I, Van Steirteghem A. Epigenetic risks related to assisted reproductive technologies. Risk analysis and epigenetic inheritance. Hum Reprod 2002; 17: 2487–94.
135. Cox GF, Burger J, Lip V, et al. Intracytoplasmic sperm injection may increase the risk of imprinting defects. Am J Hum Genet 2002; 71: 162–4.
136. Debaun MR, Niemitz EL, Feinberg AP. Association of in vitro fertilization with Beckwith-Wiedemann syndrome and epigenetic alterations of LIT1 and H19. Am J Hum Genet 2003; 72: 156–60.
137. Maher ER, Brueton LA, Bowdin SC, et al. Beckwith-Wiedemann syndrome and assisted reproduction technology (ART). J Med Genet 2003; 40: 62–4.
138. Moll AC, Imhof SM, Cruysberg JRM, et al. Incidence of retinoblastoma in children born after in-vitro fertilisation. Lancet 2003; 361: 309–10.
139. Diaz-Garcia C, Estella C, Perales-Puchalt A, et al. Reproductive medicine and inheritance of infertility by offspring: the role of fetal programming. Fertil Steril 2011; 96: 536–45.
140. Weksberg R, Shuman C, Wilkins-Haug L, et al. Workshop report: evaluation of genetic and epigenetic risks associated with assisted reproductive technologies and infertility. Fertil Steril 2007; 88: 27–31.
141. Ko K, Schöler HR. Embryonic stem cells as a potential source of gametes. Semin Reprod Med 2006; 24: 322–9.
142. Ehmcke J, Wistuba J, Schlatt S. Spermatogonial stem cells: questions, models and perspectives. Hum Reprod Update 2006; 12: 275–82.
143. Kubota H, Brinster RL. Technology insight: in vitro culture of spermatogonial stem cells and their potential therapeutic uses. Nat Clin Pract Endocrinol Metab 2006; 2: 99–108.
144. Nagy ZP, Chang CC. Artificial gametes. Theriogenology 2007; 67: 99–104.
145. Wyns C, Curaba M, Vanabelle B, et al. Options for fertility preservation in prepubertal boys. Hum Reprod Update 2010; 16: 312–28.

26

Polar body biopsy and its clinical application

Markus Montag

INTRODUCTION

Polar body (PB) biopsy with subsequent analysis of chromosomal abnormalities was introduced in 1990 by Verlinsky et al. (1). This technique opened the era of preconception genetic diagnosis as an alternative to preimplantation genetic diagnosis (PGD) of the embryo which was proposed earlier by Handyside et al. (2). It is important to note, that PB diagnosis gives direct information about the first and second PB and therefore only allows an indirect diagnosis of the maternal genetic or chromosomal constitution of the corresponding oocyte. In contrast, PGD of the embryo gives a direct diagnosis for the embryo and allows detecting both maternally and paternally derived genetic or chromosomal contributions.

Consequently embryo biopsy at the six- to eight-cell stage on day 3 was widely used, especially for preimplantation genetic screening (PGS) (3). However, since 2007, numerous randomized controlled trials reported that PGS by blastomere biopsy does not result in increased success rates (4–14) and several organizations published statements where they no longer recommend using biopsy at the blastomere stage at least for PGS (15,16). Since then the overall trend goes in two different directions: PB biopsy and blastocyst biopsy (17). Obviously PB biopsy does have limitations for the diagnosis of genetic diseases. But in view of aneuploidy screening to detect numerical chromosomal disorders which predominantly arise during meiosis in the oocyte (18), PB biopsy is a viable alternative, especially if combined with comparative genomic hybridization (CGH) for detecting all chromosomes (19). The present article gives an overview about the expectations and limitations of PB diagnosis and relevant technical details, with special emphasis on aneuploidy screening.

CLINICAL APPLICATION OF POLAR BODY DIAGNOSIS

PB biopsy has been successfully used for the detection of numerical and structural chromosomal abnormalities in human oocytes (20,21) and for the diagnosis of monogenetic diseases (22).

PB Biopsy and Detection of Numerical Chromosomal Abnormalities: PGS

Numerical chromosomal abnormalities are characterized by a wrong distribution of chromosomes or chromatids in the first or second PB. These errors are strongly correlated to maternal age. Up to 70% of oocytes from women beyond 40 years can possess such a disorder (23). This explains why women with advanced maternal age have a lower chance for pregnancy and a higher risk to miscarry once they are pregnant. One possibility to reduce these risks and probably to increase the success rates is a screening for maternally derived chromosomal abnormalities of the oocyte. This can be achieved by PB diagnosis.

During the first meiotic division the diploid chromosome content of an oocyte is reduced to two haploid chromosome sets, which both consist of paired chromatids. One paired chromatid set is extruded as part of the first PB. Sperm entry into an oocyte initiates the second meiotic division whereby the set of paired chromatids is separated and a single chromatid set becomes part of the second PB. After the first meiotic division, the number of the chromosomes in the oocyte and the first PB should be identical and the same holds true for the number of chromatids following the second meiotic division. Numerical chromosomal abnormalities can be caused by nondisjunction, meaning that a whole chromosome is not directed to the proper compartment (either oocyte or PB). Another mechanism is premature chromatid segregation into two single, separated chromatids, which has been suggested to occur frequently prior to the first meiotic division (24). Premature chromatid segregation during meiosis I can either lead to a balanced situation, where both chromatids remain in the same compartment, or to an unbalanced situation, where the two chromatids are finally allocated to different compartments. Some of the unbalanced segregations which originate in meiosis I in the oocyte can be corrected in meiosis II during the formation of the second PB (25).

PB biopsy and subsequent analysis of the first and second PB by FISH or array-CGH offers the possibility to detect numerical chromosome aberrations and to establish an indirect diagnosis for the corresponding oocyte. Alterations in the copy number in the first and second PB indicate a trisomy for the resulting embryo if one copy is missing in the PBs, or a monosomy if one signal is found in excess. Distinctions of copy numbers are easily detected in FISH and array-CGH following the introduction of single channel analysis (see below). Array-CGH has the advantage that all chromosomes can be investigated at once, whereas FISH has its limitations as only five to six chromosomes can be used in one hybridization round (26) and the efficacy of hybridization is reduced with each additional round (27).

PB biopsy and FISH for PGS is clinically used since the early 1990s and the clinical outcome has been described in numerous publications (Table 26.1). PB biopsy and array-CGH have been used clinically only recently and further results are still awaited (19,28,29).

PB Biopsy and Detection of Structural Chromosomal Aberrations

Structural chromosomal aberrations, for example balanced translocations, were found at a higher rate among infertile couples compared with the normal population (30–32). During meiosis the pairing of homolog chromosomes is disturbed by a structural aberrant chromosome and this may result in a partial aneuploidy in the oocyte. The risk for the extent of abnormal gametes is dependent on the size of the chromosome region involved in the translocation.

Usually only 10–20% of all oocytes from a translocation carrier are either balanced or normal.

Provided that the female is a carrier of a balanced translocation, PB biopsy allows selecting against abnormal oocytes using a reliable method for the genetic analysis. In the past this has been achieved by FISH probes which were designed for each individual patient and covered the chromosomal breakpoints (33). Later another technique was presented based on the combined use of centromeric and telomeric probes for FISH analysis of the chromosomes involved in the translocation (21). Recently structural chromosomal disorders were successfully investigated by whole-genome amplification and array-CGH (29). This approach offers the advantage of a combined screening for structural as well as numerical aberrations which seems to be beneficial especially for translocation patients (34).

PB Biopsy and Detection of Monogenetic Aberrations

The detection of monogenetic disorders by PB biopsy requires that the DNA of interest (e.g., the region containing the mutation) from the first and second PB is accurately amplified by polymerase chain reaction (PCR). In addition to the general risk of contamination of PCR reagents and products with foreign DNA with a potential resulting misdiagnosis, specific problems need to be addressed in the case of PB biopsy. A major problem in single cell PCR is the correct amplification of the region of interest and it is known from numerous reports that in diploid cells, occasionally one allele will not amplify, also known as allele-drop out (ADO, (35–39)). Although this phenomenon will not lead to a misdiagnosis in homozygous mutant or homozygous wild-type single cells, the situation is different in heterozygous single cells and especially, in PB diagnosis. Recombination and crossing-over of homologous chromatids frequently occur during meiosis. As a result, the first PB may consist of one chromatid carrying the mutation of interest and one chromatid carrying the wild-type or normal sequence. In this case, ADO may directly lead to a misdiagnosis, if crossing over and ADO remain undetected. Only in the case that the analysis of the second PB, which carries either a mutant or a normal chromatid reveals a discrepant result from that of the first PB, the problem would be recognized. Although ADO seems to be a frequent phenomenon in PID (between 1 and 25% and up to 40%) (40), the frequency of ADO in PB diagnosis is mainly unknown due to the low number of cases. Verlinsky (41) reported a frequency of ADO of 6% in 100 polar bodies which were analyzed.

Several strategies have been proposed to overcome this diagnostic problem, mainly coamplification of polymorphic markers which are closely linked to the region of

Table 26.1 Success Rates of Polar Body Biopsy and Aneuploidy Screening in the International Literature

Reference	Biopsy-material	No. of chromosomes	No. of cycles	No. embryos per transfer	Clinical pregnancy rate
Biopsy using zona drilling by acidic Tyrode solution					
Verlinsky et al. (60)	PB I / I+II	3	45	3.1	21.7%
Dyban et al. (61)	PB I / I+II	3	161	2.6	14.8%
Verlinsky et al. (62)	PB I / I+II	3	235	2.5	16.0%
Verlinsky et al. (63)	PB I / I+II	3	598	2.6	21.4%
Verlinsky et al. (64)	PB I / I+II	3	659	2.1	22.3%
Verlinsky et al. (65)	PB I / I+II	3/5	821	2.5	22.2%
Kuliev et al. (20)	PB I / I+II	3/5	1297	2.35	21.9%[a]
Biopsy using a 1.48 μm diode laser					
Montag et al. (55)	PB I	5	50	1.9	30.9%
Montag et al. (59)	PB I	5/6	110	1.8	26.6%
van der Ven et al. (66)	PB I / I+II	5/6	170	1.7	23.3%[b]

Abortion rate: [a] 23.7%; [b] 14.3%.

interest or the improvement of amplification efficiency through the use of nested primers (42). The use of PCR conditions which allow for continuous quantification of the PCR product for example, with fluorescent primers will help to determine ADO or cases of preferential amplification of alleles. Although ADO has for long been recognized to be a substantial problem in PGD and especially PB diagnosis, a systematic evaluation of this phenomenon which might eventually lead to strategies to decrease ADO rates has only recently been begun (40).

Because in PB diagnosis, only the maternal contribution to a potential genetic disease can be investigated, the isolated application of this technique is limited to selected genetic scenarios, for example autosomal dominant diseases with an affected mother or X-linked recessive and dominant disease where the mother is a mutation carrier. In view of the increasing use of blastocyst biopsy, the majority of cases with a genetic disease will be offered this approach which also has the advantage, that usually several trophectoderm cells are biopsied and thus the amplification is much more robust for a reliable genetic diagnosis.

PB BIOPSY TECHNIQUES

For PB biopsy, timing is a crucial point. The first PB degenerates with time and doing a biopsy later than 10 hours after ICSI may result in lower hybridization efficiency. The second PB is formed around two to four hours after ICSI but as it is firmly attached to the oolemma with a cytoplasmic strand and spindle remnants up to six hours after ICSI (43), the optimal time for biopsy is 8–16 hours after ICSI. Recent data show that for testing of second PB in array-CGH the amplification efficiency of the isolated DNA is lower if biopsy is done before eight hours after ICSI (44). Based on this one may conclude that the optimal timing for sequential biopsy is 4–10 hours after ICSI for the first and 8–16 hours after ICSI for the second PB. For simultaneous biopsy of the first and second PB an optimal time window is at 8–10 hours after ICSI.

Removal of polar bodies requires access to the perivitelline space through the zona pellucida. For PB biopsy, acidic Tyrode solution as a chemical means (45) cannot be used as it has a negative impact on further development if applied at the oocyte stage. Another method based on three-dimensional zona dissection was proposed by Cieslak et al. (46). Although this method can be performed with simple glass tools, multiple steps including dissection, release, and rotation of the oocyte are needed and the procedure definitely requires skill and time.

The use of a 1.48 μm diode laser drilling for PB biopsy was proposed already in 1997 (47). Animal experimentation showed the potential of this method for PB biopsy and for assisted hatching (48) and allowed to investigate its proper mode of application (49). For example the size and position of laser-drilled openings can influence further embryonic development and in particular the mode of hatching at the blastocyst stage (50). Due to its ease, laser-assisted biopsy is now widely used for biopsy of blastomeres (51,52) and blastocyst cells (53) and its advantage over the use of acidic Tyrode solution was reported (54).

For laser-assisted PB biopsy, the size of the drilled opening is usually in the range of 20 μm but it can be easily adjusted to the diameter of the aspiration capillary (Fig. 26.1). As the capillary can be introduced through the laser-drilled opening, there is no need for a sharp aspiration needle. This allows the use of flame-polished, blunt-ended aspiration needles and greatly reduces the risk of damaging the PB, the blastomere, or the remaining oocyte or embryo. The procedure becomes safer, more accurate, and more reliable thus allowing to significantly reducing the number of cells which cannot be reliably diagnosed as a result of technical problems during the biopsy procedure (55). The performance of laser-assisted PB biopsy is shown in (Table 26.2).

Another benefit is that laser drilling and subsequent biopsy can be performed without changing the culture dish or the capillaries in contrast to zona drilling using acidic Tyrode solution. This may help prevent the contamination of samples to be diagnosed by sensitive techniques such as PCR.

The simultaneous removal of the first and second PB is best accomplished if the oocyte is affixed to the holding capillary with the first PB at the 12 o'clock position and the second PB is right to the first one but in the same focal plane. An opening is drilled at 2–3 o'clock, and by shoving the biopsy capillary into the perivitelline space, both polar bodies can be removed simultaneously, provided that the cytoplasmic bridge between the second PB and the oocyte is not too firm (Fig. 26.1).

In all manipulation steps and zona opening techniques it is important to drill only one opening, as two openings, for example to retrieve both polar bodies through separate openings, may cause problems at the time of hatching because the embryo could hatch through both openings simultaneously and therefore may get trapped within the zona (49). Another important point is to generate a sufficient opening which allows consecutive hatching at the blastocyst stage, because smaller openings (<15 μm) may also cause the trapping of the embryo followed by degeneration (49). Laser drilled openings will stay permanently in the zona and therefore gentle handling during subsequent transfer of oocytes to other media droplets and even during the embryo transfer is recommended.

A position paper with relevant best-practice guidelines for PB biopsy for PGD/PGS has been published by ESHRE (56).

TRANSFER OF PBs FOR ANEUPLOIDY SCREENING BY FISH

Once both PBs are biopsied, the first and second PB of an oocyte are placed together in a neighboring droplet of medium until all oocytes are biopsied. A special pretreatment of polar bodies like hyoosmotic swelling in water or proteinase/pronase treatment is not necessary due to the small cytoplasmic content of PBs. For transfer onto

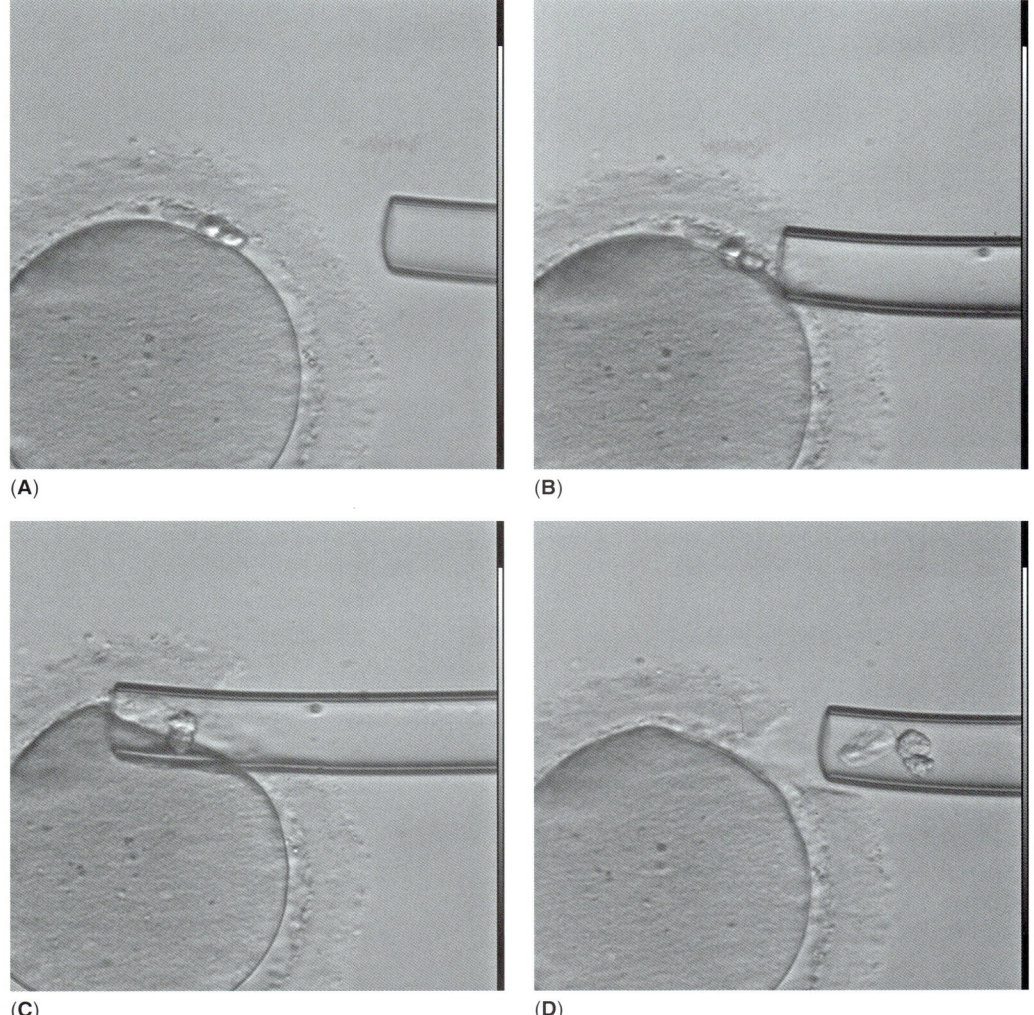

Figure 26.1 Simultaneous biopsy of the first and second polar body (PB). For removal of the first and second PB the oocyte is held in a position where the PBs are located at 12 o'clock (**A**). An opening is drilled at 1–2 o'clock (**B**) which allows to retrieve both PBs by sliding the capillary over them (**C**). If the second PB is still firmly fixed to the oolemma, the capillary with the second PB already inside is slowly forced toward to the left in order to rupture the cytoplasmic bridge. Note the sharp border of the laser drilled opening (**D**).

Table 26.2 Efficacy of Laser-Assisted Polar Body Biopsy

Treatment cycles with polar body biopsy	174
No. of oocytes with biopsy	1245
No. of oocytes degenerated due to biopsy	5 (0.4%)
No. of polar bodies lost during biopsy/ transfer	20 (1.6%)
No. of polar bodies without hybridization signals	27 (2.2%)
No. of oocytes with FISH results	1193 (95.8%)

the glass slide, the first and second PB of one oocyte are removed from the medium drop and transferred with the biopsy capillary into a tiny drop (0.2 µL) of either water placed on a clean glass slide (Fig. 26.2). It is important to release the PBs at the bottom of the slide and to avoid floating in the droplet. The small volume guarantees that the PBs will attach to the slide within a small area and that the fluid will dry out very fast, which reduces the risk of a dislocation of the PBs on the slide. Nevertheless, the drying process must be observed under a stereo microscope and the final location of the PBs after air-drying must be marked on top of the slide by encircling with a suitable marker (diamond marker or Tungsten pen). It is not absolutely required to distinguish the first and second PB at that stage, as this becomes obvious during FISH analysis. With some experience, the first and second PBs from up to 12 oocytes can be placed within a round area of 10 mm, each PB pair encircled with a marker. Fixation is performed with 2 to 3 drops of 10 µL methanol:acetic acid (3:1, ice cold −20°C) followed by a second fixation after air-drying using methanol at room temperature for five minutes. Once the slides are air-dried, 2.5 µL of hybridization solution are placed onto a 12 mm round cover slip, which is then inverted onto the area where the polar bodies are located. The cover slip should be sealed with rubber cement and additionally covered with a stretch of parafilm which facilitates later removal of the

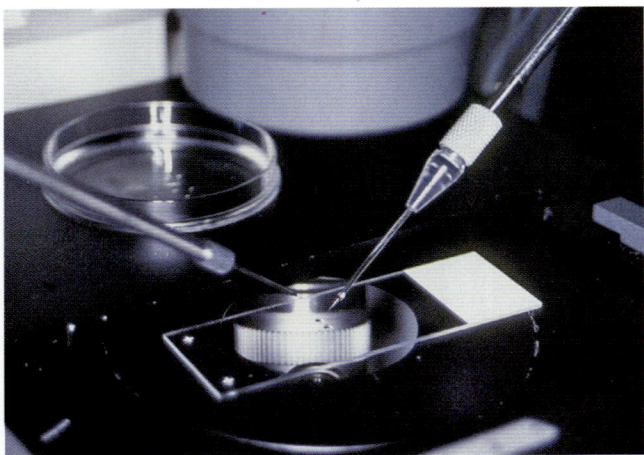

Figure 26.2 Transfer of isolated PBs onto a slide. Transfer of isolated PBs from the dish (seen in the background) into the droplet on the slide must be performed on the microscope stage. The set-up shown here allows sliding the dish used for biopsy backwards. Therefore, the aspiration capillary only needs to be lowered into the droplet for release of the PB.

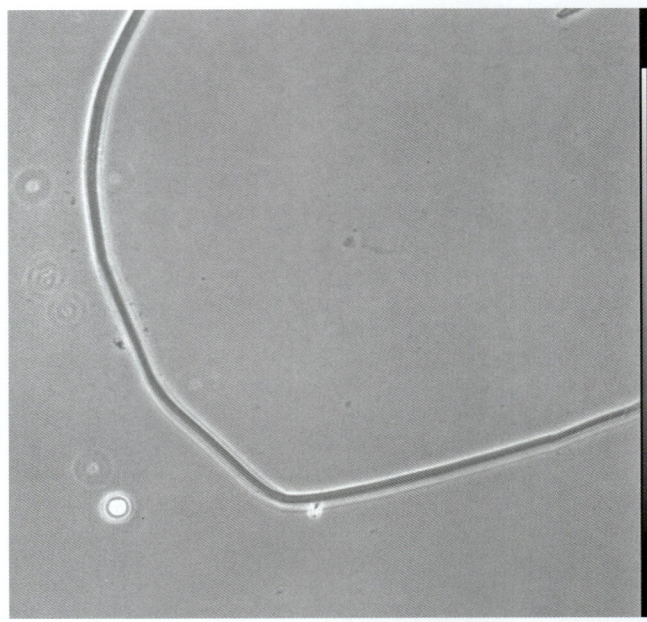

Figure 26.3 Identification of the polar body on the slide. This photograph is taken with a 10× phase contrast objective and the diamond circle surrounding the polar body can be partially seen. The polar body appears gray-shaded and is marked by an arrow.

cover slip after hybridization. The slide is then placed into a hybridization oven, where co-denaturation of the probe and the DNA of the PB occur at a temperature suitable for the probes used (usually around 68–73°C for up to 10 minutes). Hybridization is usually performed at 37°C. Centromeric probes require only 20–30 minutes of hybridization, whereas locus-specific probes require longer times. Commercially available multi-probe kits are usually hybridized for four to eight hours, followed by two rapid washing steps (73°C, 0.7xSSC and 0.3% NP-40 for 7 minutes followed by 2xSSC, 0.1 % NP-40 for 1 minute) which should be carried out exactly as described by the manufacturer. Following washing, a cover slip and anti-fade mounting medium must be applied to the slide, which should then be stored immediately in the dark until FISH analysis.

FISH ANALYSIS AND INTERPRETATION OF RESULTS

Prior to the analysis of the FISH results, the polar bodies located on the glass slide must be positioned under the microscope. This is rather easy if a circle is made around the area of PB deposition on top of the slide. The use of a 10× phase contrast objective usually allows for identification of the diamond circle and even the PBs can be identified in most cases (Fig. 26.3). For FISH analysis, a 100× oil immersion objective with good transmission properties for the necessary wavelengths must be used. In the fluorescence viewing mode, the right focal plane can be easily adjusted by focusing the diamond line followed by searching the PBs within the encircled area. Once the PBs are allocated, it is recommended to view the different chromosome signals in the order which is proposed by the

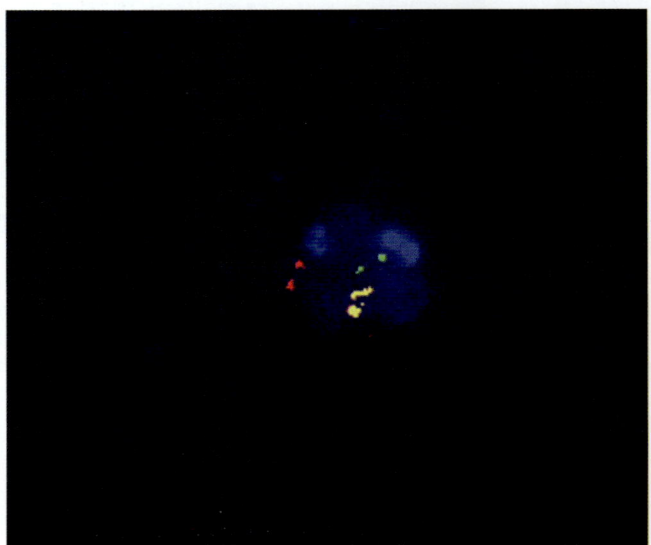

Figure 26.4 First polar body with correct signals for chromosomes 13, 16, 18, 21, and 22. This polar body shows two signals for each of the chromosomes under investigation. This picture is a composite overlay, where initially each chromosome probe was assembled as black and white using the appropriate filter set and prior to overlay signals were colored using a software program (13: red, 16 + 18: blue, 21: green, 22: yellow). The signals for 16 and 18 are taken by a dual band pass filter set and therefore cannot be labeled with different colors. This mode of presentation also applies for the following figures in color.

manufacturer of the kit, as certain fluorophores will fade more quickly compared with others.

Each chromosome should give two signals in the first PB and one signal in the second. An example of a first PB with a correct number of signals for chromosomes 13, 16, 18, 21, and 22 is shown (Fig. 26.4), where chromosomes

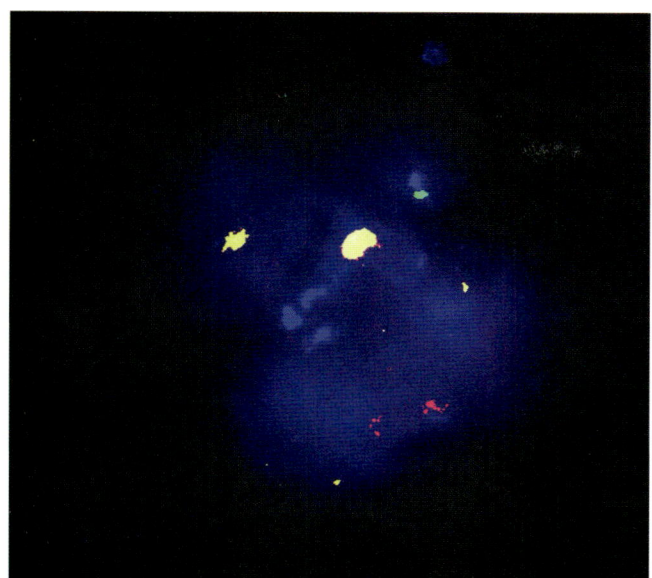

Figure 26.5 Chromosome segregation and trisomy 21. This polar body displays several common features which can be observed during the evaluation of fluorescence signals. First, only signals for chromosome 18 are located side by side (blue dotted signals on the left), whereas all other chromosomes have undergone predivision of chromatids. Only one signal is present for chromosome 21 (green) which indicates that one additional chromatid 21 is present in the oocyte, and the embryo can develop a trisomy 21 (chromosome 13: red, 16 + 18: blue, 21: green, 22: yellow – small dots, X: yellow – large dots).

16 and 18 are detected by centromer-specific probes and chromosomes 13, 21, and 22 by locus-specific probes. It can be seen that the signals for chromosomes 16 and 18 can be clearly distinguished, despite the centromeric location of the probe. This is due to an early onset of chromatid separation within the first PB which seems to start soon after oocyte retrieval, probably due to in vitro culture (57). In contrast, locus-specific probes will usually give good signals which are easy to evaluate, as the loci are located on the arms of the chromosome.

As mentioned earlier, most signals in the first PB are split signals due to premature chromatin segregation and as demonstrated by several studies, unbalanced predivision of chromatids is the most common origin of aneuploidy (24). The example on display (Fig. 26.5) depicts a first PB where only the two signals for the two chromatids 18 are located side by side, whereas chromosomes 13, 16, 22, and X show a balanced predivision and chromosome 21 an unbalanced predivision with only one signal in the PB. The corresponding oocyte contains one additional chromatid 21 and therefore can develop a trisomy 21.

A frequent problem in the analysis of the first PB is the degeneration of chromatin which may lead to speckled signals. This is most frequently observed for chromosomes 13 and 22. A diagnosis of aneuploidy or malsegregation is still possible, provided that the speckled regions are well separated from each other due to predivision.

Another problem is the high degree of fragmentation observed in first PBs (Fig. 26.6). Obviously, all fragments can contain chromatin material and therefore it is obligatory to remove all fragments. In such a case the drying process on the slide must be watched very carefully. Even if only one fragment is overlooked during the FISH analysis, one may easily risk a misdiagnosis if one of the chromosomes under investigation is located in the missing fragment.

Finally, PBs which are very advanced in the process of degeneration possess weak membranes which are likely to rupture during the fixation process. However, usually the chromatin will still affix to the glass slide after drying of the transfer droplet, although the signal will be spread and look like an elongated strand or a bundle of DNA. Therefore FISH analysis is still possible but the signals are scattered all over the encircled area, making interpretation of the results rather difficult.

TRANSFER OF POLAR BODIES FOR ANEUPLOIDY SCREENING BY ARRAY-CGH

For array-CGH the first and the second PB must be transferred separately into individual PCR reaction tubes. This step should be performed in a laminar flow cabinet in order to avoid any contamination of the sample. Transfer can be easily accomplished by a 0.1–2.5 µL micropipette or by a stripping pipette used for oocyte denudation. Taking the PB into the pipette tip must be done under visual control at a stereomicroscope. Release of the PB in the PCR tube is best accomplished if the tube is prefilled with phosphate buffered saline (PBS), the amount of which depends on the requirements of the subsequent amplification protocol. A usual protocol is 2.5 µL of PBS and in this case the tube should be prefilled with 2.2 µL of PBS and the transfer of a single PB is done in 0.3 µL medium. After transfer, tubes must be kept or stored in an upright position until amplification. Whole genome amplification, labeling of amplified DNA, hybridization, and subsequent washing are usually performed according to the instructions provided by the manufacturer.

The standard procedure for array-CGH is the labeling of the sample (PB) DNA by Cy3 and by labeling of a male reference DNA with Cy5. Both labeled DNAs are then combined and co-hybridized on an array. For evaluation the ratio of Cy3 versus Cy5 from that array is calculated by specific software. An example of such an analysis is shown in Figure 26.7A. Another recent approach uses a different strategy by which two samples, for example the first PB labeled with Cy3 and the second PB labeled with Cy5 are co-hybridized on one array and a male and female reference DNA labeled in Cy3/Cy5 and Cy5/Cy3 are co-hybridized as a dye-swap set up on two control arrays. The software hence calculates the Cy3 signal to both the Cy5 from the male control as well as to the Cy5

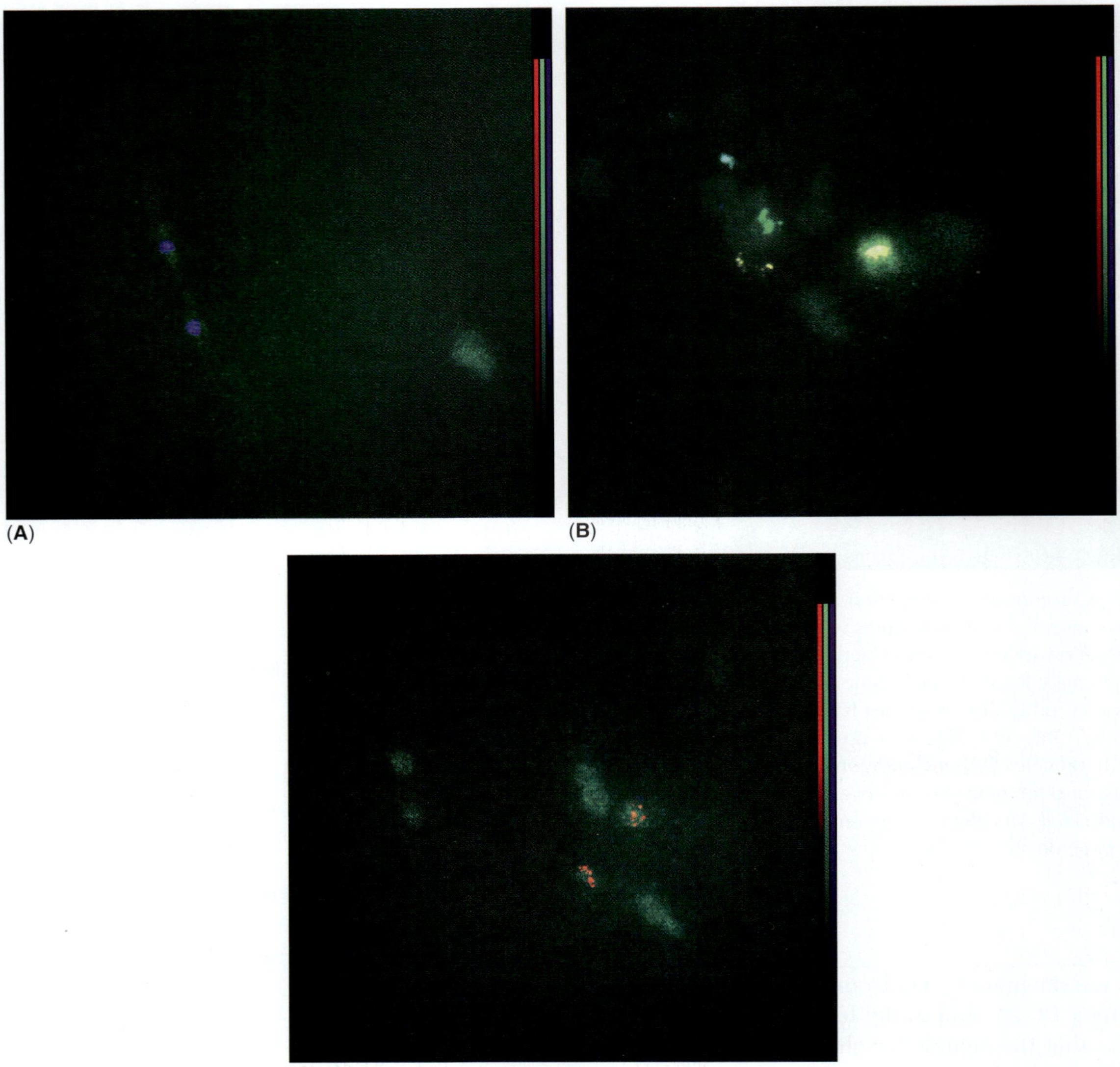

Figure 26.6 FISH analysis of a fragmented polar body. This example shows a highly fragmented polar body, where the fragments were located on the slide within a large area and consequently not all fragments could be viewed within one field. Following predivision both chromatids 18 (blue) are present in separated fragments (**A**). Two neighboring signals can be found for chromosomes 21 (green), 22 (yellow) and X (bright yellow, – very close), but only one signal 16 (blue) (**B**). Chromosome 13 (red) again is located in two different fragments (**C**).

from the female control array which gives a much better resolution and supports a highly accurate analysis (Fig. 26.7B, C).

CONCLUSIONS

The pioneering work in PB diagnosis was performed by Yuri Verlinsky and Santiago Munné and efficient biopsy techniques were elaborated by Cieslak et al. (46) and Montag et al. (47,48). This has led to a variety of (genetic and chromosomal) diagnostic applications following PB biopsy. Most cases of PB diagnosis have been performed for PGS and by FISH. More recently PB biopsy followed by array-CGH has been introduced for PGS (17,19,28,29,44) and the feasibility of this approach for a reliable diagnosis has been proven in a concordance analysis (19,44). However, still to date there is no prospective randomized controlled trial to prove the benefit of PB diagnosis for aneuploidy screening in terms of higher pregnancy and birth rates. This underlines the fact that such studies are still needed and that the procedure itself must be continuously evaluated. Consequently, the use of PB diagnosis and aneuploidy screening should be primarily offered to patients at a high risk for chromosomal aberrations and patients who are more likely to benefit from this therapy (58). The relevant data should be published continuously in order to enable an evaluation of this technique in the view of evidence-based medicine. Finally, we may conclude, that the use of a non-contact laser for PB biopsy is a safe and efficient approach (44,59).

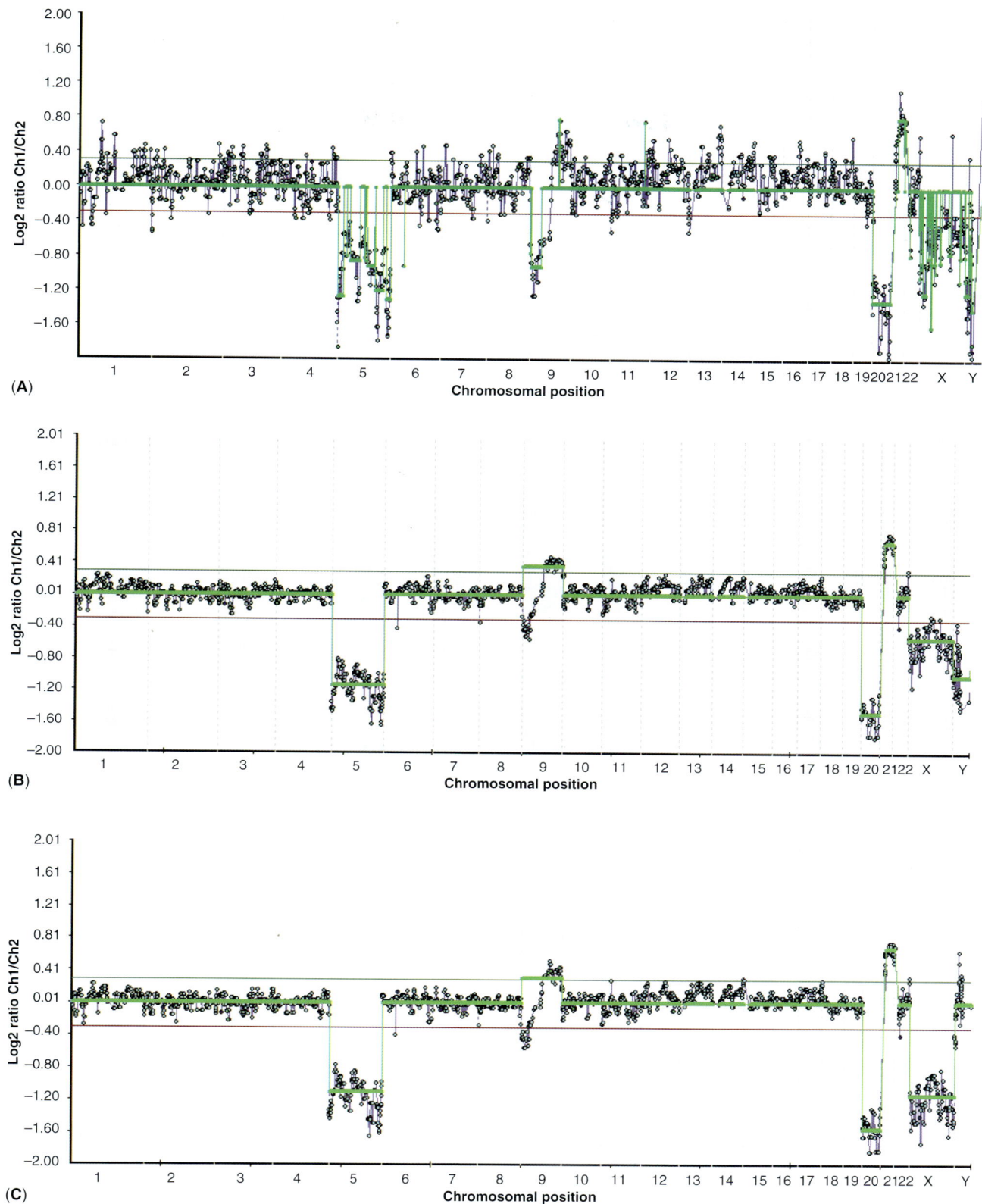

Figure 26.7 Array-CGH of polar bodies: conventional versus single channel CGH. A standard evaluation of an array-CGH experiments with PB-1 DNA labeled with Cy3 and co-hybridized with a male reference DNA labeled with Cy5. The ratio of Cy3 versus Cy5 from the array is shown in (**A**). Signals for chromosomes 5, 20, 21 and 9p and 9Q are out of the mean ratio and indicate a loss or gain of chromosomes or chromatids. The same sample DNA was used in a single channel experiment and the ratio of the PB-1 DNA deviations was calculated with a male (**B**) or female control DNA (**C**). The comparison shows that the single channel experiment gives a highly reduced background noise and that especially the quoting of the gonosomal aneuploidies becomes much easier.

REFERENCES

1. Verlinsky Y, Ginsberg N, Lifchez A, et al. Analysis of the first polar body: Preconception genetic diagnosis. Hum Reprod 1990; 5: 826–9.
2. Handyside AH, Kontogianni EH, Hardy K, Winston RML. Pregnancies from biopsied human preimplantation embryos sexed by Y-specific DNA amplification. Nature 1990; 244: 768–70.
3. Harper J. Introduction to preimplantation genetic diagnosis. In: Harper J, ed. Preimplantation Genetic Diagnosis. 2nd edn. Cambridge: Cambridge University Press, 2010: 1–47.
4. Staessen C, Platteau P, Van Assche E, Michiels A. Comparison of blastocyst transfer with or without preimplantation genetic diagnosis for aneuploidy screening in couples with advanced maternal age: a prospective randomized controlled trial. Hum Reprod 2004; 19: 2849–58.
5. Stevens J, Wale P, Surrey ES, Schoolcraft WB. Is aneuploidy screening for patients aged 35 or over beneficial? A prospective randomized trial. Fertil Steril 2004; 82(Suppl 2): 249.
6. Mastenbroek S, Twisk M, Van Echten-Arends J, et al. In Vitro Fertilization with Preimplantation Genetic Screening. N Engl J Med 2007; 357: 9–17.
7. Blockeel C, Schutyser V, De Vos A, et al. Prospectively randomized controlled trial of PGS in IVF/ICSI patients with poor implantation. Reprod Biomed Online 2008; 17: 848–54.
8. Hardarson T, Hanson C, Lundin K, et al. Preimplantation genetic screening in women of advance maternal age decrease in clinical pregnancy rate: a randomized controlled trial. Hum Reprod 2008; 23: 2806–12.
9. Jansen RP, Bowman MC, de Boer KA, et al. What next for preimplantation genetic screening (PGS)? Experience with blastocyst biopsy and testing for aneuploidy. Hum Reprod 2008; 23: 1476–8.
10. Mersereau JE, Pergament E, Zhang X, Milad MP. Preimplantation genetic screening to improve in vitro fertilization pregnancy rates: a prospective randomized controlled trial. Fertil Steril 2008; 90: 1287–9.
11. Debrock S, Melotte C, Spiessens C, et al. Preimplantation genetic screening for aneuploidy in embryos after in vitro fertilization (IVF) does not improve reproductive outcome in women over 35: a prospective controlled randomized trial. Fertil Steril 2010; 93: 364–73.
12. Staessen C, Verpoest W, Donoso P, et al. Preimplantation genetic screening does not improve delivery rate in women under the age of 36 following single-embryo transfer. Hum Reprod 2008; 23: 2818–25.
13. Anderson R, Pickering S. The current status of preimplantation genetic screening: British Fertility Society Policy and Practice Guidelines. Hum Fertil 2008; 11: 71–5.
14. Meyer L, Klipstein S, Hazlett W, et al. A prospective randomized controlled trial of preimplantation genetic screening in the "good prognosis" patient. Fertil Steril 2009; 91: 1731–8.
15. American Society for Reproductive Medicine (ASRM). Preimplantation genetic testing: a practice committee opinion. Fertil Steril 2008; 90(Suppl): S136–43.
16. Schoolcraft WB, Katz-Jaffe MG, Stevens J, et al. Preimplantation aneuploidy testing for infertile patients of advanced maternal age: a randomized prospective trial. Fertil Steril 2009; 92: 157–62.
17. Geraedts J, Collins J, Gianaroli L, et al. What next for preimplantation genetic screening? A polar body approach! Hum Reprod 2010; 25: 575–7.
18. Nicolaidis P, Petersen MB. Origin and mechanisms of non-disjunction in human autosomal trisomies. Hum Reprod 1998; 13: 313–19.
19. Geraedts J, Montag M, Magli MC, et al. Polar body array CGH for prediction of the status of the corresponding oocyte. I. Clinical results. Hum Reprod 2011; 26: 3173–80.
20. Kuliev A, Cieslak J, Ilkevitch Y, Verlinsky Y. Chromosomal abnormalities in a series of 6733 human oocytes in preimplantation diagnosis for age-related aneuploidies. Reprod Biomed Online 2002; 6: 54–9.
21. Munné S, Sandalinas M, Escudero T, et al. Outcome of preimplantation genetic diagnosis of translocations. Fertil Steril 2000; 73: 1209–18.
22. Verlinsky Y, Cieslak J, Ivakhenko V, et al. Chromosomal abnormalities in the first and second polar body. Mol Cell Endocrinol 2001; 183S: 47–9.
23. Hassold T, Chiu D. Maternal age-specific rates of numerical chromosome abnormalities with special reference to trisomy. Hum Genet 1985; 70: 11–17.
24. Angell RR. Predivision in human oocytes at meiosis 1: a mechanism for trisomy formation in man. Hum Genet 1991; 86: 383–7.
25. Angell RR. Possible pitfalls in preimplantation diagnosis of chromosomal abnormailities based on polar body biopsy. Hum Reprod 1994; 9: 181–2.
26. Montag M, Limbach N, Sabarstinski M, et al. Polar body biopsy and aneuploidy testing by simultaneous detection of six chromosomes. Prenatal Diag 2005; 25: 867–71.
27. Munné S. Preimplantation genetic diagnosis for infertility (preimplantation genetic screening). In: Harper J, ed. Preimplantation Genetic Diagnosis. 2nd edn. Cambridge: Cambridge University Press, 2010: 203–9.
28. Wells D, Escudero T, Levy B, et al. First clinical application of comparative genomic hybridization and polar body testing for preimplantation genetic diagnosis of aneuploidy. Fertil Steril 2002; 78: 543–9.
29. Montag M, Köster K, van der Ven K, et al. Kombinierte Translokations- und Aneuploidieuntersuchungen nach Polkörperbiopsie und array-Comparative Genomic Hybridisation. J Reproduktionsmed Endokrinol 2010a; 6: 498–502.
30. Stern C, Pertile M, Norris H, et al. Chromosome translocations in couples with in-vitro fertilization implantation failure. Hum Reprod 1999; 14: 2097–101.
31. Van der Ven K, Peschka B, Montag M, et al. Increased frequency of constitutional chromosomal aberrations in female partners of couples undergoing intracytoplasmic sperm injection (ICSI). Hum Reprod 1998; 13: 48–54.
32. Peschka B, Leygraaf J, van der Ven K, et al. Type and frequency of chromosome aberrations in 551 couples undergoing intracytoplasmic sperm injection. Hum Reprod 1999; 14: 2257–63.
33. Munne S, Fung J, Cassel MJ, et al. Preimplantation genetic analysis of translocations: case-specific probes for interphase cell analysis. Hum Genet 1998; 102: 663–74.
34. Fiorentino F, Spizzichino L, Bono S, et al. PGD for reciprocal and Robertsonian translocations using array comparative genomic hybridization. Hum Reprod 2011; 26: 1925–35.

35. Gitlin SA, Lanzendorf SE, Gibbons WE. Polymerase chain reaction amplification specifity: incidence of allele-dropout using different DNA preparation methods for heterozygous single cells. J Assisted Reprod Genet 1996; 13: 107–11.
36. Sermon K, Lissens W, Joris H, et al. Clinical application of preimplantation diagosis for myotonic dystrophy. Prenat Diagn 1997; 17: 925–32.
37. Ray PF, Ao A, Taylor DM, et al. Assessment of single blastomere analysis for preimplantation diagnosis of the delta F508 deletion causing cystic fibrosis in clinical practice. Prenat Diagn 1994; 18: 1402–12.
38. Rechitsky S, Strom C, Verlinsky O, et al. Allele dropout in polar bodies and blastomeres. J Assisted Reprod Genet 1998; 15: 253–7.
39. Hussey ND, Davis T, Hall JR, et al. Preimplantation genetic diagnosis for b-thalassaemia using sequencing of single cell PCR products to detect mutations and polymorphic loci. Mol Hum Reprod 2002; 8: 1136–43.
40. Fiorentino F, Magli MC, Podini D, et al. The minisequencing method: an alternative strategy for preimplantation genetic diagnosis of single gene disorders. Reprod Biomed online 2003; 9: 399–410.
41. Verlinsky Y. Polar body-based preimplantation diagnosis for x-linked disorders. Reprod Biomed online 2001; 4: 38–42.
42. Sermon K. Preimplantation genetic diagnosis for monogenic disorders: multiplex PV Three dimensional partial zona dissection for preimplantation genetic diagnosis and assisted hatching PCR and whole-genome amplification for gene analysis at the single cell level. In: Harper J, ed. Preimplantation Genetic Diagnosis. 2nd edn. Cambridge: Cambridge University Press, 2010: 237–46.
43. Montag M, van der Ven K, van der Ven H. Polar body diagnosis. In: Harper J, ed. Preimplantation Genetic Diagnosis. 2nd edn. Cambridge: Cambridge University Press, 2010: 166–74.
44. Magli C, Montag M, Köster M, et al. Polar body array CGH for prediction of the status of the corresponding oocyte. I. Technical aspects. Hum Reprod 2011; 26: 3181–85.
45. Gordon JW, Talansky BE. Assisted fertilization by zona drilling: a mouse model for correction of oligospermia. J Exp Zool 1987; 239: 347–81.
46. Cieslak J, Ivakhenko V, Wolf G, et al. Three-dimensional partial zona dissection for preimplantation genetic diagnosis and assisted hatching. Fertil Steril 1999; 71: 308–13.
47. Montag M, van der Ven K, Delacrétaz G, et al. Efficient preimplantation genetic diagnosis using laser assisted microdissection of the zona pellucida for polar body biopsy followed by primed in situ labelling (PRINS). J Assisted Reprod Genet 1997; 14: 455–6.
48. Montag M, van der Ven K, Delacrétaz G, et al. Laser assisted microdissection of zona pellucida facilitates polar body biopsy. Fertil Steril 1998; 69: 539–42.
49. Montag M, van der Ven H. Laser-assisted hatching in assisted reproduction. Croat Med J 1999; 40: 398–403.
50. Montag M, Koll B, Holmes P, van der Ven H. Significance of the number of embryonic cells and the state of the zona pellucida for hatching of mouse blastocysts in vitro versu in vivo. Biol Reprod 2000; 62: 1738–44.
51. Licciardi F, Gonzalez A, Tang YX, et al. Laser ablation of the mouse zona pellucida for blastomere biopsy. J Assist Reprod Genet 1995; 12: 462–6.
52. Boada M, Carrera M, De La Iglesia C, et al. Successful use of a laser for human embryo biopsy in preimplantation genetic diagnosis: report of two cases. J Assist Reprod Genet 1997; 15: 301–5.
53. Veiga A, Sandalinas M, Benkhalifa M, et al. Laser blastocyst biopsy for preimplantation diagnosis in the human. Zygote 1997; 5: 351–4.
54. Joris H, de Vos A, Janssens R, et al. Comparison of the results of human embryo biopsy and outcome of preimplantation genetic diagnosis (PGD) after zona drilling using acid Tyrode of a laser. Hum Reprod 2000; 15S: 53–4.
55. Montag M, van der Ven K, van der Ven H. Erste klinische Erfahrungen mit der Polkörperdiagnostik in Deutschland. J Fertil Reprod 2002; 4: 7–12.
56. Harton GL, Magli MC, Lundin K, et al. ESHRE PGD Consortium/Embryology Special Interest Group–best practice guidelines for polar body and embryo biopsy for preimplantation genetic diagnosis/screening (PGD/PGS). Hum Reprod 2011; 26: 41–6.
57. Munne S, Dailey T, Sultan KM, et al. The use of first polar bodies for preimplantation diagnosis of aneuploidy. Mol Hum Reprod 1995; 10: 1014–20.
58. Munne S, Sandalinas M, Escudero T, et al. Improved implantation after preimplantation genetic diagnosis of aneuploidy. Reprod Biomed Online 2003; 7: 91–7.
59. Montag M, van der Ven K, Dorn C, van der Ven H. Outcome of laser-assisted polar body biopsy. Reprod Biomed Online 2004; 9: 425–9.
60. Verlinsky Y, Cieslak J, Freidin M, et al. Pregnancies following pre-conception diagnosis of common aneuploidies by FISH. Hum Reprod 1995; 10: 1923–7.
61. Dyban A, Freidine M, Severova E, et al. Detection of aneuploidy in human oocytes and corresponding first polar body by fluorescent in situ hybridisation. J Assisted Reprod Genet 1996; 13: 73–8.
62. Verlinsky Y, Cieslak J, Ivakhenko V, et al. Birth of healthy children after preimplantation diagnosis of common aneuploidies by polar body fluorescent in situ hybridization analysis. Fertil Steril 1996; 66: 126–9.
63. Verlinsky Y, Cieslak J, Ivakhenko V, et al. Prepregnancy genetic testing for age-related aneuploidies by polar body analysis. Genetic Testing 1997/98; 4: 231–5.
64. Verlinsky Y, Cieslak J, Ivakhenko V, et al. Prevention of age-related aneuploidies by polar body testing. J Assisted Reprod Genet 1999; 16: 165–9.
65. Verlinsky Y, Cieslak J, Ivakhenko V, et al. Chromosomal abnormalities in the first and second polar body. Mol Cell Endocrinol 2001; 183S: 47–9.
66. van der Ven K, Montag M, van der Ven H. Polar body diagnosis – a step in the right direction? Dtsch Arztebl Int 2008; 105: 190–6.

27

Preimplantation genetic diagnosis for infertility

Dagan Wells and Elpida Fragouli

INTRODUCTION

There are various approaches for preimplantation genetic diagnosis (PGD), but in essence all share the same principal aim—to allow healthy embryos to be distinguished from those affected by genetic abnormalities. Depending on the exact protocol used, inherited mutations affecting the function of specific genes or abnormalities of chromosome copy number can be detected. The preferential transfer of genetically "normal" embryos to the uterus provides a high probability that any resulting pregnancy will be healthy. In some respects PGD can be considered an alternative to conventional prenatal diagnosis, with the advantage that pregnancy termination is avoided.

Genetic diagnosis at the preimplantation stage was first attempted in humans more than 20 years ago (1). Procedures involve the generation of embryos using in vitro fertilization (IVF) techniques, followed by biopsy and testing of embryonic material. Sampling can take place at four different developmental stages: on the day of oocyte retrieval by removing the first polar body (PB) from the mature oocyte; on day 1 by biopsying the second PB from the zygote (the first PB may also be taken at this time); on day 3 by removing one to two cells (blastomeres) from the cleavage-stage embryo; or on days 5–6 by removing a small clump of trophectoderm (TE) cells from the blastocyst (reviewed in (2)).

The diagnosis of single gene disorders relies on use of the polymerase chain reaction (PCR) to amplify DNA from the biopsied cell(s) to a sufficient level for standard genetic techniques of mutation detection to be employed. The main challenges facing this form of PGD are achieving efficient, accurate amplification of the disease locus and avoiding contamination with non-embryonic sources of DNA. A detailed overview of the techniques developed for PGD of inherited disorders is beyond the scope of this chapter; instead this review will focus on the detection of chromosome abnormalities using PGD technologies and their use by infertile patients undergoing IVF to try and improve treatment outcomes.

Aneuploidy, the situation in which an abnormal number of chromosomes is present in the cell, is extremely common in human oocytes and embryos. It is thought that most aneuploid embryos undergo developmental arrest, fail to implant, or miscarry (3,4). Since the transfer of a chromosomally abnormal embryo is unlikely to result in a healthy live birth, it has been suggested that efforts should be made to identify and preferentially transfer chromosomally normal (euploid) embryos. There are several theoretical advantages of such an approach for infertile patients: Implantation and pregnancy rates achieved after IVF should be improved since the embryos chosen for transfer are more likely to be viable; miscarriages should be less frequent for the same reason; the incidence of Down syndrome and other disorders related to aneuploidy should also be reduced. The use of chromosome screening strategies to assist in the identification and transfer of viable embryos is sometimes referred to as *PGD for infertility*, but is perhaps more commonly known as preimplantation genetic screening (PGS). In most cases PGS is used for patients considered to be at elevated risk of producing oocytes and/or embryos affected by aneuploidy, specifically couples who have experienced repeated implantation failure, or recurrent pregnancy loss, or where the female partner is of advanced reproductive age (5).

For PGS, embryos are generated using IVF techniques, and PBs, blastomeres, or TE samples are taken for analysis (6–8). Traditionally, fluorescence in situ hybridization (FISH) has then been utilized to examine a subset of the chromosomes in the biopsied material (7,9,10). Although widely used during the last two decades, FISH has significant limitations in terms of the amount of information it provides and accuracy. Using the FISH approach most laboratories specializing in PGD have only been able to assess a maximum of 12 chromosomes per embryo, leaving at least half of the chromosomes untested. Increasingly, FISH is now being replaced by techniques that allow the copy number of all of the chromosomes to be evaluated, such as metaphase or array-CGH (aCGH), real-time PCR, and single nucleotide polymorphism (SNP) microarrays (8,11–16).

CHROMOSOME SCREENING AT THE CLEAVAGE STAGE OF PREIMPLANTATION DEVELOPMENT

Historically, the most common time to perform PGS has been at the cleavage stage. Numerous studies using FISH to examine the chromosome content of preimplantation embryos have shown that in addition to meiotically derived aneuploidy, mostly originating from the oocyte, postzygotic chromosome segregation errors are also often seen during the first few mitotic divisions (3,7,17). Chromosome malsegregation occurring after fertilization leads to a phenomenon called "mosaicism," which can be defined as the presence of two or more karyotypically (i.e., chromosomally) distinct cell lines within the same embryo. The degree of mosaicism tends to vary. Some embryos have no mosaicism, while others may become karyotypically unstable and highly mosaic, with abnormalities affecting multiple different chromosomes in each of their cells. Embryos of this type are termed "chaotic mosaics" (3).

With the development of methods to examine the copy number of every chromosome it has become possible to quantify the true frequency of mosaicism at the cleavage stage. Only a quarter of cleavage-stage embryos tested using CGH (Fig. 27.1) were found to be composed entirely of normal cells (4,18). Approximately two-thirds of embryos were mosaic. In some embryos a mixture of aneuploid and normal cells was seen as a potential problem for diagnosis based upon the analysis of a single cell. However, the majority of mosaic embryos were devoid of any normal cells, suggesting that in most cases mosaicism would not lead to a serious diagnostic error. Follow-up studies of embryos tested using aCGH have confirmed that the misdiagnosis rate is low (<5%) despite the issue of mosaicism (9).

The results of studies using FISH for the purpose of PGS were initially encouraging. Data were suggestive of improved implantation and pregnancy rates for women of advanced reproductive age (37 years or more) and recurrent miscarriage (RM) (19–24). Additionally miscarriage rates were reduced for these patient groups. However, no benefits were observed for younger women, and no clear advantage was seen for couples with a history of repeated implantation failure. Unfortunately, it was several years before large scale randomized controlled trials (RCTs) of the technology were undertaken. Most of the early data were derived from studies in which control groups were either assembled retrospectively from historical data or, at best, were case controlled but not randomized.

Staessen and colleagues (25) were the first to report results from an RCT using PGS. The principal indication for screening was advanced reproductive age (>37 years). Two blastomeres from each embryo were biopsied and seven chromosomes were screened. At first glance, PGS appeared to be associated with superior results, but the study had insufficient statistical power to determine whether this was a truly significant difference (implantation rate 17.1% vs 11.5% for the control group and clinical pregnancy rate of 16.5% vs 10.4%). The conclusion was that PGS made no difference to outcome. The decision to sample two blastomeres was taken to ensure maximum accuracy. However, while testing of two cells can potentially lead to small improvements in the diagnostic reliability, there is now conclusive evidence that this strategy has a detrimental effect on subsequent implantation (26–28). Thus it seems highly likely that PGS outcomes would have been better if single cell biopsy had been employed.

The debate about the clinical efficacy of PGS using FISH reached a crescendo with the publication of a multicenter, double-blind RCT in 2007 (29). Embryos from women ≥35 years of age underwent single blastomere biopsy and 8 chromosomes were examined. The study found that, rather than improve pregnancy rates, PGS

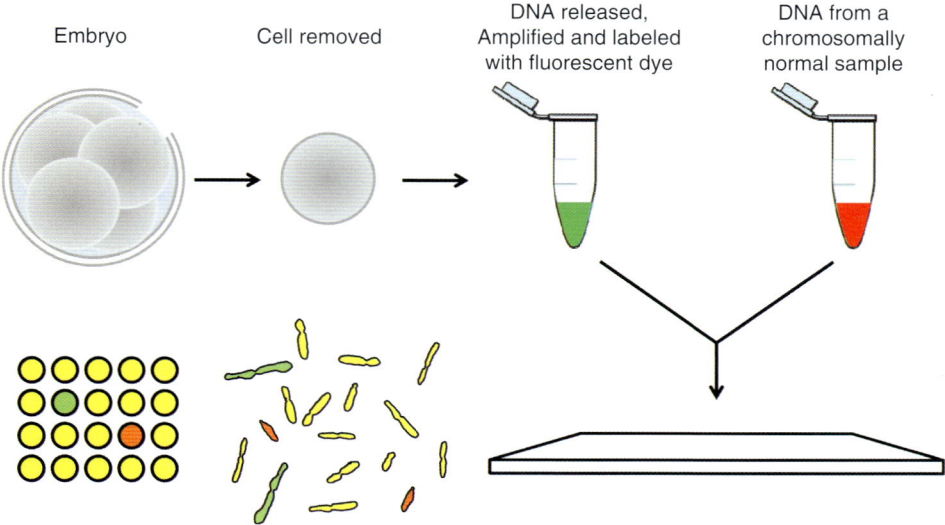

Figure 27.1 Comprehensive chromosome screening using comparative genomic hybridization. The material for analysis (polar body, blastomere, or trophectoderm biopsy) is placed in a microcentrifuge tube. Its DNA is then released, subjected to whole genome amplification, and labeled with a fluorescent dye. The sample DNA is mixed with a reference DNA, derived from a chromosomally normal individual, labeled in a different color. The mixture of differentially labeled DNA samples is then applied to a glass slide upon the surface of which are many metaphase chromosomes, or alternatively a microarray (multiple spots, each containing a DNA probe specific for a small region of chromosome). Each of the DNA samples hybridizes to complementary sequences on the chromosomes or on the microarray probes. The relative intensity of the two colors gives an indication of the chromosome copy number in the test sample relative to the euploid reference sample.

had a detrimental effect (25% pregnancy rate in the test group compared to 37% in the control group). A detailed evaluation of the methodology employed during this study has highlighted the major shortcomings of the study, with particular criticism of the level of proficiency in biopsy and genetic analysis (26,30–32). Despite the numerous deficiencies of the study, it did succeed in highlighting the difficulties in improving IVF outcomes using the technologies available at the time. More studies followed, resulting in a total of eight RCTs using cleavage-stage FISH analysis published in peer-reviewed journals. None was able to demonstrate a benefit of chromosome screening (33–40). Some experts still maintain that FISH applied to blastomeres can lead to improved IVF outcomes, and point to technical deficiencies affecting all of the RCTs undertaken thus far. However, for most observers, the case for performing PGS using FISH on day 3 now seems weak.

Technological advances now allow a comprehensive chromosomal analysis of human oocytes and embryos and provide superior accuracy and reproducibility compared with FISH. The principal techniques used for this purpose are microarray CGH (array-CGH or aCGH) and SNP microarrays. CGH and aCGH have been extensively tested and validated using cells from aneuploid cell lines, PBs, and cells from embryos (12,13,18,41–46). Microarray CGH (aCGH) is the most widely used of the new PGS methodologies (Fig. 27.2). The technique involves simultaneous hybridization of differentially labeled DNA samples (e.g., the DNA from the test sample: green; a chromosomally normal reference DNA: red) to chromosome-specific DNA probes affixed on a microscope slide. The ratio of green:red fluorescence on each chromosome-specific probe indicates whether there has been any gain or loss of chromosomal material in the test sample (an excess of green fluorescence is indicative of a gain; an excess of red fluorescence is indicative of a loss). Microarray CGH is a robust methodology that, importantly for PGS, provides results within 24 hours. Follow-up analysis of embryos that underwent single blastomere biopsy and aCGH revealed a 98% accuracy rate when the most well optimized methodology was used (47).

SNP microarrays detect aneuploidy by interrogating 10,000–500,000 individual polymorphisms scattered throughout the human genome. Aneuploidy is detected either by an increase/decrease in fluorescence intensity for all of the probes on a specific chromosome or by using informative polymorphisms on each chromosome to track their inheritance from parents to embryos (15,16). The latter approach requires analysis of parental DNAs in addition to those from the embryos.

Amongst other studies, one investigation validated the SNP microarray approach using 99 single cells derived from 9 aneuploid cell lines, and 335 blastomeres, obtained from a total of 235 cleavage-stage embryos (16,48). As with the aCGH methodology, SNP microarrays were shown to accurately detect chromosome abnormalities in both types of single cells (concordance rate: 96.5–99.8%). The same group also compared the accuracy of SNP

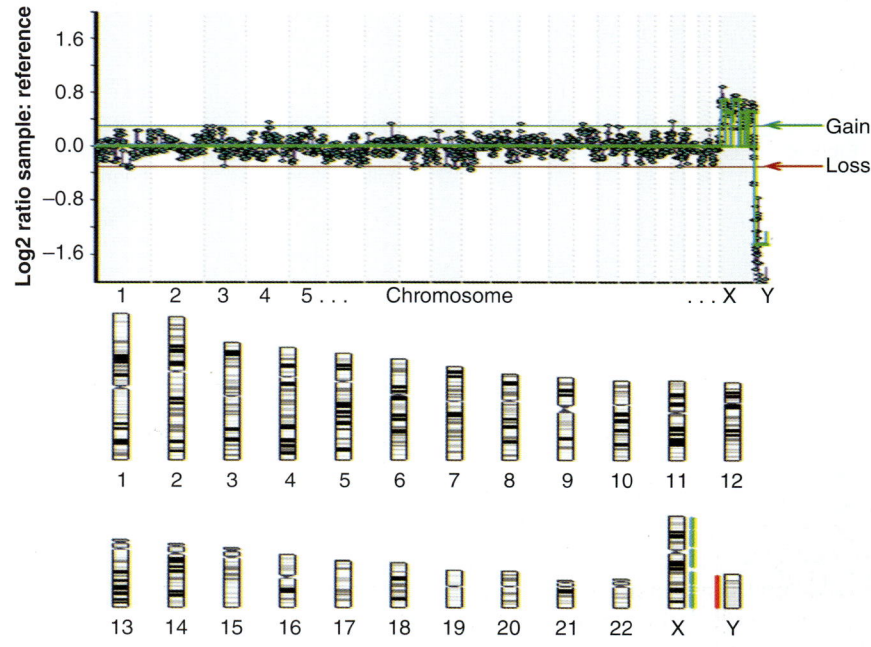

Figure 27.2 Microarray-comparative genomic hybridization (CGH) result of a microarray-CGH experiment. The approach is essentially identical to metaphase-CGH except that labeled DNA samples are hybridized to DNA probes affixed (spotted) onto a glass slide. The image shows the ratio of fluorescence for the differentially labeled test (embryo) and reference (normal male) DNA samples, as detected on each of the probes. The probes have been displayed in the order that they appear along the length of each chromosome, beginning with chromosome 1 and ending with the Y chromosome. An equal amount of fluorescence was recorded for test and reference DNAs on all probes for all chromosomes, the only exceptions being the X and Y chromosomes. The sample contained more X chromosome material than the normal male reference and less Y chromosome material. In other words the embryo was a normal female (XX *vs.* XY).

microarrays with that of FISH, examining a total of 160 blastomeres from 13 arrested cleavage-stage embryos with the use of one of the two methods (16). This study, carried out in a prospective randomized blinded manner, showed that FISH may have a tendency to overestimate aneuploidy.

To date, no RCTs using comprehensive chromosome screening technologies have been published (although at the time of writing several are underway). However, the available clinical data do seem encouraging. Despite this fact, the possibility of damage to the embryo, caused by cleavage-stage biopsy, and the issue of chromosomal mosaicism, have led to interest in testing at times other than day 3: either earlier (PB sampling) or later (TE sampling).

CHROMOSOME SCREENING OF THE FEMALE GAMETE

Female meiosis consists of two separate divisions, meiosis I (MI) and II (MII). During MI, one set of 23 chromosomes (each comprised of two chromatids) enters the first PB while the other set remains in the much larger oocyte. The cell cycle of the oocyte then arrests until fertilization, after which MII is completed. During MI, sister chromatids are held together and it is only at the end of MII that they are finally separated, one of the chromatids passing into the second PB, the other remaining in the oocyte. Molecular analysis of samples from chromosomally abnormal pregnancies and miscarriages has shown that most aneuploidies occur during female meiosis (reviewed in (49)). Various cytogenetic methods, such as G or R-banding, FISH, spectral karyotyping, and CGH, have been employed to examine the chromosomes of a large number of human oocytes. These studies have demonstrated a clear relationship between advancing maternal age and increasing aneuploidy rates. The expected aneuploidy rate seen in oocytes generated by women below the age of 25 years is approximately 5–10%, increasing to 10–25% in the early 30s, and exceeding 50% for women of 40 years or more (13,44,49–53).

Since the polar bodies are not required for oocyte competence, their removal should not have any negative effect on subsequent embryo development. Additionally, any abnormality seen in a PB is expected to be reciprocated in the corresponding oocyte (e.g., a chromosome loss seen in the 1st PB is expected to result in a gain of chromosomal material in the oocyte). As the abnormality is present from the moment of fertilization, it should theoretically be present in every cell of the resulting embryo and consequently, chromosomal mosaicism is less of an issue for diagnosis using PBs than for blastomere-based analyses. The principal disadvantage of PB examination is that chromosome errors of paternal and/or postzygotic origin cannot be detected.

For almost two decades FISH was the main method used for the examination of PBs (51,54,55). In most cases analysis was restricted to just five chromosomes (13,16,18,21) and (22). Examination of over 20,000 oocytes from reproductively older women, confirmed the extraordinarily high rate of abnormality in the human female gamete, 46.8% carrying chromosome errors (51,54,55). As far as clinical outcomes were concerned, it was often stated that PB screening improved implantation and pregnancy rates and led to a reduction in spontaneous abortion and improved the take-home baby rates (37), but no detailed clinical data were presented and no RCTs were ever carried out. Apart from concerns over the paucity of well-controlled clinical data, the methodology had significant limitations. Eighteen of the 23 oocyte chromosomes were not examined and both PBs had to be spread onto microscope slides, a process that can lead to artifactual loss of chromosomes, impacting accuracy.

The issues associated with the use of FISH for the examination of oocytes encouraged development of more comprehensive cytogenetic methods for PB analysis. Wells and colleagues (56) were the first to describe an accelerated metaphase CGH protocol, compatible with an embryo transfer on day 3 of preimplantation development. Although the method was successfully clinically applied, it remained too labour intensive for routine application. Conventional CGH was further optimized and validated in a large number of metaphase II oocyte-first PB pairs (43,44) and was clinically applied again as part of a "double-factor" PGD approach, combining chromosome screening (using CGH) and PGD for a single gene disorder (using PCR-based methods) (Fig. 27.3) (57).

A clinical study using metaphase CGH to analyze the first and second PBs of 70 women of advanced reproductive age (average age 40.8 years), and with a history of unsuccessful IVF treatments, revealed an oocyte abnormality rate of 70% (8,13). Overall, a similar incidence of errors occurring in MI and MII were observed, although for women over 40 years of age MII errors were the most common. This finding suggests that the biopsy and analysis of not only the first but also the second PB is advisable, particularly for women of advanced reproductive age. Nineteen (27%) of the couples who underwent PGS received no transfer, as chromosome abnormalities were detected for all examined oocytes. For those patients who received a transfer, the pregnancy rate was 25% (16.3% per initiated cycle) (unpublished data and (8)). Thus, the pregnancy rate obtained remained relatively low, but is nevertheless almost double the rate expected for such poor prognosis patients. However, it is difficult to draw definitive conclusions from this study due to an inadequate control group.

Both aCGH and SNP microarrays have been used clinically for the analysis of first and sometimes second PBs and are now preferred to metaphase CGH due to their superior speed and ease of use (58,59). The ESHRE-PGS Task Force has also been exploring the feasibility of using aCGH, examining first and second PBs, as well as the corresponding oocytes, allowing the true reliability of this approach to be evaluated. The initial data are encouraging, indicating an accuracy rate of 94% (60). This investigation is the first part of a planned

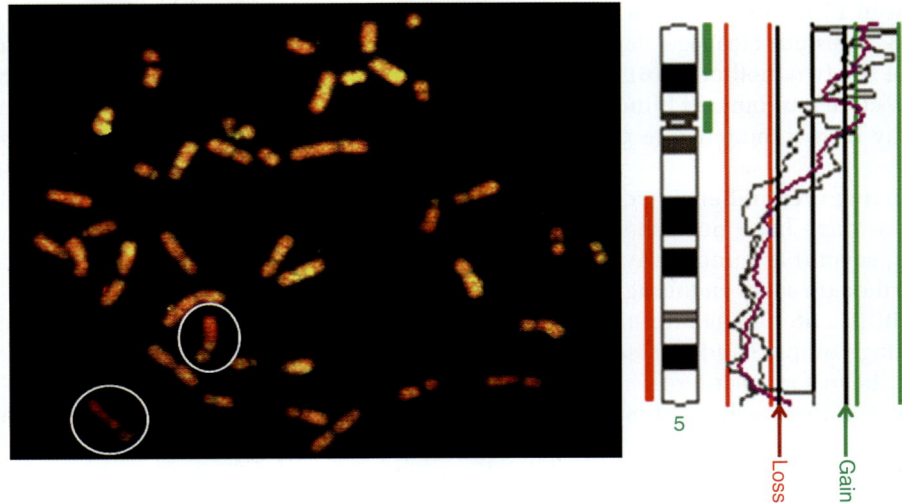

Figure 27.3 Metaphase-comparative genomic hybridization (CGH). Result of a metaphase-CGH experiment. A chromosomally normal cell in the metaphase of the cell cycle has been hybridized with DNA from an embryo (green) and DNA from a euploid reference sample (red). Most chromosomes appear yellow, indicating an equal (i.e., normal) copy number in the sample compared with the reference. However, chromosome 5 displays increased green coloration on the short arm and increased red on the long arm. This is more clearly displayed by the computer assisted analysis of red and green ratio (*right hand panel*). The pink line shows the mean ratio of red and green along the length of the chromosome, while the gray lines show the ratios for each of the 2 copies of chromosome 5 assessed in this cell. For such analyses it is typical to average the results obtained from 10 cells hybridized with the same DNA samples. In this case, a structural anomaly (duplication of the 5p and deletion of 5q) has been clearly detected.

multicenter randomized clinical trial that ESHRE is undertaking to assess the efficacy of PGS via PB analysis (2). At the time of writing, this RCT is about to begin and the obtained results will hopefully determine whether PB analysis is capable of enhancing the pregnancy rates.

CHROMOSOME SCREENING AT THE BLASTOCYST STAGE OF PREIMPLANTATION DEVELOPMENT

Although data using new cytogenetic methodologies, such as aCGH, suggest that comprehensive screening at the zygote or cleavage stages may improve IVF outcomes, the optimal time to apply such analyses may well turn out to be the blastocyst stage. It is possible to remove several cells (typically about five) from the TE of blastocysts. Although a greater number of cells are taken, the relative proportion of the embryo volume removed is smaller than that associated with single blastomere biopsy at the cleavage stage. Additionally, the cells removed are derived from a tissue that does not contribute to the fetus. Thus far, we have been unable to detect any impact of TE biopsy on subsequent embryo development. Unlike cleavage-stage embryos, blastocysts are very robust.

An RCT using TE biopsy for the purpose of PGS conducted a few years ago yielded disappointing results (61). However, this was probably related to the strategy employed. Only five chromosomes were examined using FISH (13, 18, 21, X, and Y) and the detection of a single aneuploid cell could have led to an embryo being discarded even if the other cells from the same biopsy were apparently normal. The detection of a mixture of normal and abnormal cells in a single biopsy specimen could be due to errors of the FISH technique or mosaicism. It was therefore clear that a more robust cytogenetic method was needed for the screening of blastocysts.

At the time of writing, four different investigations have reported optimization and validation of CGH (metaphase or array) or SNP microarrays for the analysis of TE samples (13,45,62,63). The first two studies involved single or double TE biopsy of a total of 64 spare nontransferred blastocysts, followed by CGH and/or aCGH analysis. The remaining embryo cells were spread onto microscope slides and a minimum of nine chromosomes were analyzed via FISH. Another 10 blastocysts were disaggregated and parts of their TE and ICM were individually analyzed by CGH (13,45). These cytogenetic methods showed that 39% of blastocysts were normal in every cell, 37% were uniformly aneuploid due to one or more meiotic chromosome errors, and 24% were mosaic containing a mixture of different cell lines. Most of the mosaic blastocysts did not contain any chromosomally normal cells. Indeed, mosaic embryos in which more than a third of the cells were normal accounted for less that 6% of analyzed blastocysts. This suggests that most mosaic embryos have few normal cells and are therefore likely to have significantly reduced viability, providing reassurance that potentially viable embryos will rarely be discarded due to mosaicism. Additionally, 100% concordance was seen for the TE and ICM pairs (13,45). The other two blastocyst studies used SNP microarrays to examine the chromosome complement of nontransferred blastocysts, which were also disaggregated into separate TE and ICM samples (62,63). Varying degrees of mosaicism were seen in 24% of the embryos investigated, with the remaining 76% being either uniformly euploid or aneuploid. Concordance between results for the TE and corresponding ICMs was good (62,63).

Improvements in clinical outcomes after the use of comprehensive chromosome screening applied to TE biopsies have been seen during two different investigations. In the first study, carried out by our group (11), clinical outcome data obtained from 45 infertile couples who underwent blastocyst biopsy, followed by vitrification, CGH analysis, and transfer of euploid embryos in a subsequent cycle, were compared with outcomes from 113 couples receiving blastocyst transfer in the same IVF clinic during the same time period. Results obtained from this comparison showed that 68.9% of blastocysts transferred after CGH testing led to clinical pregnancies, whereas the figure was 44.8% for the cycles without aneuploidy screening. It was therefore concluded that the probability of an embryo selected for transfer producing a child is increased 1.5-fold (11). An RCT is currently being planned, to confirm these preliminary observations.

The second study was an actual RCT, which employed comprehensive aneuploidy screening of 24 chromosomes with the use of quantitative PCR (Q-PCR) (64). A total of 28 patients whose characteristics were <43 years of age and with one or more prior failed cycles participated in the trial. Thirteen of these patients (average maternal age 34 ± 3.2 years) generated blastocysts which underwent chromosome analysis via Q-PCR (test group), whereas the remaining 15 (average maternal age 32 ± 6.0 years) comprised the control group and did not receive the test. Fresh embryo transfers took place for both the test and the control groups. Clinical outcome comparisons between the two groups showed that the pregnancy rates were significantly higher in the test group (92%), than those seen in the control group (60%). Implantation rates were also improved in the test group, compared with the control (75% vs. 56%, respectively), but the difference was not statistically significant. The authors stated that this was an ongoing study (64).

Chromosome screening during the final stage of preimplantation development has given very promising preliminary results, but data from large RCTs (preferably multicenter) will be necessary to substantiate these observations.

CONCLUSIONS

Aneuploidy screening for embryo selection has come a long way ever since it was initially proposed as a means to improve clinical outcomes for infertile patients. It is obvious from published data that PGS approaches using FISH to screen blastomeres, PBs, or TE samples are hampered by a variety of technical issues, which could potentially lead to increased risks of misdiagnosis. Although there is evidence that day 3 PGS with the use of FISH may be capable of reducing the incidence of spontaneous abortion and aneuploid pregnancy, most laboratories have been unable to achieve any enhancement of implantation or pregnancy rates for patients undergoing IVF. The deficiencies of the early PGS methods have led a number of research groups to develop alternative molecular cytogenetic methods that examine the entire chromosome complement of single cells. These methods have been optimized and validated, and are increasingly employed in a clinical setting. As cleavage-stage analysis may suffer occasional diagnostic errors due to mosaicism and risks the possibility of damage to the embryo, many IVF clinics have chosen to sample oocytes (via PB biopsy) or blastocyst-stage embryos (via TE biopsy) instead. Preliminary results are encouraging, especially for the combination of comprehensive chromosome screening with TE cell biopsy, which has yielded remarkable pregnancy rates in a couple of published studies. Several RCTs are now underway, taking place both in the United States and Europe, using comprehensive molecular cytogenetic methods for PGS. The results obtained from these RCTs will hopefully clarify the extent to which chromosome screening can assist infertile couples in establishing a successful pregnancy and ultimately a healthy live birth.

ACKNOWLEDGMENTS

DW is funded by the NIHR Biomedical Research Centre Programme.

REFERENCES

1. Handyside AH, Kontogianni EH, Hardy K, Winston RM. Pregnancies from biopsied human preimplantation embryos sexed by Y-specific DNA amplification. Nature 1990; 344: 768–70.
2. Harper JC, Harton G. The use of arrays in preimplantation genetic diagnosis and screening. Fertil Steril 2010; 94: 1173–7.
3. Delhanty JD, Harper JC, Ao A, et al. Multicolour FISH detects frequent chromosomal mosaicism and chaotic division in normal preimplantation embryos from fertile patients. Hum Genet 1997; 99: 755–60.
4. Wells D, Delhanty JD. Comprehensive chromosomal analysis of human preimplantation embryos using whole genome amplification and single cell comparative genomic hybridization. Mol Hum Reprod 2000; 6: 1055–62.
5. Munne S, Lee A, Rosenwaks Z, Grifo J, Cohen J. Diagnosis of major chromosome aneuploidies in human preimplantation embryos. Hum Reprod 1993; 8: 2185–91.
6. Kuliev A, Cieslak J, Verlinsky Y. Frequency and distribution of chromosome abnormalities in human oocytes. Cytogenet Genome Res 2005; 111: 193–8.
7. Mantzouratou A, Mania A, Fragouli E, et al. Variable aneuploidy mechanisms in embryos from couples with poor reproductive histories undergoing preimplantation genetic screening. Hum Reprod 2007; 22: 1844–53.
8. Fragouli E, Katz-Jaffe M, Alfarawati S, et al. Comprehensive chromosome screening of polar bodies and blastocysts from couples experiencing repeated implantation failure. Fertil Steril 2010; 94: 875–87.
9. Colls P, Escudero T, Cekleniak N, et al. Increased efficiency of preimplantation genetic diagnosis for infertility using "no result rescue." Fertil Steril 2007; 88: 53–61.
10. Munné S, Fragouli E, Colls P, et al. Improved detection of aneuploid blastocysts using a new 12-chromosome FISH test. RBM Online 2010; 20: 92–7.

11. Schoolcraft WB, Fragouli E, Stevens J, et al. Clinical application of comprehensive chromosomal screening at the blastocyst stage. Fertil Steril 2010; 94: 1700–6.
12. Fragouli E, Alfarawati S, Daphnis DD, et al. Cytogenetic analysis of human blastocysts with the use of FISH, CGH and aCGH: Scientific data and technical evaluation. Hum Reprod 2011; 26: 480–90.
13. Fragouli E, Alfarawati S, Goodall NN, et al. The cytogenetics of polar bodies: Insights into female meiosis and the diagnosis of aneuploidy. Mol Hum Reprod 2011; 17: 286–95.
14. Gutierrez-Mateo C, Colls P, Sanchez-Garcıa J, et al. Validation of microarray comparative genomic hybridization for comprehensive chromosome analysis of embryos. Fertil Steril 2011; 95: 953–8.
15. Handyside AH, Harton GL, Mariani B, et al. Karyomapping: A universal method for genome wide analysis of genetic disease based on mapping crossovers between parental haplotypes. J Med Genet 2010; 47: 651–8.
16. Treff NR, Levy B, Su J, et al. SNP microarray-based 24 chromosome aneuploidy screening is significantly more consistent than FISH. Mol Hum Reprod 2010; 16: 583–9.
17. Munne S, Sandalinas M, Escudero T, et al. Chromosome mosaicism in cleavage-stage human embryos: Evidence of a maternal age effect. RBM Online 2002; 4: 223–32.
18. Voullaire L, Slater H, Williamson R, Wilton L. Chromosome analysis of blastomeres from human embryos by using comparative genomic hybridization. Hum Genet 2000; 106: 210–17.
19. Gianaroli L, Magli C, Ferraretti A Munné S. Preimplantation diagnosis for aneuploidies in patients undergoing in vitro fertilization with a poor prognosis: Identification of the categories for which it should be proposed. Fertil Steril 1999; 72: 837–44.
20. Munné S, Magli C, Cohen J, et al. Positive outcome after preimplantation diagnosis of aneuploidy in human embryos. Hum Reprod 1999; 14: 2191–9.
21. Munné S, Sandalinas M, Escudero T, et al. Improved implantation after preimplantation genetic diagnosis of aneuploidy. RBM Online 2003; 7: 91–7.
22. Munne S, Chen S, Fischer J, et al. Preimplantation genetic diagnosis reduces pregnancy loss in women aged 35 years and older with a history of recurrent miscarriages. Fertil Steril 2005; 84: 331–5.
23. Munne S, Fischer J, Warner A, et al. Preimplantation genetic diagnosis significantly reduces pregnancy loss in infertile couples: A multicenter study. Fertil Steril 2006; 85: 326–32.
24. Platteau P, Staessen C, Michiels A, et al. Preimplantation genetic diagnosis for aneuploidy screening in women older than 37 years. Fertil Steril 2005; 84: 319–24.
25. Staessen C, Platteau P, Van Assche E, et al. Comparison of blastocyst transfer with or without Preimplantation genetic diagnosis for aneuploidy screening in couples with advanced maternal age: A prospective randomized controlled trial. Hum Reprod 2004; 19: 2849–58.
26. Munne S, Gianaroli L, Tur-Kaspa I, et al. Substandard application of preimplantation genetic screening may interfere with its clinical success. Fertil Steril 2007; 88: 781–4.
27. Cohen J, Wells D, Munné S. Removal of 2 cells from cleavage stage embryos is likely to reduce the efficacy of chromosomal tests that are used to enhance implantation rates. Fertil Steril 2007; 87: 496–503.
28. De Vos A, Staessen C, De Rycke M, et al. Impact of cleavage-stage embryo biopsy in view of PGD on human blastocyst implantation: A prospective cohort of single embryo transfers. Hum Reprod 2009; 24: 2988–96.
29. Mastenbroek S, Twisk M, Van Echten-Arends J, et al. Preimplantation genetic screening in women of advanced maternal age. N Engl J Med 2007; 357: 9–17.
30. Braude P, Flinter F. Use and misuse of preimplantation genetic testing. BMJ 2007; 335: 752–4.
31. Cohen J, Grifo J. Multicentre trial of preimplantation genetic screening reported in the New England Journal of Medicine: An in-depth look at the findings. RBM Online 2007; 15: 365–6.
32. Kuliev A, Verlinsky Y. Impact of PGD for chromosome disorders on reproductive outcome. RBM Online 2008; 16: 9–10.
33. Stevens J, Wale P, Surrey ES, Schoolcraft WB, Gardner DK. Is aneuploidy screening for patients aged 35 or over beneficial? A prospective randomized trial. Fertil Steril 2004; 82: S249–9.
34. Blockeel C, Schutyser V, De Vos A, et al. Prospectively randomised controlled trial of PGS in IVF/ICSI patients with poor implantation. Reprod Biomed Online 2008; 17: 848–54.
35. Hardarson T, Hanson C, Lundin K, et al. Preimplantation genetic screening in women of advanced maternal age caused a decrease in clinical pregnancy rate: A randomised controlled trial. Hum Reprod 2008; 23: 2806–12.
36. Mersereau JE, Pergament E, Zhang X, Milad MP. Preimplantation genetic screening to improve in vitro fertilization pregnancy rates: A prospective randomized controlled trial. Fertil Steril 2008; 90: 1287–8.
37. Staessen C, Verpoest W, Donoso P, et al. Preimplantation genetic screening does not improve delivery rate in women under the age of 36 following single-embryo transfer. Hum Reprod 2008; 23: 2818–25.
38. Meyer LR, Klipstein S, Hazlett WD, et al. A prospective randomized controlled trial of preimplantation genetic screening in the "good prognosis" patients. Fertil Steril 2009; 91: 1731–8.
39. Schoolcraft WB, Katz-Jaffe MG, Stevens J, Rawlins M, Munne S. Preimplantation aneuploidy testing for infertile patients of advanced maternal age: A randomized prospective trial. Fertil Steril 2009; 92: 57–62.
40. Debrock S, Melotte C, Spiessens C, et al. Preimplantation genetic screening for aneuploidy of embryos after in vitro fertilization in women aged at least 35 years: A prospective randomized trial. Fertil Steril 2010; 93: 364–73.
41. Wells D, Sherlock JK, Handyside AH, Delhanty JD. Detailed chromosomal and molecular genetic analysis of single cells by whole genome amplification and comparative genomic hybridisation. Nucleic Acids Res 1999; 27: 1214–18.
42. Wilton L, Williamson R, McBain J, et al. Birth of a healthy infant after preimplantation confirmation of euploidy by comparative genomic hybridization. N Engl J Med 2001; 345: 1537–41.
43. Gutierrez-Mateo C, Benet J, Wells D, et al. Aneuploidy study of human oocytes first polar body comparative genomic hybridization and metaphase II fluorescence in situ hybridization analysis. Hum Reprod 2004; 19: 2859–68.

44. Fragouli E, Wells D, Thornhill A, et al. Comparative genomic hybridization analysis of human oocytes and polar bodies. Hum Reprod 2006; 21: 2319–28.
45. Fragouli E, Lenzi M, Ross R, et al. Comprehensive molecular cytogenetic analysis of the human blastocyst stage. Hum Reprod 2008; 23: 2596–608.
46. Voullaire L, Wilton L, McBain J, et al. Chromosome abnormalities identified by comparative genomic hybridization in embryos from women with repeated implantation failure. Mol Hum Reprod 2002; 8: 1035–41.
47. Gutierrez-Mateo C, Colls P, Sanchez-Garcia J, et al. Validation of microarray comparative genomic hybridization for comprehensive chromosome analysis of embryos. Fertil Steril 2011; 95: 953–8.
48. Treff NR, Su J, Tao X, Levy B, Scott RT Jr. Accurate single cell 24 chromosome aneuploidy screening using whole genome amplification and single nucleotide polymorphism microarrays. Fertil Steril 2010; 94: 2017–21.
49. Hassold T, Hall H, Hunt P. The origin of human aneuploidy: Where we have been, where we are going. Hum Mol Genet 2007; 16: R203–8.
50. Sandalinas M, Marquez C, Munne S. Spectral karyotyping of fresh, non-inseminated oocytes. Mol Hum Reprod 2002; 8: 580–5.
51. Kuliev A, Cieslak J, Ilkevitch Y, Verlinsky Y. Chromosomal abnormalities in a series of 6,733 human oocytes in preimplantation diagnosis for age-related aneuploidies. RBM Online 2003; 6: 54–9.
52. Pellestor F, Andreo B, Arnal F, Humaeu C, Demaille J. Maternal ageing and chromosomal abnormalities: New data drawn from in vitro unfertilized human oocytes. Hum Genet 2003; 112: 195–203.
53. Fragouli E, Escalona A, Gutiérrez-Mateo C, et al. Comparative genomic hybridization of oocytes and first polar bodies from young donors. RBM Online 2009; 19: 228–37.
54. Kuliev A, Verlinsky Y. Meiotic and mitotic nondisjunction: Lessons from preimplantation genetic diagnosis. Hum Reprod Update 2004; 10: 401–7.
55. Kuliev A, Zlatopolsky Z, Kirillova I, et al. Meiosis errors in over 20,000 oocytes studied in the practice of preimplantation aneuploidy testing. RBM Online 2011; 2: 2–8.
56. Wells D, Escudero T, Levy B, et al. First clinical application of comparative genomic hybridization and polar body testing for preimplantation genetic diagnosis of aneuploidy. Fertil Steril 2002; 78: 543–9.
57. Obradors A, Fernandez E, Oliver-Bonet M, et al. Birth of a healthy boy after a double factor PGD in a couple carrying a genetic disease and at risk for aneuploidy: Case Report. Hum Reprod 2008; 23: 1949–56.
58. Fishel S, Gordon A, Lynch C, et al. Live birth after polar body array comparative genomic hybridization prediction of embryo ploidy-the future of IVF? Fertil Steril 2010; 93: 1006–e7–1006.e10.
59. Treff NR, Su J, Kasabwala N, et al. Robust embryo identification using first polar body single nucleotide polymorphism microarray-based DNA fingerprinting. Fertil Steril 2010; 93: 2453–5.
60. Geraedts J, Collins J, Gianaroli L, et al. What next for preimplantation genetic screening? A polar body approach! Hum Reprod 2010; 25: 575–7.
61. Jansen RPS, Bowman MC, de Boer KA, et al. What next for preimplantation genetic screening (PGS)? Experience with blastocyst biopsy and testing for aneuploidy. Hum Reprod 2008; 23: 1476–8.
62. Northrop LE, Treff NR, Levy B, Scott RT. SNP microarray based 24 chromosome aneuploidy screening demonstrates that cleavage stage FISH poorly predicts aneuploidy in embryos that develop to morphologically normal blastocysts. Mol Hum Reprod 2010; 16: 590–600.
63. Johnson DS, Cinnioglu C, Ross R, et al. Comprehensive analysis of karyotypic mosaicism between trophectoderm and inner cell mass. Mol Hum Reprod 2010; 16: 944–9.
64. Scott R, Tao X, Taylor D, Ferry KM, Treff NR. A prospective randomized controlled trial demonstrating significantly increased clinical pregnancy rates following 24 chromosome aneuploidy screening: Biopsy and analysis on day 5 with fresh transfer. Feril Steril 2010; 94: S2.

28

Genetic analysis of the embryo

Yuval Yaron, Veronica Gold, Sagit Peleg-Schalka, and Mira Malcov

INTRODUCTION

For couples at risk of transmitting a genetic disease, preimplantation genetic diagnosis (PGD) and transfer of disease-free embryos offer an alternative to prenatal diagnosis by chorionic villous sampling or amniocentesis, followed by therapeutic abortion of affected fetuses. Molecular PGD was initially employed for embryo sexing in couples at risk for X-linked diseases. The technique used polymerase chain reaction (PCR) to amplify Y-chromosome specific sequences, and only embryos diagnosed as females were transferred (1). During the last two decades, the range of genetic abnormalities that can be detected by PGD has increased exponentially and in fact it may be performed for virtually any genetic disorder for which the mutation has been detected. PGD can also be employed in carriers of cancer predisposition genes and other late-onset genetic conditions. This however raises many ethical and practical questions. For instance, familial adenomatous polyposis (FAP) is an autosomal dominant syndrome with almost 100% risk of colorectal cancer without prophylactic colectomy. In a study including 20 individuals with FAP, 95% would consider undergoing prenatal testing and 90% would consider PGD (2). In comparison, carriers of BRCA 1/2 mutations are at risk for breast and/or ovarian cancer, but this at a comparatively lower risk of developing malignancy. A similar survey conducted among such carriers revealed that 75% felt it was acceptable to offer PGD for this indication but only 14% of patients contemplating a future pregnancy would consider PGD themselves (3).

Moreover, it is possible to perform combined PGD and HLA typing. This may prove beneficial in cases where the parents already have a child affected with a genetic disease amenable to bone marrow transplantation. In this approach, any future sibling produced by PGD may be not only free of the familial disease but will also be a suitable bone marrow donor for the affected child. This approach has been successfully employed in assessing Fanconi anemia (4) and has been coined "savior sibling." However, the use of PGD for HLA-typing, particularly in the absence of a genetic disease, and its use in screening embryos for susceptibility to cancer and late-onset diseases as well as for gender selection raise important ethical concerns.

Lastly, PGD for chromosomal imbalances, such as in balanced translocation carriers, has been traditionally performed using fluorescence in situ hybridization. It has recently been suggested that this can also be performed using PCR-based techniques (5). Additionally, comparative genomic hybridization (CGH) has been introduced to PGD, particularly for aneuploidy screening (discussed in chap. 26). However, CGH may also be used for diagnosis of embryos with unbalanced reciprocal or Robertsonian translocation (6).

Despite its promise, PGD is still limited by technical difficulties due to the minute amount of genetic material, and the inherent pitfalls of the PCR, such as amplification failure, allele drop-out (ADO), and foreign DNA contamination. There is also a rather narrow window of opportunity to perform diagnosis within hours to enable embryo transfer without jeopardizing pregnancy rates. This chapter will review the various aspects of the genetic analysis of preimplantation embryos.

BASIC PRINCIPLES OF PGD

Polymerase Chain Reaction

Single cell molecular analysis for PGD was made possible by the PCR, first introduced in the mid-1980s (7,8). The technique enriches a DNA sample for one specific oligonucleotide fragment, the *PCR product* or *amplicon*. The technique uses a pair of short oligonucleotide fragments, *primers*, which are homologous to stretches of genomic DNA at a locus of interest. The PCR thermocycler is programmed to perform successive cycles consisting of *denaturation*, at temperatures >90°C, during which the double-stranded template DNA melts into two separate single strands; *annealing*, in which the primers attach to their region of homology; and *extension*, during which new nucleotides (dNTPs) are added in succession to recreate a double-stranded DNA molecule by the enzymatic action of the thermo stable *Taq* polymerase. The resulting new strands serve as templates for the subsequent cycles. After 30–40 such cycles, the initial minute quantity of DNA is amplified to the extent that it can actually be visualized by methods such as radioactive-labeling, ethidium bromide, or silver staining. The PCR products may further be subjected to a variety of analytic techniques that determine the presence of point mutations, small deletions, or insertions, or for analysis of linked polymorphic genetic markers. Finally, the precise composition of the amplified fragment may be studied by direct sequencing.

The number of cycles that may be performed in standard PCR is limited by a gradual decline in amplification efficiency with each subsequent cycle. This is partly due to the decrease in the activity of the *Taq* polymerase over time. Another reason is the "fraying" of the amplicon edges by the exonuclease activity of *Taq* polymerase. This causes the amplicons to become unsuitable templates for further amplification because their primer annealing sites become eroded.

Due to these limitations, when the number of initial DNA template molecules is limited, as in a single cell PGD analysis, the quantity of amplified DNA may be insufficient for a complete molecular analysis. The two-step, *nested-primer PCR* approach offers a solution to this problem, by allowing sufficient amplification of even a single DNA copy. The method employs a first pair of *outer primers*, designed to amplify the region of interest in the *primary* PCR reaction. The PCR product of the primary PCR reaction is then further amplified using a second set of inner- or *nested primers*. The use of nested primers proximal to the annealing site of the outer primers increases amplification efficiency, since the nested primers anneal to sites that have not been eroded. This technique also decreases the rate of nonspecific amplification.

Pitfalls of PCR in PGD

The precise diagnosis by PCR relies on several key elements: adequately functioning reagents such as primers, dNTPs, and *Taq* polymerase; the presence of an adequate tested DNA template; and the lack of any DNA contamination. Perturbations in any of these elements may lead to misdiagnosis (9). In particular, PCR for PGD has three potential pitfalls: amplification failure, ADO, and contamination.

Amplification Failure

Amplification by PCR is unsuccessful in approximately 10% of isolated blastomeres, regardless of their genotype. The main reasons for amplification failure include biopsy technique, premature cell lysis, lysis protocol used, and PCR conditions (10,11). There appears to be an association between embryo or blastomere morphology and the success rate of PCR amplification. Cells that appear to be anucleate and those derived from arrested or fragmented embryos have low amplification efficiency (12,13). In such cells, the DNA may be degraded or entirely absent. Adequate positive and negative controls must be used, to establish and fine-tune the PCR protocol and to ensure the integrity of the results. This is of particular importance in cases where the diagnosis is based on detection of deletions, such as in Duchenne muscular dystrophy (DMD). When in such cases an allele is not amplified, one must be certain that this is indeed due to a deletion and not secondary to amplification failure.

Allele Drop-Out

ADO occurs when only one of the two alleles present in a cell is amplified to a detectable level. ADO is equally likely to affect either of the alleles in a heterozygous cell and thus it is not possible to predict which allele will be 'dropped out' in a given reaction. The most significant implication of ADO is misdiagnosis of heterozygous embryos, particularly in PGD of dominant disorders. In such cases, the absence of the mutated allele due to ADO may result in the misdiagnosis of an affected fetus as a normal one. Likewise, ADO may be responsible for misdiagnosis of recessive disorders in affected compound heterozygotes, where if only one of the mutations is detected, the embryo may be mistaken for a heterozygote (14). The reported frequency of ADO varies widely. In most experiments the rate of ADO is reported to be 5–20%, although, in some cases ADO has been shown to affect over 30% of single cell amplifications (13,15–19), or none of the cells (20).

The causes of ADO are still not fully understood. Current hypotheses include inaccessibility of the DNA template due to imperfect denaturing temperature or incomplete cell lysis and DNA degradation prior to PCR. Ray and Handyside (17) demonstrated that an increase in denaturing temperature from 90°C to 96°C during PCR may be associated with a four-fold reduction in ADO at the cystic fibrosis locus and an 11-fold reduction at the beta-globin locus. The use of alkaline lysis buffer or lysis buffer containing proteinase K and detergents has also been suggested to reduce ADO (17,21). Degenerated and apoptotic cells show increased ADO probably due to partial degradation of the DNA strands. It has been suggested that ADO is higher in blastomeres than in other cell types (18). This may be explained, at least partly, by the higher rate of haploidy of blastomeres (22).

In cases of diagnosis of dominant disorders or recessive diseases when both parents carry different mutations, measures should be taken to avoid or reduce the risk of ADO. A number of PGD protocols have been suggested that achieve this goal, most based on advanced techniques such as multiplex PCR in order to include flanking polymorphic markers, quantitative-fluorescent (QF) PCR, reverse transcription PCR, and others, as will be described in the following sections. Other less sensitive detection methods may "overlook" the minimally amplified allele, resulting in ADO (16,19,23). The significant frequency of ADO resulting in misdiagnosis has led many PGD centers to use two cells from each embryo for genetic analysis.

Contamination

Contamination is one of the greatest obstacles in the analysis of specific genes in single cells (24). In the setting of PGD, there may be three main sources for possible contamination. First, paternal genome contamination may rise from the fact that many spermatozoa are still embedded in the zona pellucida after IVF, and may thus be mistakenly sampled with the blastomere, second polar body, or trophectoderm cells during embryo biopsy. Intracytoplasmic sperm injection (ICSI) using a single sperm that is injected into the oocyte completely abolishes this possibility. Accordingly, most PGD units are routinely using ICSI for all PGD cases in which diagnosis relies on PCR. The second source of possible contamination may arise from maternal cumulus cells adherent to the oocytes. Stripping of the cumulus cells from the zona pellucida is performed mechanically and/or by enzymes to reduce this risk. Finally, external contamination either from laboratory technicians or from PCR products generated during previous experiments is yet another source of contamination. The risk of external contamination is influenced by the number of PCR cycles required for sufficient amplification of the DNA. Thus, with a starting template of only one genome, the risk of contamination with exogenous DNA sequences is a particularly concerning problem that must be avoided by the use of adequate safety measures, as will be described next.

ADVANCED MOLECULAR METHODS FOR PGD

Multiplex PCR

Multiplex PCR refers to the simultaneous amplification of more than one fragment in the same PCR reaction using more than one pair of unrelated primers (16,18,19,25). One or more primer pairs amplify the DNA fragment containing the locus to be tested, while the other(s) serve as a positive control within the same reaction. Amplification of multiple loci within the same multiplex PCR reaction is possible in single blastomeres. This requires careful primer design and reaction optimization to ensure that all primers sets amplify efficiently under the same conditions including annealing temperatures and concentrations of the different reagents in the PCR buffer, such as $MgCl_2$. Careful design of primers is mandated in order to avoid primer-dimer formation, interaction between different PCR products, and interaction of primers with products. The primers should be designed such that the product of each PCR primer pair is of a different size so that it may be distinguished by gel electrophoresis. Alternatively, different fluorescent tags can be used for each primer pair.

Successful multiplex PCR reactions enable simultaneous assessment of numerous loci (25,26). Multiplex PCR reaction may include assays for specific gene defects, unique sequences of specific chromosomes, and linked-informative polymorphic markers. This allows both the analysis of the disease mutation, assessment of aneuploidy, as well as reduction in the risk of contamination and ADO (15,18,27–30). This strategy is particularly useful for the PGD of dominant disorders, in which one primer set amplifies the region of mutation, while the other amplifies a polymorphic marker that is linked with the tested gene (28,31). The probability of ADO affecting both mutation site and the linked polymorphic site is very low, and decreases as more polymorphic markers are tested. This decreases both false-positive and false-negative results (32).

Fluorescent PCR

The PCR products are commonly separated by gel electrophoresis, and their migration depends chiefly on their size. The standard visualization techniques include radioactive labeling, ethidium bromide, or silver staining. These techniques are rather insensitive, requiring a relatively large amount of DNA. Moreover, they cannot distinguish between products of a relatively similar size nor provide an adequate estimate of quantity. Fluorescent PCR employs primers tagged with a fluorescent dye, which label the resulting amplicons, enabling detection by florescence-based DNA sequencers using a module such as GeneScan™ (3130XL Genetic Analyzer, Applied Biosystems (AB) CA, USA). A laser beam scans the acrylamide gel as the fluorescent products pass across the laser path by means of electrophoresis. The different fluorescent dyes absorb the light at a particular wavelength and emit fluorescence at a different wavelength. The emitted light passes through a filter, digitally amplified, and analyzed by a computer. With this technique, it is possible to separate, detect, and analyze the fluorescent-labeled PCR products with sensitivity 1000 times greater than that achieved using conventional methods (33). This method also has a higher fragment-size resolution and is able to distinguish between products having a size difference of even 1–2 bp. Thus, several primer sets can be multiplexed even if their product sizes only vary slightly.

This approach significantly reduces the likelihood of ADO resulting from preferential amplification, since even minimally amplified alleles are detected (16,19,23). In addition, since the detection efficiency is several magnitudes higher, fewer PCR cycles are required, thereby reducing the risk of contamination. Moreover, since fewer cycles are needed, less time is required for the complete analysis. Using this approach, Sermon et al. (23) have successfully reduced the rate of ADO by a factor of four in the diagnosis of myotonic dystrophy, and Findlay et al. (16) reported an accurate diagnosis in as much as 97% of the cases.

Quantitative Fluorescent PCR

QF PCR provides information on the ploidy of the cell (34). It amplifies specific DNA sequences unique for each chromosome, such as short tandem repeat (STR) markers which are composed of a varying number of nucleotide repeats (2–5 bp) and are highly polymorphic. Normal individuals are usually heterozygous for such polymorphic markers, that is, they have a different number of repeats, and therefore have different-sized alleles. During the initial exponential phase of PCR amplification, the amount of DNA product is proportional to the original number of repeats (35,36). Disomic individuals thus produce different sized alleles with a ratio of 1:1, whereas trisomic DNA samples produce either three alleles of different lengths at a ratio of 1:1:1 (trisomic tri-allelic), or two alleles of the same size at a ratio of 2:1 (trisomic di-allelic) (34). This method has been successfully used in prenatal diagnosis of aneuploidy (37). In PGD, however, QF-PCR is only reliable in identifying tri-allelic trisomies, since the interpretation of di-allelic trisomies is problematic due to the possibility of preferential amplification (19).

Whole Genome Amplification

The most significant limitation of single cell analysis is the small amount of DNA. As mentioned previously, multiplex PCR is one way to overcome this problem. In addition, methods designed to achieve nonspecific amplification of the entire genome, that is, whole genome amplification (WGA), have been developed (24,38). These techniques amplify a large proportion of the entire genome, thereby allowing further analyses by specific PCR reactions, allowing confirmation of diagnosis by alternative methods or the analysis of other genes.

There are several WGA techniques:

Primer Extension Preamplification

Primer extension preamplification (PEP) is a WGA method designed mainly for single cells. Using random-sequence primers of 15 bp it has been claimed to amplify at least 70% of the genome in more than 30 copies (38). This, however, is likely to be a rather conservative estimate since Paunio et al. (39) reported that PEP yields at least 1000 copies of the genome, and Wells et al. (24) have suggested that more than of 90% of genomic sequences are represented in PEP amplification products. One of the drawbacks of PEP is the time required, which is usually more than 12 hours. Sermon et al. (40) have successfully adopted a modified protocol that requires less than 6 hours, and Tsai (41) have improved the efficiency by further technical modifications. Several autosomal recessive, dominant, and X-linked disorders have been successfully detected in single cells using PEP, including Tay–Sachs disease, cystic fibrosis, hemophilia A, DMD and FAP coli (15,42,43).

Degenerate Oligonucleotide Primed PCR

A second form of WGA called degenerate oligonucleotide primed (DOP) PCR has been recently applied to PGD (24,44). DOP-PCR amplifies a similar proportion of the genome as does PEP, but to a greater extent, providing sufficient DNA for over 100 subsequent PCR amplifications (20), or for other analytical procedures such as CGH. It has been shown that using a combination of DOP-PCR, CGH, and QF-PCR it is possible to determine the copy number of each chromosome and conduct various molecular studies on single cells and blastomeres (24,45,46).

Multiple Displacement Amplification

Multiple displacement amplification (MDA) is a recently developed non PCR-based method that has been utilized for clinical samples with limited DNA content, providing high yield of relatively long fragments (>10 kb) with uniform and reliable representation across the genome (47).

In MDA, annealing of exonuclease-resistant random hexamers to DNA template is followed by strand-displacement DNA synthesis at a constant temperature of 30°C, without the need of cyclic DNA denaturation (47,48). The strand-displacing mechanism is accomplished by the Φ29 DNA polymerase (47) or the *Bacillus stearothermophilus* (Bst) DNA polymerase large fragment (49). This mechanism allows increasing random priming events that form a network of hyper-branched DNA structures which generate thousands of copies of the original DNA in only few hours (49,50). It appears that MDA is more advantageous due to decreased rates of unspecific amplification artifacts (51), incomplete coverage of loci (39), strong amplification bias (47), and short length of the DNA products (52).

The Φ29 enzyme has been widely preferred over B*st* DNA polymerase due to its superior sequence fidelity (48,53), and its higher processivity (number of nucleotides incorporated per single DNA polymerase/DNA-binding event), the highest one described for a DNA polymerase (47,54,55). This attribute explains its low amplification bias (less than threefold) compared with DOP and PEP-PCR methods (10^2 and 10^6 fold) (47).

Hellani et al. (56) and Handyside et al. (57) published the first successful reports of single-cell MDA from lymphocytes and blastomeres with further analysis of array-CGH and nested PCR for 20 different loci, respectively. Despite these advantages, ADO is not completely eliminated (53), with ADO rates 10–31%.

In the setting of PGD, MDA has significant advantages: It obviates the need to set up unique single cell protocols, such that following MDA, second round PCR may employ standard PCR protocols commonly used in molecular labs. In addition, the large quantity of DNA uniformly representing the entire genome, allows subsequent analyses of a variety of other loci (53) both for diagnosis as well as research. Yet, the technique is not widely used in established PGD units. This may be due to higher rates of ADO, cost, and time required.

In 2006 Renwick et al. (58) coined the term "preimplantation genetic haplotyping" (PGH), which utilizes MDA with subsequent multiplex PCR of a fixed set of numerous disease-associated polymorphic markers. This helps determine the high-risk haplotype by linkage analysis using a single protocol for each disease, without the need to establish a specific protocol for each different mutation (58). Although the same test can be applied to several couples without considering or even identifying the mutation they carry, it has several limitations: It requires additional informative family members to determine the phase (i.e., to determine the mutation-associated parental haplotype). It requires the use of various informative disease-linked markers and the occurrence of recombination events could lead to misdiagnosis (53).

Polymorphic Markers

Multiplex PCR and WGA allow both the analysis of the tested gene for mutation, as well as analyzing polymorphic genetic markers such as STRs, also known as microsatellites, in a process referred to as "DNA fingerprinting." This technique is useful for ruling out contamination from various sources described earlier, and thus improves reliability of the diagnosis. The amplification of one or more highly polymorphic STRs allows the determination of the source of DNA amplified (59). As mentioned previously, polymorphic STRs consist of a varying number of repeats of a 2–5 bp motif, present in introns throughout the genome. At each informative STR locus, each parent has two alleles of varying repeat number, resulting in two amplicons of different lengths in each individual. The resulting embryo will have inherited only one allele from each parent. Any deviation from the expected inheritance of one allele from each parent is indicative of contamination, maternal, paternal, or external (16,19,59).

Polymorphic STRs can also be used in the actual diagnosis when the exact mutation causing the disease is unknown. In such cases, polymorphic markers in close proximity or within the disease locus are used to evaluate whether the embryo has inherited the affected allele. Intragenic markers and tightly linked ones are preferred as they are unlikely to be separated from the mutation by recombination during meiosis. In order to perform such linkage analysis, the parents and both healthy and affected siblings are analyzed to determine which polymorphic marker is inherited along with the disease. Such a strategy has been used for the diagnosis of Marfan syndrome, the first autosomal dominant disorder to be tested by PGD (60) and DMD. In the latter, only 60% of DMD patients exhibit detectable large-scale deletions in the dystrophin gene. Since it is the largest known human gene, spanning more than 2 million bp, it is often impossible to detect small deletions or point mutations (61). Linkage analysis has also been suggested for the diagnosis of disease with large tri-nucleotide repeat expansions, such as fragile X and myotonic dystrophy (23,62). Single cell analysis of the expanded portion of the expanded repeat region may lead to misdiagnosis due to difficulty in PCR amplification. Alternatively, it is possible to diagnose with certainty unaffected embryos by the detection of the normal maternal and paternal FMR1 repeat region (63). In addition, polymorphic markers may be used in combination with direct mutation analysis to increase precision and reliability of the diagnosis. Search for suitable polymorphic markers is possible using available publications/NCBI-STS databases as well as on-line programs such as GeneLoc, HapMap, etc.

PCR-Based PGD for Translocation Carriers

Traditionally, PGD for reciprocal and Robertsonian translocations were performed using FISH approaches. While generally successful, these techniques are subject to errors due to problems of signal and cell overlap, suboptimal hybridization, interpretation difficulties due to the presence of mosaicism etc. In contrast, molecular methods are usually associated with a lower error rate and are more reproducible. In addition, multiple polymorphic markers may be employed to increase precision and reliability, and decrease the rate of ambiguous results. In addition, with Robertsonian translocation cases where there is the risk of uniparental disomy, the use of PCR-based methods with informative markers can assure the choice of embryos demonstrating biparental inheritance (5).

Mutation Analysis

All the above-mentioned PCR techniques amplify the DNA of a single cell to a detectable level. In disorders caused by large-scale deletions, such as DMD or spinal muscular atrophy (SMA), the actual PCR amplification reaction is sufficient for making a diagnosis since it is based on the lack of amplification of the corresponding deleted portion of the gene. In other disorders caused by trinucleotide expansion, such as fragile X or myotonic dystrophy, the disease allele is significantly larger than the normal one, and amplicon size may also be diagnostic. More commonly however, the amplified fragment harboring the mutation is indistinguishable from the normal one using the standard visualization methods such as gel electrophoresis. In such cases, further analysis of the amplified fragment is required for mutation detection. Whenever the targeted mutation is precisely known, specific methods can be devised for the detection of the particular mutation. This is preferred to scanning methods that are used to search for mutations that have not been characterized. Scanning methods include heteroduplex analysis, single-strand conformational polymorphism, denaturant gradient gel electrophoresis, and others. These methods are based on the fact the normal DNA strands, mutant DNA strands, and various combinations thereof, often have varying electrophoretic migratory properties under different conditions, allowing to distinguish between them. These techniques often assist in scanning for a mutation in diseases that are caused by numerous different mutations. While PGD using these techniques has been reported in conditions such as beta-thalassemia (64–66), it is preferred to limit their use to initial mutation screen in the affected family members. Once the specific fragment of the gene harboring the mutation has been detected by these methods, further analysis is mandated using direct sequencing. The latter provides bona fide evidence of the mutation, and also facilitates the development of direct diagnostic techniques such as restriction endonuclease digestion of DNA or amplification refractory mutation system.

Restriction Endonuclease Digestion

Alteration in the DNA sequence caused by mutations, may often lead to a creation or abolition of specific restriction endonuclease recognition sites. These bacterially-derived enzymes recognize specific DNA sequences and cleave the DNA strand at or near to the recognition site. When the precise mutation is known, a restriction enzyme may be selected which differentially cleaves the normal DNA strand but not the mutant one, or vice versa. Following electrophoresis, it is possible to distinguish the digested from the non-digested products and thereby detect the presence or absence of the mutation. Many mutations alter the recognition site of at least one of the many possible, commercially available, restriction enzymes.

As an example, the ZFX and ZFY genes located on the X and Y chromosome respectively, can be distinguished according to difference in the size of the fragments produced by the restriction enzyme *HaeIII*. This allows sex determination to be performed more accurately then based on the presence or lack of amplification of the Y-chromosome specific SRY gene.

Amplification Refractory Mutation System

Amplification refractory mutation system employs three primers in the PCR reaction: A common primer which anneals upstream of the mutation site and two other primers, which differ slightly, each specific for either the normal or mutant alleles. The site-specific primers may be designed to vary in length, to contain a restriction site, or are tagged by different fluorescent markers (19). Any of these methods would facilitate the distinction of amplicons produced by either the normal or mutant allele. Since this test results in selective amplification of both the mutant and normal alleles, it is considered to be a safer method than the detection of the mutant allele alone. Using this technique in the multiplex PCR approach, it is possible to identify several different mutations, such as for cystic fibrosis, in a single-cell PCR reaction (67).

Minisequencing

Minisequencing SnaPshot™ (SNaPshot™ kit (AB) CA, USA) permits analysis of very small DNA fragments amplified by PCR, based on primer extension. It has been suggested that smaller amplicons have a lower rate of ADO rates. This would potentially improve the reliability of PGD without the need for extensive optimization for individual mutations. Bermudez et al. report single-cell protocols for the diagnoses of cystic fibrosis, sickle cell anemia, and β-thalassemia using this technique (68).

DNA Microarray Technology

DNA microarrays or "chips" allow the simultaneous detection of up to thousands of different polymorphism or mutations in defined genes. Numerous oligonucleotide probes (usually 20–25 bp) are arrayed in microscopic predefined regions on a solid surface such as a thumbnail-sized glass slide. The probes are complementary to known mutations in defined genes or single nucleotide polymorphisms throughout the genome. The microarray is hybridized with a fluorescent-labeled tested DNA and the fluorescent signal is detected and digitally analyzed. Hybridization is indicative of a match between the tested DNA and the specific oligonucleotide probe. For each possible mutation, several slightly varied probes may be used to increase sensitivity.

Array CGH

Aneuploidy, chromosome number imbalance, represents a major cause of spontaneous abortions (69–71). Fluorescence *in situ* hybridization (FISH) for detection of aneuploidy is discussed elsewhere in this textbook. The major drawback of FISH, however, lies in the fact that only a limited set of chromosomes can be analyzed in a single cell, usually 5–10. CGH following WGA is an alternative to interphase FISH (72) that may be used to screen for all aneuploidies in single blastomeres (73–75) and polar bodies (76,77). In CGH, *test* and *reference* DNA samples are labeled with two different fluorochromes and co-hybridized to normal human metaphase spread on a microscope slide (78,79). A computerized imaging system calculates the fluorescence ratio for each fluorochrome at each chromosomal locus. Deviation from a 1:1 ratio indicates a change in DNA copy number (i.e., deletion, duplication, trisomy, etc.) (79).

Array CGH is a simpler, more uniform technique that employs selected genomic regions printed onto a solid surface as hybridization probes. This eliminates the use of metaphase spreads that are un-uniform, and enable higher resolution, depending on the number, density, and size of the genomic probes printed on the array (78–81).

Le Caignec et al. (78) detected chromosomal imbalances from single lymphoblasts, fibroblasts, and blastomeres by array CGH following WGA by MDA. This approach may be preferable to array CGH following DOP-PCR that was reported by Hu et al. (82).

Array CGH has the potential to become an important method for aneuploidy diagnosis and screening in the setting of PGD (or alternatively preimplantation genetic screening–PGS; see chap. 27 by Wells), to a greater extent than standard FISH, allowing a larger number of abnormalities to be detected Wells et al. (96). It has been suggested that full genome aneuploidy screening for embryo selection would enhance implantation rates (78).

LABORATORY TECHNIQUES IN PGD

PGD at the single-cell level is a multistep complex procedure. The various pitfalls outlined previously necessitate adequate calibration of the techniques employed to avoid misdiagnosis. Due to ethical limitations, single human blastomeres are difficult to obtain, therefore different PGD centers have developed different protocols, and there is as yet no uniform method. Because of the numerous genetic disorders amenable to PGD it is impossible to provide suitable protocols for all. Instead, some of the commonly used laboratory methods will be described in the following section.

General Safety Measures

It is highly recommended that a physically separated site be used for template preparation, PCR assembly, and product analysis. Equipment and reagents used for single-cell PCR should be solely reserved for this purpose and should never be allowed to come into contact with previously amplified DNA samples. To avoid contamination, lab technicians should wear disposable outer clothing, caps, masks, shoe covers, and powder-free gloves that are kept in the room. In order to avoid external contamination from previously amplified DNA, some centers use a room kept under constant positive pressure. All equipment and required disposable supplies such as tubes, racks, and pipettes are to be kept in the room.

Glassware should be sterilized and aerosol-resistant pipette tips should be used. All reagents and solutions should be DNA free, sterilized by autoclaving, filtered through a 0.22 mM filter or by UV irradiation. All reagents should be prepared in a fume hood equipped with UV light. These safety measures, however, should not be considered a substitute for efforts to avoid the possibility of external contamination occurring in the first place.

The PCR reagents should be rigorously tested prior to any clinical case to ensure that they have not become contaminated. It is recommended that all PCR reagents (minus *Taq* polymerase) be prepared in excess and aliquoted to reduce the number of pipetting and sampling from the stock preparation. Sample aliquots may then be tested while the remaining is frozen until use.

To detect contamination in the analyzed sample, a negative control should be used consisting of all PCR reagents, substituting the template DNA or blastomere with an aliquot of the final blastomere wash buffer. To eliminate contamination by sperm, ICSI is employed.

The Choice of Positive Controls

A variety of cells harboring the mutation of interest may be used as positive controls, such as buccal cells, cumulus cells, lymphocytes, or lymphoblasts. To reduce the chance of misdiagnosis due to ADO, it is possible to biopsy and analyze two blastomeres from the same embryo (15,16,83). The isolated single cells may also be used for calibration of the PGD techniques and for testing the precision, sensitivity, and reliability of the single-cell PCR strategy.

Buccal cells may be obtained from patients by mouth-washing with double-distilled water or by scraping the inside of the cheek with a sterile cotton swab and suspending the smear in PBS. The suspension is centrifuged at 7.5 g for five minutes. The cell pellet is washed three times in PBS, and cells are resuspended and isolated using a pulled glass micro-pipette under an inverted microscope. Single cells are then washed several times in PBS microdrops to ensure that indeed only a single cell is aspirated and transferred to sterile PCR tubes for further use (84–86).

Cumulus cells may be obtained by incubating the retrieved oocyte in IVF culture medium supplemented with 80 IU hyaluronidase. Separated cumulus cells are then rinsed with IVF culture medium, washed in PBS, and transferred to sterile PCR tubes using pulled glass micropipette under a stereomicroscope (39)

Lymphocytes may be isolated from peripheral blood by the Ficoll-Paque method, washed three times in PBS, resuspended, and diluted in culture medium on a glass slide. Individual cells are then selected using pulled glass micropipette under an inverted microscope, washed three times in PCR buffer (50 mM KCl, 10 mM Tris-HCl pH 8.3) supplemented with 0.01% polyvinylpyrrolidone (PVP), and transferred to sterile PCR tubes for further use. Lymphocytes may be used fresh or frozen-thawed. For freezing, lymphocytes are washed three times in PBS, resuspended in autologous plasma, and 20 µL of concentrated lymphocytes is added to 40 µL of fetal calf serum, 120 µL of RPMI medium and 20 µL of dimethyl sulfoxide (DMSO) and kept in liquid nitrogen until required. Cells can be stored for up to a year. Thawing is performed by several washes with culture medium (87).

A lymphoblast cell-line carrying the known mutation is probably the best choice, since its establishment provides a perpetual source of cells with a known genetic composition. The cell-line is achieved by transformation of peripheral blood lymphocytes with the Ebstein–Barr virus (EBV) (88). Once the cell-line is established, single cells may be aspirated and transferred to 1.5 mL Eppendorf tubes, washed three times with PBS, resuspended in 50 µL PBS, and kept at 4°C until use (89).

Embryonic Cell Isolation

Embryo biopsy is described in detail in chapter 14. For the purpose of genetic analysis of the embryo, the single biopsied nucleated cells are washed several times in droplets of PCR buffer (50 mM KCl, 10 mM Tris-HCl pH 8.3) supplemented with 0.01% polyvinylpyrrolidone (PVP) or 4 mg/mL bovine serum albumin (BSA) in a Petri dish using a pulled micro-pipette. PVP or BSA is used in order to prevent adherence of the cells to the pipette. The isolated cell is transferred in a minimal volume of washing buffer to a PCR tube containing lysis buffer or water, and can be frozen immediately at −80°C until use. Alternatively, the cells can be lysed immediately and then frozen (16,17,62,87,90,91).

Cell Lysis

Lysis of the single embryonic ells and exposure of their genetic material to the PCR reagents is one of the most critical steps, and greatly affects ADO rates, and efficiency and reliability of PGD (El-Hashemite and Delhanty 1997). Among the several options, the three most commonly used lysis solutions are water, alkaline lysis buffer, and proteinase K/SDS buffer. There is yet no consensus as to which is superior.

Water

Single blastomeres are washed three times in PBS transferred under visual control by pulled micropipettes to PCR tubes containing 60 µL of biotechnology grade water. An aliquot from the last washing droplet is added to a PCR tube containing 60 µL of water, which is to serve as a negative control. Lysis is accomplished by two cycles of freezing in liquid nitrogen and thawing, and then boiling for 10 minutes. Lysates can be stored until use at −20°C (16).

Alkaline Lysis Buffer

Single cells are transferred as above to PCR tubes containing 5 μL alkaline lysis buffer (200 mM KOH, 50 mM dithiothreitol). For immediate use, samples are placed at −80°C for at least 30 minutes and undergo immediate lysis by incubation at 65°C for 10 minutes. Alternatively, samples may be immediately lysed, frozen, and stored (not longer than one week) at −80°C until further processing (15,92). After lysis, 5 μL neutralization buffer (300 mM/L KCl, 900 mM/L Tris-HCl pH 8.3, 200 mM/L HCl) is added. Lysates are centrifuged briefly and placed on ice for immediate use or stored at −20°C until use (93).

Proteinase K/SDS Buffer

Single blastomeres are washed three times in PBS or PCR buffers supplemented with 0.01% PVP or BSA and transferred individually to PCR tubes containing 5 μL proteinase K/ sodium dudecyl sulfate (SDS) buffer (17 mM SDS and 400 ng/mL proteinase K) (85,94). Samples are incubated at 50°C for one hour followed by denaturation at 99°C for 15 minutes to inactivate the enzyme. Lysates can be stored at −80°C until used (El-Hashemite et al. 1997), (86).

Primary and Nested PCR Conditions

For the primary PCR reaction, the following are mixed with the biopsied cell lysate to a final volume of 50 μL: PCR buffer (10 mM Tris-HCl, 50 mM KCl and 2.5 mM $MgCl_2$ pH 8.3), 0.3 mM dNTP, 1–2 U *Taq* polymerase, and 0.5 mM outer primers. It is recommended to perform optimization of the reaction by using different $MgCl_2$ concentrations and different pH conditions. Amplification efficiency can be improved by addition of one or more of the following ingredients: glycerol, gelatin, betaine, DMSO, $(NH_4)SO_4$ or detergents.

The PCR-thermocycler program begins with a prolonged stage of initial denaturation at 95°C for 6 minutes. This has been shown to correlate with reduction in ADO rates (92). This is followed by 30 cycles of denaturation at 94°C for one minute, annealing at 52–65°C (according to the primers melting temperature) for one minute, and extension at 72°C for one minute. Final extension at 72°C for 10 minutes is usually performed. Specificity of the reaction can be improved by using "hot start."

For the secondary or nested PCR, 2–5 μL of the primary PCR product serves as template to be used with the nested primers. In the nested-PCR reaction, the duration and temperature of the initial denaturation step may be reduced and $MgCl_2$ concentration can be lowered. DMSO is not requested for this step. Other reagents and PCR conditions may be similar to those used in the primary PCR reaction (20,95).

Multiplex PCR

According to the standard protocol, each 50 μL reaction includes 1–1.5 units of *Taq* polymerase, 0.3 mM for each dNTP, 0.5–2.5 mM $MgCl_2$, and 0.1–0.5 mM of each primer. The reaction 10x PCR buffer is usually composed of 500 mM KCl, 100 mM Tris-HCl pH 8.3 but at least one of the following ingredients is usually added: glycerol, gelatin, betaine, DMSO, $(NH4)SO_4$ and detergents. The PCR-thermocycler program begins with initial denaturation at 96°C for five minutes (ensuring appropriate accessibility to the DNA strands). This is followed by 30 cycles of 94°C for 45 seconds, 52–56°C for 60 seconds, and 72°C for 60 seconds. Final extension of 5–15 minutes at 72°C is usually performed.

If ethidium bromide gel electrophoresis analysis is performed, a nested PCR is usually required. After primary PCR is performed, a 2–5 μL aliquot of the product serves as DNA template for a nested-PCR reaction.

Primer Extension Preamplification

This method is based on multiple rounds of extensions using a random mixture of 15-base oligonucleotides as primers. Theoretically, the mixture contains up to 1×10^9 different primers. The PEP–PCR reaction in a final volume of 60 μL includes 33 mM random primers, 10 × PCR buffer (100 mM Tris-HCl pH 8.3, 25 mM $MgCl_2$, 1 mg/mL gelatin and 500 mM KCl), 0.1 mM dNTPs, and 5 U of *Taq* polymerase. The PCR buffer should be free of K^+ if the cell was lysed by an alkaline lysis buffer. The reaction is carried out in 50 cycles of the following: denaturation at 92°C for one minute, annealing at 37°C for two minutes, a programmed ramping step of 10 seconds/°C until 55°C, and extension at 55°C for 4 minutes (38,39,42).

Improvement of amplification can be achieved by raising the denaturation temperature, elongating the denaturation period, raising the pH buffer from 8.3 to 8.8, modifying the $MgCl_2$ and gelatin concentrations, reducing the KCl concentration and using a more thermo stable DNA polymerase, and one that has minimal exonuclease activity. Addition of glycerol, betaine, BSA, detergents, spermidine, and $(NH_4)SO_4$ may also improve the product yield. Primers should be dissolved in Tris-HCl 5–10 mM pH 8.3 and not in TE buffer to prevent the chelation of Mg^{+2} ions by EDTA. The PEP-PCR product should produce an even smear on ethidium bromide gel electrophoresis. A 2–10 L aliquot of the PEP product serves as a template for subsequent PCR reactions amplifying the mutation containing fragment, linked polymorphic markers, and for sex determination.

Degenerate Oligonucleotide Primed PCR

DOP-PCR is based on multiple rounds of extensions using a universal primer containing a 6 bp degenerate region representing all possible nucleotide combinations, flanked with GC-rich short sequence to improve hybridization to genomic DNA.

DOP–PCR reaction mixture in a final volume of 100 L contains 2.0 mM degenerated primers, 10 × PCR buffer (100 mM Tris-HCl pH 8.3, 25 mM $MgCl_2$, and 500 mM KCl). However, the buffer should be K^+ free if the cell was lysed by alkaline lysis buffer). Thermal cycling conditions are as follows: prolonged initial denaturation step at 94°C for nine minutes, then eight cycles of denaturation at 94°C for 1 minute, annealing at 30°C for 1.5 minutes, and extension at 72°C for three minutes, followed by 50 cycles of denaturation at 94°C for one minute, annealing at 62°C for one minute, and extension at 72°C for one and one-half minutes. Final extension at 72°C for eight minutes (24). As for PEP, amplification efficiency may be improved by adding and changing the reaction ingredients and by gradually increasing the extension time after the first 10 cycles.

Multiple Displacement Amplification

MDA is based on DNA amplification using a bacteriophage DNA polymerase and exonuclease-resistant phosphorothioate-modified random hexamer oligonucleotide primers in an isothermal strand displacement reaction. It is achieved using bacteriophage Φ29 DNA polymerase, hexamers primers, and reaction buffer, according to the manufacturer's instructions (GenomiPhi v2 DNA Amplification Kit, GE Healthcare or Repli-G kit, Qiagen, Crawley, UK). The samples are incubated at 30°C for two to six hours, followed by a 3–10 minute incubation at 65°C to inactivate the enzyme. Amplified products can undergo subsequent diverse analyses as CGH.

Fluorescent PCR

Fluorescent PCR is performed in a final volume of 25 L of 10× PCR buffer containing 15 mM $MgCl_2$ and 0.2 mM of each dNTP, and fluorescent-tagged primers at a final concentration of 0.05 mM. After a "hot-start," 0.6–1.5 U of Taq polymerase is added to the reaction mix. Initial denaturation is first performed at 95°C for 5 minutes, followed by 36 cycles of denaturation at 94°C for 60 seconds, annealing at 60°C for 60 seconds, and extension at 72°C for 60 seconds. The reaction completed with a final extension at 70°C for 10 minutes. Due to its high sensitivity, nested PCR is usually not necessary (19,83,97).

Restriction Enzyme Digestion

For each different restriction enzyme, different conditions such as buffer, temperature, and concentration are specified in the commercially available kits. Some PCR reagents may interfere with the digestion reaction. To avoid this, PCR products can be purified by absorption of the DNA fragments onto glass fibers in the presence of chaotropic salts, then washed and eluted with a low-salt buffer or water. The isolated fragment may then be subjected to the restriction enzyme and buffer, incubated for one to two hours at 37°C, resolved by electrophoresis on agarose or acrylamide gels.

Product Detection

Ethidium Bromide Gel Electrophoresis

An aliquot of the PCR products is applied to an agarose or acrylamide gel containing 0.05% ethidium bromide, and visualized under UV light. One lane is provided for a "DNA ladder" containing a mixture of DNA fragments of known sizes. This allows the determination of the size, presence, and a measure of quantity of the resulting fragments. This technique, however, is neither sensitive nor accurate because it does not detect PCR products if the amplification yield is low, nor does it allow distinguishing between alleles differing in length by a few base pairs.

GeneScan™

Following fluorescent PCR, size-separation is performed on an acrylamide gel or using a capillary method available in some sequencers. Fragment sizes are automatically determined for each PCR product. Each primer set is labeled with a different fluorescent marker therefore the products may be distinguished according to their specific emission wavelengths. The relative quantity of each PCR product may also be determined by the relative intensities of their fluorescence. Using a weight marker standard within each lane makes it possible to distinguish between products with a size difference of as little as 1–2 bp. The results are demonstrated as a diagram with colored peaks (16,19).

REFERENCES

1. Handyside AH, Kontogianni EH, Hardy K, Winston RM. Pregnancies from biopsied human preimplantation embryos sexed by Y-specific DNA amplification. Nature 1990; 344: 768–70.
2. Kastrinos F, Stoffel EM, Balmaña J, Syngal S. Attitudes toward prenatal genetic testing in patients with familial adenomatous polyposis. Am J Gastroenterol 2007; 102: 1284–90.
3. Menon U, Harper J, Sharma A, et al. Views of BRCA gene mutation carriers on preimplantation genetic diagnosis as a reproductive option for hereditary breast and ovarian cancer. Hum Reprod 2007; 22: 1573–7.
4. Verlinsky Y, Rechitsky S, Schoolcraft W, Strom C, Kuliev A. Preimplantation diagnosis for Fanconi anemia combined with HLA matching. JAMA 2001; 285: 3130–3.
5. Traversa MV, Carey L, Leigh D. A molecular strategy for routine preimplantation genetic diagnosis in both reciprocal and Robertsonian translocation carriers. Mol Hum Reprod 2010; 16: 329–37.
6. Alfarawati S, Fragouli E, Colls P, Wells D. First births after preimplantation genetic diagnosis of structural chromosome abnormalities using comparative genomic hybridization and microarray analysis. Hum Reprod 2011; 26: 1560–74.
7. Saiki RK, Gelfand DH, Stoffel S, et al. Primer-directed enzymatic amplification of DNA with a thermostable DNA polymerase. Science 1988; 239: 487–91.
8. Saiki RK, Scharf S, Faloona F, et al. Enzymatic amplification of beta-globin genomic sequences and restriction

site analysis for diagnosis of sickle cell anemia. Science 1985; 230: 1350–4.
9. Navidi W, Arenhim N. Using PCR in preimplantation genetic disease diagnosis. Hum Reprod 1991; 6: 836–48.
10. Kontogianni EH, Griffin DK, Handyside AH. Identifying the sex of human preimplantation embryos in X-linked disease: amplification efficiency of a Y-specific alphoid repeat from single blastomeres with two lysis protocols. J Assist Reprod Genet 1996; 13: 125–32.
11. Sermon K, Lissens W, Nagy ZP, Van Steirteghem A, Liebaers I. Simultaneous amplification of the two most frequent mutations of infantile Tay-Sachs disease in single blastomeres. Hum Reprod 1995; 10: 2214–17.
12. Cui KH, Matthews CD. Nuclear structural conditions and PCR amplification in human preimplantation diagnosis. Mol Hum Reprod 1996; 2: 63–71.
13. Ray PF, Ao A, Taylor DM, Winston RM, Handyside AH. Assessment of the reliability of single blastomere analysis for preimplantation diagnosis of the delta F508 deletion causing cystic fibrosis in clinical practice. Prenat Diagn 1998; 18: 1402–12.
14. Grifo JA, Tang YX, Munne S, et al. Healthy deliveries from biopsied human embryos. Hum Reprod 1994; 9: 912–16.
15. Ao A, Wells D, Handyside AH, Winston RM, Delhanty JD. Preimplantation genetic diagnosis of inherited cancer: familial adenomatous polyposis coli. J Assist Reprod Genet 1998; 15: 140–4.
16. Findlay I, Ray P, Quirke P, Rutherford A, Lilford R. Allelic drop-out and preferential amplification in single cells and human blastomeres: implications for preimplantation diagnosis of sex and cystic fibrosis. Hum Reprod 1995; 10: 1609–18.
17. Ray PF, Handyside AH. PCR from single cells for preimplantation diagnosis. In: Elles R, ed. Methods in Molecular Biology: Molecular Diagnosis of Genetic Disease. New Jersey, USA: Humana Press Inc, 1996.
18. Rechitsky S, Strom C, Verlinsky O, et al. Allele dropout in polar bodies and blastomeres. J Assist Reprod Genet 1998; 15: 253–7.
19. Sherlock J, Cirigliano V, Petrou M, Tutschek B, Adinolfi M. Assessment of diagnostic quantitative fluorescent multiplex polymerase chain reaction assays performed on single cells. Ann Hum Genet 1998; 62: 9–23.
20. Dreesen JC, Bras M, de Die-Smulders C, et al. Preimplantation genetic diagnosis of spinal muscular atrophy. Mol Hum Reprod 1998; 4: 881–5.
21. El-Hashemite N, Delhanty JD. A technique for eliminating allele specific amplification failure during DNA amplification of heterozygous cells for preimplantation diagnosis. Mol Hum Reprod 1997; 3: 975–8.
22. Harper JC, Coonen E, Handyside AH, et al. Mosaicism of autosomes and sex chromosomes in morphologically normal, monospermic preimplantation human embryos. Prenat Diagn 1995; 15: 41–9.
23. Sermon K, De Vos A, Van de Velde H, et al. Fluorescent PCR and automated fragment analysis for the clinical application of preimplantation genetic diagnosis of myotonic dystrophy (Steinert's disease). Mol Hum Reprod 1998; 4: 791–6.
24. Wells D, Sherlock JK. Strategies for preimplantation genetic diagnosis of single gene disorders by DNA amplification. Prenat Diagn 1998; 18: 1389–401.
25. Eggerding FA. A one-step coupled amplification and oligonucleotide ligation procedure for multiplex genetic typing. PCR Methods Appl 1995; 4: 337–45.
26. Malcov M, Naiman T, Yosef DB, et al. Preimplantation genetic diagnosis for fragile X syndrome using multiplex nested PCR. Reprod Biomed Online 2007; 14: 515–21.
27. Blake D, Tan SL, Ao A. Assessment of multiplex fluorescent PCR for screening single cells for trisomy 21 and single gene defects. Mol Hum Reprod 1999; 5: 1166–75.
28. Kuliev A, Rechitsky S, Verlinsky O, et al. Preimplantation diagnosis of thalassemias. J Assist Reprod Genet 1998; 15: 219–25.
29. Fragouli E. Preimplantation genetic diagnosis: present and future. J Assist Reprod Genet 2007; 24: 201–7.
30. Wells D. Advances in preimplantation genetic diagnosis. Eur J Obstet Gynecol Reprod Biol 2004; 115: S97–101.
31. Xu K, Shi ZM, Veeck LL, Hughes MR, Rosenwaks Z. First unaffected pregnancy using preimplantation genetic diagnosis for sickle cell anemia. JAMA 1999; 281: 1701–6.
32. Findlay I, Mathews P, Quirke P. Preimplantation genetic diagnosis using fluorescent polymerase chain reaction: results and future developments. J Assist Reprod Genet 1999; 16: 199–206.
33. Hattori M, Yoshioka K, Sakaki Y. High-sensitive fluorescent DNA sequencing and its application for detection and mass-screening of point mutations. Electrophoresis 1992; 13: 560–5.
34. Mansfield ES. Diagnosis of Down syndrome and other aneuploidies using quantitative polymerase chain reaction and small tandem repeat polymorphisms. Hum Mol Genet 1993; 2: 43–50.
35. Ferre F. Quantitative or semi-quantitative PCR: reality versus myth. PCR Methods Appl 1992; 2: 1–9.
36. Pinkel D, Straume T, Gray JW. Cytogenetic analysis using quantitative, high-sensitivity, fluorescence hybridization. Proc Natl Acad Sci USA 1986; 83: 2934–8.
37. Verma L, Macdonald F, Leedham P, et al. Rapid and simple prenatal DNA diagnosis of Down's syndrome. Lancet 1998; 352: 9–12.
38. Zhang L, Cui X, Schmitt K, et al. Whole genome amplification from a single cell: implications for genetic analysis. Proc Natl Acad Sci USA 1992; 89: 5847–51.
39. Paunio T, Reima I, Syvanen AC. Preimplantation diagnosis by whole-genome amplification, PCR amplification, and solid-phase minisequencing of blastomere DNA. Clin Chem 1996; 42: 1382–90.
40. Sermon K, Lissens W, Joris H, Van Steirteghem A, Liebaers I. Adaptation of the primer extension preamplification (PEP) reaction for preimplantation diagnosis: single blastomere analysis using short PEP protocols. Mol Hum Reprod 1996; 2: 209–12.
41. Tsai YH. Cost-effective one-step PCR amplification of cystic fibrosis delta F508 fragment in a single cell for preimplantation genetic diagnosis. Prenat Diagn 1999; 19: 1048–51.
42. Kristjansson K, Chong SS, Van den Veyver IB, et al. Preimplantation single cell analyses of dystrophin gene deletions using whole genome amplification. Nat Genet 1994; 6: 19–23.
43. Snabes MC, Chong SS, Subramanian SB, et al. Preimplantation single-cell analysis of multiple genetic loci by whole-genome amplification. Proc Natl Acad Sci USA 1994; 91: 6181–5.
44. Telenius H, Pelmear AH, Tunnacliffe A, et al. Cytogenetic analysis by chromosome painting using DOP-PCR

amplified flow-sorted chromosomes. Genes Chromosomes Cancer 1992; 4: 257–63.
45. Voullaire L, Wilton L, Slater H, Williamson R. Detection of aneuploidy in single cells using comparative genomic hybridization. Prenat Diagn 1999; 19: 846–51.
46. He ZY, Liu HC, Mele CA, et al. Recycling of a single human blastomere fixed on a microscopic slide for sexing and diagnosis of specific mutations by various types of polymerase chain reaction. Fertil Steril 1999; 72: 341–8.
47. Dean FB, Hosono S, Fang L, et al. Comprehensive human genome amplification using multiple displacement amplification. Proc Natl Acad Sci USA 2002; 99: 5261–6.
48. Spits C, Le Caignec C, De Rycke M, et al. Whole-genome multiple displacement amplification from single cells. Nat Protoc 2006; 1: 1965–70.
49. Lage JM, Leamon JH, Pejovic T, et al. Whole genome analysis of genetic alterations in small DNA samples using hyperbranched strand displacement amplification and array-CGH. Genome Res 2003; 13: 294–307.
50. Hughes S, Lim G, Beheshti B, et al. Use of whole genome amplification and comparative genomic hybridisation to detect chromosomal copy number alterations in cell line material and tumour tissue. Cytogenet Genome Res 2004; 105: 18–24.
51. Cheung VG, Nelson SF. Whole genome amplification using a degenerate oligonucleotide primer allows hundreds of genotypes to be performed on less than one nanogram of genomic DNA. Proc Natl Acad Sci USA 1996; 93: 14676–9.
52. Telenius H, Carter NP, Bebb CE, et al. Degenerate oligonucleotide-primed PCR: general amplification of target DNA by a single degenerate primer. Genomics 1992; 13: 718–25.
53. Coskun S, Alsmadi O. Whole genome amplification from a single cell: a new era for preimplantation genetic diagnosis. Prenat Diagn 2007; 27: 297–302.
54. Blanco L, Bernad A, Lazaro JM, et al. Highly efficient DNA synthesis by the phage phi 29 DNA polymerase. Symmetrical mode of DNA replication. J Biol Chem 1989; 264: 8935–40.
55. Rodríguez I, Lázaro JM, Blanco L, et al. A specific subdomain in phi29 DNA polymerase confers both processivity and strand-displacement capacity. Proc Natl Acad Sci USA 2005; 102: 6407–12.
56. Hellani A, Coskun S, Benkhalifa M, et al. Multiple displacement amplification on single cell and possible PGD applications. Mol Hum Reprod 2004; 10: 847–52.
57. Handyside AH, Robinson MD, Simpson RJ, et al. Isothermal whole genome amplification from single and small numbers of cells: a new era for preimplantation genetic diagnosis of inherited disease. Mol Hum Reprod 2004; 10: 767–72.
58. Renwick PJ, Trussler J, Ostad-Saffari E, et al. Proof of principle and first cases using preimplantation genetic haplotyping–a paradigm shift for embryo diagnosis. Reprod Biomed Online 2006; 13: 110–19.
59. Pickering SJ, McConnell JM, Johnson MH, Braude PR. Use of a polymorphic dinucleotide repeat sequence to detect non-blastomeric contamination of the polymerase chain reaction in biopsy samples for preimplantation diagnosis. Hum Reprod 1994; 9: 1539–45.
60. Harton GL, Tsipouras P, Sisson ME, et al. Preimplantation genetic testing for Marfan syndrome. Mol Hum Reprod 1996; 2: 713–15.
61. Lee SH, Kwak IP, Cha KE, et al. Preimplantation diagnosis of non-deletion Duchenne muscular dystrophy (DMD) by linkage polymerase chain reaction analysis. Mol Hum Reprod 1998; 4: 345–9.
62. Sermon K, Lissens W, Joris H, et al. Clinical application of preimplantation diagnosis for myotonic dystrophy. Prenat Diagn 1997; 17: 925–32.
63. Daniels R, Holding C, Kontogianni E, Monk M. Single-cell analysis of unstable genes. J Assist Reprod Genet 1996; 13: 163–9.
64. El-Hashemite N, Wells D, Delhanty JD. Single cell detection of beta-thalassaemia mutations using silver stained SSCP analysis: an application for preimplantation diagnosis. Mol Hum Reprod 1997; 3: 693–8.
65. Kanavakis E, Vrettou C, Palmer G, et al. Preimplantation genetic diagnosis in 10 couples at risk for transmitting beta-thalassaemia major: clinical experience including the initiation of six singleton pregnancies. Prenat Diagn 1999; 19: 1217–22.
66. Vrettou C, Palmer G, Kanavakis E, et al. A widely applicable strategy for single cell genotyping of beta-thalassaemia mutations using DGGE analysis: application to preimplantation genetic diagnosis. Prenat Diagn 1999; 19: 1209–16.
67. Scobie G, Woodroffe B, Fishel S, Kalsheker N. Identification of the five most common cystic fibrosis mutations in single cells using a rapid and specific differential amplification system. Mol Hum Reprod 1996; 2: 203–7.
68. Bermudez MG, Piyamongkol W, Tomaz S, et al. Single-cell sequencing and mini-sequencing for preimplantation genetic diagnosis. Prenat Diagn 2003; 23: 669–77.
69. Chandley AC. Infertility and chromosome abnormality. Oxf Rev Reprod Biol 1984; 6: 1–46; Review.
70. Hassold T, Chen N, Funkhouser J, et al. A cytogenetic study of 1000 spontaneous abortions. Ann Hum Genet 1980; 44: 151–78.
71. Jacobs PA. The chromosome complement of human gametes. Oxf Rev Reprod Biol 1992; 14: 47–72.
72. Kallioniemi A, Kallioniemi OP, Sudar D, et al. Comparative genomic hybridization for molecular cytogenetic analysis of solid tumors. Science 1992; 258: 818–21.
73. Voullaire L, Slater H, Williamson R, Wilton L. Chromosome analysis of blastomeres from human embryos by using comparative genomic hybridization. Hum Genet 2000; 106: 210–17.
74. Wells D, Delhanty JD. Comprehensive chromosomal analysis of human preimplantation embryos using whole genome amplification and single cell comparative genomic hybridization. Mol Hum Reprod 2000; 6: 1055–62.
75. Wilton L, Williamson R, McBain J, Edgar D, Voullaire L. Birth of a healthy infant after preimplantation confirmation of euploidy by comparative genomic hybridization. N Engl J Med 2001; 345: 1537–41.
76. Fragouli E, Wells D, Thornhill A, et al. Comparative genomic hybridization analysis of human oocytes and polar bodies. Hum Reprod 2006; 21: 2319–28.
77. Wells D, Escudero T, Levy B, et al. First clinical application of comparative genomic hybridization and polar body testing for preimplantation genetic diagnosis of aneuploidy. Fertil Steril 2002; 78: 543–9.
78. Le Caignec C, Spits C, Sermon K, et al. Single-cell chromosomal imbalances detection by array CGH. Nucleic Acids Res 2006; 34: e68.

79. Wilton L. Preimplantation genetic diagnosis and chromosome analysis of blastomeres using comparative genomic hybridization. Hum Reprod Update 2005; 11: 33–41.
80. Bejjani BA, Shaffer LG. Application of array-based comparative genomic hybridization to clinical diagnostics. J Mol Diagn 2006; 8: 528–33.
81. Pinkel D, Segraves R, Sudar D, et al. High resolution analysis of DNA copy number variation using comparative genomic hybridization to microarrays. Nat Genet 1998; 20: 207–11.
82. Hu DG, Webb G, Hussey N. Aneuploidy detection in single cells using DNA array-based comparative genomic hybridization. Mol Hum Reprod 2004; 10: 283–9.
83. Findlay I, Quirke P, Hall J, Rutherford A. Fluorescent PCR: a new technique for PGD of sex and single-gene defects. J Assist Reprod Genet 1996; 13: 96–103.
84. Findlay I, Lilford R. Sources and detection of contamination in preimplantation diagnosis. Proceedings of the XII Annual Scientific Meeting of the Fertility Society of Australia, 1994: 101.
85. Holding C, Bentley D, Roberts R, Bobrow M, Mathew C. Development and validation of laboratory procedures for preimplantation diagnosis of Duchenne muscular dystrophy. J Med Genet 1993; 30: 903–9.
86. Ioulianos A, Wells D, Harper JC, Delhanty JD. A successful strategy for preimplantation diagnosis of medium-chain acyl-CoA dehydrogenase (MCAD) deficiency. Prenat Diagn 2000; 20: 593–8.
87. Hussey ND, Donggui H, Froiland DA, et al. Analysis of five Duchenne muscular dystrophy exons and gender determination using conventional duplex polymerase chain reaction on single cells. Mol Hum Reprod 1999; 5: 1089–94.
88. Ventura M, Gibaud A, Le Pendu J, et al. Use of a simple method for the Epstein-Barr virus transformation of lymphocytes from members of large families of Réunion Island. Hum Hered 1988; 38: 36–43.
89. Van de Velde H, Sermon K, De Vos A, et al. Fluorescent PCR and automated fragment analysis in preimplantation genetic diagnosis for 21-hydroxylase deficiency in congenital adrenal hyperplasia. Mol Hum Reprod 1999; 5: 691–6.
90. Ao A, Handyside AH. Cleavage stage human embryo biopsy. Hum Reprod Update 1995; 1: 3.
91. Salido EC, Yen PH, Koprivinkar K, Yu LC, Shapiro LJ. The human enamel protein gene amelogenin is expressed from both X and Y chromosomes. Am J Hum Genet 1992; 50: 303–16.
92. Ao A, Ray P, Harper J, et al. Clinical experience with preimplantation genetic diagnosis of cystic fibrosis (delta F508). Prenat Diagn 1996; 16: 137–42.
93. Cui XF, Li HH, Goradia TM, et al. Single-sperm typing: determination of genetic distance between the G gamma-globin and parathyroid hormone loci by using the polymerase chain reaction and allele-specific oligomers. Proc Natl Acad Sci USA 1989; 86: 9389–93.
94. Han S, Zhong XY, Troeger C, et al. Current application of single-cell PCR. Cell Mul Life Sci 2000; 57: 96–105.
95. Cui KH, Haan EA, Wang LJ, Matthews CD. Optimal polymerase chain reaction amplification for preimplantation diagnosis in cystic fibrosis (delta F508). BMJ 1995; 311: 536–40.
96. Wells D, Sherlock JK, Handyside AH, Delhanty JD. Detailed chromosomal and molecular genetic analysis of single cells by whole genome amplification and comparative genomic hybridization. Nucleic Acids Res 1999; 27: 1214–18.
97. Findlay I, Quirke P. Fluorescent polymerase chain reaction: Part I. A new method allowing genetic diagnosis and DNA fingerprinting of single cells. Human Reprod Update 1996a; 2: 137–52.

29

The analysis of endometrial receptivity

Tamara Garrido-Gomez, Francisco Domínguez, Maria Ruiz, Felip Vilella, and Carlos Simon

INTRODUCTION

The human endometrium is a complex, multicellular tissue that is primarily regulated by steroid hormones [estrogens (E), progesterone (P), androgens, and glucocorticoids]. Endometrial receptivity is a self-limited period in which the endometrium acquires a functional and transient ovarian steroid-dependent status that allows a blastocyst to attach to the endometrial epithelium and to invade further into the decidualized stroma through mediation by immune cells, cytokines, growth factors, chemokines, and adhesion molecules (1–3). This specific period, known as the window of implantation (WOI), opens five days after endogenous or exogenous progesterone action and closes two days later (4,5).

Despite increasing interest in regulation of endometrial receptivity in recent years, the role of the endometrium in successful implantation remains a challenge. During the WOI, the endometrium displays a receptive phenotype which, at the morphological level, implies that endometrial epithelial cells undergo plasma membrane transformation (6). Pinopodes are formed during this period and they have been proposed to be morphological markers of the receptive status (7), although their functional role is questionable (8). Using the single molecule approach, a myriad of biochemical markers has been proposed, ranging from cytokines and their receptors (9), adhesion molecules and their receptors, to cyclins (10–12), and classical hormonal receptors (13–15) although none of them has been clinically consolidated as diagnostic tools (15).

The application of new techniques, such as genomics, proteomics, and secretomics, and the interrogation of the vast amount of data obtained with complex bioinformatics have led to a new understanding of endometrial receptivity and its relation to infertility treatment.

In this chapter, we will analyze the transcriptomics of human endometrial receptivity and will place emphasis on its clinical translation by means of the endometrial receptivity array (ERA) test. In the second part, we will focus on the proteomics of human receptivity, first the endometrium with special attention paid to annexin A2, C98, and CD147, and then the development of noninvasive biomarkers of endometrial receptivity in endometrial fluid.

TRANSCRIPTOMICS OF ENDOMETRIAL RECEPTIVITY

The transcriptome reflects the genes that are being actively expressed at any given time in a specific cell population. Gene expression is the most fundamental level at which the genotype gives rise to the phenotype. The genetic code stored in DNA is "interpreted" by gene expression, and the properties of this expression give rise to the organism's phenotype.

The study of endometrial *transcriptomics*, also referred to as expression profiling, examines the mRNAs levels in the endometrium throughout the menstrual cycle using high-throughput techniques based on DNA microarray technology. In the last decade, this development has favored research to reveal the existence of specific expression profiles relating to the different menstrual cycle phases (Table 29.1). This finding initiated the possibility of classifying the molecular status of the endometrium according to its transcriptomic profile (16,17) in an attempt to overcome the problems of subjectivity that produce the inter- and intracycle variations of endometrial dating.

This transcriptomic signature has been investigated in multiple studies by using gene expression arrays and by comparing endometrial biopsies taken at the WOI (Table 29.1). One of the pioneer publications of our group (Riesewijk et al. (18)) compared the gene expression profiles of pre-receptive (LH + 2) versus receptive (LH + 7) endometrium obtained from the same fertile woman. We found 211 genes to be differentially expressed between both groups of samples (some of them previously related with receptiveness). Other works have focused on endometrial gene expression profiling, but they differ in experimental design terms (19–23). The results of these works vary, except for one gene which is consistently upregulated in them all: osteopontin. However, the list of consensus genes increases when we reduce the works compared. In this case, there are several important molecules which have been highlighted such as proteins previously identified in the endometrium, genes involved in lipid metabolism, immune response, and regulation of cell cycle, ion binding, and enzymes (24). All these data are complementary because the variability among them is due to the differences in experimental designs (pooling

Table 29.1 Summary of Studies Performed in Human Endometrium Using Microarray Analysis

Process studied	Microarray	Company	Number of gene targets	Study
Decidualization	Clontech	Atlas array Stanford University	588	Popovici et al. (2000) (99)
Decidualization	Incyte human GEM-V	Incyte Genomics	6918	Brar et al. (2001) (100)
Endometrial cancer	Hu6800	Affymetrix	6000	Mutter et al. (2001) (101)
WOI	HG-U95A	Affymetrix	12,686	Carson et al. (2002) (19)
Endometriosis	Human genes GeneFilter GF211	Research Genetics	4133	Eyster et al. (2002) (102)
WOI	HG-U95A	Affymetrix	12,686	Kao et al. (2002) (20)
Endometriosis	Atlas human cDNA expression Array	Clontech	597	Lebovic et al. (2002) (103)
Endometriosis	Home-made	University of Tokyo	23,040	Arimoto et al. (2003) (104)
WOI	HG-U95A-E	Affymetrix	>60,000	Borthwick et al. (2003) (21)
RU486	Home-made	University of Cambridge	~1000	Catalano et al. (2003) (105)
WOI	Human cytokine expression array	R&D Systems	375	Domínguez et al. (2003) (106)
Endometriosis	HG-U95A	Affymetrix	12,686	Kao et al. (2003) (86)
Endometrial cancer	Oncochip	Centro Nacional de Investigaciones Oncológicas	6386	Moreno-Bueno et al. (2003) (107)
Progesterone effect	Human Chip 1K set 1	Takara Shuzo	1000	Okada et al. (2003) (108)
WOI	HG-U95A	Affymetrix	12,686	Riesewijk et al. (2003) (18)
Endometrial cancer	Home-made	National Cancer Institute	9984	Risinger et al. (2003) (109)
Decidualization	HG-U95A	Affymetrix	12,686	Tierney et al. (2003) (110)
Endometrial cancer	GEMarray clones	Incyte Genomics	18,098	Cao et al. (2004) (111)
Endometrial cancer	HG-U133A	Affymetrix	>22,000	Ferguson et al. (2004) (112)
Endometriosis	Atlas human 1.2 cDNA expression array	Clontech	1176	Matsuzaki et al. (2004) (113)
Stimulated cycles	HG-U95Av2	Affymetrix	12,686	Mirkin et al. (2004) (30)
Menstrual cycle	Home-made	Peter MacCallum Cancer Institute	10,000	Ponnampalam et al. (2004) (16)
Endometrial cancer	Home-made	University of Cambridge	1056	Saidi et al. (2004) (114)
In vitro models	1-cDNA Array	Agilent	12,814	Barbier et al. (2005) (115)
Endometrial cancer	HG-U133A	Affymetrix	>22,000	Ferguson et al. (2005) (116)
Stimulated cycles	HG-U133A	Affymetrix	>22,000	Horcajadas et al. (2005) (27)
In vitro models	HG-U133A 2.0	Affymetrix	18,400	Krikun et al. (2005) (117)
Endometriosis	Atlas human 1.2 cDNA expression array	Clontech	1176	Matsuzaki et al. (2005) (118)
Endometrial cancer	HG-U133A – U133B	Affymetrix	>22,000	Maxwell et al. (2005) (119)
WOI	HG-U95Av2	Affymetrix	12,686	Mirkin et al. (2005) (22)
Menstrual cycle	HG-U133A	Affymetrix	>22,000	Punyadeera et al. (2005) (120)
In vitro models	Home-made	University of Cambridge	>15,000	Rossi et al. (2005) (121)
RU486	Home-made	University of Cambridge	>15,000	Sharkey et al. (2005) (122)
Stimulated cycles	HG-U133A	Affymetrix	>22,000	Simón et al. (2005) (123)
Menstrual cycle	HG-U133 Plus 2.0	Affymetrix	>47,000	Talbi et al. (2005) (124)
In vitro models	Home-made	University of Cambridge	>15,000	White et al. (2005) (125)
Proliferative phase	BD Atlas nylon cDNA expression array	BD Biosciences Clontech	588	Yanahiara et al. (2005) (126)
Endometrial cancer	Human Unigen1	Incyte Genomics	9600	Gielen et al. (2006) (127)
Endometriosis	HG-U133 Plus 2.0	Affymetrix	>47,000	Hever et al. (2006) (128)
IUD	Home-made	University of Cambridge	>16,000	Horcajadas et al. (2006) (33)
In vitro models	HG-U133 Plus 2.0	Affymetrix	>47,000	Huang et al. (2006) (129)
Endometrial cancer	UniGEM V cDNA microarray	Incyte Genomics	7800	Matsumura et al. (2006) (130)
In vitro models	HG-U133 Plus 2.0	Affymetrix	>47,000	Sarno et al. (2006) (131)
Endometriosis	Home-made	Medical College of Wisconsin	9600	Wu et al. (2006) (132)
Endometrial cancer	HG-U133A – U133B	Affymetrix	>22,000	Dainty et al. (2007) (133)

(Continued)

Table 29.1 Summary of Studies Performed in Human Endometrium Using Microarray Analysis (Continued)

Process studied	Microarray	Company	Number of gene targets	Study
Endometriosis	CodeLink Whole Human Genome Bioarrays	GE-Amersham Biosciences	45,674	Eyster et al. (2007) (134)
WOI	Home-made	University of Cambridge	>16,000	Feroze-Zaidi et al. (2007) (135)
In vitro models	HG-U133 Plus 2.0	Affymetrix	>47,000	Gielen et al. (2007) (136)
Endometriosis	Atlas human 1.2 Array	Clontech	1176	Mettler et al. (2007) (137)
Endometriosis	miRNA Bioarray	Ambion	287	Pan et al. (2007) (138)
Endometrial cancer	35K Human oligo microarray	Norwegian Microarray Consortium	24,650	Paulssen et al. (2008) (139)
Endometriosis	HG-U133A 2.0	Affymetrix	14,500	Van Langendonckt et al. (2007) (140)
Endometrial cancer	HG-U133 Plus 2.0	Affymetrix	>47,000	Wong et al. (2007) (141)
Pregnancy	HG-U133A 2.0	Affymetrix	14,500	Bersinger et al. (2008) (142)
Menstrual cycle	Sentrix Human Illumina 6V1 Expression Bead chip	Illumina	>47,000	Cloke et al. (2008) (143)
Pregnancy	HG-U133 Plus 2.0	Affymetrix	>47,000	Evans et al. (2008) (144)
Signaling	HG-U133 Plus 2.0	Affymetrix	>47,000	Gielen et al. (2008) (145)
Endometrial cancer	Cancer profiling array	Clontech	241	Hamm et al. (2008) (146)
Stimulated cycles	HG-U133A	Affymetrix	>22,000	Horcajadas et al. (2008) (147)
Decidualization	HG-U133 Plus 2.0	Affymetrix	>47,000	Horne et al. (2008) (148)
Endometriosis	HG-U95Av2	Affymetrix	12,686	Hull et al. (2008) (149)
Stimulated cycles	HG-U133A	Affymetrix	>22,000	Liu et al. (2008) (150)
Menstrual cycle	HG-U133 Plus 2.0	Affymetrix	>47,000	Lu et al. (2008) (151)
Menstrual cycle	HG-U133 Plus 2.0	Affymetrix	>47,000	Macklon et al. (2008) (152)
Pregnancy	HG-U133 Plus 2.0	Affymetrix	>47,000	Savaris et al. (2008) (153)
Endometriosis	Home-made	University of Cambridge	22,000	Sherwin et al. (2008) (154)
WOI	Home-made	National Cancer Institute	9128	Tapia et al. (2008) (155)
Stimulated cycles	HG-U133 Plus 2.0	Affymetrix	>47,000	Zhou et al. (2008) (156)
Menstrual cycle	HG-U133A	Affymetrix	>22,000	Ball et al. (2009) (157)
Paracrine effects	Home-made	University of Cambridge	>15,000	Germeyer et al. (2009) (158)
WOI	HG-U133 Plus 2.0	Affymetrix	>47,000	Haouzi et al. (2009) (23)
Stimulated cycles	HG-U133 Plus 2.0	Affymetrix	>47,000	Van Vaerenbergh et al. (2009) (159)
Adenomyosis	HG-U133 Plus 2.0	Affymetrix	>47,000	Chen et al. (2010) (160)
WOI	Whole Human Genome Oligo Microarray	Agilent	>40,000	Labarta et al. (2011) (35)

All the gene information from these studies are available at http://www.endometrialdatabase.com.

or not pooling the isolated RNA, sample size, data analysis, statistical methods, sampling time during the cycle, type of microarrays used, and patient inclusion criteria) (23,25,26).

An interesting approach is the comparative investigation on the gene expression profile between natural and controlled ovarian stimulation cycles (27–32). Even the impact of agonist versus antagonist on the endometrial gene profile (30–32) has been investigated. Moreover, the gene expression profiling of the refractory endometrium induced by an intra uterine device (IUD) has also been addressed (33), and the same may be said of the effect of a pathological condition such as obesity (34) or the presence of high progesterone levels (>1.2 ng/mL) at the end of the follicular phase on controlled ovarian stimulation (35). Recently, the comparative genomic profile of fertile women versus those with unexplained infertility has been published (36).

All these studies have demonstrated the existence of different gene expression profiles related to the phase of the menstrual cycle and therefore hormonally regulated (26). Because of this, in recent years, functional genomics of endometrial receptivity has been widely investigated to find transcriptomic markers of receptiveness during the WOI with a view to employing them as molecular tools for the molecular diagnosis of endometrial receptivity (23,37,38). This new advance would imply the substitution of other biochemical and morphological markers whose effectiveness has been questioned (25,39,40).

The ERA is a customized array that describes the transcriptomic signature of receptivity or non-receptivity of the human endometrium during the WOI (41). In order to design this diagnostic tool, all the available studies were analyzed and a study was designed to differentially analyze the expression profile of endometrial samples taken during the secretory phase (LH + 1, +3, +5, +7). From the

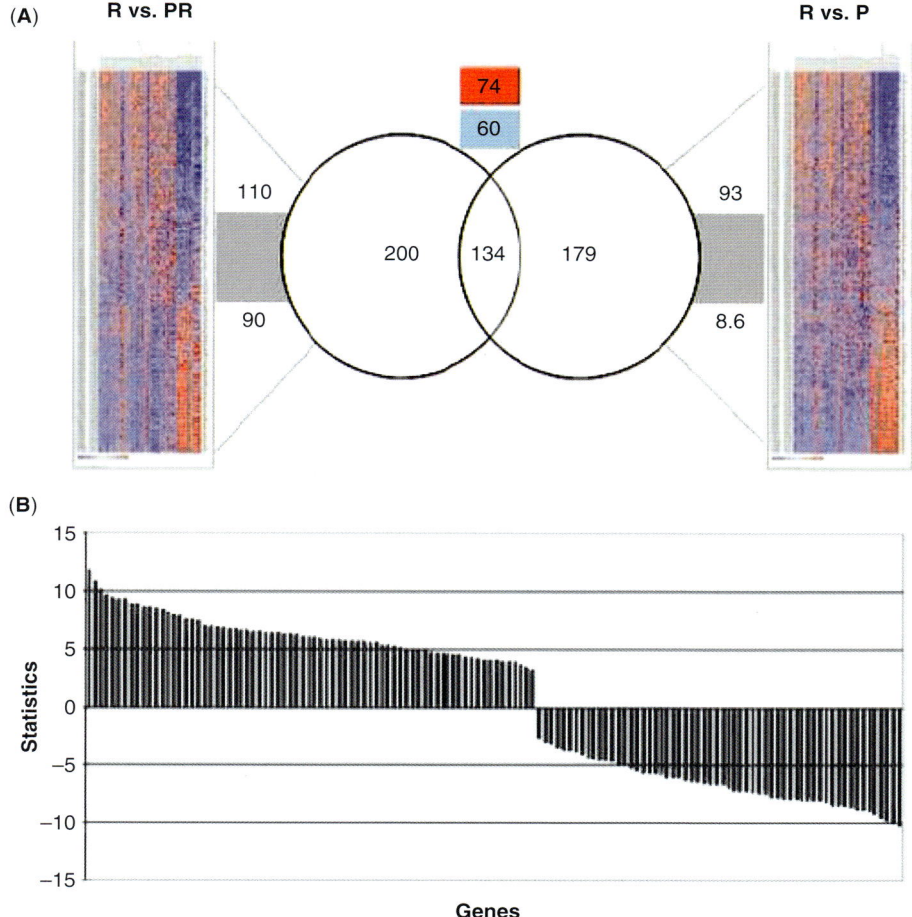

Figure 29.1 Endometrial receptivity transcriptomic signature. (**A**) Gene selection: intersection among 578 genes statistically significant in Receptive versus Pre-receptive (R vs. PR) and Receptive versus Proliferative (R vs. P). Number of genes up- and downregulated in each 579 comparison and in the intersection is indicated. (**B**) T-statistic average for the 134 genes of the 580 endometrial receptivity signature (74 up- and 60 downregulated).

data obtained, 238 genes with differential expressions (fold change >3; and false discovery rate <0.05) were selected. Three statistical approaches were followed: the union of the T-Rex gene list (GEPAS) and the SAM gene list intersected with the multitest gene list. Moreover, an informatics predictor was designed to analyze the data obtained with the array and to classify an endometrial sample as "Receptive" or "Non Receptive." Once the array and the predictor were designed, a cohort of samples taken in the pre-receptive phase (LH + 3, +5), the receptive phase (LH + 7) and the proliferative phase (days 8–12 of the menstrual cycle) were used to train the predictor and to define the transcriptomic signature. Of all the genes present in the customized array, 134 defined the transcriptomic signature of the receptive endometrium (Fig. 29.1). In this study (41), endometrial dating has attempted to classify an LH + 7 endometrium in transcriptomic terms with a specificity and sensitivity of 0.8857 and 0.99758, respectively. This diagnostic tool (array plus predictor) can be used clinically in reproductive medicine and gynecology since the transcriptomic signature has been shown to be a potential endometrial receptivity biomarker cluster. The ERA works by dating an endometrial biopsy at LH + 7 as "Receptive" (expression profile compatible for the WOI) or "Non Receptive" (expression profiles not compatible for the WOI). Currently, more than 150 clinical analyses have been carried out on patients with implantation failure, 65% of women with a "Receptive" result have become pregnant, and all the women (100%) who obtained a "Non–Receptive" result did not become pregnant. Moreover, the consistency of the results has been proven in alternative cycles. This tool is useful not only for clinical diagnosis, but also for research based on the analysis of variation in receptive expression profiles due to different treatment methods or conditions. An improved version of ERA2 is being prepared by concentrating efforts on the knowledge of genes and pathways relating to the nonreceptive profile.

PROTEOMICS OF ENDOMETRIAL RECEPTIVITY AND DECIDUALIZATION

Proteomics is often considered the next step in the study of biological systems (42). Unlike genomics, proteomics is a true reflection of cellular function. An initial attempt to identify differential protein markers between a proliferative and a secretory endometrium was published by De Souza et al. (43). This group employed the first quantitative approximation to assess the proteomic repertoire using isotope-coded affinity tags (ICAT), affinity purification, and liquid chromatography coupled online with mass spectrometry (LC-MS) between a proliferative and a secretory endometrium. Five proteins were found with significant differential expressions, where FRAT1 and the glutamate NMDA receptor subunit zeta 1 precursor were the most interesting. The utility of these proteins as biomarkers of endometrial receptivity still remains unknown.

Parmar et al. (44) published a prospective study by identifying the proteins with differential expression throughout the menstrual cycle. Image analysis software was used to compare the two-dimensional protein maps of midsecretory endometrial phase (MSE) versus maps of proliferative endometrium and midsecretory phase uterine fluids. Matrix-assisted laser desorption/ionization time of flight in tandem (MALDI-TOF-TOF) analysis revealed upregulation of calreticulin, the beta chain of fibrinogen, adenylate kinase isoenzyme 5, and transferrin in the proliferative endometrium and of annexin A5, annexin V, alpha1-antitrypsin, creatine kinase, and peroxidoxin 6 in MSE if compared with the other phase. The midsecretory-phase endometrial tissue 2D map was also compared with that of uterine fluid from the same phase to reveal the presence of heat-shock protein 27, transferrin, and alpha1-antitrypsin precursor in both endometrial tissues and uterine secretions.

Our group investigated the proteomics of endometrial receptivity by comparing the pre-receptive (LH + 2) versus the receptive (LH + 7) human endometrium proteome (45). For this purpose, endometrial biopsies obtained from the same fertile woman (n = 6) in the same menstrual cycle were used. Protein extracts were analyzed using two-dimensional fluorescence difference gel electrophoresis (2D-DIGE) and matrix-assisted laser desorption/ionization time-of-flight mass spectrometry (MALDI-TOF-MS). The results show 32 differentially expressed proteins in the receptive versus the pre-receptive endometrium, with 12 and 23 up- and downregulated spots, respectively. It is interesting to emphasize two of the most consistently and differentially expressed proteins: annexin A2 and stathmin 1. These cytoskeleton-related proteins display a consistent opposite regulation in the receptive versus the pre-receptive endometrium. This is not surprising since the endometrial receptive phenotype is associated with the remodeling of the epithelial organization, primarily as a result of the disruption of the cytoskeleton in response to an external stimulus (46). These proteins were tested functionally in an endometrial refractoriness model induced by inserting an IUD. Our results demonstrate that the staining pattern of these proteins was similar to the pre-receptive stage when an IUD was present. This evidence suggests that annexin A2 and stathmin 1 are functionally implied in endometrial receptivity. Therefore, both molecules could be important to predict the receptivity status and could be possible targets for interception (45). We are now investigating whether annexin A2 could be directly involved in the first stages of human embryo adhesion into the maternal endometrium using an in vitro model of adhesion to simulate the embryo implantation process.

Decidualization is a P-dependent event that occurs in the endometrial stroma and commences during the mid-late secretory phase immediately after the WOI closes (47). In humans, it is independent of the presence of a blastocyst in the uterine cavity. Decidualized stromal cells exhibit increased local production of proteins, including prolactin, insulin-like growth factor-binding protein-1, relaxin, and tissue factor (48–51) as well as local production of extracellular matrix proteins, including laminin and fibronectin (52).

Although previous studies have established that P plays a central role in regulating decidualization (53), the role of estradiol (E2) in this process has not received much attention. An earlier study showed that administration of P alone to ovariectomized mice sustained the decidual response, indicating a noncompulsory role of exogenous E in regulating this process (54). Conversely, it has been reported that administration of ICI 182780, an ER antagonist, severely impairs the formation of decidual tissue in mice, hinting that E acting via ER regulates this process (55).

Our group (56) investigated the proteome and secretome repertoire of decidualized in vitro cells. The proteomic analysis revealed 60 differentially expressed proteins (36 over- and 24 underexpressed) in decidualized versus control ESCs, including known decidualization markers (cathepsin B) and new biomarkers (transglutaminase 2, peroxiredoxin 4, and the ACTB protein). In the secretomic analysis, a total of 13 secreted proteins (11 up- and 2 downregulated) were identified, including well-recognized markers (IGFBP-1 and PRL) and novel ones (MPIF-1 and PECAM-1). These data were combined and integrated with complex bioinformatics to model the human decidualization interactome for the first time (Fig. 29.2).

C98 AND CD147 AS KEY MOLECULES IN ENDOMETRIAL RECEPTIVITY

Endometrial receptivity is probably not determined exclusively by the expression of selective adhesion molecules, and a series of cytoskeletal rearrangements are also likely to be important. Microvilli and specialized adhesive structures, such as endothelial docking structures, are enriched in tetraspanin microdomains (57). Tetraspanins are a group of hydrophobic proteins with four transmembrane domains and two extracellular loops. The association of tetraspanins with some integrins and other membrane proteins is well characterized (58). Mice deficient in tetraspanin CD9 display severely reduced fertility due to sperm–egg fusion defects (59–61); however, CD9's function in implantation remains undetermined. Different in vitro and ex vivo models and culture systems have been used to mimic endometrial receptivity and implantation

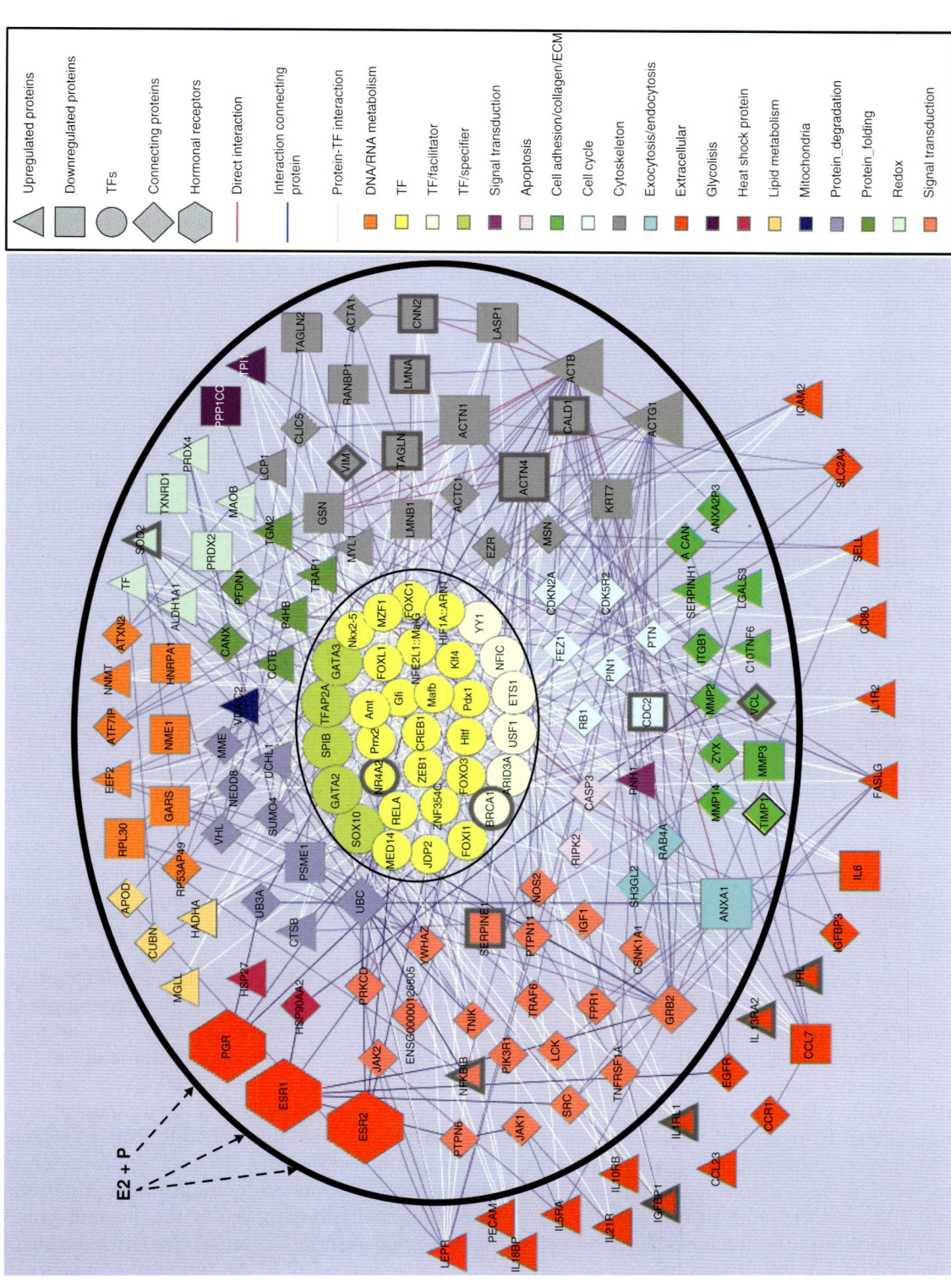

Figure 29.2 Model of the human decidual interactome. Decidualization interactome including the proteins detected in our study as differentially regulated, both intra- and extracellularly together with the information present in public databases and data repositories. Triangle, the significantly overexpressed proteins in our proteomic analysis. Squaring, the significantly under expressed proteins in our proteomic analysis. Circle, transcription factors. Rhombus, connecting proteins added to construct the interaction network. Pink line, direct interactions among the deregulated proteins found in our proteomic analysis. Blue line, indirect interactions among the deregulated proteins through connecting proteins. White line, interactions among the proteins and transcription factors. Proteins are classified into 19 different functional categories, indicated by different colors in the legend (cytoskeleton, redox, exocytosis/endocytosis, cell adhesion/collagen/ECM, protein folding, protein degradation, DNA/RNA metabolism, lipid metabolism, heat shock protein, glycolysis, mitochondria, extracellular, signal transduction, cell cycle, and angiogenesis). The remarked proteins correspond to the identified gene whose differential expression was observed at both the gene expression and protein levels. Source: Adapted from Ref. 56.

(62,63), ranging from the use of endometrial cell lines (64) or endometrium explants, (65) to artificial ex vivo uterus (66). Our group has employed two human endometrial cell lines distinguished by different adhesiveness. RL95–2 is a human epithelial cell line derived from a moderately differentiated endometrial adenocarcinoma (61,62) which exhibits a more pronounced adhesiveness than any other human endometrial epithelial cell line for trophoblast-derived cells (JAR cells) (63) and mouse blastocysts (64). HEC-1-A, in contrast, is only weakly adhesive, but exhibits a polarized distribution of integrins and a more epithelial morphology (64). Screening of these cell lines has identified the upregulated expression of CD98 and CD147 molecules in the high-receptivity cell line RL95–2. CD98 is a multifunctional type II glycoprotein involved in amino acid transport(65), cell fusion (66) and integrin-dependent spreading (67), whose gene deletion is embryonically lethal (68). CD147-deficient mice have implantation defects (69); however, the CD147 expression in humans is not that restricted to the WOI (70). We analyzed the expression of these molecules in the human endometrium throughout the menstrual cycle. Thus, CD9 and CD147 both occur in the luminal epithelium, while CD98 might function as a receptivity determinant since its expression is undetectable outside the WOI (Fig. 29.3). In contrast to what has been described in renal and intestinal epithelial cells (71,72), CD98 is polarized to the apical surface of endometrial epithelium by co-localizing at apical microvillae with tetraspanin CD9. CD98 has been shown to form molecular complexes with CD147 (73), β1 and β3 integrins (67), and ICAM-1 (71) in different cell types. This suggests that CD98 forms two independent complexes with CD147 and with tetraspanins. Insertion into tetraspanin-enriched microdomains might regulate CD98 polarity and an association with β3 integrin. Progesterone treatment did not significantly alter the plasma membrane expression of CD98, while exposure to 17-b-estradiol induced a significant increase of CD98 in primary endometrial cells (74). To directly assess whether CD98 is able to confer receptivity to the endometrial epithelium, cells of the poorly adhesive endometrial cell line HEC-1-A were transiently transfected with GFP-tagged constructs of different adhesion molecules. Mouse hatching blastocysts were allowed to adhere onto transfected endometrial monolayers, and the number of adhered blastocysts after 24 hours or 48 hours were analyzed. Overexpression of CD9 led to a significant increase in blastocyst adhesion, while siRNA and lentiviral infection with CD98 and CD9-specific shRNA was able to significantly reduce the blastocyst adhesion rate (74). Moreover, reducing CD98 plasma membrane expression levels by 30% had a clear inhibitory effect on blastocyst adhesion. An analysis of the role of endometrial CD98 in implantation in mice has not yet been reported since the gene deletion of CD98 is embryonically lethal (68). Mating of heterozygous animals showed empty decidual swellings, indicative of resorption after implantation. However, CD98 mRNA levels did not significantly lower in heterozygous animals if compared with the wild-type ones (67). Therefore, the complete deletion by conditional knockouts in endometrial epithelial tissue would help explore this issue. Association of adhesion receptors with tetraspanins has been demonstrated to be important for avidity regulation of their adhesive functions (75). Our data reveal that the overexpression of tetraspanin CD9 in HEC-1-A cells greatly enhances blastocyst adhesion. Although CD9 is constitutively expressed in luminal epithelial cells throughout the menstrual cycle, the levels of this tetraspanin in HEC-1-A were significantly lower than those of primary EEC. Restoration of the CD9 levels in transfected HEC-1-A cells might facilitate the adhesive function of associated receptors, such as CD98. Moreover in mice, the CD9 expression has also been reported to be upregulated by steroid hormones and found to be highly expressed in the epithelial cells surrounding the implanted embryo (76). CD98 has also been proposed to be functionally linked to CD147 (73). However, CD98 only partially co-localized with CD147 in primary endometrial epithelial cells, and appears to engage in two independent molecular interactions with CD147 and with CD9. CD147 is strongly expressed in the mouse embryo trophectoderm and uterine endometrium (77), and embryo transfer to the uterus of CD147 null females demonstrates that CD147 is necessary for implantation in mouse (78). In humans, however, CD147 is expressed in both the stroma and epithelium in the secretory phase (79). Our biochemical, immunohistological, and functional data demonstrate that CD98 (possibly linked to CD147) is a key determinant of human endometrial receptivity, whose expression is tightly regulated during the WOI.

SECRETOMICS AND LIPIDOMICS OF ENDOMETRIAL RECEPTIVITY

Proteomic and lipidomic techniques have been applied to analyze endometrial fluid to study endometrial receptivity. This viscous liquid is a complex biological fluid secreted by the endometrial glands, which provides nutrients for blastocyst survival and constitutes the microenvironment where the embryo-endometrial dialog occurs prior to implantation (80–82). The advantage of working with endometrial fluid is that it can be collected easily and painlessly by aspiration using noninvasive methods (83). Furthermore, uterine secretions are less complex in terms of their protein repertoire, and may serve as a pool of biomarkers for functional endometrial operation.

Endometrial secretion has been shown to contain products of apoptotic epithelial cells, and the proteins originating from the transudation of serum and proteins secreted from the glandular epithelium. This secretion undergoes significant changes in protein content during the transition from the proliferative phase to the secretory phase (84). Endometrial secretion composition varies during the menstrual cycle as a result of the changes in ovarian steroid serum concentration (85). In the past, electrophoresis was the technique used to analyze the protein patterns of uterine secretions throughout the menstrual cycle. These studies revealed three different protein patterns that are typical of the equivalent phases of the menstrual cycle: intermediate phase, proliferative phase, and secretory

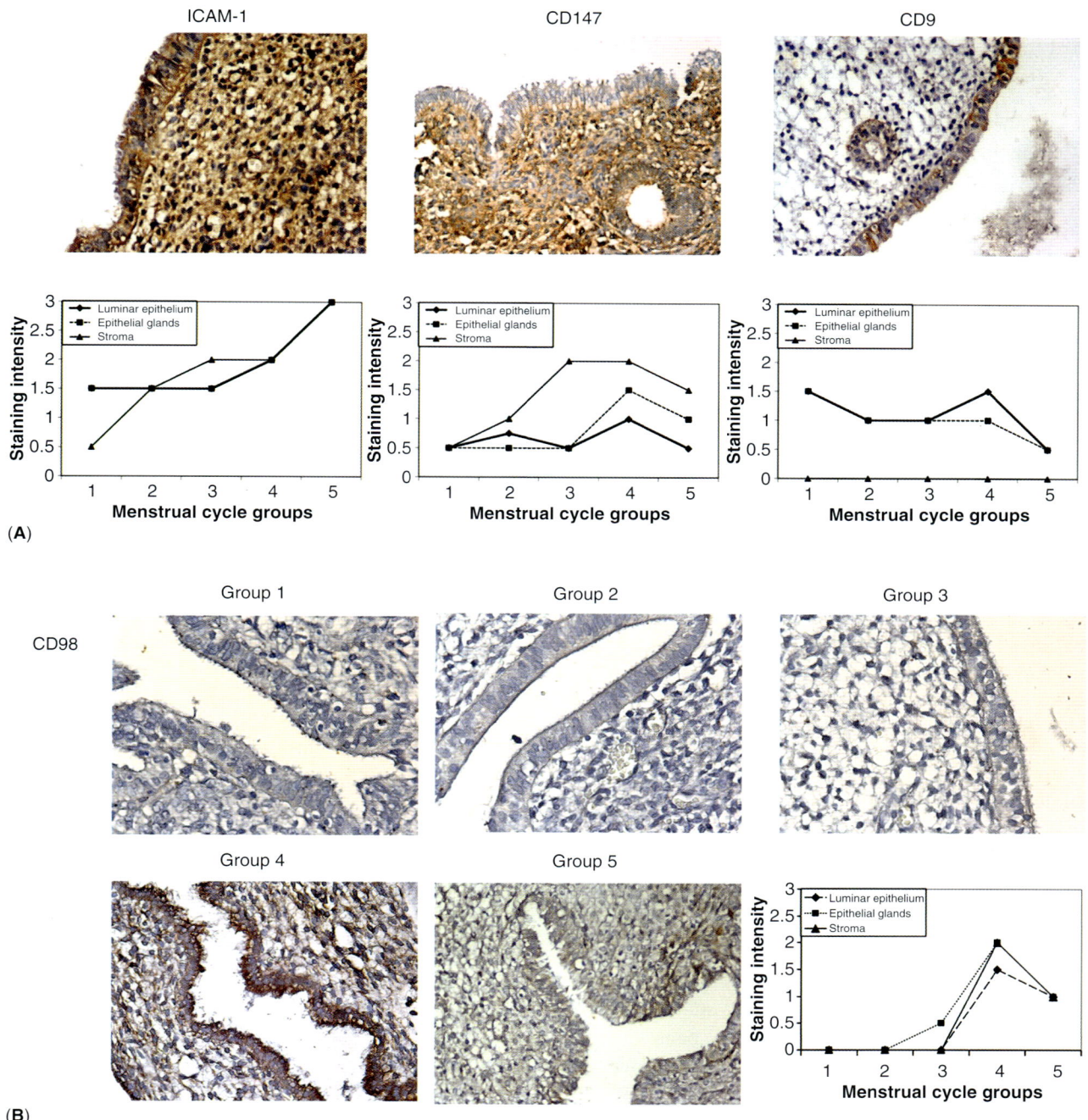

Figure 29.3 CD98 is expressed in the implantation window in human endometrium. (**A**) Immunolocalization of ICAM-1, CD147, and CD9 in human endometrium throughout the menstrual cycle. The micrographs show representative immunohistochemical stains of luminal epithelium on day 20, corresponding to the implantation window. Images correspond to a 200× magnification. The chart plot expression based on semi-quantitative staining analysis throughout the menstrual cycle in 3–5 endometrial samples per group in epithelial glands (square), luminar epithelium (rhombus), or stroma (triangle). (**B**). Immunolocalization of CD98 (anti-CD98 pAb) in human endometrium throughout the menstrual cycle. Micrographs depict the luminar epithelium in the 5 menstrual cycle groups in sequence: group1, = day 5, group 2 = day 9, group 3 = day 15, group 4 = day 20, and group 5 = day 25. Images correspond to a 200× magnification. The chart plots semi-quantitative analysis of the stainings throughout the menstrual cycle in 3–5 endometrial samples per group as in (A).

phase. The results present characteristic "families" of protein bands corresponding to 63 proteins, some of which are identified by their molecular weight (80).

In another work (86), endometrial fluid obtained transcervically by aspiration immediately prior to embryo transfer was analyzed and the protein profile in each sample was determined. These studies also demonstrated that endometrial secretion can be obtained for analysis immediately prior to embryo transfer in IVF cycles without lowering implantation rates. Although uterine fluid aspiration is a safe method, sometimes the material obtained is not enough for its analysis or it may be diluted as a result of uterine washing, thus making it difficult to interpret the results (87).

Van der Gaast et al. (88) investigated the effect of ovarian stimulation in IVF on endometrial secretion and markers of receptivity in the mid-luteal phase. The endometrial fluids obtained in this period in the stimulated cycle were compared with the spontaneous cycle. Protein composition was analyzed by sodium dodecyl sulfate-polyacrylamide gel electrophoresis (SDS-PAGE), and gels were stained with Coomassie brilliant blue. The protein pattern was obtained by measuring the relative density of each band by means of scanning laser densitometer and the GelScan XL software package. In this pilot study, ovarian stimulation did not alter the investigated markers of endometrial maturation in the mid-luteal phase.

More recently, an integral work was presented (89) to identify the catalog of proteins present in an endometrial fluid aspirate during the secretory phase of the menstrual cycle. To accomplish this objective, three different, but complementary, strategies were used: first, in-solution digestion followed by reverse phase high-performance liquid chromatography coupled with tandem mass spectrometry (HPLC-MS/MS); second, protein separation by denaturing one-dimensional electrophoresis (SDS-PAGE) followed by HPLC-MS/MS analysis. Finally, two-dimensional polyacrylamide gel electrophoresis (2D-PAGE) followed by MALDI-TOF/TOF analysis. The combination of the three strategies led to the successful identification of 803 different proteins in the International Protein Index human database (v3.48). This catalog of proteins presented here proves a valuable reference for the study of embryo implantation and for future discovery of the biomarkers involved in pathologic alterations of an endometrial function.

The current technical limitations of applying proteomics to the study of protein patterns in endometrial fluid lies in that the majority of identified proteins correspond to serum proteins, thus masking the identification of those proteins present at low concentrations, which is of great interest, such as biomarkers for endometrial receptivity, embryo development, diseases and/or interception.

The endometrium contains lipid compounds whose importance in reproduction has long since been known. However, the vast majority of studies have investigated the lipid content using morphological observations in endometrial biopsies and not in endometrial fluids (90). This diagnostic technique is dependent on the observer's subjectivity and, for this reason, the efficiency of histological methods as a predictor of endometrial receptivity has been questioned in different publications (91,92). This scenario opens up a gap in our understanding of endometrial biology, which entails a handful of missing opportunities in diagnoses. Lipidomics can serve to unravel the specific lipid composition of endometrial fluid throughout the menstrual cycle and to also elucidate whether a particular lipid makeup is predictive of endometrial receptivity (93).

Unlike proteomics, lipidomics has not been consistently applied to the field of human reproduction. Yet, synthesis of defective endometrial prostaglandins (PGs) in humans has been linked with repeated implantation failure in patients undergoing IVF (94), indicating how lipids intervene as important mediators in early pregnancy. Most of these studies have concentrated on the role of PGs in the endometrium, where they cause increased vascular permeability and decidualization (95). Nevertheless, their importance in influencing embryo maturation and acquisition of implantation competency has also been suggested (96,97).

Some recent reports have put into practice lipidomics to study the reproductive function by assessing the lipid content of endometrial biopsies during pregnancy (96). However, these works neither refer to endometrial fluid in humans nor assess whether a particular lipid profile is distinctive of the WOI in relation to the rest of the cycle. Our lab has carried out preliminary lipidomics analyses of endometrial fluid from patients at different stages of their natural menstrual cycles (98). Briefly, a total of 39 endometrial fluid samples were obtained throughout the menstrual cycle and were analyzed for changes in lipid content and concentration in two independent single-blind experiments. In the first experiment, we found that the concentration of two specific lipids, PGE2 and PGF2α, significantly increased between days 19 and 21 of the menstrual cycle, which is coincident with the so-called WOI. None of the remaining lipids identified in our samples (N-arachidonoyl ethanolamine, N-palmitoyl ethanolamine, N-oleoyl ethanolamine, 2-arachidonoyl glycerol, N-stearoyl ethanolamine, N-linoleoyl ethanolamine, PGF1) underwent significant changes during the menstrual cycle. The results from these preliminary experiments show twofold and 20-fold increase peaks in the concentration of PGE2 and PGF2α, respectively, during the clinical WOI (Mann–Whitney U test, $p < 0.01$) (98).

The results provided above are meaningful for two reasons; first, they represent proof-of-principle that endometrial fluids are suitable for lipidomic analyses, a possibility which has never been investigated before; second, they illustrate how lipid changes actually occur in endometrial fluid throughout the cycle by increasing the likelihood of developing noninvasive methods to assess endometrial receptivity.

CONCLUSION

The significant histological, biological, and physiological features which occur in the endometrial WOI are ultimately the result of the changes occurring at the gene transcription level, together with post-transcriptional modifications and epigenetic changes. In recent years, "omics" techniques and complex models, such as leukocyte transendothelial migration, have advanced and these help speed up the identification of those genes/proteins of interest. Technical limitations still exist which complicate the unification of the results obtained. Proteomics together with genomics and secretomics are complementary approaches that provide diverse but comparable perspectives which will improve our understanding of the complexity of this process and the identification of key biomarkers. The next step will be to integrate this information into a system biology approach to develop models for functions of interest, such as embryo viability, endometrial receptivity, and the embryo-endometrial dialog.

In conclusion, the application of new technologies and models to the endometrium can be used to search new biomarkers to determine endometrial receptivity and possible causes in infertility and to investigate interceptive molecules to prevent embryo implantation.

REFERENCES

1. Kämmerer U, von Wolff M, Markert UR. Inmunology of human endometrium. Inmunobiology 2004; 209: 569–74.
2. Giudice LC. Implantation and endometrial function. In: Fauser BCJM, ed. Molecular Biology in Reproductive Medicine. New York, NY, USA, London, UK: Parthenon Publishing Group, 1999.
3. Dimitriadis E, White CA, Jones R, et al. Cytokines, chemokines and growth factors in endometrium related to implantation. Hum Reprod Update 2005; 11: 613–30.
4. Finn CL, Martin L. The control of implantation. J Reprod Fertil 1974; 39: 195–206.
5. Martín J, Dominguez F, Avila S, et al. Human endometrial receptivity: gene regulation. J Reprod Immunol 2002; 55: 131–9.
6. Murphy CR. Uterine receptivity and the plasma membrane transformation. Cell Res 2004; 14: 259–67.
7. Nikas G. Cell-surface morphological events relevant to human implantation. Hum Reprod 1999; 14: 37–44.
8. Quinn CE, Casper RF. Pinopodes: a questionable role in endometrial receptivity. Hum Reprod Update 2009; 15: 229–36.
9. Giudice LC, Saleh W. Growth factors in reproduction. Trends Endocrinol Metab 1995; 6: 60–9.
10. Lessey BA. Endometrial integrins and the establishment of uterine receptivity. Hum Reprod 1998; 13: 247–58.
11. Dubowy RL, Feinberg RF, Keefe DL, et al. Improved endometrial assessment using cyclin E and p27. Fertil Steril 2003; 80: 146–56.
12. Kliman HJ, Honig S, Walls D, et al. Optimization of endometrial preparation results in a normal endometrial function test (EFT) and good reproductive outcome in donor ovum recipients. J Assist Reprod Genet 2006; 23: 299–303.
13. Lessey BA, Killam AP, Metzger DA, et al. Immunohistochemical analysis of human uterine estrogen and progesterone receptors throughout the menstrual cycle. J Clin Endocrinol Metab 1988; 67: 334–40.
14. Develioglu OH, Hsiu JG, Nikas G, et al. Endometrial estrogen and progesterone receptor and pinopode expression in stimulated cycles of oocyte donors. Fertil Steril 1999; 71: 1040–7.
15. Aghajanova L, Simon C, Horcajadas JA. Are favourite molecules of endometrial receptivity still in favour? Expert Rev Obstet Gynecol 2008; 3: 487–501.
16. Ponnampalam AP, Weston GC, Trajstman AC, Susil B, Rogers PA. 2004; Molecular classification of human endometrial cycle stages by transcriptional profiling. Mol Hum Reprod 2004; 10: 879–93.
17. Talbi S, Hamilton AE, Vo KC, et al. Molecular phenotyping of human endometrium distinguishes menstrual cycle phases and underlying biological processes in normo-ovulatory women. Endocrinology 2006; 147: 1097–121.
18. Riesewijk A, Martín J, van Os R, et al. Gene expression profiling of human endometrial receptivity on days LH + 2 versus LH + 7 by microarray technology. Mol Hum Reprod 2003; 9: 253–64.
19. Carson DD, Lagow E, Thathiah A, et al. Changes in gene expression during the early to mid-luteal (receptive phase) transition in human endometrium detected by high-density microarray screening. Mol Hum Reprod 2002; 8: 871–9.
20. Kao LC, Tulac S, Lobo S, et al. Global gene profiling in human endometrium during the window implantation. Endocrinology 2002; 143: 2119–38.
21. Borthwick JM, Charnock-Jones DS, Tom BD, et al. Determination of the transcript profile of human endometrium. Mol Hum Reprod 2003; 9: 19–33.
22. Mirkin S, Arslan M, Churikov D, et al. In search of candidate genes critically expressed in the human endometrium during the window of implantation. Hum Reprod 2005; 20: 2104–17.
23. Haouzi D, Mahmoud K, Fourar M, et al. Identification of new biomarkers of human endometrial receptivity in the natural cycle. Hum Reprod 2009; 24: 198–205.
24. Horcajadas JA, Martínez-Conejero JA, Simón C. Endometrial receptivity in natural and controlled ovarian-stimulated cycles. Biennial Rev Infertility 2011; 1: 43–55.
25. Horcajadas JA, Riesewijk A, Martín J, et al. Global gene expression profiling of human endometrial receptivity. J Reprod Immunol 2004; 63: 41–9.
26. Horcajadas JA, Pellicer A, Simón C. Wide genomic analysis of human endometrial receptivity: new times, new opportunities. Hum Reprod Update 2007; 13: 77–86.
27. Horcajadas JA, Riesewijk A, Polman J, et al. Effect of controlled ovarian hyperstimulation in IVF on endometrial gene expression profiles. Mol Hum Reprod 2005; 11: 195–205.
28. Horcajadas JA, Mínguez P, Dopazo J, et al. Controlled ovarian stimulation induces a functional genomic delay of the endometrium with potential clinical implications. J Clin Endocrinol Metab 2008; 93: 4500–10.
29. Martínez-Conejero JA, Simón C, Pellicer A, et al. Is ovarian stimulation detrimental to the endometrium? Reprod Biomed Online 2007; 15: 45–50.
30. Mirkin S, Nikas G, Hsiu JG, et al. Gene expression profiles and structural/functional features of the peri-implantation endometrium in natural and gonadotropin-stimulated cycles. J Clin Endocrinol Metab 2004; 89: 5742–52.
31. Simon C, Oberyé J, Bellver J, et al. Similar endometrial development in oocyte donors treated with either high- or standard-dose GnRH antagonist compared to treatment with a GnRH agonist or in natural cycles. Hum Reprod 2005; 20: 3318–27.
32. Liu Y, Lee KF, Ng EH, et al. Gene expression profiling of human peri-implantation endometria between natural and stimulated cycles. Fertil Steril 2008; 90: 2152–64.
33. Horcajadas JA, Sharkey AM, Catalano RD, et al. Effect of an intrauterine device on the gene expression profile of the endometrium. J Clin Endocrinol Metab 2006; 91: 3199–207.

34. Bellver J, Martínez-Conejero JA, Labarta E, et al. Endometrial gene expression in the window of implantation is altered in obese women especially in association with polycystic ovary syndrome. Fertil Steril 2011; 95: 2335–41.
35. Labarta E, Martínez-Conejero JA, Alamá P, et al. Endometrial receptivity is affected in women with high circulating progesterone levels at the end of the follicular phase: a functional genomics analysis. Hum Reprod 2011; 26: 1813–25.
36. Altmäe S, Martínez-Conejero JA, Salumets A, et al. Endometrial gene expression analysis at the time of embryo implantation in women with unexplained infertility. Mol Hum Reprod 2010; 16: 178–87.
37. Aghajanova L, Simón C, Horcajadas JA. Are favorite molecules of endometrial receptivity still in favor? Expert Rev Obstetrics Gynecol 2008; 3: 487–501.
38. Tapia A, Vilos C, Marín JC, et al. Bioinformatic detection of E47, E2F1 and SREBP1 transcription factors as potential regulators of genes associated to acquisition of endometrial receptivity. Reprod Biol Endocrinol 2011; 27: 9–14.
39. Martín J, Domínguez F, Ávila S, et al. Human endometrial receptivity: gene regulation. J Reprod Immunol 2002; 55: 131–9.
40. Coutifaris C, Myers ER, Guzick DS, et al. Histological dating of timed endometrial biopsy tissue is not related to fertility status. Fertil Steril 2004; 82: 1264–72.
41. Díaz-Gimeno P, Horcajadas JA, Martínez-Conejero JA, et al. A genomic diagnostic tool for human endometrial receptivity based on the transcriptomic signature. Fertil Steril 2011; 95: 50–60.
42. Shankar R, Cullinane F, Brennecke SP, et al. Applications of proteomics methodologies to human pregnancy research: a growing gestation approaching delivery? Proteomics 2004; 4: 1909–17.
43. DeSouza L, Diehl G, Yang EC, et al. Proteomic analysis of the proliferative and secretory phases of the human endometrium: protein identification and differential protein expression. Proteomics 2005; 5: 270–81.
44. Parmar T, Gadkar-Sable S, Savardekar L, et al. Protein profiling of human endometrial tissues in the midsecretory and proliferative phases of the menstrual cycle. Fertil Steril 2009; 92: 1091–103.
45. Domínguez F, Garrido-Gomez T, Lopez JA, et al. Proteomic analysis of the human receptive versus nonreceptive endometrium using differential in-gel electrophoresis and MALDI-MS unveils stathmin 1 and annexin A2 as differentially regulated. Human Reprod 2009; 24: 2607–17.
46. Martin JC, Jasper MJ, Valbuena D, et al. Increased adhesiveness in cultured endometrial-derived cells is related to the absence of moesin expression. Biol Reprod 2000; 63: 1370–6.
47. King A. Uterine leukocytes and decidualization. Hum Reprod Update 2000; 6: 28–36.
48. Goldsmith LT, Weiss G. Relaxin in human pregnancy. Ann N Y Acad Sci 2009; 1160: 130–5.
49. Daly DC, Maslar IA, Riddick DH. Prolactin production during in vitro decidualization of proliferative endometrium. Am J Obstet Gynecol 1983; 145: 672–8.
50. Giudice LC, Dsupin BA, Irwin JC. Steroid and peptide regulation of insulin-like growth factor-binding proteins secreted by human endometrial stromal cells is dependent on stromal differentiation. J Clin Endocrinol Metab 1992; 75: 1235–41.
51. Lockwood CJ, Nemerson Y, Guller S, et al. Progestational regulation of human endometrial stromal cell tissue factor expression during decidualization. J Clin Endocrinol Metab 1993; 76: 231–6.
52. Irwin JC, Kirk D, King RJ, Quigley MM, Gwatkin RB. Hormonal regulation of human endometrial stromal cells in culture: an in vitro model for decidualization. Fertil Steril 1989; 52: 761–8.
53. Lydon JP, DeMayo FJ, Funk CR, et al. Mice lacking progesterone receptor exhibit pleiotropic reproductive abnormalities. Genes Dev 1995; 9: 2266–78.
54. Paria BC, Das N, Das SK, et al. Histidine decarboxylase gene in the mouse uterus is regulated by progesterone and correlates with uterine differentiation for blastocyst implantation. Endocrinology 1998; 139: 3958–66.
55. Curtis SH, Korach KS. Steroid receptor knockout models: phenotypes and responses illustrate interactions between receptor signaling pathways in vivo. Adv Pharmacol 2000; 47: 357–80.
56. Garrido-Gomez T, Dominguez F, Lopez JA, et al. Modeling human endometrial decidualization from the interaction between proteome and secretome. J Clin Endocrinol Metab 2011; 96: 706–16.
57. Barreiro O, Yanez-Mo M, Sala-Valdes M, et al. Endothelial tetraspanin microdomains regulate leukocyte firm adhesion during extravasation. Blood 2005; 105: 2852–61.
58. Berditchevski F. Complexes of tetraspanins with integrins: more than meets the eye. J Cell Sci 2001; 114: 4143–51.
59. Le Naour F, Rubinstein E, Jasmin C, et al. Severely reduced female fertility in CD9-deficient mice. Science 2000; 287: 319–21.
60. Miller BJ, Georges-Labouesse E, Primakoff P, et al. Normal fertilization occurs with eggs lacking the integrin alpha6beta1 and is CD9- dependent. J Cell Biol 2000; 149: 1289–96.
61. Miyado K, Yamada G, Yamada S, et al. Requirement of CD9 on the egg plasma membrane for fertilization. Science 2000; 287: 321–4.
62. Lindenberg S. Experimental studies on the initial trophoblast endometrial interaction. Dan Med Bull 1991; 38: 371–80.
63. Mercader A, Valbuena D, Simon C. Human embryo culture. Methods Enzymol 2006; 420: 3–18.
64. Bentin-Ley U, Pedersen B, Lindenberg S, et al. Isolation and culture of human endometrial cells in a three-dimensional culture system. J Reprod Fertil 1994; 101: 327–32.
65. Landgren BM, Johannisson E, Stavreus-Evers A, et al. A new method to study the process of implantation of a human blastocyst in vitro. Fertil Steril 1996; 65: 1067–70.
66. Bulletti C, Jasonni VM, Tabanelli S, et al. Early human pregnancy in vitro utilizing an artificially perfused uterus. Fertil Steril 1988; 49: 991–6.
67. Tinel H, Denker HW, Thie M. Calcium influx in human uterine epithelial RL95-2 cells triggers adhesiveness for trophoblast-like cells. Model studies on signalling events during embryo implantation. Mol Hum Reprod 2000; 6: 1119–30.

68. Way DL, Grosso DS, Davis JR, et al. Characterization of a new human endometrial carcinoma (RL95-2) established in tissue culture. In Vitro 1983; 19: 147–58.
69. John NJ, Linke M, Denker HW. Quantitation of human choriocarcinoma spheroid attachment to uterine epithelial cell monolayers. In Vitro Cell Dev Biol Anim 1993; 29A: 461–468.
70. Martin JC, Jasper MJ, Valbuena D, et al. Increased adhesiveness in cultured endometrial-derived cells is related to the absence of moesin expression. Biol Reprod 2000; 63: 1370–6.
71. Fenczik CA, Sethi T, Ramos JW, et al. Complementation of dominant suppression implicates CD98 in integrin activation. Nature 1997; 390: 81–5.
72. Tsumura H, Suzuki N, Saito H, et al. The targeted disruption of the CD98 gene results in embryonic lethality. Biochem Biophys Res Commun 2003; 308: 847–51.
73. Kuno N, Kadomatsu K, Fan QW, et al. Female sterility in mice lacking the basigin gene, which encodes a transmembrane glycoprotein belonging to the immunoglobulin superfamily. FEBS Lett 1998; 425: 191–4.
74. Noguchi Y, Sato T, Hirata M, et al. Identification and characterization of extracellular matrix metalloproteinase inducer in human endometrium during the menstrual cycle in vivo and in vitro. J Clin Endocrinol Metab 2003; 88: 6063–72.
75. Liu X, Charrier L, Gewirtz A, et al. CD98 and intracellular adhesion molecule I regulate the activity of amino acid transporter LAT-2 in polarized intestinal epithelia. J Biol Chem 2003; 278: 23672–7.
76. Palacin M, Kanai Y. The ancillary proteins of HATs: SLC3 family of amino acid transporters. Pflugers Arch 2004; 447: 490–4.
77. Xu D, Hemler ME. Metabolic activation-related CD147-CD98 complex. Mol Cell Proteomics 2005; 4: 1061–71.
78. Domínguez F, Simón C, Quiñonero A, et al. Human endometrial CD98 is essential for blastocyst adhesion. PLoS One 2010; 15: 5–13380.
79. Wakabayashi T, Craessaerts K, Bammens L, et al. Analysis of the gamma-secretase interactome and validation of its association with tetraspanin-enriched microdomains. Nat Cell Biol 2009; 11: 1340–6.
80. Lessey BA, Killam AP, Metzger DA, et al. Immunohistochemical analysis of human uterine estrogen and progesterone receptors throughout the menstrual cycle. J Clin Endocrinol Metab 1988; 67: 334–40.
81. Develioglu OH, Hsiu JG, Nikas G, et al. Endometrial estrogen and progesterone receptor and pinopode expression in stimulated cycles of oocyte donors. Fertil Steril 1999; 71: 1040–7.
82. Lessey BA. Endometrial integrins and the establishment of uterine receptivity. Hum Reprod 1998; 13: 247–58.
83. Aghajanova L, Simon C, Horcajadas JA. Are favourite-molecules of endometrial receptivity still in favour? Expert Rev Obstet Gynecol. 2008; 3: 487–501.
84. Horcajadas JA, Pellicer A, Simón C. Wide genomic analysis of human endometrial receptivity: new times, new opportunities. Hum Reprod Update 2007; 13: 77–86.
85. Carson D, Lagow E, Thathiah A, et al. Changes in gene expression during the early to mid-luteal (receptive phase) transition in human endometrium detected by high-density microarray screening. Mol Hum Reprod 2002; 8: 971–9.
86. Kao LC, Germeyer A, Tulac S, et al. Expression profiling of endometrium from women with endometriosis reveals candidate genes for disease based implantation failure and infertility. Endocrinology 2003; 144: 2870–81.
87. Borthwick J, Charnock-Jones S, Tom BD, et al. Determination of the transcript profile of human endometrium. Mol Hum Reprod 2003; 9: 19–33.
88. Van der Gaast MH, Classen-Linke I, Krusche CA, et al. Impact of ovarian stimulation on mid-luteal endometrial tissue and secretion markers of receptivity. Reprod Biomed Online 2008; 17: 553–63.
89. Mirkin S, Arslan M, Churikov D, et al. In search of candidate genes critically expressed in the human endometrium during the window of implantation. Hum Reprod 2005; 20: 2104–17.
90. Noyes RW, Hertig AT, Rock J. Dating the endometrial biopsy. Am J Obstet Gynecol 1975; 122: 262–3.
91. Coutifaris C, et al. Histological dating of timed endometrial biopsy tissue is not related to fertility status. Fertil Steril 2004; 82: 1264–72.
92. Murray MJ, et al. A critical analysis of the accuracy, reproducibility, and clinical utility of histologic endometrial dating in fertile women. Fertil Steril 2004; 81: 1333–43.
93. Wenk MR. The emerging field of lipidomics. Nat Rev Drug Discov 2005; 4: 594–610.
94. Achache H, Tsafrir A, Prus D, et al. Defective endometrial prostaglandin synthesis identified in patients with repeated implantation failure undergoing in vitro fertilization. Fertil Steril 2010; 94: 1271–8.
95. Ye X, et al. LPA3-mediated lysophosphatidic acid signalling in embryo implantation and spacing. Nature 2005; 435: 104–8.
96. Durn JH, et al. Lipidomic analysis reveals prostanoid profiles in human term pregnant myometrium. Prostaglandins Leukot Essent Fatty Acids 2010; 82: 21–6.
97. Huang JC, et al. Stimulation of embryo hatching and implantation by prostacyclin and peroxisome proliferator-activated receptor delta activation: implication in IVF. Hum Reprod 2007; 22: 807–14.
98. Berlanga O, Bradshaw HB, Vilella-Mitjana F, et al. How endometrial secretomics can help in predicting implantation. Placenta 2011; 32(Suppl 3): S271–5.
99. Popovici RM, Kao LC, Giudice LC. Discovery of new inducible genes in in vitro decidualized human endometrial stromal cells using microarray technology. Endocrinology 2000; 141: 3510–13.
100. Brar AK, Handwerger S, Kessler CA, Aronow BJ. Gene induction and categorical reprogramming during in vitro human endometrial fibroblast decidualization. Physiol Genomics 2001; 7: 135–48.
101. Mutter GL, Baak JPA, Fitzgerald JT, et al. Global expression changes of constitutive and hormonally regulated genes during endometrial neoplasic transformation. Gynecol Oncol 2001; 83: 177–85.
102. Eyster KM, Boles AL, Brannian JD, Hansen KD. DNA microarray analysis of gene expression markers of endometriosis. Fertil Steril 2002; 77: 38–42.
103. Lebovic DI, Baldocchi RA, Mueller MD, Taylor RN. Altered expression of a cell-cycle suppressor gene, Tob-1, in endometriotic cells by cDNA array analyses. Fertil Steril 2002; 78: 849–54.

104. Arimoto T, Katagiri T, Oda K, et al. Genome-wide cDNA microarray analysis of gene-expression profiles involved in ovarian endometriosis. Int J Oncol 2003; 22: 551–60.
105. Catalano RD, Yanaihara A, Evans AL, et al. The effect of RU486 on the gene expression profile in an endometrial explant model. Mol Hum Reprod 2003; 9: 465–73.
106. Domínguez F, Avila S, Cervero A, et al. A combined approach for gene discovery identifies insulin-like growth factor-binding protein-related protein 1 as a new gene implicated in human endometrial receptivity. J Clin Endocrinol Metab 2003; 88: 1849–57.
107. Moreno-Bueno G, Sanchez-Estevez C, Cassia R, et al. Differential gene expression profile in endometrioid and nonendometrioid endometrial carcinoma: STK15 is frequently overexpressed and amplified in nonendometrioid carcinomas. Cancer Res 2003; 63: 5697–702.
108. Okada H, Nakajima T, Yoshimura T, Yasuda K, Kanzaki H. Microarray analysis of genes controlled by progesterone in human endometrial stromal cells in vitro. Gynecol Endocrinol 2003; 17: 271–80.
109. Risinger JI, Maxwell GL, Chandramouli GV, et al. Microarray analysis reveals distinct gene expression profiles among different histologic types of endometrial cancer. Cancer Res 2003; 63: 6–11.
110. Tierney EP, Tulac S, Huang ST, Giudice LC. Activation of the protein kinase a pathway in human endometrial stromal cells reveals sequential categorical gene regulation. Physiol Genomics 2003; 16: 47–66.
111. Cao QJ, Belbin T, Socci N, et al. Distinctive gene expression profiles by CDNA microarrays in endometrioid and serous carcinomas of the endometrium. Int J Gynecol Pathol 2004; 23: 321–9.
112. Ferguson SE, Olshen AB, Viale A, et al. Gene expression profiling of tamoxifen-associated uterine cancers: evidence for two molecular classes of endometrial carcinoma. Gynecol Oncol 2004; 92: 719–25.
113. Matsuzaki S, Canis M, Vaurs Barriere C, et al. DNA microarray analysis of gene expression profiles in deep endometriosis using laser capture microdissection. Mol Hum Reprod 2004; 10: 719–28.
114. Saidi SA, Holland CM, Kreil DP, et al. Independent component analysis of microarray data in the study of endometrial cancer. Oncogene 2004; 23: 6677–83.
115. Barbier CS, Becker KA, Troester MA, Kaufman DG. Expression of exogenous Human telomerase in cultures of endometrial stromal cells does not alter their hormone responsiveness. Biol Reprod 2005; 73: 106–14.
116. Ferguson SE, Olshen AB, Viale A, Barakat RR, Boyd J. Stratification of intermediate-risk endometrial cancer patients into groups at high risk or low risk for recurrence based on tumor gene expression profiles. Clin Cancer Res 2005; 11: 2252–7.
117. Krikun G, Schatz F, Taylor R, et al. Endometrial endothelial cell steroid receptor expression and steroid effects on gene expression. J Clin Endocrinol Metab 2005; 90: 1812–18.
118. Matsuzaki S, Canis M, Vaurs-Barrière C, et al. DNA microarray analysis of gene expression in eutopic endometrium from patients with deep endometriosis using laser capture microdissection. Fertil Steril 2005; 84: 1180–90.
119. Maxwell GL, Chandramouli GV, Dainty L, et al. Microarray analysis of endometrial carcinomas and mixed mullerian tumors reveals distinct gene expression profiles associated with different histologic types of uterine cancer. Clin Cancer Res 2005; 11: 4056–66.
120. Punyadeera C, Dassen H, Klomp J, et al. Oestrogen-modulated gene expression in the human endometrium. Cell Mol Life Sci 2005; 62: 239–50.
121. Rossi M, Sharkey AM, Vigano P, et al. Identification of genes regulated by interleukin-1beta in human endometrial stromal cells. Reproduction 2005; 130: 721–9.
122. Sharkey AM, Catalano R, Evans A, Charnock-Jones DS, Smith SK. Novel antiangiogenic agents for use in contraception. Contraception 2005; 71: 263–71.
123. Simón C, Bellver J, Vidal C, et al. Similar endometrial development in oocyte donors treated with high- or low-dose GnRHantagonist compared to GnRH-agonist treatment and natural cycles. Hum Reprod 2005; 12: 3318–27.
124. Talbi S, Hamilton AE, Vo KC, et al. Molecular phenotyping of human endometrium distinguishes menstrual cycle phases and underlying biological processes in normo-ovulatory women. Endocrinology 2005; 147: 1097–121.
125. White CA, Dimitriadis E, Sharkey AM, Salamonsen LA. Interleukin- 11 inhibits expression of insulin-like growth factor binding protein-5 mRNA in decidualizing human endometrial stromal cells. Mol Hum Reprod 2005; 11: 649–58.
126. Yanaihara A, Otsuka Y, Iwasaki S, et al. Differences in gene expression in the proliferative human endometrium. Fertil Steril 2005; 83: 1206–15.
127. Gielen SCJP, Hanekamp EE, Hanifi-Moghaddam P, et al. Growth regulation and transcriptional activities of estrogen and progesterone in human endometrial cancer cells. Int J Gynecol Cancer 2006; 16: 110–20.
128. Hever A, Roth RB, Hevezi PA, et al. Molecular characterization of human adenomyosis. Mol Hum Reprod 2006; 12: 737–48.
129. Huang SJ, Schatz F, Masch R, et al. Regulation of chemokine production in response to pro inflammatory cytokines in first trimester decidual cells. J Reprod Immunol 2006; 72: 60–73.
130. Matsumura N, Mandai M, Miyanishi M, et al. Oncogenic property of acrogranin in human uterine leiomyosarcoma: direct evidence of genetic contribution in In vivo tumorigenesis. Clin Cancer Res 2006; 12: 1402–11.
131. Sarno JL, Schatz F, Lockwood CJ, Huang ST, Taylor HS. Thrombin and interleukin-1beta; regulate HOXA10 expression in human term decidual cells: implications for preterm labor. J Clin Endocrinol Metab 2006; 91: 2366–72.
132. Wu Y, Kajdacsy-Balla A, Strawn E, et al. Transcriptional characterizations of differences between eutopic and ectopic endometrium. Endocrinology 2006; 147: 232–46.
133. Dainty LA, Risinger JI, Morrison C, et al. Overexpression of folate binding protein and mesothelin are associated with uterine serous carcinoma. Gynecol Oncol 2007; 105: 563–70.
134. Eyster KM, Klinkova O, Kennedy V, Hansen KA. Whole genome deoxyribonucleic acid microarray

analysis of gene expression in ectopic versus eutopic endometrium. Fertil Steril 2007; 88: 1505–33.
135. Feroze-Zaidi F, Fusi L, Takano M, et al. Role and regulation of the serum- and glucocorticoid-regulated kinase 1 in fertile and infertile human endometrium. Endocrinology 2007; 2148: 5020–9.
136. Gielen SC, Santegoets LA, Kühne LC, et al. Genomic and nongenomic effects of estrogen signaling in human endometrial cells: involvement of the growth factor receptor signaling downstream AKT pathway. Reprod Sci 2007; 14: 646–54.
137. Mettler L, Salmassi A, Schollmeyer T, et al. Comparison of c-DNA microarray analysis of gene expression between eutopic endometrium and ectopic endometrium (endometriosis). Assist Reprod Genet 2007; 24: 249–58.
138. Pan Q, Luo X, Toloubeydokhti T, Chegini N. The expression profile of micro-RNA in endometrium and endometriosis and the influence of ovarian steroids on their expression. Mol Hum Reprod 2007; 13: 797–806.
139. Paulssen RH, Moe B, Grønaas H, Orbo A. Gene expression in endometrial cancer cells (Ishikawa) after short time high dose exposure to progesterone. Steroids 2008; 73: 116–28.
140. Langendonckt AV, Punyadeera C, Kamps R, et al. Identification of novel antigens in blood vessels in rectovaginal endometriosis. Mol Hum Reprod 2007; 13: 875–86.
141. Wong YF, Cheung TH, Lo KWK, et al. Identification of molecular markers and signaling pathway in endometrial cancer in Hong Kong Chinese women by genome-wide gene expression profiling. Oncogene 2007; 26: 1971–82.
142. Bersinger NA, Wunder DM, Birkhäuser MH, Mueller MD. Gene expression in cultured endometrium from women with different outcomes following IVF. Mol Hum Reprod 2008; 14: 475–84.
143. Cloke B, Huhtinen K, Fusi L, et al. The androgen and progesterone receptors regulate distinct gene networks and cellular functions in decidualizing endometrium. Endocrinology 2008; 149: 4462–74.
144. Evans J, Catalano RD, Morgan K, et al. Prokineticin 1 signaling and gene regulation in early human pregnancy. Endocrinology 2008; 149: 2877–87.
145. Gielen SC, Santegoets LA, Hanifi-Moghaddam P, Burger CW, Blok LJ. Signaling by estrogens and tamoxifen in the human endometrium. J Steroid Biochem Mol Biol 2008; 109: 219–23.
146. Hamm A, Veeck J, Bektas N, et al. Frequent expression loss of inter-alpha-trypsin inhibitor heavy chain (ITIH) genes in multiple human solid tumors: a systematic expression analysis. BMC Cancer 2008; 8: 25.
147. Horcajadas JA, Mínguez P, Dopazo J, et al. Controlled ovarian stimulation induces a functional genomic delay of the endometrium with potential clinical implications. J Clin Endocrinol Metab 2008; 93: 4500–10.
148. Horne AW, van den Driesche S, King AE, et al. Endometrial inhibin/activin beta-B subunit expression is related to decidualization and is reduced in tubal ectopic pregnancy. J Clin Endocrinol Metab 2008; 93: 2375–82.
149. Hull ML, Escareno CR, Godsland JM, et al. Endometrial-Peritoneal Interactions during Endometriotic Lesion Establishment. Am J Pathol 2008; 173: 700–15.
150. Liu Y, Lee KF, Ng EH, Yeung WS, Ho PC. Gene expression profiling of human peri implantation endometria between natural and stimulated cycles. Fertil Steril 2008; 90: 2152–64.
151. Lu Z, Hardt J, Kim JJ. Global analysis of genes regulated by HOXA10 in decidualization reveals a role in cell proliferation. Mol Hum Reprod 2008; 14: 357–66.
152. Macklon NS, van der Gaast MH, Hamilton A, Fauser BC, Giudice LC. The impact of ovarian stimulation with recombinant FSH in combination with GnRH antagonist on the endometrial transcriptome in the window of implantation. Reprod Sci 2008; 15: 357–65.
153. Savaris RF, Hamilton AE, Lessey BA, Giudice LC. Endometrial gene expression in early pregnancy: lessons from human ectopic pregnancy. Reprod Sci 2008; 15: 797–816.
154. Sherwin JR, Sharkey AM, Mihalyi A, et al. Global gene analysis of late secretory phase, eutopic endometrium does not provide the basis for a minimally invasive test of endometriosis. Hum Reprod 2008; 23: 1063–8.
155. Tapia A, Gangi LM, Zegers-Hochschild F, et al. Differences in the endometrial transcript profile during the receptive period between women who were refractory to implantation and those who achieved pregnancy. Hum Reprod 2008; 23: 340–51.
156. Zhou L, Li R, Wang R, Huang HX, Zhong K. Local injury to the endometrium in controlled ovarian hyperstimulation cycles improves implantation rates. Fertil Steril 2008; 89: 1166–76.
157. Ball LJ, Levy N, Zhao X, et al. Cell type- and estrogen receptor-subtype specific regulation of selective estrogen receptor modulator regulatory elements. Mol Cell Endocrinol 2009; 299: 204–11.
158. Germeyer A, Sharkey AM, Prasadajudio M, et al. Paracrine effects of uterine leucocytes on gene expression of human uterine stromal fibroblasts. Mol Hum Reprod 2009; 15: 39–48.
159. Van Vaerenbergh I, Van Lommel L, Ghislain V, et al. In GnRH antagonist/rec-FSH stimulated cycles, advanced endometrial maturation on the day of oocyte retrieval correlates with altered gene expression. Hum Reprod 2009; 24: 1085–91.
160. Chen YJ, Li HY, Chang YL, et al. Suppression of migratory/invasive ability and induction of apoptosis in adenomyosis-derived mesenchymal stem cells by cyclooxygenase-2 inhibitors. Fertil Steril 2010; 94: 1972–9.

30

Human embryonic stem cells

Rachel Eiges, Michal Avitzour, and Benjamin Reubinoff

INTRODUCTION

A pluripotent stem cell is an undifferentiated cell, which has the potential to develop into virtually any cell type in the body. Pluripotent stem cells are transiently present during embryogenesis, in preimplantation embryos and fetal gonads. They can also be maintained as established cell lines, derived from preimplantation embryos, primordial germ cells, or germ cell tumors.

Embryonic stem (ES) cell lines are certain types of pluripotent stem cell lines, which have been derived by the isolation and propagation of inner cell mass (ICM) cells of blastocyst-stage embryos. These unique cell lines can develop into a wide range of cell types in vitro and in vivo. In addition, they are immortal. They can be grown continuously in culture without losing their properties or their wide developmental potential. These two features, pluripotency and unlimited self-renewal, have made ES cells extremely interesting and important to basic and applied research, especially to cell-based therapy and the study of early embryonic development.

The derivation of ES cell lines in mammals was first demonstrated in mice (1,2) in which basic methods for their isolation, propagation, and genetic manipulation were established. The accumulated experience in the mouse has allowed scientists to better define the properties of ES cells that:

- Are derived from ICMs of blastocysts
- Are capable of undergoing unlimited number of symmetrical cell divisions without differentiating
- Maintain a normal karyotype
- Can give rise to differentiated cells of ectoderm, mesoderm, and endoderm origin in vitro and in vivo within teratoma/teratocarcinoma tumors following engraftment into immunodeficient mice
- Can colonize all fetal tissues, including the germ line, during embryonic development following their injection into host blastocysts
- Clonogenic, each single cell can give rise to many other genetically identical cells that share the same properties and potentials as the original
- Specifically express the transcription factors Oct-4, Nanog, and Rex1 regulatory molecules characteristic of pluripotent cells

Based on the accumulated experience both with mouse ES cells and with human embryonal carcinoma (EC) cells (3), which are pluripotent and resemble ES cells in many respects, ES cell lines were successfully derived from nonhuman primates (common marmoset and rhesus monkeys) (4,5). These studies have set the stage for the derivation of human ES cells (hESCs) in human, first by J. Thomson (1998) (5) and Benjamin Reubinoff (2000) (6), and later by other groups. The described cell lines were derived from ICM cells of normal surplus blastocysts donated by couples undergoing IVF. The hESCs proliferate for extended periods in vitro, maintain a normal karyotype, differentiate spontaneously into somatic cell lineages of all three primary germ layers, and form teratomas when injected into immunodeficient mice. Moreover, they express a panel of markers that are typical to nonhuman primate ES cells as well as to other types of human pluripotent stem cells lines [embryonic carcinoma (EC) cells and embryonic germ (EG) cells] (7). As hESCs research advances, scientists and clinicians better appreciate the far-reaching potential of these cells. Therefore, it is not surprising that many of the IVF clinics worldwide are now aiming to set the required system and skills for the establishment of new ES cell lines from human embryos.

ORIGIN OF EMBRYOS

The increasing use of IVF for the treatment of infertility has led to the development of improved methods for handling and growing human embryos in culture. The availability of such embryos, combined with the skills obtained in the derivation of ES cells in nonhuman primates, has set the ground for the success in the establishment of hESCs lines from blastocyst stage embryos. However, the use of human embryos for research purposes has always been controversial. In general, most people consider the creation of embryos solely for research purposes immoral. Yet, harvesting stem cells from surplus embryos that were created during IVF treatments and are no longer required for assisted reproduction is also controversial. Consequently, during the past few years several methods for hESCs derivation have been developed (Fig. 30.1). Some provide an alternative source to the methods that are based on conventional

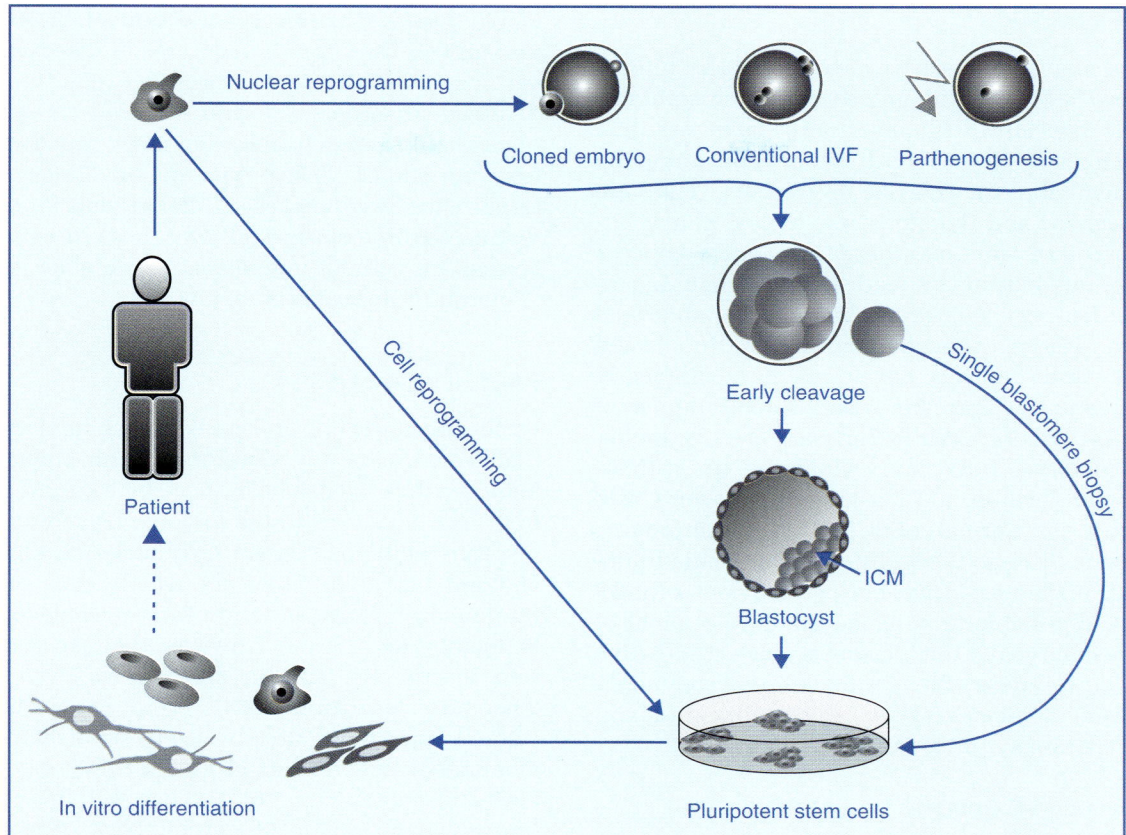

Figure 30.1 Origin and derivation of pluripotent stem cell lines. *Abbreviations*: ICM, inner cell mass; IVF, in vitro fertilization.

IVF, and therefore may be more acceptable on those who oppose to destruction of living embryos for the benefit of hESCs derivation.

CONVENTIONAL IVF

High Quality Embryos

Preimplantation Stage Embryos (Blastocyst and Early Cleavage)

In some countries it is permitted to use surplus human embryos for research. In such cases potential providers of high quality diploid embryos would be couples that have completed their IVF treatments and family planning. It is possible to obtain high quality embryos for hESCs derivation, under appropriate informed consent and ethical approval. By optimizing culture conditions, high-quality blastocysts can be obtained on day 5 postfertilization at a fairly reasonable rate. Such embryos, which were originally created for assisted reproduction, were used for the derivation of hESCs lines, first by Thomson (1998) (5) and later by many others. Although the most commonly used method for hESCs derivation employs high quality blastocysts, successful derivation from other stages of preimplantation development, such as morulas, have also been employed (8). There is an enormous amount of surplus human embryos in long-term storage in fertility clinics. These cryopreserved embryos pose hard dilemmas for couples that have completed IVF treatment and do not want any more children. They are also hard on the fertility clinics, which are short in storage place for unclaimed embryos. These surplus embryos provide ample supply of biological material for hESCs derivation. Yet, in practice, few couples donate their surplus embryos for research. Nevertheless, studies indicate that tailored education and counseling will encourage potential donors to provide more embryos for hESCs derivation (9).

Single Blastomere

An alternative approach to the commonly used methods for creating new stem cell lines that might be ethically more acceptable relies on the ability to propagate in culture a single cell removed from an early cleavage stage embryo. This technique, which is based on using single cell biopsies similar to that used in preimplantation genetic diagnosis (PGD), does not interfere with the embryo's developmental potential. The derivation of ES cells from single blastomere biopsies (SBB) was originally developed in mouse, where multiple pluripotent stem cell lines were established (10). A proof of principle experiment for this strategy was reported in humans, where 19 ES-cell-like outgrowths and two stable hESC lines were obtained (11). The later maintained undifferentiated growth in culture for more than eight months, had a normal karyotype, differentiated to embryoid bodies (EBs) in vitro and teratomas in vivo, and expressed a panel of markers that are typical to hESCs.

Low Quality Embryos

A different source for early cleavage stage human embryos may be low quality grade ones. Such embryos, which show over 50% fragmentation or have less than four blastomeres by day 3 in culture, are considered by many as unsuitable for transfer or freezing. They are usually discarded and therefore may be less controversial for use. Yet, in rare cases these low quality embryos may develop into blastocysts if allowed to remain in culture (12). In fact, it has been established that abnormal fertilization, degree of fragmentation, multinucleated blastomeres, and delayed development at the early cleavage stage tightly correlate with ICM cell number at day 5 postfertilization. While early-arrested or highly fragmented embryos only rarely yield cell lines, those that achieve to develop into blastocysts may serve as a robust source for normal hESCs (13). By improving embryo culture through the addition of Leukemia inhibitory factor (LIF) and basic fibroblast growth factor (bFGF or FGF2), it is possible to enhance the development of poor quality embryos to the blastocyst stage (14). At the same time, since low quality grade embryos commonly contain several viable cells, they can be utilized for single blastomere biopsy (SBB, see above) (15,16).

Genetically Aberrant Embryos

One potential cell source for pluripotent cell lines are genetically abnormal embryos that are routinely put aside by the IVF clinicians. Such embryos are obtained as part of preimplantation genetic screening (PGS) programs. PGS is a tailor-made assisted reproduction technique (ART) especially designed for infertile couples experiencing recurrent miscarriages or IVF failure. It involves aneuploidy screening by FISH analysis of single blastomeres, biopsied from IVF derived embryos. As such, it allows to selectively transfer embryos with a normal karyotype and occasionally results in discarding embryos with numerical chromosomal abnormalities, such as lethal trisomies and nullisomies. Yet, several reports indicate that chromosome self-correction occurs in a significant proportion of embryos, as they continue to grow in culture (17) since most of these aneuploid embryos are actually mosaic mixtures of normal and chromosomally abnormal cells (18). These embryos may serve as a potential source of cells for hESCs derivation, as was demonstrated by Peura et al. (2007) (19) and Lavon et al. (20). Moreover, it is possible to establish hESC lines that naturally carry specific gene defects. Such mutant pluripotent cell lines can be established directly from genetically affected embryos, obtained through PGD. PGD is an ART that benefits couples at high risk of transmitting a genetic defect. In PGD, embryos diagnosed to be free of the disease are selectively transferred for implantation while the affected ones are discarded. The genetically aberrant embryos can be used for the establishment of novel ES cell lines, which naturally inherit mutations associated with particular genetic disorders. To date, over 150 different HESC lines have been established from genetically affected embryos through PGD (19–24). This large collection of hESCs includes mutant cell lines for a wide range of diseases including various dominant and recessive conditions, many X-linked disorders, several chromosomal rearrangements, and even cell lines that carry cancer predisposition mutations. These type of cell lines have great importance by serving as cellular models for the study of distinct disorders, especially for those in which no good animal or cellular models are available (see section "Potential Applications" below).

PARTHENOGENESIS

Parthenogenesis is a process by which an oocyte is stimulated to divide and develop into an embryo without being fertilized. It can be induced by triggering the oocyte to resume meiosis without undergoing cell division. The resulting embryos contain only maternal chromosomes and are unviable. They are usually lost at the peri-implantation stage, suffering from poor development of extraembryonic tissues. However, they can easily develop into blastocysts, and in some cases even reach the 25-somite stage (in mice) (25). Indeed, parthenogenetic ES cell lines have already been established in several mammalian species including mice (26), macaque monkeys (27), and human (28,29). These cell lines display the typical characteristic of normal hESC lines. They are immortal; express the typical markers of undifferentiated cells, differentiate into many different cell types in vitro, and form teratomas in severe combined immunodeficient (SCID) mice. The great advantage of generating parthenogenetic hESCs is that it involves egg manipulation, rather than embryo destruction. Moreover, they may be more acceptable for the production of new cell lines since they naturally lack a full potential for embryo development. Another advantage of parthenogenetic hESC lines over conventional cell lines is that they have two identical sets of chromosomes, that is, they are predominantly homozygous. Homozygosity reduces the complexity of tissue matching of the cells and therefore may be a favorable cell source for hESCs when considered for cell-based therapy (28). Yet, it remains to be shown if these cells are indistinguishable from wild-type cells in terms of their function and safety due to their unusual epigenetic status, which reflects the status of the chromosomes in the oocyte, lacking paternal imprints.

SOMATIC CELL REPROGRAMMING

Nuclear Transfer-Derived Embryos

It might be possible to obtain ES cell lines from blastocysts that have been established by somatic cell nuclear transfer (SCNT). In this method, a nucleus from a somatic cell of an adult is introduced into an enucleated oocyte, resulting in a cloned embryo. The SCNT-derived blastocyst may be used for the establishment of an ES cell line perfectly matched to the donor of the nucleus, which can serve as an unlimited source of cells for autologous transplantation. In addition, this approach is especially advantageous for the derivation of affected hESC lines for a wide range of multifactorial disorders, such as heart disorders, diabetes, and cancer, which result from mutations in multiple genes. The complicated bases of these diseases make them especially difficult to model, study, and treat. Although sophisticated, the procedure termed therapeutic cloning is not unreasonable, as it has been previously demonstrated to be feasible in mice (30,31) and primates (32). Moreover, it has been shown that human oocytes are capable of supporting embryo development following somatic cell nuclear transfer to the blastocyst stage using nuclei of undifferentiated hESCs (33) and even fully differentiated fibroblasts (34). However, so far, the derivation of ES cells from human SCNT embryos was not reported. In addition, before therapeutic cloning can be considered for clinical use, safety concerns should be carefully addressed and it should be determined how well a somatic nucleus can be reprogrammed without being transmitted through the germ line (35). Moreover, the problem of egg supply must be resolved to make it practical for clinical application. Although in vitro matured oocytes can be used as recipients for human SCNT, they can support embryonic development only to the four- to eight-cell stage, the stage at which embryonic genome activation normally takes place (36). Further research is required to reveal whether culture conditions alone can improve human embryonic development to the blastocyst stage following SCNT using in vitro maturation of oocytes.

Transcription Factor Induced Pluripotent Stem (iPS) Cells

If an efficient method for de-differentiating somatic cells directly in culture was available, the technical and ethical complications associated with embryo availability and destruction, egg donation for research purposes, and cloning would have been resolved. Moreover, it would allow the derivation of many different cell clones from a single individual. In addition, it may have particular advantages for producing disease models directly from somatic cells of patients, specifically in cases where the gene defect underlying the disease is extremely rare, has not yet been identified, results from multiple genes simultaneously, is highly variable in expression, or is of low penetrance. Indeed, recent studies in mice and human show that differentiated cells can be induced to reprogram to an ES-like pluripotent state by over-expression of only few defined transcription factors (Oct4, Sox2, Nanog, c-Myc, and Klf4) (37–40). These artificially induced pluripotent stem (iPS) cell lines can be employed as cellular models for a wide range of disorders including amyotrophic lateral sclerosis (ALS) (41), familial dysautonomia (42), type 1 diabetes (43), Long QT syndrome (44), Rett syndrome (45) and even Hutchinson Gilford Progeria (46) and Dyskeratosis congenital (47). The iPS cells display all characteristics typical to ES cells including cell morphology, self-renewal ability, developmental potential (teratomas and germ-line transmitting chimeras), and gene expression pattern. The iPS cells can be derived from many different types of somatic cells in human, including fibroblasts, keratinocytes, blood, and even pancreas (48–51). Yet, although iPS cells are easier to obtain and may even complement hESCs under particular conditions, they still need to be thoroughly compared with hESCs, which are still considered the gold standard by which all other pluripotent stem cells are judged. If these cells prove to be indistinguishable from hESCs in terms of their biological potential and epigenetic state, and safety issues related to their production are resolved, then this approach would bypass the technical and ethical difficulties that are involved with hESCs derivation.

DERIVATION OF HUMAN ES CELLS

The same methodologies that were developed for the derivation of mouse ES cell lines were used for the initial derivation of human lines, with some modifications. According to these methodologies, human embryos are cultured to the expanded blastocyst stage by using the standard commercially available media. The importance of blastocyst quality for the successful derivation of ES cell lines has not been studied in a systematic manner. Data from various stem cell centers, regarding the success rates of ES cells derivation from blastocysts, demonstrate a 13–50% efficiency (5,7,15,52).

The zona pellucida of the blastocyst is first removed by either enzymatic (6) or chemical digestion (15). To isolate the ICM, the outer trophectoderm layer is removed, most commonly by immunosurgery (5,6), although gentle mechanical (using 27 G needles) (15) or laser-assisted (53) removal is also possible. The ICM is then plated on mitotically inactivated feeders that support the proliferation and prevent the differentiation of the stem cells. In an alternative approach, isolation of the ICM is not performed and the intact blastocyst is plated on feeders (54). While successful derivation of hESCs lines has been reported following plating of intact blastocysts, further studies are required to compare the efficiencies of deriving new lines from isolated ICMs versus intact blastocysts.

So far, mouse embryonic fibroblasts (MEFs) were most commonly used in the derivation of human ES cells, though human fibroblasts derived from fetal muscle (55), placenta (56), foreskin (57), lung (16), marrow cells (58,) and from hESCs themselves were also utilized.

Derivation of the most commonly used MEFs follows the methods that were originally described for the mouse ES cell system (3), and the fibroblasts are maintained in culture according to standard tissue culture techniques. Similar to the mouse ES cell system, to maintain the potential of the fibroblasts to support undifferentiated proliferation of hESCs, it is important to avoid overcrowded cultures (3). In addition, minimizing the digestion by trypsin during routine subculture may also improve the efficiency of the fibroblasts to support undifferentiated growth. A relatively low concentration of trypsin (0.05%) is recommended. Only low passage cells (up to passage 5) are used to prepare feeder layers within gelatin treated tissue culture dishes.

Human feeders are commercially available (CRL-2429; ATCC, Manassas, VA) (57,59). Mitotic inactivation of feeders may be accomplished either by irradiation (5) or by treatment with mitomycin C (6). There may be a significant variability between various batches of MEFs, which were derived according to the same protocol, with respect to their capability of supporting undifferentiated proliferation of hESCs. To overcome this problem, the competence of various batches of MEFs to support undifferentiated cultures of established mouse or primate ES cell lines may be tested prior to their use in the derivation of new hESC lines. It has been suggested that human foreskin feeders are more potent than mouse feeders in preventing spontaneous differentiation (57).

The composition of the culture medium that was initially used for the derivation of hESC was similar to the traditional serum containing composition that was developed for the mouse ES cell system. High quality water and serum with low endotoxin levels are required for successful derivation and propagation of hESCs. Serum free media are now more commonly used to derive new hESC lines (53,60) (Appendix C). Variability in the competence of serum replacement preparations to promote undifferentiated propagation of hESCs may exist and comparing the competence of few batches on existing hESC lines to select the most competent batch for the derivation of new hESC lines may be considered.

Within several days following plating of ICMs or intact blastocysts on feeders, groups of small tightly packed cells may be identified proliferating from the ICMs. Seven to eight days after plating, clumps of these small cells may be mechanically isolated from outgrowths of differentiated cells by using the sharp edge of a glass micropipette. Following replating on fresh feeders, they give rise to round flat colonies of cells with well-defined borders (Fig. 30.2). The cells within the colonies have a large nucleus, a high nuclear cytoplasmic ratio, and prominent nucleoli (Fig. 30.2). The colonies are further propagated about every seven days.

To exploit the potential of hESCs for regenerative medicine, they should preferably be derived and propagated in an animal-free defined culture system, under clean room conditions, utilizing good manufacture practice (GMP)–grade reagents. The process of derivation should be strictly documented. Numerous studies reported on various improvements toward the development of hESC lines under the above conditions (clinical-grade hESCs). So far, only a single group reported the derivation of hESC lines under GMP conditions, though animal-derived reagents were still utilized for culturing both the feeders and hESCs (61).

Derivation of hESCs raises moral concerns due to the destruction of the ex utero preimplantation early human embryos. To avoid these moral issues, methodology to derive hESCs from single blastomeres, which may be removed from the cleavage-stage embryo by biopsy, as performed during PGD, without interfering with the embryo's developmental potential was established (11,62). Following initial overnight culture and proliferation of the single blastomere, the resulting cells may serve for both PGD and stem cell derivation. Thus the procedure does not interfere with the process of PGD, or the developmental competence of the embryo. It addresses the ethical concerns of many, and allows the generation of matched tissue for children born from transferred PGD embryos.

MAINTENANCE OF HUMAN ES CELLS IN CULTURE

Human ES cell cultures usually include a variable level of background spontaneous differentiation. To minimize this process, selective propagation of predominantly undifferentiated colonies or of undifferentiated areas (usually in the periphery of the colonies) may be required to maintain the culture at an undifferentiated state. Human ES cells are highly sociable cells and the survival of single cells is low, therefore, propagation of clumps of 50 cells is most commonly used (Appendix D).

In addition to the traditional serum containing culture system, an alternative serum-free culture method has been developed and is commonly used (Appendix C). A commercially available supplement is used to replace the serum, and FGF2 is required to promote undifferentiated proliferation (63). The serum-free culture system is more effective in supporting the survival of single hESCs. While the cloning efficiency is extremely low in the presence of serum, it is improved to 0.83% in the serum-free culture system (63). The addition of Rho-associated kinase (ROCK) inhibitor to the growth medium was shown to further improve hESCs cloning efficiency (64).

The requirement for feeder cells may be eliminated by culturing the stem cells on laminin, fibronectin, or Matrigel-coated plastic surfaces in the presence of mouse embryonic fibroblasts-conditioned medium (65–67). The development of feeder-independent culture systems improves the capability of growing the hESCs on a large scale and manipulating them in vitro. Great efforts by many research groups have been directed to identify the growth factors that will support the maintenance of hESCs in the absence of feeders or their conditioned medium. FGF2 (68), and factors from the transforming growth factor (TGF) superfamily (activin and TGFβ1 (69,70)) were most commonly reported to support undifferentiated propagation of hESCs. In addition, Wnt signaling (71), insulin growth factor (IGF) signaling (72), as well as blocking of Bone morphogenic protein (BMP) signaling (68) have been shown to have a role in maintaining pluripotency of hESCs without feeders. Various combinations of growth factors including FGF2, noggin, TGFβ1, activin A, pipecolic acid, γ-aminobutyric acid (GABA), LiCl, with various media, and culturing the cells on various extracellular matrices were shown to promote feeder-free cultures of undifferentiated hESCs (70,73–82). Derivation and propagation of hESCs in suspension, with or without microcarriers, provides another feeder-free culture system, which may pave the way to large-scale expansion of hESCs (83–90). Further studies are required to identify the ideal chemically defined, feeder and animal reagent-free culture system that will support prolonged self-renewal of genetically stable pluripotent hESCs.

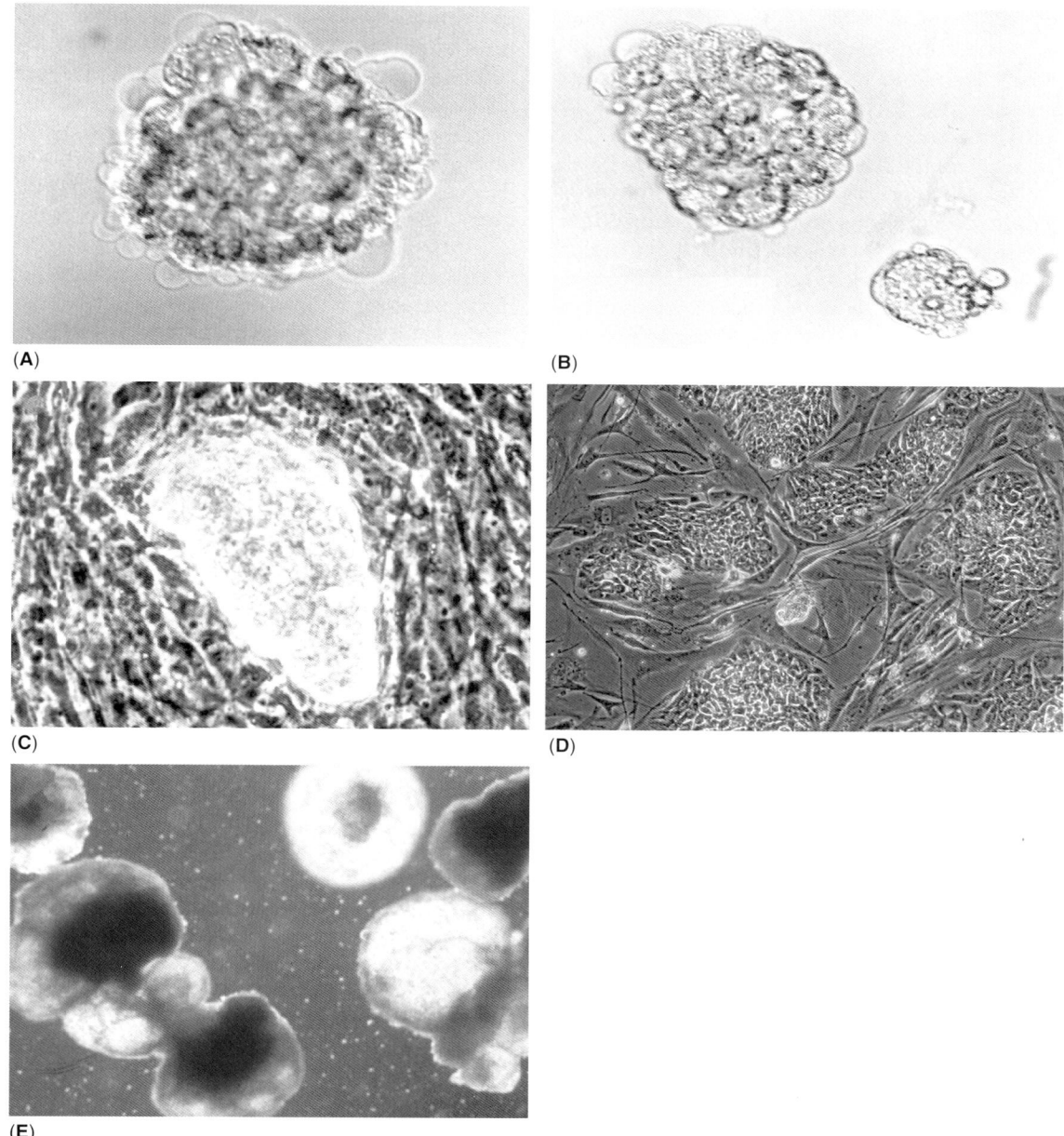

Figure 30.2 Human ES cells – derivation, propagation, and in vitro differentiation. Phase contrast images of six-day-old human blastocysts undergoing immunosurgery. Note lysis of trophectodermal cells (**A**) Isolated inner cell mass (ICM) near the remnants of the trophectodermal cells (**B**) An ICM three days after plating on MEFs (**C**) Human embryonic stem (ES) colonies four days after plating on mouse embryonic fibroblasts (MEFs) (**D**) Twenty-day-old cystic embryoid bodies (EBs) (**E**) Figures A and B with the courtesy of A. Bongso and CY Fong, Figures D and E with the courtesy of N Benvenisty, and Figure C with the permission of Nature Publishing Group.

The niche that regulates self-renewal and pluripotency of hESCs has been extensively studied. It has been suggested (72) that the niche is comprised of autologous fibroblast-like cells, which originate from the hESCs themselves. In response to FGF signaling, the hESCs-derived fibroblasts secrete IGF-II, which acts directly on hESCs through IGF1 receptor and promotes self-renewal. While the expression of IGF1 receptor is restricted to the hESCs, the fibroblasts exclusively express FGF receptor. Activation of FGF signaling in the fibroblasts also induces the secretion of TGFβ, which prevents differentiation of hESCs. Thus it was suggested that FGF factors do not act directly on hESCs but rather through the autologously derived fibroblasts that secrete IGF-II and TGFβ factors.

In line with these data, it has been shown that IGF-II can promote the undifferentiated propagation of hESCs in the absence of feeders (72). Others challenged this concept and showed evidence for direct effect of FGF signaling on hESCs (91).

Human ES cells may be cryopreserved by the conventional slow rate freezing and rapid thawing method (using hESC serum-free culture medium supplemented with 10% Dimethyl sulfoxide (DMSO) and 30% serum replacement) (67). However, given the relatively low effectiveness of this approach (92), a large number of cells should be frozen to achieve successful and reliable thawing. It has been reported that the addition of ROCK inhibitor to the pre-freezing and post-thawing medium increases cell survival (93,94).

In the initial steps of derivation of new hES cells lines, or when the culture conditions are not ideal, large numbers of undifferentiated hES cells may not be available. Under these circumstances, vitrification with the opened pulled-straw method (OPS), allows reliable cryopreservation. The cells retain their key properties following thawing (92).

It should be noted that under optimal culture conditions, when the level of background differentiation is low, nonselective propagation of the cultures in bulk by using gentle enzymatic digestion (with collagenase IV or trypsin) is possible. However, changing the culture conditions and methods of propagation may be associated with the acquirement of genetic abnormalities by the cells. Therefore, it is essential to monitor the genetic stability of the cells by routine repeated cytogenetic analyses (95). The genetic stability of hESCs can also be analyzed by array-CGH (96,97) or Single nucleotide polymorphism (SNP) analysis (98,99), which have higher resolution compared to conventional karyotyping. These molecular assays can identify small genetic abnormalities, however, the interpretation of the significance of these findings needs further research and clarification.

CHARACTERIZATION OF HUMAN ES CELLS

Establishing a consensus regarding the exact uniform criteria and standards that should be used to characterize and define hESCs would be extremely useful in comparing the characteristics of different hESC lines (100). So far, the hESC lines that were derived by a number of groups were characterized by demonstrating the key properties of ES cells (as above) that were applicable to the human system. Given the potential unlimited self-renewal capability of hESCs, an important part of the characterization process is to repeatedly demonstrate the key properties during prolonged propagation of the cells in culture. Here, we will summarize the properties that were most commonly used to define the reported hESC lines in the literature.

Colonies of hESCs are flat with well-defined borders distinct from the surrounding fibroblasts. In the presence of serum, undifferentiated cells have distinct borders, a large nucleus with prominent nucleoli and a high nuclear cytoplasmic ratio (Fig. 30.2) (5,7). In serum free-culture conditions, the colonies tend to become more tightly packed, with less distinct borders between the cells (63).

The International Stem Cell Initiative (ISCI) characterized 59 hESC lines from a large number of laboratories worldwide (101). Despite diverse genotypes and the different techniques that were used for derivation and maintenance, all lines exhibited remarkably similar phenotypes. All cell lines strongly expressed the glycolipid antigens SSEA3 and SSEA4, the keratin sulphate antigens TRA-1–60, TRA-1–81, GCTM2, and GCT343, and the protein antigens CD9 and Thy1 (CD90). In addition, they were all positive for tissue-nonspecific alkaline phosphatase and class 1 Human leukocyte antigen (HLA), and strongly expressed the developmentally regulated genes NANOG, OCT4 (POU5F1), TDGF, DNMT3B, GABRB3, and GDF3.

The characterization of hESCs further includes the demonstration of key properties of ES cells. Standard cytogenetic analysis methods are used to show that the stem cells retain a normal karyotype along propagation in culture (5,6,102). Although most hESC lines have a normal diploid karyotype during their initial growth period, accumulated data suggests that the cells tend to acquire chromosomal abnormalities during prolonged culture (103,104). The most frequent karyotype changes observed were gains of chromosomes 12 and 17, and to a lesser extent chromosome X, aberrations which are typical to testicular germ cell tumors. The nonrandom nature of the observed changes in the hESCs culture strongly points toward a selection pressure that drives to the appearance of these specific chromosomal abnormalities. These changes most probably reflect the progressive adaptation of self-renewing cells to their culture conditions, evidenced by increased growth rate, enhanced cloning efficiency, reduced tendency for apoptosis, and decrease in differentiation capacity in high passage cultures. Suboptimal culture conditions, including cell harvesting technique (manual as opposed to bulk), cell density, type of growth media, supporting feeder layer, and multiple rounds of thawing, appear to favor a drift toward chromosomally abnormal cells, which may overtake the culture. Therefore, regardless of what the selection driving factors are, it is absolutely essential to regularly monitor the karyotype of the cells at frequent intervals.

The pluripotent potential of hESCs is demonstrated by showing the potential of the cells to differentiate into progeny representing the three germ layers both in vitro and in vivo within teratoma tumors. Induction of differentiation in vitro is described in details in the following section. Teratoma tumors are generated following engraftment (intramuscular (5), under the testicle, or kidney capsule (6,) and subcutaneously (105)) of undifferentiated cells into SCID mice (4–6 weeks old) (63) (Fig. 30.3). The utilization of variable amounts of undifferentiated cells ($10^3 - 5 \times 10^6$) (67,106) was reported to produce teratomas within six to 16 weeks following engraftment. Histological analysis of the tumors reveals a variety of differentiated tissues including gut-like, primitive bronchus (endoderm) bone, cartilage, striated muscle, and fetal glomeruli (mesoderm) squamous epithelium and primitive neural tissue (ectoderm) (Fig. 30.3) (5,6,107).

Clonal expansion of a pluripotent cell population from a single cell is required to verify that the cultures are not mixtures of early progenitors of multiple lineages but truly include pluripotent cells.

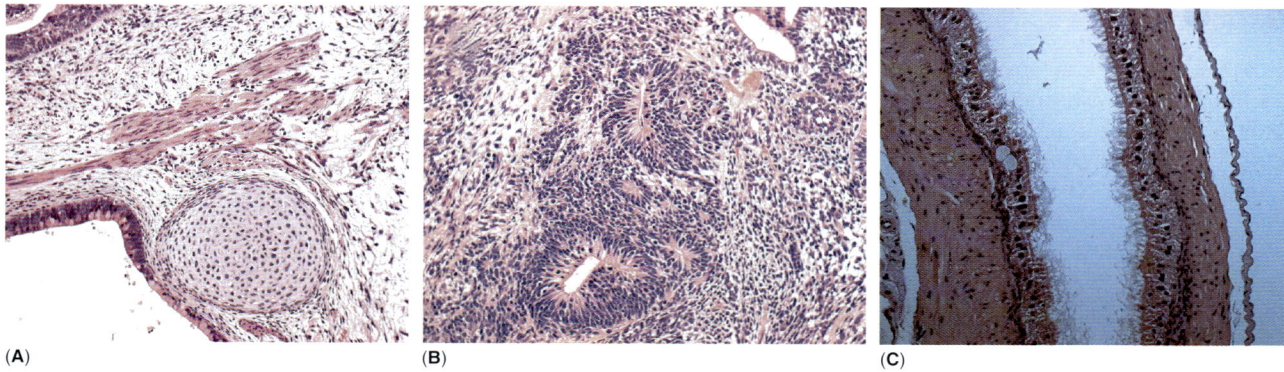

Figure 30.3 Histology of differentiated tissues within teratoma tumors. Shown cartilage and squamous epithelium [(**A**) mesoderm and ectoderm), neuronal rosettes [(**B**) ectoderm)], and ciliated columnar epithelium [(**C**)endoderm)].

IN VITRO DIFFERENTIATION

Spontaneous Differentiation

Spontaneous Differentiation by Cell Aggregation

It is possible to trigger the differentiation of hESCs in vitro by growing them in suspension culture. In suspension, the cells tend to aggregate, forming multicellular structures termed EBs (108). As these cell structures form, they undergo spontaneous differentiation to produce terminally differentiated cells of mesoderm, ectoderm, and endoderm origin. The formation of EBs is a gradual process and is accompanied by morphological changes. It begins with the formation of small bodies of densely packed cells (simple EBs), which by day 7 begin to cavitate (cavitated EBs) and eventually accumulate fluid within cysts. By day 20, the cystic EBs, which are a product of spontaneous and disorganized differentiation, are considered to be mature and are composed of various terminally differentiated cell types, including nerve (109–111), blood (112), endothelial (113), heart (114), and pancreatic (115) cells. Some have even been shown to be functional as in the case of nerve cells (109).

The EBs can easily be obtained by growing the cells under conditions that prevent their adherence to the culture dish. This is performed by growing the cells in bacterial petri dishes in the absence of feeders, thereby promoting their aggregation (see Appendix E). However, this method entails large variations in size and shape of the EBs, and therefore, also in the differentiation status of the cells. To obtain a more homogeneous cell culture, the "hanging drop" method may be applied (see Appendix E).

Spontaneous Differentiation by Prolonged Culture on Feeders

An alternative method for inducing spontaneous differentiation is to obtain high-density cultures. The hESCs are cultivated to high density for extended periods (four weeks) in the presence of serum, without replacement of the feeder layer. High-density cultures lead to the piling up of cells, forming three dimensional multicellular and vesicular structures (6). Progeny representing the three embryonic germ layers, as well as differentiated cells from the extra embryonic lineages are generated within high density cultures (6,107). While, in general, differentiation within high-density cultures is disorganized, areas within these cultures that are comprised predominantly from one committed progenitor cell type may be identified. By dissecting these areas out from the cultures it is possible to isolate and develop highly enriched cultures of early progenitors from a specific lineage such as the neural one (107).

INDUCED DIFFERENTIATION

Spontaneous differentiation of ES cells in vitro is a stochastic process that results in the production of heterogeneous cell populations. However, the development of a highly purified population of a specific cell type is required for most of the scientific and therapeutic applications of hESCs. Thus, it is necessary to direct the differentiation of the cells in vitro and/or to combine it with a lineage-based selection approach. There are several strategies that can be utilized for this purpose:

Growth Factors

Exogenic factors can augment the process of differentiation toward a specific cell fate (110). For example, it has been well established that the addition of retinoic acid (RA) (110), Noggin, and/or TGFβ inhibitor (116,117) induces the differentiation of ES cells into neurons, and that BMP4 can direct their differentiation into trophoblast cells (118).

The growth or differentiation inducing factors can be supplemented continuously or sequentially to the media, according to the requested cell type and protocol. They may be used to promote differentiation into a specific fate within EBs or in flat feeder-dependent (119) or feeder-free (82) cultures. Since the cultures that are obtained following treatments with differentiation-inducing factors are still relatively heterogeneous, at present, this approach should be combined with additional strategies such as lineage selection, selective culture conditions, and overexpression of key transcription factors.

Lineage Selection

The lineage selection approach allows the obtaining of a highly purified population of cells by performing selection for or against a specific cell type. Cells of a specific type may be sorted from heterogeneous populations of differentiated cells based on the expression of lineage-specific cell surface markers, or by genetic selection. The latter approach is based on the genetic introduction of a selectable marker gene under the regulation of a tissue specific promoter. The marker gene may either be a selectable reporter, such as Green fluorescent protein (GFP), which can be selected for by fluorescence-activated cell sorter (FACS) (120,121) or the insertion of a drug resistance gene such as the neomycin resistance gene, which allows the direct isolation of the desired cells by the presence of G418 in the media (122).

Overexpression of Key Regulator Genes

It is possible to force the differentiation of ES cells into specific lineages by over-expressing transcription factors which play major roles in early commitment of cells into specific lineages. This has been previously demonstrated to be feasible in the mouse ES cell system, where over-expression of MyoD resulted in the induction of skeletal myocytes, which fused to create multinuclear contractile myotubes (123). Similar experiments demonstrated the effect of Hepatocyte nuclear factor (HNF) on the generation of hepatocytes (124), and of Nurr1 in the production of dopaminergic neurons (125).

POTENTIAL APPLICATIONS AND FUTURE GOALS

Cell Source for Transplantation

The establishment of ES cell lines was achieved in many mammalian species since the first derivation of such cells in mice. Yet, none drew as much attention as the human derived cells due to their enormous biomedical potential. Since hESCs can be grown indefinitely in culture without losing their basic properties, and have the potential to develop into practically any cell type in vitro, they may be used as an unlimited cell source for cell transplantation. Once efficient protocols for induced differentiation are established, it will be possible to generate specific cell types in large numbers for the repair of degenerating or damaged tissues in humans. This will reduce the current supply problems of tissues available for transplantation. Indeed, it has been demonstrated that both mouse and human ES cell-derived progeny can integrate following their transplantation into adult animals. The transplanted differentiated cells were shown to provide a therapeutic effect in animal models of various conditions (107,111,122,125–131).

Following extensive studies showing safety and therapeutic effectiveness in animal models, the first two Phase I clinical trials using hESCs derivatives are currently in progress. One using oligodendrocyte progenitor cells (GRNOPC1) to treat spinal cord injury (132), and the other uses retinal pigment epithelial (RPE) cells to treat Stargardt macular dystrophy (SMD), and dry age-related macular degeneration (dry AMD).

Immune rejection is expected after transplantation of hESC-derived progeny, which are shown to express major histocompatibility complex (MHC) class I antigens (133). There are several possibilities that can be applied for minimizing graft rejection of ES cell derivatives. One possibility is to establish a bank that will include a large number of ES cell lines that differ in their MHC expressed molecules, thus allowing MHC matching between the donor cell line and the recipient. Alternatively, it may be possible to generate a "universal" donor cell line by "knocking out" the genes that are responsible for graft rejection. Finally, it might be feasible in the future to generate genetically identical ES cell lines, either by somatic cell nuclear transfer or by de-differentiating somatic cells directly in culture through genetic manipulation, as described earlier in this chapter, to provide the patients with autologous grafts.

Gene Therapy

One of the great advantages of ES cells over other cell types is their accessibility for genetic manipulation. They can easily be induced to genetic modifications and can be selectively propagated, allowing the clonal expansion of genetically altered cells in culture (134). Genetic manipulation of hESCs can therefore be utilized for monitoring, selecting, and even directing the differentiation of the cells into specific lineages. Moreover, the hESC-derived progenitors may be used as delivery vectors for the regulated release of drugs and therapeutic proteins at the site of the damaged tissue. Such a cell-based delivery system will permit the production of a therapeutic agent at a steady state level and in consistent physiological concentrations, overcoming current limitations caused by incomplete drug accessibility. Furthermore, it may be possible sometime in the future to repair the genetic defect by replacing the aberrant gene with an intact sequence. This can be accomplished by coupling embryo cloning with gene therapy, so that the genetic manipulation will be carried out on the genome of SCNT-derived isogenic hESC lines obtained from patients. Using this technique, it is possible to cure the disease by providing the patients with genetically engineered autologous grafts, overcoming the difficulties in graft rejection as a result of the immune response. This approach of combining gene therapy with therapeutic cloning has been previously shown to be feasible in mice, where immune-deficient Rag2-/- mutant mice were used as nuclear donors for generating blastocysts from which an isogenic ES cell line was isolated (31). The mutant ES cells were corrected for Rag2-/- gene activity by homologous recombination and used as a source for hematopoietic committed cells. The genetically engineered blood cells were then grafted into the Rag2-/- mutant mice, resulting in the rescue of the immune-deficient phenotype (31).

Drug Screening and Toxicology

Much effort is invested in the development of new drugs by trying to understand the pathology of a disease and its underlying treatment. This approach, which is disease-oriented, requires model systems that are based on human cells, rather than animals, which, in many cases, are inadequate. Obviously, the best model system would be specific cell types of humans that display the appropriate phenotype. However, the currently available cellular models in humans are limited in their potential by the lack of relevant and validated cell types. Most are suboptimal since they are based on the use of abnormal cancer cell lines or on primary cell cultures. Human ES cells, however, may be exceptionally useful for drug screening and development, as they have the capacity to self-renew in culture and can potentially differentiate into all cell types in the body. Provided that efficient protocols for induced differentiation of hESCs are established, it will be possible to generate specific cell types in large numbers so that the targeted tissues will be accessible for large-scale drug screening and development. Moreover, hESCs can be genetically modified relatively easily. This should allow the introduction of reporter genes, under appropriate regulation, that will facilitate the analysis of examined compounds. In addition, establishing mutant cell lines will allow generating specific terminally differentiated impaired cells in large numbers so that diseased tissues of patients will be accessible for research. Finally, since differentiating hESCs can recapitulate, to some extent, early human embryogenesis, they may have great value in assessing the potential toxicity of new drug candidates and their teratogenic effect.

Embryo Development

The study of early human development is restricted by ethical constrains on research of human embryos. Moreover, apart from the early stages of preimplantation development, human embryos are inaccessible for research. The use of animal models, specifically the mouse, has allowed overcoming these obstacles, taking advantage of their well-defined genetics and reproductive characteristics. Yet, despite the strong conservation throughout evolution, there are still major differences in critical developmental events as a product of genetic variation across species. The limitation of the currently available models has emphasized the need for an alternative system that would better mimic certain aspects of early human embryo development. hESCs may have great value for basic research as well, since they recapitulate early events in embryo development as they are induced to spontaneously differentiate in vitro. The concept of using differentiating ES cells as an in vitro model system to study developmentally regulated biological phenomena has been originally practiced in the mouse, where growing EBs were used for studying X inactivation (135) and globin gene switching (136). In humans, gene expression microarray studies have shown that spontaneously differentiating hESCs mimic, in terms of gene transcription, developmental stages in the embryo which are otherwise unattainable for research (137). Moreover, gene profiling has allowed recovering known molecular pathways during human EBs formation, as they occur in the embryo. Hence, hESCs can serve as a model to study early human development.

Genetic Disorders in Human

The limitations of the currently available animal and cellular models, as described above, have emphasized the need of an alternative system that will better mimic certain genetic anomalies. The availability of mutant hESCs that harbor a specific mutation at a discrete site should be most valuable for the study of some pathologies in man. Basically, there are two strategies by which mutant hESCs can be established. One is to artificially induce a specific modification in the DNA of a preexisting cell line by homologous recombination. Using this approach, a cellular model system for Lesch–Nyhan syndrome was generated by targeting the HPRT gene in XY wild-type hESCs (138,139). The other approach is to establish an hESC line directly from a genetically affected embryo so that the resulting cell lines will naturally inherit the genetic defect (see section Conventional IVF under Genetically aberrant embryos). The great advantage of this approach, as compared to the former, is that it does not require to genetically engineer the cells. In addition, it allows introducing genetic modifications that are otherwise inaccessible such as triplet repeat expansions as well as numerical and structural chromosomal abnormalities. To date, mutant hESC lines have been established for various disorders including Cystic fibrosis (CF) (21), myotonic dystrophy (24), Huntington disease (24), Duchenne muscular dystrophy (22), thalassemia (22), Fragile X syndrome (140), Hemophilia A (53) as well as trisomies 16 and 5 (20,52,53,90,141–144). These type of cell lines have great importance by serving as cellular models for the study of distinct disorders, especially for those in which no good animal or cellular models are available (see section Potential Applications above). It will enable to generate large amounts of the desired cells that are directly impaired by the genetic lesion. Availability of such cells will allow studying the abnormal phenotype at the cellular and molecular levels, providing greater understanding of the pathology of the disease. Moreover, there are some disorders that are developmentally regulated and their genetic abnormality exerts its effect during the early stage of embryogenesis. In such cases, mutant hESCs will have an extremely important role in investigating the underlying mechanism that leads to the manifestation of disease. Using this approach, a fragile X affected hESC line was used to investigate the molecular events that are involved in the pathogenesis of this disease, demonstrating that the inactivation of the associated gene is a multistep process that is developmentally regulated and is triggered by cell differentiation (140). Finally, the availability of mutant hESC lines will allow carrying out disease-oriented drug screenings and may serve as a powerful tool for gene manipulation and therapy, as described above.

CONCLUSIONS

The derivation of ES cell lines from human embryos has initiated a new era in the fields of biotechnology, pharmacology, basic scientific research, and regenerative medicine. It is now well established that hESC lines can be readily and reproducibly derived. Yet, there still exists a need to increase the number of cell lines that are available to the research community and to generate more lines with a broader genetic and ethnic background. New lines from genetically abnormal embryos are also required, as well as lines suitable for clinical purposes. Much more research and development is required to exploit the remarkable potential of hESCs. Appropriate public support and adequate legislation are crucial for the realization of the far-reaching applications of hESCs.

PROTOCOLS

Appendix A: Immunosurgery

1. Reconstitute antihuman serum (Sigma, St. Louis, MO; Cat number H-3383) with 2 ml DDW. Dilute 1:5 in blastocyst culture medium.
2. Reconstitute guinea pig complement (Invitrogen, Rockville, MD) with 5 ml of PBS. Dilute 1:5 in blastocyst culture medium.
3. Prepare a four-well dish with a 10 µl drop of the antihuman serum under pre-equilibrated sterile mineral oil. Place 0.5 ml of blastocyst culture medium in the other wells.
4. Transfer the blastocyst to the antihuman serum drop for 30 minutes incubation in 5% CO_2.
5. Prepare a four-well dish with a 50 µl drop of the complement solution under pre-equilibrated mineral oil. Place 0.5 ml blastocyst culture media in other wells. Incubate 10–15 minutes in 37°C, 5% CO_2.
6. Transfer the embryo after three washes in blastocyst medium into the complement drop and incubate 30 minutes.
7. Wash × 3 in blastocyst medium.
8. Remove the damaged trophectodermal cells by pipetting the blastocyst through a small-bore glass pipette.
9. Plate the resulting ICM clump on a MEF feeder layer that was plated the previous day and cultured with the culture medium for hESCs.
10. If there are indications of low ICM viability, (low plating efficiency and/or low colony formation), all washes should be extended to 5 minutes.

Appendix B: Preparation of MEF cells

Isolation of MEFS

1. Collect 13.5-day-old fetuses from pregnant mice using sterile equipment: Sacrifice pregnant mice and dissect the embryos by removing the uterus and transferring it into a sterile PBS-containing petri dish.
2. Rinse twice in PBS and relocate all work to laminar flow hood.
3. Using sterile tweezers and scissors, remove the fetuses from the uterus, separate them from extra-embryonic tissues (amniotic and yolk sacs), and transfer them to a clean petri dish with PBS.
4. Count the number of collected fetuses and prepare, for later use, 1× 10-cm tissue culture dish for every three fetuses.
5. Remove head and internal parts (liver, heart, kidney, lung, and intestine) with sterile tweezers under a stereomicroscope.
6. Cut the remaining tissues into small pieces in a minimal volume of PBS (1–2 mL) and transfer into a sterile 50-mL Falcon tube.
7. Disaggregate the cell clumps obtained by cutting them into tiny pieces with sterile knife scalpels.
8. Add MEF media to reach 10 mL per three embryos, distribute cell suspension evenly into 10-cm tissue culture dishes and incubate.
9. Change media the following day. When plates are confluent (2–3 days after dissection) split 1:3 by trypsinization.
10. Change media (10 mL) every two days. When cell density reaches confluence, trypsinize the cells and freeze each 10-cm plate in one cryovial, store in liquid nitrogen.

Mitomycin-c Inactivation of MEFs

1. Thaw contents of one cryotube into 3× 10-cm culture dishes.
2. Grow the cells to confluence by changing the media every other day.
3. Further propagate the cells by splitting them twice at a 1:3 dilution (sums to 27 plates).
4. To inactivate the cells, add 40 µL of mitomycin-C stock solution (1 mg/mL) to 5 mL culture media (final concentration of 8 µg/mL) and incubate at 37°C, 5% CO_2, for three hours.
5. Aspirate the mitomycin-containing medium and wash the plates twice with 6 mL PBS.
6. Trypsinize cells by adding 1 mL of trypsin-EDTA and incubate at 37°C, 5% CO_2, for 5 minutes.
7. Add 5 mL medium and suspend the cells by vigorous pipetting.
8. Collect cell suspension into a 50-mL Falcon tube.
9. Centrifuge mitomycin-treated cell pool at 1000 g for 5 minutes.
10. Aspirate supernatant and add fresh medium to reach a final cell concentration of 4×10^6 cells/10-cm dish. Feeder plates can be stored in the incubator for three to four days, but should be examined under the microscope before use.
11. It is possible to freeze mitomycin-C treated MEFs and keep them for later use. For this purpose freeze $1.5–7 \times 10^6$ cells in each cryotube and later thaw and plate to give 1–5 × 10 cm dishes, respectively.

Appendix C: Composition of Serum-Free Medium for Undifferentiated Growth of hES Cells (63)

- Knockout Dulbecco's Modified Eagle's Medium – 80% (Invitrogen)
- Knockout serum replacement (SR) – 20% (Invitrogen)
- Basic fibroblast growth factor (bFGF) – 4 ng/ml (Invitrogen)
- β-mercaptoethanol – 0.1 mM (Invitrogen, keep in original bottle at 4°C)
- Nonessential amino acids – 1% (Invitrogen)
- L-Glutamine 2 mM (Invitrogen)
- Penicillin – 50 u/ml, streptomycin 50 μg/ml (Invitrogen)

Appendix D: Selective Propagation of Clumps of Undifferentiated hES Cells

1. Use a dark field stereomicroscope in a laminar flow hood.
2. Identification of the morphology of areas within colonies (usually at the periphery of colonies) that are predominantly undifferentiated is easily learned by comparing the morphology of colonies between phase contrast and stereomicroscopy.
3. Replace the culture medium with PBS containing Ca^{2+} and Mg^{2+}.
4. Slice the colonies into small areas containing about 50 undifferentiated cells by using the sharp edge of a micropipette.
5. Replace the PBS with the regular pre-equilibrated stem cell medium containing Dispase (Invitrogen, 10 mg/ml).
6. Incubate the dish for approximately 5 minutes at 37°C in a humidified atmosphere containing 5% CO_2.
7. As soon as the sliced clumps of undifferentiated cells detach from the culture dish, pick them up with a wide bore micropipette, wash them twice in PBS containing Ca^{2+} and Mg^{2+}, and plate them onto a fresh fibroblast feeder layer.

Appendix E: EB Formation

To obtain cystic EBs, it is essential to minimize the disruption of the cells as they aggregate and expand. They should be gently manipulated using wide pipettes and kept in an unchanged position in the incubator as they grow.

Mass Culture in Suspension

1. Passage human ES cells once on gelatin-coated plates to avoid the presence of residual MEF cells in the EBs.
2. Harvest cells using trypsin, centrifuge and resuspend in EB medium (human ES cells serum-free media in the absence of bFGF).
3. Place 10^7 cells into a UV irradiated 10-cm^2 petri dish.
4. Incubate the cells for two days without moving the plates.
5. Following two days small cell clumps are formed. It is essential that these aggregates are not disturbed. At this stage, change media once in two to three days, according to its color. This is achieved by placing the plate at an angle, allowing the growing EBs to concentrate at the bottom end of the plate. Gently aspirate as much of the media as possible and replace it with the same amount of fresh media. Alternatively, it is possible to use a wide pipette to collect and transfer the EBs in the media into a conical tube. The EBs tend to concentrate at the bottom of the tube without centrifugation, allowing for the careful aspiration of the media and the addition of fresh media. Following resuspension, the cells are transferred gently back to the dish using a wide pipette.

Hanging Drops

1. Passage human ES cells once on gelatin-coated plates to avoid the presence of residual MEF cells in the EBs.
2. Harvest cells using trypsin, centrifuge, and resuspend in EB medium (see above).
3. Count and resuspend cells to 1–10×10^6/ml (400–4000 cells/40 μl).
4. Place 40 μl drops on the inner side of a cover of a 35 mm tissue culture dish (no more than 25 drops per lid).
5. Put 10 ml PBS in the dish to avoid the evaporation of the drops.
6. Place lid back on the plate so that the drops hang downward from the cover of the dish.
7. Place in the incubator and do not touch or move for the next two days.
8. By day three, collect all drops very gently with a wide 1 ml cut tip and place in a petri dish with 10 ml media.
9. Change media every two to three days as described above.

REFERENCES

1. Evans MJ, Kaufman MH. Establishment in culture of pluripotential cells from mouse embryos. Nature 1981; 292: 154–6.
2. Martin GR. Isolation of a pluripotent cell line from early mouse embryos cultured in medium conditioned by teratocarcinoma stem cells. Proc Natl Acad Sci USA 1981; 78: 7634–8.
3. Lovell-Badge RH, Bygrave A, Bradley A, et al. Tissue-specific expression of the human type II collagen gene in mice. Proc Natl Acad Sci USA 1987; 84: 2803–7.
4. Marshall VS, Waknitz MA, Thomson JA. Isolation and maintenance of primate embryonic stem cells. Methods Mol Biol 2001; 158: 11–18.
5. Thomson JA, Itskovitz-Eldor J, Shapiro SS, et al. Embryonic stem cell lines derived from human blastocysts. Science 1998; 282: 1145–7.
6. Reubinoff BE, Pera MF, Fong CY, Trounson A, Bongso A. Embryonic stem cell lines from human blastocysts: somatic differentiation in vitro. Nat Biotechnol 2000; 18: 399–404.
7. Pera MF, Reubinoff B, Trounson A. Human embryonic stem cells. J Cell Sci 2000; 113(Pt 1): 5–10.

8. Strelchenko N, Verlinsky O, Kukharenko V, Verlinsky Y. Morula-derived human embryonic stem cells. Reprod Biomed Online 2004; 9: 623–9.
9. McMahon CA, Gibson FL, Leslie GI, et al. Embryo donation for medical research: attitudes and concerns of potential donors. Hum Reprod 2003; 18: 871–7.
10. Chung Y, Klimanskaya I, Becker S, et al. Embryonic and extraembryonic stem cell lines derived from single mouse blastomeres. Nature 2006; 439: 216–19.
11. Klimanskaya I, Chung Y, Becker S, Lu SJ, Lanza R. Human embryonic stem cell lines derived from single blastomeres. Nature 2006; 444: 481–5.
12. Alikani M, Munne S. Nonviable human pre-implantation embryos as a source of stem cells for research and potential therapy. Stem Cell Rev 2005; 1: 337–44.
13. Lerou PH, Yabuuchi A, Huo H, et al. Human embryonic stem cell derivation from poor-quality embryos. Nat Biotechnol 2008; 26: 212–14.
14. Fan Y, Luo Y, Chen X, Sun X. A modified culture medium increases blastocyst formation and the efficiency of human embryonic stem cell derivation from poor-quality embryos. J Reprod Dev 2010; 56: 533–9.
15. Mitalipova M, Calhoun J, Shin S, et al. Human embryonic stem cell lines derived from discarded embryos. Stem Cells 2003; 21: 521–6.
16. Zhang X, Stojkovic P, Przyborski S, et al. Derivation of human embryonic stem cells from developing and arrested embryos. Stem Cells 2006; 24: 2669–76.
17. Munne S, Velilla E, Colls P, et al. Self-correction of chromosomally abnormal embryos in culture and implications for stem cell production. Fertil Steril 2005; 84: 1328–34.
18. Evsikov S, Verlinsky Y. Mosaicism in the inner cell mass of human blastocysts. Hum Reprod 1998; 13: 3151–5.
19. Peura TT, Bosman A, Stojanov T. Derivation of human embryonic stem cell lines. Theriogenology 2007; 67: 32–42.
20. Lavon N, Narwani K, Golan-Lev T, et al. Derivation of euploid human embryonic stem cells from aneuploid embryos. Stem Cells 2008; 26: 1874–82.
21. Pickering SJ, Minger SL, Patel M, et al. Generation of a human embryonic stem cell line encoding the cystic fibrosis mutation deltaF508, using preimplantation genetic diagnosis. Reprod Biomed Online 2005; 10: 390–7.
22. Verlinsky Y, Strelchenko N, Kukharenko V, et al. Human embryonic stem cell lines with genetic disorders. Reprod Biomed Online 2005; 10: 105–10.
23. Ben-Yosef D, Amit A, Malcov M, et al. Female sex bias in human embryonic stem cell lines. Stem Cells Dev. 2012; 21: 363–72.
24. Mateizel I, De Temmerman N, Ullmann U, et al. Derivation of human embryonic stem cell lines from embryos obtained after IVF and after PGD for monogenic disorders. Hum Reprod 2006; 21: 503–11.
25. Surani MA, Barton SC. Development of gynogenetic eggs in the mouse: implications for parthenogenetic embryos. Science 1983; 222: 1034–6.
26. Lin H, Lei J, Wininger D, et al. Multilineage potential of homozygous stem cells derived from metaphase II oocytes. Stem Cells 2003; 21: 152–61.
27. Cibelli JB, Grant KA, Chapman KB, et al. Parthenogenetic stem cells in nonhuman primates. Science 2002; 295: 819.
28. Kim K, Lerou P, Yabuuchi A, et al. Histocompatible embryonic stem cells by parthenogenesis. Science 2007; 315: 482–6.
29. Revazova ES, Turovets NA, Kochetkova OD, et al. Patient-specific stem cell lines derived from human parthenogenetic blastocysts. Cloning Stem Cells 2007; 9: 432–49.
30. Munsie MJ, Michalska AE, O'Brien CM, et al. Isolation of pluripotent embryonic stem cells from reprogrammed adult mouse somatic cell nuclei. Curr Biol 2000; 10: 989–92.
31. Rideout WM 3rd, Hochedlinger K, Kyba M, Daley GQ, Jaenisch R. Correction of a genetic defect by nuclear transplantation and combined cell and gene therapy. Cell 2002; 109: 17–27.
32. Byrne JA, Pedersen DA, Clepper LL, et al. Producing primate embryonic stem cells by somatic cell nuclear transfer. Nature 2007; 450: 497–502.
33. Stojkovic M, Stojkovic P, Leary C, et al. Derivation of a human blastocyst after heterologous nuclear transfer to donated oocytes. Reprod Biomed Online 2005; 11: 226–31.
34. French AJ, Adams CA, Anderson LS, et al. Development of human cloned blastocysts following somatic cell nuclear transfer with adult fibroblasts. Stem Cells 2008; 26: 485–93.
35. Hochedlinger K, Jaenisch R. Nuclear transplantation, embryonic stem cells, and the potential for cell therapy. N Engl J Med 2003; 349: 275–86.
36. Heindryckx B, De Sutter P, Gerris J, Dhont M, Van der Elst J. Embryo development after successful somatic cell nuclear transfer to in vitro matured human germinal vesicle oocytes. Hum Reprod 2007; 22: 1982–90.
37. Meissner A, Wernig M, Jaenisch R. Direct reprogramming of genetically unmodified fibroblasts into pluripotent stem cells. Nat Biotechnol 2007; 25: 1177–81.
38. Nakagawa M, Koyanagi M, Tanabe K, et al. Generation of induced pluripotent stem cells without Myc from mouse and human fibroblasts. Nat Biotechnol 2008; 26: 101–6.
39. Okita K, Ichisaka T, Yamanaka S. Generation of germline-competent induced pluripotent stem cells. Nature 2007; 448: 313–17.
40. Takahashi K, Yamanaka S. Induction of pluripotent stem cells from mouse embryonic and adult fibroblast cultures by defined factors. Cell 2006; 126: 663–76.
41. Dimos JT, Rodolfa KT, Niakan KK, et al. Induced pluripotent stem cells generated from patients with ALS can be differentiated into motor neurons. Science 2008; 321: 1218–21.
42. Lee G, Papapetrou EP, Kim H, et al. Modelling pathogenesis and treatment of familial dysautonomia using patient-specific iPSCs. Nature 2009; 461: 402–6.
43. Maehr R, Chen S, Snitow M, et al. Generation of pluripotent stem cells from patients with type 1 diabetes. Proc Natl Acad Sci USA 2009; 106: 15768–73.
44. Itzhaki I, Maizels L, Huber I, et al. Modelling the long QT syndrome with induced pluripotent stem cells. Nature 2011; 471: 225–9.
45. Cheung AY, Horvath LM, Grafodatskaya D, et al. Isolation of MECP2-null Rett Syndrome patient hiPS cells and isogenic controls through X-chromosome inactivation. Hum Mol Genet 2011; 20: 2103–15.
46. Zhang J, Lian Q, Zhu G, et al. A human iPSC model of Hutchinson Gilford Progeria reveals vascular smooth

muscle and mesenchymal stem cell defects. Cell Stem Cell 2011; 8: 31–45.
47. Batista LF, Pech MF, Zhong FL, et al. Telomere shortening and loss of self-renewal in dyskeratosis congenita induced pluripotent stem cells. Nature 2011; 474: 399–402.
48. Aasen T, Raya A, Barrero MJ, et al. Efficient and rapid generation of induced pluripotent stem cells from human keratinocytes. Nat Biotechnol 2008; 26: 1276–84.
49. Bar-Nur O, Russ HA, Efrat S, Benvenisty N. Epigenetic memory and preferential lineage-specific differentiation in induced pluripotent stem cells derived from human pancreatic islet Beta cells. Cell Stem Cell 2011; 9: 17–23.
50. Loh YH, Agarwal S, Park IH, et al. Generation of induced pluripotent stem cells from human blood. Blood 2009; 113: 5476–9.
51. Takahashi K, Tanabe K, Ohnuki M, et al. Induction of pluripotent stem cells from adult human fibroblasts by defined factors. Cell 2007; 131: 861–72.
52. Tropel P, Tournois J, Come J, et al. High-efficiency derivation of human embryonic stem cell lines following pre-implantation genetic diagnosis. In Vitro Cell Dev Biol Anim 2010; 46: 376–385.
53. Turetsky T, Aizenman E, Gil Y, et al. Laser-assisted derivation of human embryonic stem cell lines from IVF embryos after preimplantation genetic diagnosis. Hum Reprod 2008; 23: 46–53.
54. Heins N, Englund MC, Sjoblom C, et al. Derivation, characterization, and differentiation of human embryonic stem cells. Stem Cells 2004; 22: 367–76.
55. Richards M, Fong CY, Chan WK, Wong PC, Bongso A. Human feeders support prolonged undifferentiated growth of human inner cell masses and embryonic stem cells. Nat Biotechnol 2002; 20: 933–6.
56. Genbacev O, Krtolica A, Zdravkovic T, et al. Serum-free derivation of human embryonic stem cell lines on human placental fibroblast feeders. Fertil Steril 2005; 83: 1517–29.
57. Ellerstrom C, Strehl R, Moya K, et al. Derivation of a xeno-free human embryonic stem cell line. Stem Cells 2006; 24: 2170–6.
58. Cheng L, Hammond H, Ye Z, Zhan X, Dravid G. Human adult marrow cells support prolonged expansion of human embryonic stem cells in culture. Stem Cells 2003; 21: 131–42.
59. Inzunza J, Gertow K, Stromberg MA, et al. Derivation of human embryonic stem cell lines in serum replacement medium using postnatal human fibroblasts as feeder cells. Stem Cells 2005; 23: 544–9.
60. Cowan CA, Klimanskaya I, McMahon J, et al. Derivation of embryonic stem-cell lines from human blastocysts. N Engl J Med 2004; 350: 1353–6.
61. Crook JM, Peura TT, Kravets L, et al. The generation of six clinical-grade human embryonic stem cell lines. Cell Stem Cell 2007; 1: 490–4.
62. Klimanskaya I, Chung Y, Becker S, Lu SJ, Lanza R. Derivation of human embryonic stem cells from single blastomeres. Nat Protoc 2007; 2: 1963–72.
63. Amit M, Carpenter MK, Inokuma MS, et al. Clonally derived human embryonic stem cell lines maintain pluripotency and proliferative potential for prolonged periods of culture. Dev Biol 2000; 227: 271–8.
64. Watanabe K, Ueno M, Kamiya D, et al. A ROCK inhibitor permits survival of dissociated human embryonic stem cells. Nat Biotechnol 2007; 25: 681–6.
65. Darr H, Mayshar Y, Benvenisty N. Overexpression of NANOG in human ES cells enables feeder-free growth while inducing primitive ectoderm features. Development 2006; 133: 1193–201.
66. Brimble SN, Zeng X, Weiler DA, et al. Karyotypic stability, genotyping, differentiation, feeder-free maintenance, and gene expression sampling in three human embryonic stem cell lines derived prior to August 9, 2001. Stem Cells Dev 2004; 13: 585–97.
67. Xu C, Inokuma MS, Denham J, et al. Feeder-free growth of undifferentiated human embryonic stem cells. Nat Biotechnol 2001; 19: 971–4.
68. Xu RH, Peck RM, Li DS, et al. Basic FGF and suppression of BMP signaling sustain undifferentiated proliferation of human ES cells. Nat Methods 2005; 2: 185–90.
69. Amit M, Shariki C, Margulets V, Itskovitz-Eldor J. Feeder layer- and serum-free culture of human embryonic stem cells. Biol Reprod 2004; 70: 837–45.
70. Vallier L, Alexander M, Pedersen RA. Activin/Nodal and FGF pathways cooperate to maintain pluripotency of human embryonic stem cells. J Cell Sci 2005; 118: 4495–509.
71. Sato N, Meijer L, Skaltsounis L, Greengard P, Brivanlou AH. Maintenance of pluripotency in human and mouse embryonic stem cells through activation of Wnt signaling by a pharmacological GSK-3-specific inhibitor. Nat Med 2004; 10: 55–63.
72. Bendall SC, Stewart MH, Menendez P, et al. IGF and FGF cooperatively establish the regulatory stem cell niche of pluripotent human cells in vitro. Nature 2007; 448: 1015–21.
73. Amit M, Itskovitz-Eldor J. Feeder-free culture of human embryonic stem cells. Methods Enzymol 2006; 420: 37–49.
74. Derda R, Musah S, Orner BP, et al. High-throughput discovery of synthetic surfaces that support proliferation of pluripotent cells. J Am Chem Soc 2010; 132: 1289–95.
75. Klim JR, Li L, Wrighton PJ, Piekarczyk MS, Kiessling LL. A defined glycosaminoglycan-binding substratum for human pluripotent stem cells. Nat Methods 2010; 7: 989–94.
76. Kolhar P, Kotamraju VR, Hikita ST, Clegg DO, Ruoslahti E. Synthetic surfaces for human embryonic stem cell culture. J Biotechnol 2010; 146: 143–6.
77. Lu J, Hou R, Booth CJ, Yang SH, Snyder M. Defined culture conditions of human embryonic stem cells. Proc Natl Acad Sci USA 2006; 103: 5688–93.
78. Ludwig TE, Bergendahl V, Levenstein ME, et al. Feeder-independent culture of human embryonic stem cells. Nat Methods 2006; 3: 637–46.
79. Melkoumian Z, Weber JL, Weber DM, et al. Synthetic peptide-acrylate surfaces for long-term self-renewal and cardiomyocyte differentiation of human embryonic stem cells. Nat Biotechnol 2010; 28: 606–10.
80. Rajala K, Lindroos B, Hussein SM, et al. A defined and xeno-free culture method enabling the establishment of clinical-grade human embryonic, induced pluripotent and adipose stem cells. PLoS One 2010; 5: e10246.
81. Villa-Diaz LG, Nandivada H, Ding J, et al. Synthetic polymer coatings for long-term growth of human embryonic stem cells. Nat Biotechnol 2006; 28: 581–3.
82. Yao S, Chen S, Clark J, et al. Long-term self-renewal and directed differentiation of human embryonic

stem cells in chemically defined conditions. Proc Natl Acad Sci USA 2006; 103: 6907–12.
83. Amit M, Chebath J, Margulets V, et al. Suspension culture of undifferentiated human embryonic and induced pluripotent stem cells. Stem Cell Rev 2010; 6: 248–59.
84. Fernandes AM, Marinho PA, Sartore RC, et al. Successful scale-up of human embryonic stem cell production in a stirred microcarrier culture system. Braz J Med Biol Res 2009; 42: 515–22.
85. Nie Y, Bergendahl V, Hei DJ, Jones JM, Palecek SP. Scalable culture and cryopreservation of human embryonic stem cells on microcarriers. Biotechnol Prog 2009; 25: 20–31.
86. Oh SK, Chen AK, Mok Y, et al. Long-term microcarrier suspension cultures of human embryonic stem cells. Stem Cell Res 2009; 2: 219–30.
87. Olmer R, Haase A, Merkert S, et al. Long term expansion of undifferentiated human iPS and ES cells in suspension culture using a defined medium. Stem Cell Res 2010; 5: 51–64.
88. Phillips BW, Horne R, Lay TS, et al. Attachment and growth of human embryonic stem cells on microcarriers. J Biotechnol 2008; 138: 24–32.
89. Singh H, Mok P, Balakrishnan T, Rahmat SN, Zweigerdt R. Up-scaling single cell-inoculated suspension culture of human embryonic stem cells. Stem Cell Res 2010; 4: 165–79.
90. Steiner D, Khaner H, Cohen M, et al. Derivation, propagation and controlled differentiation of human embryonic stem cells in suspension. Nat Biotechnol 2010; 28: 361–4.
91. Yu P, Pan G, Yu J. Thomson JA FGF2 sustains NANOG and switches the outcome of BMP4-induced human embryonic stem cell differentiation. Cell Stem Cell 2011; 8: 326–34.
92. Reubinoff BE, Pera MF, Vajta G, Trounson AO. Effective cryopreservation of human embryonic stem cells by the open pulled straw vitrification method. Hum Reprod 2001; 16: 2187–94.
93. Li X, Meng G, Krawetz R, Liu S, Rancourt DE. The ROCK inhibitor Y-27632 enhances the survival rate of human embryonic stem cells following cryopreservation. Stem Cells Dev 2008; 17: 1079–85.
94. Martin-Ibanez R, Unger C, Stromberg A, et al. Novel cryopreservation method for dissociated human embryonic stem cells in the presence of a ROCK inhibitor. Hum Reprod 2008; 23: 2744–54.
95. Huang J, Wei W, Zhang J, et al. Whole genome DNA copy number changes identified by high density oligonucleotide arrays. Hum Genomics 2004; 1: 287–99.
96. Elliott AM, Elliott KA, Kammesheidt A. High resolution array-CGH characterization of human stem cells using a stem cell focused microarray. Mol Biotechnol 2010; 46: 234–42.
97. Wu H, Kim KJ, Mehta K, et al. Copy number variant analysis of human embryonic stem cells. Stem Cells 2008; 26: 1484–9.
98. Maitra A, Arking DE, Shivapurkar N, et al. Genomic alterations in cultured human embryonic stem cells. Nat Genet 2005; 37: 1099–103.
99. Josephson R, Sykes G, Liu Y, et al. A molecular scheme for improved characterization of human embryonic stem cell lines. BMC Biol 2006; 4: 28.
100. Brivanlou AH, Gage FH, Jaenisch R, et al. Stem cells. Setting standards for human embryonic stem cells. Science 2003; 300: 913–16.
101. Adewumi O, Aflatoonian B, Ahrlund-Richter L, et al. Characterization of human embryonic stem cell lines by the international stem cell initiative. Nat Biotechnol 2007; 25: 803–16.
102. Carpenter MK, Rosler E, Rao MS. Characterization and differentiation of human embryonic stem cells. Cloning Stem Cells 2003; 5: 79–88.
103. Baker DE, Harrison NJ, Maltby E, et al. Adaptation to culture of human embryonic stem cells and oncogenesis in vivo. Nat Biotechnol 2007; 25: 207–15.
104. Draper JS, Smith K, Gokhale P, et al. Recurrent gain of chromosomes 17 q and 12 in cultured human embryonic stem cells. Nat Biotechnol 2004; 22: 53–4.
105. Prokhorova TA, Harkness LM, Frandsen U, et al. Teratoma formation by human embryonic stem cells is site dependent and enhanced by the presence of Matrigel. Stem Cells Dev 2009; 18: 47–54.
106. Hovatta O, Mikkola M, Gertow K, et al. A culture system using human foreskin fibroblasts as feeder cells allows production of human embryonic stem cells. Hum Reprod 2003; 18: 1404–9.
107. Reubinoff BE, Itsykson P, Turetsky T, et al. Neural progenitors from human embryonic stem cells. Nat Biotechnol 2001; 19: 1134–40.
108. Itskovitz-Eldor J, Schuldiner M, Karsenti D, et al. Differentiation of human embryonic stem cells into embryoid bodies compromising the three embryonic germ layers. Mol Med 2000; 6: 88–95.
109. Carpenter MK, Inokuma MS, Denham J, et al. Enrichment of neurons and neural precursors from human embryonic stem cells. Exp Neurol 2001; 172: 383–97.
110. Schuldiner M, Eiges R, Eden A, et al. Induced neuronal differentiation of human embryonic stem cells. Brain Res 2001; 913: 201–5.
111. Zhang SC, Wernig M, Duncan ID, Brustle O, Thomson JA. In vitro differentiation of transplantable neural precursors from human embryonic stem cells. Nat Biotechnol 2001; 19: 1129–33.
112. Kaufman DS, Hanson ET, Lewis RL, Auerbach R, Thomson JA. Hematopoietic colony-forming cells derived from human embryonic stem cells. Proc Natl Acad Sci USA 2001; 98: 10716–21.
113. Levenberg S, Golub JS, Amit M, Itskovitz-Eldor J, Langer R. Endothelial cells derived from human embryonic stem cells. Proc Natl Acad Sci USA 2002; 99: 4391–6.
114. He JQ, Ma Y, Lee Y, Thomson JA, Kamp TJ. Human embryonic stem cells develop into multiple types of cardiac myocytes: action potential characterization. Circ Res 2003; 93: 32–9.
115. Assady S, Maor G, Amit M, et al. Insulin production by human embryonic stem cells. Diabetes 2001; 50: 1691–7.
116. Chambers SM, Fasano CA, Papapetrou EP, et al. Highly efficient neural conversion of human ES and iPS cells by dual inhibition of SMAD signaling. Nat Biotechnol 2009; 27: 275–80.
117. Itsykson P, Ilouz N, Turetsky T, et al. Derivation of neural precursors from human embryonic stem cells in the presence of noggin. Mol Cell Neurosci 2005; 30: 24–36.
118. Xu RH, Chen X, Li DS, et al. BMP4 initiates human embryonic stem cell differentiation to trophoblast. Nat Biotechnol 2002; 20: 1261–4.

119. D'Amour KA, Bang AG, Eliazer S, et al. Production of pancreatic hormone-expressing endocrine cells from human embryonic stem cells. Nat Biotechnol 2006; 24: 1392–401.
120. Eiges R, Schuldiner M, Drukker M, et al. Establishment of human embryonic stem cell-transfected clones carrying a marker for undifferentiated cells. Curr Biol 2001; 11: 514–18.
121. Li M, Pevny L, Lovell-Badge R, Smith A. Generation of purified neural precursors from embryonic stem cells by lineage selection. Curr Biol 1998; 8: 971–4.
122. Klug MG, Soonpaa MH, Koh GY, Field LJ. Genetically selected cardiomyocytes from differentiating embronic stem cells form stable intracardiac grafts. J Clin Invest 1996; 98: 216–24.
123. Dekel I, Magal Y, Pearson-White S, Emerson CP, Shani M. Conditional conversion of ES cells to skeletal muscle by an exogenous MyoD1 gene. New Biol 1992; 4: 217–24.
124. Dushnik-Levinson M, Benvenisty N. Embryogenesis in vitro: study of differentiation of embryonic stem cells. Biol Neonate 1995; 67: 77–83.
125. Kim JH, Auerbach JM, Rodriguez-Gomez JA, et al. Dopamine neurons derived from embryonic stem cells function in an animal model of Parkinson's disease. Nature 2002; 418: 50–6.
126. Brustle O, Jones KN, Learish RD, et al. Embryonic stem cell-derived glial precursors: a source of myelinating transplants. Science 1999; 285: 754–6.
127. Soria B, Roche E, Berna G, et al. Insulin-secreting cells derived from embryonic stem cells normalize glycemia in streptozotocin-induced diabetic mice. Diabetes 2000; 49: 157–62.
128. Idelson M, Alper R, Obolensky A, et al. Directed differentiation of human embryonic stem cells into functional retinal pigment epithelium cells. Cell Stem Cell 2009; 5: 396–408.
129. Kelly OG, Chan MY, Martinson LA, et al. Cell-surface markers for the isolation of pancreatic cell types derived from human embryonic stem cells. Nat Biotechnol 2011; 29: 750–6.
130. Keirstead HS, Nistor G, Bernal G, et al. Human embryonic stem cell-derived oligodendrocyte progenitor cell transplants remyelinate and restore locomotion after spinal cord injury. J Neurosci 2005; 25: 4694–705.
131. Lu B, Malcuit C, Wang S, et al. Long-term safety and function of RPE from human embryonic stem cells in preclinical models of macular degeneration. Stem Cells 2009; 27: 2126–35.
132. Mayor S. First patient enters trial to test safety of stem cells in spinal injury. BMJ 2010; 341: c5724.
133. Drukker M, Katz G, Urbach A, et al. Characterization of the expression of MHC proteins in human embryonic stem cells. Proc Natl Acad Sci USA 2002; 99: 9864–9.
134. Capecchi MR. Altering the genome by homologous recombination. Science 1989; 244: 1288–92.
135. Heard E, Chaumeil J, Masui O, Okamoto I. Mammalian X-chromosome inactivation: an epigenetics paradigm. Cold Spring Harb Symp Quant Biol 2004; 69: 89–102.
136. Lindenbaum MH, Grosveld F. An in vitro globin gene switching model based on differentiated embryonic stem cells. Genes Dev 1990; 4: 2075–85.
137. Dvash T, Mayshar Y, Darr H, et al. Temporal gene expression during differentiation of human embryonic stem cells and embryoid bodies. Hum Reprod 2004; 19: 2875–83.
138. Urbach A, Schuldiner M, Benvenisty N. Modeling for Lesch-Nyhan disease by gene targeting in human embryonic stem cells. Stem Cells 2004; 22: 635–41.
139. Zwaka TP, Thomson JA. Homologous recombination in human embryonic stem cells (2003). Nat Biotechnol 2004; 21: 319–21.
140. Eiges R, Urbach A, Malcov M, et al. Developmental study of fragile X syndrome using human embryonic stem cells derived from preimplantation genetically diagnosed embryos. Cell Stem Cell 2007; 1: 568–77.
141. Bradley CK, Scott HA, Chami O, et al. Derivation of Huntington's disease-affected human embryonic stem cell lines. Stem Cells Dev 2011; 20: 495–502.
142. Candan ZN, Kahraman S. Establishment and characterization of human embryonic stem cell lines, Turkey perspectives. In Vitro Cell Dev Biol Anim 2010; 46: 345–55.
143. Narwani K, Biancotti JC, Golan-Lev T, et al. Human embryonic stem cells from aneuploid blastocysts identified by pre-implantation genetic screening. In Vitro Cell Dev Biol Anim 2010; 46: 309–16.
144. Taei A, Gourabi H, Seifinejad A, et al. Derivation of new human embryonic stem cell lines from preimplantation genetic screening and diagnosis-analyzed embryos. In Vitro Cell Dev Biol Anim 2010; 46: 395–402.

31

Microfluidics in ART: Current progress and future directions

Jason E. Swain, Thomas B. Pool, Shuichi Takayama, and Gary D. Smith

INTRODUCTION

Optimized production of preimplantation embryos for use in assisted reproductive techniques (ART) has been a central goal of reproductive scientists since the inception of the field, and, subsequently, methodologies have continually been refined to aid in this endeavor. For example, skilled technicians meticulously handle gametes and embryos in prescribed manners, extensive research has refined culture media formulations to cater to the changing metabolic needs of gametes and embryos, and commercial manufacturers have even produced specialized equipment to meet the specific needs of cells in ART. Though approached from different perspectives, the commonality between these advancements is the pursuit to minimize external stresses imposed upon gametes and embryos due to artificial manipulation within the in vitro fertilization (IVF) laboratory. Environmental and intracellular factors influenced by these manipulations, such as osmotic imbalances, shifts in temperature, and pH fluctuations, can all have devastating effects on embryo quality. However, even with these tremendous improvements, relatively little attention has been paid to the platform on which gametes and embryos are cultured and manipulated.

In regard to culture platform, clinical embryology laboratories have historically selected between polystyrene test tubes, Petri dishes, organ culture wells, or four-well plates to accommodate varying number of cells and volumes of media used. The vast majority of these approaches are largely static in regard to their ability to actively regulate media flow, though new dynamic culture systems are emerging (1). Although each of these approaches offer certain advantages, it remains evident that environmental conditions offered by all of these culture platforms are in extreme contrast to what is observed in vivo.

In the quest to optimize embryo development in vitro, a "back to nature" ideology has been adopted by some to formulate embryo culture media (2). To the best of its ability, this approach attempts to base culture media formations on composition of fluids in the female reproductive tract to chemically manipulate embryo development in vitro. Similarly, this same naturalist approach may also be applied to culture platforms. Exploration of the differential effects of physical and structural environment experienced by gametes and embryos in vitro versus in vivo may provide a means to further improve clinical IVF. In vivo, gametes and embryos are exposed to the constricted "moist" environment of the female reproductive tract, surrounded by various oriented glycoproteins as they are gently moved via ciliated epithelium. This is in stark contrast to the expansive, largely static environment gametes and embryos are exposed to in vitro, resting on inert synthetic polymers, bathed in a relative ocean of media. Microfluidic technology offers a platform on which to further manipulate culture conditions in vitro by pheno-mimicking physiologic conditions in vivo, thereby conveying any potential benefit of this gentle stimulation, in the hopes of creating an environment more suitable to gamete and embryo development and function.

BASIS AND APPEAL OF MICROFLUIDICS

Though new dynamic embryo culture devices are emerging, many utilizing fluid movement on the macro level, the focus of this review will be largely on the those approaches or platforms employing microfluidics. The term "microfluidic" refers to technology utilizing characteristics of fluid movement in a micro- or nano-environment. These characteristics, discussed in depth elsewhere (3), rely heavily on variables such as fluid density, viscosity, velocity, and size/geometry of the environment. Taken together, these variables are used to calculate Reynolds number. At the macro level, fluid flow results in chaotic particle movement within the fluid stream, resulting in turbulence, as indicated by a high Reynolds number. In contrast, in the decreasing dimensions of microfluidic channels, Reynolds's number decreases and fluid is imparted with streamlined and predictable flow patterns. These predictable flow patterns conferred by microfluidic devices impose laminar flow upon fluids, allowing parallel movement of multiple streams of media through the same microchannel with no mixing, except by diffusion across the fluid–fluid interface (Fig. 31.1). It is at these extremely small scales that fluid viscosity and surface tension become increasingly important considerations for fluid flow. As a result, microfluidic approaches offer certain advantages, as well as disadvantages, over larger

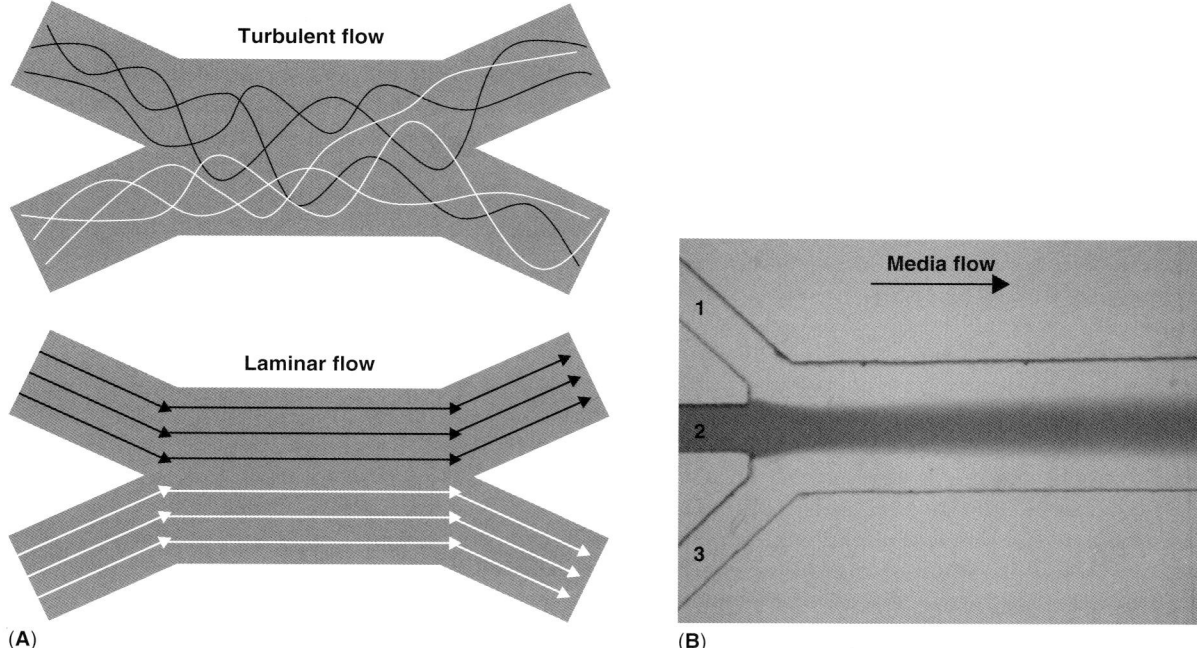

Figure 31.1 (**A**) Illustration of turbulent versus laminar flow. Laminar flow is one of the inherent properties of microfluidic platforms that allows for unique applications in ART. (**B**) Microfluidic device demonstrating laminar flow. Fluid from channels 1, 2, and 3 flow in parallel with no mixing, except by simple diffusion.

dynamic fluid movement approaches, and may also yield differing results in regard to gamete and embryo culture.

Characteristic fluid flow patterns in microfluidic devices are amenable to applications requiring precise fluid sampling or manipulations; including examination of cellular behavior and interactions. Thus, microfluidics carries immense potential for improving clinical ART by offering the ability to seamlessly adjust composition of media flowing to developing gametes and embryos, without the external stresses currently experienced through manual manipulation as required with current sequential culture systems. In addition, microfluidic technology utilizes minimal amounts of media in a constrictive environment, similar to that experienced by gametes and embryos in vivo. Thus, a microfluidic platform allows clinical IVF to pursue physiologic mimicry through both chemical and physical manipulations to the in vitro culture environment. Furthermore, and perhaps more importantly, the scale of microfluidic platforms grants the ability to implement multiple procedural steps of IVF on the same device. This "lab-on-a-chip" would not only save space, but also time, as it allows for automation of processes as well as inclusion of diagnostic assays aimed at noninvasively identifying the healthiest cells for subsequent use.

FABRICATION OF MICROFLUIDIC DEVICES FOR ART

Fabrication of microfluidic devices for use in ART has been covered elsewhere, discussing biocompatible materials, as well as manufacturing approaches (4–6). A practical guide of considerations in regard to fabricating perfusion-based microfluidic platforms for adherent cell-culture also exists (7), and key issues that must be addressed for functional application also largely apply to applications in ART. To summarize, various materials have been found to be adequate for gamete and embryo culture, and currently tested devices are composed of polydimethylsiloxane (PDMS), silicone, borosilicate glass, Pyrex, quartz, or combinations of these materials (8–17). Materials selected for construction of microfluidic channels may differ from material selected for cell substrate, or the actual surface on which cells lie. Though cell substrate surface is a critical consideration for adherent cell culture to insure cell attachment, it is not as crucial a factor for culture of nonadherent oocytes or embryos. Manufacturing techniques for microchannels involve molding, photolithography, and chemically or mechanically etching channels into suitable materials. The most commonly used material for microchannel fabrication is the polymer PDMS; selected due to inherent use and fabrication advantages, such as flexibility, ease of soft-lithography patterning, and low autofluoresence for use with microscopy (7). Subsequently, compatible microchannel components are bonded to companion components/platforms with nontoxic adhesives or epoxies. Benefits of these materials and manufacturing processes include rapid, repeatable, precise, and inexpensive production; a necessity for use in clinical ART, as devices should be disposable to ensure sterility.

MEDIA FLOW AND DYNAMIC APPROACHES IN ART MICROFLUIDIC DEVICES

As mentioned, one benefit of microfluidics for use in ART is the ability to achieve dynamic media flow on a culture platform. Although the approach of dynamic media flow in embryo culture is not new, prior attempts at perfusion systems, which remove or renew media on the macroscale, has proved inefficient and subsequently not been implemented on a large scale (18–20). Other simplified approaches using gentle media agitation on the macroscale are receiving more widespread attention, but lack the power for media removal or renewal, and associated potential benefits. Fortunately, the unique nature of microfluidic platforms allows for alternate approaches to accomplish media perfusion and movement that are more amenable for widespread use. These methods are often dictated by constraints of platform design, which is dependent upon whether perfusion systems are recirculating or non-recirculating. Furthermore, ability of perfusion systems to operate over long periods of time with minimal manipulation is essential. In adherent cell systems, perfusion devices have been operated successfully for over one week (21,22).

Early devices for ART applications have employed gravity driven passive flow, with hydrostatic pressure in media reservoirs as an important variable to drive media flow down microchannels (10,11,14,17,23,24). While simplicity of the approach is advantageous, it is difficult to regulate flow speed or volume changes, especially over time when height of media columns diminishes. Others have utilized manually applied pressure via externally attached syringes to input/output ports to cause media flow through microfluidic devices (25). Again, simplicity of this approach is attractive, however, it is difficult to regulate pressure precisely and manual methods to regulate flow are not feasible for use over the long periods of time required for embryo culture. A variation of the syringe-driven flow approach has been further adapted through use of Hamilton syringes attached to a programmable infusion pump (16). Although more precise and feasible for use over time, the required external tubing and machinery is problematic for use within a closed incubator environment. Additionally, at least one study has used a tilting culture system in conjunction with microfluidic channels, which, while still using gravity, offers more consistent control over flow gravity-driven hydrostatic pressure approaches. Titling devices may offer an improved means of provided gentle media and embryo movement, thereby possibly conveying any associated benefits, but have only been examined with use of larger volume microdrops (26,27). Furthermore, tilting approaches and simple agitation don't necessarily remove or replenish the existing media. Regardless, this approach appears promising and warrants future study. Similar methods of combining simplified, constrictive microchannels with other dynamic methods of inducing fluid movement/flow, such as vibration (28–30) may be helpful, as gentle agitation appears to beneficial for human embryos. Application of shaking or rotating platform (31–35) with constrictive culture approaches remains to be explored and offer a seemingly simple way of introducing gentle physical stimulation to developing embryos. Finally, a Braille pumping system using tiny electric piezo actuators has been used successfully to peristaltically move media along microchannels during embryo culture (36–39). This approach not only allows for precise computerized regulation of speed and flow patterns, but devices are compact enough to fit multiple units within a single incubator. It should be noted, however, that the Braille system, like most other dynamic culture devices, is an electronic device and special precautions must be taken to account for the humid incubator environment. Modified Braille systems have now been utilized in human clinical trials and it will be interesting to note what benefits exist. Other possible approaches yet to be explored for ART to regulate fluid flow in microfluidic devices include pneumatics or magnetic gates/actuators. In addition, perhaps the most intriguing concept for regulating media flow within microfluidic devices entails use of expansive characteristics of a three-dimensional matrix, hydrogel, to regulate flow through channels (40). This technology offers the ability to control media flow through mechanical responses in the hydrogel due to external stimuli such as temperature, light, pH, and biological cues.

Regardless of the perfusion approach adopted, a culture environment enabling dynamic media flow on the microlevel will allow chemical manipulation of cells by permitting gradual change of media flowing toward the gamete/embryo. One could imagine a progressive sequential or multistep culture media supplemented with varying chemical treatments or energy substrates being deployed to cells at prescribed time-points, in a gradually changing manner, without the need for an embryologist to physically move embryos to new culture dishes. In addition, dynamic media flow also permits physical manipulation of gametes/embryos, either transporting cells to desired locations or imparting physical changes. Indeed, both chemical and physical manipulation of oocytes/embryos has been achieved in microfluidic devices through manipulations of flowing media. Removal of cumulus cells has been achieved in a microfluidic device through suction applied via an attached syringe, drawing cumulus cells away from the oocyte down a small adjacent channel (41). Syringe driven flow has also been used to position oocytes to allow removal of zona pellucida by flowing a bolus of acidified media over the cell (42). Finally, a microfluidic device has been designed utilizing suction and electorotation to isolate and manipulate a single embryo in a manner that may be suitable for intracytoplasmic sperm injection (ICSI) (43). These integrated activities further serve to demonstrate potential for microfluidic technology for ART.

In additional to various methods of achieving media flow, shape of the culture area may be another important consideration. Sheer forces applied to cells may be impacted by the shape of the culture area, as well as disruption of any local gradients that may accumulate around embryos when in culture (39). Thus, as mentioned previously, examination of other dynamic culture approaches, in conjunction with various novel static constrictive culture platforms, may prove insightful and beneficial for improved embryo development in vitro.

REQUIREMENTS OF MICROFLUIDICS FOR ART

Although theoretical advantages for microfluidics platforms in ART should be now readily apparent, it is important to recognize that several potential issues must be addressed to achieve widespread acceptance. Many of these issues exist regardless of the cell system cultured within microfluidic devices; however, reproductive applications of microfluidic platforms also carry unique considerations. These considerations can be grouped into four major categories:

1. Material/design biocompatibility
2. Device operation/failure
3. Manipulation/handling of embryos
4. IVF laboratory compatibility

Material/Design Biocompatibility

As with other embryo culture dishes, it must be shown that microfluidic devices are nontoxic and pass quality control assays. Though initial testing has identified suitable fabrication materials, in-house testing must also verify biocompatibility of individual lots, ensuring contaminants were not introduced during production. Paramount in assuring biocompatibility is the ability to sterilize devices following fabrication. Current studies have utilized devices treated with UV light, ethanol or ethylene oxide, or autoclaving (16,17). Although these approaches do not appear to affect properties of PDMS (7,44), high heat or chemical sterilization can warp or change biochemical properties of other polymers. Future exploration of more traditional sterilization methods, such as gamma irradiation should be explored.

Fabrication materials used in current microfluidic devices display unique properties that must also be addressed before implementation into IVF labs. Although these properties may be conducive for fabrication purposes, materials such as PDMS are absorptive and can alter media characteristics, including media flow and osmolarity, thereby impeding subsequent embryo development (45). Fortunately, surface modification to fabrication materials, including parylene coating or bonding with poly(ethylene glycol) methyl ether methacrylate (PEG-MA), may alleviate some of these concerns (46,47).

Furthermore, unique properties of microfluidics may require development of specialized culture media to accommodate the technology and optimize embryo production. Due to extremely small channel dimensions, media viscosity is an essential variable to maintain laminar flow. Therefore, protein amounts or sources should be explored for compatibility. Additionally, small volumes of media utilized in microfluidics may result in rapid and damaging shift in pH. This is extremely important when considering use of microfluidic platforms with oocytes, as oocytes appear to lack porters/antiporters to regulate their intracellular pH (48–51). Thus, specialized culture media with increased buffering capacity may also prove beneficial.

Finally, determination of optimal media volumes, as well as optimal numbers of gametes and embryos cultured in each microfluidic device is very important, as depletion of factors or build-up of wastes is potentially problematic at such a small scale, a problem more pronounced if media flow is not present. These would appear to be crucial recommendations that should accompany devices if/when they are commercially available. Future examination of these factors, and others, is essential to demonstrate efficacy of microfluidic devices in ART.

Device Operation/Failure

Microfluidic devices employing dynamic culture must incorporate reliable mechanisms imparting media flow. This requires a safe and effective interface between the microchannel platform and the perfusion regulatory device. Furthermore, a key consideration in regard to operation of dynamic flow is the ability to avoid bubble formation within microchannels. Construction of a bubble trap along the microfluidic channel may help alleviate this concern (52). Alternatively, larger scale dynamic platforms may be used, though this may ameliorate benefits of the small scale. Fortunately, if devices fail and media flow halts, the result is the current default static system. However, it is essential that devices possess methods to easily determine if flow has been interrupted, and if so, easy correction or repair should be available.

Manipulation/Handling of Embryos

Perhaps the most difficult criterion to address in regard to construction and implementation of microfluidic technology in the IVF lab is the ability to easily manipulate or remove gametes/embryos, a limitation not often considered with devices currently used for adherent somatic cell culture or diagnostic assays. Furthermore, daily observation and manipulation of embryos cannot be a labor intensive process, as increased time to view, add, or remove embryos will adversely stress blastomeres. Detriments with prolonged manipulation are exacerbated by the inherent problems that exist when dealing with extremely small volumes of liquid in microfluidics, such as rapid evaporation, resulting osmolarity shifts, as well as rapid shifts in pH and temperature. Thus, design must incorporate a user-friendly interface through which the embryologist can access cells. A current approach that seems to work well is to culture cells within funnels (40), or to simply place a larger traditional static culture dish on a platform that moves or agitates the media. Furthermore, paramount in minimizing risks with prolonged handling is the ability to easily visualize cells within the device. Therefore, materials used must possess optical properties to visualize and track individual cells within the device for grading purposes. Optical properties should also be compatible with emerging technologies, such as polarized microscopy. PDMS appears to be adequate for these purposes. Finally, device designs should accommodate different laboratory practices, perhaps offering various constructions, adjusting design to allow both individual and group culture.

IVF Laboratory Compatibility

Importantly, to gain widespread acceptance in clinical IVF, microfluidic devices need to be compatible initially with current IVF lab set up and practices. Thus, devices must fit into contemporary incubators without external or bulky tubing or apparatus. Though much of the prospective power of microfluidic technology resides in more advanced analytical and automated processes that can be resident on the platform, these advancements cannot be realized without strong initial acceptance by the practicing embryologist.

MICROFLUIDICS IN ANDROLOGY

Though future refinement is still required, progress addressing key issues of microfluidics has progressed enough to begin to take advantage of unique applications offered by microfluidic platforms in areas of reproduction, such as andrology (53). As early as 1993, microchannel devices made of silicone were used to evaluate sperm function via interactions with cervical mucus, hyaluronan, spermicide and antisperm antibody beads (54). The same group later published a report demonstrating sperm count and motility assessment performed on etched glass microchannel devices (55). More recent devices composed of PDMS have proven useful for computerized analysis of pig sperm linear velocity and head displacement (56).

The first peer-reviewed publication on the use of microfluidic technology for separation of motile sperm from semen samples utilized a PDMS passive gravity-driven device where the hydrostatic pressure of two separate inlet reservoirs drove media flow down a converging microfluidic channel (Fig. 31.2) (23). The principle of the device took advantage of the fact that only motile sperm can traverse the border that separates the parallel streams of diluted semen and fresh medium. Thus, the laminar flow properties exhibited by media in microchannels allowed motile sperm to swim away from nonmotile sperm, debris, and seminal plasma and collect in a separate outlet reservoir. Follow-up experiments demonstrated that this microfluidic device design was not only biocompatible with human sperm, but that it could isolate motile, morphologically normal cells (10). Furthermore, surface modification of PDMS microfluidic sperm sorter devices to increase hydrophilicy with coating such as PEG-MA may further improve this technology (46). Although limitations exist with the current device, including inability to process large sample sizes, clogging, and sample viscosity issues; this novel approach provides a feasible alternative to isolate sperm from oligozoospermic patients for use in ICSI.

Another approach employing microfluidics for sperm sorting utilized mouse sperm placed into a PDMS/glass device, to isolate sperm based on motility, but also via chemotaxis toward cumulus cells (57). Sperm were placed into an inlet reservoir (2 mm radius), allowed to

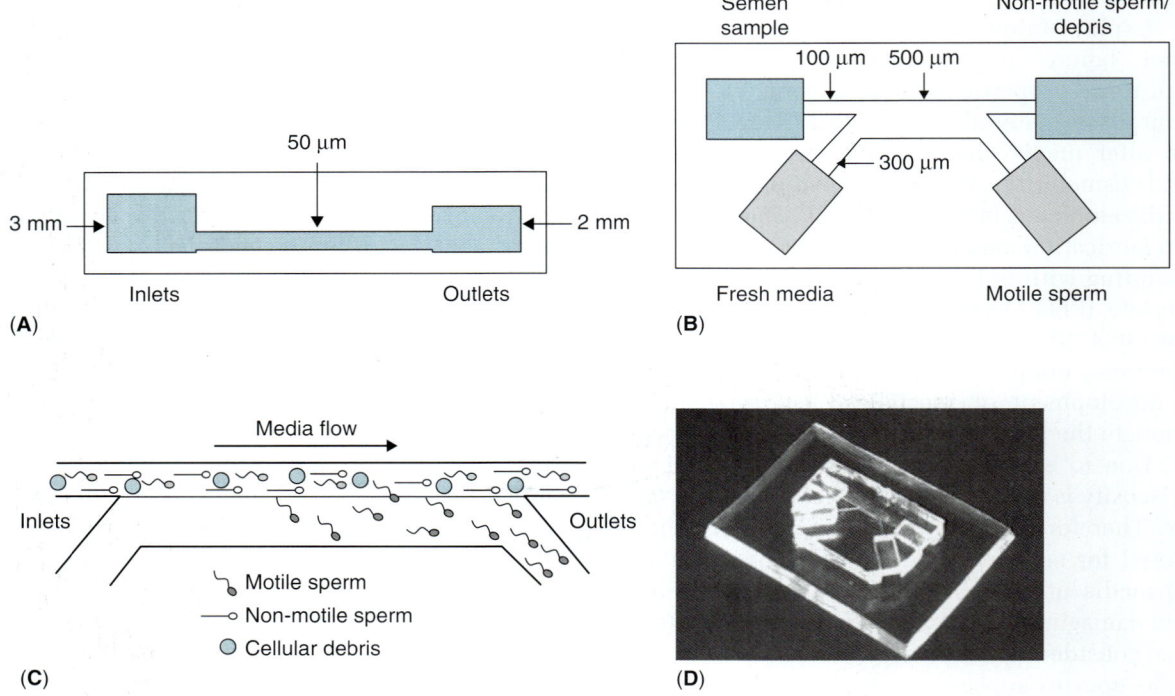

Figure 31.2 Illustration of a microfluidic sperm sorter. (**A**) *Top view*. (**B**) *Side view*. (**C**) Illustration demonstrating how laminar flow allows motile sperm to swim away from nonmotile sperm and debris to collect in a separate reservoir. (**D**) Image of sperm sorter device composed of PDMS.

swim down a straight channel, whose dimensions were optimized for motile sperm recovery at 1 × 7 mm (w × l). Sperm then collected in a small central reservoir (1.25 mm radius), where video imaging could occur, before swimming onward into one of two branching channels (1 × 5 mm, w × l), each leading to separate collection reservoir (2 mm radius) (Fig. 31.3). Other microfluidic devices to explore sperm chemotaxis also exist and offer further methods to explore sperm function (58).

In another use of microfluidic technology for andrology, a PDMS/glass device has been constructed that directs sperm flow within oriented microchannels to separate, align, and orient sperm of mouse, bull, and human (59) (Fig. 31.4), providing potential applications for ICSI. Utilizing that fact that motile sperm orient themselves against media flow within these devices, and that motile sperm can swim against media flow of certain velocity, a series of three reservoirs and four microfluidic channels allow processing of sperm via hydrostatic media flow. Though this device requires precise regulation of media volumes to regulate hydrostatic pressure, such devices were designed with the future intent of exploring implementation of a means to sort X- and Y-bearing sperm, and the ability to add a "laser cutting" component to separate sperm heads from tails for ICSI.

Due to the limitations inherent in a microfluidic sperm-sorting device, utilization of the technology must provide some added benefit over conventional processing methods. Conventional sperm preparation methods such as serial centrifugation, density gradient separation, or swim-up, are reported to induce sperm DNA damage, perhaps to exposure to reaction oxygen species (ROS) (60–62). Preliminary data indicate that sperm isolated using a microfluidic sperm-sorting device had significantly lower levels of DNA damage and higher motility compared to these more conventional approaches (24). Thus, microfluidic sperm sorting may allow for selection of higher quality sperm, potentially leading to improved embryo quality.

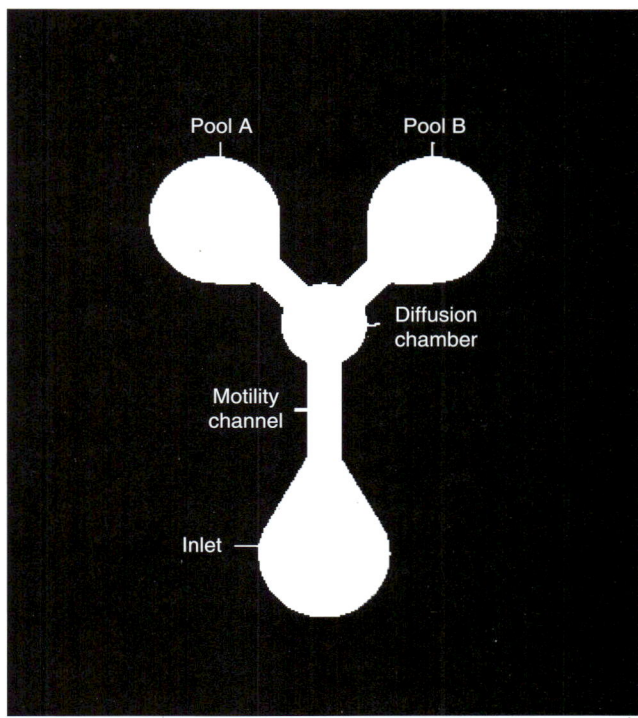

Figure 31.3 Image of a microfluidic sperm sorter that integrates isolation of sperm based on motility and chemotaxis toward cumulus cells. Final enriched sperm populations are obtained from pools A and B.

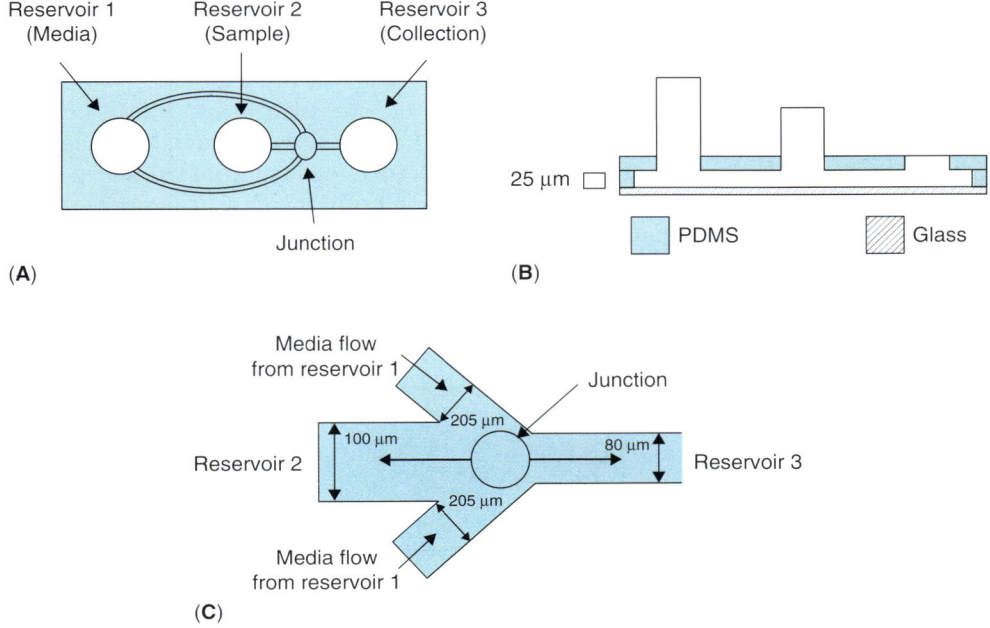

Figure 31.4 Diagram illustrating microfluidic device for separation, orientation, and alignment of motile sperm from bull, mouse, and human. The device was constructed from PDMS and glass. Fresh media is loaded into reservoir 1, while semen samples are loaded in reservoir 2. Hydrostatic pressure differences, due to differences in height of media columns in the three reservoirs, cause media flow in various indicated directions. These media streams converge at a point known as the "junction." Motile spermatozoa orient themselves against direction of media flow and are able to swim through the current to collect in reservoir 3. Abbreviation: PDMS, polydimethylsiloxane.

Utilizing these advantages of a microfluidic device for sperm isolation, implementation of a microfluidic sperm sorter manufactured out of quartz has begun in clinical IVF. A preliminary report indicates human semen can be processed rapidly and isolated motile sperm can be used to successfully fertilize human oocytes following ICSI (11). Continued research will determine if this technology results in improved embryo development and/or implantation rates.

MICROFLUIDICS IN EMBRYOLOGY

As mentioned, employing microfluidic technology for embryology applications requires considerations unique from microfluidic devices utilizing adherent cells, including the ability to isolate or manipulate individual cells. In addition, sensitivity of reproductive cells demands specialized precautions. Thus, progress in implementing devices has been slow. However, as with andrology applications, refinement of microfluidic designs has resolved several long-standing issues and platforms have begun to receive initial testing in all aspects of embryology, including in vitro oocyte maturation (IVM), IVF, and embryo culture.

In Vitro Maturation

IVM is an especially appealing approach for human ART considering tremendous advantages offered, including reduced cost and reduced health risk to disorders such as ovarian hyperstimulation syndrome (OHSS) (63). However, IVM is still an inefficient practice. Fortunately, microfluidic approaches offer the potential to improve current IVM success rates. Preliminary data suggest that while porcine oocytes do not mature efficiently in silicone devices (2% Metaphase MII), they can indeed be matured successfully in PDMS microchannels (2% vs. 71% development to MII) (12). Oocytes matured in 200 μm wide PDMS microchannels, containing approximately 8 μl of media, displayed comparable development to MII as control oocytes matured in 8 μl or 500 μl drops. However, oocyte maturation consists of two components; nuclear and cytoplasmic maturation. Interestingly, cumulus cell expansion was noticeably diminished in oocytes matured in microchannels and 8 μl microdrops. This observation may be indicative of quality oocyte cytoplasmic maturation, as oocytes regulate cumulus cell development and function (64). Thus, size and/or volume limitations of microchannels may have some limiting effect on porcine oocyte cytoplasmic properties, or physically restrict cumulus expansion. In contrast, subsequent follow-up experiments by Walters and coworkers from the same research group suggest oocyte cytoplasmic maturation may actually be enhanced in static microchannels. Pig oocytes matured in 250 μm wide PDMS/borosilicate glass microchannels produced significantly higher numbers of two-cell embryos following IVF and embryo culture in microdrops compared to oocytes matured in 500 μl drops (67% vs. 49%) (15). Unfortunately, pronuclear formations, embryo development past the maternal-zygotic transition, or blastocyst cell numbers were not reported. Additionally, it should be noted that chips utilized in these studies were not engineered with active media flow. Though some passive gravity-driven media flow may have been present, this parameter was not measured nor recorded in experiments. Interestingly, preliminary studies indicate bovine oocytes matured in dynamic microfluidic devices with Braille pin regulated media flow, actually yields improved blastocyst development following IVF compared to static matured oocytes (personal communication, Dr. Gary Smith). Despite these preliminary findings, the field awaits peer-reviewed publications examining effects of fluid flow in microfluidic devices on more informative markers of oocyte cytoplasmic maturation; including genomic, proteomic, or metabolomic profiles.

In Vitro Fertilization

Another demonstration of microfluidic application in ART can be seen in IVF performed "on chip." The first attempt at this procedural step was performed using porcine oocytes placed into PDMS/borosilicate microchannels. Sperms were added in a manner where pressure differences created from volume of media added resulted in gravity-driven flow of sperm past oocytes (Fig. 31.5). It was shown that oocyte numbers used in experiments had

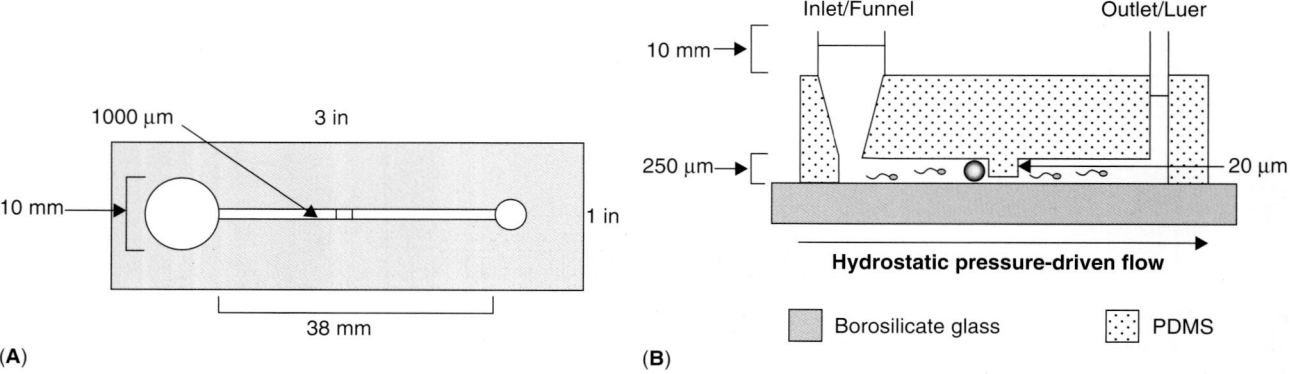

Figure 31.5 Illustration of a PDMS/borosilicate microfluidic device used to perform IVF "on chip": (**A**) *top view*; (**B**) *side view*. *Abbreviation*: PDMS, polydimethylsiloxane.

no effect on sperm penetration. Further, fertilization in microchannels resulted in significantly lower rates of polyspermic penetration compared to fertilization in control microdrops (14). Reduced polyspermic penetration rates were attributed to the physical characteristics of the microfluidic device, mimicking the environment in utero. It is thought that microfluidic devices serve to limit time of oocyte exposure to sperm, as sperm were not confined to the vicinity of the oocytes, as in microdrop culture, but allowed to flow past the eggs along the length of the microchannel. Further examination of sperm motility characteristics and interactions with oocytes during attempted fertilization in microfluidic channels demonstrated that flow rate is extremely important in regulating sperm motion, as a threshold exists where sperm are no longer capable of independent movement (65). Furthermore, sperm motion paths were influenced by the contours of the device. These qualities have immense implications for success of fertilization in microfluidic device.

Utilizing cleavage of mouse embryos to two-cell as an indicator of successful fertilization, Suh and colleagues (17) demonstrated that fertilization of mouse oocytes can occur in a microfluidic device (Fig. 31.6). Although initial experiments utilizing high concentrations of sperm revealed that overall fertilization rates were decreased on the microfluidic device compared to controls, subsequent experiments demonstrated that, by lowering sperm concentration, fertilization rates in microfluidic devices were actually higher than fertilization in control drops. Fertilization rates obtained at these lower sperm concentrations in microfluidic devices were comparable to rates obtained with higher sperm concentrations in control microdrops. These results appear to be the result of chip design, as authors observed increased concentration of sperm in the vicinity of the oocyte in microfluidic devices. This increased concentration may not only explain increased rates of fertilization at reduced sperm concentration, but may also explain reduced fertilization rates at high concentrations of sperm. Increased sperm concentration may potentially result in decreased availability of local metabolic substrates, or result in detrimental shifts in culture conditions, such as pH or localized build up of metabolic byproducts.

Clark and coworkers presented preliminary data demonstrating that both IVM and IVF of porcine oocytes could be performed on the same microfluidic device without removal of the cells between procedures (13). Media within devices were changed and sperm added via manual pipetting without disturbing oocytes. Although there were no observable benefits achieving cleavage to two-cell compared to control treatments (49% vs. 51%), this was the first demonstration of multiple tasks of in vitro embryo production performed upon the same microfluidic platform. Such a realization has tremendous potential for performing multiple sequential steps "on chip" and minimization of stress to gametes/embryos.

More recently, fertilization has been performed on a microfluidic microwell device (66,67). Devices made of PDMS were constructed that consisted of an inlet and outlet reservoir, which generated media flow using gravity. Microchannels, (1 mm × 200 µm w × h), leading from each reservoir connect to a larger microchamber (3 × 10 mm, w × l), which houses individual square microwells (200 × 200 × 200 µm, l × w × h), which contain individual oocytes (Fig. 31.7). Microwell depth was optimized to permit retention of oocytes while allowing adequate debris removal and sperm interaction with oocytes. Media and sperm (1 × 10^6/ml) could then be flowed over the microwell housing the oocytes at ~2.5 mm/s. With oocytes settled at the bottom of microwells and out of the direct fluid stream, sheer forces are reduced, while permitting retention of any local autocrine/paracrine factors. Using this approach, similar rates of mouse oocyte fertilization were obtained compared to controls (69.0% vs. 71.4%)

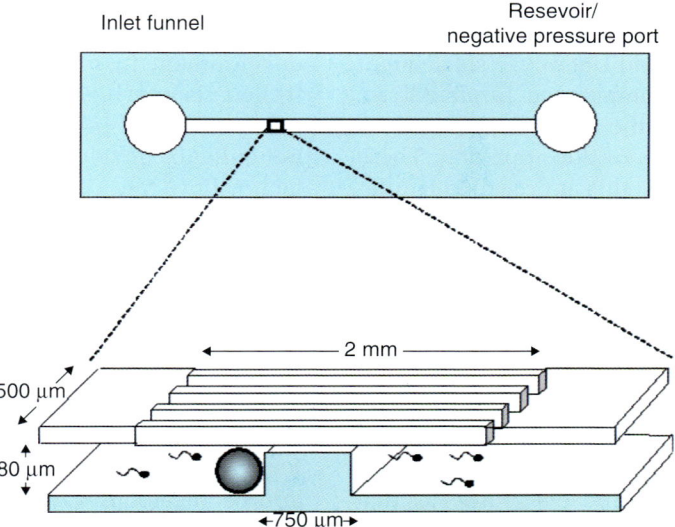

Figure 31.6 Microfluidic device composed of PDMS utilized to perform mouse IVF "on chip." *Abbreviation*: PDMS, polydimethylsiloxane.

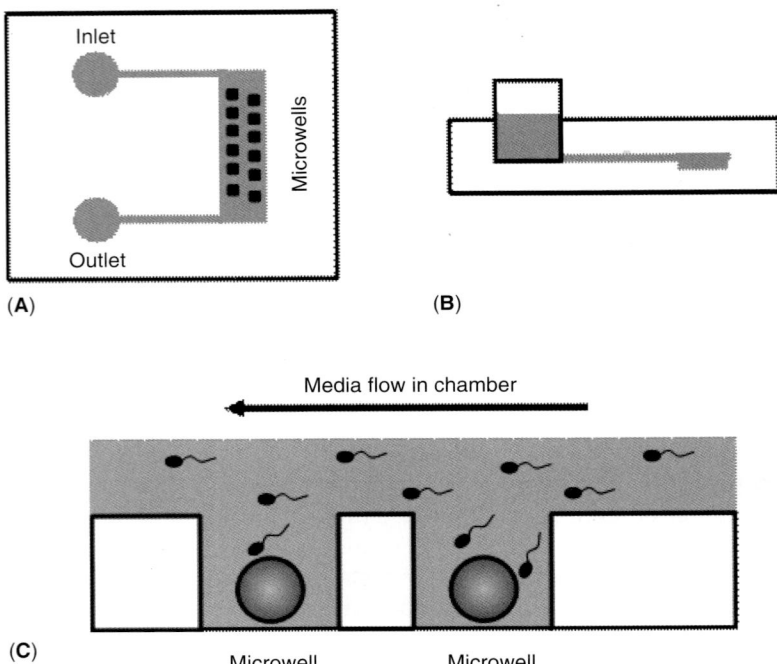

Figure 31.7 Microfluidic PDMS device utilizing gravity-driven media flow to pass sperm over mouse oocytes for in vitro fertilization (IVF). Oocytes are housed individually within microwells (200 × 200 × 200 μm, l × w × h) to prevent sheer stress, maintain autocrine/paracrine factors, and permit tracking of individual cells. (**A**) *Top view*; (**B**) *side view*; (**C**) close-up of microwells.

(66). An alternate device from the same research group with differing design also yielded promising fertilization results and is discussed later (67).

IVF not only entails mixing of sperm and eggs, but also required manipulation of presumptive zygotes to move cumulus cells to visualize pronuclei. As previously mentioned, cumulus cells (41,68), and even zona pellucida (42) can be removed using a microfluidic device with flow driven manually via attached syringes, exposing oocytes to chemical and physical manipulation. Inclusion of these abilities on the same device where IVF is performed would be extremely advantageous in minimizing stress imposed upon the embryo. Regardless, it is evident that chip design is extremely important to efficacy of the fertilization process and refinement with further testing of various designs is essential to advance IVF on microfluidic devices. Additionally, subsequent assessment of developmental competence, implantation, and live birth rates of microfluidic derived IVF embryos is required to determine efficacy of this approach. These efforts, though, are important, as this approach may offer substantial benefit to patients undergoing infertility treatment due to conditions such as oligozoospermia.

Embryo Culture

Exhaustive studies have been conducted aimed at optimizing preimplantation embryo culture in vitro, and, similar to IVM and IVF, a microfluidic platform may aid in this endeavor. The initial report on embryo culture using microfluidics by Raty and colleagues indicates that two-cell mouse embryos can be cultured to the blastocyst stage within static microchannels (9,69) (Fig. 31.8). These experiments demonstrate that, compared to 30 μl control microdrops, culture within microchannel containing about 500 μl of media (10 μl within the actual channel itself) resulted in significantly greater 16-cell/morula formation at 24 hours, greater blastocyst formation at 48 hours and 72 hours, and a greater portion of hatched blastocysts at 72 hours and 96 hours. Subsequent experiments utilizing a similar device by Walters and coworkers from the same research group showed that in vivo derived four-cell porcine embryos could be cultured to blastocyst and transferred, resulting in live birth (70). However, in these experiments, no observable beneficial effects on embryo development were seen when compared to culture in control organ well dishes.

Building upon the initial chip-based static embryo culture studies, Hickman et al. examined mouse embryo development in microchannels with media flow, controlled via a syringe infusion pump (16) (Fig. 31.9). Flow rates examined in this study (0.1 and 0.5 μl/hour) did not enhance development compared to static culture. In fact, a flow rate of 0.5 μl/hour resulted in significantly lower development of two-cell mouse embryos to morula and blastocyst stages, while producing higher numbers of abnormal embryos compared to controls. Thus, flow rate and manner of flow delivery may be important variables for embryo culture in microfluidic devices. Indeed, embryos sense sheer stress, which can induce apoptosis and be detrimental to embryo development (71). However, it is questionable if flow rates necessary for dynamic fluid flow in microfluidic channels would approach velocities high enough to cause concern. Additionally, it should be noted that these data on the impact of media flow and flow rate on embryo development

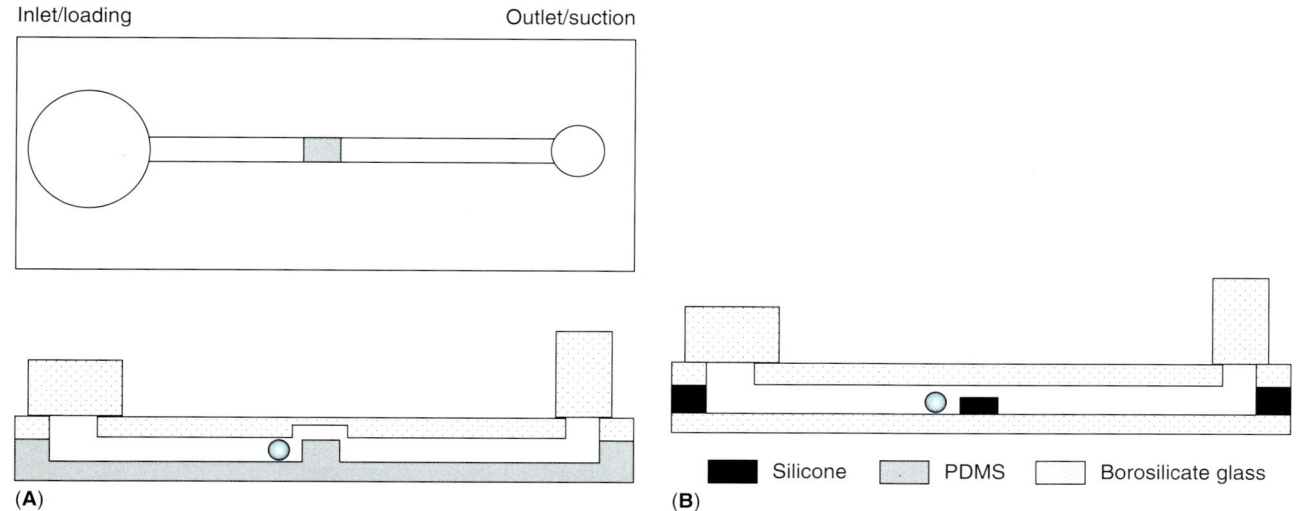

Figure 31.8 Illustration of the first microfluidic device created to culture preimplantation mouse embryos. (**A**) *Top view* and (**B**) *side view* of devices made out of differing materials. *Abbreviation*: PDMS, polydimethylsiloxane.

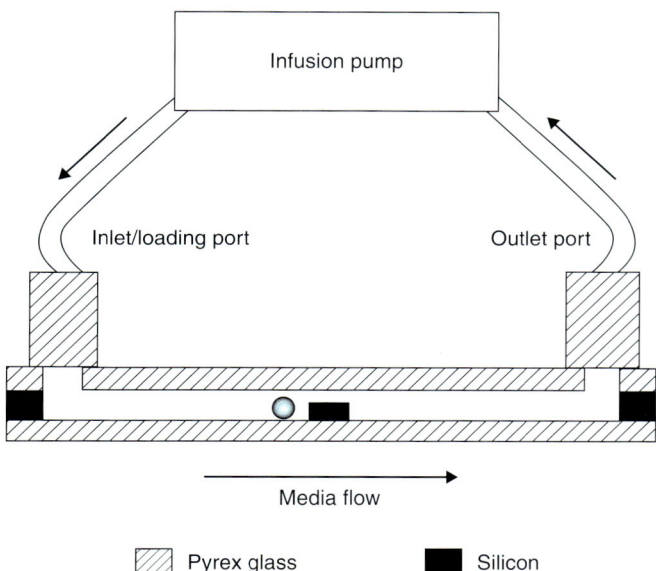

Figure 31.9 Diagram depicting a microfluidic perfusion system utilizing a syringe infusion pump to regulate media flow to culture preimplantation embryos.

should be re-assessed, as culture conditions may have been suboptimal. In this particular study, control mouse embryos cultured in control static microchannels did not improve embryo development as previously reported by Raty and colleagues from the same research group (9). One possible source of variation requiring future study was the increased number of embryos cultured in each device.

Interestingly, utilizing an alternate chip design, Cabrera and coworkers presented preliminary data that one-cell mouse embryos could be cultured efficiently within microfluidic devices offering media flow (38). Embryos were loaded into a funnel reservoir, while medium was added and removed via a microfluidic channel connected to the bottom of the funnel via actions of a Braille actuator (Fig. 31.10). It was demonstrated that regardless of media flow pattern (back and forth vs. flow through) or speed (fast vs. slow), one-cell mouse embryos cultured in dynamic devices showed greater hatching of blastocysts and significantly higher cell number than static controls, yielding numbers similar to those obtained from in vivo derived blastocysts.

Bormann and colleagues subsequently presented preliminary data validating beneficial effects of Braille driven media flow in a microfluidic device on murine and bovine embryo development (37). Greater number of mouse embryos reached morula stage at 48 hours, blastocyst at 72 hours, and hatched blastocyst at 96 hours compared to control static chips, while significantly more bovine embryos reached the blastocyst stage at 144 hours in microfluidic devices compared to control static devices. Follow-up experiments by Bormann and colleagues indicated that beneficial effects of embryo culture in the dynamic culture device are additive and require a minimum 48 hours of culture at the beginning or end of 96 hour–culture periods (36). Importantly, more recent studies indicate that not only is there a benefit on preimplantation embryo development, but that quality of embryos cultured in a microfluidic device with media flow are superior to those grown in static systems, as evidenced by increased implantation rates, lower rates of absorption, and higher ongoing pregnancy rates in mouse (39) (Fig. 31.11).

Yet another approach to culturing embryos within microfluidic devices has employed not only dynamic media flow, but also coculture. Mizuno and coworkers have adopted a "womb-on-a-chip" design, where endometrial cells are grown in a lower chamber, while embryos are cultured in an upper chamber, separated from the lower by a thin membrane (8,72), thus allowing embryos to interact with secreted factors from the endometrial cells (Fig. 31.12). In this preliminary report,

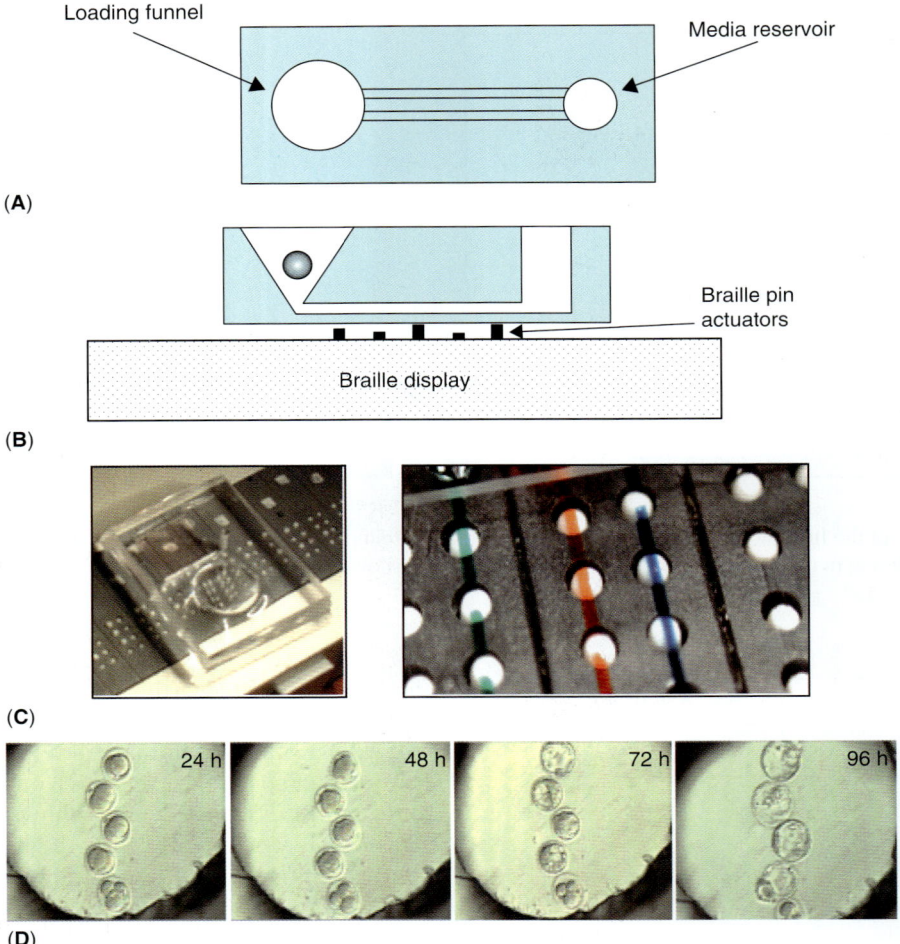

Figure 31.10 Microfluidic device composed of polydimethylsiloxane (PDMS) utilizing Braille actuators to drive media flow through two microchannels. Media flow is accomplished via Braille pin deflection of the thin bottom of the PDMS platform. Coordinated pin rise/fall allows peristaltic movement of a media bolus along the length of the microfluidic channels. (**A**) *Top view;* (**B**) *side view;* (**C**) image of Braille pin PDMS device and demonstration of Braille pin rise/fall used to control fluid flow through microfluidic channels; (**D**) Images of mouse embryos grown over 96 h within the microwell that is fed by media from the attached microchannels.

authors demonstrated that mouse ova fertilized on and resulting embryos cultured in these devices showed similar cleavage to two-cell and similar blastocyst formation rates compared to 50 μl control microdrops (72). Furthermore, cell number was significantly higher in blastocysts fertilized/cultured in microfluidic devices. Subsequently, blastocysts obtained from microfluidic devices were transferred to recipient female mice and resulted in live offspring at rates similar to embryo cultured in static microdrops. Though these experiments are still preliminary, they add to the advancement of microfluidic technology in ART, showing that both IVF and embryo culture can be performed on the same device, and that the resulting embryos yield live offspring. A similar coculture approach was taken by the same group, culturing two-cell mouse embryos to blastocyst stage on the refined OptiCell microfluidic device. OptiCell microfluidic coculture culture yielded chromosomally normal embryos, capable of yielding live offspring (73).

Mizuno and colleagues published an abstract reporting the first instance of human embryo culture within microfluidic devices. Donated two- to four-stage frozen human embryos were cultured to the blastocyst stage, resulting in significantly higher rates of blastocyst development from microfluidic devices compared to control microdrops (8). Additionally, visual scoring of microfluidic-derived blastocyst development revealed higher quality blastocysts with significantly higher cell numbers compared to static controls. Unfortunately, coculture confounds interpretation of results obtained, as it is impossible to discern if effects are attributed to coculture or microfluidic design. As the goal of embryo culture has been development of defined culture media, it will be interesting to see if similar studies can be performed without the use of coculture.

Recently, mouse embryos have been cultured successfully in microwells housed on the same microfluidic device where fertilization occurred. Han et al. (66) demonstrated that oocytes could be fertilized in microwells using media and sperm movement via gravity-driven hydrostatic pressure (Fig. 31.7). Fertilization media was then replaced with embryo culture media by flowing media though the channels on the same device and embryos cultured. Though there was no active media

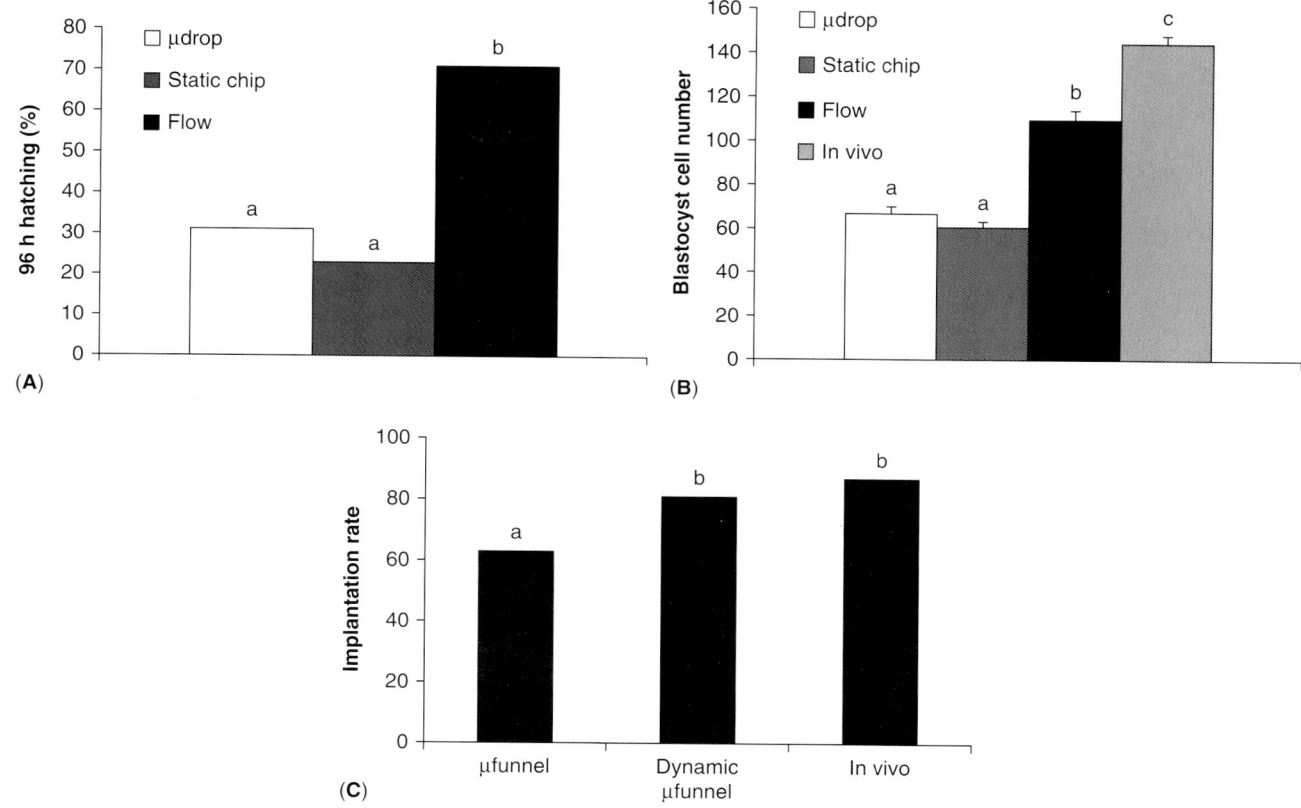

Figure 31.11 Microfluidic culture in a microfunnel improves mouse embryo development compared to static culture techniques resulting in (**A**) increased rates of blastocyst hatching at 96 hours, (**B**) resulting blastocyst cell number, (**C**) as well as implantation rates following embryo transfer. *Source*: Adapted from Ref. 39. Different superscripts between treatments indicate a statistically significant difference, $p < 0.05$.

flow during the 96 hours of embryo development, similar high rates of blastocyst formation were obtained following culture in microwells compared to controls (87.5% vs. 87.8%). Similarly, using a revised device design employing the "octacolumn" to house oocytes/embryos rather than microwells, the same group again demonstrated mouse oocyte fertilization and subsequent embryo development on the same microfluidic platform, yielding high rates of blastocyst formation, similar to controls (86.9% vs. 85.3%) (67). This approach of combining multiple steps successfully on the same platform offers tremendous potential to minimize cell handling and associated stress.

Finally, at least one study has used a tilting culture system in conjunction with microfluidic channels to gently agitate embryos during culture. Bovine embryos were tilted 10° over 1 min and cultured inside straight microchannels (200 μm × 50 mm × 200 μm, w × l × h) or microchannels with a 150–160 μm constriction. Though no difference in blastocyst formation was observed or reported, and the influence of the tilting system alone was not examined, authors suggest that combining an embryo tilting system with a 169 μm constricted microchannels may offer a means of improving bovine embryo cleavage, yielding higher rates of eight-cell development after 44 hours or culture compared to straight channels (56.7% vs. 23.9%) (74). It should be pointed out, however, that tilting approaches simply agitate and don't necessarily remove or replenish the existing media like perfusion systems. Similar methods of combining a simplified microchannel or microfluidic devices with other dynamic methods of inducing fluid movement, generally used at the macro-level, such as vibration or agitation, may be helpful, as gentle agitation appears to beneficial for human embryos (29,30). Though more recent dynamic culture platforms that agitate media and embryos by simply placing traditional culture dishes with microdrops or larger volumes of media on a moving or vibrating platforms have been examined and appear promising (26–31), in the context of this review, these aren't considered microfluidic culture platforms and may not utilize the full potential of the constrictive environment offered by other microfluidic approaches.

WHY DO OOCYTES/EMBRYOS BENEFIT FROM MICROFLUIDICS?

How do microfluidic approaches work to improve embryo development? It has been hypothesized that unknown autocrine/paracrine factors secreted by gametes or embryos are localized due to the confining nature of microfluidic devices, and that this localization of factors may carry certain benefits. Indeed, oocytes and embryos do secrete various factors, and research is ongoing to identify components of this secretome as noninvasive markers of embryo developmental competence (75,76). If secretion of beneficial factors from cultured cells is responsible for

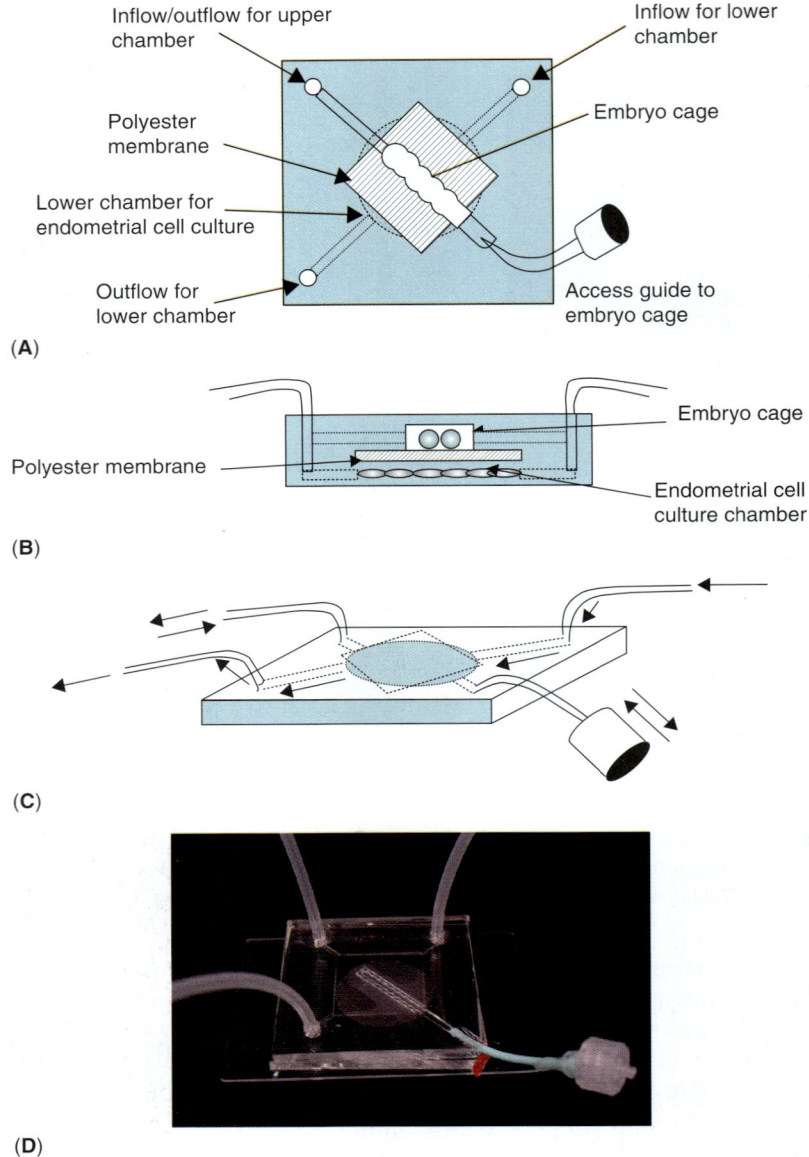

Figure 31.12 Illustrations of the "womb-on-a-chip" microfluidic perfusion system. Embryos are grown in a coculture system, separated from endometrial cells by a thin polyester membrane. (**A**) *Top view*; (**B**) *side view*; (**C**) Indication of media flow; (**D**) Image of polydimethylsiloxane (PDMS) "womb-on-a-chip" microfluidic device. *Source*: Photo courtesy of Dr. Teruo Fujii.

improved development, then quantity of embryos, volume of media, and surface area occupied would be extremely important factors to consider. Discussion of these issues in traditional culture platforms has been eloquently reviewed (77). Indeed, several studies have examined beneficial effects of group embryo culture and media volume on traditional static culture platforms of several species, including human (78–81). Though direct comparisons are difficult due to differences in experimental parameters, it appears that in certain instances group culture does provide beneficial effects. Furthermore, in dealing with group culture, another important variable to consider is quality of companion embryos (82,83). However, experiments exploring effects of embryo density within microfluidic devices are lacking.

Although the autocrine/paracrine debate offers an attractive means by which embryo development may benefit from microfluidic culture, secretion of trophic factors from embryos does not necessary explain improved embryo development within microfluidic devices with dynamic conditions. With media flow, trophic factors would presumably be diluted or removed, yet advanced development is still observed. Alternatively, benefits within dynamic devices could be the result of removal of harmful embryo metabolic byproducts, such as ammonia (84), or disruption of any gradients that may form (85,86). Shape of culture area can impact media flow characteristics (87) and may be important in this respect. If this is indeed the case, then undoubtedly a delicate balance exists on the correct number of embryos to culture in static devices to not negate any potential benefit of group autocrine/paracrine factors. However, it should be noted that studies removing spent culture media and replacing with fresh media from microdrops at various intervals shows no benefit to embryo development (88,89). Thus, removal of byproducts or disruption of gradients may not be the sole reason for improved embryo development within microfluidic devices.

A common denominator of static and flow devices is the constrictive nature of the micro devices, confining embryos to a very small area. Thus, benefits may somehow be related to cell proximity and spacing. Indeed, spacing of embryos during group culture affects development. Two innovative studies attached either pig or cattle embryos to culture dishes at measurable distances and demonstrated if embryo spacing was too great, blastocyst development was not achieved (90,91). This spacing theory is supported by studies showing advanced embryo development in confining ultra-microdrops (89), culture within glass capillary tubes (80,92), culture within small concave wells (GPS dish) (1), as well as culture within extremely small volumes/area in the "well of a well" or WOW technique (93). If spacing is important and can improve embryo development when cultured in groups, then another variable to consider in designing microfluidic devices for ART is shape of the culture area (77), which can dictate if embryos are in direct contact or maintain physical separation. It remains to be seen if microfluidic embryo culture improves development of individually cultured embryos.

In terms of gradients formed in culture, it has been suggested by some that benefits of culturing embryos within extremely small volumes, including microfluidic culture, may result from a reduction in localized oxygen tension due to culture in these confined spaces. In traditional culture approaches, reduced oxygen levels from atmospheric levels of around 20% to around 5–7% is beneficial for embryo development and quality (94–96). Interestingly, the majority of reported microfluidic culture experiments were performed in 5% CO_2 in air, and thus, reduction in localized oxygen would appear to be a plausible theory. However, bovine embryos cultured in dynamic microfluidic devices in 5% O_2 still showed improved development over static culture in the same device (37). Also, it should also be noted that hypoxic conditions are detrimental to oocytes and embryos (95,97). Thus, if localized oxygen depletion is occurring in microdevices, culturing in reduced oxygen tension could in fact result in hypoxia, decreasing embryo development. Fortunately, as the bovine study by Bormann and colleagues indicated, this does not appear to be the case. In support of this, mathematical modeling suggests oxygen depletion does not appear to be a factor in microdrops, regardless of the number of mouse embryos cultured, as diffusion and convection currents mix the environment to prevent anoxic regions (98). Thus, localized reduction in oxygen levels is questionable, especially when one considers the microfluidic devices used in ART studies are composed of PDMS, which is extremely gas permeable. However, at least one mathematical modeling study by Byatt-Smith et al. (19) suggested that, due to slightly larger size, culture of human embryos within static microdrops may become marginally hypoxic, especially when cultured in 5% O_2 (99). As a preventative measure to hypoxia, these same authors hypothesized that "embryos may develop more successfully in stirred, as opposed to still medium." Therefore, in studies utilizing dynamic microfluidic devices, media renewal due to flow should prevent any localized build-up or depletion of factors, including oxygen, thereby alleviating the possibility that advanced development is due to oxygen depletion.

Yet another possibility for benefits of microfluidic culture, at least in dynamic flow devices, is gentle agitation of embryos or media surrounding embryos. When considering the growing amount of data from both micro, as well as macro dynamic culture devices, this seems like a plausible explanation. Embryos can sense sheer stress and activate various intracellular signaling pathways in response (71,100). While high rates of agitation or pathway activation may be detrimental, there may be a range of gentle agitation that permits intermediate activation of relevant signaling cascades that promote embryo development. Physiologically, this makes sense, as gentle stimulation may be mimicking the vibrating actions of the ciliated epithelium within the female reproductive tract (28,29).

Unfortunately, each microfluidic device utilized to date is different in its construction (culturing in channels, culturing in funnels, culturing with/without flow, using coculture, utilizing different number of embryos/volume), thereby making it difficult to ascertain where the benefit to embryo development actually lies. Regardless, it is obvious that a culmination of factors is dictating embryo development and quality within any culture device, including microfluidic platforms. Further research examining divergence of gene expression patterns, molecular signaling pathways, or other biochemical endpoint are required to begin to elucidate possible explanations for observed effects in microfluidic culture and to optimize this promising technology for use in ART (Table 31.1).

MICROFLUIDICS AND NONINVASIVE VIABILITY ASSESSMENT

Perhaps the most important benefit of implementing a microfluidic platform for ART is the ability to integrate diagnostic tools to monitor gamete and embryo environmental conditions and physiologic processes. Though environmental monitoring has not yet received attention in ART, as examples, using a nano-sized optical sensor, it is possible to monitor pH of interstitial fluid flowing through a microfluidic device (101). Using nano- or microsensors, one can monitor temperature fluctuations (102,103), media flow rate (104), and volume of the cell to indicate shifts in media osmolarity (105). Additionally, electrical sensors have been developed to measure real-time changes in levels of ROS as indicators of oxidative stress on microfluidic devices (106,107). Conceivably, any one, or a combination of these approaches could be adapted for use with ART microfluidic devices, as measurement of any of these environmental parameters may

Table 31.1 Practical Considerations Which Must Be Addressed in Order for Microfluidic Devices to Gain Widespread Acceptance into IVF Laboratories

Biocompatibility	Operation	Manipulation of cells	Lab compatibility
Nontoxic fabrication materials	Perfusion system (recirculation vs. non)	Easy visualization	Fit in conventional incubators
Sterilization of device	Ability to be used over 5–6 days	Rapid loading/unloading	User friendly external apparatus
Packaging to pass "in-house" QC	Easy rectification of failure	Ability to isolate/monitor Individual cells	Short set-up time
Disposable	Easy rectification of failure		
Design issues (volume, embryo no.)			

provide insight into improvement of culture conditions and current IVF lab practices.

Furthermore, it has long been the goal of reproductive investigators to discover a means by which to interrogate gametes and embryos to identify markers of physiologic processes as a noninvasive means of predicting developmental competence and implantation potential. Current research is examining secreted proteins from embryos in the hopes of relating this information to cell quality (75,76). Implementation of ELISA assays "on-chip" have met with some success in adherent cell systems (108,109), and may prove useful in analyzing embryo secretomic profiles. Additionally, examination of oocyte or embryo metabolomic activity and profiles has also showed promise in offering a noninvasive predictor of embryo quality (110–112). A silicone microfluidic device has been designed to measure oxygen consumption rates as an indicators of mouse preimplantation embryo metabolic activity (113) and preliminary data measuring glucose, lactate, and pyruvate levels of spent embryo culture media in a pneumatic controlled microfluidic device exists (114). Although embryos were not grown in microfluidic devices in these studies, ideally these types of analysis systems will be constructed on the same device as cultured cells, allowing rapid, real-time analysis without additionally stressing embryos by additional manipulation or removing them from the incubator environment.

FUTURE DIRECTIONS

In a now increasingly used quote, Bavister stated "Ideally, the culture medium should change progressively during development to keep pace with the embryo's needs, but continuous flow or perfusion culture systems are difficult to maintain on a microscale and may be impractical" (115). It is apparent that advances in microfluidic technology may offer a solution to this impasse, as designs are quickly approaching a stage where continuous flow of media will no longer be problematic. Microfluidic chip design and technology has progressed dramatically, ensuring compatibility with essential requirements of the IVF lab. In fact, at least one report exists reporting culture of human embryos on chip (8), and at least one commercial company has refined their system enough to begin testing microfluidic culture devices with donated human embryos. The attributes of microfluidics allows the pursuit of a more in vivo–like culture environment, culturing embryos in confined spaces, in small volumes of media, as well as allowing for media flow and progressive substrate change to meet the evolving nutritional requirements of the developing embryo.

Finally, microfluidic design allows embryologist to explore spatial considerations not afforded by a two-dimensional surface of a dish. Thus, the scale of microfluidic devices offers the ability to shuttle in a new area in embryo culture. Emerging technological advancements offer the capability of not only regulating embryo culture fluid dynamics, but also substrate compositional dynamics, essentially marking the end of "fixed" chemistry in media. By combining a microfluidic platform with three-dimensional matrices of oriented macromolecules to create a "moist" rather than a fluid environment, more like that of the female reproductive tract, embryos may benefit in ways previously unavailable in standard culture systems. Through chemical–physical interactions, oriented macromolecules within the female reproductive tract are hypothesized to support embryo cellular homeostatic mechanisms, imparting responsiveness or plasticity to the embryo (116,117). Thus, implementation of oriented three-dimensional matrices for in vitro embryo culture may render embryos more competent to compensate for encountered homeostatic imbalances. This approach has shown some promise on a macroscale for follicle and oocyte culture (118,119). However, as pointed out, the physical presentation of these macromolecules to gametes or embryos is problematic. Pool stated "to mimic the physical–chemical conditions present in vivo, a potential culture system must be able to present an array of macromolecules, an assemblage that changes qualitatively, with time, from fixed sites in a minimum volume of water" (117). Microfluidics offers a platform that can alleviate these previous limitations and offer certain benefits over macro systems. One can imagine a microfluidic device housing multiple individual chambers in which a single embryo is encapsulated within a transparent three-dimensional oriented organic matrix, perfused with culture media that changes composition over time to meet the changing metabolic needs of the cell. Appropriate selection criterion would allow subsequent transfer of the

Table 31.2 Suggested Variables That Should Receive Future Study to Assist in Widespread Implementation of Microfluidic Platforms in ART

- Effects of embryo/gamete density
- Importance of embryo/gamete spacing
- Effects on cell transcriptome, proteome, metabolome, and secretome
- Influences on embryo developmental competence, implantation, and pregnancy
- Optimization of media flow rates/patterns
- Development of specialized culture media

biodegradable scaffold and enclosed embryo. Suitable biodegradable matrixes, such as poly(DL-lactide-co-glycolide) (PLGA) (120) and poly(glycerol-sebacate) (PGS) (121), have received recent attention in other cell systems. Furthermore, with continued advancement and use of three-dimensional matrices, such as hydrogels, it is even imaginable to have an organic, self-regulating microfluidic device providing peristaltic media flow (40,122), truly embracing a physiologic pheno-mimetic approach to embryo culture.

Perhaps more importantly, not only can microfluidic devices be used to manipulate gametes and culture embryos more efficiently, but they also lend themselves to integration with other systems. Microfluidic chips have been designed that can perform multiple aspects of in vitro embryo production (13,43,72) and it is extremely feasible to imagine a microfluidic device–integrated multiparametric, real-time, on-chip-diagnostic assays to assist in selection of the most viable gametes/embryos. Eventually, automation of such microfluidic devices may allow for reduced manipulation and prevent unneeded imbalances in embryo homeostasis, even alerting embryologist and taking preventive actions if monitored variables fall out of a specified range. However, diligence in these pursuits is called for. Although the field has received tremendous initial interest, the lack of peer-reviewed publications demonstrates the infancy of the technology. Continued research and exacting experimentation are required to realize the full potential of microfluidic technology for ART (Table 31.2).

REFERENCES

1. Swain JE, Smith GD. Advances in embryo culture platforms: novel approaches to improve preimplantation embryo development through modifications of the microenvironment. Hum Reprod Update 2011; 17: 541–57.
2. Leese HJ. Human embryo culture: back to nature. J Assist Reprod Genet 1998; 15: 466–8.
3. Beebe D, Wheeler M, Zeringue H, et al. Microfluidic technology for assisted reproduction. Theriogenology 2002; 57: 125–35.
4. Bormann C, Wheeler M, Beebe D, et al. Microfluidics for assisted reproductive technologies. In: Khademhosseini A, Borenstein J, Toner M, Takayama S, Eds. Micro- and nanoengineering of the cell microenvironment: technologies and applications 2008; Chapter 11 Artech House.
5. Wheeler MB, Walters EM, Beebe DJ. Toward culture of single gametes: the development of microfluidic platforms for assisted reproduction. Theriogenology 2007; 68(Suppl 1): S178–89.
6. Glasgow IK, Zeringue HC, Beebe DJ, et al. Handling individual mammalian embryos using microfluidics. IEEE Trans Biomed Eng 2001; 48: 570–8.
7. Kim L, Toh YC, Voldman J, et al. A practical guide to microfluidic perfusion culture of adherent mammalian cells. Lab Chip 2007; 7: 681–94.
8. Mizuno J, Ostrovidov S, Sakai Y, et al. Human ART on chip: improved human blastocyst development and quality with IVF-chip. Fertil Steril 2007; 88–S101.
9. Raty S, Walters EM, Davis J, et al. Embryonic development in the mouse is enhanced via microchannel culture. Lab Chip 2004; 4: 186–90.
10. Schuster TG, Cho B, Keller LM, et al. Isolation of motile spermatozoa from semen samples using microfluidics. Reprod Biomed Online 2003; 7: 75–81.
11. Shibata D, Ando H, Iwase A, et al. Analysis of sperm motility and fertilization rates after the separation by microfluidic sperm sorter made of quartz. Fertil Steril 2007; 88: S110.
12. Walters E, Beebe D, Wheeler M. In vitro maturation of pig oocytes in polydimethylsiloxane (PDMS) and silicon microfluidic devices. Theriogenology 2001; 55: 497.
13. Clark S, Walters E, Beebe D, et al. A novel integrated in vitro maturation and in vitro fertilization system for swine. Theriogenology 2003; 59: 441.
14. Clark SG, Haubert K, Beebe DJ, et al. Reduction of polyspermic penetration using biomimetic microfluidic technology during in vitro fertilization. Lab Chip 2005; 5: 1229–32.
15. Hester P, Roseman H, Clark S, et al. Enhanced cleavage rates following in vitro maturation of pig oocytes within polydimehtylsiloxane-borosilcate microchannels. Theriogenology 2002; 57: 723.
16. Hickman D, Beebe D, Rodriguez-Zas S, et al. Comparison of static and dynamic medium enviornments for culturing of pre-implantation mouse embryos. Comp Med 2002; 52: 122–6.
17. Suh RS, Zhu X, Phadke N, et al. IVF within microfluidic channels requires lower total numbers and lower concentrations of sperm. Hum Reprod 2006; 21: 477–83.
18. Lim JM, Reggio BC, Godke RA, et al. Perifusion culture system for bovine embryos: improvement of embryo development by use of bovine oviduct epithelial cells, an antioxidant and polyvinyl alcohol. Reprod Fertil Dev 1997; 9: 411–18.
19. Lim JM, Reggio BC, Godke RA, et al. Development of in-vitro-derived bovine embryos cultured in 5% CO_2 in air or in 5% O_2, 5% CO_2 and 90% N_2. Hum Reprod 1999; 14: 458–64.
20. Goverde HJ, Peeters RH, Willems PH. The development of a superfusion system for studying intracellular and secretory processes in embryos. In Vitro Cell Dev Biol Anim 1994; 30A: 819–21.
21. Chung BG, Flanagan LA, Rhee SW, et al. Human neural stem cell growth and differentiation in a gradient-generating microfluidic device. Lab Chip 2005; 5: 401–6.

22. Hung PJ, Lee PJ, Sabounchi P, et al. A novel high aspect ratio microfluidic design to provide a stable and uniform microenvironment for cell growth in a high throughput mammalian cell culture array. Lab Chip 2005; 5: 44–8.
23. Cho BS, Schuster TG, Zhu X, et al. Passively driven integrated microfluidic system for separation of motile sperm. Anal Chem 2003; 75: 1671–5.
24. Schulte R, Chung Y, Ohl D, et al. Microfluidic sperm sorting device provides a novel method for selecting motile with higher DNA integrity. Fertil Steril 2007; 88: S76.
25. Davis J, Raty S, Eddington D, et al. Development of microfluidic systems for the culture of mammalian embryos. First International IEEE EMBS Special Topic Conference on Microtechnology in Medicine and Biology. Lyons, France, 2000.
26. Matsuura K, Hayashi N, Kuroda Y, et al. Improved development of mouse and human embryos using a tilting embryo culture system. Reprod Biomed Online 2010; 20: 358–64.
27. Koike T, Matsuura K, Naruse K, et al. In-vitro culture with a tilting device in chemically defined media during meiotic maturation and early development improves the quality of blastocysts derived from in-vitro matured and fertilized porcine oocytes. J Reprod Dev 2010; 56: 552–7.
28. Mizobe Y, Yoshida M, Miyoshi K. Enhancement of cytoplasmic maturation of in vitro-matured pig oocytes by mechanical vibration. J Reprod Dev 2010; 56: 285–90.
29. Isachenko V, Maettner R, Sterzik K, et al. In-vitro culture of human embryos with mechanical microvibration increases implantation rates. Reprod BioMed Online 2011; 22: 536–44.
30. Isachenko E, Maettner R, Isachenko V, et al. Mechanical agitation during the in vitro culture of human preimplantation embryos drastically increases the pregnancy rate. Clin Lab 2010; 56: 569–76.
31. Hoppe PC, Pitts S. Fertilization in vitro and development of mouse ova. Biol Reprod 1973; 8: 420–6.
32. Isachenko V, Montag M, Isachenko E, et al. Effective method for in-vitro culture of cryopreserved human ovarian tissue. Reprod Biomed Online 2006; 13: 228–34.
33. Oakes M, Cabrera L, Nanadivada H, et al. Effects of 3-dimensional topography, dynamic fluid movement and an insoluble glycoprotein matrix on murine embryo development. In: Proceedings from the SGI Annual Meeting. Glasgow, Scotland, 2009.
34. Zeilmaker GH. Fusion of rat and mouse morulae and formation of chimaeric blastocysts. Nature 1973; 242: 115–16.
35. Cohen J, Ooms MP, Vreeburg JT. Reduction of fertilizing capacity of epididymal spermatozoa by 5 alpha-steroid reductase inhibitors. Experientia 1981; 37: 1031–2.
36. Bormann C, Cabrera L, Heo Y, et al. Dynamic microfluidic embryo dynamic microfluidic embryo culture enhances blastocyst development of murine and bovine embryos. In: Proceedings from the 14th World Congress on In Vitro Fertilization. Montreal, CA, 2007: 84.
37. Bormann C, Cabrera L, Heo Y, et al. Dynamic microfluidic embryo culture enhances blastocyst development of murine and bovine embryos. Biol Reprod 2007; 1: 89.
38. Cabrera L, Heo Y, Ding J, et al. Improved blastocyst development with microfluidics and braille pin actuator enabled dynamic culture. Fertil Steril 2006; 87: S43.
39. Heo YS, Cabrera LM, Bormann CL, et al. Dynamic microfunnel culture enhances mouse embryo development and pregnancy rates. Hum Reprod 2010; 25: 613–22.
40. Eddington DT, Beebe DJ. Flow control with hydrogels. Adv Drug Deliv Rev 2004; 56: 199–210.
41. Zeringue HC, Rutledge JJ, Beebe DJ. Early mammalian embryo development depends on cumulus removal technique. Lab Chip 2005; 5: 86–90.
42. Zeringue HC, Wheeler MB, Beebe DJ. A microfluidic method for removal of the zona pellucida from mammalian embryos. Lab Chip 2005; 5: 108–10.
43. Park J, Jung SH, Kim YH, et al. Design and fabrication of an integrated cell processor for single embryo cell manipulation. Lab Chip 2005; 5: 91–6.
44. Simmons A, Hyvarinen J, Poole-Warren L. The effect of sterilisation on a poly(dimethylsiloxane)/poly(hexamethylene oxide) mixed macrodiol-based polyurethane elastomer. Biomaterials 2006; 27: 4484–97.
45. Toepke MW, Beebe DJ. PDMS absorption of small molecules and consequences in microfluidic applications. Lab Chip 2006; 6: 1484–6.
46. Wu JM, Chung Y, Belford KJ, et al. A surface-modified sperm sorting device with long-term stability. Biomed Microdevices 2006; 8: 99–107.
47. Heo YS, Cabrera LM, Song JW, et al. Characterization and resolution of evaporation-mediated osmolality shifts that constrain microfluidic cell culture in poly(dimethylsiloxane) devices. Anal Chem 2007; 79: 1126–34.
48. Lane M, Baltz JM, Bavister BD. Bicarbonate/chloride exchange regulates intracellular pH of embryos but not oocytes of the hamster. Biol Reprod 1999; 61: 452–7.
49. Lane M, Baltz JM, Bavister BD. Na+/H+ antiporter activity in hamster embryos is activated during fertilization. Dev Biol 1999; 208: 244–52.
50. Fitzharris G, Baltz JM. Granulosa cells regulate intracellular pH of the murine growing oocyte via gap junctions: development of independent homeostasis during oocyte growth. Development 2006; 133: 591–9.
51. Phillips KP, Petrunewich MA, Collins JL, et al. The intracellular pH-regulatory HCO3-/Cl- exchanger in the mouse oocyte is inactivated during first meiotic metaphase and reactivated after egg activation via the MAP kinase pathway. Mol Biol Cell 2002; 13: 3800–10.
52. Kim L, Vahey MD, Lee HY, et al. Microfluidic arrays for logarithmically perfused embryonic stem cell culture. Lab Chip 2006; 6: 394–406.
53. Suh R, Takayama S, Smith GD. Microfluidic applications for andrology. J Androl 2005; 26: 664–70.
54. Kricka LJ, Faro I, Heyner S, et al. Micromachined analytical devices: microchips for semen testing. J Pharm Biomed Anal 1997; 15: 1443–7.
55. Kricka LJ, Nozaki O, Heyner S, et al. Applications of a microfabricated device for evaluating sperm function. Clin Chem 1993; 39: 1944–7.
56. Matsuura K, Kuroda Y, Yamashita K, et al. Hydrophobic silicone elastomer chamber for recording trajectories of

motile porcine sperms without adsorption. J Reprod Dev 2011; 57: 163–7.
57. Xie L, Ma R, Han C, et al. Integration of sperm motility and chemotaxis screening with a microchannel-based device. Clin Chem 2010; 56: 1270–8.
58. Koyama S, Amarie D, Soini HA, et al. Chemotaxis assays of mouse sperm on microfluidic devices. Anal Chem 2006; 78: 3354–9.
59. Seo D, Agca Y, Feng Z, et al. Development of sorting, aligning, and orienting motile sperm using microfluidic device operated by hyrdostatic pressure. Microfluid Nanofluid 2007; 3: 561–70.
60. Agarwal A, Ikemoto I, Loughlin KR. Effect of sperm washing on levels of reactive oxygen species in semen. Arch Androl 1994; 33: 157–62.
61. Shekarriz M, DeWire DM, Thomas AJ Jr, et al. A method of human semen centrifugation to minimize the iatrogenic sperm injuries caused by reactive oxygen species. Eur Urol 1995; 28: 31–5.
62. Fraczek M, Sanocka D, Kurpisz M. Interaction between leucocytes and human spermatozoa influencing reactive oxygen intermediates release. Int J Androl 2004; 27: 69–75.
63. Chian RC, Lim JH, Tan SL. State of the art in in-vitro oocyte maturation. Curr Opin Obstet Gynecol 2004; 16: 211–19.
64. Gilchrist RB, Ritter LJ, Myllymaa S, et al. Molecular basis of oocyte-paracrine signalling that promotes granulosa cell proliferation. J Cell Sci 2006; 119: 3811–21.
65. Lopez-Garcia MD, Monson RL, Haubert K, et al. Sperm motion in a microfluidic fertilization device. Biomed Microdevices 2008; 10: 709–18.
66. Han C, Zhang Q, Ma R, et al. Integration of single oocyte trapping, in vitro fertilization and embryo culture in a microwell-structured microfluidic device. Lab Chip 2010; 10: 2848–54.
67. Ma R, Xie L, Han C, et al. In vitro fertilization on a single-oocyte positioning system integrated with motile sperm selection and early embryo development. Anal Chem 2011; 83: 2964–70.
68. Zeringue HC, Beebe DJ. Microfluidic removal of cumulus cells from Mammalian zygotes. Methods Mol Biol 2004; 254: 365–74.
69. Raty S, Davis J, Beebe D, et al. Culture in microchannels enhances in vitro embryonic development of preimplantation mouse embryos. Theriogenology 2001; 55: 241.
70. Walters E, Clark S, Roseman H, et al. Production of live piglets following in vitro embryo culture in a microfluidic environment. Theriogenology 2003; 59: 441.
71. Xie Y, Wang F, Zhong W, et al. Shear stress induces preimplantation embryo death that is delayed by the zona pellucida and associated with stress-activated protein kinase-mediated apoptosis. Biol Reprod 2006; 75: 45–55.
72. Mizuno J, Ostrovidov S, Nakamura H, et al. Human ART on chip: development of microfluidic device for IVF and IVC. Hum Reprod 2007; 22: I169–70.
73. Nakamura H, Mizuno J, Akaishi K, et al. New embryo co-culture sytstem for human assisted reproductive technology (ART) by OptiCell. Hum Reprod 2007; 22: i170.
74. Kim MS, Bae CY, Wee G, et al. A microfluidic in vitro cultivation system for mechanical stimulation of bovine embryos. Electrophoresis 2009; 30: 3276–82.
75. Bormann C, Swain J, Ni Q, et al. Preimplantation embryo secretome identification. Fertil Steril 2006; 86(Suppl 2): s116.
76. Katz-Jaffe MG, Schoolcraft WB, Gardner DK. Analysis of protein expression (secretome) by human and mouse preimplantation embryos. Fertil Steril 2006; 86: 678–85.
77. Reed M. Communication skills of embryos maintained in group culture-the autocrine paracrine debate. Clin Embryologist 2006; 9: 5–19.
78. Moessner J, Dodson WC. The quality of human embryo growth is improved when embryos are cultured in groups rather than separately. Fertil Steril 1995; 64: 1034–5.
79. Almagor M, Bejar C, Kafka I, et al. Pregnancy rates after communal growth of preimplantation human embryos in vitro. Fertil Steril 1996; 66: 394–7.
80. Lane M, Gardner DK. Effect of incubation volume and embryo density on the development and viability of mouse embryos in vitro. Hum Reprod 1992; 7: 558–62.
81. Canseco RS, Sparks AE, Pearson RE, et al. Embryo density and medium volume effects on early murine embryo development. J Assist Reprod Genet 1992; 9: 454–7.
82. Spindler RE, Crichton EG, Agca Y, et al. Improved felid embryo development by group culture is maintained with heterospecific companions. Theriogenology 2006; 66: 82–92.
83. Spindler RE, Wildt DE. Quality and age of companion felid embryos modulate enhanced development by group culture. Biol Reprod 2002; 66: 167–73.
84. Lane M, Gardner DK. Ammonium induces aberrant blastocyst differentiation, metabolism, pH regulation, gene expression and subsequently alters fetal development in the mouse. Biol Reprod 2003; 69: 1109–17.
85. Trimarchi JR, Liu L, Smith PJ, et al. Noninvasive measurement of potassium efflux as an early indicator of cell death in mouse embryos. Biol Reprod 2000; 63: 851–7.
86. Trimarchi JR, Liu L, Porterfield DM, et al. Oxidative phosphorylation-dependent and -independent oxygen consumption by individual preimplantation mouse embryos. Biol Reprod 2000; 62: 1866–74.
87. Heo YS, Cabrera LM, Bormann CL, et al. Dynamic microfunnel culture enhances mouse embryo development and pregnancy rates. Hum Reprod 2010; 25: 613–22.
88. Fukui Y, Lee ES, Araki N. Effect of medium renewal during culture in two different culture systems on development to blastocysts from in vitro produced early bovine embryos. J Anim Sci 1996; 74: 2752–8.
89. Ali J. Continuous ultra micro drop culture yields higher pregnacy and implation rates than either large-drop culture or fresh-medium replacement. Clin Embryologist 2004; 7: 2): 1–23.
90. Stokes PJ, Abeydeera LR, Leese HJ. Development of porcine embryos in vivo and in vitro; evidence for embryo 'cross talk' in vitro. Dev Biol 2005; 284: 62–71.
91. Gopichandran N, Leese HJ. The effect of paracrine/autocrine interactions on the in vitro culture of bovine

preimplantation embryos. Reproduction 2006; 131: 269–77.
92. Thouas GA, Jones GM, Trounson AO. The 'GO' system—a novel method of microculture for in vitro development of mouse zygotes to the blastocyst stage. Reproduction 2003; 126: 161–9.
93. Vajta G, Peura TT, Holm P, et al. New method for culture of zona-included or zona-free embryos: the Well of the Well (WOW) system. Mol Reprod Dev 2000; 55: 256–64.
94. Gardner DK, Lane M. Alleviation of the '2-cell block' and development to the blastocyst of CF1 mouse embryos: role of amino acids, EDTA and physical parameters. Hum Reprod 1996; 11: 2703–12.
95. Feil D, Lane M, Roberts CT, et al. Effect of culturing mouse embryos under different oxygen concentrations on subsequent fetal and placental development. J Physiol 2006; 572: 87–96.
96. Rinaudo PF, Giritharan G, Talbi S, et al. Effects of oxygen tension on gene expression in preimplantation mouse embryos. Fertil Steril 2006; 86(Suppl 4): 1252–65; 1265 e1251–1236.
97. Banwell KM, Lane M, Russell DL, et al. Oxygen concentration during mouse oocyte in vitro maturation affects embryo and fetal development. Hum Reprod 2007; 22: 2768–75.
98. Baltz JM, Biggers JD. Oxygen transport to embryos in microdrop cultures. Mol Reprod Dev 1991; 28: 351–5.
99. Byatt-Smith JG, Leese HJ, Gosden RG. An investigation by mathematical modelling of whether mouse and human preimplantation embryos in static culture can satisfy their demands for oxygen by diffusion. Hum Reprod 1991; 6: 52–7.
100. Xie Y, Wang F, Puscheck EE, et al. Pipetting causes shear stress and elevation of phosphorylated stress-activated protein kinase/jun kinase in preimplantation embryos. Mol Reprod Dev 2007; 74: 1287–94.
101. Baldini F, Giannetti A, Mencaglia AA. Optical sensor for interstitial pH measurements. J Biomed Opt 2007; 12: 024024.
102. Chang YH, Lee GB, Huang FC, et al. Integrated polymerase chain reaction chips utilizing digital microfluidics. Biomed Microdevices 2006; 8: 215–25.
103. Lucchetta EM, Munson MS, Ismagilov RF. Characterization of the local temperature in space and time around a developing Drosophila embryo in a microfluidic device. Lab Chip 2006; 6: 185–90.
104. Lien V, Vollmer F. Microfluidic flow rate detection based on integrated optical fiber cantilever. Lab Chip 2007; 7: 1352–6.
105. Ateya DA, Sachs F, Gottlieb PA, et al. Volume cytometry: microfluidic sensor for high-throughput screening in real time. Anal Chem 2005; 77: 1290–4.
106. Amatore C, Arbault S, Bouton C, et al. Monitoring in real time with a microelectrode the release of reactive oxygen and nitrogen species by a single macrophage stimulated by its membrane mechanical depolarization. Chembiochem 2006; 7: 653–61.
107. Amatore C, Arbault S, Chen Y, et al. Electrochemical detection in a microfluidic device of oxidative stress generated by macrophage cells. Lab Chip 2007; 7: 233–8.
108. Eteshola E, Balberg M. Microfluidic ELISA: on-chip fluorescence imaging. Biomed Microdevices 2004; 6: 7–9.
109. Herrmann M, Roy E, Veres T, et al. Microfluidic ELISA on non-passivated PDMS chip using magnetic bead transfer inside dual networks of channels. Lab Chip 2007; 7: 1546–52.
110. Gardner DK, Wale P, Collins R, Lane M. Glucose consumption by human embryos on day 4 and day 5 is predictive of pregnancy and sex. Hum Reprod 2011; 26: 1981–6.
111. Lane M, Gardner DK. Selection of viable mouse blastocysts prior to transfer using a metabolic criterion. Hum Reprod 1996; 11: 1975–8.
112. Seli E, Sakkas D, Scott R, et al. Noninvasive metabolomic profiling of embryo culture media using Raman and near-infrared spectroscopy correlates with reproductive potential of embryos in women undergoing in vitro fertilization. Fertil Steril 2007; 88: 1350–7.
113. O'Donovan C, Twomey E, Alderman J, et al. Development of a respirometric biochip for embryo assessment. Lab Chip 2006; 6: 1438–44.
114. Urbanski JP, Johnson MT, Craig DD, et al. Noninvasive metabolic profiling using Microfluidics for analysis of single preimplantation embryos. Anal Chem 2008; 80: 6500–7.
115. Bavister BD. Culture of preimplantation embryos: facts and artifacts. Hum Reprod Update 1995; 1: 91–148.
116. Pool TB, Martin JE. High continuing pregnancy rates after in vitro fertilization-embryo transfer using medium supplemented with a plasma protein fraction containing alpha- and beta-globulins. Fertil Steril 1994; 61: 714–19.
117. Pool TB. Recent advances in the production of viable human embryos in vitro. Reprod Biomed Online 2002; 4: 294–302.
118. Pangas SA, Saudye H, Shea LD, et al. Novel approach for the three-dimensional culture of granulosa cell-oocyte complexes. Tissue Eng 2003; 9: 1013–21.
119. Combelles CM, Fissore RA, Albertini DF, et al. In vitro maturation of human oocytes and cumulus cells using a co-culture three-dimensional collagen gel system. Hum Reprod 2005; 20: 1349–58.
120. Vozzi G, Flaim C, Ahluwalia A, et al. Fabrication of PLGA scaffolds using soft lithography and microsyringe deposition. Biomaterials 2003; 24: 2533–40.
121. Fidkowski C, Kaazempur-Mofrad MR, Borenstein J, et al. Endothelialized microvasculature based on a biodegradable elastomer. Tissue Eng 2005; 11: 302–9.
122. Eddington DT, Liu RH, Moore JS, et al. An organic self-regulating microfluidic system. Lab Chip 2001; 1: 96–9.

Index

Page numbers in bold indicate Figures, page number in italic indicate Tables

abortive apoptosis, 76–77
accreditation. *See* laboratory accreditation
acidic aniline blue (AAB) stain, 79–80, 125–26
acid Tyrode's assisted hatching, 188
acridine orange (AO) assay, 82–83
acridine orange-stained spermatozoa, **127**
acrosome-reacted sperm, **56**
aggressive immobilization procedure, 175, **175**
airborne toxic agents, 21
air-filled syringe, **167**
alkaline lysis buffer, 361
allele drop-out (ADO), 201, 355
American Society for Reproductive Medicine (ASRM), 10, *13*
amino acids
    embryo culture systems, *221*, 221–22
    embryo morphology, 247
amplification failure, 355
amplification refractory mutation system, 359
andrology, 400–402
aneuploidy screening
    by array-CGH, 341–42
    fluorescence in situ hybridization, 338–40
    preimplantation genetic diagnosis, 330
    success rates of, *337*
aniline blue staining, **125–26**
anti-Müllerian hormone (AMH), 98
array comparative genomic hybridization, **343**, 359
assay
    acridine orange, 82–83
    chromomycin A_3, 80–81
    comet, 84–85
    DBD-FISH assay, 81–82
    hemizona, 57, **58**
    mannose binding, 58, **58**
    in situ nick translation, 82
    sperm chromatin structure, 85–86
    sperm DNA integrity, 58
    TUNEL, 85, **86**
assisted hatching (AH)
    acid Tyrode's method, 188
    benefits, 192–93
    blastocyst assisted hatching, 190
    contact lasers, 188–89
    laser-assisted hatching, 188
    microtools, 187
    noncontact lasers, 189
    partial zona dissection method, 188
    reasons for, 187
    results by authors, 190–92, *191–92*
    ZP thinning, 189–90
audits, 39
augmented pregnancy rate, 300
azoospermia, 324

Bartoov IMSI classification, 139
base fresh pregnancy rate, 300
Beckwith-Wiedemann syndrome, 181
bench-top incubators, 165
bioassay methods
    hamster sperm motility assay, 22–23
    human sperm survival assay, 23–24
    mouse embryo assay, 24–25
biochemical pregnancy rate (BPR), 257, **258**
BioStation®, 255
blastocyst
    day 3 embryos, 232–33
    embryo morphology development, 242–44
    embryo transfer, 228–30
    grading system, *243*
    human, **244**
    mouse, **248**
blastocyst assisted hatching, 190
blastocyst-stage biopsy, 204–6
buccal cells, 360

carbon dioxide, embryo culture systems, 225
Cassuto and Barak IMSI classification, 139–40, **140**
cell aggregation, 387
cell lysis
    alkaline lysis buffer, 361
    proteinase K buffer, 361
    sodium dudecyl sulfate buffer, 361
    water, 360–61
cell strainer, **157**
chablon, 137, **137**
chaotic mosaics, 347
chaperone protein, 122–23
chilling injury, 286
chromomycin A_3 (CMA_3) assay, 80–81
chromosomal aberrations, 324, *325*
chromosome screening
    blastocyst stage, 350–51
    cleavage stage, 346–49
    comparative genomic hybridization, **347**
    female gamete, 349–50
cleavage-stage embryos
    cell selection, 203–4
    diagnostic efficiency, 204
    embryo morphology, 242
    preparation before biopsy, 202, 207
    removal of cells, 202–3
    safety and success rates, 203
    timing of biopsy, 202, 207
Clinical and Laboratory Standards Institute (CLSI), 32
clinical embryology, 40
Clinical Laboratory Improvement Amendments of 1988 (CLIA '88), 10, *12*
clinical pregnancy, 179, *180*, **242**
clinical pregnancy rate (CPR), 257, **258**
comet assay, 84–85
comparative genomic hybridization (CGH). *See* chromosome screening
computer-assisted semen analysis (CASA), 53–54
congenital bilateral absence of the vas deferens (CBAVD), 326, *326*
contact lasers, 188–89
containment systems, 165
contamination, 355–56

controlled rate cooling
  biophysics of, 275–77
  frozen-thawed oocytes, 278–79, 281
  oocyte cryopreservation, 281–83
  oocyte preparation for freezing, 280–81
  oocyte selection, 277–78
  reproducibility, 278
  timing of freezing, 279–80
  timing of insemination, 279–80
controlled zona dissection, 188
conventional in vitro fertilization
  genetically aberrant embryos, 382
  low quality embryos, 382
  preimplantation stage embryos, 381
  single blastomere, 381
Cornell replacement strategies
  natural cycle replacement, 295–96
  programmed cycle replacement, 296
Cryoloop approach, 311
Cryopette, 311
cryopreservation
  clinical efficiency of oocyte, 281–83
  cumulative pregnancy rates per retrieval, 230
  human embryo, 307–8
  injury and prevention during, 308–10
cryoprotectant agents (CPAs), 275
cryoprotectants, 294–95, 309–10
Cryotop vitrification
  additional tools, 287
  device, 286, **287**
  equilibration and cooling, 287–89
  of human oocytes, 291
  preparation steps, 286–87
  solutions, *287*
  timing, 286
  warming and dilution, 289–90
  working environment, 286–87
Cryovials, 303
Cumulase®, 174
cumulus cells, 98, 360
cumulus-oocyte complexes (COCs), **154, 156**
cystic fibrosis, 326, *326*
cytoplasmic halo effect, 214–15
cytoplasmic inclusions, 103–4, **104, 117**

decidualization, 369–71, **371**
defective sperm chromatin packaging, 76
degenerate oligonucleotide primed polymerase chain reaction
    (DOP-PCR), 361–62
direct assays
  comet assay, 84–85
  TUNEL assay, 85
DNA breakage detection-Fluorescent in situ hybridization
    (DBD-FISH) assay, 81–82
DNA fingerprinting, 358
DNA microarray technology, 359
drug screening applications, 389

embryo biopsy
  benefits, limitations, and factors, *199*
  blastocyst-stage biopsy, 204–6
  cleavage-stage embryos (*see* cleavage-stage embryos)
  micromanipulation, 168–69
  penetration of zona pellucida, 197–200
  polar body biopsy, 200–1
embryo composition
  amino acids, 221–22
  macromolecules, 222–23
embryo culture components
  carbon dioxide, 225
  embryo:volume ratio, 226–27
  incubation chamber, 224–25
  incubation vessel, 226–27
  medium storage, 227
  oxygen, 225–26
  pH, 225
  quality control, 227–28
embryo culture systems
  blastocyst transfer, 228–30
  components, 224–28
  composition of embryo, 221–23
  cumulative pregnancy rates per retrieval, 230
  dynamics of embryo, 219–20
  future developments, 230–31
  human embryonic stem cells, 384–86
  implantation rate, *181*
  maternal physiology, 219–20, *220*
  microfluidics, 404–7
  monoculture/sequential media, 223–24
  pronucleate oocytes, 232
  protocols, 231–32
  randomized trials, *229*
  single embryo transfer, 218–19, 230
  susceptibility of preimplantation embryo, 220–21
  in vivo *vs.* in vitro, 224
EmbryoGuard®, 255
embryology applications
  embryo culture, 404–7
  in vitro fertilization, 402–4
  in vitro maturation, 402
embryology laboratory
  access rules, 36
  air quality, 37
  cleanliness, 37
  facilities, 36
  general laboratory layout, 36
  health and safety, 36
  light exposure, 37
  temperature, 36–37
embryo morphokinesis
  intracellular dynamics, 255–56
  kinetics development, 255–56
  time-lapse imaging (*see* time-lapse imaging technology)
embryo morphology
  amino acid utilization, 247
  as assessment tool, 240–41
  blastocyst development, 242–44
  carbohydrate utilization, 247
  cleavage-stage embryos, 242
  metabolomics, 249–50
  noninvasive analysis, 245, **247**
  pronucleate oocytes, 241–42
  specific factors, 247–49
  strategy selection, 244–45
Embryonic cell isolation, 360
Embryonic proteome, 266–69
Embryonic secretome
  embryo quality, 269–72
  protein profiling protocol, 272
embryo perfusion culture system, **231**
EmbryoScope™, 255, **258**
embryo vitrification
  cooling rates, 311–12
  cryopreservation approach, 307–8
  cryoprotectants, 310
  influencing factors, 313–16
  injury and prevention during cryopreservation, 308–10
  traditional tools of cryopreservation, 310–11
  transmission of infectious agents, 312–13
endometrial receptivity
  CD98, CD147, 370, 372
  decidualization, 369–71
  definition, 366
  lipidomics, 372–74

proteomics, 369–70
secretomics, 372–74
transcriptomics, 366, 368–69, **369**
endometrial receptivity array (ERA), 368
endotoxin testing, 302
equipments
　bench-top incubators, 165
　containment systems, 165
　glass microtools, 167
　heated stages, 165
　for IVF laboratory, 168–69
　laser-assisted micromanipulation, 168
　manipulators, 164–65
　microsyringes, 166
　optics, 165
　stereomicroscope, 165
　tool chucks, 167
　tubing, 166–67
　vibration, 167
　See also micromanipulation
ethidium bromide gel electrophoresis, 362
European Cooperation for Accreditation, 39
European Society of Human Reproduction and Embryology (ESHRE), 32
European Union Tissue and Cells Directive (EUTCD), 32
Express® Software, 272
external audits, 39
eye-selected conventional intracytoplasmic sperm injection, 131–32

failure mode and effects analysis (FMEA), *44*, 44–45
familial adenomatous polyposis (FAP), 354
Fertilase®, **189–90**
Fertility Clinic Success Rate and Certification Act of 1992, 10
fertilization
　abnormal pronuclear formation and patterns, **213**, 214–15
　cytoplasmic halo, 215
　microfluidics, 402–4
　pronuclear grading, 212–14
　timing of events, 212
fluorescence in situ hybridization (FISH), 359
fluorescent polymerase chain reaction, 356, 362
follicle stimulating hormone (FSH), 78, 96
freezing
　oocyte preparation for, 280–81
　timing of, 279–80
　traditional, 286
frozen-thawed oocytes
　developmental performance of, 281
　survival and insemination of, 278–79
FSH priming, 151–52
Fyrite®, 225

GeneScan™, 356, 362
gene therapy applications, 388
genetically aberrant embryos, 382
genetic causes, male infertility
　chromosomal aberrations, 324
　congenital bilateral absence of the vas deferens, 326
　cystic fibrosis, 326
　globozoospermia, 328
　Kallmann syndrome, 327
　Kennedy's disease, 327
　microdeletions on Y chromosome, 324–26
　myotonic dystrophy, 326–27
　primary ciliary dyskinesia, 327
genetic diagnosis. *See* preimplantation genetic diagnosis (PGD)
genetic evaluation, male infertility
　of infertile males, 328–29
　of pregnancies, 329–30
genetic screening, 330
genetic testing
　consequences and recommendations, 329
　vs. genetic screening, 330
G85 from K-Systems, **166**
giant oocytes, 104, **104**
glass microtools, 167
globozoospermia, 328
glutamine, 227
gradient separation procedures, 63–65

Halosperm®, 83
Hamster sperm motility assay, 22–23
hatching. *See* assisted hatching
hCG priming, 152
heated stages, 165
hemizona assay, 57, **58**
high-speed vitrification, **309**, **312**
HIV-infected men, semen preparation, 65, **66**
homemade microsyringe, 166, **167**
hormonal stimulation protocols, 119
HspA2. *See* chaperone protein
human blastocysts, **244**
human embryonic stem cells (hESCs)
　cell source for transplantation, 388
　characterization of, 386
　conventional in vitro fertilization, 381–82
　in culture systems, 384–86
　derivation of, 383–84
　drug screening applications, 389
　embryo development applications, 389
　gene therapy applications, 388
　human genetic disorders, 389–90
　induced differentiation, 387–88
　nuclear transfer-derived embryos, 382–83
　origin of embryos, 380–81
　parthenogenesis, 382
　properties of, 380
　protocols of, 390–91
　toxicology applications, 389
　transcription factor induced pluripotent stem cells, 383
　in vitro differentiation, 387
human endometrium
　CD98, **373**
　microarray analysis, *367–68*
human genetic disorders, 389–90
human leukocyte antigen G (HLA-G), 248
human proteome, 266
human sperm survival assay, 23–24, 302
hyaluronan-bound sperm, 124–25, 127
hyaluronic acid (HA) binding-mediated sperm selection
　clinical results, 131–32
　hyaluronan-bound sperm, 124–25, 127
　intracytoplasmic morphologically selected sperm injection, 127–28
　large vacuoles with IMSI, 129–31
　nuclear abnormalities, 129–31
　PICSI dish methods, 124
　scientific basis of, 122–23
　sperm plasma membrane remodeling, 123
　zona pellucida and HA receptor, 123–24
8-hydroxy-2-deoxyguanosine (8-OHdG), 86–87
hypo-osmotic swelling test (HOST), 55–56

immotile cilia syndrome, 327
immotile sperm, 65
immunobead binding test, 55
incubation chamber, 224–25
incubation vessel, 226–27
indirect assay, 82–83
induced differentiation
　growth factors, 387
　key regulator genes, 388
　lineage selection, 388

induced pluripotent stem (iPS) cells, 383
infectious agents transmission, 312–13
infertility
    blastocyst stage, 350–51
    cleavage stage, 346–49
    female gamete, 349–50
    See also male infertility
in situ nick translation (NT) assay, 82
internal audits, 39
International Organization for Standardization (ISO), 31
International Standards and Regulatory Frameworks, 31–32
International Stem Cell Initiative (ISCI), 386
intracytoplasmic morphologically selected sperm injection (IMSI)
    Bartoov classification, 139
    Cassuto and Barak classification, 139–40
    chablon calculation, 137
    dish preparation, 137
    and DNA integrity, 143–46
    equipment, **136,** 136–37
    vs. eye-selected conventional ICSI, 131–32
    hyaluronic acid binding-mediated sperm selection, 127–28
    laboratory and clinical outcomes, *142*
    magnification calculation, 137
    and nuclear abnormalities, 129–31
    reproductive outcomes, 140–41, 143
    sample preparation, 138
    Vanderzwalmen classification, 139
intracytoplasmic sperm injection (ICSI)
    children's health, 180–81
    clinical outcomes, 178–80
    embryo development and replacement, 176–77
    extended sperm search, 177
    eye-selected conventional, 131–32
    fertilization evaluation, 176–77
    hyaluronic acid binding-mediated sperm selection (*see* hyaluronic acid binding-mediated sperm selection)
    immobilization procedures, 175
    oocytes collection and preparation, 173–74
    oocytes preparation and evaluation (*see* oocytes preparation and evaluation)
    ooplasmic injection, 175–76
    optional sperm selection techniques, 177–78
    semen collection, 172–73
    semen processing, 173
    setting microinjection, 174
    spermatozoon selection, 174–75
    sperm cryopreservation, 173
in vitro differentiation, 387
in vitro fertilization (IVF)
    conventional (*see* conventional in vitro fertilization)
    microfluidics, 402–4
    risk management, *43*
in vitro maturation (IVM)
    chronological procedures, **153**
    clinical outcome and malformation rate, 156–58
    donor oocyte sources, 159
    FSH priming, 151–52
    hCG priming, 152
    history of, 151
    indications of, 151
    Metformin, 155–56
    microfluidics, 402
    mitochondrial distribution, 159
    oocyte identification, 154–55
    oocytes maturation, 158
    oocyte status, 152–54
    ovum pickup, 155
    preimplantation genetic diagnosis, 159
    ultrastructural investigation, 158–59
ion exchange chromatography, 272
ISO 9001:2008, 31, 34
ISO 15189:2007
    advisory services, 39
    audits, 39
    culture medium, devices, and disposables, 37–38
    equipment, 38
    examination procedures, 34–35
    key performance indicators, 38
    laboratory facilities, 36
    pre- and post-examination procedures, 35
    quality assurance, 38–39
    reporting results, 35–36
    table of contents, *34*
    training and accreditation of embryologists, 40
ISO 17025:2005, 31
Isolate™, 63
ISolate®, 173
IVF-OSAKA IVM needle, 155, **157**

Joint Commission International (JCI), 32

Kallmann syndrome, 327
Kartagener syndrome, 327
Kennedy's disease, 327
key performance indicators (KPIs), 38
kinematic measurements, CASA, **54**

laboratory accreditation, 33–34
laboratory PGD techniques
    cell lysis, 360–61
    degenerate oligonucleotide primed PCR, 361–62
    embryonic cell isolation, 360
    fluorescent PCR, 362
    general safety measures, 359–60
    multiple displacement amplification, 362
    multiplex PCR, 361
    positive controls, 360
    primer and nested PCR, 361
    primer extension preamplification, 361
    product detection, 362
    restriction enzyme digestion, 362
laboratory protocol
    cumulus cells removal, 116, 119
    microscopic evaluation, 116–19
    oocyte denudation, 116, 119
laboratory settings
    building materials, 5–6
    "burning-in" of facility, 6–7
    construction and renovation, 5–6
    design requirements, 3
    design types, 2
    equipment, 4
    insurance issues, 7
    maintenance planning, 7
    microscopes, 5
    personnel and experiences, 1
    staff requirements, 2
    sterilization, 7
    storage, 5
    supervision of construction, 3
    visualization of cells, 5
laboratory staffing norms, 13–15, *14*
laminar flow, **397**
laser-assisted hatching, 188, **190**
laser-assisted micromanipulation, 168
laser-assisted polar body biopsy, 338, *339*
lineage selection approach, 388
lipidomics, 372–74
lipocalin-1, 270, **272**
liquid nitrogen-mediated disease transmission, 290–91
low quality embryos, 382
lymphoblast cell-line, 360
lymphocytes, 360

macromolecules, 222–23
magnetic cell separation, 88
Makler®, 173
male infertility
    consequences and recommendations, 328–30
    controversies, 330
    diagnosis of, 78
    future findings, 330–31
    genetic causes (*see* genetic causes, male infertility)
    See also infertility
mammalian embryology, *314*
manipulators, 164–65
mannose binding assay, 58, **58**
maternal physiology, 219–20, *220*
mature spermatozoa, 178
McGill Cryoleaf, **309**
mechanical micromanipulator, **164**
MediCult IVM® system, 154, *155*
metabolomics, 249–50, *250*
metaphase-comparative genomic hybridization, **350**
metformin, 155–56
microarray-comparative genomic hybridization, **348**
microfluidic perfusion system, **405**, **408**
microfluidics
    in andrology, 400–402
    basis and appeal of, 396–97
    device operation/failure, 399
    dynamic approaches, 397–98
    in embryology, 402–7
    fabrication of devices, 397
    future directions, 410–11
    IVF laboratory compatibility, 400
    manipulation/handling of embryos, 399–400
    material/design biocompatibility, 399
    media flow, 397–98
    noninvasive viability assessment, 409–10
    oocytes/embryos benefits from, 407–9
microfluidic sperm sorter, **400–401**
micromanipulation
    air quality conditions, 163
    applications of, 163
    equipments (*see* equipments)
    media and, 163–64
    plate set-up, 169
    principles of, 163
    procedures, 169–70
    set-up station, **165**
    techniques, 169–70
    temperature conditions, 163
microsurgical epididymal sperm aspiration (MESA), 65, 71
microsyringes, 166
minisequencing, 359
Mitochondria, 328
mixed agglutination reaction, 55
monogenetic disorders detection, 337–38
mosaicism, 347
motile sperm organellar morphology examination (MSOME),
    135–36, 138, **138**, 177
mouse blastocysts, **248**
mouse embryo assay (MEA), 24–25
mouse embryo bioassay, 302
multiple displacement amplification (MDA), 362
multiplex polymerase chain reaction, 356, 361
mutation analysis, 358
myotonic dystrophy, 326–27

Narishige IM 6 syringe, **166**
Narishige micromanipulator, **164**
National Committee for Clinical Laboratory Standards (NCCLS),
    15, *15*
National/Regional Standards, 32–33
natural cycle replacement, 295–96

nested polymerase chain reaction, 361
noncontact laser systems, 189
nonpermeable cryoprotectants, 310
noonan syndrome, 328
nuclear transfer-derived embryos, 382–83
numerical chromosomal abnormalities, 336–37

oligo-astheno-teratozoospermia (OAT), 324
One-Phor-All®, 85
oocyte-Corona-Cumulus complex (OCCC), 98–99
oocyte donor model, *224*
oocytes
    cryopreservation, *278*, 281–83, *282*
    giant, 104, **104**
    handling of, 115
    laboratory protocol (*see* laboratory protocol)
    morphological characteristics, 114–15
oocytes controlled rate cooling
    biophysics of, 275–77
    freezing time, 279–80
    frozen-thawed oocytes, 278–79, 281
    oocyte cryopreservation, 281–83
    oocyte preparation for freezing, 280–81
    oocyte selection, 277–78
    reproducibility, 278
    timing of insemination, 279–80
oocytes Cryotop vitrification
    additional tools, 287
    device, 286–87
    equilibration and cooling, 287–89
    preparation steps, 286–87
    protocol, **288**
    results, 291
    solution equilibration procedure, **288–89**
    solutions, 287
    timing, 286
    warming and dilution, 289–90
    working environment, 286–87
oocytes preparation and evaluation
    cumulus cells removal, 116, 119
    handling of oocytes, 115
    microscopic evaluation, 116–19
    morphological abnormalities, **117**
    morphological characteristics, 114–15, **115**
    oocyte denudation, 116, 119
oocytes selection and retrieval
    metaphase II morphological features, 102–5
    nuclear maturity evaluation, 99–102
    Oocyte-Corona-Cumulus complex evaluation, 98–99
    ovarian stimulation protocols, 97–98
    perifollicular vascularization, 98
    serum and follicular anti-Müllerian hormone, 98
ooplasmic injection, 175–76
Oosafe®, 37
Open pulled straw (OPS), **309**, 311
ovarian stimulation protocols, 97–98
oxidative stress (OS), 77
oxygen, embryo culture systems, 225–26

parthenogenesis, 382
partial zona dissection (PZD), 188
pentoxifylline (POF), 65, 72
Percoll™, 63
percutaneous epididymal sperm aspiration (PESA), 65, 71
perifollicular vascularization, 98
pH, embryo culture systems, 225
physiologic intracytoplasmic sperm injection (PICSI), 124
pinopodes, 366
pluripotent stem cells, 380
polar body (PB) biopsy
    detection of monogenetic disorders, 337–38
    FISH analysis, 340–42, **342**

polar body (PB) biopsy (*Continued*)
  human embryo, 200–1
  laser-assisted, 338, *339*
  numerical chromosomal abnormalities, 336–37
  structural chromosomal aberrations, 337
  success rates of, *337*
  techniques, 338
  transfer of polar bodies, 338–42
polydimethylsiloxane (PDMS), 397
polymerase chain reaction (PCR)
  allele drop-out, 355
  amplification failure, 355
  contamination, 355–56
preimplantation genetic diagnosis (PGD)
  amplification refractory mutation system, 359
  array CGH, 359
  biopsy at developmental stages, *198*
  chromosome screening (*see* chromosome screening)
  DNA microarray technology, 359
  fluorescent polymerase chain reaction, 356
  minisequencing, 359
  multiplex polymerase chain reaction, 356
  mutation analysis, 358
  polymerase chain reaction, 355–56
  polymorphic markers, 357–58
  principles of, 354–56
  quantitative fluorescent polymerase chain reaction, 356–57
  restriction endonuclease digestion, 358–59
  strategic considerations, *198*
  translocation carriers, 358
  in vitro maturation, 159
  whole genome amplification, 357
preimplantation genetic screening (PGS), 346, 382
primary ciliary dyskinesia, 327
primer extension preamplification (PEP), 361
primer polymerase chain reaction, 361
Primo Vision®, 255
process testing
  comparison of sensitivities, 25–26
  hamster sperm motility assay, 22–23
  human sperm survival assay, 23–24
  mouse embryo assay, 24–25
  sensitivity *vs.* sensibility, 26–27
product detection, 362
programmed cycle replacement, 296
projected augmented pregnancy rate, 300
pronuclear grading, 212–14
pronucleate oocytes
  embryo culture systems, 232
  embryo morphology, 241–42
proteinase K buffer, 361
proteomics, 369–70
PureCeption™, 63
PureSperm™, 63

quality assurance, 11, 38–39
quality control
  definition, 11
  of embryo and specimen identification, 27
  introductory comments, 10–11
  laboratory personnel, 11, 13
  laboratory staffing norms, 13–15
  materials and supplies, 21–22
  new legislation, 10
  new procedures, 9–10
  new products, 9
  procedures, 15
  process testing, 22–27
  record keeping, 11
quality control equipments
  CO_2 levels, 17–18
  computerized semen analyzers, 18
  computers, 20–21
  daily temperature, 16–17
  humidity of incubator, 18
  lasers, 18–19
  microscopes, 18
  parameters and frequency of, *16*
  periodic review of control records, 19–20
quality standards
  International Standards and Regulatory Frameworks, 31–32
  laboratory accreditation, 33–34
  National/Regional Standards, 32–33
  risk management, 43–45
  sample identification, witnessing, and prevention of misidentification, 41–43
  See also embryology laboratory; ISO 15189:2007
quantitative fluorescent polymerase chain reaction, 356–57

reactive oxygen species (ROS), 77
reproducibility, 278
Research Instruments (RI), 164
restriction endonuclease digestion, 358–59
restriction enzyme digestion, 362
risk management, *43*, 43–45

Scientists in Reproductive Technologies (SIRT), 40
screw-actuated syringe (SAS), **166**
secretomics, 372–74
seeding, 295
Serum Substitute Supplement (SSS™), 154
setting up of laboratory
  building materials, 5–6
  "burning-in" of facility, 6–7
  construction and renovation, 5–6
  design requirements, 3
  design types, 2
  equipment, 4
  insurance issues, 7
  maintenance planning, 7
  microscopes, 5
  personnel and experiences, 1
  staff requirements, 2
  sterilization, 7
  storage, 5
  supervision of construction, 3
  visualization of cells, 5
Sil-Select™, 64
single blastomere, 381
single embryo transfer, 218–19, 230
single pronucleate (1PN) zygotes, 214
slow cooling rate protocol, *279*
slow freezing
  blastocysts freezing, 295
  blastocysts thawing, 295
  in childhood, 301
  complications, 302–3
  embryos freezing, 295
  embryos thawing, 295
  natural cycle replacement, 295–96
  pregnancy potential, 299–301
  programmed cycle replacement, 296
  quality control issues, 302
  results, 296–99
  thawing of embryo, 295
  vs. vitrification, 301
SnaPshot™, 359
sodium dudecyl sulfate buffer, 361
somatic cell nuclear transfer (SCNT), 382–83
somatic cell reprogramming
  nuclear transfer-derived embryos, 382–83
  transcription factor induced pluripotent stem cells, 383
sperm acrosome assays, 56–57

spermatozoa
  acridine orange-stained, **127**
  agarose microgel, **83**
  quick-stained, **53**
sperm chromatin assessment
  abortive apoptosis, 76–77
  assisted reproductive techniques, 78
  cancer patients, 78–79
  chromatin structure, 75–76
  contributing factors, 77–78
  defective sperm chromatin packaging, 76
  deficiencies in recombination, 77
  embryonal loss, 78
  male infertility diagnosis, 78
  oxidative stress, 77
  strategic DNA damage methods, 87–88
sperm chromatin dispersion (SCD) test, 83–84
sperm chromatin structure assay (SCSA), 85–86
sperm cryopreservation, 173
sperm DNA integrity assay, 58
sperm DNA integrity tests, *146*
sperm evaluation
  biochemical tests, 57
  cell types, 51
  computer-assisted semen analysis, 53–54
  container labeling, 49
  hemizona assay, 57
  hypo-osmotic swelling test, 55–56
  liquefaction and viscosity, 49–50
  mannose binding assay, 58
  patient history, 48
  progression, 50–51
  semen analysis, 48–49
  semen volume, 50
  specimen care, 49
  specimen collection, 49
  sperm acrosome assays, 56–57
  sperm antibodies, 54–55
  sperm concentration, 50
  sperm DNA integrity assay, 58
  sperm malformations, **52**
  sperm morphology, 51, 53
  sperm motility, 50
  sperm penetration assay, 57
  sperm vitality, 51, 55
SpermGrad™, 63
sperm nuclear DNA damage
  acidic aniline blue stain, 79–80
  AO assay, 82–83
  chromomycin A$_3$ assay, 80–81
  comet assay, 84–85
  DBD-FISH assay, 81–82
  8-hydroxy-2-deoxyguanosine, 86–87
  in situ NT assay, 82
  SCD test, 83–84
  sperm chromatin structure assay, 85–86
  toluidine blue stain, 80
  TUNEL assay, 85
sperm penetration assay (SPA), 57
sperm plasma membrane remodeling, 123
sperm preparation techniques
  comparison of results, 67–69
  complications, 69
  future directions and controversies, 69
  gradient separation procedures, 63–65
  HIV-infected men semen, 65
  immotile samples, 65

  semen collection, 62
  surgical aspirates, 65
  swim-up procedures, 63
  tissue samples, 65
SpermSlow™, 145
spinal and bulbar muscular atrophy, 327
spontaneous differentiation, 387
severe male factor. *See* oligo-astheno-teratozoospermia (OAT)
stereomicroscope, 165
structural chromosomal aberrations, 337
subfertility, 48
SupraSperm™, 63
swim-up sperm procedures, 63

Taq polymerase, 354–55
TE biopsy. *See* blastocyst-stage biopsy
teratoma tumors, **387**
terminal deoxynucleotidyl transferase (TdT)-mediated deoxyuridine triphosphate (dUTP) nick end labeling (TUNEL) assay, 85, **86**
testicular biopsy, 71
Testsimplets®, 173
time-lapse imaging technology
  applications in embryology, 254–55
  embryo implantation and variables measurement, 257–60
  establishing kinetic markers, 260–61
  experimental studies, 256–57
  noninvasive analysis, 263
toluidine blue (TB) stain, 80, **81**
tool chucks, 167
total reached magnification, 137
toxicology applications, 389
transcription factor induced pluripotent stem cells, 383
transcriptomics, 366, 368–69
translocation carriers, 358
trophectoderm cell, **190**
trophoblast cells, 169, **169**
turbulent *vs.* laminar flow, 396–97, **397**
two-dimensional polyacrylamide gel electrophoresis (2D-PAGE), 266–67
Tygerberg morphology, 128, 131

vacuolated spermatozoon, **145**
vacuoles, **140**
Vanderzwalmen IMSI classification, 139
vitrification
  Cryotop (*see* Cryotop vitrification)
  human embryo (*see* embryo vitrification)
  liquid nitrogen-mediated disease transmission, 290–91
  vs. slow freezing, 301
  techniques in embryology, *308*
  vs. traditional freezing, 286

whole genome amplification (WGA), 357
window of implantation (WOI), 366
womb-on-a-chip, 405, **408**
written protocol, *15*

zander bench-top antivibration table, **163**
zeptoproteomics, 266
ZILOS-tk® Laser, 168
zona pellucida (ZP)
  in assisted hatching, 186
  and HA receptor, 123–24
  penetration of, 197–200
  thinning, 189–90
zygotes, 212–15, **213–15**, 260